D1758305

University of Liverpool

Withdrawn from stock

Veterinary Parasitology

Veterinary Parasitology

Third Edition

M.A. Taylor BVMS, PhD, MRCVS, DipEVPC, CBiol, MIBiol
R.L. Coop BSc, PhD
R.L. Wall BSc, MBA, PhD, FRES

Blackwell Publishing

© 2007 by M.A. Taylor, R.L. Coop & R.L. Wall

Blackwell Publishing editorial offices:
Blackwell Publishing Ltd, 9600 Garsington Road, Oxford OX4 2DQ, UK
Tel: +44 (0)1865 776868
Blackwell Publishing Professional, 2121 State Avenue, Ames, Iowa 50014-8300, USA
Tel: +1 515 292 0140
Blackwell Publishing Asia Pty Ltd, 550 Swanston Street, Carlton, Victoria 3053, Australia
Tel: +61 (0)3 8359 1011

The right of the Authors to be identified as the Authors of this Work has been asserted in accordance with the Copyright, Designs and Patents Act 1988.

All rights reserved. No part of this publication may be reproduced, stored in a retrieval system, or transmitted, in any form or by any means, electronic, mechanical, photocopying, recording or otherwise, except as permitted by the UK Copyright, Designs and Patents Act 1988, without the prior permission of the publisher.

Designations used by companies to distinguish their products are often claimed as trademarks. All brand names and product names used in this book are trade names, service marks, trademarks or registered trademarks of their respective owners. The Publisher is not associated with any product or vendor mentioned in this book.

This publication is designed to provide accurate and authoritative information in regard to the subject matter covered. It is sold on the understanding that the Publisher is not engaged in rendering professional services. If professional advice or other expert assistance is required, the services of a competent professional should be sought.

First Edition published 1987 by Longman Scientific & Technical
Second Edition published 1996 by Blackwell Science Ltd
Third Edition published 2007 by Blackwell Publishing Ltd
3 2008

ISBN: 978-1-4051-1964-1

Library of Congress Cataloging-in-Publication Data
Taylor, M.A. (Mike A.)
Veterinary parasitology / M.A. Taylor, R.L. Coop, R.L. Wall. — 3rd ed.
p. cm.
Rev. ed. of: Veterinary parasitology / G.M. Urquhart . . . [et al.]. 2nd ed. 1996.
Includes bibliographical references and index.
ISBN: 978-1-4051-1964-1 (pbk. : alk. paper)
1. Veterinary parasitology. I. Coop, R.L. II. Wall, Richard, Ph.D. III. Title.

SF810.A3V425 2007
636.089′696—dc22

2007008603

A catalogue record for this title is available from the British Library

Set in 9/10pt Times
by Graphicraft Limited, Hong Kong
Printed and bound in Singapore
by C.O.S. Printers Pte Ltd

The publisher's policy is to use permanent paper from mills that operate a sustainable forestry policy, and which has been manufactured from pulp processed using acid-free and elementary chlorine-free practices. Furthermore, the publisher ensures that the text paper and cover board used have met acceptable environmental accreditation standards.

For further information on Blackwell Publishing, visit our website:
www.BlackwellVet.com

Contents

(*Contents list continues on pages vi–xx*)

Introduction

Unlike previous editions, parasites are now organised under the hosts and organ systems in which they are found. As many parasites have features in common, the first chapter of this book provides a background to the taxonomic classification and common morphological features of the many groups of parasites found in domestic animals. More detailed individual descriptions are then provided under the respective host chapters. Throughout the book extensive indexing and cross-referencing are provided both in the overview that follows, and at the end of each host chapter. Non-obligate ectoparasites, that may be found on several hosts, are now grouped in a separate chapter, Chapter 11: Facultative parasites and arthropod vectors.

Further general chapters are provided on The epidemiology of parasitic diseases (Chapter 12); Resistance to parasitic diseases (Chapter 13); Antiparasitics (Chapter 14); and The laboratory diagnosis of parasitism (Chapter 15).

1 PARASITE TAXONOMY AND MORPHOLOGY

A. VETERINARY HELMINTHOLOGY

Phylum	**Class**	**Superfamily** Family Sub-family	**Genus**	**Chapters**
Nemathelminthes	Nematoda	**Trichostrongyloidea**	*Ostertagia*	***1, 2, 3, 8***
			Teladorsagia	***1, 3, 8***
			Haemonchus	***1, 2, 3, 8***
			Marshallagia	***1, 3, 8***
			Mecistocirrus	***1, 2, 3, 5***
			Hyostrongylus	***1, 5***
			Trichostrongylus	***1, 2, 3, 4, 5, 7, 8, 9, 10***
			Cooperia	***1, 2, 3, 8***
			Nematodirus	***1, 2, 3, 8***
			Dictyocaulus	***1, 2, 3, 4, 8***
			Amidostomum	***1, 7***
			Ollulanus	***1, 5, 6***
			Ornithostrongylus	***1, 10***
			Impalaia	***1, 8***
			Graphinema	***8***
			Spiculopteragia	***8***

(*continued*)

Phylum	Class	Superfamily Family Sub-family	Genus	Chapters
			Apteragia	***8***
			Rinadia	***8***
			Camelostrongylus	***8***
			Nematodirella	***8***
			Lamanema	***8***
			Graphidium	***9***
			Obeliscoides	***9***
			Nippostrongylus	***9***
			Nematospiroides	***9***
			Libyostrongylus	***10***
			Epomidiostomum	***7***
		Strongyloidea	*Strongylus*	***1, 4***
		Strongylinae	*Triodontophorus*	***1, 4***
			Chabertia	***1, 2, 3, 8***
			Oesophagostomum	***1, 2, 3, 5, 8***
			Stephanurus	***1, 2, 5***
			Syngamus	***1, 2, 7, 10***
			Mammomonogamus	***1, 2, 3, 6***
			Globocephalus	***5***
			Deletrocephalus	***10***
			Paradeletrocephalus	***10***
			Kalicephalus	***10***
			Codiostomum	***10***
			Poteriostomum	***4***
			Craterostomum	***4***
			Oesophagodontus	***4***
			Cyathostoma	***4, 10***
		Cyathostominae	*Cyathostomum*	***1, 4***
			Cylicocyclus	***1, 4***
			Cylicodontophorus	***1, 4***
			Cylicostephanus	***1, 4***
		Ancylostomatoidea	*Ancylostoma*	***1, 6***
			Uncinaria	***1, 6***
			Bunostomum	***1, 2, 3, 8***
			Gaigeria	***1, 3***
			Agriostomum	***2***
			Necator	***1, 1***
		Metastrongyloidea	*Metastrongylus*	***1, 5***
			Muellerius	***1, 3, 8***
			Protostrongylus	***1, 3, 8***
			Cystocaulus	***1, 3, 8***
			Spiculocaulus	***1, 3***
			Neostrongylus	***1, 3***

(*continued*)

Phylum	Class	Superfamily Family Sub-family	Genus	Chapters
			Oslerus	***1, 6***
			Filaroides	***1, 6***
			Aelurostrongylus	***1, 6***
			Angiostrongylus	***1, 6, 9***
			Crenosoma	***1, 6***
			Anafilaroides	***1, 6***
			Vogeloides	***6***
			Gurltia	***1***
			Parelophostrongylus	***1, 8***
			Elaphostrongylus	***1, 8***
			Varestrongylus	***3, 8***
		Rhabditoidea	*Strongyloides*	***1, 2, 3, 5, 6, 7***
			Halicephalobus	***1, 4***
			Rhabditis	***1, 4***
			Rhabdias	***10***
		Ascaridoidea	*Ascaris*	***1, 5***
			Toxocara	***2, 6***
			Toxascaris	***1, 6***
			Parascaris	***1, 4***
			Ascaridia	***1, 7, 10***
			Heterakis	***1, 7, 10***
			Paraspidodera	***9***
			Sulcascaris	***10***
			Ophidascaris	***10***
			Porrocaecum	***7***
			Polydelphus	***10***
		Anisakidae	*Anisakis*	***1***
			Contracaecum	***1, 7***
			Hysterothylacium	***1***
			Pseudoterranova	***1***
			Angusticaecum	***1, 10***
		Oxyuroidea	*Oxyuris*	***1, 4***
			Probstmayria	***1, 4***
			Skrjabinema	***1, 2, 3, 8***
			Paraspidodera	***1, 9***
			Enterobius	***1***
			Aspicularis	***9***
			Passalurus	***9***
			Syphacia	***9***
		'Subuluroidea'	*Subulura*	***1, 7***
		Spiruroidea	*Spirocerca*	***1, 6***
			Habronema	***1, 4***

(*continued*)

Phylum	Class	Superfamily Family	Genus	Chapters
			Draschia	***1, 4***
			Parabronema	***1, 2, 3, 8***
			Thelazia	***1, 2, 4, 6, 8***
			Gnathostoma	***1, 5, 6***
			Gongylonema	***1, 2, 3, 5, 7, 8***
			Ascarops	***1, 5***
			Physocephalus	***1, 5***
			Simondsia	***1, 5***
			Physaloptera	***1, 6***
			Spirura	***1, 6, 10***
			Echinuria	***1, 7***
			Dispharynx	***1, 7, 10***
			Tetrameres	***1, 7, 10***
			Streptocara	***1, 7***
			Cheilospirura	***1, 7***
			Histiocephalus	***1, 7***
			Hartertia	***1, 7***
			Oxyspirura	***1, 7***
			Odontospirura	***10***
		Filarioidea	*Parafilaria*	***1, 2, 4***
			Stephanofilaria	***1, 2***
			Dirofilaria	***1, 6***
			Dipetalonema	***1, 6, 8***
			Onchocerca	***1, 2, 4, 8***
			Setaria	***1, 2, 4***
			Elaeophora	***1, 2, 3, 4, 8***
			Ornithofilaria	***1***
			Pelecitus	***1***
			Brugia	***1***
			Loa	***1***
			Wuchereria	***1***
			Mansonella	***1***
			Suifilaria	***5***
			Paronchocercaria	***10***
		Trichuroidea	*Trichuris*	***1, 2, 3, 5, 6, 8, 9***
			Capillaria	***1, 2, 3, 6, 7, 8, 9, 10***
			Trichinella	***1, 4, 5, 6***
			Trichosomoides	***9***
		Dioctophymatoidea	*Dioctophyma*	***1, 5, 6***
			Hystrichis	***1, 7***
			Eustrongylides	***1, 7***
		Dracunculoidea	*Dracunculus*	***1, 2***
			Avioserpens	***1, 7***
Acanthocephala		**Oligacanthorhynchidae**	*Macracanthorhynchus*	***1, 4, 5***
		Polymorphidae	*Polymorphus*	***1, 7***
			Filicollis	***1, 7***

(*continued*)

Phylum	Class Sub-class	Family	Genus	Chapters
Platyhelminthes	Trematoda			
	Digenea	Fasciolidae	*Fasciola*	***1, 2, 3, 4, 5, 6, 8***
			Fascioloides	***1, 2, 3, 8***
			Fasciolopsis	***1, 5***
		Dicrocoeliidae	*Dicrocoelium*	***1, 2, 3, 8***
			Eurytrema	***1, 2, 3, 5, 6, 8***
			Platynosomum	***1, 6***
		Paramphistomatidae	*Paramphistomum*	***1, 2, 3, 8***
			Orthocoelium (syn *Ceylonocotyle*)	***1, 2, 3, 8***
			Cotylophoron	***1, 2, 3***
			Bothriophoron	***1***
			Gastrodiscus	***1, 4, 5***
			Homologaster	***1, 2***
			Explanatum (syn *Gigantocotyle*)	***1***
			Pseudodiscus	***4***
	Digenea	Troglotrematidae	*Paragonimus*	***1, 6***
			Nanophyetus	***1, 6***
			Collyriclum	***1, 7***
		Cyclocoelidae	*Typhlocoelum*	***1, 7***
			Hyptiasmus	***1, 7***
		Opisthorchiidae	*Opisthorchis* (syn *Clonorchis*)	***1, 6***
			Metorchis	***1, 6***
			Parametorchis	***1, 6***
			Pseudamphistomum	***1, 6***
		Schistosomatidae	*Schistosoma*	***1, 2, 3, 4, 5, 6, 8***
			Bilharziella	***1, 7***
			Trichobilharzia	***1***
			Orientobilharzia	***1, 3***
			Ornithobilharzia	***1***
			Heterobilharzia	***1***
			Austrobilharzia	***1***
		Diplostomatidae	*Alaria*	***1, 6***
			Diplostomum	***1***
		Echinostomatidae	*Echinostoma*	***1, 6, 7, 10***
			Echinoparyphium	***1, 7, 10***
			Hypoderaeum	***1, 7, 10***
			Echinochasmus	***1, 6***
			Euparyphium	***1, 6***
		Notocotylidae	*Notocotylus*	***1, 7***
			Catatropis	***1, 7***
			Cymbiforma	***1, 2, 3***
		Brachylaemidae	*Brachylaemus*	***1, 7, 10***
			Skrjabinotrema	***1, 3***
		Plagiorchiidae	*Plagiorchis*	***1, 7***
		Prosthogonimidae	*Prosthogonimus*	***1, 7***

(*continued*)

Phylum	Class Sub-class	Family	Genus	Chapters
		Heterophyidae	*Heterophyes*	***1, 6***
			Metagonimus	***1, 6***
			Apophallus	***6***
			Cryptocotyle	***6***
			Haplorchis	***1, 6***
		Strigeidae	*Apatemon*	***7***
			Cotylurus	***7***
			Parastrigea	***7***

Phylum	Class Order	Family	Genus	Chapters
Platyhelminthes	**Cestoda**			
	Cyclophyllidea	Taeniidae	*Taenia* *(syn Multiceps)*	***1, 2, 3, 5, 6, 8, 9***
			Echinococcus	***1, 2, 3, 4, 5, 6, 8***
		Anoplocephalidae	*Anoplocephala*	***1, 4***
			Paranoplocephala	***1, 4***
			Moniezia	***1, 2, 3, 8***
			Cittotaenia	***9***
		Dilepididae	*Dipylidium*	***1, 6***
			Amoebotaenia	***1, 7***
			Choanotaenia	***1, 7***
			Metroliasthes	***1, 7***
		Davaineidae	*Davainea*	***1, 7, 10***
			Raillietina	***1, 7, 10***
			Cotugnia	***1, 7***
			Huttuynia	***10***
		Hymenolepididae	*Hymenolepis*	***1, 7***
			Fimbriaria	***1, 7***
			Rodentolepis	***1, 9***
		Mesocestoididae	*Mesocestoides*	***1, 6***
		Thysanosomidae	*Stilesia*	***1, 2, 3, 8***
			Thysanosoma	***1, 2, 3***
			Thysaniezia	***1, 2, 3, 8***
			Avitellina	***1, 2, 3, 8***
	Pseudophyllidea	Diphyllobothriidae	*Diphyllobothrium*	***1, 6***
			Spirometra	***1, 6***

(*continued*)

B. VETERINARY ENTOMOLOGY

Phylum	CLASS Order Sub-order	Family	Genus	Chapters
Arthropoda	**Insecta**			
	Hemiptera	Cimicidae	*Cimex*	***1***
		Reduviidae	*Triatoma*	***1, 11***
			Rhodnius	***1, 11***
			Panstrongylus	***1***
	Diptera			
	Nematocera	Ceratopogonidae	*Culicoides*	***1, 11***
		Simuliidae	*Simulium*	***1, 11***
		Psychodidae	*Phlebotomus*	***1, 11***
			Lutzomyia	***1, 11***
		Culicidae	*Aedes*	***1, 11***
			Anopheles	***1, 11***
			Culex	***1, 11***
	Brachycera	Tabanidae	*Chrysops*	***1, 11***
			Haematopota	***1, 11***
			Tabanus	***1, 11***
	Cyclorrhapha	Muscidae	*Musca*	***1, 11***
			Hydrotaea	***1, 11***
			Stomoxys	***1, 11***
			Haematobia	***1, 11***
		Fanniidae	*Fannia*	***1, 11***
		Hippoboscidae	*Hippobosca*	***1, 11***
			Melophagus	***1, 3***
			Lipoptera	***11***
		Glossinidae	*Glossina*	***1, 11***
		Calliphoridae	*Lucilia*	***1, 2, 3, 11***
			Calliphora	***1, 3, 11***
			Protophormia	***1, 3, 11***
			Phormia	***1, 3, 11***
			Cochliomyia (syn *Callitroga*)	***1, 11***
			Chrysomya	***1, 11***
			Cordylobia	***1, 11***
		Sarcophagidae	*Sarcophaga*	***11***
			Wohlfahrtia	***1, 11***
		Oestridae	*Hypoderma*	***1, 2, 8***
			Oestrus	***1, 3, 8***
			Dermatobia	***1, 11***
			Przhevalskiana (syn *Crivellia*)	***1, 3***
			Cephenemyia	***1, 8***
			Oedemagena	***1, 8***
			Gedoelstia	***1, 3***
			Cephalopina (syn *Cephalopsis*)	***1, 8***
			Rhinoestrus	***1, 4***
			Pharyngomyia	***8***
			Cuterebra	***1, 9***
			Gasterophilus	***1, 4***

(*continued*)

Phylum	CLASS Order Sub-order	Family	Genus	Chapters
	Phthiraptera			
	Anoplura	Haematopinidae	*Haematopinus*	***1, 2, 4, 5***
		Microthoraciidae	*Microthoracius*	***1, 8***
		Linognathidae	*Linognathus*	***1, 2, 3, 6***
			Solenopotes	***1, 2***
		Polyplacidae	*Polyplax*	***1, 9***
	Amblycera	Menoponidae	*Menacanthus*	***1, 7***
			Menopon	***1, 7***
			Holomenopon	***1, 7***
			Ciconiphilus	***7***
			Trinoton	***7***
			Amyrsidea	***1, 7***
			Mecanthus	***7***
		Boopidae	*Heterodoxus*	***1, 6***
		Gyropidae	*Gyropus*	***1, 9***
			Gliricola	***1, 9***
		Trimenoponidae	*Trimenopon*	
	Ischnocera	Philopteridae	*Cuclotogaster*	***1, 7***
			Lipeurus	***1, 7***
			Goniodes	***1, 7***
			Goniocotes	***1, 7***
			Anaticola	***7***
			Acidoproctus	***7***
			Anatoecus	***7***
			Ornithobius	***7***
			Columbicola	***1, 10***
		Trichodectidae	*Bovicola* (*syn Damalinia*)	***1, 2, 3, 4***
			Felicola	***1, 6***
			Trichodectes	***1, 6***
		Degeeriellidae	*Lagopoecus*	***7***
	Siphonaptera	Ceratophyllidae	*Ceratophyllus*	***1, 11***
			Nosopsyllus	***1, 9***
		Pulicidae	*Ctenocephalides*	***1, 6, 11***
			Spilopsyllus	***1, 11***
			Echidnophaga	***1, 11***
			Pulex	***1, 11***
			Xenopsylla	***1, 9***
			Archaeopsylla	***1, 11***
			Tunga	***1, 11***
		Leptopsyllidae	*Leptopsylla*	***1, 9***

(*continued*)

Phylum	CLASS Sub-class Sub-order	Family	Genus	Chapters
Arthropoda	**Arachnida**			
	Acari			
	Ixodida (Metastigmata)	Ixodidae	*Ixodes*	***1, 10, 11***
			Dermacentor	***1, 11***
			Rhipicephalus	***1, 11***
			Haemaphysalis	***1, 10, 11***
			Boophilus	***1, 11***
			Amblyomma	***1, 10, 11***
			Hyalomma	***1, 10, 11***
			Aponomma	***1, 10***
		Argasidae	*Argas*	***1, 10, 11***
			Otobius	***1, 11***
			Ornithodoros	***1, 10, 11***
	Sarcoptiformes (Astigmata)	Sarcoptidae	*Sarcoptes*	***1, 2, 3, 4, 5, 6, 8***
			Notoedres	***1, 6, 9***
			Trixacarus	***1, 9***
		Psoroptidae	*Psoroptes*	***1, 2, 3, 4, 8***
			Chorioptes	***1, 2, 3, 4, 8***
			Otodectes	***1, 6***
		Knemidokoptidae	*Knemidokoptes*	***1, 7***
		Listeropheridae	*Mycoptes*	***1, 9***
		Cytoditidae	*Cytodites*	***1, 7, 10***
		Laminosioptidae	*Laminosioptes*	***1, 7***
		Analgidae	*Megninia*	***1, 7***
		Atopomelidae	*Chirodiscoides*	***1, 9***
		Dermoglyphidae	*Dermoglyphus*	***1, 7***
		Freyanidae	*Freyana*	***1, 7***
		Epidermoptidae	*Epidermoptes*	***1, 7***
			Microlichus	***1, 7***
			Promyialges	***1, 7***
		Pterolichidae	*Pterolichus*	***1, 7***
			Sideroferus	***1, 7***
		Hypoderidae	*Hypodectes*	***1, 7***
	Trombidiformes (Prostigmata)	Demodicidae	*Demodex*	***1, 2, 3, 4, 5, 6, 9***
		Cheyletidae	*Cheyletiella*	***1, 6***
		Trombiculidae	*Neotrombicula*	***1, 11***
			Eutrombicula	***1, 11***
			Leptotrombidium	***1, 9***
			Neoschongastia	***1, 7***
		Psorergatidae	*Psorergates*	***1, 2, 3, 9***
		Pyemotidae	*Pyemotes*	***1, 11***
		Myobidae	*Myobia*	***1, 9***
			Radfordia	***1, 9***
		Syringophilidae	*Syringophilus*	***1, 7***
		Pterygosomatidae	*Geckobiella*	***1, 10***
			Pimeliaphilus	***1, 10***
			Hirstiella	***1, 10***
			Ixodiderma	***1, 10***

(*continued*)

Phylum	CLASS Sub-class Sub-order	Family	Genus	Chapters
			Scapothrix	***1, 10***
			Zonurobia	***1, 10***
	Mesostigmata	Macronyssidae	*Ornithonyssus*	***1, 7, 9***
	(Gamesid Mites)		*Neoliponyssus*	***10***
			Ophionyssus	***1, 10***
		Dermanyssidae	*Dermanyssus*	***1, 7, 9***
			Liponyssoides	***1, 9***
		Halarachnidae	*Pneumonyssus*	***1, 6***
		Entonyssidae	*Entonyssus*	***1, 10***
			Entophionyssus	***1, 10***
			Mabuyonysus	***1, 10***
		Rhinonyssidae	*Sternosoma*	***1, 7***
		Laelapidae	*Hirstionyssus*	***1, 9***
			Haemogamasus	***1, 9***
			Eulaelaps	***1, 9***
			Laelaps	***1, 9***
			Androlaelaps	***1, 9***
Arthropoda	**Pentastomida**			
		Linguatulidae	*Linguatula*	***1, 10***

C. VETERINARY PROTOZOOLOGY

Phylum Sub-phylum	Order Sub-order	Family	Genus	Chapters
PROTISTA				
Sarcomastigophora				
Sarcodina	**Amoebidorida**	**Endamoebidae**	*Entamoeba*	***1, 2, 3, 4, 5, 6, 9, 10***
			Endolimax	***1***
Mastigophora	**Kinetoplastorida**	**Trypanosomatidae**	*Leishmania*	***1, 6***
			Trypanosoma	***1, 2, 3, 4, 5, 6, 7, 8, 10***
	Trichomonadorida	**Trichomonadidae**	*Tritrichomonas*	***1, 2, 5, 7, 9***
			Trichomonas	***1, 6, 7, 10***
			Tetratrichomonas	***1, 2, 3, 5, 6, 7, 9***
			Trichomitus	***1, 5***
			Pentatrichomonas	***1, 6, 10***
			Chilomastix	***7, 10***
			Enteromonas	***10***
			Eutrichomonas	***10***
			Herpatomonas	***10***
			Leptomonas	***10***
			Proteromonas	***10***
		Monocercomonadidae	*Histomonas*	***1, 7***
			Monocercomonas	***1, 2, 10***
		Retortamonadorididae	*Retortamonas*	***1, 2, 3, 9***

(continued)

Phylum Sub-phylum	Order Sub-order	Family	Genus	Chapters
	Diplomonadorida	**Diplomonadidae**	*Giardia*	***1, 2, 3, 4, 5, 6, 9***
			Spironucleus (syn Hexamita)	***1, 7, 9, 10***
			Caviomonas	***1, 9***
			Monocercomonoides	***1, 9***
			Protomonas	***1, 9***
			Hexamastix	***1, 9***
			Chilomitus	***1, 9***
		Cochlosomatidae	*Cochlosoma*	***1, 7***
Apicomplexa	**Eucoccidiorida**			
	Eimeriorina	**Eimeriidae**	*Eimeria*	***1, 2, 3, 4, 5, 7, 8, 9, 10***
			Isospora	***1, 5, 6, 8, 10***
			Cyclospora	***1, 10***
			Tyzzeria	***1, 7, 10***
			Wenyonella	***1, 7, 10***
			Caryospora	***1, 10***
			Hoarella	***1, 10***
			Octosporella	***1, 10***
			Pythonella	***1, 10***
			Dorisella	***1, 10***
		Cryptosporidiidae	*Cryptosporidium*	***1, 2, 3, 4, 5, 6, 7, 8, 9, 10***
		Sarcocystiidae	*Besnoitia*	***1, 2, 3, 6, 8, 10***
			Hammondia	***1, 6***
			Sarcocystis	***1, 2, 3, 4, 5, 6, 7, 8, 9, 10***
			Neospora	***1, 2***
			Frenkelia	***1***
			Toxoplasma	***1, 2, 3, 4, 5, 6, 7, 8, 9, 10***
		Lankesterellidae	*Lankesterella*	***1***
			Schellakia	***1, 10***
		Atoxoplasmatidae	*Atoxoplasma*	***1***
		Klossiellidae	*Klossiella*	***1, 4, 9, 10***
		Hepatozoidae	*Hepatozoon*	***1, 6, 9, 10***
		Haemogregarinidae	*Haemogregarina*	***10***
	Haemosporida	**Plasmodiidae**	*Haemoproteus*	***1, 7, 10***
			Hepatocystis	***1***
			Leucocytozoon	***1, 7, 10***
			Plasmodium	***1, 7, 10***
	Piroplasmorida	**Babesiidae**	*Babesia*	***1, 2, 3, 4, 5, 6, 8***
		Theileriidae	*Theileria*	***1, 2, 3, 4, 8***
			Cytauxzoon	***1, 6***

(*continued*)

Phylum Sub-phylum	**Order** Sub-order	**Family**	**Genus**	**Chapters**
Microspora	**Microspororida**	**Nosematidae**	*Encephalitozoon*	***1, 6, 9***
		Enterocytozoonidae	*Enterocytozoon*	***1***
Ciliophora	**Trichostomatorida**	**Balantidiidae**	*Balantidium*	***1, 5, 10***
		Pycnotrichidae	*Buxtonella*	***2, 8***
		Nyctotheridae	*Nyctotherus*	***1, 10***
Bigyra Blastocysta	**Blastocystida**	**Blastocystidae**	*Blastocystis*	***1***
Ascomycota	**Pneumocystida**	**Pneumocystidaceae**	*Pneumocystis*	***1, 2***

D. RICKETTSIAE

Kingdom	**Order**	**Family** Sub-family	**Genus**	**Chapters**
Monera	**Rickettsiales**	**Rickettsiaceae**		
		Rickettsieae	*Rickettsia*	***1, 2, 3, 6, 9***
			Rochalimaea	***1***
			Coxiella	***1***
			Neorickettsia	***4***
		Ehrlichieae	*Ehrlichia*	***1, 2, 3, 6***
			*'Cowdria'**	***1, 2, 3***
		Bartonellaceae	*Bartonella*	***1***
			Grahamella	***1***
		Anaplasmataceae	*Anaplasma*	***1, 2, 3, 4, 6, 8***
			Aegyptianella	***1, 7***
			Eperythrozoon	***1, 2, 3, 5***
			Haemobartonella (syn Mycoplasma)	***1, 6***

* Genus *Cowdria* now classified as *Ehrlichia*.

Foreword to the first edition

This book is intended for students of veterinary parasitology, for practising veterinarians and for others requiring information on some aspect of parasitic disease.

Originally intended as a modestly expanded version of the printed notes issued to our students in the third and fourth years of the course, the text, perhaps inevitably, has expanded. This was due to three factors. Firstly, a gradual realization of the deficiencies in our notes; secondly, the necessity of including some of the comments normally imparted during the lecture course; and thirdly, at the suggestion of the publishers, to the inclusion of certain aspects of parasitic infections not treated in any detail in our course.

We should perhaps repeat that the book is primarily intended for those who are directly involved in the diagnosis, treatment and control of parasitic diseases of domestic animals. The most important of these diseases have therefore been discussed in some detail, the less important dealt with more briefly and the uncommon either omitted or given a brief mention, Also, since details of classification are of limited value to the veterinarian we have deliberately kept these to the minimum sufficient to indicate the relationships between the various species. For a similar reason, taxonomic detail is only presented at the generic level and, occasionally, for certain parasites, at species level. We have also trod lightly on some other areas such as, for example, the identification of species of tropical ticks and the special significance and epidemiology of some parasites of regional importance. In these cases, we feel that instruction is best given by an expert aware of the significance of particular species in that region.

Throughout the text we have generally referred to drugs by their chemical, rather than proprietary, names because of the plethora of the latter throughout the world. Also, because formulations are often different, we have avoided stating doses; for these, reference should be made to the data sheets produced by the manufacturer. However, on occasions when a drug is recommended at an unusual dose, we have noted this in the text.

In the chapters at the end of the book we have attempted to review five aspects of veterinary parasitology, epidemiology, immunity, anthelmintics, ectoparasiticides and laboratory diagnosis. We hope that this broader perspective will be of value to students, and particularly to those dismayed by the many complexities of the subject.

There are no references in the text apart from those at the end of the chapter on diagnosis. This was decided with some regret and much relief on the grounds that it would have meant the inclusion, in a book primarily intended for undergraduates, of hundreds of references. We hope that those of our colleagues throughout the world who recognize the results of their work in the text will accept this by way of explanation and apology.

We would, however, like to acknowledge our indebtedness to the authors of several source books on veterinary parasitology whose work we have frequently consulted. These include *Medical and Veterinary Protozoology* by Adam, Paul & Zaman, *Veterinaermedizinische Parasitologie* by Boch & Supperer, Dunn's *Veterinary Helminthology*, Euzéby's *Les Maladies Vermineuses des Animaux Domestiques*, Georgi's *Parasitology for Veterinarians*, Reinecke's *Veterinary Helminthology*, Service's *A Guide to Medical Entomology* and Soulsby's *Helminths, Arthropods and Protozoa of Domesticated Animals*.

Any student seeking further information on specific topics should consult these or, alternatively, ask his or her tutor for a suitable review.

The ennui associated with repeated proofreading may occasionally (we hope, rarely) have led to some errors in the text. Notification of these would be welcomed by the authors. Finally we hope that the stresses endured by each of us in this collaborative venture will be more than offset by its value to readers.

Acknowledgements to the first edition

We would like to express our gratitude to the following individuals and organizations who assisted us in the preparation of this book.

Firstly, to Drs R. Ashford and W. Beesley of Liverpool; Dr J. Bogan, Glasgow; Dr W. Campbell, Rahway, USA; Dr R. Dalgleish, Brisbane; Dr L. Joyner, Weybridge, England; Dr T. Miller, Florida; Dr M. Murray, Nairobi; Dr R. Purnell, Sandwich, England; Dr S.M. Taylor, Belfast; Professor K. Vickerman, Glasgow. Each of these read and commented on sections of the text in which they are expert. Any errors in these areas are, however, solely the responsibility of the authors.

Secondly, to the following individuals and companies who kindly allowed us to use their photographs or material as illustrations or plates:

Dr E. Allonby, Nairobi (Plate I d, e, f); Dr K. Angus, Edinburgh (Fig. 167); Dr J. Arbuckle, Guildford, England (Fig. 61); Dr E. Batte, North Carolina, USA (Plate IIIf); Dr I. Carmichael, Johannesburg, S. Africa (Fig. 142); Dr L. Cramer, Sao Paulo (Fig. 126b); Crown Copyright, UK (Plate XIVb); Dr J. Dunsmore, Murdoch, W. Australia (Plate IVd); Professor J. Eckert, Zurich (Fig. 96); Glaxovet, Harefield, England (Plate IIf); Dr I. Herbert, Bangor, Wales (Fig. 172); Dr A. Heydorn, W. Berlin (Figs 170, 171); Professor F. Hörning, Berne (Fig. 82; Plate Ve); Dr B. Iovanitti, Balcarce, Argentina (Figs 22, 23); Dr D. Jacobs, London (Fig. 38); Drs D. Kelly and A. Longstaffe, Bristol (Figs 156, 157); The late Dr I. Lauder, Glasgow (Fig. 65, Plate XIc, e, XIIb); Drs B. Lindemann and J. McCall, Georgia, USA (Fig. 67); Dr N. McEwan, Glasgow (Plate XId, XIIe); Dr G. Mitchell, Ayr, Scotland (Plate VIe); Professor M. Murray, Glasgow (Figs 68, 84, 152); Dr A. Nash, Glasgow (Fig. 138b, Plate XIIc); Dr Julia Nicholls, Adelaide, Australia (Figs 6, 14c, d); Dr R. Purnell, Sandwich, England (Fig. 173, Plate VIIId, e, f); Professor H. Pirie, Glasgow (Fig. 40); Dr J. Reid, Brussels (Plate XIIa); Dr Elaine Rose, Houghton Poultry Research Station, Huntingdon, England (Figs 160, 163b, 164a, b); Professor I. Selman, Glasgow (Plate XIf); Dr D. Taylor, Glasgow (Plate XIVc); Dr M. Taylor, London (Fig. 85); Dr S. Taylor, Belfast (Plate IIa); Dr H. Thompson, Glasgow (Fig. 92, Plate IVb, c, VId); Dr R. Titchener, Ayr, Scotland (Fig. 113b, Plate VIIIa); Dr A. Waddell, Brisbane, Australia (Fig. 66, Plate IVe); Wellcome Research Laboratories, Berkhamsted, England (Plate VIIIc); Dr A. Wright, Bristol (Plate VIb, XIb, XIId, f). In this context we are also extremely grateful to Miss E. Urquhart, Wrexham, Wales who prepared many of the line drawings.

Thirdly, to the pharmaceutical companies of Crown Chemical, Kent, England; Hoechst UK, Bucks; Merck Sharp & Dohme, Herts; Pfizer, Kent; Schering, New Jersey; Syntex Agribusiness, California. Their generosity enabled us to present many of the photographs in colour, thus enhancing their value.

Finally, to those members of the Faculty of Veterinary Medicine, Glasgow, whose cooperation was essential in the production of this book. We would especially like to thank Kenneth Bairden, our chief technician, who prepared much of the material for photography, often at inordinately short notice; Archie Finnie and Allan May, of the Photographic Unit, who, almost uncomplainingly, undertook the extra work of photographing many specimens; our two departmental secretaries, Elizabeth Millar and Julie Nybo, without whose skill and attention to detail this book would certainly not have been written.

G.M. Urquhart
J. Armour
J.L. Duncan
A.M. Dunn
F.W. Jennings
September 1985

Foreword and acknowledgements to the second edition

The first edition of this book was published in 1987 and the authors considered that a second edition is now necessary for several reasons.

Firstly, the widespread use of drugs such as avermectins and milbemycins, which have had a significant effect on anthelmintic prophylaxis and control. At the time of the first edition only one, ivermectin, was marketed whereas at the present time there are now several such products, supplemented by a number of new, long-acting chemoprophylactic devices.

Secondly, in many countries the production of a number of older anthelmintics and insecticides has largely ceased or many are difficult to find.

Thirdly, several parasitic diseases have now been described, about which little was known at the time of the first edition. Notably these are neosporosis and Lyme disease. Also included is a short description of the nasal mite of dogs, *Pneumonyssus caninum*, kindly provided by Professor Arvid Uggla of The National Veterinary Institute and Swedish University of Agricultural Sciences, Uppsala, Sweden.

Fourthly, we have taken the opportunity of rewriting some parts of the text, which on reflection, were less clear than we had hoped. In many cases, this has been supplemented by new diagrams or photographs.

Another change in this edition is the adoption of the standardized nomenclature of animal parasitic diseases (SNOAPAD) proposed by an expert committee appointed by the World Association for the Advancement of Veterinary Parasitology (WAAVP) published in *Veterinary Parasitology* (1988) **29**, 299–326. Although this may have a discomforting effect on those who have used certain familiar terms for animal parasitic diseases for many years, it is designed to improve the clarity of scientific communication by the general use of uniform terminology and should, in the long term, prove particularly beneficial in facilitating the retrieval of computerized data related to veterinary parasitology.

At the end of the book we have given a list of books and journals, which should be useful to anyone who wishes to pursue a specific subject in greater detail. This is confined to publications, which are readily available in most libraries of universities and research institutes.

We wish to thank Drs Ken Bairden, Quintin McKellar and Jacqueline McKeand for helpful comments on the text, also Mr Stuart Brown who assisted in the preparation of some of the new illustrations and Una B. Shanks RSW who prepared all of the new drawings.

We should mention, with great regret, the death of our co-author Dr Angus M. Dunn, who died in 1991 before this review was started, but we are reasonably certain that he would have approved of all the alterations we have made.

At the start of this revision we had intended to include new sections on parasitic disease of both fish and laboratory animals. However, a subsequent review of the literature currently available on these two subjects indicated that both were adequately covered in existing publications and it seemed more sensible to include the titles of these in the list of suggested reading.

Finally we wish to express our appreciation of the reception accorded to the first edition by reviewers, colleagues and students; we hope this second edition will be equally well received.

Foreword to the third edition

On behalf of the original authors of the first and second editions of *Veterinary Parasitology*, I would like to congratulate the new team of authors responsible for the third edition, which has expanded considerably from the previous two in order to include new areas of interest in the subject at local, national and international levels.

It is worth reflecting that the first edition was essentially a written and illustrated expansion of the printed notes issued to undergraduate veterinary students at the University of Glasgow. These notes very much mirrored the research interests of the staff within the Department of Veterinary Parasitology, which were principally in the helminthology branch of the subject, and to a lesser extent the protozoology and entomology components. Understandably this bias was reflected in the first edition, which was aimed at a readership of veterinary undergraduates and practising veterinary surgeons.

In the second edition, apart from the inclusion of some new and emerging diseases, the main change was the adoption of the standardised nomenclature of animal parasitic diseases (SNAOPAD) proposed by an expert committee of the World Association for the Advancement of Veterinary Parasitology (WAAVP).

By the time edition three was sought there was a clamour from the ever expanding population of those interested in the subject to produce a book that was not only suitable for students and practitioners but also provided more detailed information required by those researching the subject whether in academia, government institutions or industry.

This was a difficult task to undertake but the current authors have managed to produce a well illustrated text suitable for those studying and researching the subject. I particularly liked the re-vamped sections on entomology and protozoology and the updating of that on helminthology. The new chapters on parasites of laboratory animals and exotic pets were needed and the highlighting of zoonotic potential, where appropriate, was a welcome feature.

Despite the wealth of new material the original flavour of the first edition can still be detected, which gives great pleasure to myself, and my former colleagues at Glasgow.

I am sure the new edition will command great interest and respect from the international community of veterinary students, researchers and practitioners.

Professor Sir James Armour

Preface and acknowledgements to the third edition

The third edition has been written to accommodate a wider readership which includes teachers and students in veterinary schools, research groups in universities and institutes, veterinarians in practice and in government service and others who are involved in aspects of parasitic disease. In producing the new edition of *Veterinary Parasitology* the authors had several aims.

The first was to preserve the spirit of the first and second editions, which had been compiled by eminent and respected veterinary parasitologists in their field and which provided a solid background on which to consolidate.

The second aim was to expand the sections on protozoa and ectoparasites and to incorporate a larger selection of parasites, which are of veterinary significance in other parts of the world. The book focuses mainly on core information relating to parasites of livestock and companion animals but new sections on parasites of poultry and gamebirds, laboratory animals, exotic pets and 'farmed' species have been included. The majority of parasitic diseases are now covered in detail using a standardised format for each parasite to allow easy referencing and for comparison between species within a genus. Where appropriate, reference is made to human infections where there is natural transmission of parasitic disease between vertebrate animals and man (zoonoses).

The third aim was to present the information in a format which is compatible with the current parasitology teaching modules used within many university veterinary schools. This inevitably has had to be a compromise, as approaches to teaching veterinary parasitology differ throughout the world, but, by arranging the parasites under host species and their predilection site within the host and providing a comprehensive check list for each section and extensive cross-referencing, it is hoped that information on particular parasites can be easily located. Taxonomy of the main parasitic phyla and classes are provided within an introductory chapter along with generic descriptions and anatomical features of the parasite orders and families. Additional detailed sections are provided at the back of the book on veterinary antiparasitics, with a section on laboratory diagnosis, including numerous tables and identification charts. In keeping with previous editions a series of brief overviews of topics relevant to veterinary parasitology have been included to provide the non-expert with basic background information and to also highlight additional sources of reading.

The classification of parasites has been updated to reflect many of the systematic changes introduced, particularly where molecular genetics-based taxonomic reorganisation has been introduced. Throughout, synonyms have been provided reflecting older taxonomic nomenclature or where controversy remains. As with the previous edition, parasitic infections are described according to the Standardised Nomenclature of Animal Parasitic Diseases guidelines (SNOAPAD, 1988; *Veterinary Parasitology* 29, 299–326). In considering treatment of parasitic infections we have used the generic names of drugs to avoid listing the wide range of products, which are currently marketed in different countries. Dose rates of drugs are not always stated as many vary from country to country, being influenced by the relevant regulatory authorities. In all cases, readers are advised to consult the manufacturer's data sheets for current information and local regulations.

The authors are extremely grateful to Professor Sir James Armour and Professor James Duncan for their interest and support and for reading through the drafts of the text and their constructive comments. Any errors in the book are solely the responsibility of the authors. In order to assist the reader and for clarification we took the decision to produce much of the book and illustrations in colour and we are most grateful for the generous financial support of the following pharmaceutical companies which made this possible:

Fort Dodge Animal Health; Pfizer Animal Health Division of Pfizer Ltd; Merial Animal Health; Novartis Animal Health; Schering-Plough Animal Health; Bayer Animal Health; Virbac Ltd.

The new edition has benefited considerably from the range of expertise of the three authors:

Professor Mike Taylor is a veterinary graduate of Glasgow University Veterinary College, having studied under the authors of the first and second editions, whose enthusiasm for their subject greatly influenced his interest in veterinary parasitology. After 6 years in general veterinary practice, a large part of his career was spent at the Central Veterinary Laboratory, Weybridge, later to become the VLA, where he worked on the epidemiology and control of parasitic helminths, protozoa and ectoparasites of domestic animals, and in particular parasite chemotherapy and anthelmintic resistance. During this time he studied for a PhD at the Royal Veterinary College (RVC), London, under the expert guidance of Professor Dennis Jacobs. He is currently head of Veterinary Surveillance at the Central Science Laboratory York, a visiting Professor of Parasitology at the Royal Veterinary College, London and at the University of Wales, Bangor, a Fellow of Edinburgh University, a Diplomate of the European College of Veterinary Parasitology and Editor-in-Chief of *Veterinary Parasitology*.

Dr Bob Coop graduated in biochemistry from the University of Liverpool and then undertook a PhD in large animal parasitology at the University of Wales, Bangor. He has spent over 35 years in veterinary parasitology research, initially working with lungworm infection in pigs and then on the epidemiology and pathogenesis of gastrointestinal nematode infection in small ruminants, and in particular the nutrition–parasite interaction and sustainable control strategies. Formerly as Head of the Division of Parasitology at the Moredun Research Institute, and now as a Fellow of the Moredun Foundation, he has considerable experience of knowledge transfer to end-user groups and veterinarians in practice.

Professor Richard Wall graduated in zoology from the University of Durham followed by a PhD in insect population ecology at the University of Liverpool. He is now Professor of Zoology at the University of Bristol, where he teaches and heads a research group studying a diverse range of arthropods, focusing particularly on ectoparasites of veterinary importance and insect colonisers of dung and carrion. His research ranges widely from fundamental studies of arthropod taxonomy and physiology, through to field population ecology and farm-level investigations of the application of sustainable control technologies.

Finally, the help and support of the following list of people is acknowledged in producing this textbook. Professor Quintin McKellar (previous scientific director) and Professor Julie Fitzpatrick (current scientific director) of the Moredun Research Institute provided support to Dr Coop allowing him full access to the library facilities following his retirement. Dr Frank Jackson for comments on the manuscript. Michelle Moore, Matthew Carroll and Caroline Chaffer provided invaluable assistance with setting up much of the initial file documentation required to develop the re-organised structure of the book. Ralph Marshall at the Veterinary Laboratories Agency provided information on coccidial species of camelids and gamebirds. The technical support of Shelagh Wall is gratefully acknowledged.

The following individuals kindly allowed us to use their photographs or material as illustrations or figures: Dr L. Gibbons – Fig. 8.2; Dr J. McGarry – Figs. 2.10, 7.1, 7.4 and 8.1.

1
Parasite taxonomy and morphology

PRINCIPLES OF CLASSIFICATION

When examined, living organisms can be seen to form natural groups with features in common. These similarities may be morphological, but increasingly may be based on DNA analysis. Groups of organisms are combined into biologically meaningful groups, usually attempting to represent evolutionary pathways. A group of this sort is called a **taxon**, and the study of this aspect of biology is called **taxonomy**. The study of the complex systems of inter-relationship between living organisms is called **systematics**.

The taxa into which organisms may be placed are recognised by international agreement; the primary ones are: **kingdom**, **phylum**, **class**, **order**, **family**, **genus** and **species**. The intervals between these are large, and some organisms cannot be allocated to them precisely, so intermediate taxa, prefixed appropriately, have been formed; examples of these are the **suborder** and the **superfamily**. As an example, the taxonomic status of one of the common abomasal parasites of ruminants may be expressed as shown below

Kingdom	Animalia
Phylum	Nemathelminthes
Class	Nematoda
Order	Strongylida
Suborder	Strongylina
Superfamily	Trichostrongyloidea
Family	Trichostrongylidae
Subfamily	Haemonchinae
Genus	*Haemonchus*
Species	*contortus*

The names of taxa must follow a set of internationally agreed rules, but it is permissible to anglicise the endings, so that members of the superfamily Trichostrongyloidea in the example above may also be termed trichostrongyloids.

The names of the genus and species are expressed in Latin form, the generic name having a capital letter, and they must be in grammatical agreement. It is customary to print Latin names in italics. Accents are not permitted. If an organism is named after a person, amendment may be necessary; the name of Müller, for example, has been altered in the genus *Muellerius*.

HELMINTHOLOGY

The higher taxa containing helminths of veterinary importance are:

Major
Nemathelminthes (roundworms)
Platyhelminthes (flatworms)

Minor
Acanthocephala (thornyheaded worms)

Phylum NEMATHELMINTHES

The phylum Nemathelminthes has six classes but only one of these, the **nematoda**, contains worms of parasitic significance. The nematodes are commonly called **roundworms**, from their appearance in cross-section.

Class NEMATODA

A system of classification of nematodes of veterinary importance is given in Table 1.1. It must be emphasised that this is not an exact expression of the general system for parasitic nematodes, but is a simplified presentation intended for use in the study of veterinary parasitology. It is based on the ten superfamilies in which nematodes of veterinary importance occur, and which are conveniently divided into **bursate** and **non-bursate** groups.

STRUCTURE AND FUNCTION

Most nematodes have a cylindrical form, tapering at either end, and the body is covered by a colourless, somewhat translucent, layer: the cuticle.

The cuticle is secreted by the underlying hypodermis, which projects into the body cavity forming two lateral

Table 1.1 Parasitic Nematoda of veterinary importance: simplified classification.

Superfamily	Typical features
Bursate nematodes	
Trichostrongyloidea *Trichostrongylus, Ostertagia, Dictyocaulus, Haemonchus* etc.	Buccal capsule small. Life cycle **direct**; infection by L_3
Strongyloidea *Strongylus, Syngamus* etc.	Buccal capsule well developed; leaf crowns and teeth usually present. Life cycle **direct**; infection by L_3
Ancylostomatoidea *Ancylostoma, Uncinaria* etc.	
Metastrongyloidea *Metastrongylus, Muellerius, Protostrongylus* etc.	Buccal capsule small. Life cycle **indirect**; infection by L_3 in intermediate host
Non-bursate nematodes	
Rhabditoidea *Strongyloides, Rhabditis* etc.	Very small worms; buccal capsule small. Free-living and parasitic generations. Life cycle **direct**; infection by L_3
Ascaridoidea *Ascaris, Toxocara, Parascaris* etc.	Large white worms. Life cycle **direct**; infection by L_2 in egg
Oxyuroidea *Oxyuris, Skrjabinema* etc.	Female has long, pointed tail. Life cycle **direct**; infection by L_3 in egg
Spiruroidea *Spirocerca, Habronema, Thelazia* etc.	Spiral tail in male. Life cycle **indirect**; infection by L_3 from insect
Filarioidea *Dirofilaria, Onchocerca, Parafilaria* etc.	Long thin worms. Life cycle **indirect**; infection by L_3 from insect
Trichuroidea *Trichuris, Capillaria, Trichinella* etc.	Whip-like or hair-like worms. Life cycle **direct** or **indirect**; infection by L_1
Dioctophymatoidea *Dioctophyma* etc.	Very large worms. Life cycle **indirect**; infection by L_3 in aquatic annelids

cords, which carry the excretory canals, and a dorsal and ventral cord carrying the nerves (Fig. 1.1). The muscle cells, arranged longitudinally, lie between the hypodermis and the body cavity. The latter contains

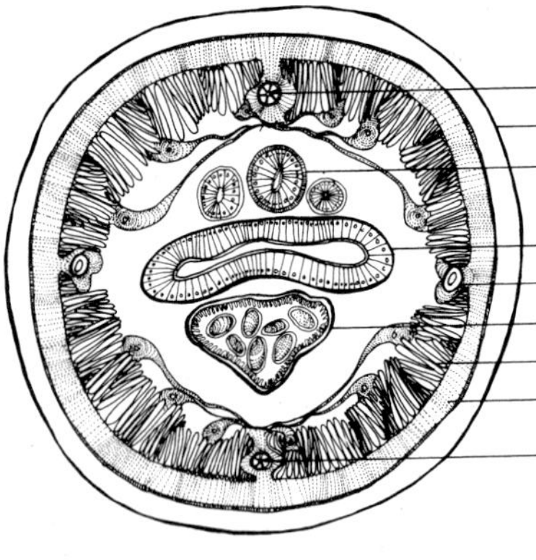

Fig. 1.1 Transverse section of a generalised female nematode.

fluid at a high pressure, which maintains the turgidity and shape of the body. Locomotion is effected by undulating waves of muscle contraction and relaxation that alternate on the dorsal and ventral aspects of the worm. Most of the internal organs are filamentous and suspended in the fluid-filled body cavity (Fig. 1.1).

The **digestive system** is tubular (Fig. 1.2a). The mouth of many nematodes is a simple opening, which may be surrounded by two or three lips, and leads directly into the oesophagus. In others, such as the strongyloids, it is large, and opens into a **buccal capsule**, which may contain teeth. Such parasites, when feeding, draw a plug of mucosa into the buccal capsule, where it is broken down by the action of enzymes, which are secreted into the capsule from adjacent glands. Some of these worms may also secrete anticoagulant, and small vessels, ruptured in the digestion of the mucosal plug, may continue to bleed for some minutes after the worm has moved to a fresh site.

Those with very small buccal capsules, like the trichostrongyloids, or simple oral openings, like the

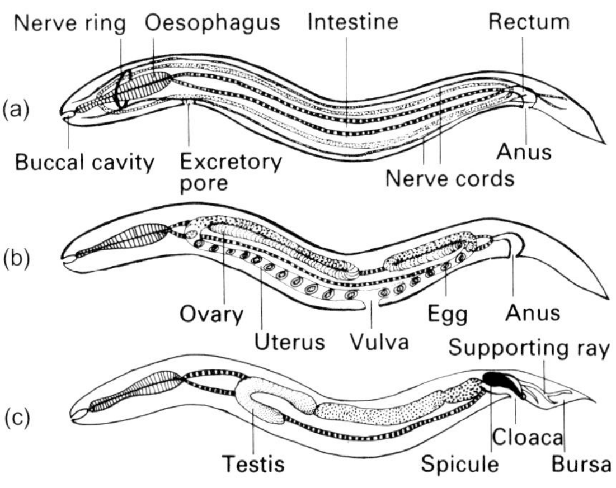

Fig. 1.2 Longitudinal sections of a generalised nematode. (a) Digestive, excretory and nervous system. (b) Reproductive system of a female nematode. (c) Reproductive system of a male nematode.

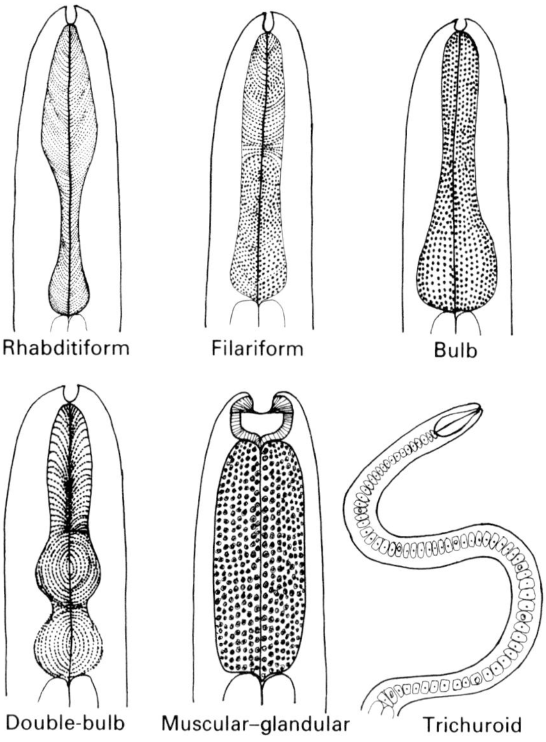

Fig. 1.3 The basic forms of oesophagus found in nematodes.

ascaridoids, generally feed on mucosal fluid, products of host digestion and cell debris, while others, such as the oxyuroids, appear to scavenge on the contents of the lower gut. Worms living in the bloodstream or tissue spaces, such as the filarioids, feed exclusively on body fluids.

The **oesophagus** is usually muscular and pumps food into the intestine. It is of variable form (Fig. 1.3), and is a useful preliminary identification character for groups of worms. It may be **filariform**, simple and slightly thickened posteriorly, as in the bursate nematodes; **bulb-shaped**, with a large posterior swelling, as in the ascaridoids; or **double bulb-shaped**, as in the oxyuroids. In some groups this wholly muscular form does not occur: the filarioids and spiruroids have a **muscular–glandular** oesophagus which is muscular anteriorly, the posterior part being glandular; the **trichuroid** oesophagus has a capillary form, passing through a single column of cells, the whole being known as a stichosome. A **rhabditiform** oesophagus, with slight anterior and posterior swellings, is present in the preparasitic larvae of many nematodes, and in adult free-living nematodes.

The **intestine** is a tube whose lumen is enclosed by a single layer of cells or by a syncytium. The luminal surfaces possess microvilli, which increase the absorptive capacity of the cells. In female worms the intestine terminates in an anus, while in males there is a cloaca which functions as an anus, and into which opens the vas deferens and through which the copulatory spicules may be extruded.

The so-called '**excretory system**' is very primitive, consisting of a canal within each lateral cord joining at the excretory pore in the oesophageal region.

The **reproductive systems** consist of filamentous tubes. The **female organs** comprise ovary, oviduct and uterus, which may be paired, ending in a common short vagina, which opens at the vulva (Fig. 1.2b). At the junction of uterus and vagina in some species there is a short muscular organ, the ovejector, which assists in egg laying. A vulval flap may also be present.

The **male organs** consist of a single continuous testis and a vas deferens terminating in an ejaculatory duct into the cloaca (Fig. 1.2c). Accessory male organs are sometimes important in identification, especially of the trichostrongyloids, the two most important being the spicules and gubernaculum (Fig. 1.4). The **spicules** are chitinous organs, usually paired, which are inserted in the female genital opening during copulation. The **gubernaculum**, also chitinous, is a small structure, which acts as a guide for the spicules. With the two sexes in close apposition the amoeboid sperm are transferred from the cloaca of the male into the uterus of the female.

The **cuticle** may be modified to form various structures (Figs 1.5a and 1.5b), the more important of which are:

Leaf crowns consisting of rows of papillae occurring as fringes round the rim of the buccal capsule (external leaf crowns) or just inside the rim (internal leaf crowns). They are especially prominent in certain nematodes of horses. Their function is not known, but it is suggested that they may be used to pin a patch of mucosa in position during feeding, or that they may

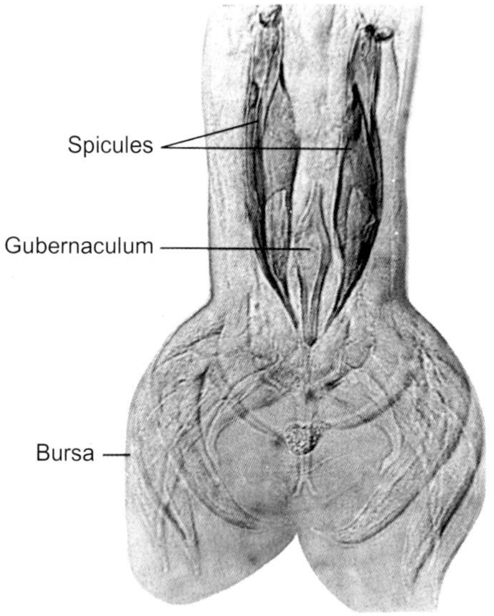

Fig. 1.4 Male trichostrongylid nematode bursa showing spicules and bursa.

prevent the entry of foreign matter into the buccal capsule when the worm has detached from the mucosa.

Cervical papillae occur anteriorly in the oesophageal region, and **caudal papillae** posteriorly at the tail. They are spine-like or finger-like processes, and are usually diametrically placed. Their function may be sensory or supportive.

Cervical and **caudal alae** are flattened wing-like expansions of the cuticle in the oesophageal and tail regions.

Cephalic and **cervical vesicles** are inflations of the cuticle around the mouth opening and in the oesophageal region.

The **copulatory bursa**, which embraces the female during copulation, is important in the identification of certain male nematodes and is derived from much expanded caudal alae, which are supported by elongated caudal papillae called **bursal rays**. It consists of two lateral lobes and a single small dorsal lobe.

Plaques and **cordons** are plate-like and cord-like ornamentations present on the cuticle of many nematodes of the superfamily Spiruroidea.

BASIC NEMATODE LIFE CYCLE

In the Nematoda, the sexes are separate and the males are generally smaller than the females, which lay eggs or larvae. During development, a nematode moults at intervals, shedding its cuticle. In the complete life cycle there are four moults, the successive larval stages being designated L_1, L_2, L_3, L_4 and finally L_5, which is the immature adult.

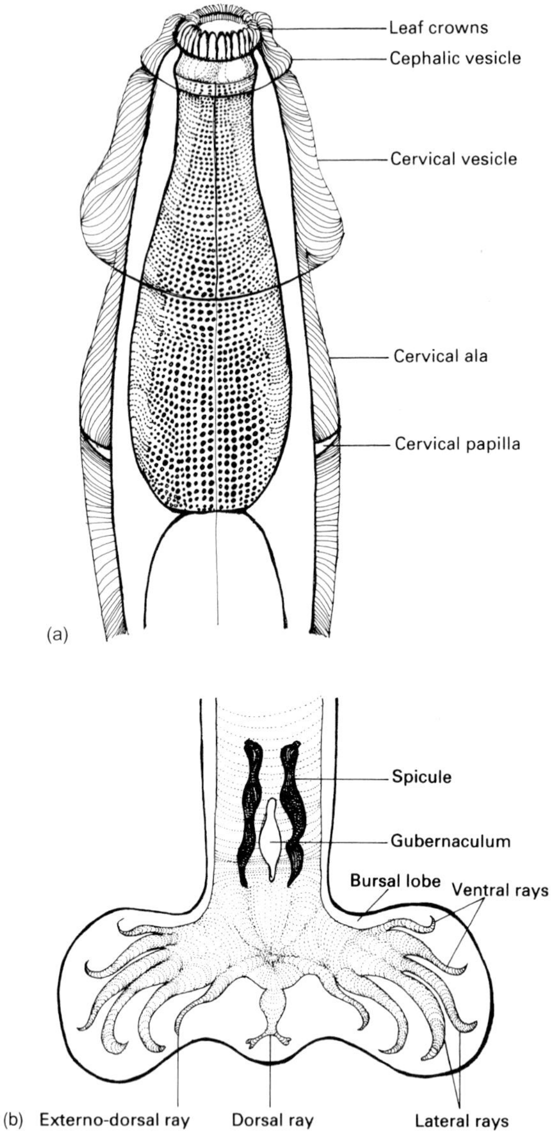

Fig. 1.5 Cuticular modifications of a generalised nematode. (a) Anterior region. (b) Posterior region of a male.

One feature of the basic nematode life cycle is that immediate transfer of infection from one **final host** to another rarely occurs. Some development usually takes place either in the faecal pat or in a different species of animal, the **intermediate host**, before infection can take place.

In the common form of **direct** life cycle, the free-living larvae undergo two moults after hatching and infection is by ingestion of the free L_3. There are some important exceptions however, infection sometimes being by larval penetration of the skin or by ingestion of the egg containing a larva.

In **indirect** life cycles, the first two moults usually take place in an intermediate host and infection of the final host is either by ingestion of the intermediate host or by inoculation of the L_3 when the intermediate host, such as a blood-sucking insect, feeds.

After infection, two further moults take place to produce the L_5 or immature adult parasite. Following copulation a further life cycle is initiated.

In the case of gastrointestinal parasites, development may take place entirely in the gut lumen or with only limited movement into the mucosa.

However, in many species, the larvae travel considerable distances through the body before settling in their final (predilection) site and this is the migratory form of life cycle. One of the most common routes is the **hepatic–tracheal**. This takes developing stages from the **gut** via the portal system to the **liver** then via the hepatic vein and posterior vena cava to the **heart** and from there via the pulmonary artery to the **lungs**. Larvae then travel via the bronchi, trachea and oesophagus to the **gut**. It should be emphasised that the above is a basic description of nematode life cycles and that there are many variations.

DEVELOPMENT OF THE PARASITE

EGG

Nematode eggs differ greatly in size and shape, and the shell is of variable thickness, usually consisting of three layers.

The inner membrane, which is thin, has lipid characteristics and is impermeable. A middle layer, which is tough and chitinous gives rigidity and, when thick, imparts a yellowish colour to the egg. In many species this layer is interrupted at one or both ends with an operculum (lid) or plug. The third outer layer consists of protein, which is very thick and sticky in the ascaridoids and is important in the epidemiology of this superfamily.

In contrast, in some species the eggshell is very thin and may be merely present as a sheath around the larva.

The survival potential of the egg outside the body varies, but appears to be connected with the thickness of the shell, which protects the larva from desiccation. Thus parasites whose infective form is the larvated egg usually have very thick-shelled eggs which can survive for years on the ground.

HATCHING

Depending on the species, eggs may hatch outside the body or after ingestion.

Outside the body, hatching is controlled partly by factors such as temperature and moisture and partly by the larva itself. In the process of hatching, the inner impermeable shell membrane is broken down by enzymes secreted by the larva and by its own movement. The larva is then able to take up water from the environment and enlarges to rupture the remaining layers and escape.

When the larvated egg is the infective form, the host initiates hatching after ingestion by providing stimuli for the larva, which then completes the process. It is important for each nematode species that hatching should occur in appropriate regions of the gut and hence the stimuli will differ, although it appears that dissolved carbon dioxide is a constant essential.

LARVAL DEVELOPMENT AND SURVIVAL

Three of the important superfamilies, the trichostrongyloids, the strongyloids and the rhabditoids, have a completely free-living preparasitic phase. The first two larval stages usually feed on bacteria, but the L_3, sealed off from the environment by the retained cuticle of the L_2, cannot feed and must survive on the stored nutrients acquired in the early stages. Growth of the larva is interrupted during moulting by periods of lethargus in which it neither feeds nor moves.

The cuticle of the L_2 is retained as a sheath around the L_3; this is important in larval survival with a protective role analogous to that of the eggshell in egg-infective groups.

The two most important components of the external environment are temperature and humidity. The optimal temperature for the development of the maximum number of larvae in the shortest feasible time is generally in the range 18–26°C. At higher temperatures, development is faster and the larvae are hyperactive, thus depleting their lipid reserves. The mortality rate then rises, so that few will survive to L_3. As the temperature falls the process slows, and below 10°C the development from egg to L_3 usually cannot take place. Below 5°C movement and metabolism of L_3 is minimal, which in many species favours survival.

The optimal humidity is 100%, although some development can occur down to 80% relative humidity. It should be noted that even in dry weather where the ambient humidity is low, the microclimate in faeces or at the soil surface may be sufficiently humid to permit continuing larval development.

In the trichostrongyloids and strongyloids, the embryonated egg and the ensheathed L_3 are best equipped to survive in adverse conditions such as freezing or desiccation; in contrast, the L_1 and L_2 are particularly vulnerable. Although desiccation is generally considered to be the most lethal influence in larval survival, there is increasing evidence that by entering a state of anhydrobiosis, certain larvae can survive severe desiccation.

On the ground most larvae are active; although they require a film of water for movement and are stimulated by light and temperature, it is now thought that larval movement is mostly random and encounter with grass blades accidental.

INFECTION

As noted previously, infection may be by ingestion of the free-living L_3, and this occurs in the majority of trichostrongyloid and strongyloid nematodes. In these, the L_3 sheds the retained sheath of the L_2 within the alimentary tract of the host, the stimulus for exsheathment being provided by the host in a manner similar to the hatching stimulus required by egg-infective nematodes. In response to this stimulus the larva releases its own exsheathing fluid, containing an enzyme leucine aminopeptidase, which dissolves the sheath from within, either at a narrow collar anteriorly so that a cap detaches, or by splitting the sheath longitudinally. The larva can then wriggle free of the sheath.

As in the preparasitic stage, growth of the larva during parasitic development is interrupted by two moults, each of these occurring during a short period of lethargus.

The time taken for development from infection until mature adult parasites are producing eggs or larvae is known as the **prepatent period** and this is of known duration for each nematode species.

METABOLISM

The main food reserve of preparasitic nematode larvae, whether inside the egg shell or free-living, is lipid, which may be seen as droplets in the lumen of the intestine. The infectivity of these stages is often related to the amount present; larvae which have depleted their reserves are not as infective as those which still retain quantities of lipid.

Apart from these reserves the free-living first and second stage larvae of most nematodes feed on bacteria. However, once they reach the infective third stage, they are sealed in the retained cuticle of the second stage, cannot feed and are completely dependent on their stored reserves.

In contrast, the adult parasite stores its energy as glycogen, mainly in the lateral cords and muscles, and this may constitute 20% of the dry weight of the worm.

Free-living and developing stages of nematodes usually have an aerobic metabolism, whereas adult nematodes can metabolise carbohydrate by both glycolysis (anaerobic) and oxidative decarboxylation (aerobic). However, in the latter, pathways may operate which are not present in the host and it is at this level that some antiparasitic drugs operate.

The oxidation of carbohydrates requires the presence of an electron transport system, which in most nematodes can operate aerobically down to oxygen tensions of 5.0 mmHg or less. Since the oxygen tension at the mucosal surface of the intestine is around 20 mmHg, nematodes in close proximity to the mucosa normally have sufficient oxygen for aerobic metabolism. Otherwise, if the nematode is temporarily or permanently some distance from the mucosal surface, energy metabolism is probably largely anaerobic.

As well as the conventional cytochrome and flavoprotein electron transport system, many nematodes have 'haemoglobin' in their body fluids which gives them a red pigmentation. This nematode haemoglobin is chemically similar to myoglobin and has the highest affinity for oxygen of any known animal haemoglobin. The main function of nematode haemoglobin is thought to be to transport oxygen, acquired by diffusion through the cuticle or gut, into the tissues; blood-sucking worms presumably ingest a considerable amount of oxygenated nutrients in their diet.

The end products of the metabolism of carbohydrates, fats or proteins are excreted through the anus or cloaca, or by diffusion through the body wall. Ammonia, the terminal product of protein metabolism, must be excreted rapidly and diluted to non-toxic levels in the surrounding fluids. During periods of anaerobic carbohydrate metabolism, the worms may also excrete pyruvic acid rather than retaining it for future oxidation when aerobic metabolism is possible.

The 'excretory system' terminating in the excretory pore is almost certainly not concerned with excretion, but rather with osmoregulation and salt balance.

Two phenomena which affect the normal parasitic life cycle of nematodes and which are of considerable biological and epidemiological importance are **arrested larval development** and the **periparturient rise** in faecal egg counts.

ARRESTED LARVAL DEVELOPMENT

(synonyms: inhibited larval development, hypobiosis) This phenomenon may be defined as the temporary cessation in development of a nematode at a precise point in its parasitic development. It is usually a facultative characteristic and affects only a proportion of the worm population. Some strains of nematodes have a high propensity for arrested development while in others this is low.

Conclusive evidence for the occurrence of arrested larval development can only be obtained by examination of the worm population in the host. It is usually recognised by the presence of large numbers of larvae at the same stage of development in animals withheld from infection for a period longer than that required to reach that particular larval stage.

The nature of the stimulus for arrested development and for the subsequent maturation of the larvae is still a matter of debate. Although there are apparently different circumstances which initiate arrested larval development, most commonly the stimulus is an environmental one received by the free-living infective stages prior to ingestion by the host. It may be seen as a ruse by the parasite to avoid adverse climatic conditions for its progeny by remaining sexually immature in the host until more favourable conditions return. The name commonly applied to this seasonal arrestment is **hypobiosis**. Thus the accumulation of arrested larvae often coincides with the onset of cold autumn/winter conditions in the northern hemisphere, or very dry conditions in the subtropics or tropics. In contrast, the maturation of these larvae coincides with the return of environmental conditions suitable to their free-living development, although it is not clear what triggers the signal to mature and how it is transmitted.

The degree of adaptation to these seasonal stimuli and therefore the proportion of larvae which do become arrested seems to be a heritable trait and is affected by various factors, including grazing systems and the degree of adversity in the environment. For example, in Canada where the winters are severe, most trichostrongyloid larvae ingested in late autumn or winter become arrested, whereas in southern Britain with moderate winters, about 50–60% are arrested. In the humid tropics where free-living larval development is possible all the year round, relatively few become arrested.

However, arrested development may also occur as a result of both acquired and age immunity in the host and, although the proportions of larvae arrested are not usually so high as in hypobiosis, they can play an important part in the epidemiology of nematode infections. Maturation of these arrested larvae seems to be linked with the breeding cycle of the host and occurs at or around parturition.

The epidemiological importance of arrested larval development from whatever cause is that, first, it ensures the survival of the nematode during periods of adversity; secondly, the subsequent maturation of arrested larvae increases the contamination of the environment and can sometimes result in clinical disease.

PERIPARTURIENT RISE (PPR) IN FAECAL EGG COUNTS

(Synonyms: post-parturient rise, spring rise.)

This refers to an increase in the numbers of nematode eggs in the faeces of animals around parturition.

This phenomenon is most marked in ewes, goats and sows and recent data supports the hypothesis that there is competition between the immune system, the rapidly growing fetus in late pregnancy and the udder during lactation, for nutrients, particularly metabolisable protein. This relaxation of immunity can be largely restored by supplementation with rumen-undegradable protein and is also influenced by the body protein status of the ewe.

The source of the PPR is three-fold:

(1) Maturation of larvae arrested due to host immunity.
(2) An increased establishment of infections acquired from the pastures and a reduced turnover of existing adult infections.
(3) An increased fecundity of existing adult worm populations.

Contemporaneously, but not associated with the relaxation of host immunity, the PPR may be augmented by the maturation of hypobiotic larvae.

The importance of the PPR is that it occurs at a time when the numbers of new susceptible hosts are increasing and so ensures the survival and propagation of the worm species. Depending on the magnitude of infection, it may also cause a loss of production in lactating animals and, by contamination of the environment, lead to clinical disease in susceptible young stock.

NEMATODE SUPERFAMILIES

Superfamily TRICHOSTRONGYLOIDEA

The trichostrongyloids are small, often hair-like, worms in the bursate group, which, with the exception of the lungworm *Dictyocaulus*, parasitise the alimentary tract of animals and birds. Structurally they have few cuticular appendages and the buccal capsule is vestigial. The males have a well developed bursa and two spicules, the configuration of which is used for species differentiation. The life cycle is direct and usually non-migratory and the ensheathed L_3 is the infective stage.

The trichostrongyloids, including *Dictyocaulus*, are responsible for considerable mortality and widespread morbidity, especially in ruminants. The most important alimentary genera are *Ostertagia*, *Teladorsagia*, *Haemonchus*, *Trichostrongylus*, *Cooperia*, *Nematodirus*, *Hyostrongylus*, *Marshallagia* and *Mecistocirrus*. Other genera of lesser importance are *Amidostomum*, *Ollulanus*, *Ornithostrongylus* and *Impalaia*.

Superfamily STRONGYLOIDEA

There are several important parasites of domestic mammals and birds in this superfamily of bursate nematodes.

Most are characterised by a large buccal capsule, which often contains teeth or cutting plates, and in some there are prominent leaf crowns surrounding the mouth opening. The adults occur on mucosal surfaces of the gastrointestinal and respiratory tracts and feeding is generally by the ingestion of plugs of mucosa.

With the exception of three genera, *Syngamus*, *Mammomonogamus* and *Cyathostoma*, which are parasitic in the trachea and major bronchi, and *Stephanurus* found in the peri-renal area, all other genera of veterinary importance in this superfamily are found in the intestine and can be conveniently divided into two groups, the **strongyles** and **hookworms**.

The strongyles are parasitic in the large intestine and the important genera are *Strongylus*, *Triodontophorus*, *Chabertia* and *Oesophagostomum*. The cyathostomins (cyathostomes or trichonemes) of horses include the genera *Cyathostomum*, *Cylicocyclus*, *Cylicodontophorus* and *Cylicostephanus*.

Syngamus and *Cyathostoma* are important parasites of the respiratory tract of birds. *Mammomonogamus* are parasites of the respiratory tract of cattle, sheep and goats.

Superfamily ANCYLOSTOMATOIDEA

Hookworms are parasites of the small intestine and the genera of veterinary importance are *Ancylostoma*, *Uncinaria*, *Bunostomum* and to a lesser extent, *Gaigeria* and *Agriostomum*.

In humans important hookworm genera are *Ancylostoma* and *Necator*.

Superfamily METASTRONGYLOIDEA

Most worms in this superfamily inhabit the lungs or the blood vessels adjacent to the lungs. The typical life cycle is indirect, and the intermediate host is usually a mollusc.

They may be conveniently divided into three groups according to host: those occurring in pigs (*Metastrongylus*), in sheep and goats (*Muellerius*, *Protostrongylus*, *Cystocaulus*, *Spiculocaulus* and *Neostrongylus*), and in the domestic and wild carnivores (*Oslerus*, *Filaroides*, *Aelurostrongylus*, *Angiostrongylus*, *Crenosoma*, *Anafilaroides*, *Metathelazia* and *Gurltia*).

Elaphostrongylus occurs in deer in Europe; *Parelaphostrongylus* occurs in deer and camelids in North America.

Superfamily RHABDITOIDEA

This is a primitive group of nematodes which are mostly free-living, or parasitic in lower vertebrates and invertebrates. Although a few normally free-living genera such as *Halicephalobus* (*Micronema*) and *Rhabditis* occasionally cause problems in animals, the only important genus from the veterinary point of view is *Strongyloides*.

Superfamily ASCARIDOIDEA

The ascaridoids are among the largest nematodes and occur in most domestic animals, both larval and adult stages being of veterinary importance. While the adults in the intestine may cause unthriftiness in young animals, and occasional obstruction, an important feature of the group is the pathological consequences of the migratory behaviour of the larval stages.

With a few exceptions the genera have the following characters in common. They are large, white opaque worms, which inhabit the small intestine. There is no buccal capsule, the mouth consisting simply of a small opening surrounded by three lips. The common mode of infection is by ingestion of the thick-shelled egg containing the L_2. However, the cycle may involve transport and paratenic hosts.

Genera of veterinary interest are *Ascaris*, *Toxocara*, *Toxascaris*, *Parascaris*, *Ascaridia*, *Heterakis* and to a lesser extent the anisakids (*Anisakis*, *Contracaecum*, *Hysterothylacium*, *Pseudoterranova*, *Angusticaecum*).

Superfamily OXYUROIDEA

Adult oxyuroids of animals inhabit the large intestine and are commonly called pinworms because of the pointed tail of the female parasite. They have a double bulb oesophagus and a direct life cycle. The genera of veterinary interest are *Oxyuris* and *Probstmayria*, both parasitic in the horse; *Skrjabinema*, which is a parasite of ruminants; *Paraspidodera* in guinea pigs; and *Subulura* (Subuluroidea) which are parasites of poultry. Oxyurids include the common human pinworm, *Enterobius*.

Superfamily SPIRUROIDEA

The precise classification of a number of genera currently assigned to this superfamily is controversial, but there are some of significance in veterinary medicine: *Spirocerca*, *Habronema*, *Draschia*, *Parabronema*, *Thelazia*, *Gnathostoma*, *Gongylonema* and to a lesser extent *Ascarops*, *Physocephalus*, *Simondsia*, *Physaloptera*, *Spirura*, *Echinuria*, *Dispharynx*, *Tetrameres*, *Streptocara*, *Cheilospirura*, *Histiocephalus*, *Hartertia* and *Oxyspirura*. A major characteristic of this group is the tight spirally coiled tail of the male. The life cycles are indirect involving arthropod intermediate hosts.

Members of the genus *Thelazia* are principally found in or around the eyes of animals and can be responsible for keratitis. Unlike most spiruroids, the

L_1 stage is not ingested from the faeces, but by flies feeding on ocular secretions.

The genus *Gongylonema* is unusual among the spiruroids in having a very wide final host range, which includes all the domesticated animals, though it is most prevalent in ruminants. Like most spiruroids the favoured location of the adults is in the upper alimentary tract, in the oesophagus, and in the forestomachs and stomach of mammals and the crop of birds.

Superfamily FILARIOIDEA

This superfamily is closely related to the Spiruroidea and, as in the latter, all its genera have indirect life cycles. None of them inhabits the alimentary tract, and they depend upon insect vectors for transmission.

Within the superfamily, differences in biological behaviour are seen, the more primitive forms laying eggs, which are available to the vectors in dermal exudates, and the more highly evolved forms laying larvae, termed microfilariae. The latter, which may be enclosed in a flexible, sheath-like 'egg shell' are taken up by parasitic insects feeding on blood and tissue fluids. In some species, the microfilariae only appear in the peripheral blood and tissues at regular intervals, some appearing in the daytime and others at night; this behaviour is termed diurnal or nocturnal periodicity.

Genera of interest in veterinary medicine include *Parafiliaria*, *Stephanofilaria*, *Dirofilaria*, *Dipetalonema*, *Onchocerca*, *Setaria*, *Elaeophora*, *Ornithofilaria* and *Pelecitus*. Of greater importance in human medicine are the genera *Onchocera*, *Brugia*, *Loa*, *Wuchereria* and *Mansonella*.

FILARIOSIS IN MAN

Though they are probably the most important group of helminth infections in humans, filarioid nematodes are of only marginal concern to the veterinarian, since domestic animals are of little significance in their epidemiology. The following are the most important species in man:

1. *Onchocerca volvulus*. Human onchocercosis due to *O. volvulus* occurs around the world in the equatorial zone, and is transmitted by *Simulium* spp (black flies). The adult worms live in subcutaneous nodules, and almost the entire pathogenic effect is caused by the microfilariae; dermatitis and elephantiasis are common, but the most important effect is ocular onchocercosis ('river blindness'), so-called because of its distribution along the habitats of *Simulium* spp. Dying microfilariae cause a sclerosing keratinitis in the cornea that leads to corneal opacification and retinochorioiditis. It has been estimated that in Africa there are about 20 million people affected by onchocercosis. The only other animals to which it is transmissible are the higher primates, chimpanzee and gorilla. Ivermectin is effective in reducing skin microfilarial counts in *O. volvulus* infection and repeated treatment should help reduce transmission. The onchocercosis associated pathology in the eye and skin has also been shown to be reduced with ivermectin treatment.
2. *Brugia* spp are carried by many species of mosquito and occur in Southeast Asia, notably in Malaysia, causing elephantiasis. The most important species, *B. malayi*, is also infective for monkeys and domestic and wild carnivores, and has been transmitted experimentally to the cat and dog. The lesser species occurring in man, *B. pahangi*, has a reservoir in many species of domestic and wild animals, including the dog and cat. Adult parasites inhabit lymph nodes and afferent lymphatic vessels.
3. *Wuchereria bancrofti* is also mosquito borne and affects the lymphatic system causing elephantiasis in Africa, Asia and South America. It is exclusive to man. As with *Brugia* spp, the main pathogenic effects are associated with adult worms rather than with microfilariae.
4. *Loa loa* is transmitted by *Chrysops* spp (tabanid flies), and occurs in west, central and east Africa, where it causes the transient subcutaneous enlargements known as 'Calabar swellings'. It is confined to man, apes and monkeys. Longevity can be up to 20 years.
5. *Mansonella ozzardi*, carried by *Culicoides* spp and *Simulium* spp, occurs in the Caribbean, and in Central and South America. It lives in the fat and on the mesentery or pleural cavity, and is usually considered to be non-pathogenic, though recently it has been associated with allergic signs. The prevalence is extremely high in endemic areas, where parasites closely resembling *M. ozzardi* are commonly found in monkeys and in horses and cattle. There is, however, reluctance to presume that these animals may be reservoir hosts until positive identification is made.

Superfamily TRICHUROIDEA

The members of this superfamily are found in a wide variety of domestic animals. A common morphological feature is the 'stichosome' oesophagus that is composed of a capillary-like tube surrounded by a single column of cells.

There are three genera of interest. The first, *Trichuris*, is found in the caecum and colon of mammals; the second, *Capillaria*, is most commonly present in the alimentary or respiratory tract of mammals or birds. Both lay eggs with plugs at both poles. The adults of the third genus, *Trichinella*, are found in the small intestine of mammals and produce larvae, which immediately invade the tissues of the same host.

Superfamily DIOCTOPHYMATOIDEA

Species of veterinary interest in this superfamily are the 'kidney worm', *Dioctophyma renale*; *Hystrichis* and *Eustrongylides* occur in aquatic fowl.

Superfamily DRACUNCULOIDEA

Members of this superfamily are parasites of the subcutaneous tissues. The two genera of veterinary significance are *Dracunculus* and *Avioserpens*. The life cycle involves development in a species of *Cyclops* before becoming infective to the final host.

Phylum ACANTHOCEPHALA

This is a separate class, closely related to the Nematoda, which contains a few genera of veterinary importance. They are generally referred to as 'thorny-headed worms' due to the presence of a hook-covered proboscis anteriorly, and most are parasites of the alimentary tract of vertebrates. The hollow proboscis armed with recurved hooks, which aid in attachment, is retractable and lies in a sac. There is no alimentary canal, with absorption taking place through the thick cuticle, which is often folded and invaginated to increase the absorptive surface. The sexes are separate, males being much smaller than females. Posteriorly, the male has a muscular bursa and penis and, after copulation, eggs, discharged by ovaries into the body cavity of the female, are fertilised and taken up by a complex structure called the uterine bell, which only allows mature eggs to pass out. These are spindle-shaped, thick-shelled and contain a larva which has an anterior circlet of hooks and spines on its surface and is called an **acanthor**. The life cycle is indirect, involving either an aquatic or terrestrial arthropod intermediate host. On ingestion by the intermediate host, the egg hatches and the acanthor migrates to the haemocoel of the arthropod where it develops to become a **cystacanth** after 1–3 months. The definitive host is infected by ingestion of the arthropod intermediate host, and the cystacanth, which is really a young adult, attaches and grows to maturity in the alimentary canal. The prepatent period varies from 5–12 weeks.

Family OLIGACANTHORHYNCHIDAE

The major genus of veterinary significance is *Macracanthorhynchus*, which is found in pigs.

Family POLYMORPHIDAE

A few genera are parasites of rodents (*Moniliformis*) aquatic birds (*Polymorphus*, *Filicollis*) and fishes (*Echinorhynchus*, *Acanthocephalus*).

Phylum PLATYHELMINTHES

This phylum contains the two classes of parasitic flatworms, the **Trematoda** and the **Cestoda**.

Class TREMATODA

The class Trematoda falls into two main subclasses, the **Monogenea**, which have a direct life cycle, and the **Digenea**, which require an intermediate host. The former are found mainly as external parasites of fish, while the latter are found exclusively in vertebrates and are of considerable veterinary importance.

The adult digenetic trematodes, commonly called 'flukes', occur primarily in the bile ducts, alimentary tract and vascular system. Most flukes are flattened dorsoventrally, have a blind alimentary tract, suckers for attachment and are hermaphrodite. Depending on the predilection site, the eggs pass out of the final host, usually in faeces or urine, and the larval stages develop in a molluscan intermediate host. For a few species, a second intermediate host is involved, but the mollusc is essential for all members of the group.

There are many families in the class Trematoda, and those which include parasites of major veterinary importance are the Fasciolidae, Dicrocoeliidae, Paramphistomidae and Schistosomatidae. Of lesser importance are the Troglotrematidae and Opisthorchiidae. The most important group by far are the Fasciolidae and the discussion below of structure, function, and life cycle is largely orientated towards this group.

Subclass DIGENEA

STRUCTURE AND FUNCTION OF DIGENETIC TREMATODES

The adult possesses two muscular suckers for attachment. The oral sucker at the anterior end surrounds the mouth, and the ventral sucker, as the name indicates, is on that surface. The body surface is a tegument, which is absorptive and is often covered with spines. The muscles lie immediately below the tegument. There is no body cavity and the organs are packed in a parenchyma (Fig. 1.6).

The digestive system is simple, the oral opening leading into a pharynx, oesophagus and a pair of branched intestinal caeca, which end blindly. Undigested material is presumably regurgitated. The

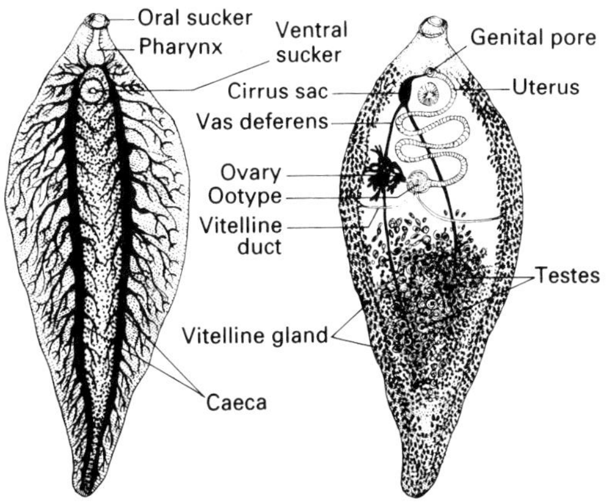

Fig. 1.6 Internal structure of a generalised digenetic trematode.

excretory system consists of a large number of ciliated flame cells, which impel waste metabolic products along a system of tubules, which ultimately join and open to the exterior. The nervous system is simple, consisting of a pair of longitudinal trunks connecting anteriorly with two ganglia.

The trematodes are usually hermaphrodite and both cross- and self-fertilisation may occur. The male reproductive system consists of a pair of testes each leading into a vas deferens; these join to enter the cirrus sac containing a seminal vesicle and the cirrus, a primitive penis which terminates at the common genital opening (Fig. 1.6). The female system has a single ovary leading into an oviduct, which is expanded distally to form the ootype. There the ovum acquires a yolk from the secretion of the vitelline glands and ultimately a shell. As the egg passes along the uterus, the shell becomes hardened and toughened and is finally extruded through the genital opening adjacent to the ventral sucker. The mature egg is usually yellow because of the tanned protein shell and most species have an operculum.

Food, generally blood or tissue debris, is ingested and passed into the caeca where it is digested and absorbed. Metabolism appears to be primarily anaerobic.

LIFE CYCLE OF DIGENETIC TREMATODES

The essential point of the life cycle is that whereas one nematode egg can develop into only one adult, one trematode egg may eventually develop into hundreds of adults. This is due to the phenomenon of asexual multiplication, **parthenogony**, in the molluscan intermediate host, i.e. the production of new individuals by single larval forms.

The adult flukes are always oviparous and lay eggs with an operculum or lid at one pole. In the egg the embryo develops into a pyriform (pear-shaped), ciliated larva called a **miracidium**. Under the stimulus of light, the miracidium releases an enzyme, which attacks the proteinaceous cement holding the operculum in place. The latter springs open like a hinged lid and the miracidium emerges within a few minutes.

The miracidium, propelled through the water by its cilia, does not feed and must, for its further development, find a suitable snail within a few hours. It is believed to use chemotactic responses to 'home' in on the snail and, on contact, it adheres by suction to the snail and penetrates its soft tissues aided by a cytolytic enzyme. The entire process of penetration takes about 30 minutes, after which the cilia are lost and the miracidium develops into an elongated sac, the **sporocyst**, containing a number of germinal cells. These cells develop into **rediae**, which migrate to the hepato-pancreas of the snail; rediae are also larval forms possessing an oral sucker, some flame cells and a simple gut. From the germinal cells of the rediae arise the final stages, the **cercariae**, although if environmental conditions for the snail are unsuitable, a second or daughter generation of rediae is often produced instead. The cercariae, in essence young flukes with long tails, emerge actively from the snail, usually in considerable numbers. The actual stimulus for emergence depends on the species, but is most commonly a change in temperature or light intensity. Once a snail is infected, cercariae continue to be produced indefinitely, although the majority of infected snails die prematurely from gross destruction of the hepato-pancreas.

Typically the cercariae swim for some time, utilising even a film of water, and within an hour or so attach themselves to vegetation, shed their tails and encyst. This stage is called a **metacercaria**.

Encysted metacercariae have great potential for survival extending to months. Once ingested, the outer cyst wall is removed mechanically during mastication. Rupture of the inner cyst occurs in the intestine and depends on a hatching mechanism, enzymatic in origin, triggered by a suitable oxidation–reduction potential and a carbon dioxide system provided by the intestinal environment. The emergent juvenile fluke then penetrates the intestine and migrates to the predilection site where it becomes adult after several weeks.

Family FASCIOLIDAE

These are large leaf-shaped flukes. The anterior end is usually prolonged into the shape of a cone and the anterior sucker is located at the end of the cone. The ventral sucker is placed at the level of the 'shoulders' of the fluke. The internal organs are branched while the cuticle is covered in spines. There are three important genera: *Fasciola*, *Fascioloides* and *Fasciolopsis*.

Family DICROCOELIIDAE

These trematodes are small, lancet-like flukes occurring in the biliary and pancreatic ducts of vertebrates. Miracidia are present in the eggs when they are passed in the faeces; there is no redial stage during development in the snail and two to three intermediate hosts may be involved in the life cycle. Members of this family are found in ruminants (*Dicrocoelium*, *Eurytrema*), and cats (*Platynosomum*).

Family PARAMPHISTOMATIDAE

Adult paramphistomes are mainly parasitic in the forestomachs of ruminants, although a few species occur in the intestine of ruminants, pigs and horses. Their shape is not typical of the trematodes, being conical rather than flat. All require a water snail as an intermediate host. There are several genera: *Paramphistomum*, *Cotylophoron*, *Bothriophoron*, *Orthocoelium* (syn *Ceylonocotyle*), *Gastrodiscus*, *Homologaster* and *Explanatum* (syn *Gigantocotyle*), of which *Paramphistomum* is the most common and widespread.

Family TROGLOTREMATIDAE

Several genera are of local veterinary interest. *Paragonimus*, commonly referred to as the 'lung fluke', is found in cats, dogs and other carnivores and in man in North America and Asia. The cycle involves a water snail and a crayfish or fresh water crab. Pulmonary signs are comparatively rare in cats or dogs and the veterinary interest is in the potential reservoir of infection for man.

The genus *Nanophyetus* is a fluke found mainly in the small intestine of dogs, mink and other fish-eating mammals. It occurs in the northwest United States and parts of Siberia and is of importance because the flukes are vectors of the rickettsial, *Neorickettsia helminthoeca*, which causes a severe haemorrhagic enteritis of dogs, the so-called 'salmon poisoning'. This name is derived from the cycle of the fluke, which involves a water snail and a fish that is often one of the salmonid type.

The genus *Collyriclum* are parasites occurring within subcutaneous cysts in chickens, turkeys and wild birds. Intermediate hosts are snails and dragonflies.

Family CYCLOCOELIDAE

These are medium-sized to large fluke, parasites of aquatic birds in the body cavity, air sacs or nasal cavities. Genera include *Typhlocoelum* in the respiratory tract of ducks, and *Hyptiasmus* in the nasal and orbital sinuses of ducks and geese.

Family OPISTHORCHIIDAE

The members of this family require two intermediate hosts, the first being water snails and the second a wide variety of fish, in which the metacercariae are encysted. The final hosts are fish-eating mammals in which they inhabit the bile ducts.

Opisthorchis (syn *Clonorchis*) is by far the most important genus, with *Metorchis*, *Parametorchis* and *Pseudamphistomum* being of lesser importance.

Family SCHISTOSOMATIDAE

This family is primarily parasitic in the blood vessels of the alimentary tract and bladder. In man, schistosomes are often responsible for severe and debilitating disease and veterinary interest lies in the fact that they can cause a similar disease in animals, some of which may act as reservoirs of infection for man. The schistosomes differ from other flukes in that the sexes are separate, the small adult female lying permanently in a groove, the gynaecophoric canal, in the body of the male (see Fig. 2.12). The most important genus is *Schistosoma* with *Bilharziella*, *Trichobilharzia*, *Orientobilharzia*, *Ornithobilharzia*, *Heterobilharzia* and *Austrobilharzia* other genera of lesser importance.

Family DIPLOSTOMATIDAE

The family Diplostomatidae includes the genera *Alaria* and *Diplostomum*. The life cycle involves two intermediate hosts, namely freshwater snails and frogs. The definitive host is infected through eating frogs containing encysted metacercariae (mesocercariae).

Family ECHINOSTOMATIDAE

The family Echinostomatidae includes the genera *Echinostoma*, *Echinoparyphium* and *Hypoderaeum*, which are parasites of birds, and *Echinochasmus* and *Euparyphium*, which are parasites of fish-eating mammals. The life cycle involves two intermediate hosts, namely freshwater snails and fish or frogs. The definitive host is infected through eating the second intermediate host containing encysted metacercariae (mesocercariae).

Family NOTOCOTYLIDAE

The family Notocotylidae includes the genera *Notocotylus*, *Paramonostomum* and *Catatropis*, which are parasites of birds, and *Cymbiforma*, which occur in sheep, goats and cattle. The small eggs are characterised by long filaments at the poles. The intermediate hosts are snails.

Family BRACHYLAEMIDAE

Members of this family are parasites of birds (*Brachylaemus*) or sheep (*Skrjabinotrema*). The intermediate hosts are snails.

Family PLAGIORCHIIDAE

Plagiorchis are parasites of birds. The life cycle involves two intermediate hosts, namely freshwater snails and larvae of dragonflies. The definitive host is infected through eating the dragonflies or their nymphs containing encysted metacercariae.

Family PROSTHOGONIMIDAE

Prosthogonimus are also parasites of birds with life cycles similar to *Plagiorchis*.

Family HETEROPHYIDAE

These are small trematodes found in the intestines of mammals and birds. The life cycle generally involves two intermediate hosts, namely freshwater snails and fishes or frogs. Genera of veterinary interest are *Heterophyes* found in dogs, cats, foxes and man; *Metagonimus* in the small intestines of dogs, cats, pigs and man; and *Rossicotrema* in cats, dogs, foxes and seals.

Family STRIGEIDAE

These worms are characterised by a constriction dividing the body into an anterior flattened adhesive organ and a posterior cylindrical part. They are parasites of the alimentary tract of birds. The life cycle involves two intermediate hosts, freshwater snails and a second host that may be a fish or leech. Genera include *Apatemon* and *Cotylurus* in the intestine of pigeons and ducks; and *Parastrigea* in ducks.

Class CESTODA

This class differs from the Trematoda in having a tape-like body with no alimentary canal. The body is segmented, each segment containing one and sometimes two sets of male and female reproductive organs. Almost all the tapeworms of veterinary importance are in the order Cyclophyllidea, the two exceptions being in the order Pseudophyllidea.

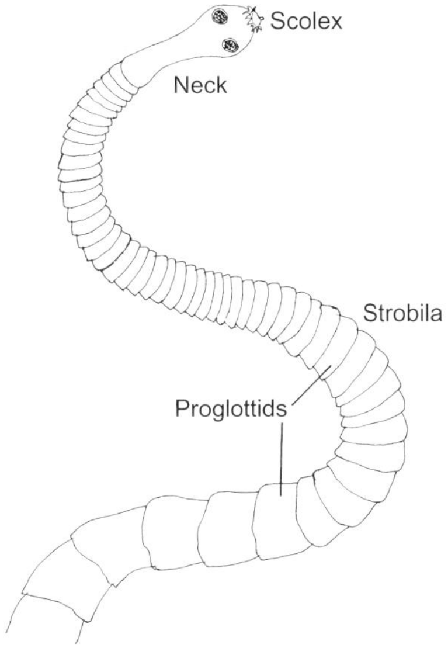

Fig. 1.7 Structure of a typical cyclophyllidean cestode.

Order CYCLOPHYLLIDEA

STRUCTURE AND FUNCTION

The adult cestode (Fig. 1.7) consists of a head or **scolex** bearing attachment organs, a short unsegmented neck and a chain of segments. The chain is known as a **strobila** and each segment as a **proglottid**.

The organs of attachment are four suckers on the sides of the scolex and these may bear hooks. The scolex usually bears anteriorly a mobile protrusible cone or rostellum and in some species this may be also armed with one or more concentric rows of hooks, which aid in attachment.

The proglottids are continuously budded from the neck region and become sexually mature as they pass down the strobila. Each proglottid is hermaphrodite with one or two sets of reproductive organs, the genital pores usually opening on the lateral margin or margins of the segment (Fig. 1.8); both self-fertilisation and cross-fertilisation between proglottids may occur. The structure of the genital system is generally similar to that of the trematodes. As the segment matures, its internal structure largely disappears and the fully ripe or gravid proglottid eventually contains only remnants of the branched uterus packed with eggs. The gravid segments are usually shed intact from the strobila and pass out with the faeces. Outside the body the eggs are liberated by disintegration of the segment or are shed through the genital pore.

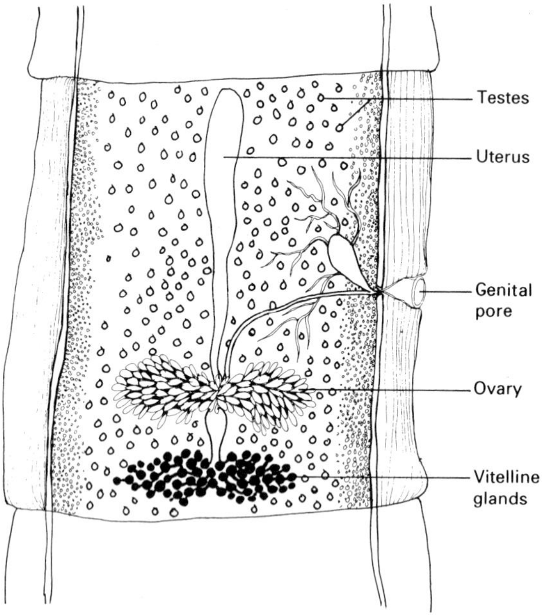

Fig. 1.8 Mature segment illustrating the reproductive organs.

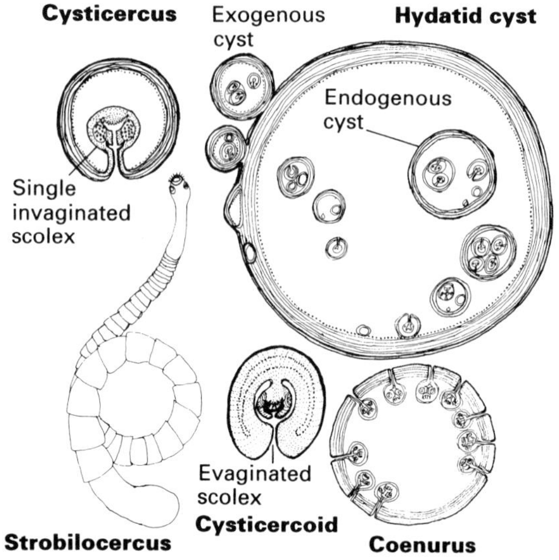

Fig. 1.9 Larval stages of cyclophyllidean cestodes.

The fully embryonated egg consists of:

(1) The hexacanth (six-hooked) embryo or **oncosphere**.
(2) A thick, dark, radially striated 'shell' called the **embryophore**.
(3) A true shell, which is a delicate membrane and is often lost while still in the uterus.

The tegument of the adult tapeworm is highly absorptive, the worm deriving all its nourishment through this structure. Below the tegument are muscle cells and the parenchyma, the latter a syncytium of cells, which fills the space between the organs. The nervous system consists of ganglia in the scolex from which nerves enter the strobila. The excretory system, as in the Trematoda, is composed of flame cells leading to efferent canals, which run through the strobila to discharge at the terminal segment.

LIFE CYCLE

The typical life cycle of these cestodes is indirect with one or more intermediate hosts. With few exceptions, the adult tapeworm is found in the small intestine of the final host, the segments and eggs reaching the exterior in the faeces.

When the egg is ingested by the intermediate host, the gastric and intestinal secretions digest the embryophore and activate the oncosphere. Using its hooks, it tears through the mucosa to reach the blood or lymph stream or, in the case of invertebrates, the body cavity. Once in its predilection site the oncosphere loses its hooks and develops, depending on the species, into one of the following larval stages, often known as **metacestodes** (Fig. 1.9):

- **Cysticercus:** Fluid-filled cyst containing an attached single invaginated scolex, sometimes called a protoscolex.
- **Coenurus:** Similar to a cysticercus, but with numerous invaginated scolices.
- **Strobilocercus:** The scolex is evaginated and is connected to the cyst by a chain of asexual proglottids. The latter are digested away after ingestion by the final host, leaving only the scolex.
- **Hydatid:** This is a large fluid-filled cyst lined with germinal epithelium from which are produced invaginated scolices which lie free or in bunches, surrounded by germinal epithelium (brood capsules). The contents of the cysts other than the fluid, i.e. scolices and brood capsules, are frequently described as 'hydatid sand'. Occasionally also, daughter cysts complete with cuticle and germinal layer are formed endogenously or, if the cyst wall ruptures, exogenously.
- **Cysticercoid:** A single evaginated scolex embedded in a small solid cyst. Typically found in very small intermediate hosts such as arthropods.
- **Tetrathyridium:** Worm-like larva with an invaginated scolex; found only in Mesocestoididae.

When the metacestode is ingested by the final host the scolex attaches to the mucosa, the remainder of the structure is digested off, and a chain of proglottids begins to grow from the base of the scolex.

The seven main families of veterinary interest in the order Cyclophyllidea are the *Taeniidae*, *Anoplocephalidae*, *Dilepididae*, *Davaineidae*, *Hymenolepididae*, *Mesocestoididae* and *Thysanosomidae*.

Family TAENIIDAE

The adults are found in domestic carnivores and man. The scolex has an armed rostellum with a concentric double row of hooks (the important exception is *Taenia saginata* whose scolex is unarmed). The gravid segments are longer than they are wide.

The intermediate stage is a cysticercus, strobilocercus, coenurus or hydatid cyst and these occur only in mammals.

Genera of importance are *Taenia* (syn *Multiceps*) and *Echinococcus*.

Family ANOPLOCEPHALIDAE

These are essentially tapeworms of horses (*Anoplocephala*, *Paranoplocephala*) and ruminants (*Moniezia*). The scolex has neither rostellum nor hooks and the gravid segments are wider than they are long. The intermediate stage is a cysticercoid present in forage mites of the family Oribatidae.

Family DILEPIDIDAE

These are tapeworms of the dog, cat (*Dipylidium*), and the fowl (*Amoebotaenia*, *Choanotaenia*, *Metroliasthes*). The scolex usually has an armed rostellum with several rows of hooks. The intermediate stage is a cysticercoid.

Family DAVAINEIDAE

These are mainly parasites of birds (*Davainea*, *Raillietina*, *Cotugnia*). These tapeworms usually have rows of hooks on both rostellum and suckers. The intermediate stage is a cysticercoid.

Family HYMENOLEPIDIDAE

These parasites are of minor veterinary importance. Members of this family, which have a characteristically slender strobila, infect birds, man and rodents (*Hymenolepis*, *Rodentolepis*, *Fimbriaria*). The intermediate stage is a cysticercoid present in an arthropod host.

Family MESOCESTOIDIDAE

Also of minor veterinary importance, these cestodes of carnivorous animals and birds have two metacestode stages. The first is a cysticercoid in an insect or mite, and the second a solid larval form, a tetrathyridium, in a vertebrate. Genera include *Mesocestoides* found in dogs, cats and wild mammals, and *Dithyridium* in chickens, turkeys and wild birds.

Family THYSANOSOMIDAE

Closely related to the Anoplocephalidae, this family contains several tapeworms of veterinary importance found mainly in sheep and other ruminants (*Stilesia*, *Thysanosoma*, *Thysaniezia* and *Avitellina*).

The intermediate stage is a cysticercoid present in forage mites of the family Oribatidae.

Order PSEUDOPHYLLIDEA

The morphology of the Pseudophyllidea is generally similar to that of the Cyclophyllidea, but there are two distinct features. First, the scolex has no suckers and instead has two longitudinal grooves or **bothria**, which become flattened to form organs of attachment. Secondly, the egg shell is thick, brown and operculate, and the **coracidium**, which emerges after hatching, is an oncosphere with an embryophore which is ciliated for mobility in water.

The pseudophyllidean life cycle utilises two intermediate hosts. The coracidium must first be ingested by a crustacean in whose body cavity a larval **procercoid** develops. Subsequently, if the crustacean is eaten by a freshwater fish, the procercoid is liberated, and in the muscles of the new host develops into a second larval stage, a **plerocercoid**, which possesses the characteristic scolex; it is only this stage which is infective to the final host.

This order contains only two genera of veterinary importance, *Diphyllobothrium* and *Spirometra*.

Family DIPHYLLOBOTHRIIDAE

The genus *Diphyllobothrium* is an important cestode of humans and fish-eating mammals. They are long tapeworms with an unarmed scolex, with two muscular bothria.

Spirometra are tapeworms of dogs, cats and wild carnivores and an occasional human zoonosis (sparganosis).

ENTOMOLOGY

Veterinary entomology, in its literal sense, means a study of insects of veterinary importance. This term, however, is commonly used to describe the wider study of all arthropods parasitic on animals, including arachnids such as ticks and mites.

Phylum ARTHROPODA

The phylum Arthropoda contains over 80% of all known animal species and consists of invertebrates whose major characteristics are a hard chitinous exoskeleton, a segmented body and jointed limbs.

CLASSIFICATION

There are two major classes of arthropods of veterinary importance, namely the Insecta and Arachnida, and the important orders in these classes are shown in Figs 1.10 and 1.11.

The two major classes can be differentiated by the following general characteristics:

Insecta: These have three pairs of legs, the head, thorax and abdomen are distinct, and they have a single pair of antennae.

Arachnida: The adults have four pairs of legs, the body is divided into the gnathosoma (mouthparts) and idiosoma (fused cephalo-thorax and abdomen); there are no antennae.

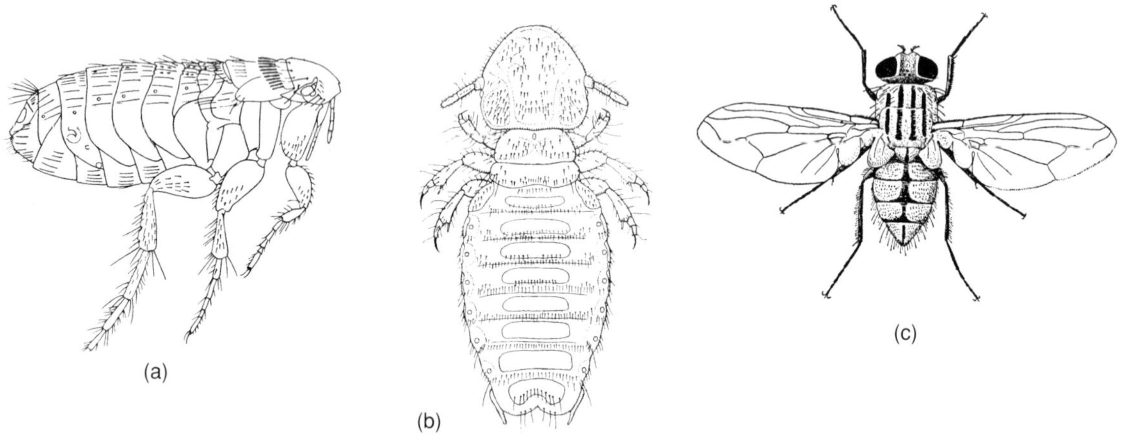

Fig. 1.10 A flea (Siphonaptera) (a), louse (Phthiraptera) (b) and adult fly (Diptera) (c), showing the general morphological features of insect ectoparasites.

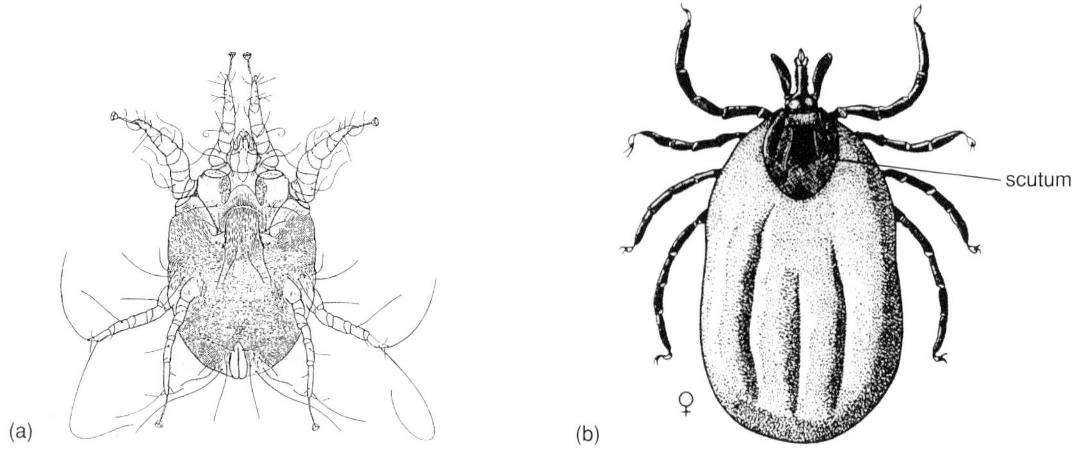

Fig. 1.11 A mite (a) and tick (b) showing the general morphological features of arachnid ectoparasites (from Baker *et al.*, 1956).

A third class of arthropod, the **Pentastomida**, is of lesser veterinary importance. The adults are found in the respiratory passages of vertebrates and resemble annelid worms rather than arthropods.

STRUCTURE AND FUNCTION

SEGMENTATION

Arthropods are **metameric**, that is they are divided into segments. However, within a number of arthropod classes, particularly the arachnids, there has been a tendency for segmentation to become greatly reduced and, in many of the mites for example, it has almost disappeared. Segments have become fused into clusters, such as the head, thorax and to a lesser extent the abdomen. Each group of segments is specialised for functions different from those of the other parts of the body.

EXOSKELETON

The **exoskeleton** is the outer covering, which provides support and protection to the living tissues of arthropods. The exoskeleton is non-cellular. Instead it is composed of a number of layers of **cuticle**, which are secreted by a single outer cell layer of the body known as the **epidermis** (Fig. 1.12). The outer layer of cuticle, the **epicuticle**, is composed largely of proteins and, in many arthropods, is covered by a waxy layer. The next two layers are the outer **exocuticle** and the inner **endocuticle**. Both are composed of a protein and a polysaccharide called **chitin**, which has long, fibrous molecules containing nitrogen. For extra strength the exocuticle may be tanned, or **sclerotised**. This is where proteins, interwoven between the chitin bundles, become tightly cross-linked giving it extra strength. The sclerotised cuticle is hard and dark in colour.

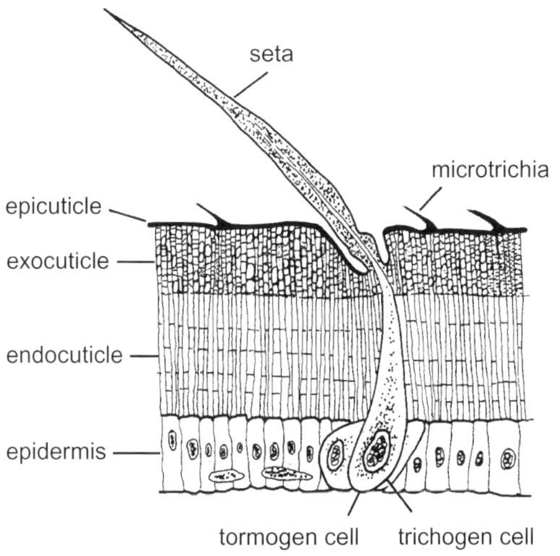

Fig. 1.12 Diagrammatic section through the arthropod integument.

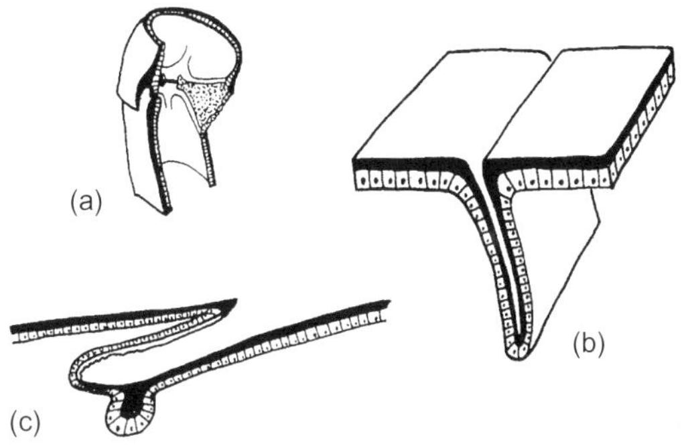

Fig. 1.13 (a) Articulation of a generalised arthropod leg joint. (b) A multicellular apodeme. (c) Intersegmental articulation, showing intersegmental membrane folded beneath the exoskeleton (after Snodgrass, 1935).

The cuticle is often penetrated by fine pore canals, which allow the passage of secretions from the epidermis to the surface. The cuticle has many outgrowths in the form of scales, spines, hairs and bristles.

Movement is made possible by the division of the cuticle into separate plates, called **sclerites**. Plates are connected by **intersegmental membranes**, where the cuticle is soft and flexible (Fig. 1.13). The muscles attach on the inside of the exoskeleton to rod-like invaginations of the cuticle called **apodemes**. The soft, flexible, unsclerotised cuticle present at the joints of the adult arthropod exoskeleton also occurs in the integument of larval arthropods.

APPENDAGES

Primitively each arthropod segment bears a pair of leg-like appendages. However, the number of appendages has frequently been modified through loss or structural differentiation. In insects there are always three pairs of legs in the adult stage. In mites and ticks there are three pairs of legs in the larval life cycle stage and four pairs in the nymphal and adult stages. The cuticular skeleton of the legs is divided into tube-like segments connected to one another by soft articular membranes, creating joints at each junction.

GAS EXCHANGE

For some small arthropods the exoskeleton is thin and lacks a waxy epicuticle. For these animals oxygen and carbon dioxide simply diffuse directly across the cuticle. However, this method of gas exchange is only functional over very short distances and for very small animals. In most of the terrestrial groups of arthropod ectoparasite, the protective cuticle is punctured by a

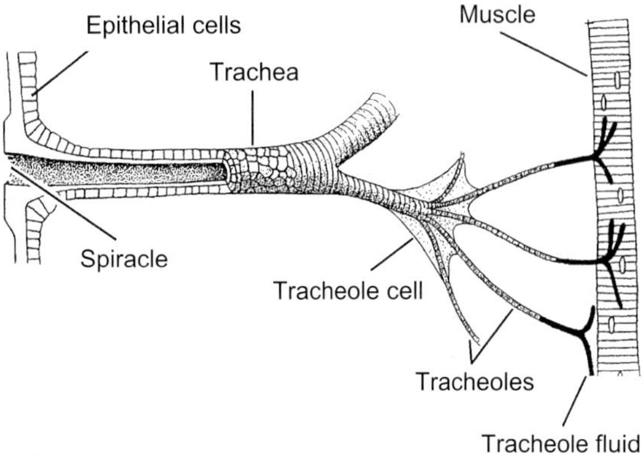

Fig. 1.14 A spiracle, trachea and tracheoles (after Snodgrass, 1935).

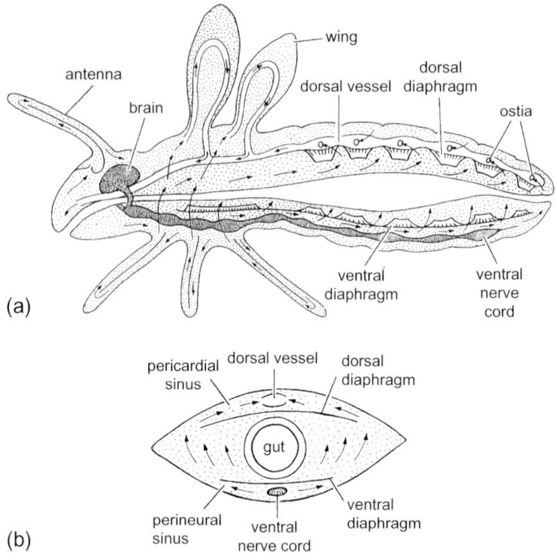

Fig. 1.15 Generalised arthropod circulatory system. (a) Longitudinal section through the body. (b) Transverse section through the abdomen (reproduced from Gullan and Cranston, 1994, after Wigglesworth, 1972).

number of openings. In the insects these openings are called **spiracles**; in the mites and ticks they are called **stigmata** (Fig. 1.14).

Typically spiracles or stigmata open into cuticle-lined air-conducting tubes called **tracheae**, which form longitudinal and transverse tracheal trunks that interconnect among the segments. The tracheae branch repeatedly as they extend to all parts of the body. The branches of the tracheae end within the cells of muscles and other tissues in extremely fine **tracheoles**, which are the principal sites of gas exchange. The ends of the tracheoles contain fluid and are usually less than 1 µm in diameter. Tracheoles are particularly numerous in tissues with high oxygen requirements.

Oxygen enters through the respiratory openings and passes down the trachea, usually by diffusion along a concentration gradient. Carbon dioxide and (in terrestrial insects) water vapour move in the opposite direction. Water loss is a major problem for most terrestrial arthropds and for them gas exchange is often a compromise between getting enough oxygen into the body while making sure that they do not desiccate. Hence in periods of inactivity the respiratory openings are often kept closed by valves which open only periodlically. In large and highly mobile insects active pumping movements of the thorax and or abdomen may be used to help to ventilate the outer parts of the tracheal system.

CIRCULATORY SYSTEM

The arthropod circulatory system is relatively simple, consisting of a series of central cavities or sinuses, called a **haemocoel** (Fig. 1.15). The haemocoel contains blood, called **haemolymph**, in which hormones are transported, nutrients are distributed from the gut and wastes removed via the excretory organs. The haemolymph is not involved in gas exchange.

In most mites the circulatory system consists only of a network of sinuses and circulation probably results from contraction of body muscles. Insects, on the other hand have a functional equivalent of the heart, the **dorsal vessel**. This is essentially a tube running along the length of the body. The dorsal vessel is open at its anterior end, closed at its posterior end and is perforated by pairs of lateral openings called **ostia**. The ostia only permit a one-way flow of haemolymph into the dorsal vessel. The dorsal vessel pumps haemolymph forward eventually into sinuses of the haemocoel in the head. Haemolymph then percolates back through the haemocoel, until it is again picked up by the dorsal vessel through the ostia.

NERVOUS SYSTEM

Arthropods have a complex nervous system associated with the well developed sense organs, such as eyes and antennae, and behaviour that is often highly elaborate. The central nervous system consists of a dorsal brain in the head which is connected by a pair of nerves which run around the foregut to a series of ventral nerve cord ganglia.

DIGESTIVE SYSTEM

The gut of an arthropod is essentially a simple tube that runs from mouth to anus. The precise shape of

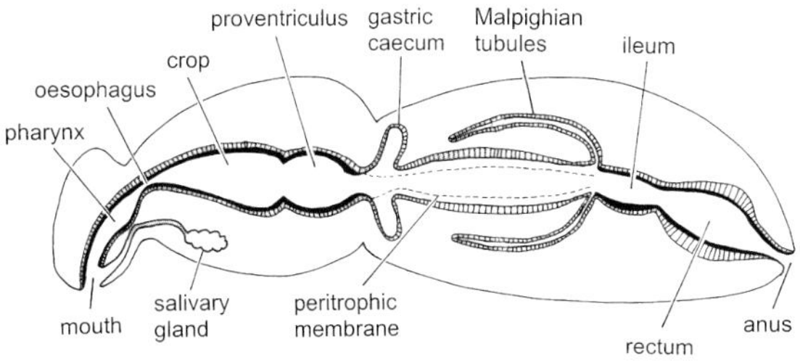

Fig. 1.16 Digestive tract of a generalised arthropod, showing the fore-, mid- and hindgut. The cuticular linings of the fore and hind gut are indicated by thickend lines.

the gut varies between arthropods depending on the nature of their diet.

The gut is divided into three sections: the foregut, midgut and hindgut (Fig. 1.16). The foregut and hindgut are lined with cuticle. In fluid-feeding arthropods there are prominent muscles, which attach to the walls of the pharynx, to form a pump. The foregut is concerned primarily with the ingestion and storage of food, the latter usually taking place in the **crop**. Between the foregut and the midgut is a valve called the **proventriculus** or **gizzard**. The midgut is the principal site of digestion and absorption. It has a cellular lining, which secretes digestive enzymes. Absorption takes place largely in the anterior of the midgut, in large outpockets called **gastric caecae**. The hindgut terminates in an expanded region, the **rectum**, which functions in the absorption of water and the formation of faeces. Nitrogenous wastes are eliminated from the haemocoel by long, thin projections called the **Malpighian tubules**, which open into the gut at the junction of the mid- and the hindgut. In mites and ticks the gut follows a broadly similar plan, but may be simplified, often with only one pair of Malpighian tubules.

ARTHROPOD SENSE ORGANS

The sensory receptors of arthropods are usually associated with modifications of the chitinous exoskeleton. The most common type of receptor is associated with hairs, bristles and setae. Bristles may act as mechanoreceptors, movement triggering the receptor at its base. Alternatively, the bristle may carry chemoreceptors, which may be senstive to specific chemical cues. The sensory hairs and bristles are distributed most densely at particular locations such as the antennae or legs.

Most arthropods have eyes, but these can vary greatly in complexity. Simple eyes, known as **stemmata** consisting of only a few sensory cells, are found in many larval insects. More complex **ocelli**, which contain between 1 and 1000 sensory cells and an overlying corneal lens, are found in many larval and adult insects. These simple eyes do not form images but are very sensitive at low light intensities and to changes in light intensity. The most complex type of arthropod eye, known as a compound eye, is large with thousands of long, cylindrical units called **ommatidia**, each covered by a translucent cornea, called a **facet**. There is no mechanism for accommodation, the compound eye does not form an effective image and its principal function is in detecting movement. In the female of some species of insect the eyes are distinctly separated (**dichoptic**) while in the males they may be very close together (**holoptic**). Ocelli and compound eyes may both occur in the same animal. In some arthropods, such as the ticks and lice, eyes may be greatly reduced or absent. In others such as some blood-sucking flies, whose sight is important in locating their hosts, the eyes are well developed.

REPRODUCTIVE SYSTEM

In most arthropods the sexes are separate and mating is usually required for the production of fertile eggs. The female reproductive system is composed of a pair of **ovaries**. Each ovary is divided into egg tubes, or **ovarioles**. The ovarioles lead, via the **oviduct** to an **ovipositor**. Most arthropods lay eggs, but some retain the eggs which hatch within the oviduct, and live larvae may be deposited at various stages of development.

The male reproductive system is usually composed of a pair or **testes**, each subdivided into a set of sperm tubes, leading to the vas deferens and the external genitalia, with a penis, or **aedeagus**. Accessory glands produce secretions, which may form a packet, called a **spermatophore**, which encloses the sperm and protects it during insemination.

Sperm may be delivered directly to the female during copulation or, in some species of mite, the spermatophore is deposited on the ground and the female is induced to walk over and pick up the spermatophore with her genital opening. Sperm are usually stored by the female in organs called **spermathecae**. As an ovulated egg passes down the oviduct it is fertilised by sperm released from the spermathecae.

MOULTING

To grow, arthropods must shed the exoskeleton periodically; this is **moulting** or, more properly, **ecdysis**. Before the old exoskeleton is shed the epidermis secretes a new epicuticle. The new epicuticle is soft and wrinkled at this stage. When the old skeleton is shed the soft, whitish exoskeleton of the newly moulted animal is stretched, often by the ingestion of air or water. Once expanded, sclerotisation occurs, resulting in hardening and darkening of the cuticle. The stages between moults are known as **stages**, or **stadia**, and distinct morphological life cycle stages are known as **instars**.

Class INSECTA

GENERAL MORPHOLOGY AND LIFE CYCLE

Members of the class Insecta can be distinguished from the other arthropods by the presence of only three pairs of legs in the adults, and the broad division of the body into three sections: the head, thorax and abdomen.

The head carries the main sensory organs: the single pair of antennae, a pair of compound eyes and, often, a number of ocelli. The mouth is surrounded by mouthparts which are very variable in form. In the ancestral form, represented by living insects such as cockroaches or grasshoppers, the mouthparts are composed of the following elements (Fig. 1.17). The **labrum** or upper lip is a hinged plate attached to the face or clypeus. The paired **mandibles** (jaws) and **maxillae** (secondary jaws) have areas of their surfaces adapted for cutting, slashing or grinding. The maxillae may also carry maxillary palps, which are sensory in function and used in the monitoring of food. A **hypopharynx** arises from the floor of the mouth and bears the external opening of the salivary glands and is similar to a tongue. A **labium** or lower lip usually bears two sensory labial palps, but these may be extensively modified, especially in flies. The mouthparts of different insects show a remarkable variety of specialisation, which is related to their diet.

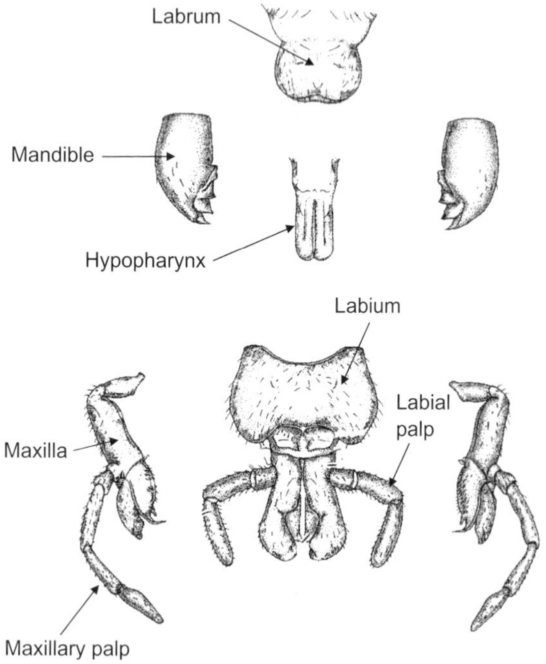

Fig. 1.17 Mouthparts of a generalised omnivorous insect.

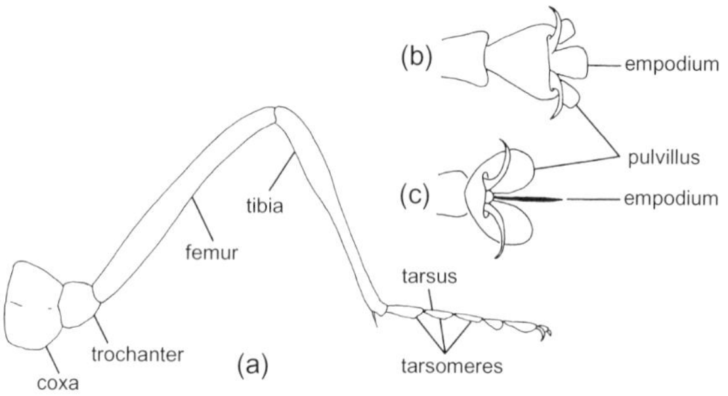

Fig. 1.18 (a) The segments of the leg, and the empodium and pulvilli of adult (b) brachycerran and (c) cyclorrhaphous Diptera.

The thorax is composed of three fused segments: the **prothorax**, the **mesothorax** and the **metathorax**. On each of these segments there is a single pair of legs. Each leg is composed of six segments. The basal section of the leg articulating with the body is the **coxa**, which is followed by a short, triangular **trochanter**. There then follows the **femur**, the **tibia**, one to five segments of the **tarsus**, the tarsomeres and, finally, the **pretarsus** composed of claws and ridged pads. Between the claws there may be two pad-like **pulvilli** surrounding a central bristle or pad, known as the **empodium** (Fig. 1.18). The legs of insects are generally adapted for walking or running but some are modified for specialised functions, such as jumping (fleas) or clinging to the hairs of their host's body (lice).

Most orders of insect have two pairs of wings articulating with the mesothorax and metathorax (pterygotes). Some orders of primitive insects have never developed wings (apterygotes), while others, such as the fleas and lice, which once had wings, have now lost them completely. Others, such as some of the hippoboscids, have wings for only a short time as adults, after which they are shed. The wing consists of a network of sclerotised veins, which enclose regions of thin, transparent cuticle called cells. The veins act as a framework to brace and stabilise the wing and may carry haemolymph and nerves. The arrangement of the veins tends to be characteristic of various groups of insect species and so is important in identification and taxonomy (Fig. 1.19). In several groups of insects, such as beetles, the front wings have been modified to various degrees as protective coverings for the hind wings and abdomen, known as **elytra**. In the true flies (the Diptera) the hind wings have been reduced to form a pair of club-like **halteres**, which are used as stabilising organs to assist in flight.

The abdomen is composed primitively of 11 segments, although the tenth and eleventh segments are usually small and not externally visible and the

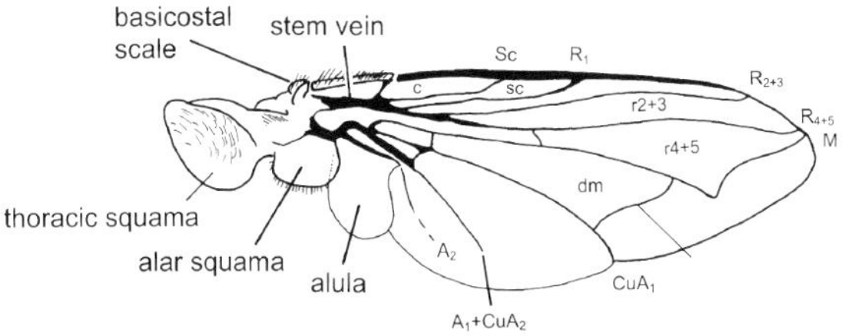

Fig. 1.19 The wing veins and cells of a typical insect, the calypterate dipteran, *Calliphora vicina*.

eleventh segment has been lost in most advanced groups. The genital ducts open ventrally on segment eight or nine of the abdomen and these segments often bear external organs that assist in reproduction. The genitalia are composed of structures which probably originated from simple abdominal appendages. In the male, the basic external genitalia consist of one or two pairs of claspers, which grasp the female in copulation, and the penis (**aedeagus**). However, there is considerable variation in the precise shape of the male genitalia in various groups of insect and these differences may be important in the identification of species. In the female the tip of the abdomen is usually elongated to form an ovipositor.

Within the class Insecta there are generally considered to be 30 orders, of which only three, the flies (Diptera), fleas (Siphonaptera) and lice (Phthiraptera), are of major veterinary importance.

INSECT LIFE CYCLES

In most insects, the juvenile stadia broadly resemble the adult, except that the genitalia and, where appropriate, wings are not developed. The juveniles, usually called **nymphs**, make new cuticle and shed the old one at intervals throughout development, typically four or five times, increasing in size before the emergence of the adult. This is often described as a simple life cycle with incomplete or partial metamorphosis, known as **hemimetabolous metamorphosis** (Fig. 1.20).

In other, more advanced, insects the juvenile and adult stages are dissimilar. The juvenile instar, which may be referred to as a **larva**, **maggot**, **grub** or **caterpillar**, has become concerned primarily with feeding and growth. In contrast, the adult, or **imago**, has become the specialised reproductive and dispersal instar. To reach the adult form, the larva must undergo complete metamorphosis, during which the entire body is reorganised and reconstructed. The transformation between the juvenile and the adult is made possible by the incorporation of a **pupal** stage, which acts as a bridge between juvenile and adult. The pupa does not feed and is generally (but not always) immobile. However, it is metabolically very active as old larval

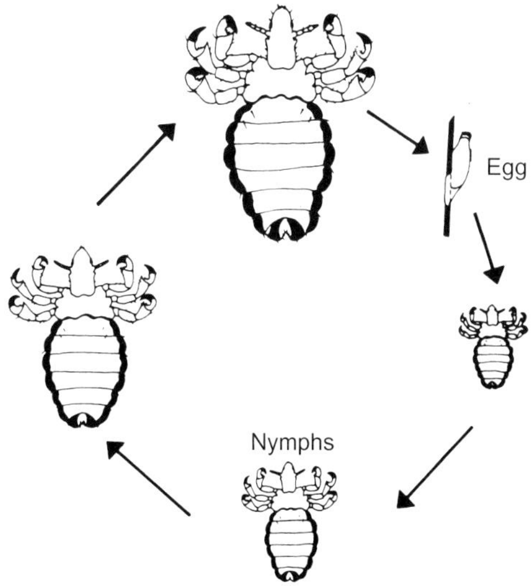

Fig. 1.20 Life cycle of a generalised louse, displaying hemimetabolous metamorphosis and passing through three nymphal stages prior to emergence as a reproductive adult.

tissues and organs are lost or remoulded and replaced by adult organs. This pattern of development is described as a **complex life cycle** with **holometabolous metamorphosis** (Fig. 1.21).

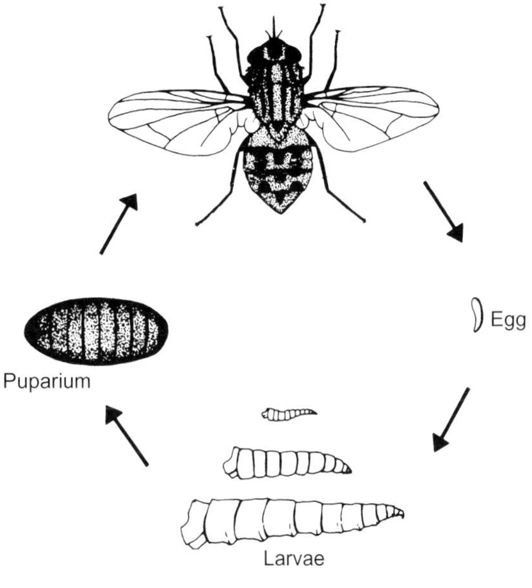

Fig. 1.21 Life cycle of a fly, *Stomoxys calcitrans*, displaying holometabolous metamorphosis, with the egg giving rise to maggot-like larva, pupa and finally reproductive adult.

Order HEMIPTERA

This order includes a large number of plant lice and bugs of considerable economic importance. Only a small number of species are of veterinary importance.

Family CIMICIDAE

Bed-bugs of the genus, *Cimex*, are blood feeders on a wide range of animals and humans.

Family REDUVIIDAE

Triatome or cone-nose bugs, sometimes called kissing or assassin bugs, of the genera *Rhodnius*, *Triatoma* and *Panstrongylus*, are blood-feeders on a wide range of animals and humans. They are vectors of the protozoan parasite *Trypanosoma cruzi* which causes Chagas' disease, in South America.

Order DIPTERA

The Diptera are the true flies; it one of the largest orders in the class Insecta, with over 120 000 described species. They have only one pair of wings, the hind pair having been reduced to become **halteres**, which help the insect to maintain stable flight. All species of Diptera have a complex life cycle with complete metamorphosis. As a result, dipterous flies can be parasites as larvae or adults, but they are rarely parasites in both life cycle stages. The adults of many members of this order are also important as vectors of disease.

The order Diptera is most commonly divided into three sub-orders, **Cyclorrhapha**, **Brachycera** and **Nematocera**, and this is the classification system that will be adopted here (Fig. 1.22). Adults of these sub-orders can be distinguished morphologically by wing venation (Fig. 1.23) and antennal structure (Fig. 1.24), and also by ecological habitats. However, recent work has suggested that the sub-order Cyclorrhapha should be replaced as an infraorder known as the Muscomorpha, within an enlarged sub-order Brachycera. This is known as the 'McAlpine classification' but is not, as yet, universally accepted.

Suborder NEMATOCERA

Flies of the sub-order Nematocera are usually small, slender and delicate with long, filamentous antennae composed of many articulating segments (Fig. 1.24).

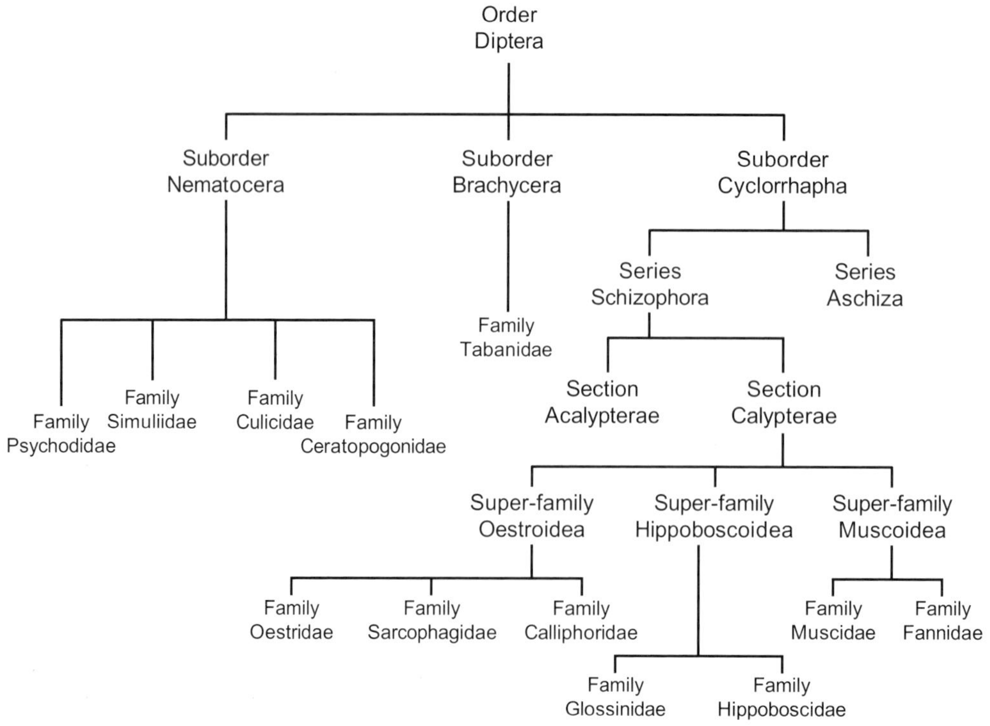

Fig. 1.22 Classification of the families of Diptera of veterinary importance.

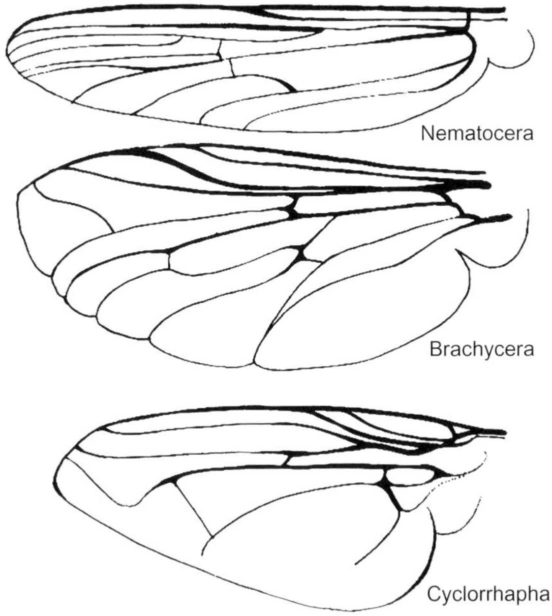

Fig. 1.23 Variations in typical wing venation found in the three suborders of Diptera.

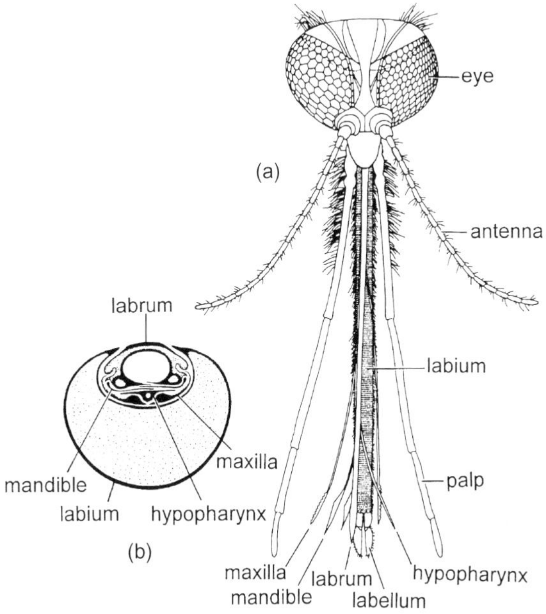

Fig. 1.25 Mouthparts of a mosquito (Diptera: Nematocera). (a) Anterior view. (b) Transverse section (reproduced from Gullan and Cranston, 1994).

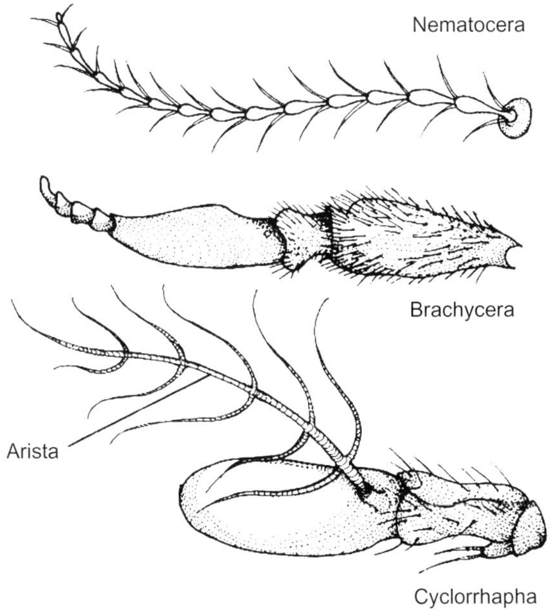

Fig. 1.24 Variations in the antennae found in the three suborders of Diptera.

The wings are often long and narrow, with conspicuous longitudinal veins (Fig. 1.23). The palps are usually pendulous, though not in mosquitoes, and usually are composed of four or five segments. Only the females are parasitic and have piercing–sucking mouthparts. Eggs are laid in or near water and develop into aquatic larvae and pupae: both of these stages have recognisable heads and are mobile.

The labium forms a protective sheath for the other mouthparts, known collectively as the stylets, and ends in two small, sensory labella (Fig. 1.25). Inside the labium lies the labrum which is curled inwards to the edges so that it almost forms a complete tube. The gap in the labrum is closed by the very fine paired mandibles to form a food canal. Behind the mandibles lies the slender hypopharynx, bearing the salivary canal, and behind this are the paired maxillae (laciniae). Both the mandibles and maxillae are finely toothed towards their tips. At the base of the mouthparts is a single pair of sensory maxillary palps. The structure of these mouthparts is essentially similar in all families of blood-feeding Nematocera. However, they are greatly elongated in the mosquitoes.

Family CERATOPOGONIDAE

This family consists of very small flies, which are commonly known as biting midges. The females feed on humans and animals and are known to transmit various viruses, protozoa and helminths. The only important genus from a veterinary standpoint is *Culicoides*.

Family SIMULIIDAE

Of the 12 genera belonging to this family of small flies, *Simulium* is the most important. Commonly referred to as 'blackflies' or 'buffalo gnats' they have a wide host range, feeding on a great variety of mammals and birds and causing annoyance due to their painful bites. In humans however, they are most important as vectors of *Onchocerca volvulus*, the filarioid nematode that causes 'river blindness' in Africa and Central and South America.

Family PSYCHODIDAE

The flies of this family are called the 'sandflies' with *Phlebotomus* the main genus of veterinary importance. In the New World the genus *Lutzomyia* is of medical importance. Both genera are important as vectors of *Leishmania*. Since, in some areas of the world, the term 'sandflies' includes some biting midges and blackflies a better term is 'phlebotomine sandflies'.

Family CULICIDAE

The Culicidae are the mosquitoes. They are small slender flies with long legs. Although their bites are a severe nuisance to humans and animals they are principally important as vectors of malaria (*Plasmodium* spp), filarial nematodes and viruses. Primarily because of their importance as vectors of human malaria there is a vast literature on their classification, behaviour and control, but the family is of limited veterinary significance and only general aspects of morphology, significance and control need be discussed. The main genera of importance are *Anopheles*, *Aedes* and *Culex*.

Suborder BRACHYCERA

These are large flies with stout antennae often consisting of only three segments, the last segment frequently bearing annulations (Fig. 1.24). The maxillary palps are usually held forwards and cross-veins are present on the wings. The females use their slashing–sponging mouthparts to pierce the skin of their host and then feed on the pool of blood created (Fig. 1.26). The eggs are laid on vegetation overhanging mud or shallow water and hatch into large carnivorous larvae with ill defined but usually retractile heads. Like the Nematocera, both larvae and pupae are mobile and aquatic, and are usually found in mud.

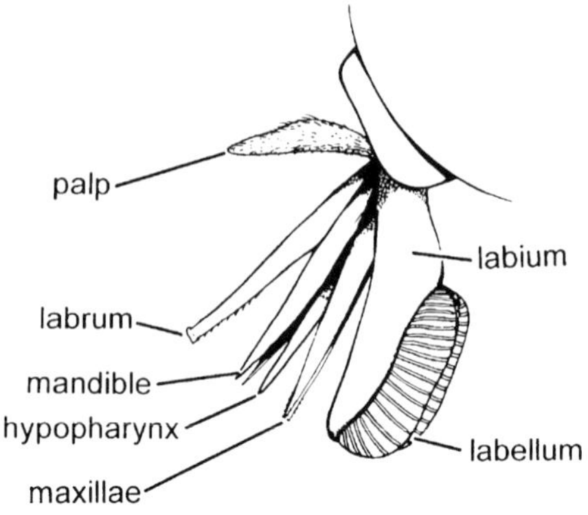

Fig. 1.26 Slashing and sponging mouthparts of a female tabanid fly.

Family TABANIDAE

There is only a single family of Brachycera of major veterinary interest, the Tabanidae, species of which are often known as horse flies, deer flies and clegs. The pain caused by their bites leads to interrupted feeding, and as a consequence, flies may feed on a succession of hosts and are therefore important in the mechanical transmission of pathogens such as trypanosomes.

The Tabanidae is one of the largest families of Diptera, containing an estimated 8000 species divided into 30 genera, only three of which are of major veterinary importance: *Tabanus* (horse flies), *Haematopota* and *Chrysops* (deer flies). Species of the genus *Tabanus* are found worldwide; the *Haematopota* are largely Palaearctic, Afrotropical and Oriental in distribution; species of the genus *Chrysops* are largely Holarctic and Oriental.

Suborder CYCLORRHAPHA

These are small to medium-sized flies with short, three-segmented antennae, the last of which often bears a feather-like attachment, the arista. The maxillary palps are small and the wings show cross-venation.

The cyclorrhaphous Diptera of veterinary interest are divided into the three superfamilies **Muscoidea**, **Hippoboscoidea** and **Oestroidea**. The Muscoidea and Hippoboscoidea, each contain two families of veterinary interest, the **Muscidae** and **Fannidae** and the **Hippoboscidae** and **Glossinidae**, respectively. The superfamily Oestroidea contains three families of veterinary interest, **Oestridae**, **Calliphoridae** and **Sarcophagidae**, species of which are primarily associated with **myiasis**, the infestation of the tissues of a living host with fly larvae.

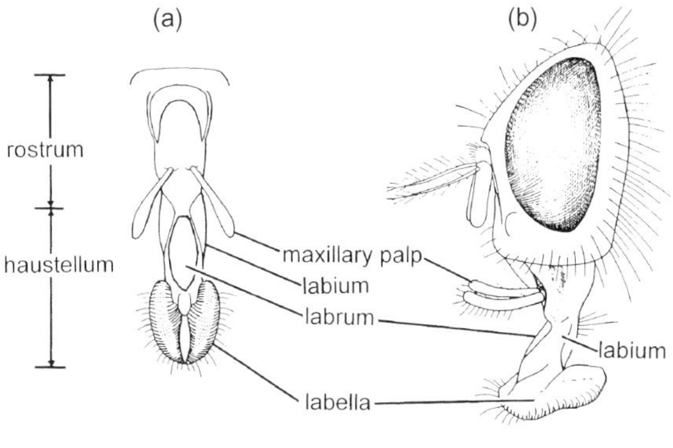

Fig. 1.27 The head and mouthparts of an adult house fly in (a) anterior and (b) lateral views (modified from Snodgrass, 1935). The mandibles and maxillae have been lost, the labrum reduced, and the labial palps expanded to form two large, fleshy labella. The labella are covered by a series of fine grooves, called pseudotracheae, along which liquid flows to the oral aperture by capillary action. The labium is flexible and the mouthparts can be retracted into the head.

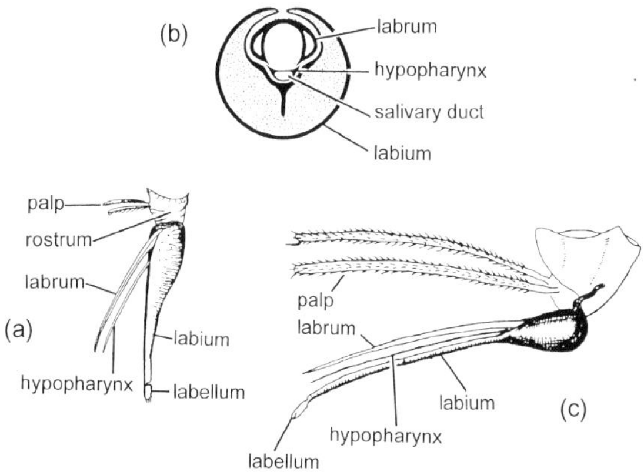

Fig. 1.28 Mouthparts and head of (a) a stable fly in lateral view and (b) cross-section. (c) Proboscis and palps of a tsetse fly (reproduced from Newstead *et al.*, 1924).

There are two basic functional types of mouthpart seen in the adult cyclorrhaphous Diptera of veterinary interest. Sponging mouthparts are used for feeding on liquid films. Such mouthparts are found in groups such as the house flies, blow flies and face flies. Biting mouthparts are used for puncturing the skin and drinking blood. They occur in groups such as the stable flies, horn flies and tsetse flies. In the sponging-type mouthparts, as seen in the house fly, the proboscis is an elongate feeding tube, composed of a basal **rostrum** bearing the maxillary palps, a median flexible **haustellum**, composed of the **labium** and flap-like **labrum**, and apical **labella** (Fig. 1.27). Mandibles and maxillae are absent. The **labrum** and the **hypopharynx** lie within the flexible anterior gutter in the labium. The labella are sponging organs, the inner surface of which are lined by grooves called **pseudotracheae**. The grooves lead towards the **oral aperture**, known as the **prestomum**. When feeding, the labella are expanded by blood pressure and opened to expose their inner surface. They are then applied to the liquid film. Liquid flows into and along the grooves by capillary action and then is drawn up the food canal by muscular pumping action. At rest, the inner surfaces of the labella are in close contact and kept moist by secretions from the labial salivary glands.

The house fly proboscis is jointed and can be withdrawn into the head capsule when not in use by the retraction of the rostrum. There are a number of minute teeth surrounding the prestomum, which can be used directly to rasp at the food. These teeth may be well developed and important in the feeding of various species of Muscidae, for example *Hydrotaea irritans*.

The ancestral cyclorrhaphous Diptera probably had the sponging mouthparts as described, without mandibles and maxillae. However, a number of species, such as stable flies and tsetse flies, have developed a blood-sucking habit and show modifications of the basic house fly mouthparts, which reflect this behaviour.

In blood-feeding Muscidae, the labella have been reduced in size and the pseudotracheae have been replaced by sharp teeth. The labium has been lengthened and surrounds the labrum and hypopharynx (Fig. 1.28). The rostrum is reduced and the rigid haustellum cannot be retracted. In feeding, the teeth of the labella cut into the skin. The entire labium and the labrum–hypopharynx, forming the food canal, are inserted into the wound. Saliva passes down a duct in the hypopharynx and blood is sucked up the food canal. Variations on this general pattern range from the robust mouthparts of stable flies to the delicate mouthparts of tsetse flies.

The larvae of cyclorrhaphous Diptera have a poorly defined head, and are mobile and worm-like, often being referred to as 'maggots' (Fig. 1.29). The mature larva pupates on or in the ground, within a hard pupal case or puparium, which is completely immobile. When the adult fly is ready to emerge, it does so by inflating a membranous ptilinal sac situated at the front of the head, which then pushes off a circular cap at the anterior end of the puparium.

Family MUSCIDAE

This family comprises many biting and non-biting genera, the latter commonly referred to as nuisance flies. As a group they may be responsible for 'fly-worry' in livestock and a number of species are vectors of important bacterial, helminth and protozoal diseases of animals. The major genera of veterinary

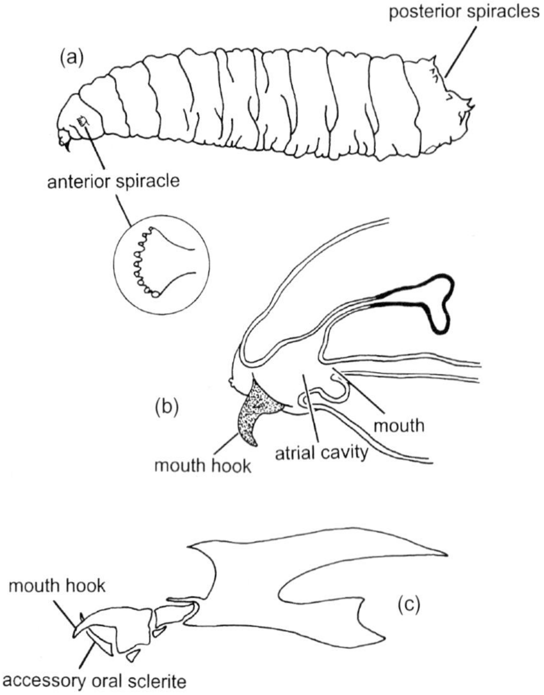

Fig. 1.29 Structure of a cyclorrhaphous fly larva. (a) Lateral view with detail of anterior spiracle (after Hall and Smith, 1993). (b) Transverse section through the head and mouthparts. (c) Cephalopharyngeal skeleton.

importance include *Musca* (house flies and related flies), *Hydrotaea* (head fly), *Stomoxys* (stable fly) and *Haematobia* (horn fly).

Family FANNIDAE

The family contains about 250 species of which species of the genus *Fannia* are of importance as nuisance pests of livestock.

Family HIPPOBOSCIDAE

The Hippoboscidae are unusual in being flattened dorsoventrally and having an indistinctly segmented abdomen, which is generally soft and leathery. They have piercing bloodsucking mouthparts, are parasitic on mammals and birds and have strong claws on the feet, which allow them to cling to hair or feathers. They tend to be either permanent ectoparasites or to remain on their hosts for long periods. The two major genera of veterinary importance are *Hippobosca* and *Melophagus*.

Family GLOSSINIDAE

The sole genus in the family Glossinidae is *Glossina*, species of which are known as tsetse flies. Tsetse flies are entirely restricted to sub-Saharan Africa, and feed exclusively on the blood of vertebrates and are of importance as vectors of trypanosomosis in animals and humans.

Family CALLIPHORIDAE

The Calliphoridae, known as blow flies, are a large family, composed of over 1000 species divided between 150 genera. At least 80 species have been recorded as causing traumatic, cutaneous myiasis. These species are found largely in five important genera: *Cochliomyia*, *Chrysomya*, *Cordylobia*, *Lucilia* and *Calliphora*. The genera *Protophormia* and *Phormia* also each contain a single species of importance. Most of these species are either primary or secondary facultative invaders. Only two species, *Chrysomya bezziana* and *Cochliomyia hominivorax*, are obligate agents of myiasis.

Family SARCOPHAGIDAE

The family Sarcophagidae, known as flesh flies, contains over 2000 species in 400 genera. Most species of Sarcophagidae are of no veterinary importance, breeding in excrement, carrion and other decomposing organic matter. The principal genus containing species which act as important agents of veterinary myiasis is *Wohlfahrtia*.

Family OESTRIDAE

This is an important family consisting of several genera of large, usually hairy, flies whose larvae are obligatory parasites of animals. All are obligate parasites, showing a high degree of host specificity. The adults have primitive, non-functional mouthparts. However, their larvae spend their entire period of larval growth and development feeding within their vertebrate hosts, causing nasopharyngeal, digestive tract, or dermal–furuncular myiases. The larvae are characterised by posterior spiracular plates containing numerous small pores.

The Oestridae contains about 150 species, known as the bots and warbles. There are four sub-families of importance: **Oestrinae**, **Gasterophilinae**, **Hypodermatinae** and **Cuterebrinae**. The sub-family Oestrinae contains one genus of major importance, *Oestrus*, and three genera of lesser importance, *Rhinoestrus*, *Cephenemyia* and *Cephalopina*. The sub-family Gasterophilinae contains a single genus of importance, *Gasterophilus*. The sub-family Hypodermatinae contains one genus of major importance, *Hypoderma*, and a second, less widespread genus, *Przhevalskiana*. The sub-family Cuterebrinae contains two genera of interest, *Cuterebra* and *Dermatobia*. Other oestrids, though of limited geographical distribution, but locally of veterinary importance are *Cephenemyia*, *Oedemagena*, *Gedoelstia* and *Cephalopina*.

Order PHTHIRAPTERA

The lice (order Phthiraptera) are permanent obligate ectoparasites, which are highly host specific, many species even preferring specific anatomical areas. They usually only leave their host to transfer to a new one. They are small insects, about 0.5–8 mm in length, dorsoventrally flattened and possess stout legs and claws for clinging tightly to fur, hair and feathers. All lice are wingless, but this is a secondary adaptation to the parasitic lifestyle, and lice are thought to be derived originally from winged ancestors. They feed on epidermal tissue debris, parts of feathers, sebaceous secretions and blood. They usually vary in colour from pale beige to dark grey, but they may darken considerably on feeding. Most are blind, but a few species have simple photosensitive eye spots.

The Phthiraptera is a small order with about 3500 described species, of which only about 20–30 are of major economic importance. The classification of the Phthiraptera is complex and remains the subject of some debate. The order is divided into four sub-orders: **Anoplura**, **Amblycera**, **Ischnocera** and **Rhynchophthirina**. However, the Rhynchophthirina is a very small sub-order, including just two African species, one of which is a parasite of elephants and the other a parasite of warthogs. The Anoplura, known as the sucking lice, are usually large, up to 5 mm, with small, pointed heads and terminal mouthparts (Fig. 1.30). They are generally slow moving, and have powerful legs, each with a single large claw. They occur exclusively on mammals. The description 'biting lice', sometimes used to describe the Anoplura, is a misnomer, because all lice bite.

In the veterinary literature, the Amblycera and Ischnocera are usually discussed together and described as the **Mallophaga** which, in older textbooks, is accorded status as a sub-order in its own right. However, Mallophaga is not a monophyletic group. Mallophaga literally means 'wool eating' and the Amblycera and Ischnocera are known as **chewing lice**.

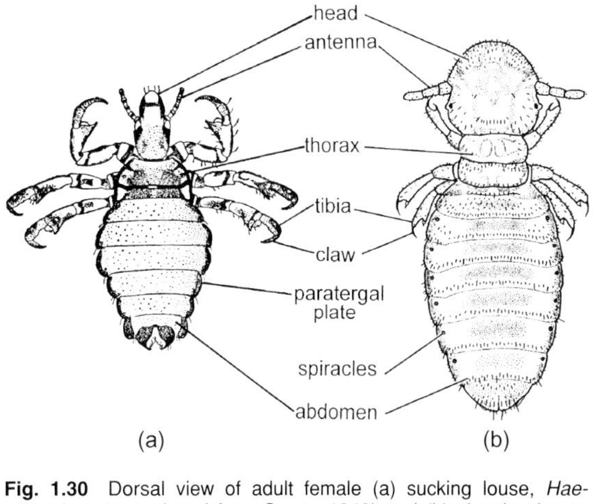

Fig. 1.30 Dorsal view of adult female (a) sucking louse, *Haematopinus* (reproduced from Smart, 1943) and (b) chewing louse, *Bovicola* (reproduced from Gullan and Cranston, 1994).

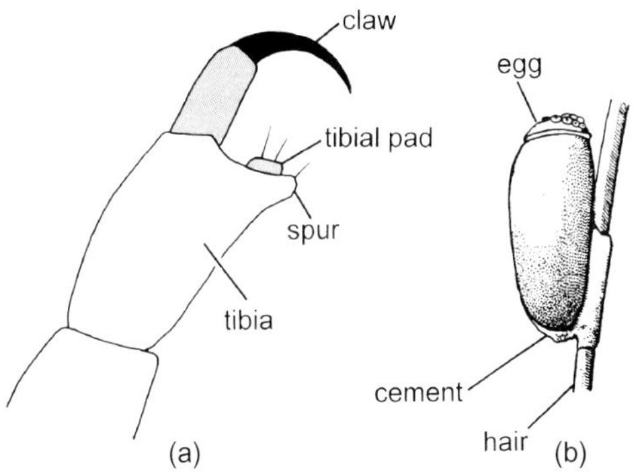

Fig. 1.31 Detail of (a) the tarsus and claw and (b) an egg attached to a hair, of an anopluran louse, *Haematopinus* (reproduced from Smart, 1943).

LOUSE LIFE CYCLES

Sucking and chewing lice have very similar life cycles. During a life span of about a month the female lays 200–300 operculate eggs ('nits'). These are usually whitish, and are glued to the hair or feathers where they may be seen with the naked eye (Fig. 1.31). There is no true metamorphosis and from the egg hatches a nymph, similar to, though much smaller than, the adult. After three moults the fully grown adult is present. The whole cycle from egg to adult usually takes 2–3 weeks.

Sucking lice, with their piercing mouthparts, feed on blood, but the chewing lice are equipped for biting and chewing and have a wider range of diet. Those on mammals ingest the outer layers of the hair shafts, dermal scales and blood scabs; the bird lice also feed on skin scales and scabs, but unlike the mammalian species, they can digest keratin, so that they also eat feathers and down.

Heavy louse infestation is known as **pediculosis**. Some species of lice may act as intermediate hosts to the tapeworm, *Dipylidium caninum*. However, despite this, lice are predominantly of veterinary interest because of the direct damage they can cause to their hosts, rather than as vectors.

The effect of lice is usually a function of their density. A small number of lice may present no problem and in fact may be a normal part of the skin fauna. However, louse populations can increase dramatically reaching high densities. Such heavy louse infestations may cause pruritus, alopecia, excoriation and self-wounding. The disturbance caused may result in lethargy and loss of weight gain or reduced egg production. Severe infestation with sucking lice may cause anaemia. Heavy infestations are usually associated with young animals or older animals in poor health, or those kept in unhygienic conditions.

Transfer of lice from animal to animal or from herd to herd is usually by direct physical contact. Because lice do not survive for long off their host, the potential for animals to pick up infestations from dirty housing is limited, although it cannot be ignored. Occasionally, lice also may be transferred between animals by attachment to flies (phoresy).

In temperate habitats, louse populations are dynamic and exhibit pronounced seasonal fluctuations. The seasonal increase in louse populations may be exacerbated by winter housing, if the animals are in poor condition and particularly if animals are deprived of the opportunity to groom themselves properly. Louse infestation may also be indicative of some other underlying problem, such as malnutrition or chronic disease.

Suborder ANOPLURA

The sub-order contains several families, two of which are of major importance in veterinary medicine, the Haematopinidae and the Linognathidae. The Polyplacidae and Hoploperidae contain species which are parasites of rodents. The Echinophthiridae contains species which are parasites of marine mammals and the Neolinagnathidae, of which there are only two species that are parasites of elephant shrews. Two other families of medical interest are the Pediculidae and Pthiridae.

Family HAEMATOPINIDAE

The family Haematopinidae contains the genus *Haematopinus* (the 'short-nosed' louse), which is the main one of veterinary importance. This is the largest louse of domestic mammals, up to 0.5 cm in length, found in cattle, pigs and horses.

Family LINOGNATHIDAE

The family Linognathidae contains two genus of veterinary importance. *Linognathus* (the 'long-nosed' louse) is bluish-black and found on cattle, sheep, goats and dogs. *Solenopotes* is a small bluish louse, which tends to occur in clusters on cattle.

Family MICROTHORACIIDAE

This family contains four species of the genus *Microthoracius*. Three species parasitise llamas and a fourth species is parasitic on camels.

Family POLYPLACIDAE

Lice of the genus *Polyplax* infest rodents and may cause problems in laboratory colonies.

Suborder AMBLYCERA

Amblycera are ectoparasites of birds, marsupials and New World mammals. Adults are medium-sized or relatively large lice, usually 2–3 mm in length. They have large, rounded heads on which the eyes are reduced or absent. They are chewing lice with mouthparts consisting of distinct mandibles on the ventral surface and a pair of two- to four-segmented maxillary palps. The four-segmented antennae are protected in antennal grooves, so that only the last segment is visible. The Amblycera contains six families, of which the families Menoponidae, Boopidae, Gyropidae and Trimenoponidae are of relevance to veterinary medicine.

Family MENOPONIDAE

Several genera are of veterinary importance on birds. *Menacanthus* can cause severe anaemia and is the most pathogenic louse of adult domestic hens and cage birds, in particular canaries. *Menopon* is found mainly on the domestic hen, but it will spread to other fowl, such as turkeys and ducks, which are in contact. *Holomenopon* is found on ducks.

Family BOOPIDAE

Members of this family occur on marsupials. *Heterodoxus* may be of importance on dogs and other canidae.

Family GYROPIDAE

Gyropus and *Gliricola* may be important in guinea pigs. Species of this family may be distinguished from other families of chewing lice because the tarsi of the mid- and hindlegs have either one or no claws.

Family TRIMENOPONIDAE

Trimenopon is found on guinea pigs.

Suborder ISCHNOCERA

The Ischnocera includes three families, two of which, the Philopteridae on domestic birds and Trichodectidae on mammals, are of major veterinary importance.

Family PHILOPTERIDAE

The family Philopteridae contains the genera *Cuclotogaster*, *Lipeurus*, *Goniodes*, *Goniocotes* and *Columbicola*, species of which are important parasites of domestic birds. The Philopteridae have five-segmented antennae and paired claws on the tarsi.

Family TRICHODECTIDAE

The family Trichodectidae contains the genera *Bovicola* (*Damalinia*), found on cattle, sheep and horses; *Felicola*, the sole species of louse found on cats; and *Trichodectes* found on dogs.

The Trichodectidae have three-segmented antennae and a single claw on the tarsi.

Suborder RHYNCHOPHTHIRINA

The Rhynchophthirina is is a very small sub-order including just two species, which are parasites of elephants and warthogs.

Order SIPHONAPTERA

Fleas (Siphonaptera) are small, wingless, obligate blood-feeding insects. Both sexes are blood-feeders and only the adults are parasitic. The order is relatively small with about 2500 described species, almost all of which are morphologically extremely similar. Over 95% of flea species are ectoparasites of mammals, whilst the others are parasites of birds.

Fleas (Fig. 1.32) are dark brown, wingless insects, usually between 1 and 6 mm in length, with females being larger than males. The body colour may vary from light brown to black. The body is laterally compressed with a glossy surface, allowing easy movement through hairs and feathers. Eyes, when present, are simply dark, photosensitive spots, and the antennae, which are short and club-like, are recessed into the head. The third pair of legs is much longer than the others, an adaptation for jumping. The head and first segment of the thorax (pronotum) may bear ventral (genal) or posterior (pronotal) rows of dark spines called ctenidia or 'combs', and these are important features used in identification.

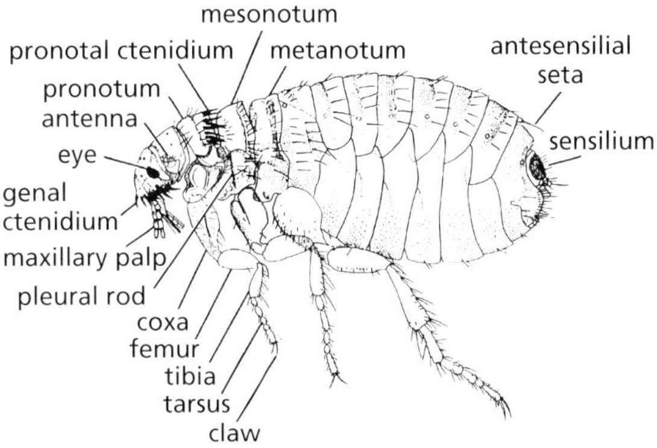

Fig. 1.32 Morphological features of an adult flea (reproduced from Gullan and Cranston, 1994).

Many species of flea are able to parasitise a range of hosts. This, combined with their mobility, which allows them to move easily between hosts, makes them parasites of considerable medical and veterinary importance and makes them difficult to control. Once on their host, fleas feed daily or every other day. Females require significantly more blood than males. Blood-feeding may have a range of damaging effects on the host animal, causing inflammation, pruritus or anaemia. Fleas may also act as vectors of bacteria, protozoa, viruses and tapeworms. However, in veterinary entomology fleas are probably of most importance as a cause of cutaneous hypersensitivity reactions. Though most important in dogs, cats and poultry, their readiness to parasitise humans as alternative hosts gives the fleas of these domestic animals a relevance in public health. Ruminants, horses and pigs do not have their own species of fleas.

FLEA LIFE CYCLES

Fleas are holometabolous and go through four stages: egg, larva, pupa and adult (Fig. 1.33). The ovoid eggs have smooth surfaces, and may be laid on the ground or on the host from which they soon drop off. Hatching occurs in 2 days to 2 weeks, depending on the temperature of the surroundings. The larvae are maggot-like, with a distinct, brownish head and have a coat of bristles. There are no appendages. They have chewing mouthparts and feed on debris and on the faeces of the adult fleas, which contain blood and give the larvae a reddish colour. The larva moults twice, the final stage being about 5.0 mm long, and then spins a cocoon, from which the adult emerges.

Moulting and pupation are dependent on the ambient temperature and humidity. Under ideal conditions, the entire cycle may take only 18 days to complete, although it can range from 6–12 months.

Two broad trends in flea life cycles can be seen. A simple association with the nest habitat is preserved

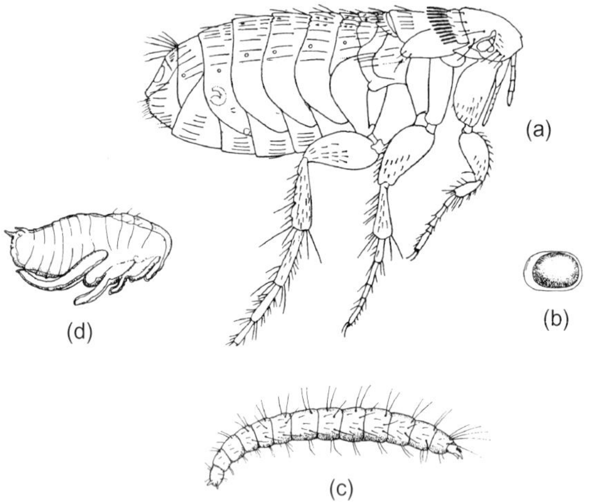

Fig. 1.33 Life cycle of a typical flea. (a) Adult. (b) Egg. (c) Larvae. (d) Pupa (after Séguy, 1944).

in many groups of the family Ceratophyllidae, characterised by infrequent and brief associations with the host and often considerable adult movement between hosts and nests. In contrast, many groups of the family Pulicidae show prolonged adult associations with the host. However, within these broad categories, a high degree of variation may exist. A few genera remain permanently attached throughout adult life. These are the burrowing, or 'stickfast', fleas, whose females are embedded in the skin, within nodules. Only the posterior part of these fleas communicates with the surface, allowing the eggs or larvae to drop to the ground and develop in the usual manner.

There are generally considered to be 15 or 16 families and 239 genera. Only two families contain species of veterinary importance: the **Ceratophyllidae** and the **Pulicidae**. The Ceratophyllidae is a large family, at present thought to contain over 500 species, of which about 80 species are parasites of birds and the remainder of which are parasites of small rodents. Most species of the family are Holarctic in distribution. The Pulicidae are parasites of a range of mammals. They are distributed worldwide.

Family CERATOPHYLLIDAE

The Ceratophyllidae is a large family containing over 500 species of which about 80 species are parasites of birds and the remainder are parasites of rodents. The genus *Nosopsyllus* are fleas of rats; *Ceratophyllus* parasitises mainly squirrels and other rodents, but contains two species of veterinary importance because they feed on poultry and other birds.

Family PULICIDAE

The Pulicidae are parasites of a range of mammals with worldwide distribution. Genera of veterinary importance include *Ctenocephalides* (dog and cat fleas), *Spilopsyllus*, *Echidnophaga*, *Pulex*, *Xenopsylla*, *Archaeopsylla*, *Tunga* and *Leptopsylla*.

Class ARACHNIDA

Members of the class Arachnida are a highly diverse group of largely carnivorous, terrestrial arthropods. The arachnids do not possess antennae or wings and they only have simple eyes. In this class there is only one group of major veterinary importance, the sub-class **Acari** (sometimes also called Acarina), containing the mites and ticks.

The sub-class Acari is an extremely diverse and abundant assembly; over 25 000 species have been described to date. They are usually small, averaging about 1 mm in length. However, some ticks may be over 3 cm in length. Segmentation is inconspicuous or absent and the sections of the body are broadly fused, so that the body appears sack-like.

The first pair of appendages, called **chelicerae**, is positioned in front of the mouth and is used in feeding. The second pair of appendages appears behind the mouth and is composed of **palps**. Their precise structure and function varies from order to order. The palps are usually short, sensory structures associated with the chelicerae. Together the chelicerae and palps form a structure called the **gnathosoma**. The body posterior to the gnathosoma is known as the **idiosoma** (Fig. 1.34). In the adult, the idiosoma is subdivided into the region that carries the legs, the podosoma, and the area behind the last pair of legs, the opisthosoma. The legs are six-segmented and are attached to the podosoma at the **coxa**, also known as the epimere. This is then followed by the trochanter, femur, genu, tibia and tarsus ending in a pair of claws and a pad-like pulvillus (Fig. 1.35).

There are three main lineages of extant mites: the Opiloacariformes, the Parasitiformes and the Acariformes. The Opiloacariformes are thought to be the most primitive of the living mites and are not parasitic. The Parasitiformes possess one to four pairs of lateral stigmata posterior to the coxae of the second pairs of legs and the coxae are usually free. The Parasitiformes include the ticks, described as the Ixodida or Metastigmata, and the gamesid mites or Mesostigmata. The Acariformes do not have visible stigmata posterior to the coxae of the second pair of legs and the coxae are often fused to the ventral body wall. The Acariformes include the mite-like mites, the Sarcoptiformes and Trombidiformes, often described as the Astigmata and Prostigmata, respectively. The terms metastigmata, mesostigmata, astigmata

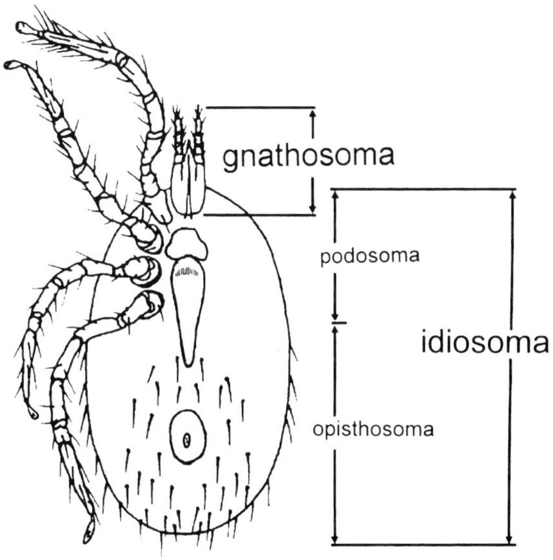

Fig. 1.34 Divisions of the body of a generalised mite.

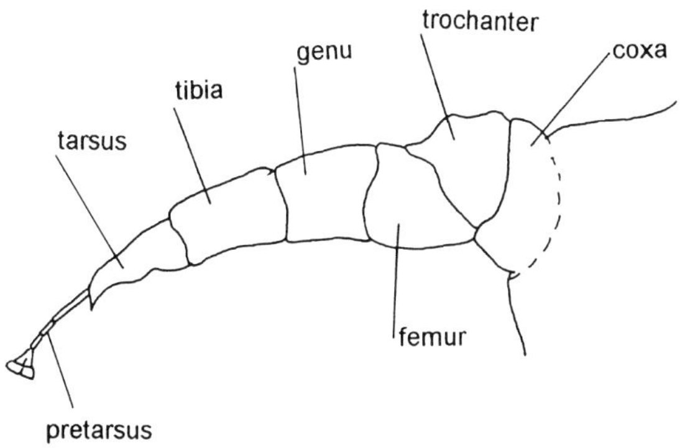

Fig. 1.35 The divisions of the leg of a generalised mite.

and prostigmata, relate to the position of the respiratory openings on the body and provide a convenient way of distinguishing the four sub-orders of parasitic importance.

LIFE CYCLES

There are four basic life cycle stages: the egg, a six-legged larva, eight-legged nymph and eight-legged adult (Fig. 1.36). But these may be further divided into pre-larva, larva, protonymph, deutonymph, tritonymph and adult. There may also be more than one moult in each of these instars. In many Acari, pre-larval and larval instars take place within the egg or have been lost. In others, one or more of the nymphal instars may be omittted.

The ticks, sub-order IXODIDA (Metastigmata)

The ticks are obligate, blood-feeding ectoparasites of vertebrates, particularly mammals and birds. They are relatively large and long-lived, feeding periodically taking large blood meals, often with long intervals between meals. Tick bites may be directly damaging to animals, causing irritation, inflammation or hypersensitivity, and, when present in large numbers, anaemia and production losses. The salivary secretions of some ticks may cause toxicosis and paralysis; however, more importantly, when they attach and feed they are

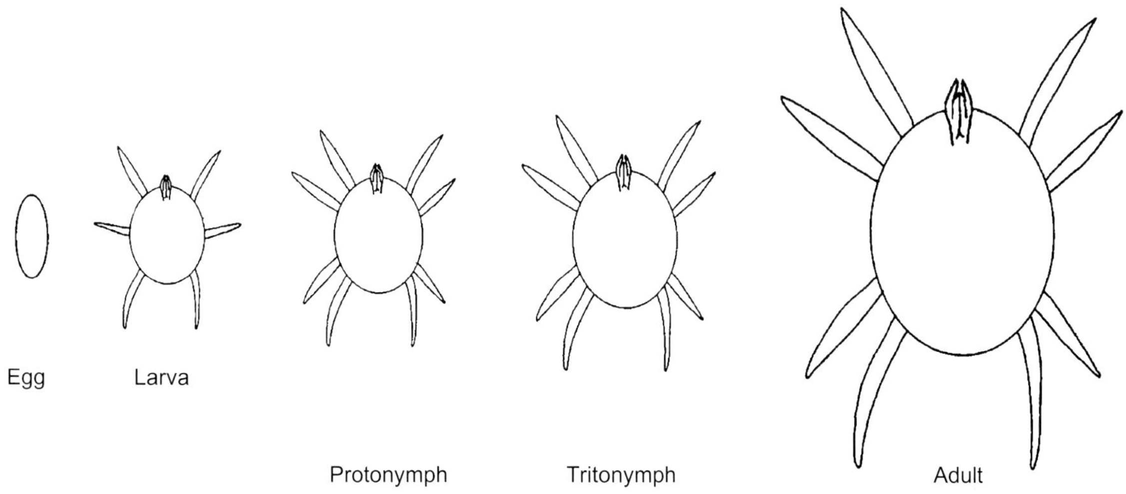

Fig. 1.36 Generalised life-cycle of a psoroptid mite.

capable of transmitting a number of pathogenic viral, bacterial, rickettsial and protozoal diseases.

Ticks belong to two families, the **Ixodidae** and **Argasidae**. The most important is the **Ixodidae**, often called the **hard ticks**, because of the presence of a rigid chitinous scutum, which covers the entire dorsal surface of the adult male. In the adult female and in the larva and nymph it extends for only a small area, which permits the abdomen to swell after feeding. The other family is the Argasidae or **soft ticks**, so-called because they lack a scutum; included in this family are the bird ticks and the tampans.

Family IXODIDAE

The Ixodidae are relatively large ticks (between 2 and 20 mm), flattened dorsoventrally. The enlarged fused **coxae** of the palps are known as the **basis capituli**, which vary in shape in the different genera. Its lower wall is extended anteriorly and ventrally to form the **hypostome**, which lies below the chelicerae (Fig. 1.37). The hypostome is armed with rows of backward barbs or teeth, and is used as an anchoring device when the tick feeds. Ventromedially there is a hypostome with recurved teeth for maintaining position; it bears a dorsal groove to permit the flow of saliva and host blood. The four-segmented sensory **palps** and heavily sclerotised **chelicerae** are anterior and visible from the dorsal surface.

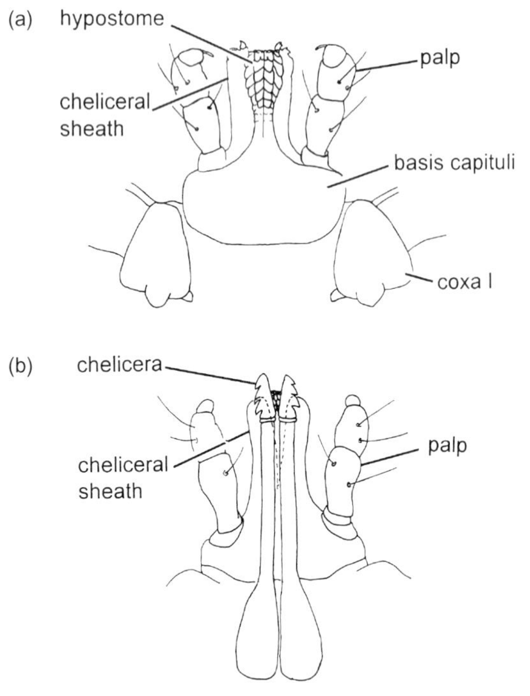

Fig. 1.37 Tick mouthparts. (a) Ventral view, showing toothed hypostome. (b) Dorsal view, showing the chelicerae behind the cheliceral sheaths.

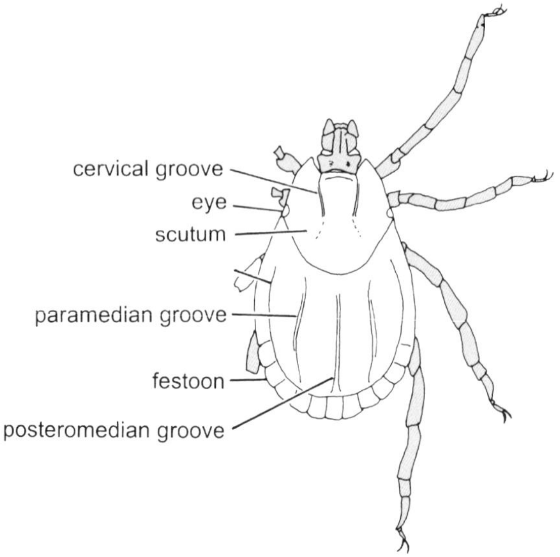

Fig. 1.38 Dorsal view of a generalised female, ixodid tick.

Ixodid ticks (Fig. 1.38) have a chitinous covering or **scutum**, which extends over the whole dorsal surface of the male, but covers only a small area behind the gnathosoma in the larva, nymph or female. Other distinguishing features are a series of grooves on the scutum and body, and, in some species, a row of notches, called **festoons**, on the posterior border of the body. Chitinous plates are sometimes present on the ventral surface of the males. Some ticks have coloured enamel-like areas on the body and these are called '**ornate** ticks'.

The coxa of the leg may be armed with internal and external **ventral spurs**; their number and size may be important in species identification (Fig. 1.39). Located on the tarsi of the first pair of legs is the Haller's organ, which is packed with chemoreceptors used for locating potential hosts. Eyes, when present, are situated on the outside margin of the scutum. Adult and nymphal ticks have a pair of respiratory openings, the **stigmata**, which lead to the tracheae. The stigmata are large and positioned posterior to the coxae of the fourth pair of legs. In adults, the genital opening, the **gonopore**, is situated ventrally behind the gnathosoma, usually at the level of the second pair of legs, and is surrounded by the **genital apron**. From the gonopore are a pair of **genital grooves** extended backwards to the **anal groove**, located ventrally, and usually posterior to the fourth pair of legs (Fig. 1.40).

The hard ticks are temporary parasites and spend relatively short periods on the host. There is a single hexapod larval stage, and a single octopod nymphal stage leading to the reproductive adut stage (Fig. 1.41).

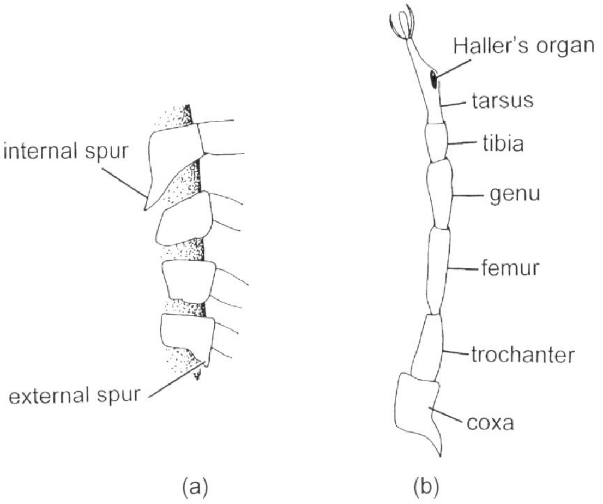

Fig. 1.39 (a) Ventral view of the coxae showing internal and external spurs and (b) segments of the leg of a generalised ixodid tick.

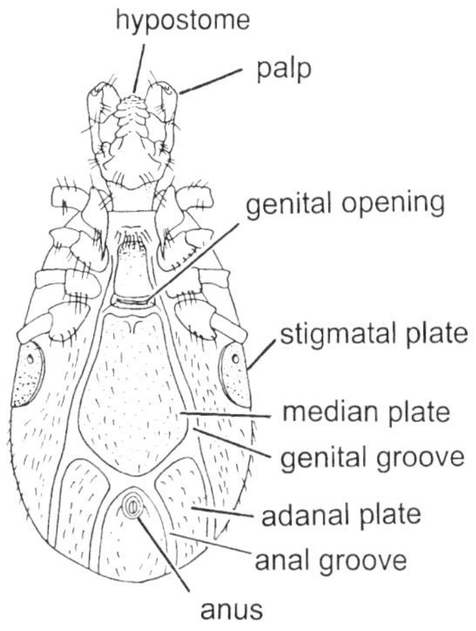

Fig. 1.40 Ventral view of a generalised male, ixodid tick.

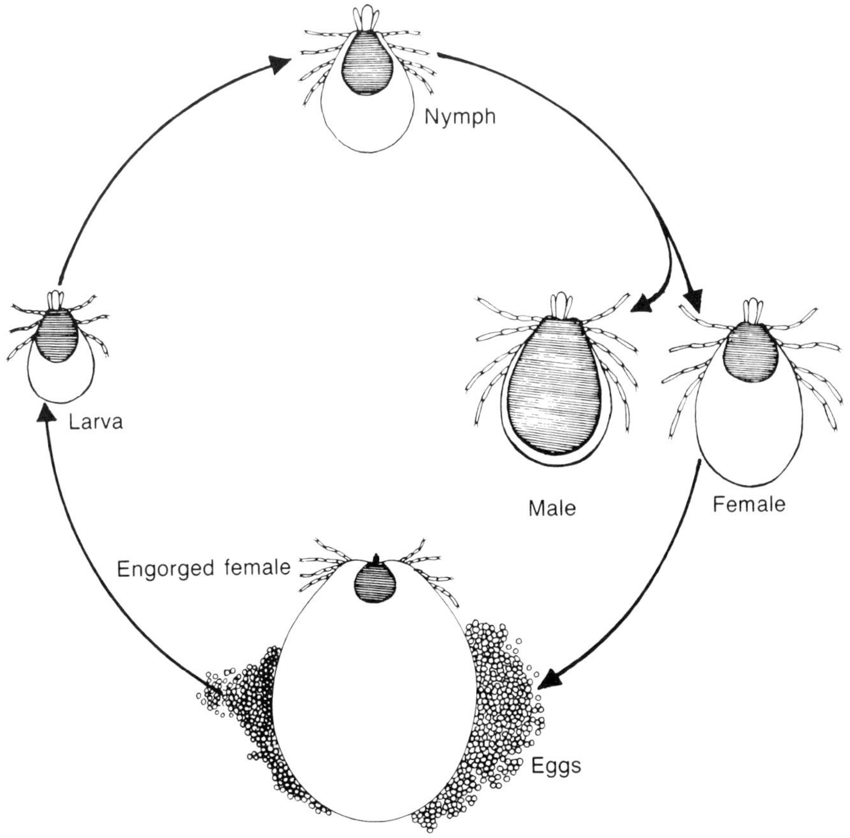

Fig. 1.41 Life cycle of an ixodid tick.

The number of hosts to which they attach during their parasitic life cycle varies from one to three. Based on this, they are classified as:

- **One-host ticks** where the entire parasitic development from larvae to adult takes place on the one host.
- **Two-host ticks** where larvae and nymphs occur on one host and the adults on another.
- **Three-host ticks** where each stage of development takes place on different hosts.

Ixodid ticks are important vectors of protozoal, bacterial, viral and rickettsial diseases. The Ixodidae contains about 650 species of ticks in thirteen genera. *Ixodes* is the largest genus containing 217 species. Other genera of veterinary importance include *Dermacentor*, *Rhipicephalus*, *Haemaphysalis*, *Boophilus*, *Amblyomma*, *Hyalomma* and *Aponomma.*

Family ARGASIDAE

Soft ticks have a leathery and unsclerotised body with a textured surface, which in unfed ticks may be characteristically marked with folds or grooves (Fig. 1.42). The integument is **inornate**. The palps appear somewhat leg-like with the third and fourth segments equal in size. The gnathosoma is located ventrally and is not visible from the dorsal view in nymphs and adults. When present, the eyes are present in lateral folds above the legs. The stigmata are small and anterior to the coxae of the fourth pair of legs. The legs are similar to those of hard ticks; the pulvulli are usually absent or rudimentary in nymphs and adults, but may be well developed in larvae.

The soft ticks have a multi-host life cycle. The larval stage feeds once before moulting to become a first-stage nymph. There are between two and seven nymphal stages, each of which feeds then leaves the host before moulting to the next stage. The adult females lay small batches of eggs after each short feed, lasting only a few minutes.

These ticks, unlike the Ixodidae, are drought resistant and capable of living for several years, and are found predominantly in deserts or dry conditions, but living in close proximity to their hosts. There are three genera of veterinary importance, *Argas*, *Otobius* and *Ornithodoros*.

THE MITES

The ectoparasitic mites of mammals and birds inhabit the skin, where they feed on blood, lymph, skin debris or sebaceous secretions, which they ingest by puncturing the skin, scavenge from the skin surface or imbibe from epidermal lesions. Most ectoparasitic mites spend their entire lives in intimate contact with their host, so that transmission from host to host is primarily by physical contact. Infestation by mites is called **acariasis** and can result in severe dermatitis, known as **mange**, which may cause significant welfare problems and economic losses. Some mites may be intermediate hosts of anoplocephalid cestodes, including *Anoplocephala*, *Moniezia* and *Stilesia*.

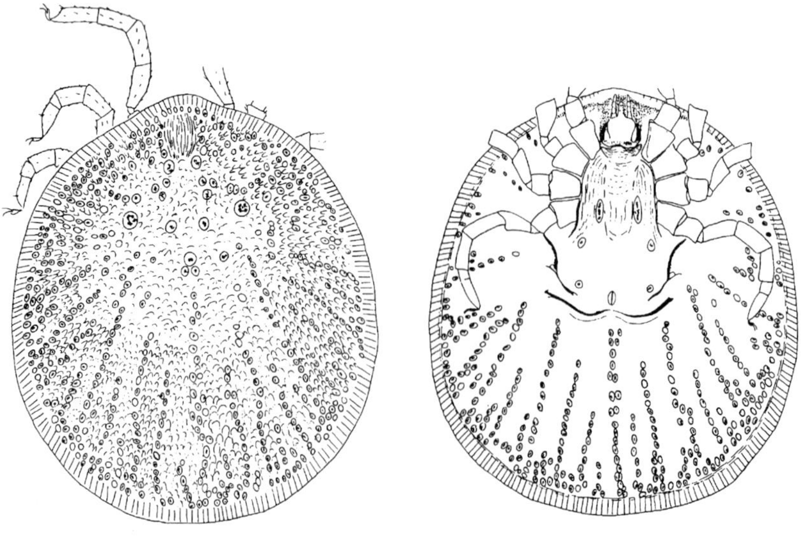

(a) (b)

Fig. 1.42 An argasid tick, *Argas vespertilonis*. (a) Dorsal view of female. (b) Ventral view of female (reproduced from Arthur, 1963).

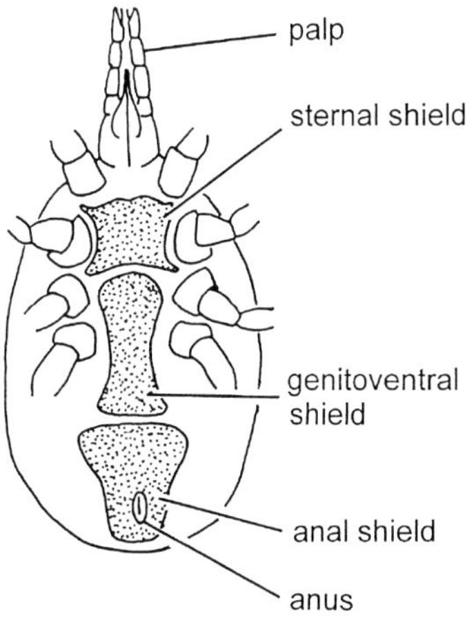

Fig. 1.43 Ventral shields of a generalised mesostigmatid mite.

Parasitic mites are small, most being less than 0.5 mm long, though a few blood-sucking species may attain several millimetres when fully engorged. The body is unsegmented but can show various sutures and grooves. The body is divided into two sections, the **gnathosoma** and **idiosoma**. The idiosoma may be soft, wrinkled and unsclerotised. However, many mites may have two or more sclerotised dorsal shields and two or three ventral shields: the **sternal**, **genitoventral** and **anal** shields (Fig. 1.43). These may be important features for mite identification. The genitoventral shield, located between the last two (posterior) pairs of legs, bears the genital orifice.

The **gnathosoma** is a highly specialised feeding apparatus bearing a pair of sensory palps and a pair of **chelicerae**, the latter sometimes bearing claw-like, or stylet-like **chelae** at their tips (Fig. 1.44). Between the chelicerae is the **buccal cone**, both of which fit within a socket-like chamber formed by enlarged coxae of the palps, ventrally and laterally and by a dorsal projection of the body wall, called the rostrum.

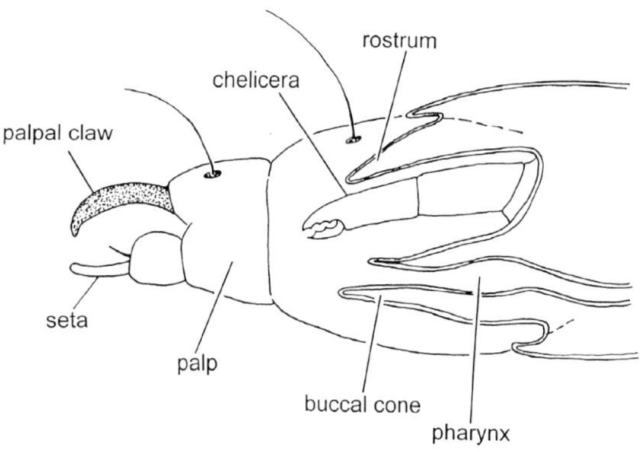

Fig. 1.44 Longitudinal section through the gnathosoma of a generalised mite.

In the mesostigmatic mites, the fused expanded coxal segments of the palps at the base of the gnathosoma are known as the **basal capituli**, from which protrudes the hypostome. The palps are one- or two-segmented in most astigmatic and prostigmatic mites, and five- or six-segmented in the Mesostigmata. The last segment of the palps usually carries a **palpal claw** or **apotele**.

Nymphal and adult mites have four pairs of legs arranged in two sets of anterior and posterior legs. Larval mites have three pairs of legs. The first pairs of legs are often modified to form sensory structures and are frequently longer and slender. At the end of the tarsus may be a pretarsus that may bear an **ambulacrum**, usually composed of paired claws, and an **empodium**, which is variable in form and may resemble a pad, sucker, claw or filamentous hair. In some parasitic astigmatic mites, the claws may be absent and replaced by stalked **pretarsi**, which may be expanded terminally into bell or sucker-like **pulvilli** (Figs 1.35 and 3.44).

In many mites, particularly astigmatic mites, gas exchange takes place through the integument. In other mites, gas exchange takes place through one to four pairs of stigmata, found on the idiosoma. The presence or absence of stigmata is used for taxonomic purposes. The stigmata in mesostigmatic mites can be associated with elongated processes called **peritremes**.

Eyes are usually absent and, hence, most mites are blind. Where they are present, however, in groups such as the trombidiformes, the eyes are simple. Hairs, or setae, many of which are sensory in function, cover the idiosoma of many species of mite. The number, position and size of the setae are extremely important in the identification of mite species.

Although, like the ticks, mites are obligate parasites, they differ from them in the important respect that most species spend their entire life cycle, from egg to adult, on the host so that transmission is mainly by contact. The life cycle of many parasitic species may be completed in less than 4 weeks and in some species as little as 8 days. Unlike the ticks, once infection is established, pathogenic populations can build up rapidly on an animal without further acquisitions. Female mites produce relatively large eggs from which a small, six-legged larva hatches. The larva moults to become an eight-legged nymph. There may be between one and three nymphal stages, known respectively as the protonymph, deutonymph and tritonymph. In many groups of mites, particularly the Astigmata, one of these nymphal instars, usually the deutonymph, is usually a facultative inactive, dispersal or protective stage, and may be omitted from the life cycle altogether. The tritonymph then moults to become an eight-legged adult.

Sub-order SARCOPTIFORMES (ASTIGMATA)

The Sarcoptiformes (Astigmata) are a large group of relatively similar mites. They are all weakly sclerotised; stigmata and tracheae are absent and respiration occurs directly through the cuticle. The order includes the families **Sarcoptidae**, **Psoroptoidae** and **Knemidocoptidae**, which are of major veterinary importance because they contain the most common mite species which cause mange and scab. Species of several other families may be important ectoparasites and species of the **Cytoditidae** and **Laminosioptidae** live in the respiratory tracts and muscles of birds and mammals.

Family SARCOPTIDAE

These are burrowing astigmatic mites with circular bodies flattened ventrally, and the cuticle covered with fine striations. The coxae are sunk into the body creating a 'short-leg' appearance with the third and fourth pairs of legs not usually visible when viewed dorsally. The legs have a claw-like empodium with the pulvillus borne on a stalk-like pretarsus. Paired claws on the tarsus are absent. The three genera of veterinary importance are *Sarcoptes*, *Notoedres* and *Trixacarus*.

Family PSOROPTIDAE

These are oval-bodied, non-burrowing, astigmatic mites. The legs are longer than those of the burrowing mites and the third and fourth pairs of legs are usually visible from above. Males have a pair of copulatory suckers, which engage the copulatory tubicles of the female deutonymph. The three genera of veterinary importance are *Psoroptes*, *Chorioptes* and *Otodectes*.

Family KNEMIDOCOPTIDAE

Twelve species of the genus *Knemidocoptes* (*Neocnemidocoptes*) have been described, of which three are of veterinary importance on poultry and domestic birds.

Family LISTEROPHERIDAE

These are parasites of fur-bearing mammals with a distinct dorsal shield, and mouthparts and legs modified for grasping hairs. The genus of veterinary interest is *Mycoptes*.

Family CYTODITIDAE

Members of the genus *Cytodites* are respiratory parasites of birds, rodents and bats. The chelicerae are absent and the palps fused to form a sucking organ.

Family LAMINOSIOPTIDAE

Laminosioptes are relatively small mites with a smooth elongated body and a few setae, affecting the muscle of chickens, turkey, geese, partridges, pigeons and wild Phasianidae.

Family ANALGIDAE

Feather mites of the genus *Megninia* are found on down and contour feathers of the chicken and other captive Galliformes.

Family ATOPOMELIDAE

Chirodiscoides is found on the fur of guinea pigs.

Family CYTODITIDAE

Members of the genus *Cytodites* are found in the respiratory system, lungs and air sacs of chickens, turkeys, canaries and a range of wild birds.

Family DERMOGLYPHIDAE

Members of the genus *Dermoglyphus* are found on the quills of chickens and cage birds.

Family FREYANITIDAE

Members of the genus *Freyana* are found on the quills of chickens and cage birds, particularly the feathers of turkeys.

Family EPIDERMOPTIDAE

Bird ked mites cause depluming mange. The genera of interest are *Epidermoptes*, found on chickens; *Microlichus* found on quail; *Promyialges* found on passeriform cage and aviary birds. Ked mites also affect hippoboscid flies affecting the bird host.

Family PTEROLICHIDAE

The two genera of veterinary significance are *Pterolichus*, found on the tail and flight feathers of chickens, and *Sideroferus*, found on the budgerigar.

Family HYPODERIDAE

The genus *Hypodectes* is of importance in pigeons, doves and other wild and captive birds.

Sub-order TROMBIDIFORMES (PROSTIGMATA)

The trombidiformes (Prostigmata) is a large and diverse group of mites existing in a wide range of forms, and occupying various ecological habitats. Prostigmatic mites usually have stigmata, which open on the gnathosoma or the anterior part of the idiosoma, known as the propodosoma. There are over 50 families, of which four contain species of veterinary importance: Demodicidae, Cheyletiellidae, Trombiculidae and Psorergatidae. Other families may be of lesser importance, not as parasites but because of the allergic responses they induce.

Family DEMODECIDAE

The Demodecidae is a family of prostigmatid mites, containing a single genus of veterinary interest, *Demodex*, species of which are found in a wide range of animals including humans. These are small mites with an elongated 'cigar-shaped' body and four pairs of 'stumpy' legs, located at the front of the body, in the adult. The striated opisthosoma forms at least half the body length.

Species of the genus *Demodex* are highly specialised mites that live in the hair follicles and sebaceous glands of a wide range of wild and domestic animals, including humans. They are believed to form a group of closely related sibling species, which are highly specific to particular hosts: *Demodex phylloides* (pig), *Demodex canis* (dog), *Demodex bovis* (cattle), *Demodex equi* (horse), *Demodex musculi* (mouse), *Demodex ratti* (rat), *Demodex caviae* (guinea pig), *Demodex cati* (cat) and *Demodex folliculorum* and *Demodex brevis* on humans.

Family CHEYLETIDAE

The majority of mites in this family are predatory, but several species of mites of the genus *Cheyletiella* are of veterinary and medical importance as ectoparasites of dogs, cats or rabbits that may transfer to humans. The body of the mite, up to 0.4 mm long, has a 'waist' and the palps are greatly enlarged, giving the appearance of an extra pair of legs. The legs terminate in 'combs' instead of claws or suckers.

Family TROMBICULIDAE

Mites of the family Trombiculidae are parasitic only at the larval stage, the nymphs and adults being free-living. There are two common genera, *Neotrombicula*, the 'harvest mite', which has a wide distribution in the Old World, and *Eutrombicula*, which occurs in North and South America, and whose larvae are known as 'chiggers'. Both of these genera will parasitise any animal, including man. Other lesser genera include *Leptotrombidium*, a vector of scrub typhus (tsutsugamushi fever) in the Far East and *Neoschongastia*, affecting chickens, quail and turkeys in North and Central America.

Family PSORERGATIDAE

Two species of the genus *Psorergates* are found on cattle and sheep; the species found on sheep is a major ectoparasite in southern hemisphere countries. The body is almost circular with the legs arranged equidistant around the body circumference, with two pairs of elongate posterior setae in the female adult mite, and single pairs in the male. The femur of each leg bears a large inwardly directed curved spine.

Family PYEMOTIDAE

These are 'forage' mites found on hay and grain predating largely on insect larvae, but they can cause dermatitis on animals and humans. Mites of the genus, *Pyemotes*, are small mites with elongated bodies, the female mites giving birth to fully formed adults.

Family MYOBIDAE

These are small blood-feeding mites found on rodents, bats and insectivores. Species of the genera *Myobia* and *Radfordia* may cause a mild dermatitis of laboratory mice and rats respectively.

Family SYRINGOPHILIDAE

Poultry quill mites, *Syringophilus*, feed on tissue fluids of feather follicles causing feather loss.

Family OPHIOPTIDAE

These mites are found beneath the scales of snakes.

Family CLOACARIDAE

These are mites found in the cloacal mucosa of reptiles. *Cloacarus* are found in aquatic terrapins.

Family PTERYGOSOMATIDAE

These are parasites of lizards including the genera *Geckobiella*, *Hirstiella*, *Ixodiderma*, *Pimeliaphilus*, *Scapothrix* and *Zonurobia*

Sub-order MESOSTIGMATA (Gamesid mites)

The Mesostigmata are a large group of mites, the majority of which are predatory, but a small number of species are important as ectoparasites of birds and mammals. Mesostigmatid mites have stigmata located above the coxae of the second, third or fourth pairs of legs. They are generally large with usually one large, sclerotised shield on the dorsal surface, and a series of smaller shields in the midline of the ventral surface. The legs are long and positioned anteriorly. Some species are host specific but the majority parasitise a range of hosts. There are two main families of veterinary interest, the Macronyssidae and Dermanyssidae, and four families of minor interest, the Halarachinidae, Entonyssidae, Rhinonyssidae and Laelapidae.

Family MACRONYSSIDAE

These are relatively large, blood-sucking ectoparasites of birds and mammals of which *Ornithonyssus*, in birds, and *Ophionyssus*, in reptiles, are of veterinary importance. Only the protonymph and adult stages feed. The mites have relatively long legs and can be seen with the naked eye.

Family DERMANYSSIDAE

Species of the genus *Dermanyssus* are blood-feeding ectoparasites of birds and mammals. They are large mites with long legs, greyish white, becoming red when engorged. *Ophionyssus* are parasites of snakes.

Family HALARACHNIDAE

Mites of the subfamily Halarachinae are obligate parasites found in the respiratory tract of mammals. *Pneumonyssus* is found in the nasal sinuses and nasal passages of dogs. Members of the subfamily Riallietiinae are obligate parasites in the external ears of mammals. *Raillietia* is found in the ears of domestic cattle.

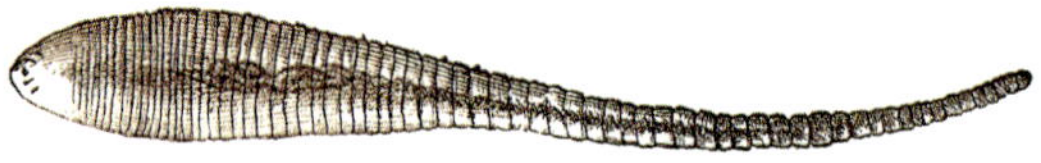

Fig. 1.45 Pentasomid: female *Linguatula serrata* (redrawn from Soulsby, 1982).

Family ENTONYSSIDAE

Mites of the family Entonyssidae are found in the respiratory tract of reptiles. *Entonyssus*, *Entophionyssus* and *Mabuyonysus* are found in the trachea and lungs of snakes.

Family RHINONYSSIDAE

Most species are parasites of the nasopharynx of birds. *Sternosoma* occurs worldwide and is found in a range of domestic and wild birds, including canaries and budgerigars.

Family LAELAPIDAE

Species of the genera, *Hirstionyssus*, *Haemogamasus*, *Haemolaelaps*, *Echinolaelaps*, *Eulaelaps* and *Laelaps* are blood-feeding parasites of rodents and are found worldwide. *Androlaelaps*, the poultry litter mite or nest mite, can occur in large numbers in chicken-house litter.

Class PENTASTOMIDA

The adults of this strange class of aberrant arthropods are found in the respiratory passages of vertebrates and resemble annelid worms rather than arthropods. The genus *Linguatula* is of some veterinary significance, with adult parasites occurring in the nasal passages and sinuses of dogs, cats and foxes. Pentastomids are up to 2.0 cm long, transversely striated, and shaped like an elongated tongue (Fig. 1.45) with a small mouth and tiny claws at the extremity of the thick anterior end.

PROTOZOOLOGY

Kingdom PROTISTA

Subkingdom PROTOZOA

The Protozoa contains unicellular organisms, which belong to the Kingdom, Protista. Protozoa are more primitive than animals, and no matter how complex their bodies may be, all the different structures are contained in a single cell.

Protozoa, like most organisms, are **eukaryotic**, in that their genetic information is stored in chromosomes contained in a nuclear envelope. In this way they differ from bacteria which do not have a nucleus and whose single chromosome is coiled like a skein of wool in the cytoplasm. This primitive arrangement, found only in bacteria, rickettsia and certain algae, is called prokaryotic and such organisms may be regarded as neither animal nor plant, but as a separate kingdom of prokaryotic organisms, the Monera.

STRUCTURE AND FUNCTION OF PROTOZOA

Protozoa, like other eukaryotic cells, have a nucleus, an endoplasmic reticulum, mitochondria and a Golgi body and lysosomes. In addition, because they lead an independent existence they possess a variety of other subcellular structures or organelles with distinct organisational features and functions.

Thus locomotion, in, for example, the genus *Trypanosoma* (Fig. 1.46) is facilitated by a single **flagellum**, and in some other protozoa by several flagella. A flagellum is a contractile fibre, arising from a structure called a basal body, and in some species is attached to the body of the protozoan along its length, so that when the flagellum beats, the cell membrane (pellicle) is pulled up to form an **undulating membrane**. Sometimes, also, it projects beyond the protozoan body as a free flagellum. During movement the shape of these organisms is maintained by microtubules in the pellicle.

Other protozoa, such as *Balantidium* (Fig. 1.47), move by means of **cilia** which are fine, short hairs, each arising from a basal body; these cover much of the body surface and beat in unison to effect movement. In such species a mouth or **cytostome** is present and the ciliary movement is also used to waft food towards this opening.

A third means of locomotion, used by protozoa such as *Entamoeba* (Fig. 1.48) are **pseudopodia**, which are prolongations of cytoplasm. Movement occurs as the rest of the cytoplasm flows into this prolongation.

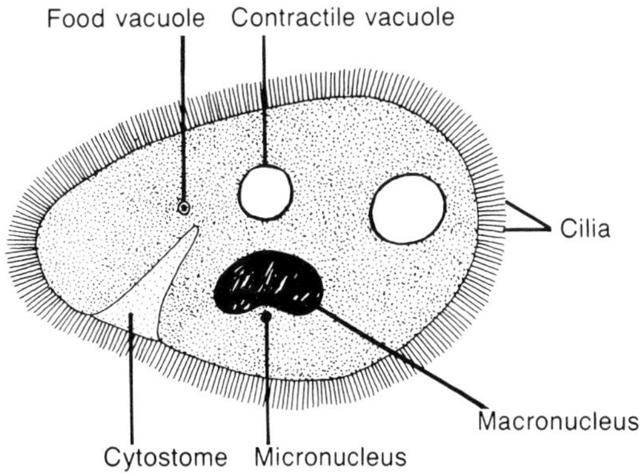

Fig. 1.47 The morphology of the intestinal protozoan *Balantidium*.

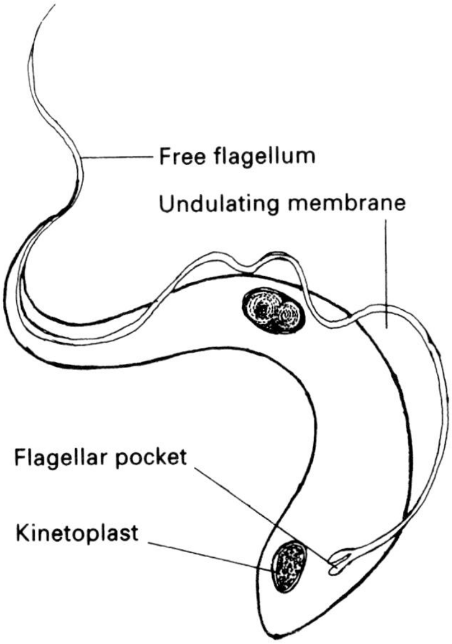

Fig. 1.46 *Trypanosoma brucei* showing the flagellum and undulating membrane.

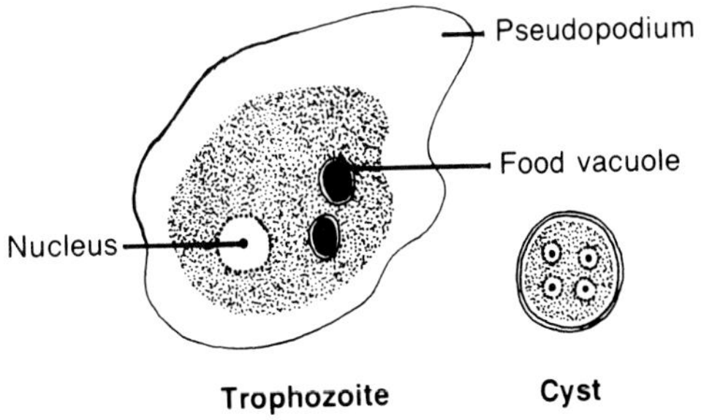

Fig. 1.48 *Entamoeba histolytica* has an amoeboid trophozoite stage and a non-motile cystic stage with four nuclei.

The pseudopodium also possesses a phagocytic capacity and can function as a cup, which closes, enveloping particulate food material in a vacuole.

Finally some protozoa, such as the extracellular stages of the *Eimeria*, have no obvious means of locomotion, but are nevertheless capable of gliding movements.

The nutrition of parasitic protozoa usually occurs by pinocytosis or phagocytosis, depending on whether tiny droplets of fluid or small objects of macromolecular dimension are taken into the cell. In both cases, the process is the same, the cell membrane gradually enveloping the droplet or object which has become adherent to its outer surface. When this is complete, the particle is carried into the cell where fusion with lysosomes effects digestion. Finally, undigested material is extruded from the cell. As noted above, some ciliated protozoa and also some stages of the organisms causing malaria obtain food through a cytostome. At the base of the cytostome the food enters a vacuole for digestion within the cell. Metabolic products are excreted by diffusion through the cell membrane.

The infective stage of some protozoa is called a **sporozoite**, while the term **trophozoite** is applied to that stage of the protozoa in the host, which feeds and grows until division commences. In most protozoa, reproduction is asexual and is accomplished by binary fission or, in the case of *Babesia* within erythrocytes, by budding. Another form of asexual reproduction, which occurs in the subphylum Sporozoa is **merogony** (**schizogony**). In the latter process, the trophozoite grows to a large size while the nucleus divides repeatedly. This structure is called a **meront** (**schizont**) and, when mature, each nucleus has acquired a portion of the cytoplasm so that the schizont is filled with a large number of elongated separate organisms called **merozoites**. The meront eventually ruptures, liberating the individual merozoites.

Protozoa that only divide asexually generally have a short generation time, and since they cannot exchange genetic material, rely on mutants to provide the variants necessary for natural selection. However, most Sporozoa at certain stages in their life cycle also have a sexual phase of reproduction, called **gametogony**, which may be followed by a free-living maturation phase, or **sporogony**. Sometimes, as in *Eimeria*, both asexual and sexual phases occur in the same host while in others, such as *Plasmodium*, the asexual phase occurs in the vertebrate host and the sexual phase in the arthropod vector.

Finally it should be noted that, although this section deals with pathogenic protozoa of veterinary importance there are many other species, particularly in the rumen, which are purely commensal or even symbiotic. These protozoa assist in the digestion of cellulose, and on being passed to the abomasum, act as a source of protein for the host.

CLASSIFICATION

Classification of the subkingdom Protozoa (kingdom Protista) is extremely complex and the classification given below is intended to give an outline of the basic differences in the structure and life cycles of the main groups. To a large extent the common characteristics of each group are reflected by similarities in the diseases they cause.

There are four phyla of protozoa of veterinary importance, the **Sarcomastigophora**, **Apicomplexa**, **Microspora** and **Ciliophora**. These and the most important genera they contain are listed in Table 1.2.

Phylum SARCOMASTIGOPHORA

Protozoa with locomotion by pseudopodia and/or flagella.

Subphylum SARCODINA

Members of the subphylum Sarcodina move by means of pseudopods, which are also used for feeding. Their cytoplasm is divided into endoplasm, containing food vacuoles and nucleus, and relatively clear ectoplasm. Reproduction is asexual by binary fission. Only a few species of the Sarcodina are pathogenic.

Family ENDAMOEBIDAE

Members of this family are parasitic in the digestive tract of vertebrates and invertebrates. Three genera contain parasites of animals and man (*Entamoeba*, *Iodamoeba*, *Endolimax*) but only *Entamoeba* contains pathogenic species of veterinary significance. Genera are differentiated on the basis of their nuclear structure.

Subphylum MASTIGOPHORA

These are flagellate protozoa having one or more flagella. Multiplication is mainly asexual by binary fission with some species producing cysts.

Class ZOOMASTIGOPHORASIDA

It is convenient for the purposes of this book to divide the Zoomastigophorasida into the **haemoflagellates**, which live in the blood, lymph and tissues (family Trypanosomatidae), and other **flagellates** (Diplomonadidae, Trichomonadidae, Monocercomonadidae) that live predominantly in the gastrointestinal tract.

Table 1.2 Classification of the protozoa.

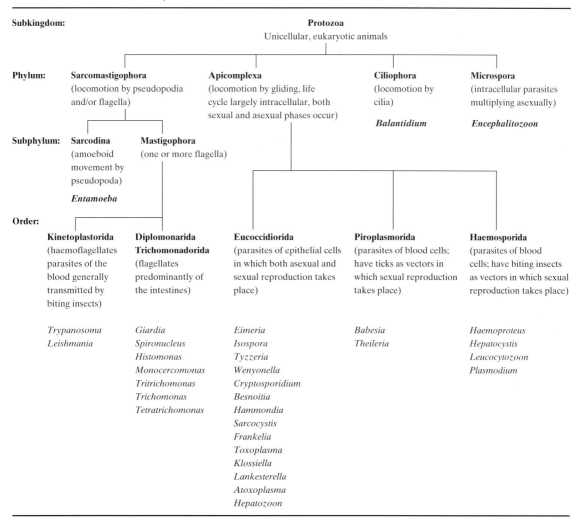

Subkingdom: **Protozoa** (Unicellular, eukaryotic animals)

Phylum:	**Sarcomastigophora** (locomotion by pseudopodia and/or flagella)	**Apicomplexa** (locomotion by gliding, life cycle largely intracellular, both sexual and asexual phases occur)	**Ciliophora** (locomotion by cilia)	**Microspora** (intracellular parasites multiplying asexually)
			Balantidium	***Encephalitozoon***

Sarcomastigophora:

Subphylum:	**Sarcodina** (amoeboid movement by pseudopoda)	**Mastigophora** (one or more flagella)
	Entamoeba	

Order:	**Kinetoplastorida** (haemoflagellates parasites of the blood generally transmitted by biting insects)	**Diplomonarida Trichomonadorida** (flagellates predominantly of the intestines)	**Eucoccidiorida** (parasites of epithelial cells in which both asexual and sexual reproduction takes place)	**Piroplasmorida** (parasites of blood cells; have ticks as vectors in which sexual reproduction takes place)	**Haemosporida** (parasites of blood cells; have biting insects as vectors in which sexual reproduction takes place)
	Trypanosoma *Leishmania*	*Giardia* *Spironucleus* *Histomonas* *Monocercomonas* *Tritrichomonas* *Trichomonas* *Tetratrichomonas*	*Eimeria* *Isospora* *Tyzzeria* *Wenyonella* *Cryptosporidium* *Besnoitia* *Hammondia* *Sarcocystis* *Frankelia* *Toxoplasma* *Klossiella* *Lankesterella* *Atoxoplasma* *Hepatozoon*	*Babesia* *Theileria*	*Haemoproteus* *Hepatocystis* *Leucocytozoon* *Plasmodium*

(Kinetoplastorida and Diplomonarida/Trichomonadorida belong to Mastigophora; Eucoccidiorida, Piroplasmorida and Haemosporida belong to Apicomplexa.)

Order KINESTOPLASTORIDA (HAEMOFLAGELLATES)

The haemoflagellates all belong to the family Trypanosomatidae, and include the trypanosomes and leishmanias.

MORPHOLOGY

Trypanosomes have a leaf-like or rounded body containing a vesicular nucleus, and a varying number of subpellicular microtubules lying beneath the outer membrane. There is a single flagellum arising from a **kinetosome** or basal granule. An undulating membrane is present in some genera and the flagellum lies on its outer border. Posterior to the kinetosome is a rod-shaped or spherical **kinetoplast** containing DNA. Members of this family were originally parasites of the intestinal tract of insects, and many are still found in insects. Others are heteroxenous, spending part of their life cycle in a vertebrate host and part in an invertebrate host.

Members of the genus *Trypanosoma* are heteroxenous and pass through amastigote, promastigote, epimastigote and tryptomastigote stages in their life cycle. In some species only tryptomastigote forms are found in the vertebrate host; in others, presumably more primitive species, both amastigote and tryptomastigote forms are present.

In the **tryptomastigote** form, the kinetoplast and kinetosome are near the posterior end and the flagellum forms the border of an undulating membrane that extends along the side of the body to the anterior end.

In the **epimastigote** form, the kinetoplast and kinetosome are just posterior to the nucleus and the undulating membrane runs forward from there.

In the **promastigote** form, the kinetoplast and kinetosome are still further anterior in the body and there is no undulating membrane.

In the **amastigote** form, the body is rounded and the flagellum emerges from the body through a wide, funnel-shaped reservoir.

THE TRANSMISSION OF TRYPANOSOME INFECTION IN ANIMALS

With one exception, all trypanosomes have arthropod vectors in which transmission is either cyclical or non-cyclical.

In **cyclical transmission** the arthropod is a necessary intermediate host in which the trypanosomes multiply, undergoing a series of morphological transformations before forms infective for the next mammalian host are produced. When multiplication occurs in the digestive tract and proboscis, so that the new infection is transmitted when feeding, the process is known as **anterior station development**; the various species of trypanosomes which use this process are often considered as a group, the **Salivaria**. All are trypanosomes transmitted by tsetse flies, the main species being *Trypanosoma congolense* (subgenus *Nanomonas*), *T. vivax* (subgenus *Duttonella*) and *T. brucei* (subgenus *Trypanozoon*).

In other trypanosomes, multiplication and transformation occurs in the gut and the infective forms migrate to the rectum and are passed with the faeces; this is **posterior station development** and the trypanosome species are grouped together as the **Stercoraria**. In domestic animals, these are all relatively nonpathogenic trypanosomes such as *Trypanosoma theileri* and *T. melophagium* transmitted by tabanid flies and sheep keds respectively. This is certainly not the case in man in which *T. cruzi*, the cause of the serious Chagas' disease in South America, is transmitted in the faeces of reduviid bugs.

Non-cyclical transmission is essentially mechanical transmission in which the trypanosomes are transferred from one mammalian host to another by the interrupted feeding of biting insects, notably tabanids and *Stomoxys*. The trypanosomes in or on the contaminated proboscis do not multiply and die quickly so that cross-transmission is only possible for a few hours. *Trypanosoma evansi*, widely distributed in livestock in Africa and Asia, is transmitted mechanically by biting flies. However, in Central and South America, *T. evansi* is also transmitted by the bites of vampire bats in which the parasites are capable of multiplying and surviving for a long period. Strictly speaking, this is more than mere mechanical transmission, since the bat is also a host, although it is certainly non-cyclical, since the multiplying trypanosomes in the bat's blood do not undergo any morphological transformation before they migrate into the buccal cavity.

It is important to note that the Salivarian trypanosomes, normally transmitted cyclically in tsetse flies, may on occasions be transmitted mechanically. Thus, in South America, *Trypanosoma vivax* has established itself, presumably by the importation of infected cattle, and is thought to be transmitted mechanically by biting flies.

Finally, apart from classical cyclical and noncyclical transmission, dogs, cats and wild carnivores may become infected by eating fresh carcasses or organs of animals that have died of trypanosomosis, the parasites penetrating oral abrasions.

The important trypanosome infections of domestic animals differ considerably in many respects and are best treated separately. The African species responsible for the 'tsetse-transmitted trypanosomoses', i.e. Salivaria, are generally considered to be the most significant.

Family TRYPANOSOMATIDAE

Members of the genus *Trypanosoma* are found in the bloodstream and tissues of vertebrates throughout the world. However, a few species are of overwhelming importance as a serious cause of morbidity and mortality in animals and man in tropical regions. With one exception, *T. equiperdum*, which is transmitted venereally, all have an arthropod vector. Trypanosomosis is one of the world's most important diseases of animals and man. Most African species are transmitted by the tsetse flies (*Glossina*).

SALIVARIAN TRYPANOSOMES

A number of species of *Trypanosoma*, found in domestic and wild animals, are all transmitted cyclically by *Glossina* in much of sub-Saharan Africa. Reproduction in the mammalian host is continuous, taking place in the tryptomastigote stage. Salivarian trypanosomes are highly pathogenic for certain mammals, such that the presence of trypanosomosis precludes the rearing of livestock in many areas, while in others, where the vectors are not so numerous, trypanosomosis is often a serious problem, particularly in cattle. The disease, sometimes known as nagana, is characterised by lymphadenopathy and anaemia accompanied by progressive emaciation and, often, death.

Salivarian trypanosomes are elongated spindle-shaped protozoa ranging from 8.0 to 39 μm long and the posterior end of the body is usually blunt. All possess a flagellum, which arises at the posterior end of the trypanosome from a basal body at the foot of a flagellar pocket. The flagellum runs to the anterior end of the body and is attached along its length to the pellicle to form an undulating membrane. Thereafter the flagellum may continue forward as a free flagellum. Within a stained specimen, a single centrally placed nucleus can be seen, and adjacent to the flagellar pocket is a small structure, the kinetoplast, which contains the DNA of the single mitochondrion.

SUBGENUS DUTTONELLA

These are monomorphic trypanosomes with a free flagellum and large kinetoplast, which is usually terminal. Development in the tsetse fly vector occurs only in the proboscis.

SUBGENUS NANNOMONAS

These are small forms usually without a free flagellum and a typically marginal medium-sized kinetoplast. Development in the tsetse fly vector occurs in the midgut and proboscis.

SUBGENUS TRYPANOZOON

These are pleomorphic (slender to stumpy) forms with or without a free flagellum and with a small subterminal kinetoplast. Development occurs in the midgut and salivary glands of the tsetse fly vector. Some forms are transmitted mechanically by tabanid vectors or by contact.

SUBGENUS PYCNOMONAS

These are stout monomorphic forms with short free flagellum and small subterminal kinetoplast. Development in the tsetse fly vector occurs in the midgut and salivary glands.

STERCORARIAN TRYPANOSOMES

The free flagellum is always present in the tryptomastigote and the kinetoplast is large and not terminal. The posterior end of the body is pointed. Multiplication in the mammalian host is discontinuous, typically taking place in the epimastigote or amastigote stages with the tryptomastigotes typically not pathogenic.

SUBGENUS MEGATRYPANUM

These are large mammalian trypanosomes with the kinetoplast typically situated near the nucleus and far from the posterior end of the body. Known vectors are hippoboscid or tabanid flies.

SUBGENUS HERPETOSOMA

These trypanosomes are of medium size with a subterminal kinetoplast, lying at some distance from the pointed end of the body. Reproduction in the mammalian host is in the amastigote and or epimastigote stages. Fleas are the main vectors.

SUBGENUS SCHIZOTRYPANUM

These are relatively small, typically 'C'-shaped trypanosomes with a large kinetoplast close to the short, pointed posterior end of the body. Multiplication in the mammalian host is typically intracellular, primarily in the amastigote form and secondarily in the epimastigote form. Known vectors are the reduviid bugs.

LEISHMANIA

Leishmania are ovoid organisms within the macrophage and possess a rod-shaped kinetoplast associated with a rudimentary flagellum, which, however, does not extend beyond the cell margin. The parasites are found in the amastigote stage in cells of the vertebrate host and in the promastigote stage in the intestine of the sandfly.

In the vertebrate host *Leishmania* is found in the macrophages and other cells of the reticuloendothelium system in the skin, spleen, liver, bone marrow, lymph nodes and mucosa. It may also be found in leucocytes in the blood.

This leishmanial, or amastigote form, after ingestion by a sandfly, transforms into a promastigote form in the insect gut in which the kinetoplast is situated at the posterior end of the body (Fig. 1.49). These divide repeatedly by binary fission, migrate to the proboscis, and when the insect subsequently feeds, are inoculated into a new host. Once within a macrophage the promastigote reverts to the amastigote form and again starts to divide.

Leishmania occur primarily in mammals, although ten species have been described in Old World lizards. They cause disease in man, dogs and various rodents. *Leishmania* have a heteroxenous life cycle, are transmitted by sandflies of the genus *Phlebotomus* in the Old World and *Lutzomyia* in the New World.

Hypopylaria are primitive species found in old world lizards, which become infected following ingestion of sandflies. Development occurs in the sandfly hindgut.

Peripylaria develop in both the hindgut and foregut of sandflies and infect both lizards and mammals. Transmission in mammals is by bite of sandflies.

Suprapylaria develop in the sandfly midgut and foregut and occur only in mammals with transmission by sandfly bite.

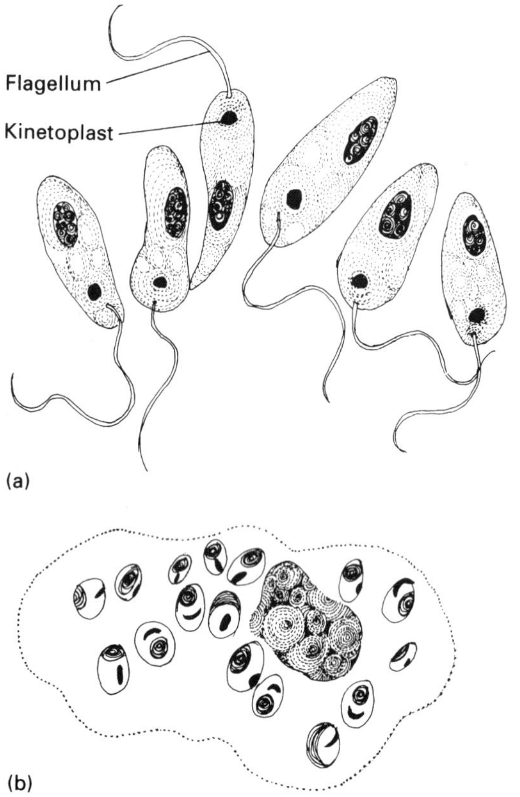

Fig. 1.49 *Leishmania*. (a) Promastigote form. (b) Amastigote form.

FLAGELLATES

Members of the families Trichomonadidae, Monocercomonadidae and Diplomonadidae occur predominantly in the gastrointestinal tract of vertebrates. Whilst many are considered to be commensals, some may be important causes of enteritis and diarrhoea.

Family TRICHOMONADIDAE

The family Trichomonadidae ('trichomonads') includes a number of genera of medical and veterinary interest: *Trichomonas*, *Tritrichomonas*, *Tetratrichomonas*, *Trichomitus* and *Pentatrichomonas*. The trichomonads have three to five flagella, of which one is usually recurrent and attached to an undulating membrane. Trichomonads have been found in the caecum and colon of virtually every species of mammals and birds, and also in reptiles, amphibians, fish and invertebrates. Specific identification and host–parasite relationships of many remain unclear.

Tritrichomonas in cattle is an important venereal disease causing infertility and abortion.

Family MONOCERCOMONADIDAE

These are similar in appearance to the trichomonads except there is no undulating membrane. The genus *Histomonas* is of veterinary importance causing major losses in turkeys and gamebirds. *Monocercomonas* occurs in a wide range of mammals, birds, reptiles, amphibians and fish and is generally considered non-pathogenic.

Family RETORTAMONADORIDIDAE

These protozoa are predominantly inhabitants of stagnant water but occur in a wide range of mammals, birds, reptiles, and insects and are generally considered non-pathogenic. Species of *Retortamonas* are found in humans, monkeys, cattle, sheep, rabbits and guinea pigs.

Family DIPLOMONADIDAE

The family Diplomonadidae contains two main genera of veterinary interest, *Giardia* and *Spironucleus*, and a few minor genera considered to be non-pathogenic in animals.

Giardia is a common cause of chronic diarrhoea in man and infection also occurs in wild and domestic animals. The organism is bilaterally symmetrical and possesses eight flagella, six of which emerge as free flagella at intervals around the body. It is unique in possessing a large adhesive disc on the flat ventral surface of the body, which facilitates attachment to the epithelial cells of the intestinal mucosa.

Spironucleus (*Hexamita*) is a cause of enteritis and diarrhoea in birds (particularly in poultry, gamebirds and pigeons) and rodents. *Caviomonas* is found in the small intestine and *Monocercomonoides*, *Protomonas*, *Hexamastix* and *Chilomitus* are found in the caecum of guinea pigs.

Family COCHLOSOMATIDAE

Cochlosoma occurs in the caeca of ducks and is of unknown pathogenicity.

Phylum APICOMPLEXA

Protozoa within the phylum Apicomplexa (Sporozoa) are characterised by occurring intracellularly and having an apical complex at some stage of their development. The trophozoites have no cilia or flagella. Reproduction involves both asexual (merogony or schizogony) and sexual (gametogony) phases. Following gametogony, a zygote is formed which divides to produce spores (sporogony).

Within the Class Sporozoasida, and Order Eucoccidiorida are three suborders of veterinary significance, the Eimeriorina (the alimentary sporozoa), and the Haemospororina and Piroplasmorina, which are blood sporozoa.

Suborder EIMERIORINA

The Eimeriorina contains parasites which occur mainly in vertebrates. Those of major veterinary importance fall into three families, the Eimeriidae, Cryptosporidiidae and Sarcocystiidae. Other families of lesser significance include the Lankesterellidae and Atoxoplasmatidae.

GENERALISED LIFE CYCLE

The life cycle is divided into three phases: sporulation, infection and merogony (schizogony), and finally, gametogony and oocyst formation (Fig. 1.50).

SPORULATION

Unsporulated oocysts, consisting of a nucleated mass of protoplasm enclosed by a resistant wall, are passed to the exterior in the faeces. Under suitable conditions of oxygenation, high humidity and optimal temperatures of around 27°C, the nucleus divides twice and the protoplasmic mass forms four conical bodies radiating from a central mass. Each of these nucleated cones becomes rounded to form a **sporoblast**, while in some species the remaining protoplasm forms the oocyst residual body. Each sporoblast secretes a wall of refractile material and becomes known as a **sporocyst**, while the protoplasm within divides into two banana-shaped **sporozoites**. In some species the remaining protoplasm within the sporocyst forms a sporocyst residual body and the sporocyst may have a knob at one end, the **Stieda body**. The time taken for these changes varies according to temperature, but under optimal conditions usually requires 2–4 days. The oocyst, now

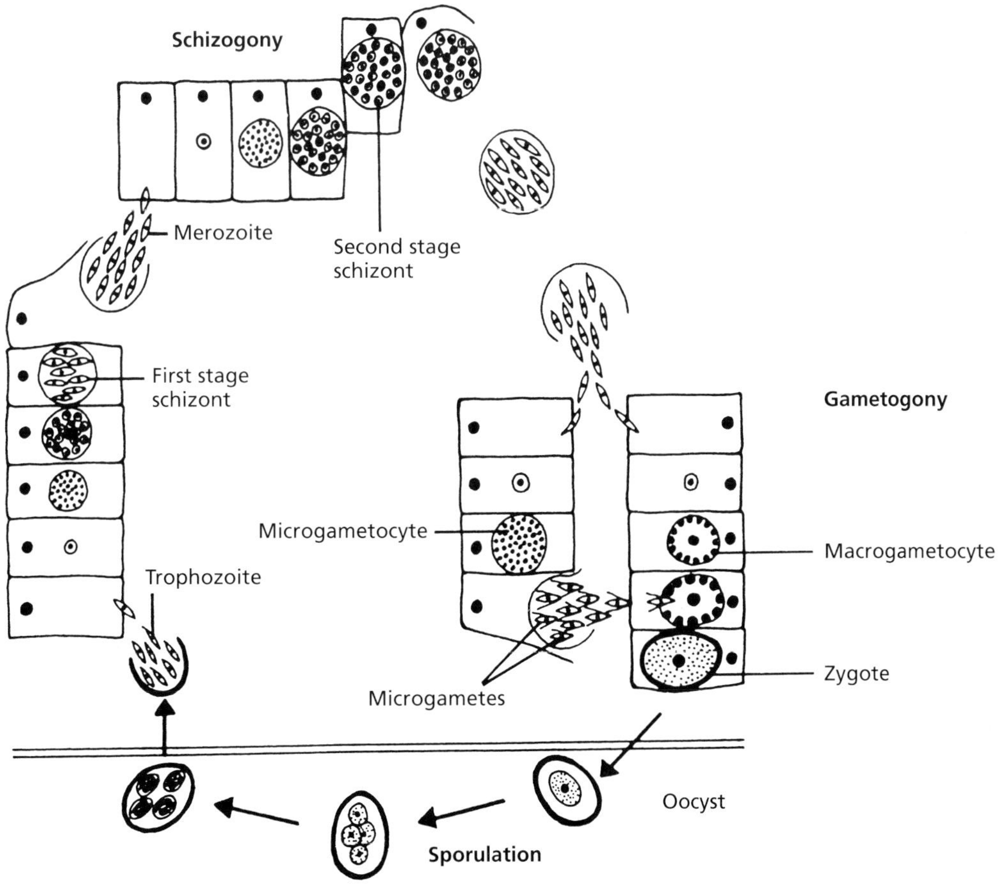

Fig. 1.50 Life cycle of *Eimeria*.

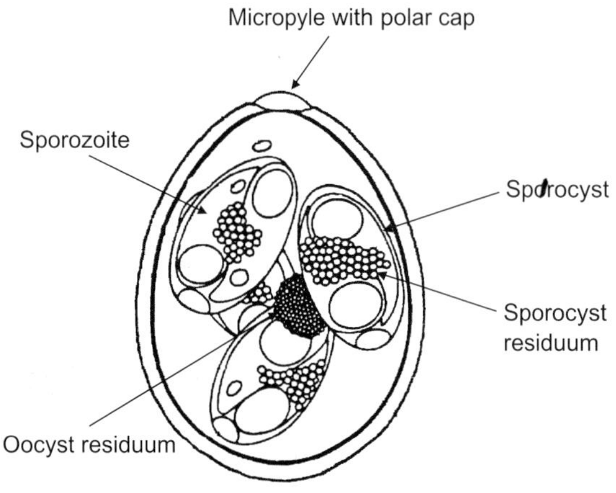

Fig. 1.51 Sporulated oocyst of *Eimeria*.

consisting of an outer wall enclosing four sporocysts each containing two sporozoites, is referred to as a **sporulated oocyst** and is the infective stage (Fig. 1.51).

INFECTION AND MEROGONY (ASEXUAL REPRODUCTION)

The host becomes infected by ingesting the sporulated oocyst. The sporocysts are then liberated either mechanically or by carbon dioxide, and the sporozoites, activated by trypsin and bile, leave the sporocyst. In most species, each sporozoite penetrates an epithelial cell, rounds up, and is then known as a **trophozoite**. After a few days each trophozoite has divided by multiple fission to form a **meront** (schizont), a structure consisting of a large number of elongated nucleated organisms known as **merozoites**. When division is complete and the meront is mature, the host cell and the meront rupture and the merozoites escape to invade neighbouring cells. Merogony may be repeated, the number of meront generations depending on the species.

GAMETOGONY AND OOCYST FORMATION (SEXUAL REPRODUCTION)

Merogony terminates when the merozoites give rise to male and female gametocytes. The factors responsible for this switch to gametogony are not fully known. The **macrogametocytes** are female and remain unicellular, but increase in size to fill the parasitised cell. They may be distinguished from trophozoites or developing meronts by the fact that they have a single large nucleus. The male **microgametocytes** each undergo repeated division to form a large number of flagellated uninucleate organisms, the **microgametes**. It is only during this brief phase that coccidia have organs of locomotion. The microgametes are freed by rupture of the host cell, one penetrates a macrogamete, and fusion of the micro- and macrogamete nuclei then takes place. A cyst wall forms around the resulting **zygote**, now known as an oocyst, and no further development usually takes place until this **unsporulated oocyst** is liberated from the body in the faeces.

Family EIMERIIDAE

This family contains 16 genera and some 1340 named species, of which the most important are *Eimeria* and *Isospora* and infections with these genera are often referred to as 'coccidiosis'. The genera are differentiated on the basis of the number of sporocysts in each oocyst and the number of sporozoites in each sporocyst (Table 1.3). Members of this family are intracellular, and most undergo merogony in the intestinal cells of their hosts. The life cycle is usually homoxenous (occuring within one host) and the majority are highly host-specific.

Eimeria is the largest genus in the family containing well over 1000 named species, with a number of important species affecting domestic mammals and birds. Oocysts contain four sporocysts, each with two sporozoites. Oocysts are unsporulated when passed in the faeces and require a period of development before becoming infective. Species of *Eimeria* are capable of causing significant morbidity and mortality and are discussed in detail under their respective hosts.

Isospora comprises about 200 species although host-specificity varies with some species. Oocysts contain two sporocysts each with four sporozoites. Species of *Isospora* can cause disease in pigs, dogs, cats and cage birds.

Table 1.3 Generic identification of coccidian parasites.

Genus	Sporocysts/ oocyst	Sporozoites/ sporocyst	Total sporozoites/ oocyst
Eimeria	4	2	8
Isospora	2	4	8
Caryospora	1	8	8
Cyclospora	2	2	4
Hoarella	16	2	32
Octosporella	8	2	16
Pythonella	16	4	64
Wenyonella	4	4	16
Dorisiella	2	8	16
Tyzzeria	0	8	8

Cyclospora has been reported in reptiles and insectivores and has recently been reported as a cause of gastrointestinal, food-borne disease in man. Oocysts consist of two sporocysts each with two sporozoites.

Caryopsora are found primarily in birds and snakes and have a two-host life cycle in which the hosts have a predator–prey relationship. Oocysts consist of a single sporocyst with eight sporozoites.

Other genera in this family are *Tyzzeria* and *Wenyonella* in birds; and *Hoarella*, *Octosporella*, *Pythonella* and *Dorisiella* in reptiles.

Family CRYPTOSPORIDIIDAE

This family contains a single genus, *Cryptosporidium*, with at least 13 species occurring in mammals, birds, reptiles and fish. Members of this family are small parasites infecting the brush border of epithelial cells mainly in the gastrointestinal tract. The life cycle is monoxenous, but some species are capable of infecting a range of vertebrate hosts. Development is intracellular but extracytoplasmic and oocysts lack sporocysts. Sporulation takes place within the host so that oocysts are immediately infective.

Family SARCOCYSTIIDAE

Five genera, *Toxoplasma*, *Sarcocystis*, *Besnoitia*, *Hammondia* and *Frenkelia*, are of veterinary interest. Their life cycles are similar to *Eimeria* and *Isospora* except that the asexual and sexual stages occur in intermediate and final hosts respectively. With the exception of the genus *Toxoplasma*, they are normally nonpathogenic to their final hosts and their significance is due to the cystic tissue stages in the intermediate hosts, which include ruminants, pigs, horses and man. The tissue phase in the intermediate host is obligatory, except in *Toxoplasma* where it is facultative.

The genus *Toxoplasma* contains a single species. Unsporulated oocysts are passed in the faeces of cats and other felids. *Toxoplasma* shows a complete lack of species-specificity in the intermediate host and is capable of infecting any warm-blooded animal and is an important zoonosis.

Sarcocystis is one of the most prevalent parasites of livestock and infects mammals, including man, birds and lower vertebrates. About 130 species have been reported. The parasites derive their name from the intramuscular cyst stage (sarcocyst) present in the intermediate (prey) host. Most *Sarcocystis* species, infecting man and domestic animals, are species-specific for their intermediate hosts and family-specific for their final hosts. *Sarcocystis* infections in the intermediate host are usually asymptomatic. Gastrointestinal disease is occasionally reported in man. The closely related genus, *Frenkelia*, differs from *Sarcocystis* in that its last generation meronts occur in the brain rather than in the muscles.

Neospora is a cause of paralysis in dogs and abortion in cattle. Recent evidence indicates members of the dog family are the final hosts.

Species of *Besniotia* have been found in cattle, horses, deer, rodents, primates and reptiles. Cats are the definitive hosts. The parasites develop in connective tissue, particularly of the skin, causing skin thickening and hair loss.

Family LANKESTERELLIDAE

Lankesterella occur in amphibians; *Schellakia* are found in reptiles. Transmission is by leeches, mites and insects.

Family ATOXOPLASMATIDAE

The genus *Atoxoplasma* occurs in birds, with about 17 named species. Transmission is by ingestion of sporulated oocysts.

Suborder ADELEORINA

Family KLOSSIELLIDAE

Klossiella is the only genus in this family. Its members are essentially non-pathogenic with most species occurring in the kidneys. The oocysts are in the kidney tubules, where they contain as many as 40 sporocysts, each with 8 to 15 sporozoites. The sporocysts pass out in the urine and infect new hosts when they are ingested.

Family HEPATOZOIDAE

The genus *Hepatozoon* has been reported from mammals, reptiles and birds and is of importance in dogs. Transmission is by ixodid ticks.

Suborder HAEMOSPORORINA

A single family, the Plasmodiidae, contains a number of genera of medical and veterinary interest. All species are heteroxenous with merogony occuring in a vertebrate host, and sporogony in an invertebrate host. There are no sporocysts with the sporozoites lying free within the oocysts.

Family PLASMODIIDAE

Three separate genera in this family, *Plasmodium*, *Haemoproteus* and *Leucocytozoon*, are the causes of avian 'malaria' in domestic and wild birds, a disease most common in the tropics and transmitted by biting dipteran flies. The vectors differ, in that avian species of *Plasmodium* are transmitted by mosquitoes; *Haemoproteus* by midges or hippoboscid flies; and *Leucocytozoon* by *Simulium* spp.

Plasmodium species are currently organised into five subgenera, which are distinguished by the morphological characteristics of the erythrocytic stages of the parasites, by the morphological changes in their host cells and by their preference for either mature erythrocytes or erythrocyte precursors. They are distinguished from the genera *Haemoproteus* and *Leucocytozoon* by the presence of merogony in circulating erythrocytes. Avian malaria is a common mosquito-transmitted disease of wild birds that infects domestic fowl and cage birds when suitable vectors and wild reservoir hosts are present. There are over 30 species of *Plasmodium* affecting birds, which differ widely in host range, geographical distribution, vectors and pathogenicity. Species that infect domestic birds occur in four of these five subgenera.

Within the family Plasmodiidae are species of *Plasmodium* which cause malaria in humans, one of the most prevalent diseases of man in the world. Sporozoites are inoculated into humans by female anopheline mosquitoes.

Hepatocystis parasitise arboreal tropical mammals such as squirrels, fruit bats and monkeys and are transmitted by midges (*Culicoides* spp).

Suborder PIROPLASMORINA

Often referred to as 'piroplasms', these parasites are found mainly in the erythrocytes or leucocytes of vertebrates. No oocysts are formed and reproduction in the vertebrate host is asexual with sexual reproduction occurring in the invertebrate host. The piroplasms are heteroxenous with known vectors ixodid or argasid ticks.

Family BABESIIDAE

The genus *Babesia* are intra-erythrocytic parasites of domestic animals and are transmitted by ticks in which the protozoan passes transovarially, via the egg, from one tick generation to the next. The disease, babesiosis, is particularly severe in naive animals introduced into endemic areas and is a considerable constraint on livestock development in many parts of the world.

Family THEILERIIDAE

The diseases caused by several species of *Theileria* are a serious constraint on livestock development in Africa, Asia and the Middle East. The parasites, which are tick-transmitted, undergo repeated schizogony in the lymphocytes, ultimately releasing small merozoites, which invade the red cells to become piroplasms. *Theileria* are widely distributed in cattle and sheep in Africa, Asia, Europe and Australia, have a variety of tick vectors and are associated with infections which range from clinically inapparent to rapidly fatal.

Various species of *Cytauxzoon* occur as theileria-like piroplasms in the red cells of wild animals. The genus differs from *Theileria* in that schizogony occurs in the reticuloendothelial cells rather than lymphocytes. *Cytauxzoon* is a cause of a fatal disease of domestic cats, characterised by fever, anaemia and icterus, in southern USA. The reservoir hosts are wild cats.

Phylum MICROSPORA

All Microspora are obligate intracellular parasites with unicellular spores, the spore possessing an extrusion apparatus and a coiled polar tube, typically filamentous, extending backwards to form a polar cap. Most are parasites of insects.

Family NOSEMATIDAE

The Nosematidae have ellipsoidal or oval spores consisting of an external wall, sporoplasm, a coiled polar tube and a polar capsule. The genus *Encephalitozoon* is of minor significance in veterinary medicine, causing disease in dogs, rabbits, other mammals and in humans.

Family ENTEROCYTOZOONIDAE

Enterocytozoon is an intestinal microsporidian frequently found in humans but has also been reported in dogs, cattle and other domestic animals. Its significance in animal hosts is unknown.

Phylum CILIOPHORA

The ciliates of domestic animals all belong to the phylum, Ciliophora. Individual organisms have a **micronucleus** containing a normal set of chromosomes and active in reproduction, and a polyploid **macronucleus**, involved in vegetative functions. Ciliates have either simple cilia or compound **cilia** in at least one stage of their life cycle. Infraciliature are found in the cortex beneath the pellicle composed of ciliary basal granules (**kinetosomes**) and associated fibrils (**kinetodesmata**). Reproduction is by transverse binary fission and sexual reproduction by conjugation, in which there is a transfer of micronuclear materials between individuals. Many species of ciliates occur as harmless commensals in the rumen and reticulum of ruminants, and the large intestine of equids. The only ciliate of importance in veterinary medicine occurs in the family Balantidiidae.

Family BALANTIDIIDAE

The only genus of importance is *Balantidium*, which has an ovoid, ellipsoidal body with elongate macronucleus and a single micronucleus with a cytosome at the base of an anterior vestibulum. *Balantidium* has worldwide distribution and is found in pigs, monkeys and man.

Family PYCNOTRICHIDAE

This family contains the genus *Buxtonella*, which has an ovoid, uniformly ciliated body with a prominent curved groove and a cyathostome near the anterior end. *Buxtonella* has worldwide distribution and is found in the caecum of cattle.

Family NYCTOTHERIDAE

The genus *Nyctotherus* are coprophilic, cilated protozoa with a peristome at the anterior end, ending in a cytosome in the middle of the body. *Nycotherus* is found in the faeces of various species of Chelonia and vegetarian lizards, such as iguanas.

MISCELLANEOUS 'PROTOZOAL' ORGANISMS

The organisms described in this section have traditionally been included in veterinary parasitology textbooks. For many of these organisms the taxonomy still remains complicated and confusing. Their inclusion in this text is for completeness and to aid differentiation from morphologically similar protozoal organisms.

Blastocystis was for many years described as a yeast, but then considered to be a protozoan in the subphylum, Blastocysta and latterly in the phylum, Bigyra. The organism is found in the intestinal tract of man and in many animals including monkeys, pigs, birds, rodents, snakes and invertebrates.

Pneumocytis is widely distributed in a wide range of healthy, domestic and wild animals. Currently it is considered to be an opportunistic mycoses of the family Pneumocystidaceae (Class: Archiascomycetes) causing infections in humans, particularly in the immunocompromised. Its significance in other hosts is not known.

RICKETTSIA

Rickettsial organisms are parasitic, Gram-negative microorganisms, associated with arthropods, which may act as vectors or primary hosts. Whilst the Rickettsia are now generally considered to be in the bacterial Kingdom, Monera, for historical reasons they are included within parasitological texts and for this reason have been retained.

Within the order, Rickettsiales, three families are recognised: the **Rickettsiaceae**, the **Bartonellaceae** and the **Anaplasmataceae**.

Family RICKETTSIACEAE

This is the most important family, which, in vertebrates, are parasites of tissue cells other than erythrocytes and are transmitted by arthropods. The two main sub-families are the Rickettsieae, which are capable of infecting suitable vertebrate hosts including humans, who may be the primary host but are more often incidental hosts, and Ehrlichieae, most of which are pathogenic in mammals.

Rickettsieae

Within the sub-family Rickettsieae three genera are recognised: *Rickettsia*, *Rochalimaea* and *Coxiella*. Species of *Rickettsia* are the important human pathogens but some species can affect dogs and cats and many have a wildlife reservoir. With the exception of louse-borne typhus and trench fever, all these human infections are zoonoses with no person-to-person or person-to-animal transmission occurring. Three groups can be distinguished within the genus: typhus group, spotted fever group and scrub typhus group.

Species of *Rochalimaea* are the cause of trench fever in humans and the disease is transmitted by lice.

The genus *Coxiella* has a single species with worldwide distribution and is the cause of Q fever. Infection is enzootic in cattle, sheep and goats but can cause severe disease in humans. The organism is widely disseminated among wild mammals and birds and has been found in ixodid and argasid ticks, gamasid mites and in human body lice (*Pediculus*).

Ehrlichieae

Ehrlichieae are minute rickettsia-like organisms, which are pathogenic for mammals, including humans. The genus of importance in veterinary medicine, *Ehrlichia* spp, are found in leucocytes in the circulating blood and are transmitted by ixodid ticks.

Family BARTONELLACEAE

Members of the Bartonellaceae are polymorphic, often rod-shaped microorganisms which are distinguished from the Anaplasmataceae, by cultural and structural characteristics. The Bartonellaceae include two genera, *Bartonella* and *Grahamella*. Several species of *Bartonella* have been described in both cats and dogs, of which one, *B. henselae*, is an important zoonosis.

Family ANAPLASMATACEAE

The Anaplasmataceae are very small, rickettsia-like particles occurring in or on the erythrocytes of vertebrates and are transmitted by arthropods. Two of the four genera, *Anaplasma* and *Aegyptianella*, are important pathogens of domestic animals. Species of the other two genera, *Eperythrozoon* and *Haemobartonella*, may also be responsible for disease. Species of *Anaplasma* are very small (0.3–1.0 μm in diameter) parasites of the erythrocytes of ruminants and are transmitted biologically by ticks and mechanically by sucking flies, especially tabanids.

Aegyptianella infect a wide range of wild and domestic birds in the warmer parts of the world and have been recorded from Africa, Asia and southern Europe. The main vectors are ticks of the genus *Argas*.

Eperythrozoon appears as rings or cocci on the erythrocytes or free in the plasma. They are worldwide in their distribution and have been found in domestic and wild mammals. Vectors include lice and mosquitoes.

Haemobartonella are coccoid or rod-shaped organisms located on or within the erythrocytes and can be spread by lice or fleas.

The taxonomy of several species is subject to much debate and there is a proposal to re-classify some species in the genera *Eperythrozoon* and *Haemobartonella* into the bacterial genus *Mycoplasma* (class Mollicutes) based on 16s rRNA gene sequences and phylogenetic analysis.

2
Parasites of cattle

ENDOPARASITES

PARASITES OF THE DIGESTIVE SYSTEM

OESOPHAGUS

Gongylonema pulchrum

Synonym: *G. scutatum*

Common name: Gullet worm

Predilection site: Oesophagus, rumen

Parasite class: Nematoda

Superfamily: Spiruroidea

Final host: Sheep, goat, cattle, pig, buffalo, horse, donkey, deer, camel, man

Intermediate host: Coprophagous beetles, cockroaches

Geographical distribution: Probably worldwide

For more details see Chapter 3 (Sheep and goats).

Hypoderma bovis

For more details see Parasites of the integument.

Hypoderma lineatum

For more details see Parasites of the integument.

RUMEN/RETICULUM

Gongylonema verrucosum

Common name: Rumen gullet worm

Predilection site: Rumen, reticulum, omasum

Parasite class: Nematoda

Superfamily: Spiruroidea

Description, gross: Long slender worms, reddish when fresh. The males are about 3.5 cm and the females 7.0–9.5 cm in length.

Description, microscopic: The adult parasites have a festooned cervical ala and cuticular bosses only on the left side of the body. The males' spicules are unequal in length with the left spicule longer than the right.

Final host: Cattle, sheep, goat, deer

Intermediate hosts: Coprophagous beetles and cockroaches

Life cycle: The life cycle is typically spiruroid. Eggs are passed in faeces and when eaten by an intermediate host they hatch and develop to the infective stage within about 4 weeks. Infection of the definitive host is through the ingestion of infected coprophagous beetles or cockroaches. The adult worms live spirally (in a zipper fashion) embedded in the mucosa or submucosa with their anterior and/or posterior ends protruding into the lumen. The prepatent period is about 8 weeks.

Geographical distribution: India, South Africa, USA

Pathogenesis: Usually regarded as non-pathogenic.

Clinical signs: Infection is usually asymptomatic.

Diagnosis: Usually an incidental finding on postmortem

Pathology: Adult worms bury in the epithelium of the forestomachs producing white or red, blood-filled zig-zag tracts in the mucosa.

Epidemiology: Infection is very much dependent on the presence and abundance of the intermediate hosts, principally coprophagous beetles of the genera *Aphodius*, *Onthophagus*, *Blaps*, *Caccobius*.

Treatment: Not reported

Control: Control is neither practical nor necessary

Paramphistomum cervi

Synonym: *Paramphistomum explanatum*

Common name: Rumen fluke

Predilection site: Rumen

Parasite class: Trematoda

Family: Paramphistomatidae

Description, gross: The adults are small, conical (pear-shaped) maggot-like flukes about 1.0 cm long and light red in colour when fresh. One sucker is visible at the tip of the cone and the other at the base. The tegument has no spines. The larval stages are less than 5.0 mm, fresh specimens having a pink colour.

Description, microscopic: The egg resembles that of *Fasciola hepatica*, being large (about 130–180 μm), and operculate, but is clear rather than yellow.

Definitive hosts: Cattle, sheep, goat, deer, buffalo, antelope

Intermediate hosts: Water snails – principally *Planorbis* and *Bulinus*

Life cycle: Development in the snail intermediate host is similar to that of *Fasciola* and under favourable conditions (26–30°C) can be completed in 4 weeks. After ingestion of encysted metacercariae with herbage, development in the final host occurs entirely in the alimentary tract. Following excystment in the duodenum the young flukes attach and feed there for about 6 weeks before migrating forward to the forestomachs where they mature. The prepatent period is between 7 and 10 weeks.

Geographical distribution: Worldwide. They are of little veterinary significance in Europe and America, but are occasionally the cause of disease in the tropics and subtropics.

Pathogenesis: The adult parasites in the forestomachs are well tolerated, even when many thousands are present and feeding on the wall of the rumen or reticulum (Fig. 2.1). Any pathogenic effect is associated with the intestinal phase of the infection.

Clinical signs: In heavy duodenal infections, the most obvious sign is diarrhoea accompanied by anorexia and intense thirst. Sometimes in cattle, there is rectal haemorrhage following a period of prolonged straining. Mortality in acute outbreaks can be as high as 90%.

Diagnosis: This is based on the clinical signs usually involving young animals in the herd and a history of grazing around snail habitats during a period of dry weather. Faecal examination is of limited value since the acute disease occurs during the prepatent period. However, large numbers of paramphistome eggs can sometimes be present in faeces during acute disease as the intestinal phase may also be accompanied by large numbers of adult flukes in the forestomach. Confirmation can be obtained by a postmortem examination and recovery of the small pink-coloured, immature flukes from the duodenal musosa and ileal contents.

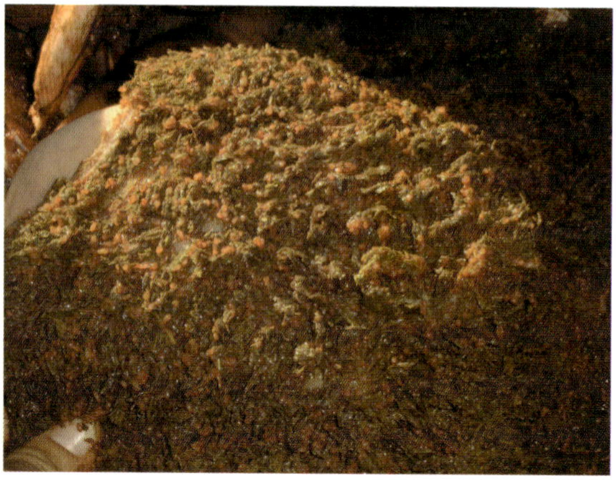

Fig. 2.1 Adult *Paramphistomum cervi* in the forestomach.

Pathology: The immature flukes are embedded in the mucosa of the upper ileum and duodenum and are plug feeders, and this can result in severe erosion of the duodenal mucosa. In heavy infections these cause enteritis characterised by oedema, haemorrhage, ulceration and associated anaemia and hypoproteinaemia. At necropsy, the young flukes can be seen as clusters of brownish pink parasites attached to the duodenal mucosa and occasionally also in the jejunum and abomasum.

Epidemiology: Paramphistomosis often depends for its continuous endemicity on permanent water masses, such as lakes and ponds, from which snails are dispersed into previously dry areas by flooding during heavy rains. Paramphistome eggs deposited by animals grazing these areas hatch and infect snails. Subsequent production of cercariae often coincides with receding water levels making them accessible to grazing ruminants. In other areas, the situation is complicated by the ability of the snails to aestivate on dry pastures and become reactivated on the return of rainfall. A good immunity develops in cattle, and outbreaks are usually confined to young stock. However, adults continue to harbour low burdens of adult parasites and are important reservoirs of infection for snails. In contrast, sheep and goats are relatively susceptible throughout their lives.

Treatment: Resorantel and oxyclozanide are considered the anthelmintics of choice against both immature and adult rumen flukes in cattle and sheep.

Control: As in *Fasciola gigantica*, the best control is achieved by providing a piped water supply to troughs and preventing access of the animals to natural water. Even then snails may gain access to watering troughs and regular application of a molluscicide at source or manual removal of snails may be necessary.

Notes: There is confusion over the classification of paramphistomes and it is likely that many described species, such as those listed below, are synonymous.

Paramphistomum microbothrium

Common name: Rumen fluke

Predilection site: Rumen

Parasite class: Trematoda

Family: Paramphistomatidae

Definitive hosts: Cattle, sheep, goat, deer, buffalo, antelope

Geographical distribution: Africa

Ceylonocotyle streptocoelium

Synonym: *Paramphistomum streptocoelium*

Common name: Rumen fluke

Predilection site: Rumen

Parasite class: Trematoda

Superfamily: Paramphistomatidae

Definitive hosts: Cattle, sheep, goat and wild ruminants

Geographical distribution: Africa

Cotylophoron cotylophorum

Synonym: *Paramphistomum cotylophorum*

Common name: Rumen fluke

Predilection site: Rumen, reticulum

Parasite class: Trematoda

Family: Paramphistomatidae

Definitive hosts: Cattle, sheep and wild ruminants

Geographical distribution: India, Australia

Monocercomonas ruminatium

Synonym: *Trichomonas ruminantium, Tritrichomonas ruminatium*

Predilection site: Rumen

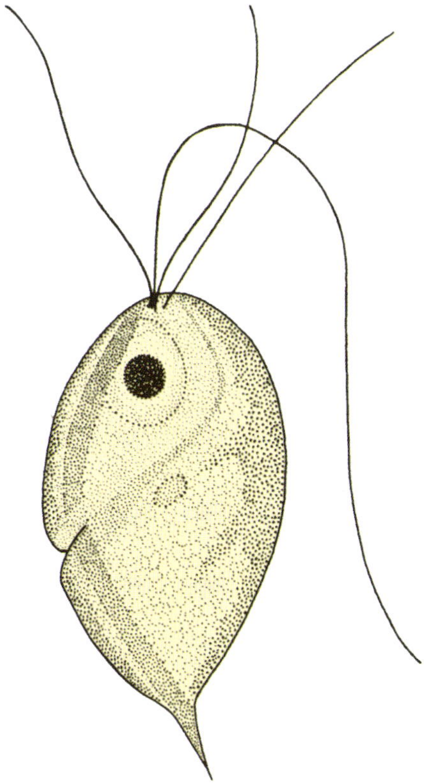

Fig. 2.2 *Monocercomonas ruminatium.*

Parasite class: Zoomastigophorasida

Family: Monocercomonadidae

Description: The trophozoite is subspherical, 3–8 × 3–7 µm, with a rounded anterior end. The axostyle is curved and may or may not extend beyond the body. A pelta and parabasal body are present. The cytosome and anterior nucleus are anterior. There are three anterior flagella and a trailing one (Fig. 2.2).

Life cycle: The life cycle is simple with trophozoites dividing by binary fission. No sexual stages are known and there are no cysts.

Geographical distribution: Worldwide

Pathogenesis: Not considered to be pathogenic

Diagnosis: Identification of trophozoites based on morphological examination.

Epidemiology: Transmission presumably occurs by ingestion of trophozoites from faeces or rumen contents.

Treatment and control: Not required

Entamoeba bovis

Predilection site: Rumen

Parasite class: Sarcodina

Family: Endamoebidae

Description: Trophozoites are 5–20 μm in diameter. The smoothly granular cytoplasm is filled with vacuoles of various sizes. The nucleus is large with a large central endostome made up of compact granules, with a row of chromatin granules of varying sizes around its periphery. The cysts are 4–14 μm in diameter and contain a single nucleus when mature with irregular clumps of chromatin granules. A large glycogen granule may or may not be present.

Hosts: Sheep, goat

Life cycle: Trophozoites divide by binary fission. Before encysting the amoebae round up, become smaller and lay down a cyst wall. Each cyst has one nucleus. Amoebae emerge from the cysts and grow into trophozoites.

Distribution: Worldwide

Pathogenicity: Non-pathogenic

Diagnosis: Identification of trophozoites, or cysts in large intestinal contents or faeces.

Treatment and control: Not required

ABOMASUM

Cattle can be parasitised by over 18 species of gastrointestinal nematodes, infection causing parasitic gastroenteritis (PGE). The most economically important gastrointestinal nematode in cattle is *Ostertagia ostertagi* and whilst the diagnosis, epidemiology, treatment and control are described in detail for this parasite, details are similar for other gastrointestinal nematodes.

Ostertagia ostertagi

Synonym: *Ostertagia lyrata, Skrjabinagia lyrata*

Common name: Brown stomach worm

Predilection site: Abomasum

Parasite class: Nematoda

Superfamily: Trichostrongyloidea

Description, gross: Adults are slender, reddish brown worms with a short buccal cavity. Males measure 6–8 mm and females 8–9 mm in length.

Description, microscopic: The cuticle in the anterior region is striated transversely whereas the rest of the body is unstriated and bears around 30 longitudinal ridges. The brown spicules are slightly curved and divided in the posterior region to terminate in three stubby hooked processes (Fig. 2.3a). In the female, the vulva is sited about 1.5 mm from the posterior and is covered with a flap. The tail tapers gradually and ends in a slender, rounded tip.

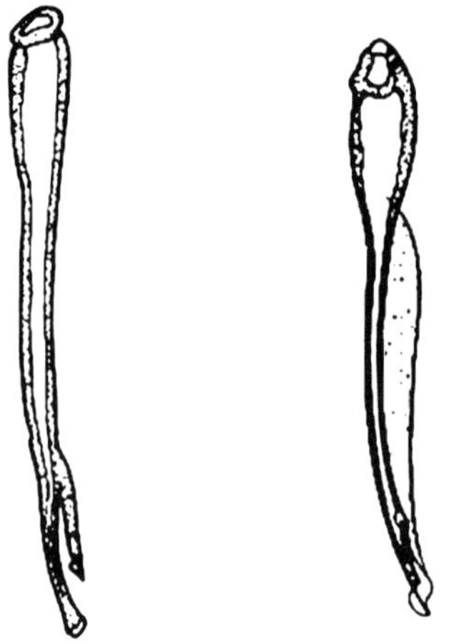

Fig. 2.3 Spicules of *Ostertagia* species. (a) *O. ostertagi*. (b) *O. leptospicularis*.

Hosts: Cattle, deer and very occasionally goats

Life cycle: The life cycle is direct. Eggs are passed in the faeces, and under optimal conditions, develop within the faecal pat to the infective third stage within 2 weeks. When moist conditions prevail, the L_3 migrate from the faeces on to the herbage. After ingestion, the L_3 exsheaths in the rumen and further development takes place in the lumen of an abomasal gland. Two parasitic moults occur before the L_5 emerges from the gland around 18 days after infection to become sexually mature on the mucosal surface. The entire parasitic life cycle usually takes 3 weeks, but under certain circumstances many of the ingested L_3 become arrested in development at the early fourth larval stage (EL_4) for periods of up to 6 months (also referred to as hypobiosis).

Geographical distribution: Worldwide. *Ostertagia* is especially important in temperate climates and in subtropical regions with winter rainfall.

Pathogenesis: Large populations of *O. ostertagi* can induce extensive pathological and biochemical changes and these are maximal when the parasites are emerging from the gastric glands (about 18 days after infection) but these may be delayed for several months when arrested larval development occurs.

In heavy infections of 40 000 or more adult worms the principal effects of these changes are first, a reduction in the acidity of the abomasal fluid, the pH increasing from 2.0 up to 7.0. This results in a failure to activate pepsinogen to pepsin. There is also a loss of bacteriostatic effect in the abomasum. Secondly, there is an enhanced permeability of the abomasal epithelium to macromolecules.

The results of these changes are a leakage of pepsinogen into the circulation, leading to elevated plasma concentrations, and the loss of plasma proteins into the gut lumen, eventually leading to hypoalbuminaemia. In addition, in response to the presence of the adult parasites, the zymogen cells secrete increased amounts of pepsin directly into the circulation.

Although reduced feed consumption and diarrhoea affect liveweight gain they do not wholly account for the loss in production. Current evidence suggests that this is primarily because of substantial leakage of endogenous protein into the gastrointestinal tract. Despite some reabsorption, this leads to a disturbance in post-absorptive nitrogen and energy metabolism due to the increased demands for the synthesis of vital proteins, such as albumin and the immunoglobulins, which occur at the expense of muscle protein and fat deposition.

Clinical signs: Bovine ostertagiosis occurs in two clinical forms. In temperate climates with cold winters the seasonal occurence of these is as follows:

Type I disease is usually seen in calves grazed intensively during their first grazing season, as the result of larvae ingested 3–4 weeks previously; in the northern hemisphere this normally occurs from mid-July onwards. In type I disease, the morbidity is usually high, often exceeding 75%, but mortality is rare provided treatment is instituted early.

Type II disease occurs in yearlings, usually in late winter or spring following their first grazing season and results from the maturation of larvae ingested during the previous autumn and subsequently become arrested in their development at the EL_4 stage. Hypoalbuminaemia is more marked, often leading to submandibular oedema. In type II the prevalence of clinical disease is comparatively low and often only a proportion of animals in the group are affected; mortality in such animals can be high unless early treatment with an anthelmintic effective against both arrested and developing larval stages is instituted.

The main clinical sign in both type I and type II disease is a profuse watery diarrhoea and in type I, where calves are at grass, this is usually persistent and has a characteristic bright green colour. In contrast, in the majority of animals with type II, the diarrhoea is often intermittent and anorexia and thirst are usually present. In both forms of the disease, the loss of body weight is considerable during the clinical phase and may reach 20% in 7–10 days.

Diagnosis: In young animals this is based on:

1. The clinical signs of inappetence, weight loss and diarrhoea.
2. The season. For example, in Europe type I occurs from July until September and type II from March to May.
3. The grazing history. In type I disease, the calves have usually been set-stocked in one area for several months; in contrast, type II disease often has a typical history of calves being grazed on a field from spring to mid-summer, then moved and brought back to the original field in the autumn. Affected farms usually also have a history of ostertagiosis in previous years.
4. Faecal egg counts. In type I disease these are usually more than 1000 eggs per gram (epg) and are a useful aid to diagnosis; in type II the count is highly variable, may even be negative and is of limited value.
5. Plasma pepsinogen levels. In clinically affected animals up to 2 years old these are usually in excess of 3.0 IU tyrosine (normal levels are 1.0 IU in non-parasitised calves). The test is less reliable in older cattle where high values are not necessarily correlated with large adult worm burdens but, instead, may reflect plasma leakage from a hypersensitive mucosa under heavy larval challenge.
6. Postmortem examination. Adult worms can be seen on close inspection of the abomasal surface. Adult worm burdens are typically in excess of 40 000, although lower numbers are often found in animals which have been diarrhoeic for several days prior to necropsy. Species differentiation is based on the structure of the male spicules (Fig. 2.3).

In older animals, laboratory diagnosis is more difficult since faecal egg counts and plasma pepsinogen levels are less reliable.

Pathology: The developing parasites cause a reduction in the functional gastric gland mass; in particular the parietal cells, which produce hydrochloric acid, are replaced by rapidly dividing, undifferentiated, non-acid-secreting cells. Initially, these cellular changes occur in the parasitised gland (Fig. 2.4), but as it becomes distended by the growing worm these changes spread to the surrounding non-parasitised glands, the end result being a thickened hyperplastic gastric mucosa.

Macroscopically, the lesion is a raised nodule with a visible central orifice; in heavy infections these nodules coalesce to produce an effect reminiscent of morocco leather (Fig. 2.5). The abomasal folds are often very oedematous and hyperaemic and sometimes necrosis and sloughing of the mucosal surface occurs (Fig. 2.6); the regional lymph nodes are enlarged and reactive.

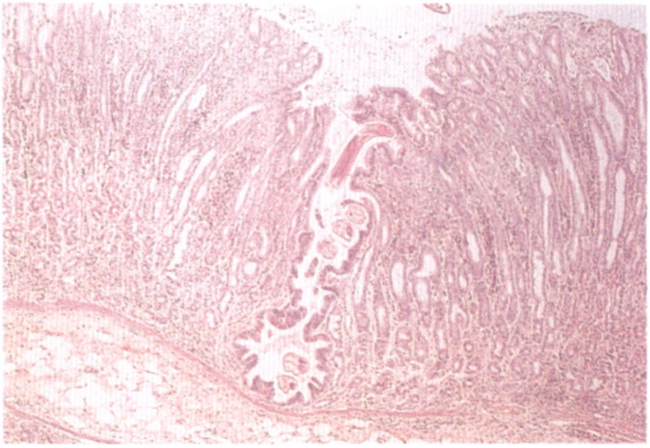

Fig. 2.4 *Ostertagia ostertagi* emerging from a gastric gland.

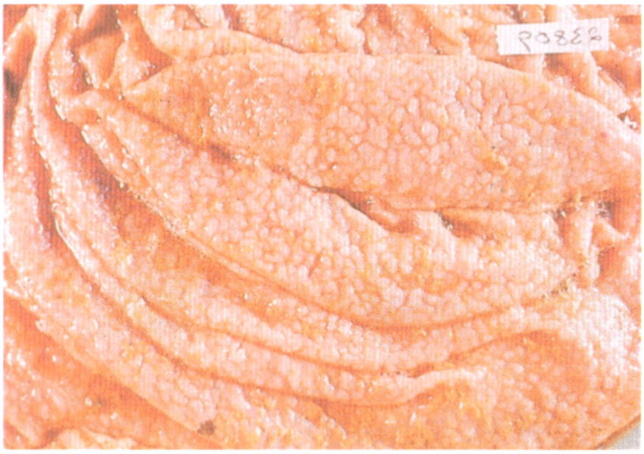

Fig. 2.5 Abomasum showing the characteristic nodules produced by the development of *O. ostertagi* larvae in the gastric glands.

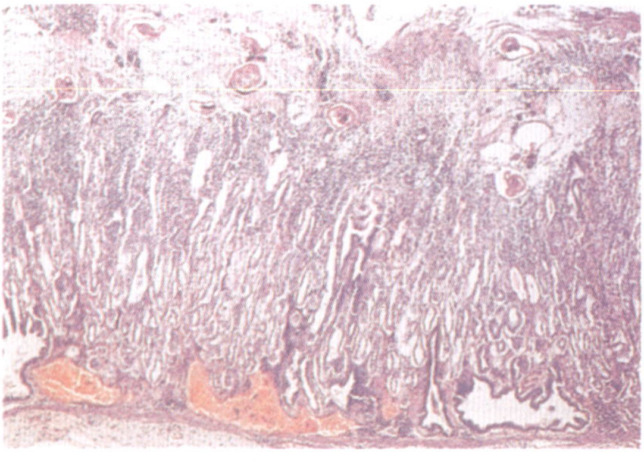

Fig. 2.6 Necrosis of mucosa in severe ostertagiosis.

Epidemiology of ostertagiosis in temperate countries of the northern hemisphere

Dairy herds

1. A considerable number of L_3 can survive the winter on pasture and in soil. Sometimes the numbers are sufficient to precipitate type I disease in calves 3–4 weeks after they are turned out to graze in the spring. However, this is unusual and the role of the surviving L_3 is rather to infect calves at a level which produces patent subclinical infection and ensures contamination of the pasture for the rest of the grazing season.
2. A high mortality of overwintered L_3 on the pasture occurs in spring and only negligible numbers can usually be detected by June. This mortality, combined with the dilution effect of the rapidly growing herbage, renders most pastures, not grazed in the spring, safe for grazing after mid-summer. However, some L_3 may survive in the soil for at least another year and can subsequently migrate on to the herbage.
3. Eggs deposited in the spring develop slowly to L_3; this rate of development becomes more rapid towards mid-summer as temperatures increase, and, as a result, the majority of eggs deposited during April to June all reach the infective stage from around mid-July onwards. If sufficient numbers of these L_3 are ingested, the type I disease occurs any time from July until October. Development from egg to L_3 slows during the autumn.
4. As autumn progresses and temperatures decline an increasing proportion (up to 80%) of the L_3 ingested become inhibited at the early fourth larval stage (EL_4). In late autumn, calves can therefore harbour many thousands of these EL_4 but few developing forms or adults. These infections are generally asymptomatic until maturation of the EL_4 takes place during winter and early spring when type II disease may materialise. Where maturation is not synchronous, clinical signs may not occur but the adult worm burdens which develop can play a significant epidemiological role by contributing to pasture contamination in the spring.

Two factors, one management and one climatic, appear to increase the prevalence of type II ostertagiosis.

First, the practice of grazing calves from May until late July on permanent pasture, then moving these to hay or silage aftermath before returning them to the original grazing in late autumn. Such pasture will still contain many L_3 and when ingested they will become arrested.

Secondly, in dry summers the L_3 are retained within the crusted faecal pat and cannot migrate on to the pasture until sufficient rainfall occurs. If rainfall is delayed until late autumn many larvae liberated on to pasture will become arrested following ingestion and so increase the chance of type II disease.

Although primarily a disease of young dairy cattle, ostertagiosis can nevertheless affect groups of older cattle in the herd, particularly if these have had little previous exposure to the parasite.

Acquired immunity is slow to develop and calves do not achieve a significant level of immunity until the end of their first grazing season. Housing over the winter allows the immunity to wane by the following spring and yearlings turned out at that time are partially susceptible to reinfection and so contaminate the pasture with small numbers of eggs. However, immunity is rapidly re-established and any clinical signs which occur are usually of a transient nature. By the second and third year of grazing, adult stock in endemic areas are usually highly immune to reinfection and of little significance in the epidemiology. However, around the periparturient period when immunity wanes, particularly in heifers, there are reports of clinical disease following calving. Burdens of adult *Ostertagia* spp in dairy cows are usually low and routine treatment of herds at calving should not be required.

Beef herds

Although the basic epidemiology in beef herds is similar to dairy herds, the influence of immune adult animals grazing alongside susceptible calves has to be considered. Thus, in beef herds where calving takes place in the spring, ostertagiosis is uncommon since egg production by immune adults is low, and the spring mortality of the overwintered L_3 occurs prior to the suckling calves ingesting significant quantities of grass. Consequently, only low numbers of L_3 become available on the pasture later in the year. However, where calving takes place in the autumn or winter, ostertagiosis can be a problem in calves during the following grazing season once they are weaned, the epidemiology then being similar to that for dairy calves.

Epidemiology of ostertagiosis in subtropical and temperate countries in the southern hemisphere

In countries with temperate climates, such as New Zealand, the seasonal pattern is similar to that reported for Europe with type I disease occurring in the summer and burdens of arrested larvae accumulating in the autumn. In those countries with subtropical climates and winter rainfall, such as parts of southern Australia, southwest Africa and some regions of Argentina, Chile and Brazil, the increase in L_3 population occurs during the winter and outbreaks of type I disease are seen towards the end of the winter period. Arrested larvae accumulate during the spring and where type II disease has been reported it has occurred in late summer or early autumn. A basically similar pattern of infection is seen in some southern parts of the USA with non-seasonal rainfall, such as Louisiana and Texas. There, larvae accumulate on pasture during winter and arrested development occurs in late winter and early spring with outbreaks of type II disease occurring in late summer or early autumn.

The environmental factors which produce arrested larvae in subtropical zones are not yet fully known.

Treatment: Type I disease responds well to treatment at the standard dosage rates with any of the modern benzimidazoles, the pro-benzimidazoles (febantel, netobimin and thiophanate), levamisole, or the avermectins/milbemycins. All of these drugs are effective against developing larvae and adult stages. Following treatment, calves should be moved to pasture which has not been grazed by cattle in the same year.

For the successful treatment of type II disease it is necessary to use drugs which are effective against arrested larvae as well as developing larvae and adult stages. Only the modern benzimidazoles (such as albendazole, fenbendazole or oxfendazole) or the avermectins/milbemycins are effective in the treatment of type II disease when used at standard dosage levels, although the pro-benzimidazoles are also effective at higher dose rates.

The field where the outbreak has originated may be grazed by sheep or rested until the following June.

In lactating dairy cattle, topical eprinomectin has the advantage that there is no milk withholding period.

Control: Traditionally, ostertagiosis has been prevented by routinely treating young cattle with anthelmintics over the period when pasture larval levels are increasing. However, it has the disadvantage that since the calves are under continuous larval challenge their performance may be impaired. With this system, effective anthelmintic treatment at housing is also necessary using a drug effective against hypobiotic larvae in order to prevent type II disease.

The prevention of ostertagiosis by limiting exposure to infection is a more efficient method of control. This may be acheived by allowing young cattle sufficient exposure to larval infection to stimulate immunity but not sufficient to cause a loss in production. The provision of this 'safe pasture' may be achieved in two ways:

1. Using anthelmintics to limit pasture contamination with eggs during periods when the climate is optimal for development of the free-living larval stages, i.e. spring and summer in temperate climates, or autumn and winter in the sub-tropics.
2. Alternatively, by resting pasture or grazing it with another host, such as sheep, which are not susceptible to *O. ostertagi*, until most of the existing L_3 on the pasture have died out.

Sometimes a combination of these methods is employed. The timing of events in the systems described below is applicable to the calendar of the northern hemisphere.

Prophylactic anthelmintic medication

Since the crucial period of pasture contamination with *O. ostertagi* eggs is the period up to mid-July, one of the efficient modern anthelmintics may be given on two or three occasions between turn-out in the spring and July to minimise the numbers of eggs deposited on the pasture. For calves going to pasture in early May two treatments, 3 and 6 weeks later, are used, whereas calves turned out in April require three treatments at intervals of 3 weeks. Where parenteral or pour-on macrocyclic lactones are used the interval after first treatment may be extended to 5 or 8 weeks (the interval depends on the anthelmintic used) due to residual activity against ingested larvae.

Several rumen boluses are available which provide either the sustained release of anthelmintic drugs over periods of 3–5 months or the pulse release of therapeutic doses of an anthelmintic at intervals of 3 weeks throughout the grazing season. These are administered to first season grazing calves at turnout and effectively prevent pasture contamination and the subsequent accumulation of infective larvae. Although offering a high degree of control of gastrointestinal nematodes there is evidence to suggest that young cattle protected by these boluses, or other highly effective prophylactic drug regimens, are more susceptible to infection in their second year at grass.

Anthelmintic prophylaxis has the advantage that animals can be grazed throughout the year on the same pasture and is particularly advantageous for the small heavily stocked farm where grazing is limited.

Anthelmintic treatment and move to safe pasture in mid-July

This system, usually referred to as 'dose and move', is based on the knowledge that the annual increase of L_3 occurs after mid-July. Therefore if calves grazed from early spring are given an anthelmintic treatment in early July and moved immediately to a second pasture such as silage or hay aftermath, the level of infection which develops on the second pasture will be low.

The one reservation with this technique is that in certain years the numbers of L_3 that overwinter are sufficient to cause heavy infections in the spring and clinical ostertagiosis can occur in calves in April and May. However, once the 'dose and move' system has operated for a few years this problem is unlikely to arise.

In some European countries the same effect has been obtained by delaying the turnout of calves until mid-summer.

Alternate grazing of cattle and sheep

This system ideally utilises a 3-year rotation of cattle, sheep and crops. Since the effective lifespan of most *O. ostertagi* L_3 is under 1 year and cross-infection between cattle and sheep in temperate areas is largely limited to *O. leptospicularis*, *Trichostrongylus axei* and occasionally *C. oncophora*, good control of bovine ostertagiosis should, in theory, be achieved. It is particularly applicable to farms with a high proportion of land suitable for cropping or grassland conservation. In marginal or upland areas reasonable control has been reported using an annual rotation of beef cattle and sheep. The drawback of alternate grazing systems is that they impose a rigorous and inflexible regimen on the use of land. Furthermore, in warmer climates where *Haemonchus* spp are prevalent, this system can prove dangerous since this very pathogenic genus establishes in both sheep and cattle.

Rotational grazing of adult and young stock

This system involves a continuous rotation of paddocks in which the susceptible younger calves graze ahead of the immune adults and remain long enough in each paddock to remove only the leafy upper herbage. The incoming immune adults then graze the lower more fibrous echelons of the herbage, which contain the majority of the L_3. Since the faeces produced by the immune adults contains few if any *O. ostertagi* eggs, the pasture contamination is greatly reduced. The optimal utilisation of permanent grassland and the control of internal parasitism without resort to therapy makes it an option for organic systems of production.

Notes: *O. ostertagi* is perhaps the most common cause of parasitic gastritis in cattle. The disease, often simply known as ostertagiosis, typically affects young cattle during their first grazing season, although herd outbreaks and sporadic individual cases have also been reported in adult cattle.

O. ostertagi is considered to be a polymorphic species with *Ostertagia lyrata* (syn. *Skrjabinagia*).

Ostertagia leptospicularis

Synonym: *Ostertagia crimensis*, *Skrjabinagia kolchida*, *Grosspiculagia podjapolskyi*

Predilection site: Abomasum

Parasite class: Nematoda

Superfamily: Trichostrongyloidea

Description, gross: Adults are slender, reddish brown worms with a short buccal cavity. Males measure 6–8 mm and females 8–9 mm in length.

Description, microscopic: Distinguished from other ostertagian species by the length of the oesophagus, which is longer than in other species (0.7 mm compared with approximately 0.6 mm). In cattle, the worms are thinner than *O. ostertagi* and males worms are differentiated on spicule morphology (Fig. 2.3b).

Hosts: Deer (roe deer), cattle, sheep, goat

Life cycle: Similar to *O. ostertagi*

Geographical distribution: Many parts of the world, particularly Europe and New Zealand.

Notes: Considered to be a polymorphic species with two male morphs, *Ostertagia leptospicularis* and *Skrjabinagia kolchida* (*Grosspiculagia podjapolskyi*).

Details of the pathogenesis, clinical signs, diagnosis, pathology, epidemiology, treatment and control are as for *O. ostertagi*.

Haemonchus contortus

Synonym: *Haemonchus placei* (see notes)

Common name: Barber's pole worm

Predilection site: Abomasum

Parasite class: Nematoda

Superfamily: Trichostrongyloidea

Notes: Until recently the sheep species was called *H. contortus* and the cattle species *H. placei*. However, there is now increasing evidence that these are the single species *H. contortus* with only strain adaptations for cattle and sheep.

For more details see Chapter 3 (Sheep and goats).

Haemonchus similis

Predilection site: Abomasum

Parasite class: Nematoda

Superfamily: Trichostrongyloidea

Description, gross: The adults are 2.0–3.0 cm and reddish in colour.

Description, microscopic: The male has an asymmetrical dorsal lobe and barbed spicules differing from *H. contortus* in that the terminal processes of the dorsal ray are longer and the spicules shorter.

Hosts: Cattle, deer

Geographical distribution: North America, Europe

Pathogenesis: As for *H. contortus*

Trichostrongylus axei

Synonym: *Trichostrongylus extenuatus*

Predilection site: Abomasum or stomach

Parasite class: Nematoda

Superfamily: Trichostrongyloidea

For more details, see Chapter 3 (Sheep and goats).

Mecistocirrus digitatus

Predilection site: Abomasum

Parasite class: Nematoda

Superfamily: Trichostrongyloidea

Description, gross: To the naked eye, the worm is indistinguishable from *Haemonchus contortus*. The males measure up to around 30 mm and the females 42 mm in length.

Description, microscopic: The male is distinguishable from *Haemonchus* by the presence of long narrow spicules that are fused together for the majority of their length (in *Haemonchus* the spicules are thicker, separate and barbed at the tips). The female differs from *Haemonchus* in that the vulva is positioned nearer to the tip of the tail and there is no vulval flap. The cuticle contains many longitudinal ridges and the cervical papillae are readily apparent. The small buccal capsule is armed with a lancet.

Hosts: Cattle, buffalo, zebu, sheep and goat; occasionally the stomach of the pig and rarely man

Life cycle: This is direct and similar to that of *Haemonchus*. The prepatent period is longer than in *Haemonchus*, being 60–80 days, partly as the result of the longer duration of the fourth stage in the abomasal mucosa.

Geographical distribution: Tropical and subtropical regions, particularly Central America and parts of Asia

Pathogenesis: In endemic areas, the pathogenesis of this haematophagous parasite is similar to that of *H. contortus* and it is of similar economic importance.

Clinical signs: Similar to *H. contortus*, inducing anaemia, weight loss and emaciation.

Diagnosis: See the description of the parasite above.

Treatment and control: See *H. contortus* for details.

Parabronema skrjabini

Predilection site: Abomasum

Parasite class: Nematoda

Superfamily: Spiruroidea

Geographical distribution: Central and east Africa, Asia, and some Mediterranean countries, notably Cyprus

For more details see Chapter 3 (Sheep and goats).

Cryptosporidium andersoni

Synonym: *Cryptosporidium muris*

Predilection site: Abomasum

Parasite class: Sporozoasida

Family: Cryptosporidiidae

Description: Oocysts, passed fully sporulated, are ellipsoid, 6.0–8.1 × 5.0–6.5 μm (mean 7.4 × 5.5 μm), with a length/width ratio of 1.35.

Life cycle: Oocysts, each with four sporozoites, are liberated in the faeces. Following ingestion, the sporozoites invade the microvillous brush border of the gastric glands and the trophozoites rapidly differentiate to form meronts with four to eight merozoites. Gametogony follows after one to two generations of meronts, and oocysts are produced in 72 hours. The prepatent period is unknown.

Geographical distribution: Reported in USA, Brazil, UK, Czech Republic, Germany, France, Japan and Iran

Pathogenesis: Generally considered to be non-pathogenic

Clinical signs: Usually asymptomatic, although depressed weight gain in calves and milk yields in milking cows have been reported.

Diagnosis: Oocysts may be demonstrated using Ziehl–Nielsen stained faecal smears in which the sporozoites appear as bright red granules. Speciation of *Cryptosporidium* is difficult, if not impossible, using conventional techniques. A range of molecular and immunological techniques has been developed, that include the use of immunofluorescence (IF) or enzyme-linked immunosorbent assays (ELISA). More recently, DNA-based techniques have been used for the molecular characterisations of *Cryptosporidium* species.

Pathology: The presence of the endogenous stages of the parasite leads to destruction of the microvilli of peptic glands, leading to elevated concentrations of plasma pepsinogen levels.

Epidemiology: The epidemiology of infection has not been studied although it is likely to be similar to *Cryptosporidium parvum* in cattle. Many calves are likely to become infected without showing clinical signs but become sources of infection for calves that follow. The primary route of infection is by the direct animal-to-animal faecal–oral route. Thus in calves, for example, overcrowding, stress of early weaning, transport and marketing, together with low levels of hygiene will increase the risk of heavy infections.

Treatment and control: There is no reported treatment. Good hygiene and management are important in preventing disease from cryptosporidiosis. Feed and water containers should be high enough to prevent faecal contamination. Young animals should be given colostrum within the first 24 hours of birth and overstocking and overcrowding should be avoided. Dairy calves should be either isolated in individual pens or kept in similar age groups and cleaned out daily.

Notes: Based on oocyst morphology, *C. muris*-like oocysts have been found in cattle in several countries around the world. Recent molecular characterisations have indicated that all bovine isolates are *C. andersoni*.

SMALL INTESTINE

Trichostrongylus colubriformis

Synonym: *Trichostrongylus instabilis*

Common name: Black scour or bankrupt worm

Predilection site: Duodenum and anterior small intestine

Parasite class: Nematoda

Superfamily: Trichostrongyloidea

For more details see Chapter 3 (Sheep and goats).

Trichostrongylus longispicularis

Predilection site: Small intestine

Parasite class: Nematoda

Superfamily: Trichostrongyloidea

Description, gross: The adults are similar in size to *T. colubriformis*.

Description, microscopic: The spicules are stout, brown, unbranched, slightly unequal in length and terminate in a tapering blunt tip that has a small semi-transparent protrusion.

Hosts: Cattle, sheep, goat, deer, camel, llama

Life cycle: This is direct and typically trichostrongyloid. See *T. colubriformis* for details.

Geographical distribution: Ruminants in Australia; and cattle in America and parts of Europe

Details of the pathogenesis, clinical signs, diagnosis, pathology, epidemiology, treatment and control are as for *T. colubriformis*.

Cooperia oncophora

Predilection site: Small intestine

Parasite class: Nematoda

Superfamily: Trichostrongyloidea

Description, gross: In size *C. oncophora* is similar to *Ostertagia* but with a large bursa. Males measure around 5.5–9 mm and females 6–8 mm in length. When fresh the worms appear pinkish white.

Description, microscopic: The main generic features are the small cephalic vesicle and the transverse cuticular striations in the oesophageal region (Fig. 2.7). The body possesses longitudinal ridges. The spicules have a distinct wing-like expansion in the middle region and often bear ridges (Fig. 2.8a); there is no gubernaculum. The females have a long tapering tail. Eggs are oval and thin-shelled.

Hosts: Cattle, sheep, goat, deer

Life cycle: This is direct and typical of the superfamily. Ingested L_3 exsheath, migrate into the intestinal crypts for two moults and then the adults develop on the surface of the intestinal mucosa. The prepatent period is around 3 weeks. The bionomic requirements of the free-living stages are similar to those of *Ostertagia*.

Geographical distribution: Worldwide

Pathogenesis: *C. oncophora* is generally considered to be a mild pathogen in calves, although in some studies it has been associated with inappetence and poor weight gains. A partial immunity to reinfection develops after about 8–12 months of exposure to infective larvae.

Clinical signs: These are loss of appetite and poor weight gains. Occasionally a heavy infection can induce intermittent diarrhoea.

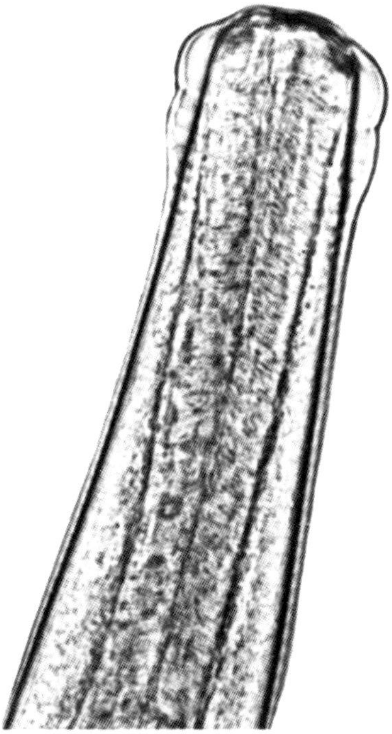

Fig. 2.7 Anterior of *Cooperia* spp showing the cephalic vesicle and cuticular striations.

Diagnosis: Eggs of *Cooperia* spp are all very similar morphologically. Faecal culture will allow identification of infective larvae.

Pathology: Moderate to heavy infections can induce a catarrhal enteritis with localised villous atrophy and oedema of the intestinal mucosa.

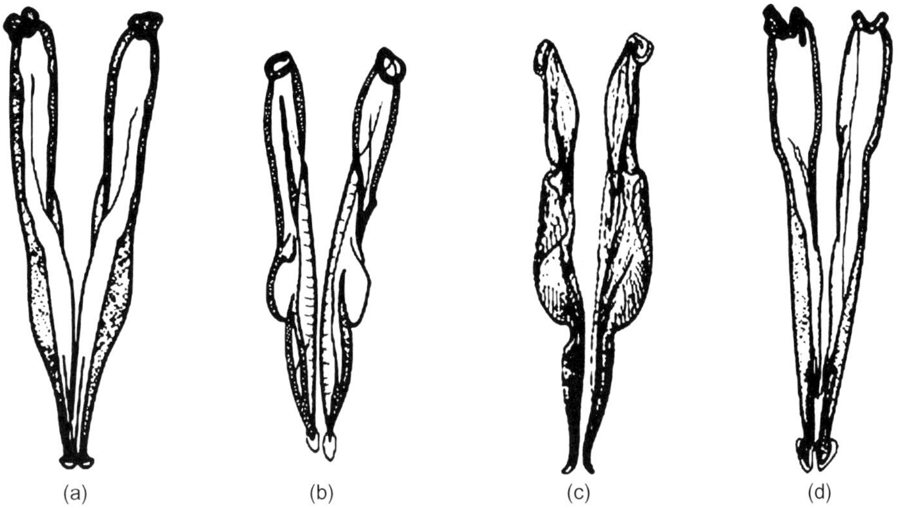

Fig. 2.8 Spicules of *Cooperia* species. (a) *C. oncophora.* (b) *C. pectinata.* (c) *C. punctata.* (d) *Cooperia surnabada.*

Epidemiology: In temperate areas, this is similar to that of *Ostertagia*. Arrested development (hypobiosis) at the EL_4 is a regular feature during late autumn and winter in the northern hemisphere, and spring and summer in the southern hemisphere. Adult animals usually show few signs of infection but act as carriers, shedding low numbers of eggs in their faeces.

In the subtropics, the epidemiology is similar to that of *Haemonchus* though *Cooperia* does not have the same high biotic potential and the L_3 survive rather better under arid conditions. Hypobiosis is also a feature during prolonged dry seasons.

Treatment: The principles are similar to those applied in bovine ostertagiosis. *Cooperia* is one of the dose-limiting species and one should consult the manufacturer's data sheets for efficacy of anthelmintics against adult and L_4 stages.

Control: Similar to that described for *Ostertagia*.

Notes: In temperate areas, members of the genus *Cooperia* usually play a secondary role in the pathogenesis of parasitic gastroenteritis of ruminants although they may be the most numerous trichostrongyle present. However, in some tropical and subtropical areas, some species are responsible for severe enteritis in calves.

Three further species of *Cooperia* are found in cattle. Details of the diagnosis, epidemiology, treatment and control are as for *C. oncophora*

Cooperia punctata

Common name: Cattle bankrupt worm

Predilection site: Small intestine

Parasite class: Nematoda

Superfamily: Trichostrongyloidea

Description, gross: Similar to *C. oncophora*. Males measure around 4.5–6.0 mm, and females 6–8 mm in length.

Description, microscopic: See *C. oncophora* and Fig. 2.8c for details.

Hosts: Cattle, deer

Life cycle: Similar to *C. oncophora* but the adults remain closely associated with the mucosa and surface epithelium. The prepatent period is around 2–3 weeks. The bionomic requirements of the free-living stages are similar to *Haemonchus*.

Geographical distribution: Worldwide

Pathogenesis: *C. punctata* is a pathogenic parasite since it penetrates the epithelial surface of the small intestine and causes a disruption similar to that of other intestinal trichostrongylid species, which leads to villous atrophy and a reduction in the area available for absorption. In heavy infections, diarrhoea has been reported.

Clinical signs: There is loss of appetite, poor weight gains and diarrhoea and there may be submandibular oedema.

Cooperia pectinata

Predilection site: Small intestine

Parasite class: Nematoda

Superfamily: Trichostrongyloidea

Description, gross: Similar to *C. oncophora*. Males measure around 7–8 mm and females 7.5–10 mm in length.

Description, microscopic: See *C. oncophora* and Fig 2.8b for details.

Hosts: Cattle, deer

Life cycle: See *C. punctata* for details

Geographical distribution: Worldwide

Pathogenesis and clinical signs: Similar to *C. punctata*. A catarrhal enteritis is often present with loss of appetite, poor weight gain, diarrhoea, and in some cases, submandibular oedema.

Cooperia surnabada

Synonym: *Cooperia mcmasteri*

Predilection site: Small intestine

Parasite class: Nematoda

Superfamily: Trichostrongyloidea

Description, gross: The males measure around 7 mm and the females 8 mm in length.

Description, microscopic: The appearance is very similar to *C. oncophora*, although the bursa is larger and the bursal rays tend to be thinner. The spicules are thinner with a posterior bifurcation and the tips possess a small conical appendage (Fig. 2.8d).

Hosts: Cattle, sheep, camel

Life cycle: Similar to that of *C. pectinata* and *C. punctata*. The bionomic requirements of the free-living stages concur with those for *Haemonchus*.

Geographical distribution: Parts of Europe, North America and Australia

Pathogenesis: Moderate pathogenicity as the worms penetrate the surface of the small intestine and can induce villous atrophy.

Clinical signs: See *C. punctata.*

Diagnosis: See *C. oncophora.*

Treatment and control: Refer to *C. oncophora.*

Nematodirus helvetianus

Common name: Thread-necked worm

Predilection site: Small intestine

Parasite class: Nematoda

Superfamily: Trichostrongyloidea

Description, gross: The adults are slender, males measuring around 11–16 mm and females 17–24 mm in length.

Description, microscopic: A small but distinct cephalic vesicle is present. The male has two sets of parallel rays in each of the main bursal lobes and the long, slender spicules end in a fused point with the surrounding membrane being lanceolate. The female has a truncate tail with a small spine, and the egg is large, ovoid and colourless and twice the size of the typical trichostrongyle egg (Fig. 2.9).

Hosts: Cattle, occasionally sheep, goat and other ruminants

Life cycle: The preparasitic phase is almost unique in the trichostrongyloids in that development to the L_3 takes place within the egg shell. *N. helvetianus* does not have the same critical hatching requirements as *N. battus* (see Chapter 3) and so the larvae often appear on the pasture within 2–3 weeks of the eggs being excreted in the faeces. More than one annual generation is therefore possible. The parasitic phase within the host is similar to that of *N. battus*. The prepatent period is around 3 weeks.

Geographical distribution: Worldwide

Pathogenesis: Although this is similar to that of *N. battus*, there is some controversy over the extent of the pathogenic effect. *N. helvetianus* has been incriminated in outbreaks of bovine parasitic gastroenteritis but experimental attempts to reproduce the disease have been unsuccessful.

Clinical signs: Low to moderate infections may produce no obvious clinical manifestations. In severe infections, diarrhoea can occur during the prepatent period and young animals may become dehydrated.

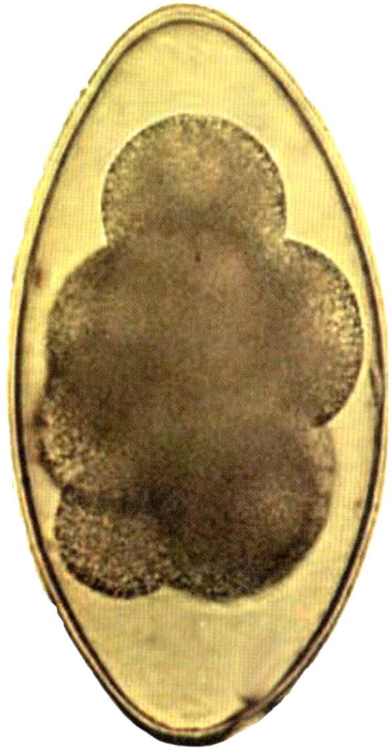

Fig. 2.9 Large egg of *Nematodirus helvetianus.*

Diagnosis: Examination of faeces will allow the large colourless eggs to be differentiated from those of *N. spathiger*. At necropsy, the tips of the male spicules will allow diagnosis from other *Nematodirus* species.

Pathology: Increased mucus production and focal compression and stunting of villi may occur in the small intestine.

Epidemiology: The eggs do not usually exhibit delayed hatching. The pattern of infection is similar to that of *Trichostrongylus* species.

Treatment: Several drugs are effective against *Nematodirus* infections; levamisole, an avermectin/milbemycin or one of the modern benzimidazoles. However, *Nematodirus* is one of the dose-limiting species and manufacturer's data sheets should be consulted as there are differences in efficacy against adults and L_4 stages between oral and parenteral administration for some macrocyclic lactones. The response to treatment is usually rapid and if diarrhoea persists coccidiosis should be considered as a complicating factor.

Control: Disease due to monospecific *Nematodirus* infections is rarely seen. They are usually part of the worm burden of trichostrongyloid species that are responsible for the syndrome of PGE in cattle and as such may be controlled by the measures outlined elsewhere.

Nematodirus battus

Common name: Thread-necked worm

Predilection site: Small intestine

Parasite class: Nematoda

Superfamily: Trichostrongyloidea
For more details see Chapter 3 (Sheep and goats).

Nematodirus spathiger

Common name: Thread-necked worm

Predilection site: Small intestine

Parasite class: Nematoda

Superfamily: Trichostrongyloidea
For more details see Chapter 3 (Sheep and goats).

Bunostomum phlebotomum

Synonym: *Monodontus phlebotomum*

Common name: Cattle hookworm

Predilection site: Small intestine, particularly the anterior jejunum and/or duodenum

Parasite class: Nematoda

Superfamily: Ancylostomatoidea

Description, gross: *Bunostomum* is one of the larger nematodes of the small intestine of ruminants, being 1–3 cm long, stout, greyish white and characteristically hooked at the anterior end with the buccal capsule opening anterodorsally (Fig. 2.10).

Description, microscopic: The large buccal capsule opens anterodorsally and bears on the ventral margin a pair of chitinous cutting plates and internally a large dorsal cone. Dorsal teeth are absent from the buccal capsule but there are two pairs of small sub-ventral lancets at its base. In the male the bursa is well developed and has an asymmetrical dorsal lobe. The right externodorsal ray arises higher up on the dorsal stem and is longer than the left. It arises near the bifurcation of the dorsal ray, which divides into two tridigitate branches. The spicules are very long and slender. In the female the vulva opens a short distance in front of the middle of the body.

The infective larva is small with 16 gut cells and a short filamentous tail. Eggs are medium-sized (97 × 50 μm) irregular broad elipse, with dissimilar sidewalls and four to eight blastomeres.

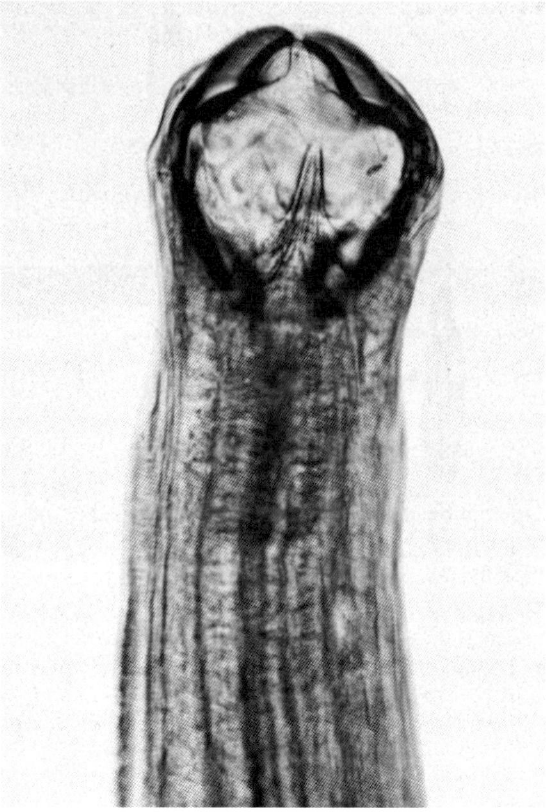

Fig. 2.10 Head of *Bunostomum phlebotomum* showing the large buccal capsule and cutting plates.

Hosts: Cattle

Life cycle: Infection with the L_3 may be percutaneous or oral. After skin penetration, the larvae travel to the lungs and moult to 4th stage larvae before re-entering the gastrointestinal tract after approximately 11 days. Ingested larvae usually develop without a migration. Further development continues in the gut. The prepatent period is about 6 weeks after skin penetration, and 7–10 weeks after ingestion.

Geographical distribution: Worldwide

Pathogenesis: The adult worms are blood-suckers and infections of 100–500 worms can produce progressive anaemia, hypoalbuminaemia, loss of weight and occasionally diarrhoea. Worm burdens of around 2000 may lead to death in cattle. In stabled cattle, pruritus of the limbs, probably caused by skin penetration by the larvae, is seen.

Clinical signs: There may be inappetence, diarrhoea and emaciation, more frequently seen in young animals. Severe infection can also induce submandibular oedema ('bottle jaw'). Postmortem examination often reveals hydrothorax and fluid within the pericardium. Older livestock frequently develop sufficient immunity to limit reinfection and in many cases *Bunostomum* is present asymptomatically. In calves, foot stamping and signs of itching may accompany skin penetration by the larvae.

Diagnosis: The clinical signs of anaemia and perhaps diarrhoea in calves are not in themselves pathognomonic of bunostomosis. However, in temperate areas, the epidemiological background may be useful in eliminating the possibility of *Fasciola hepatica* infection. In the tropics, haemonchosis must be considered, possibly originating from hypobiotic larvae. Faecal worm egg counts are useful in that these are lower than in *Haemonchus* infection while the eggs are more bluntly rounded, with relatively thick sticky shells to which debris is often adhered. For accurate differentiation, larval cultures should be prepared.

Pathology: The carcase is anaemic and cachexic. Oedema and ascites are seen. The liver is light brown and shows fatty changes. The intestinal contents are haemorrhagic and the mucosa is usually swollen, covered with mucus, and shows numerous lesions resulting from the worms feeding. The parasites may be seen still attached to the mucosa or free in the lumen.

Epidemiology: Pathogenic infections are more common in the tropics and sub-tropics and in some areas, such as Nigeria, the highest worm burdens are found at the end of the dry season, apparently due to the maturation of hypobiotic larvae. Young livestock are most susceptible. *B. phlebotomum* is often a serious pathogen in many regions such as the southern and mid-western USA, Australia and parts of Africa. In temperate countries, high worm burdens are usually uncommon. The prophylactic dosing regimes, adopted for the control of trichostrongyles, have contributed to the low prevalence of *Bunostomum*.

Treatment: Anthelmintics listed for *O. ostertagi* are effective.

Control: A combination of strategic dosing with anthelmintics and pasture management is used in the control of larvae as they are susceptible to dessication, and the infection is mainly found on permanently or occasionally moist pastures. Avoiding or draining such pastures is an effective control measure. The ground around water troughs should be kept hard and dry, or treated with liberal applications of salt. Stabled cattle should be protected by ensuring the floors and bedding are kept dry and that faeces are removed frequently, and are not allowed to contaminate food and water.

Agriostomum vryburgi

Predilection site: Small intestine

Parasite class: Nematoda

Superfamily: Ancylostomatoidea

Description, gross: Worms are stout and greyish white in colour. Males are around 9–11 mm and females 13–16 mm in length. Spicules are equal in length and a gubernaculum is present.

Description, microscopic: The shallow bucal capsule contains four pairs of large teeth on its margin and has a rudimentary leaf-crown. The large oesophageal opening houses two small subventral lancets. Eggs measure about 130–190 × 60–90 μm.

Hosts: Cattle, buffalo, ox and zebu

Life cycle: The life cycle is probably direct.

Geographical distribution: Asia and South America

Pathogenesis: The hookworms attach to the mucosa of the anterior small intestine. The pathogenicity, although unknown, presumably depends on its haematophagic habits, inducing anaemia.

Notes: *Agriostomum vryburgi* is a common hookworm of the large intestine throughout its distribution range.

Details on the diagnosis, treatment and control are likely to be similar to *B. phlebotomum*.

Strongyloides papillosus

Predilection site: Small intestine

Parasite class: Nematoda

Superfamily: Rhabditoidea

For more details see Chapter 3 (Sheep and goats).

Toxocara vitulorum

Synonym: *Neoascaris vitulorum*

Predilection site: Small intestine

Parasite class: Nematoda

Superfamily: Ascaridoidea

Description, gross: This is a very large whitish nematode, the adult male is up to 25 cm and the female 30 cm.

Description, microscopic: The cuticle is less thick than other ascarids and somewhat soft and translucent. There are three lips, broad at the base and narrowing anteriorly. The oesophagus is 3–4.5 mm long and has a posterior, granular ventriculus. The tail of the male

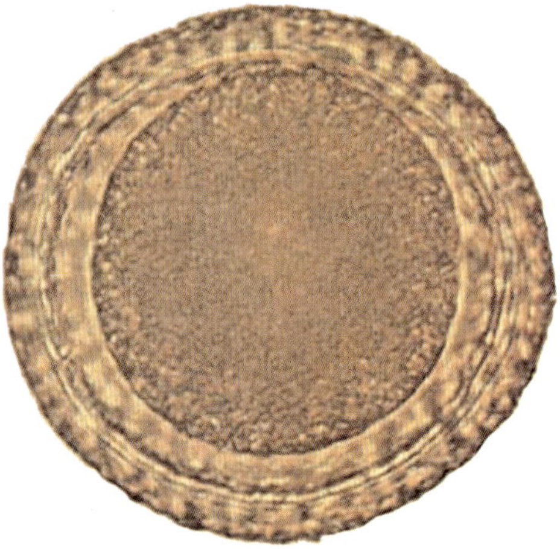

Fig. 2.11 Egg of *Toxocara vitulorum*.

usually forms a small spike-like appendage. There are about five pairs of post-cloacal papillae; the anterior pair is large and double. Pre-cloacal papillae are variable in number. The vulva is situated about one eighth of the body length from the anterior end. The egg of *T. vitulorum* is subglobular, with a thick finely pitted shell, and is almost colourless (75–95 × 60–74 μm) (Fig. 2.11).

Hosts: Cattle, buffalo and zebu, rarely sheep and goats

Life cycle: The life cycle is direct. The most important source of infection is the milk of the dam in which larvae are present for up to 3–4 weeks after parturition. There is no tissue migration in the calf following milk-borne infection and the prepatent period is 3–4 weeks. The ingestion of larvated eggs by calves over 6 months old seldom results in patency, the larvae migrating to various tissues where they remain dormant; in female animals, resumption of development in late pregnancy allows further transmammary transmission.

Geographical distribution: Africa, India, Asia

Pathogenesis: The main effects of *T. vitulorum* infection appear to be caused by the adult worms in the intestines of calves up to 6 months old. Heavy infections are often associated with unthriftyness, catarrhal enteritis and intermittent diarrhoea, and in buffalo calves particularly, fatalities may occur. Heavy burdens can be associated with intestinal obstruction and occasionally perforation may occur leading to peritonitis and death.

Clinical signs: Diarrhoea, poor condition

Diagnosis: In some instances heavily infected calves may exhale an acetone-like odour. The sub-globular eggs, with thick, pitted shells, are characteristic in bovine faeces. Egg output in young calves can be very high (>50 000 epg) but patency is short and by around 4–6 months of age, calves have expelled most of their adult worm population.

Pathology: The pathological effects of adult worms in the intestine are poorly defined. Heavy infections may obstruct the gut and lead to gut perforation. Migration up the bile or pancreatic duct may lead to biliary obstruction and cholangitis.

Epidemiology: The most important feature is the reservoir of larvae in the tissues of the cow, with subsequent milk-borne transmission ensuring that calves are exposed to infection from the first day of life. The majority of patent infections occur in calves of less than 6 months of age.

Treatment: The adult worms are susceptible to a wide range of anthelmintics, including piperazine, levamisole, macrocyclic lactones and the benzimidazoles. Many of these drugs are also effective against developing stages in the intestine.

Control: The prevalence of infection can be dramatically reduced by treatment of calves at 3 and 6 weeks of age, preventing developing worms reaching patency.

Capillaria bovis

Synonym: *Capillaria brevipes*

Predilection site: Small intestine

Parasite class: Nematoda

Superfamily: Trichuroidea

Description, gross: These are very fine filamentous worms, the narrow stichosome oesophagus occupying about one third to half the body length. Males measure around 8–9 mm and females up to 12 mm.

Description, microscopic: The males have a long thin single spicule about 0.9 mm long and often possess a primitive bursa-like structure. The eggs are barrel-shaped (similar to *Trichuris*), 45–50 × 22–25 μm, are colourless and have thick shells that are slightly striated with bipolar plugs.

Hosts: Cattle, sheep, goat

Life cycle: The life cycle is direct. The infective L_1 develops within the egg in about 3–4 weeks. Infection of the final host is through ingestion of this embryonated infective stage and development to adult worms occurs without a migration phase. The prepatent period is 3–4 weeks.

Geographical distribution: Worldwide

Pathogenesis: Considered to be of low pathogenicity and of little veterinary significance.

Clinical signs: No clinical signs have been attributed to infection with this parasite.

Diagnosis: Because of the non-specific nature of the clinical signs and the fact that, in heavy infections, these may appear before eggs are present in the faeces, diagnosis depends on necropsy and careful examination of the small intestine for the presence of the worms. This may be carried out by microscopic examination of mucosal scrapings squeezed between two glass slides; alternatively the contents should be gently washed through a fine sieve and the retained material resuspended in water and examined against a black background.

Pathology: No associated pathology

Epidemiology: Infection is by ingestion of the larvated eggs. Infection is common in sheep though not significant.

Treatment: Not usually required

Control: Not required

Moniezia benedeni

Predilection site: Small intestine

Parasite class: Cestoda

Family: Anoplocephalidae

Description, gross: These are long tapeworms, 2 metres or more, which are unarmed, possessing prominent suckers.

Description, microscopic: Segments are broader than they are long (up to 2.5 cm wide) and contain two sets of genital organs grossly visible along the lateral margin of each segment (Fig. 2.12). There is a row of inter-proglottidal glands at the posterior border of each segment, which may be used in species differentiation; in *M. benedeni* they are confined to a short row close to the middle of the segment. The irregularly quadrangular eggs have a well defined pyriform apparatus and vary from 55–75 µm in diameter.

Final host: Cattle

Intermediate hosts: Forage mites, mainly of the family Oribatidae.

Life cycle: Mature proglottids or eggs are passed in the faeces and on to pasture where the oncospheres are ingested by forage mites. The embryos migrate into the body cavity of the mite where they develop to cysticercoids in 1–4 months and infection of the final host is by ingestion of infected mites during grazing. The prepatent period is approximately 6 weeks, but the adult worms appear to be short lived, patent infections persisting for only 3 months.

Geographical distribution: Worldwide

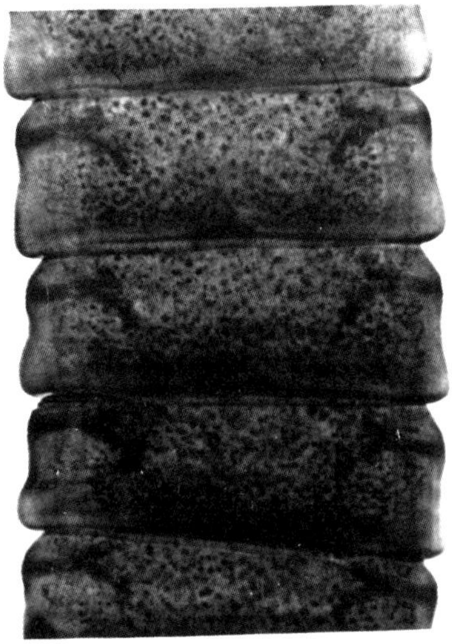

Fig. 2.12 Proglottids of *Moniezia benedeni.*

Pathogenesis: Generally regarded as of little pathogenic significance.

Clinical signs: No clinical signs have been associated with infection.

Diagnosis: This is based largely on the presence of mature proglottids in the faeces and the characteristic shape of *Moniezia* eggs (triangular, *M. expansa*; quadrangular, *M. benedeni*) that contain the oncosphere. The eggs of *M. benedeni* are slightly larger than those of *M. expansa* (see Chapter 3).

Pathology: No reported pathology.

Epidemiology: Infection is common in calves during their first year of life and less common in older animals. A seasonal fluctuation in the incidence of *Moniezia* infection can apparently be related to active periods of the forage mite vectors during the summer in temperate areas. The cysticercoids can overwinter in the mites.

Treatment: In many countries a variety of drugs, including niclosamide, praziquantel, bunamidine and a number of broad-spectrum benzimidazole compounds, which have the advantage of also being active against gastrointestinal nematodes, are available for the treatment of *Moniezia* infection. If this is carried out in calves in late spring, in temperate areas, the numbers of newly infected mites on pasture will be reduced.

Control: Ploughing and reseeding, or avoiding the use of the same pastures for young animals in consecutive years, may prove beneficial.

Notes: This genus of cestodes is common in ruminants and resembles, in most respects, *Anoplocephala* of the horse. *Moniezia* spp are the only tapeworms of ruminants in many countries of western Europe.

Thysaniezia ovilla

Synonym: *Thysaniezia giardia*

Predilection site: Small intestine

Parasite class: Cestoda

Family: Thysanosomidae

Description, gross: Adults reach 200 cm in length, varying in width up to 12 mm.

Description, microscopic: The scolex is small, measuring up to 1 mm in diameter. Segments are short, bulge outwards giving the margin of the worm an irregular appearance, and contain a single set of genital organs, rarely two, with genital pores alternating irregularly. Eggs are devoid of a pyriform apparatus and are found in groups of 10–15 in elongated paruterine organs (100 μm long), with a thick grey shell and a protruberance at one end.

Hosts: Cattle, sheep, goat, camel and wild ruminants

Intermediate hosts: Oribatid mites (*Galuma, Scheloribates*) and psocids (bark lice, dust lice)

Life cycle: Mature segments are passed in the faeces of the infected host on to pasture, where forage mites ingest the oncospheres. Cysticercoids develop within the orabatid intermediate hosts and infection of the final host is by ingestion of infected mites during grazing.

Geographical distribution: Southern Africa

Pathogenesis: Not considered pathogenic

Diagnosis: The mature segments found in the faeces are readily distinguishable from *Moniezia.*

Epidemiology: Infection is very commonly found in adult cattle in southern Africa.

Treatment and control: As for *Moniezia*.

The following species have also been reported in cattle. For more details on these species see Chapter 3 (Sheep and goats).

Moniezia expansa

Predilection site: Small intestine

Parasite class: Cestoda

Family: Anoplocephalidae

Description, gross: These are long tapeworms, 2 metres or more, which are unarmed, possessing prominent suckers.

Description, microscopic: Segments are broader than they are long (up to 1.5 cm wide) and contain two sets of genital organs grossly visible along the lateral margin of each segment. There is a row of interproglottidal glands at the posterior border of each segment, which may be used in species differentiation. In *M. expansa* they extend along the full breadth of the segment.

Final hosts: Sheep, goats, occasionally cattle

Intermediate hosts: Forage mites, mainly of the family Oribatidae

Avitellina centripunctata

Predilection site: Small intestine

Parasite class: Cestoda

Family: Thysanosomidae

Description, gross: This tapeworm resembles *Moniezia* on gross inspection except that the segmentation is so poorly marked that it appears somewhat ribbon-like. It can reach 3 metres in length by about 4 mm in width and the posterior end is almost cylindrical in appearance.

Description, microscopic: A single genitalia is present with the pores alternating irregularly. Proglottids are short. Eggs lack a pyriform apparatus and measure around 20–45 μm.

Final hosts: Sheep and other ruminants

Intermediate hosts: Thought to be oribatid mites or psocid lice

Stilesia globipunctata

Predilection site: Small intestine

Parasite class: Cestoda

Family: Thysanosomidae

Description, gross: Adults measure around 0.5 metres in length by 3–4 mm wide.

Description, microscopic: A single set of genital organs is present.

Final hosts: Sheep, cattle and other ruminants

Intermediate hosts: As for *Avitellina centripunctata*

Thysanosoma actinoides

Common name: Fringed tapeworm

Predilection site: Small intestine, bile and pancreatic ducts

Parasite class: Cestoda

Family: Thysanosomidae

Description, gross: Adult tapeworms measure 15–30 cm in length by 8 mm wide.

Description, microscopic: The scolex is up to 1.5 mm; segments are short and fringed posteriorly. Each segment contains two sets of genital organs with the testes lying medially. Several paruterine organs are present in each proglottid and the eggs have no pyriform apparatus.

Final hosts: Sheep, cattle, deer

Intermediate hosts: As for *Thysaniezia ovilla*

Geographical distribution: North and South America

Cymbiforma indica

Predilection site: Gastrointestinal tract

Parasite class: Trematoda

Family: Notocotylidae

Final hosts: Sheep, goat, cattle

Intermediate hosts: Snails

Geographical distribution: India

Bovine coccidiosis

At least 13 different species of *Eimeria* are known to infect cattle. Clinical signs of diarrhoea are associated with the presence of *E. zuernii* or *E. bovis*, which occur in the lower small intestine, caecum and colon. *E. alabamensis*, has been reported to cause enteritis in yearling calves in some European countries. Affected animals develop watery diarrhoea, shortly after turn-out in the spring on to heavily contaminated pastures previously grazed by calves.

The life cycles (where known) of the *Eimeria* species are typically coccidian (see Chapter 1, Protozoa – Phylum: Apicomplexa). Following ingestion of the sporulated oocyst there are several merogony stages within the intestinal mucosa (usually two in those in which the life cycle has been described). In some species, such as *E. bovis*, first-generation meronts are large, and are referred to as 'giant' meronts. These are followed by smaller second-generation meronts. During gametogony, fusion of macrogametocytes and microgametocytes leads to zygote formation and the excretion of unsporulated oocysts in the faeces. Sporulation outside the body may be completed in 1–4 days under ideal conditions, but can take several weeks in cold weather. Sporulated oocysts contain four sporocysts each containing two sporozoites. The life cycle takes between 1 and 4 weeks depending on the species of *Eimeria*.

Prevalence

Most cattle are infected with coccidia during their lives and in the majority of animals the parasites co-exist causing minimal damage. Disease usually only occurs if they are subjected to heavy infection or if their resistance is lowered through stress, poor nutrition or inter-current disease. The presence of infection does not necessarily lead to the development of clinical signs of disease and in many situations low levels of challenge can actually be beneficial by stimulating protective immune responses in the host.

Pathogenesis

The most pathogenic species of coccidia are those that infect and destroy the crypt cells of the large intestinal mucosa (Table 2.1). This is because the ruminant small intestine is very long, providing a large number of host cells and the potential for enormous parasite replication with minimal damage. If the absorption of nutrients is impaired, the large intestine is, to some extent, capable of compensating. Those species that invade the large intestine are more likely to cause pathological changes, particularly if large numbers of oocysts are ingested over a short period of time. Here, the rate of cellular turnover is much lower and there is no compensation effect from other regions of the gut. In calves that become heavily infected, the mucosa becomes completely denuded, resulting in severe haemorrhage and impaired water resorption

Table 2.1 Predilection sites and prepatent periods of *Eimeria* species in cattle.

Species	Predilection site	Prepatent period (days)
E. alabamensis	Small and large intestine	6–11
E. auburnensis	Small intestine	16–24
E. bovis	Small and large intestine	16–21
E. brasiliensis	Unknown	?
E. bukidnonensis	Unknown	?
E. canadensis	Unknown	?
E. cylindrica	Unknown	10
E. ellipsoidalis	Small intestine	8–13
E. pellita	Unknown	?
E. subspherica	Unknown	7–18
E. wyomingensis	Unknown	13–15
E. zuernii	Small and large intestine	15–17

leading to diarrhoea, dehydration and death. In lighter infections, the effect on the intestinal mucosa is to impair local absorption. Species that develop more superficially in the small intestines cause a change in villous architecture with a reduction in epithelial cell height and a diminution of the brush border giving the appearance of a 'flat mucosa'. These changes result in a reduction of the surface area available for absorption and consequently a reduced feed efficiency.

Clinical and pathological signs

Clinical signs are usually weight loss, anorexia and diarrhoea, often bloody. On postmortem, there may be little to see beyond thickening and petechiation of the bowel but mucosal scrapings will reveal masses of gamonts and oocysts. Giant meronts may be seen in the mucosa of the small intestine as pin-point white spots, but unless they are present in vast numbers they cause little harm. The most pathogenic stages are the gamonts.

Host resistance

Whilst animals of all ages are susceptible to infection, younger animals are generally more susceptible to disease. Occasionally, however, acute coccidiosis occurs in much older, even adult, animals with impaired cellular immunity or in those which have been subjected to stress, such as transportation, crowding in feedlot areas, extremes of temperature and weather conditions, changes in environment or severe concurrent infection.

Epidemiology

Bovine coccidiosis is primarily a disease of young animals normally occurring in calves between 3 weeks and 6 months of age but has been reported in cattle aged 1 year or more. The disease is usually associated with a previous stressful situation such as shipping, overcrowding, changes of feed, severe weather or concurrent infection with parvovirus.

Diagnosis

Diagnosis should be based on history, clinical signs (severe diarrhoea in young animals), postmortem findings (inflammation, hyperaemia and thickening of caecum with masses of gamonts and oocysts in scrapings), supported by oocyst counts and speciation to identify pathogenic species (Fig. 2.13). Counts of faecal oocysts identified to species can help to complete the picture, but oocyst numbers may be grossly misleading when considered in isolation. Healthy animals may pass more than a million oocysts per gram of faeces whereas in animals dying of coccidiosis the count may be less than 10 000. High counts of non-pathogenic species could mask significant numbers of the more pathogenic species, for instance, and give the impression that the abundant species was the cause. A key to the identification of sporulated oocysts of cattle is provided in Chapter 15: The Laboratory Diagnosis of Parasitism (Table 15.6).

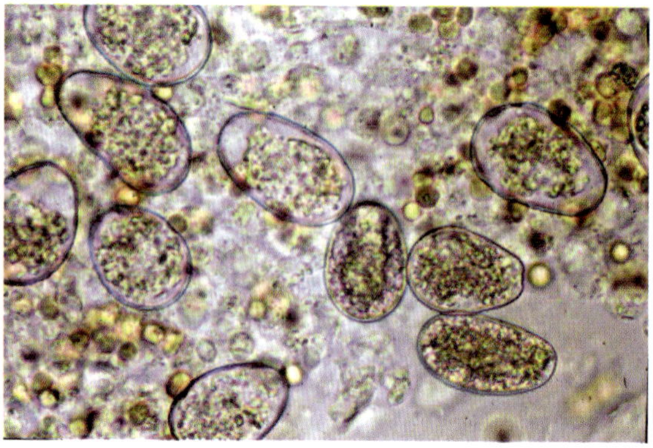

Fig. 2.13 Oocysts of *Eimeria bovis*.

Treatment

Outbreaks of clinical coccidiosis can appear suddenly and may prove troublesome to resolve as they often occur on heavily stocked farms, particularly where good husbandry and management are lacking. If deaths are occurring, early confirmation of the diagnosis is vital. Affected animals should be medicated and moved to uncontaminated pens or pasture as soon as possible.

Normally all animals in a group should be treated, as even those showing no symptoms are likely to be infected. Severely infected animals that are diarrhoeic and dehydrated may require oral or intravenous rehydration. Where non-specific symptoms of weight loss or ill-thrift are present, it is important to investigate all potential causes and seek laboratory confirmation. If coccidiosis is considered significant, much can be done through advice on management and instigation of preventative measures. Batch rearing of animals of similar ages, limits the build-up and spread of oocysts and allows targeting of treatment to susceptible age groups during the danger periods.

Prevention and control

Coccidial infections can be reduced through avoidance of overcrowding and stress, and attention to hygiene. Raising of food and water troughs, for example, can help avoid contamination by reducing the levels of infection. Young animals should be kept off heavily contaminated pastures when they are most susceptible.

Eimeria alabamensis

Predilection site: Small and large intestine

Parasite class: Sporozoasida

Family: Eimeriidae

Description: Oocysts are usually ovoid, 13–24 × 11–16 μm (mean 18.9 × 13.4 μm) with a smooth, colourless wall with no micropyle, polar body or residuum. Sporocysts are ellipsoidal, 10–16 × 4–6 μm with a tiny Stieda body and a sporocyst residuum. The sporozoites lie lengthwise head to tail in the sporocysts and have one to three clear globules. First-generation meronts are usually ovoid 7–9 × 5.5–8.0 μm, containing 8–16 merozoites. Second-generation meronts are 9–12 × 6–9 μm, ovoid or ellipsoidal in shape and contain 18–26 merozoites.

Life cycle: The life cycle is typically coccidian with the developmental stages occurring in the nucleus of epithelial cells. Sporozoites penetrate the intestinal cells as early as day 2 after infection, and meronts are visible in the nucleus from 2–8 days post infection. Parasitised cells are usually those at the tips of the villi and multiple invasion of the nucleus may occur. Two generations of meronts have been found: mature first-generation meronts are seen 2–7 days post infection, and mature second-generation meronts from the 4th to 7th days post infection. The gametocytes are found in the posterior third of the small intestine and may also occur in the mucous membrane of the caecum and colon in heavy infections. Oocysts may be seen in the cells of the lower ileum as early as 6 days post infection. The prepatent period is 6–11 days with a patent period of 1–13 days. Sporulation takes 4–8 days.

Geographical distribution: Presumed worldwide, mainly Europe

Pathogenesis: Particularly pathogenic, attacking the epithelial cells of the jejunum, ileum, and, in heavy infections, the caecum and colon.

Pathology: Infection causes catarrhal enteritis in the jejunum, ileum and caecum with petechial haemorrhages. Histologically there is necrotic inflammation and destruction of epithelial cells. There is an inflammatory response consisting predominantly of mononuclear cells with a few eosinophils and neutrophils. Numerous meronts are seen in the nuclei of villous epithelial cells, with occasional meronts in the upper colon. The mesenteric lymph nodes are enlarged, and parasite stages have been observed in the lymph nodes.

Clinical signs: Diarrhoea in calves recently turned out on to permanent paddocks. The calves become depressed and reluctant to rise. From 8 days after turnout, 850 000 to several million oocysts/g faeces are excreted. Growth rate of the calves is adversely affected. Morbidity ranges from 5–100%, average 64%, but mortality is generally low.

Treatment: Sulphonamides can be used to treat infection. Decoquinate has a prophylactic action against the parasite.

Control: Where infection is suspected to be due to oocysts overwintering on the pasture, the grazing land should be rotated to ensure that calves are not turned out on to potentially heavily infected pasture.

Infection with the following species of coccidia present in the small intestine is not usually associated with clinical signs. Specific treatment and control measures are not usually indicated for these species although they often present as mixed infections. Differentiation is based on oocyst morphology (see Table 15.5 and Figure 15.19).

Eimeria aubernensis

Predilection site: Small intestine

Parasite class: Sporozoasida

Family: Eimeriidae

Description: Oocysts are elongated, ovoid, 20–46 × 20–25 μm (mean 38.4 × 23.1 μm), yellowish brown, with a smooth or heavily granulated wall with a micropyle and polar granule, but no oocyst residuum. Sporocysts are elongate ovoid, almost ellipsoidal, 15–23 × 6–11 μm with a Stieda body and a residuum. The sporozoites are elongate, almost comma shaped, 15–18 × 3–5 μm and lie lengthwise head to tail in the sporocysts, and have a clear globule at the large end, and sometimes one to two small globules arranged randomly.

Life cycle: The first-generation meronts occur throughout the small intestine deep in the lamina propria near the muscularis mucosae. Second-generation meronts and gamonts occur in the sub-epithelium in the distal part of the villi, in the jejunum and ileum. The macrogamonts are about 18 μm in diameter when mature. The prepatent period is 16–24 days and the patent period is usually 2–8 days. The sporulation time is 2–3 days.

Geographical distribution: Worldwide

Eimeria brasiliensis

Predilection site: Unknown

Parasite class: Sporozoasida

Family: Eimeriidae

Description: Oocysts are ellipsoidal, yellowish brown, 33–44 × 24–30 μm (mean 37 × 27 μm) with a micropyle covered by a distinct polar cap. Polar granules may also be present, but there is no oocyst residuum. Sporocysts are elipsoidal, 16–22 × 7–10 μm with a residuum and sometimes a small dark Stieda body. The sporozoites are elongate and lie lengthwise, head to tail in the sporocysts and have a large posterior and a small anterior clear globule.

Life cycle: Details of the life cycle are unknown. The sporulation time is 12–14 days.

Geographical distribution: Worldwide

Eimeria bukidnonensis

Predilection site: Small and large intestine

Parasite class: Sporozoasida

Family: Eimeriidae

Description: Oocysts are pear-shaped or oval, tapering at one pole, 47–50 × 33–38 μm (mean 48.6 × 35.4 μm) yellowish brown, with a thick, radially striated wall and micropyle. A polar granule may be present but there is no oocyst residuum. Sporozoites are elongate and lie lengthwise head to tail in the sporocysts with a clear globule at each end.

Life cycle: Details of the life cycle are unknown. The sporulation time is 4–7 days.

Geographical distribution: Worldwide

Eimeria canadensis

Predilection site: Unknown

Parasite class: Sporozoasida

Family: Eimeriidae

Description: Oocysts are ovoid or ellipsoidal, colourless, or pale yellow, 28–37 × 20–22 μm (mean 32.5 × 23.4 μm) with an inconspicuous micropyle, one or more polar granules and an oocyst residuum. Sporocysts are elongate ovoid, 15–22 × 6–10 μm with an inconspicuous Stieda body and a residuum. The sporozoites are elongate, lie lengthwise head to tail in the sporocysts and have two to three clear globules each.

Life cycle: Details of the life cycle are unknown. The sporulation time is 3–4 days.

Geographical distribution: Worldwide

Eimeria cylindrica

Predilection site: Unknown

Parasite class: Sporozoasida

Family: Eimeriidae

Description: Oocysts are elongated, cylindrical, 16–27 × 12–15 μm (mean 23.3 × 12.3 μm) with a colourless, smooth wall, no micropyle, and no oocyst residuum. Sporocysts are elongate ellipsoidal, 12–16 × 4–6 μm with an inconspicuous or absent Stieda body and a residuum. The sporozoites are elongate, lie lengthwise head to tail in the sporocysts and have one or more rather indistinct clear globules.

Life cycle: Details of the life cycle are unknown. Both the prepatent and patent periods are 10 days. The sporulation time is 2–3 days.

Geographical distribution: Worldwide

Eimeria ellipsoidalis

Predilection site: Small intestine

Parasite class: Sporozoasida

Family: Eimeriidae

Description: Oocysts are ellipsoidal to slightly ovoid, colourless, 20–26 × 12–17 μm (mean 23.4 × 15.9 μm) with no discernible micropyle, polar granule or oocyst residuum. Sporocysts are ovoid, 11–17 × 5–7 μm and may have a conspicuous Stieda body, each with a residuum. The sporozoites are elongate, 11–14 × 2–3 μm and lie head to tail in the sporocysts and have two clear globules.

Life cycle: Mature gamonts lie in the terminal section of the ileum, and are seen 10 days after infection in the epithelial cells near the bottom of the crypts. The prepatent period is 8–13 days. The sporulation time is 3 days.

Geographical distribution: Worldwide

Eimeria pellita

Predilection site: Unknown

Parasite class: Sporozoasida

Family: Eimeriidae

Description: Oocysts are egg-shaped, with a very thick brown wall with evenly distributed protruberences, 36–41 × 26–30 μm (mean 40 × 28 μm) with a micropyle and polar granule consisting of several rod-like bodies but no oocyst residuum. Sporocysts are ellipsoidal, 17–20 × 7–9 μm (mean 18.5 × 8 μm), each with a small Stieda body and a small sporocyst residuum. The sporozoites are elongate and each has two clear globules.

Life cycle: Details of the life cycle are unknown. The sporulation time is 10–12 days.

Geographical distribution: Presumed worldwide

Eimeria subspherica

Predilection site: Unknown

Parasite class: Sporozoasida

Family: Eimeriidae

Description: Oocysts are round or subspherical, colourless, 9–14 × 8–13 μm (mean 11 × 10.4 μm) with no micropyle, polar granule or oocyst residuum. Sporocysts are elongate ovoid, 6–10 × 2–5 μm, each with a small Stieda body, but usually lacking a sporocyst residuum. The sporozoites are elongate and lie lengthwise head to tail in the sporocysts and each has a clear globule at the large end.

Life cycle: Details of the life cycle are unknown. The prepatent period is 7–18 days and the patent period is 4–15 days. The sporulation time is 4–5 days.

Geographical distribution: Worldwide

Eimeria wyomingensis

Predilection site: Unknown

Parasite class: Sporozoasida

Family: Eimeriidae

Description: The oocysts are ovoid, yellowish brown, 37–45 × 26–31 μm (mean 40.3 × 28.1 μm) with a thick wall, a wide micropyle but no polar granule or oocyst residuum. Sporocysts are ellipsoidal with narrowed ends (18 × 9 μm) and each has a tiny Stieda body and the residuum is generally small or absent. The sporozoites are elongate, about 7–8 × 5 μm and lie lengthwise head to tail in the sporocysts, each with a large clear globule.

Life cycle: Details of the life cycle are unknown. The prepatent period is 13–15 days and the patent period 1–7 days. The sporulation time is 5–7 days.

Geographical distribution: Worldwide

Other protozoa

Cryptosporidium parvum

Predilection site: Small intestine

Parasite class: Sporozoasida

Family: Cryptosporidiidae

Description: Mature oocysts are ovoidal or spheroidal, 4.6–5.4 × 3.8–4.7 μm (mean 5.0 × 4.5 μm) and a length:width ratio of 1.19.

Hosts: Cattle, sheep, goat, horse, deer, man

Life cycle: The life cycle of *Cryptosporidium* is basically similar to those of other intestinal coccidia although sporulation takes place within the host. The oocysts, each with four sporozoites, are liberated in the faeces. Following ingestion, the sporozoites invade the microvillous brush border of the enterocytes and the trophozoites rapidly differentiate to form meronts with four to eight merozoites. Gametogony follows after one to two generations of meronts and oocysts are produced in 72 hours. Evidence also indicates that two types of oocysts are produced. The first, the majority, are thick-walled and are passed in the faeces. The remainder are thin-walled and release their sporozoites in the intestine, causing auto-infection.

Geographical distribution: Worldwide

Pathogenesis: Cryptosporidiosis is common in young calves, although the pathogenesis of infection is not clear. It is remarkable in that, unlike other members of the Eimeriidae, *Cryptosporidium* does not enter the cells of the host and lacks host specificity so that cross-infection can occur between domestic animals and man.

Clinical signs: Clinically the disease is characterised by anorexia and diarrhoea, often intermittent, which may result in poor growth rates.

Diagnosis: Oocysts may be demonstrated using Ziehl–Nielsen stained faecal smears in which the sporozoites appear as bright red granules (Fig. 2.14). Speciation of *Cryptosporidium* is difficult, if not impossible, using conventional techniques. A range of molecular and immunological techniques has been developed, that include the use of immunofluorescence (IF) (Fig. 2.15) or enzyme-linked immunosorbent assays (ELISA). More recently, DNA-based techniques have been used for the molecular characterisations of *Cryptosporidium* species.

Pathology: The meronts and gamonts develop in a parasitophorous envelope, apparently derived from the microvilli and so the cell disruption seen with other coccidia does not apparently occur. However, mucosal changes are obvious in the ileum where there is

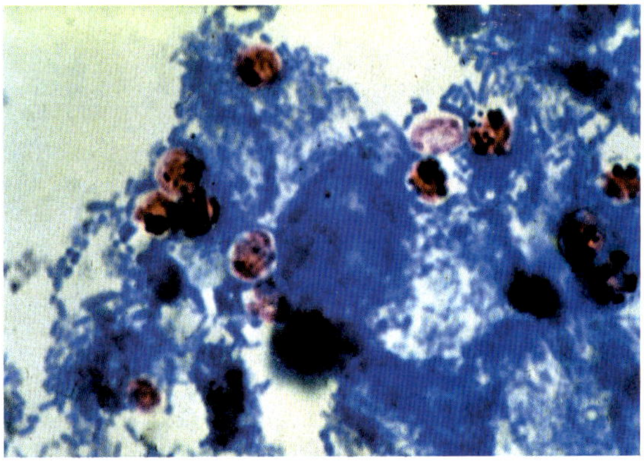

Fig. 2.14 Oocysts of *Cryptosporidium parvum* (Ziehl–Nielsen stain).

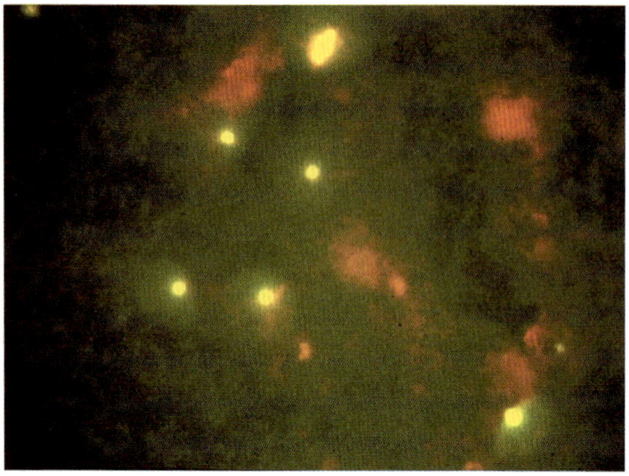

Fig. 2.15 Oocysts of *Cryptosporidium parvum* (immunofluorescent antibody test).

stunting, swelling and eventually fusion of the villi. This has a marked effect on the activity of some of the membrane-bound enzymes.

Epidemiology: A variety of mammals act as hosts to *C. parvum* but little is known of the importance of their involvement in transmitting infection to, or maintaining infection in domestic livestock. In young calves infection appears to be age related with seasonal peaks of disease reported to coincide with birth peaks in spring and autumn. The first calves to be born often become infected without showing clinical signs but become sources of infection for calves that follow. Infection spreads rapidly, and later-born calves can become so heavily infected that clinical disease results. In many instances where *Cryptosporidium* is diagnosed in animals, it appears that infections usually originate from the same host species. The primary route of infection is mainly by the direct animal-to-animal faecal–oral route. Thus in calves for example, overcrowding, stress of early weaning, transport and marketing, together with low levels of hygiene, will increase the risk of clinical infections. In lambs, chilling due to adverse weather conditions in the neonatal period, intercurrent infections or nutritional or mineral deficiencies could exacerbate or increase the likelihood of disease. Infection in these cases is likely to occur through grooming, nuzzling, coprophagy, or by faecal soiling by direct contact with infected animals. Infection may also occur indirectly through consumption of contaminated foods or environmental sources, including pasture and water.

Treatment: There is no known treatment, although spiramycin may be of some value, and the infection is difficult to control since the oocysts are highly resistant to most disinfectants except formol-saline and ammonia. Halofuginone is available for the prevention of cryptosporidiosis in calves at a dose rate of 1 mg/10 kg. Symptomatic treatment may be given in the form of anti-diarrhoeals and fluid replacement therapy.

Control: Good hygiene and management are important in preventing disease from cryptosporidiosis. Feed and water containers should be high enough to prevent faecal contamination. Young animals should be given colostrum within the first 24 hours of birth and overstocking and overcrowding should be avoided. Dairy calves should be either isolated in individual pens or kept in similar age groups and cleaned out daily. On calf-rearing farms with recurrent problems, the prophylactic use of halofuginone can be considered by treating for 7 consecutive days commencing at 24–48 hours after birth.

Notes: Recent molecular characterisations have shown that there is extensive host adaptation in *Cryptosporidium* evolution, and many mammals or groups of mammals have host-adapted *Cryptosporidium* genotypes, which differ from each other in both DNA sequences and infectivity. These genotypes are now delineated as distinct species and include, in cattle, *C. parvum, C. bovis* (also termed the bovine genotype or genotype 2) and *C. hominis* (previously termed the human genotype).

Giardia intestinalis

Synonym: *Giardia duodenalis*, *Giardia lamblia*, *Lamblia lamblia*

Predilection site: Small intestine

Parasite class: Zoomastigophorasida

Family: Diplomonadidae

Description: The trophozoite has a pyriform to ellipsoidal, bilaterally symmetrical body; 12–15 μm long by 5–9 μm wide (Fig. 2.16). The dorsal side is convex and there is a large sucking disk on the ventral side. There are two anterior nuclei, two slender axostyles, eight flagellae in four pairs and a pair of darkly staining median bodies. The median bodies are curved bars resembling the claws of a hammer. Cysts are ovoid, 8–12 × 7–10 μm and contain four nuclei (Fig. 2.17).

Hosts: Man, cattle, sheep, goat, pig, horse, alpaca, dog, cat, guinea pig, chinchilla

Life cycle: The life cycle is simple and direct, the trophozoite stage dividing by binary fission to produce further trophozoites. Intermittently, trophozoites encyst forming resistant cyst stages that pass out in the faeces of the host in the faeces.

Geographical distribution: Worldwide

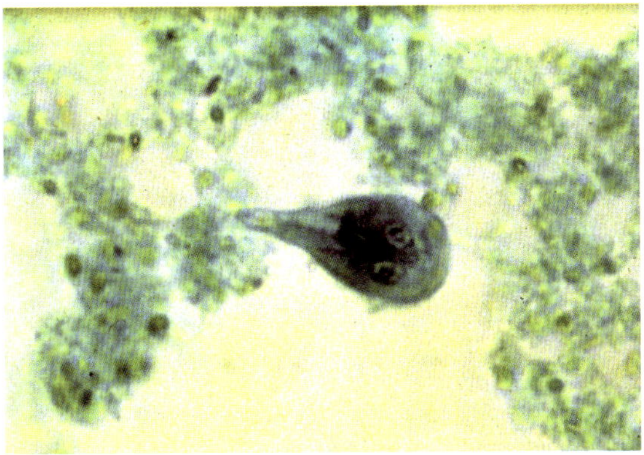

Fig. 2.16 *Giardia intestinalis* trophozoite.

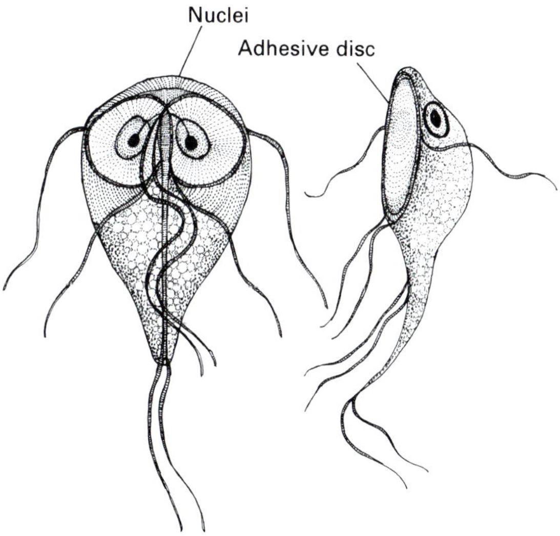

Fig. 2.17 *Giardia intestinalis.*

Pathogenesis: Infections in cattle are often asymptomatic but have been reported to cause diarrhoea in young calves.

Clinical signs: When disease does occur, the signs often include chronic, pasty diarrhoea, weight loss, lethargy and failure to thrive. The diarrhoea may be continuous or intermittent.

Diagnosis: *Giardia* cysts can be detected in faeces by a number of methods. Traditional methods of identification involve direct examination of faecal smears, or faecal concentration by formalin-ethyl acetate or zinc sulphate methods and subsequent microscopic examination. It is generally recommended that three consecutive samples be examined as cysts are excreted intermittently.

Pathology: There may be villous atrophy, crypt hypertrophy and an increased number of intraepithelial lymphocytes. Trophozoites may be seen between villi, attached by their concave surface to the brush border of epithelial cells.

Epidemiology: Molecular studies have revealed a substantial level of genetic diversity in *G. intestinalis* isolates. Human isolates fall into two major groups (assemblage A and B) with a wide host range in other mammals and it may prove to be the case that separate species names may be applicable. Other assemblages may also represent distinct species. Limited epidemiological studies suggest that in animal isolates, direct animal-to-animal contact and faecal soiling is the most likely method of transmission, although water contamination can also be considered as a possible route. The incidence of these parasites varies but can be assumed to be higher in some species than has been reported. Studies in Canada and USA indicate levels of infection in cattle of up to 20% in clinically normal animals and 100% infection rates in young diarrhoeic calves.

Treatment: There is no recommended treatment for infection in calves. Several benzimidazole anthelmintics (e.g. albendazole, fenbendazole) are effective and may prove to be of benefit.

Control: As infection is transmitted by the faecal–oral route, good hygiene and prevention of faecal contamination of feed and water is essential.

Notes: The parasite is important because of waterborne outbreaks that have occurred in human populations. There is still controversy over the classification of *Giardia* spp. The current molecular classification places isolates into eight distinct assemblages. Some authors give separate specific names to organisms isolated from different hosts, e.g. *Giardia bovis*, although species specificity of many isolates is unknown. Phylogenetic data suggest that *G. intestinalis* is a species complex composed of several species that are host specific.

LARGE INTESTINE

Oesophagostomum radiatum

Common name: Nodular worm

Predilection site: Large intestine

Parasite class: Nematoda

Superfamily: Strongyloidea

Description, gross: Adults are slender whitish worms, 1–2 cm in size, with males 12–17 mm, and females 16–22 mm long.

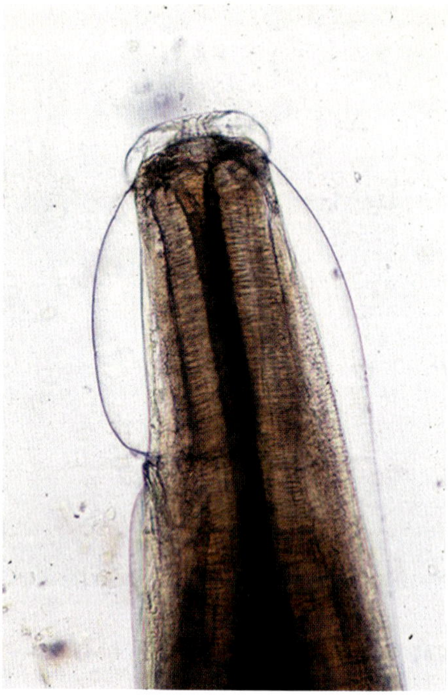

Fig. 2.18 Anterior of *Oesophagostomum radiatum* showing the large cephalic vesicle.

Description, microscopic: The cuticle forms a rounded mouth collar, and large cephalic vesicle, constricted around the middle by a shallow annular groove (Fig. 2.18). External leaf crowns are missing and the internal ring consists of 38–40 small triangular denticles. Cervical papillae are present just posterior to the cervical groove. The male bursa is well developed. The egg is a medium-sized (86 × 49 μm), regular broad elipse with barrel-shaped walls, and contains 16–32 blastomeres when passed in the faeces. The L_3 have long filamentous tails, 32 gut cells and a rounded head.

Hosts: Cattle, buffalo

Life cycle: The preparasitic phase is typically strongyloid and infection is by ingestion of L_3, which enter the mucosa of any part of the small or large intestine forming nodules in which the moult to L_4 takes place. These L_4 then emerge on to the mucosal surface, migrate to the colon, and develop to the adult stage. On reinfection, the larvae may remain arrested as L_4 in nodules for up to 1 year. The prepatent period is about 40 days.

Geographical distribution: Worldwide

Pathogenesis: In *O. radiatum* infections in cattle, the pathogenic effect is attributed to the nodules (up to 5.0 mm in diameter) in the intestine and it is one of the most damaging worms to cattle when present in high numbers, with >200 adult worms in calves and >1000 adults in adult cattle sufficient to produce clinical signs. In the later stages of the disease, anaemia and hypoalbuminaemia develop due to the combined effects of protein loss and leakage of blood through the damaged mucosa.

Clinical signs: In acute infections, there is anaemia, oedema and diarrhoea.

Diagnosis: This is based on clinical signs and postmortem examination. The presence of pea-shaped nodules in the intestinal wall on postmortem is indicative of nodular worm infection. In the chronic disease, eggs are present and L_3 can be identified following faecal culture.

Pathology: On postmortem examination, animals may be pale from anaemia, and oedematous from hypoproteinaemia. Colonic lymph nodes are enlarged and the mucosa of the colon is grossly thickened and folded by oedema and increased mixed inflammatory cell infiltrates in the lamina propria. Colonic submucosal lymphoid follicles are large and active. Effusion of tissue fluid and blood cells may be evident through small leaks between cells, or from erosions in glands or on the surface. Although repeated exposure to infective larvae may result in the accumulation of large numbers of fourth-stage worms in nodules, formation of nodules has little pathogenic significance in cattle.

Epidemiology: It is not yet known if hypobiosis occurs in *O. radiatum*. It is also capable of overwintering on pasture as L_3. In tropical and subtropical areas *O. radiatum* in cattle is especially important. Cattle develop a good immunity, partly due to age and partly to previous exposure so that it is primarily a problem in weaned calves.

Treatment: Anthelmintic therapy with broad-spectrum anthelmintics (benzimidazoles, levamisole and avermectins/milbemycins) is highly effective.

Control: Whilst not generally considered highly pathogenic, a combination of strategic dosing with anthelmintics and pasture management, as used in the control of other nematodes, will also help to control *O. radiatum*.

Trichuris globulosa

Synonym: *Trichocephalus globulosa*

Common name: Whipworms

Predilection site: Large intestine

Parasite class: Nematoda

Superfamily: Trichuroidea

Description, gross: The adults are long white worms (about 4.0–7.0 cm) with a thick broad posterior end, tapering rapidly to a long filamentous anterior end that is characteristically embedded in the mucosa.

Description, microscopic: The male tail is coiled and possesses a single spicule in a protrusible sheath. The sheath is covered with minute spines and bears a spherical appendage; the female tail is merely curved. The characteristic eggs are lemon shaped, 70 × 35 μm, with a thick smooth shell and a conspicuous polar plug (operculum) at both ends; in the faeces these eggs appear yellow or brown in colour.

Hosts: Cattle, occasionally sheep, goats, camels and other ruminants

Life cycle: The infective stage is the L_1 within the egg, which develops within 1 or 2 months of being passed in the faeces depending on the temperature. Under optimal conditions, these larvated eggs may subsequently survive and remain viable for several years. After ingestion, the plugs are digested and the released L_1 penetrate the glands of the distal ileum, caecal and colonic mucosa. Subsequently, all four moults occur within these glands, the adults emerging to lie on the mucosal surface with their anterior ends embedded in the mucosa. The prepatent period is about 7–10 weeks.

Geographical distribution: Worldwide

Pathogenesis: Most infections are light and asymptomatic. Occasionally, when large numbers of worms are present, they cause a diphtheritic inflammation of the caecal mucosa.

Clinical signs: Despite the fact that ruminants have a high incidence of light infections, the clinical significance of this genus, especially in ruminants, is generally negligible, although isolated outbreaks have been recorded.

Diagnosis: Since the clinical signs are not pathognomonic, diagnosis may depend on finding numbers of lemon-shaped *Trichuris* eggs in the faeces. Egg output is often low in *Trichuris* infections.

Pathology: In severe cases, the mucosa of the large intestine is inflamed, haemorrhagic with ulceration and formation of diptheritic membranes.

Epidemiology: The most important feature is the longevity of the eggs, which may still survive after 3 or 4 years. On pasture this is less likely since the eggs tend to be washed into the soil.

Treatment: In ruminants the benzimidazoles, the avermectins/milbemycins or levamisole by injection are very effective against adult *Trichuris*, but less so against larval stages.

Control: Prophylaxis is rarely necessary in ruminants.

Notes: The adults are usually found in the caecum but are only occasionally present in sufficient numbers to be clinically significant.

Trichuris discolor

Common name: Whipworms

Predilection site: Large intestine

Parasite class: Nematoda

Superfamily: Trichuroidea

Description, gross: Worms are similar to *T. globulosa* but the females are yellow–orange in colour.

Description, microscopic: Eggs measure about 65 × 30 μm.

Hosts: Cattle, buffalo, ox, occasionally sheep, goat

Geographical distribution: Europe, Asia, USA

Details of the life cycle, pathogenesis clinical signs, diagnosis, pathology, epidemiology, treatment and control are as for *T. globulosa.*

Homalogaster paloniae

Predilection site: Large intestine

Parasite class: Trematoda

Family: Paramphistomatidae

Description, gross: The body is divided into two with a large anterior region and small cylindrical posterior region.

Hosts: Buffalo and cattle

Intermediate hosts: Water snails

Life cycle: Presumed similar to other paramphistomes of the rumen.

Geographical distribution: Asia, Australasia

Pathogenesis: Generally considered to be non-pathogenic.

Treatment and control: Not required

Eimeria bovis

Predilection site: Small and large intestine

Parasite class: Sporozoasida

Family: Eimeriidae

Description: Oocysts are ovoid or subspherical, colourless, 23–34 × 17–23 μm (mean 27.7 × 20.3 μm) and have a smooth wall with an inconspicuous micropyle, no polar granule or oocyst residuum (see Fig. 2.13). Sporocysts are elongate ovoid, 13–18 × 5–8 μm and have an inconspicuous Stieda body and a sporocyst residuum. The sporozoites are elongate, and lie lengthwise head to tail in the sporocysts and usually have a clear globule at each end.

Life cycle: There are two asexual generations. The first-generation meronts are in the endothelial cells of the lacteals of the villi in the posterior half of the small intestine, mature at 14–18 days after infection and can be seen grossly as whitish specks in the mucosa. Second-generation meronts occur in the epithelial cells of the caecum and colon, but may extend into the last metre of the small intestine in heavy infections. The sexual stages generally occur in the caecum and colon, but may extend into the ileum in heavy infections; they appear 17 days after infection. The prepatent period is 16–21 days and the patent period usually 5–15 days. The sporulation time is 2–3 days.

Geographical distribution: Worldwide

Pathogenesis: Particularly pathogenic, attacking the caecum and colon, causing mucosal sloughing and haemorrhage.

Pathology: The most severe pathological changes occur in the caecum, colon and terminal foot of the ileum, and are due to the gamonts. The mucosa appears congested, oedematous and thickened with petechiae or diffuse haemorrhages. The gut lumen may contain a large amount of blood. Later in the infection the mucosa is destroyed and sloughs away. The submucosa may also be lost. If the animal survives, both the mucosa and submucosa regenerate.

Clinical signs: Severe enteritis and diarrhoea, or dysentery with tenesmus in heavy infections. The animal may be pyrexic, weak and dehydrated, and if left untreated, loses condition and may die.

Epidemiology: Disease is dependent on conditions, which precipitate a massive intake of oocysts, such as overcrowding in unhygienic yards or feedlots. It may also occur at pasture where livestock congregate around water troughs.

Eimeria zuernii

Predilection site: Small and large intestine

Parasite class: Sporozoasida

Family: Eimeriidae

Description: Oocysts are subspherical, colourless, 15–22 × 13–18 μm (mean 17.8 × 15.6 μm) with no micropyle or oocyst residuum. Sporocysts are ovoid, 7–14 × 4–8 μm, each with a tiny Stieda body, and a sporocyst residuum is usually absent. The sporozoites are elongate and lie head to tail in the sporocysts; each has a clear globule at the large end.

Life cycle: First-generation meronts are giant meronts and are found in the lamina propria of the lower ileum and mature at 14–16 days after infection, visible as whitish specks in the mucosa; second-generation meronts occur in the epithelial cells of the caecum and proximal colon from about 16 days after infection. The sexual stages generally occur within epithelial cells of the caecum and colon, but may extend into the ileum in heavy infections, appearing 16 days after infection. The prepatent period is 15–17 days and the patent period usually 5–17 days. The sporulation time is 2–10 days.

Geographical distribution: Worldwide

Pathogenesis: This is the most pathogenic species causing haemorrhagic diarrhoea through erosion and destruction of large areas of the intestinal mucosa. *E. zuernii* is the most common cause of 'winter coccidiosis' which occurs primarily in calves during or following cold or stormy weather in the winter months. The exact aetiology of this syndrome is uncertain.

Pathology: Generalised catarrhal enteritis involving both the large and small intestines is present. The lower small intestine, caecum and colon may be filled with semi-fluid haemorrhagic material. Large or small areas of the intestinal mucosa may be eroded and destroyed. The mucous membrane may be thickened with irregular whitish ridges in the large intestine, or smooth, dull grey areas in the small intestine or caecum. Diffuse haemorrhages are present in the intestines in acute cases, and petechial haemorrhages are seen in milder cases.

Clinical signs: In acute infections, *E. zuernii* causes haemorrhagic diarrhoea of calves. At first, the faeces are streaked with blood, but as the diarrhoea becomes more severe, bloody fluid, clots of blood and liquid faeces are passed. Tenesmus and coughing can result in the diarrhoea being spurted out up to 2–3 m. The animal's hindquarters are smeared with red diarrhoea. Secondary infections, especially pneumonia, are common. The acute phase may continue for 3–4 days. If the calf does not die in 7–10 days, it will probably recover.

E. zuernii may also cause a more chronic form of disease. Diarrhoea is present, but there is little or no blood in the faeces. The animals are emaciated, dehydrated, weak and listless. Their coats are rough, their eyes sunken and their ears droop.

Treatment: Treatment of both the above pathogenic species of coccidia is with a sulphonamide, such as sulphadimidine or sulphamethoxypyridazine, given orally or parenterally and repeated at half the initial dose level on each of the next 2 days. Alternatively, decoquinate or a combination of amprolium and ethopabate may be used.

Control: Prevention is based on good management; in particular feed troughs and water containers should be moved regularly and bedding kept dry.

Flagellate protozoa

The life cycle of the following flagellate protozoa is similar for all species found in cattle. The trophozoites reproduce by longitudinal binary fission, no sexual stages are known and there are no cysts. Transmission is thought to occur by ingestion of trophozoites from faeces. All are considered to be non-pathogenic and are generally only identified from smears taken from the large intestine of fresh carcases.

Tetratrichomonas buttreyi

Synonym: *Trichomonas buttreyi*

Predilection site: Caecum, colon

Parasite class: Zoomastigophorasida

Family: Trichomonadidae

Description: The body is ovoid or ellipsoidal, 4–7 × 2–5 μm (mean 6 × 3 μm). Cytoplasmic inclusions are frequently present. There are three or four anterior flagella, which vary in length from a short stub to more than twice the length of the body; and each ends in a knob or spatulate structure. The undulating membrane runs the full length of the body and has three to five undulations ending in a posterior free flagellum. The accessory filament is prominent, and the costa relatively delicate. The axostyle is relatively narrow, has a spatulate capitulum and extends 3–6 μm beyond the body. There is no chromatic ring at its point of exit. A pelta is present. The nucleus is frequently ovoid (2–3 × 1–2 μm) but is variable in shape and has a small endosome.

Hosts: Cattle, pig

Geographical distribution: Worldwide

Tritrichomonas enteris

Predilection site: Colon

Parasite class: Zoomastigophorasida

Family: Trichomonadidae

Description: The body is 6–12 × 5–6 μm and there are three anterior flagella of equal length, which arise from a single blepharoplast. The flagellum at the edge of the undulating membrane is single and lacks an accessory filament. The undulating membrane extends three quarters of the body length and a free flagellum extends beyond the undulating membrane. The axostyle is straight and slender, bending around the nucleus to give a spoon shape and extending at most a quarter of the body length beyond the body.

Geographical distribution: Worldwide

Tetratrichomonas pavlovi

Synonym: *Trichomonas bovis*, *Trichomonas pavlovi*

Predilection site: Caecum

Parasite class: Zoomastigophorasida

Family: Trichomonadidae

Description: The body is pyriform and is usually 11–12 × 6–7 μm. It has four anterior flagella, which are about the same length as the body. The undulating membrane is well developed and has two to four waves that extend almost to the posterior end of the body. There is a posterior free flagellum, an accessory filament and a costa. The nucleus is round or ovoid. The axostyle is slender, broadening to form a capitulum at the anterior end.

Geographical distribution: Unknown

Retortamonas ovis

Predilection site: Large intestine

Parasite class: Zoomastigophorasida

Family: Retortamonadorididae

Description: Trophozoites are pyriform and average 5.2 × 3.4 μm. There is a large cytosome near the anterior end containing a cytostomal fibril that extends across the anterior end and posteriorly along each side. An anterior flagellum and a posterior trailing flagellum emerge from the cytostomal groove. Cysts are pyriform and ovoid, containing one or two nuclei and retain the cytostomal fibril.

Geographical distribution: Worldwide

Buxtonella sulcata

Predilection site: Large intestine

Parasite class: Ciliophora

Family: Pycnotrichidae

Description: The body is ovoid, 100 × 72 μm, and uniformly ciliated with a prominent curved groove bordered by two ridges running from end to end with a cyathostome at the anterior end, and an oval or bean-shaped macronucleus, 28 × 14 μm in size.

Life cycle: The life cycle has not been described.

Geographical distribution: Worldwide

PARASITES OF THE RESPIRATORY SYSTEM

Mammomonogamus laryngeus

Synonym: *Syngamus laryngeus*

Common name: Gapeworm

Predilection site: Larynx

Parasite class: Nematoda

Superfamily: Strongyloidea

Description, gross: The worms are reddish in appearance and about 1–2 cm long. The females and males are found in permanent copulation. The buccal capsule lacks a cuticular crown.

Description, microscopic: Eggs are ellipsoid, 80–90 μm with no operculum at either end.

Hosts: Cattle, buffalo, goat, sheep, deer, rarely man

Life cycle: The life cycle is direct but the mode of transmission is unknown.

Geographical distribution: Asia, central Africa, South America and Caribbean islands

Pathogenesis: *M. laryngeus* in not very pathogenic for cattle. Worms are attached to the mucosa of the larynx and may cause laryngitis and bronchitis.

Clinical signs: Infections are usually asymptomatic but affected animals cough and lose condition. Calves may develop bronchitis and aspiration pneumonia has been recorded.

Diagnosis: This is based on clinical signs and the finding of eggs in the faeces. Disease is probably best confirmed by postmortem examination of selected cases when reddish worms will be found attached to the tracheal mucosa. The infected trachea often contains an increased amount of mucus.

Pathology: Not described

Epidemiology: Unknown

Treatment: Successful treatment has not been reported. Benzimidazoles and macrocyclic lactones are likely to be effective.

Control: No preventive or control measures have been described.

Notes: This genus, closely related to *Syngamus*, is parasitic in the respiratory passages of mammals. Infection has been reported in man causing a laryngopharyngeal syndrome.

Mammomonogamus nasicola

Synonym: *Syngamus nasicola*

Predilection site: Nasal cavities

Parasite class: Nematoda

Superfamily: Strongyloidea

Description, gross: The worms are reddish in appearance and about 1–2 cm long. Males are 4–6 mm and females 11–23 mm long and found in permanent copulation. The buccal capsule lacks a cuticular crown.

Description, microscopic: Eggs are ellipsoid, 54–98 μm with no operculum at either end.

Hosts: Sheep, goat, cattle, deer

Life cycle: The life cycle is direct but the mode of transmission is unknown.

Geographical distribution: Central and South America, central Africa, Caribbean islands

For more details on this species see under Chapter 3 (Sheep and goats).

Dictyocaulus viviparus

Common name: Bovine lungworm, husk, hoose, verminous pneumonia, parasitic bronchitis

Predilection site: Bronchi, trachea

Parasite class: Nematoda

Superfamily: Trichostrongyloidea

Description, gross: The adults are slender thread-like worms; males measure around 4.0–5.5 cm and females 6–8 cm in length.

Description, microscopic: First stage larvae are 300–360 μm with the intestinal cells containing numerous chromatin granules. There is no anterior knob (cf. *D. filaria* in sheep and goats).

Hosts: Cattle, buffalo, deer and camel

Life cycle: The female worms are ovo-viviparous, producing eggs containing fully developed larvae, which hatch almost immediately. The L_1 migrate up the trachea, are swallowed and pass out in the faeces. The larvae are unique in that they are present in fresh faeces, are characteristically sluggish, and their intestinal cells are filled with dark brown food granules (Fig. 2.19). In consequence the preparasitic stages do not require

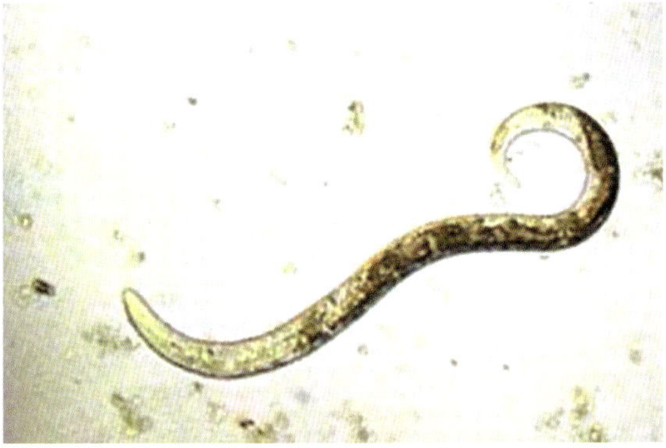

Fig. 2.19 First stage larvae of *Dictyocaulus viviparus*.

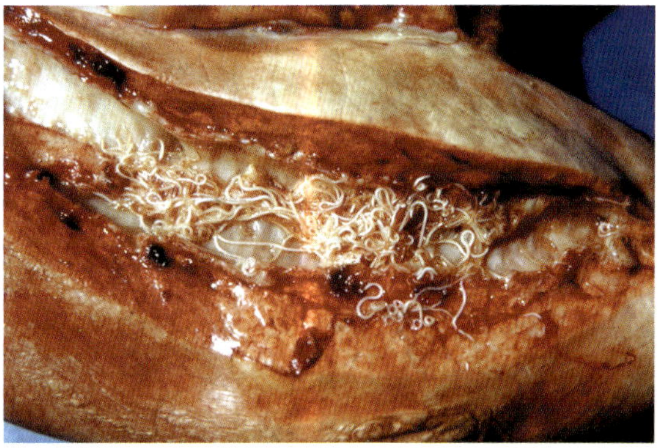

Fig. 2.20 *D. viviparus* worms in the opened bronchi of an infected calf.

to feed. Under optimal conditions the L_3 stage is reached within 5 days, but usually takes longer in the field. The L_3 leave the faecal pat to reach the herbage either by their own motility or through the agency of the ubiquitous fungus, *Pilobolus*. After ingestion, the L_3 penetrate the intestinal mucosa and pass to the mesenteric lymph nodes where they moult. The L_4 then travel via the lymph and blood to the lungs, and break out of the capillaries into the alveoli about 1 week after infection. The final moult occurs in the bronchioles a few days later and the young adults then move up the bronchi and mature. The prepatent period is around 3–4 weeks.

Geographical distribution: Worldwide, but especially important in temperate climates with a high rainfall.

Pathogenesis: Dictyocaulosis is characterised by bronchitis and pneumonia and typically affects young cattle during their first grazing season on permanent or semi-permanent pastures. Pathogensis may be divided into three phases:

(1) Pre-patent phase: around days 8–25. This phase starts with the appearance of larvae within the alveoli where they cause alveolitis. This is followed by bronchiolitis and finally bronchitis as the larvae become immature adults and move up the bronchi. Towards the end of this phase bronchitis develops, characterised by immature lungworms in the airways and by cellular infiltration of the epithelium. Heavily infected animals, whose lungs contain several thousand developing worms, may die from day 15 onwards due to respiratory failure following the development of severe interstitial emphysema and pulmonary oedema.

(2) Patent phase: around days 26–60. This is associated with two main lesions. First, a parasitic bronchitis characterised by the presence of hundreds or even thousands of adult worms in the frothy white mucus in the lumina of the bronchi (Fig. 2.20). Secondly, the presence of dark red collapsed areas around infected bronchi (Fig. 2.21). This is a parasitic pneumonia caused by the aspiration of eggs and L_1 into the alveoli.

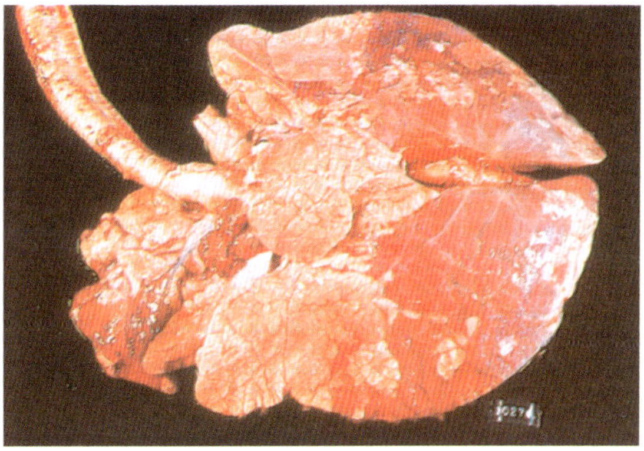

Fig. 2.21 Typical distribution of pneumonic lesions of parasitic bronchitis.

(3) Post-patent phase: around days 61–90. In untreated calves, this is normally the recovery phase after the adult lungworms have been expelled. Although the clinical signs are abating, the bronchi are still inflamed and residual lesions such as bronchial and peribronchial fibrosis may persist for several weeks or months. Eventually the bronchopulmonary system becomes completely normal and coughing ceases. However, in about 25% of animals, which have been heavily infected, there can be a flare-up of clinical signs during this phase, which is frequently fatal. This is caused by one of two entities. Most commonly, there is a proliferative lesion so that

much of the lung is pink and rubbery and does not collapse when the chest is opened. This, often described as 'epithelialisation', is due to the proliferation of type 2 pneumocytes on the alveoli giving the appearance of a gland-like organ. Gaseous exchange at the alveolar surface is markedly impaired and the lesion is often accompanied by interstitial emphysema and pulmonary oedema. The aetiology is unknown, but is thought to be due to the dissolution and aspiration of dead or dying worm material into the alveoli. The clinical syndrome is often termed postpatent parasitic bronchitis. The other cause, usually in animals convalescing indoors, is a superimposed bacterial infection of the imperfectly healed lungs leading to acute interstitial pneumonia.

Clinical signs: Within any affected group, differing degrees of clinical severity are usually apparent. Mildly affected animals cough intermittently, particularly when exercised. Moderately affected animals have frequent bouts of coughing at rest, tachypnoea (60 respirations per minute) and hyperpnoea. Frequently, squeaks and crackles over the posterior lung lobes are heard on auscultation. Severely affected animals show severe tachypnoea (80 respirations per minute) and dyspnoea and frequently adopt the classic 'air-hunger' position of mouth breathing with the head and neck outstretched. There is usually a deep harsh cough, squeaks and crackles over the posterior lung lobes, salivation, anorexia and, sometimes, mild pyrexia. Often the smallest calves are most severely affected.

Calves may show clinical signs during the prepatent period and occasionally a massive infection can cause severe dyspnoea of sudden onset often followed by death in 24–48 hours.

Most animals gradually recover, although complete return to normality may take weeks or months. However, a proportion of convalescing calves suddenly develop severe respiratory signs, unassociated with pyrexia, which usually terminates fatally 1–4 days later (postpatent parasitic bronchitis).

Diagnosis: Usually the clinical signs, the time of the year and a history of grazing on permanent or semi-permanent pastures are sufficient to enable a diagnosis to be made.

Larvae are found (50–1000/g) only in the faeces of patent cases so that faecal samples should be obtained from the rectum of a number of affected individuals. At necropsy, worms will often be apparent in the opened bronchi and their size is diagnostic. A lungworm ELISA can be used to detect antibodies to *D. viviparus*. Seroconversion takes 4–6 weeks and titres persist for 4–7 months. Serology can be helpful in cases of reinfection husk, as it will often detect larval stages. Cross-reactivity occurs with intestinal nematode species so test sensitivity and specificity requires validation and setting of appropriate optical density (OD) cut-off values when interpreting results.

Pathology:

(1) Pre-patent phase. Cellular infiltrates of inflammatory cells temporarily plug the lumina of the bronchioles and cause collapse of other groups of alveoli. This lesion is largely responsible for the first clinical signs of tachypnoea and coughing.
(2) Patent phase. The bronchial epithelium is hyperplastic and heavily infiltrated by inflammatory cells, particularly eosinophils. Aspirated eggs and larvae quickly provoke dense infiltrates of polymorphs, macrophages and multinucleated giant cells around them. There may be varying degrees of interstitial emphysema and oedema.

Epidemiology: Generally only calves in their first grazing season are clinically affected, since on farms where the disease is endemic older animals have a strong acquired immunity. In endemic areas in the northern hemisphere infection may persist from year to year in two ways:

- Overwintered larvae: L_3 may survive on pasture from autumn until late spring in sufficient numbers to initiate infection or occasionally to cause disease.
- Carrier animals: small numbers of adult worms can persist in the bronchi, particularly in yearlings, until the next grazing season. Chilling of infective larvae before administration to calves will produce arrested L_5; hypobiosis at this stage has also been observed in naturally infected calves in Switzerland, Austria and Canada, although the extent to which this occurs naturally after ingestion of larvae in late autumn and its significance in the transmission of the infection has not yet been fully established.

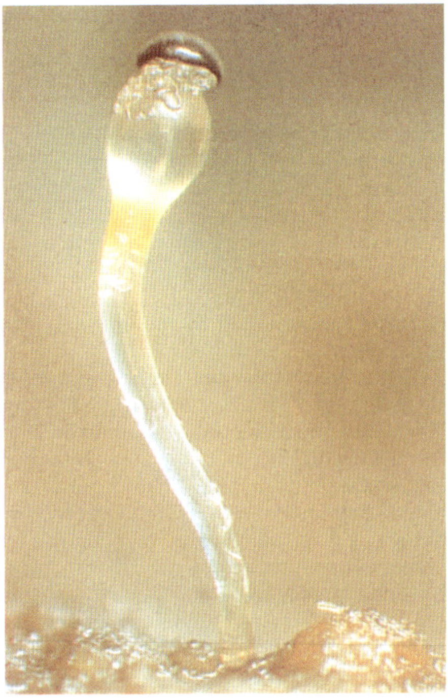

Fig. 2.22 Larvae of *Dictyocaulus viviparus* on the fungus *Pilobolus*.

The dispersal of larvae from the faecal pat appears to be effected by a fungus rather than by simple migration as the infective larvae are relatively inactive. This fungus, *Pilobolus*, is commonly found growing on the surface of bovine faecal pats about 1 week after deposition. The larvae of *D. viviparus* migrate in large numbers up the stalks of the fungi on to, and even inside, the sporangium or seed capsule (Fig. 2.22). When the sporangium is discharged it is projected a distance of up to 3 m in still air to land on the surrounding herbage.

Parasitic bronchitis is predominantly a problem in areas such as northern Europe that have a mild climate, a high rainfall and abundant permanent grass. Outbreaks of disease occur from June until November, but are most common from July until September. It is not clear why the disease is usually not apparent until calves, turned out to graze in the spring, have been at grass for 2–5 months. One explanation is that the initial infection, acquired from the ingestion of overwintered larvae in May, involves so few worms that neither clinical signs nor immunity is produced; however, sufficient numbers of larvae are seeded on to the pasture so that by July the numbers of L_3 are sufficient to produce clinical disease. Young calves, added to such a grazing herd in July, may develop clinical disease within 2–3 weeks.

An alternative explanation is that L_3 overwinter in the soil and possibly only migrate on to pasture at some point between June and October.

Although dairy or dairy-cross calves are most commonly affected, autumn-born single-suckled beef calves are just as susceptible when turned out to grass in early summer. Spring-born suckled beef calves grazed with their dams until housed or sold do not usually develop clinical signs, although coughing due to a mild infection is common. However, the typical disease may occur in weaned calves grazed until late autumn.

In tropical countries, where disease due to *D. viviparus* may occur intermittently, the epidemiology is presumably quite different and probably depends more on pasture contamination by carrier animals such as may occur during flooding when cattle congregate on damp, high areas, rather than on the prolonged survival of infective larvae.

Treatment: The modern benzimidazoles, levamisole, or the avermectin/milbemycins have been shown to be highly effective against all stages of lungworms with a consequent amelioration of clinical signs. For maximum efficiency, all of these drugs should be used as early as possible in the treatment of the disease. Where the disease is severe and well established in a number of calves one should be aware that anthelmintic treatment, while being the only course available, may exacerbate the clinical signs in one or more animals with a possible fatal termination. Whatever treatment is selected, it is advisable to divide affected calves into two groups, as the prognosis will vary according to the severity of the disease. Those calves which are only coughing and/or tachypnoeic are usually in the prepatent stage of the disease or have a small adult worm burden and treatment of these animals should result in rapid recovery. Calves in this category may not have developed a strong immunity and after treatment should not be returned to grazing which was the source of infection; if this is not possible, parenteral ivermectin, doramectin or moxidectin may be used since their residual effect prevents reinfection for an extended period.

Any calves which are dyspnoeic, anorexic and possibly pyrexic should be kept indoors for treatment and further observation. The prognosis must be guarded as a proportion of these animals may not recover while others may remain permanently stunted. In addition to anthelmintics, severely affected animals may require antibiotics if pyrexic and may be in need of hydration if they are not drinking.

Control: The best method of preventing parasitic bronchitis is to immunise all young calves with lungworm vaccine. This live attenuated vaccine is currently only available in parts of Europe and is given orally to calves aged 8 weeks or more. Two doses of vaccine are given at an interval of 4 weeks and, in order to allow a high level of immunity to develop, vaccinated calves should be protected from challenge until 2 weeks after their second dose. Dairy calves or suckled calves can be vaccinated successfully at grass provided the vaccine is given prior to encountering a significant larval challenge.

Although vaccination is effective in preventing clinical disease, it does not completely prevent the establishment of small numbers of lungworms. Consequently, pastures may remain contaminated, albeit at a very low level. For this reason it is important that all of the calves on any farm should be vaccinated whether they go to pasture in the spring or later in the year and a vaccination programme must be continued annually for each calf crop.

Control of parasitic bronchitis in first year grazing calves has been achieved by the use of prophylactic anthelmintic regimens either by strategic early season treatments or by the administration of rumen boluses, as recommended in the control of bovine ostertagiosis. The danger of these measures, however, is that through rigorous control in the first grazing season, exposure to lungworm larvae is so curtailed that cattle remain susceptible to husk during their second season; in such situations it may be advisable to consider vaccination prior to their second year at grass.

Because of the unpredictable epidemiology, the technique commonly used in ostertagiosis of 'dose and move' in midsummer does not prevent parasitic bronchitis.

Parasitic bronchitis in adult cattle

Parasitic bronchitis is only seen in adult cattle under two circumstances:

1. As a herd phenomenon, or in a particular age group within a herd, if they have failed to acquire immunity through natural challenge in earlier years. Such animals may develop the disease if exposed to heavy larval challenge, as might occur on pasture recently vacated by calves suffering from clinical husk.
2. Disease is occasionally seen where an individual adult is penned in a heavily contaminated calf paddock.

The disease is most commonly encountered in the patent phase although the other forms have been recognised. In addition to coughing and tachypnoea, a reduction in milk yield in cows is a common presenting sign.

In selecting an anthelmintic for treatment, one should consider the withdrawal period of milk for human consumption. Eprinomectin has no withdrawal period for milk.

The reinfection syndrome in parasitic bronchitis

Normally the natural challenge of adult cattle, yearlings or calves, which have acquired immunity to *D. viviparus*, whether by natural exposure, or by vaccination, is not associated with clinical signs. Occasionally, however, clinical signs do occur to produce the 'reinfection syndrome', which is usually mild, but sometimes severe. It arises when an immune animal is suddenly exposed to a massive larval challenge that reaches the lungs, and migrates to the bronchioles where the larvae are killed by the immune response. The proliferation of lymphoreticular cells around dead larvae causes bronchiolar obstruction and ultimately the formation of a macroscopically visible greyish green, lymphoid nodule about 5.0 mm in diameter. Usually the syndrome is associated with frequent coughing and slight tachypnoea over a period of a few days; less frequently there is marked tachypnoea, hyperpnoea and, in dairy cows, a reduction in milk yield. Deaths rarely occur. It can be difficult to differentiate this syndrome from the early stages of a severe primary infection. The only course of action is treatment with anthelmintics and a change of pasture.

Echinococcus granulosus

For more details see Parasites of the liver.

Pneumocystis carinii

Synonym: *Pneumocystis jiroveci*

Common name: Pneumocystosis

Predilection site: Lung

Parasite class: Archiascomycetes

Family: Pneumocystidaceae

Description: Two major forms of *P. carinii* have been consistently identified from histological and ultrastructural analysis of organisms found in human and rat lung. These are a trophic form and a larger cyst stage containing eight intracystic stages.

Hosts: Man, cattle, rat, ferret, mouse, dog, horse, pig, and rabbit

Life cycle: The life cycle of *Pneumocystis* still remains poorly understood. Information is mostly derived from histochemical and ultrastructural analysis of the lung tissue of rodents and infected humans. The presumed life cycle of *Pneumocystis* includes an asexual and a sexual growth phase. Current knowledge suggests that the trophic (trophozoite) forms are produced during asexual development. These forms are usually pleomorphic and found in clusters. They appear capable of replicating asexually by binary fission and also replicate sexually by conjugation, producing a diploid zygote, which undergoes meiosis and subsequent mitosis, resulting in the formation of a precyst initially, and then an early cyst and a mature cyst eventually. During differentiation of the organism from precyst to mature cyst, eight intracystic spores or 'daughter cells' are produced. These intracystic spores are subsequently released as the mature cyst ruptures and develop into trophic forms.

Geographical distribution: Worldwide

Pathogenesis: *Pneumocystis* is one of the major causes of opportunistic mycoses in the immunocompromised, including those with congenital immunodeficiencies, retrovirus infections such as AIDS, and cases receiving immunosuppressive therapy.

Clinical signs: Infections in animals are generally asymptomatic. In humans, pneumocystosis is observed in four clinical forms; asymptomatic infections, infantile (interstitial plasma cell) pneumonia, pneumonia in immunocompromised host and extrapulmonary infections.

Diagnosis: Gomori's methenamine silver (GMS) and Giemsa stain may be used for microscopic visualisation of *Pneumocystis*. Toluidine blue (TBO) is the most effective for cyst stages while Giemsa stains are used to show trophozoites. Axenic culture methods have been described; however, in vitro cultivation, especially from clinical samples, is not always successful. Fluorescence antibody staining techniques can be used to detect both cyst and trophozoite stages of *P. carinii*. A number of polymerase chain reactions (PCRs) have been reported which amplify specific regions of DNA from *P. carinii* and are approximately 100 times more sensitive than conventional staining techniques.

Pathology: Lesions are characterised by a massive plasma cell or histiocyte infiltration of the alveoli in which the organisms may be detected by a silver staining procedure. A foamy eosinophilic material is observed in the lungs during infection. This material is composed of masses of the organism, alveolar macrophages, desquamated epithelial alveolar cells, polymorphonuclear leucocytes and other host cells.

Epidemiology: The organism is apparently quite widely distributed in latent form in healthy individuals and in the dog, as well as a wide variety of other domestic and wild animals. The organism is thought to be transmitted by aerosol, although the natural habitats and modes of transmission of infections in humans are current areas of research. *Pneumocystis* DNA has been detected in air and water, suggesting that the free forms of the organism may survive in the environment long enough to infect a susceptible host. However, little information on the means of transmission exists currently. In humans, infections appear to spread between immunosuppressive patients colonised with *Pneumocystis*, and immunocompetent individuals transiently parasitised with the organism. Human and non-human *Pneumocystis* species have been shown to be different and host-specific, suggesting that zoonotic transmission does not occur.

The organism has been reported from a range of animals. In Denmark, examination of lungs from carcases selected randomly in an abattoir detected *P. carinii* pneumocysts in 3.8% of calves, 3.6% of sheep and 6.7% of pigs. Studies in Japan detected *P. carinii* in cattle and a wide range of other animals. The organism has also been reported to have caused pneumonia in weaning pigs.

Treatment: Trimethroprim–sulphamethoxazole is the drug of choice for treatment and prophylaxis of *Pneumocystis* infections. Pentamidine and atovaquone are the alternative therapeutic agents in humans.

Control: Control is difficult given that the details of the routes of transmission are unknown. Infection is generally asymptomatic in animals and is only likely to be detected in immunocompromised individuals.

Notes: Initially reported as a morphological form of *Trypanosoma cruzi*, this microorganism later proved to be a separate genus and was named *Pneumocystis carinii* and classified as a protozoan until the late 1980s. Following further taxonomic revision, *Pneumocystis* is now classified as a fungus, not a protozoan. The taxonomy is still complicated in that *Pneumocystis* from humans and other animals are quite different and there appear to be multiple species in this genus. Genetic variations and DNA sequence polymorphisms are often observed, suggesting the existence of numerous strains even within a single species of *Pneumocystis*.

PARASITES OF THE LIVER

Fasciola hepatica

Common name: Liver fluke

Predilection site: Liver

Parasite class: Trematoda

Family: Fasciolidae

Description, gross: The young fluke at the time of entry into the liver is 1.0–2.0 mm in length and lancet-like. When it has become fully mature in the bile ducts it is leaf-shaped, grey–brown in colour and is around 2.5–3.5 cm in length and 1.0 cm in width. The anterior end is conical and marked off by distinct shoulders from the body (Fig. 2.23a).

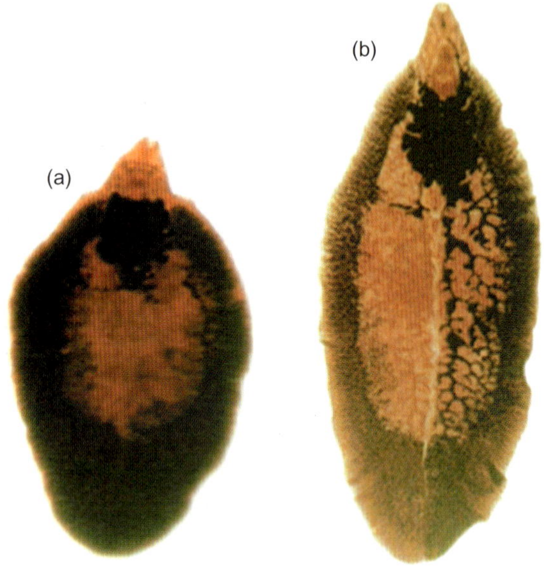

Fig. 2.23 Outline of (a) *Fasciola hepatica* and (b) *F. gigantica*. The former has broader shoulders and is shorter in length.

Description, microscopic: The tegument is covered with backwardly projecting spines. An oral and ventral sucker may be readily seen. The egg is thin-shelled, oval, operculate, browny-yellow and large (130–150 × 65–90 μm), and about twice the size of a trichostrongyle egg.

Final hosts: Sheep, cattle, goat, horse, deer, man and other mammals

Intermediate hosts: Snails of the genus *Lymnaea*. The most common, *Lymnaea (*syn *Galba) truncatula*, is an amphibious snail with a wide distribution throughout the world. Other important *Lymnaea* vectors of *F. hepatica* outside Europe are:

L. tomentosa	Australia, New Zealand
L. columella	Central and North America, Australia, New Zealand
L. bulimoides	North and Southern USA and the Caribbean
L. humilis	North America
L. viator	South America
L. diaphena	South America
L. cubensis	South America
L. viridis	China, Papua New Guinea

Life cycle: Adult flukes in the bile ducts shed eggs into the bile, which enter the intestine. Eggs passed in the faeces of the mammalian host develop and hatch, releasing motile ciliated miracidia. This takes 9–10 days at optimal temperatures of 22–26°C and little development occurs below 10°C. The liberated miracidium has a short life-span and must locate a suitable snail within about 3 hours if successful penetration of the latter is to occur. In infected snails, development proceeds through the sporocyst and redial stages to the final stage in the intermediate host, the cercaria; these are shed from the snail as motile forms, which attach themselves to firm surfaces, such as grass blades, and encyst there to form the infective metacercariae. It takes a minimum of 6–7 weeks for completion of development from miracidium to metacercaria, although under unfavourable circumstances a period of several months is required. Infection of a snail with one miracidium can produce over 600 metacercariae. Metacercariae ingested by the final host excyst in the small intestine, migrate through the gut wall, cross the peritoneum and penetrate the liver capsule. The young flukes tunnel through the liver parenchyma for 6–8 weeks, then enter the small bile ducts where they migrate to the larger ducts and occasionally the gallbladder and reach sexual maturity. The prepatent period is 10–12 weeks. The minimal period for completion of one entire life cycle of *F. hepatica* is therefore 17–18 weeks. The longevity of *F. hepatica* in untreated sheep may be years; in cattle it is usually less than 1 year.

Geographical distribution: Worldwide

Pathogenesis: This varies according to the number of metacercariae ingested, the phase of parasitic development in the liver and the species of host involved. Essentially the pathogenesis is two-fold. The first phase occurs during migration in the liver parenchyma and is associated with liver damage and haemorrhage. The second occurs when the parasite is in the bile ducts, and results from the haematophagic activity of the adult flukes and from damage to the biliary mucosa by their cuticular spines. Most studies have been in sheep and the disease in this host is discussed in more detail in Chapter 3. The seasonality of outbreaks is that which occurs in western Europe.

Although acute and subacute disease may occasionally occur under conditions of heavy challenge, especially in young calves, the chronic form of the disease is by far the most important, and as in sheep, is seen in the late winter/early spring.

The pathogenesis is similar to that in sheep but has the added features of calcification of the bile ducts and enlargement of the gallbladder. The calcified bile ducts often protrude from the liver surface, giving rise to the term 'pipe-stem liver'. Aberrant migration of the flukes is more common in cattle and encapsulated parasites are often seen in the lungs. On reinfection of adult cows, migration to the fetus has been recorded, resulting in prenatal infection. There is some experimental evidence that fasciolosis increases the susceptibility of cattle to infection with *Salmonella dublin*.

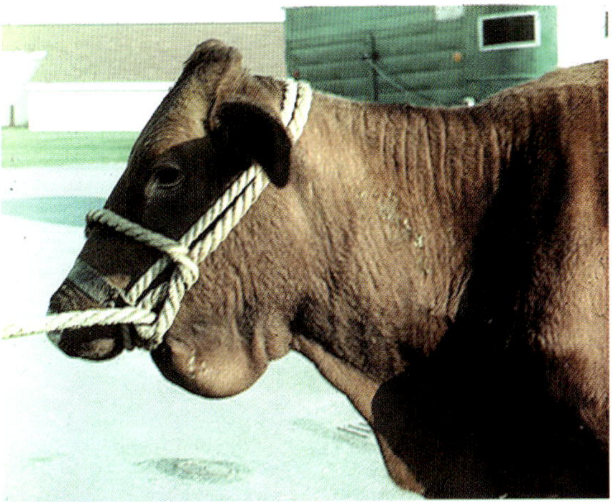

Fig. 2.24 Submandibular oedema in a cow infected with *Fasciola hepatica*.

In heavy infections, where anaemia and hypoalbuminaemia are severe, submandibular oedema frequently occurs (Fig. 2.24). With smaller fluke burdens, the clinical effect is minimal and the loss of productivity is difficult to differentiate from inadequate nutrition. It must be emphasised that diarrhoea is not a feature of bovine fasciolosis unless it is complicated by the presence of *Ostertagia* spp. Combined infection with these two parasites has been referred to as the fasciolosis/ostertagiosis complex.

Fasciola infections may cause a loss of production in milking cows during winter. Clinically, these are difficult to detect since the fluke burdens are usually low and anaemia is not apparent. The main effects are a reduction in milk yield and quality, particularly of the solids-non-fat component.

Clinical signs: In heavy infections in cattle, where anaemia and hypoalbuminaemia are severe, submandibular oedema frequently occurs. With smaller fluke burdens, the clinical effect is minimal and the loss of productivity is difficult to differentiate from inadequate nutrition. It must be emphasised that diarrhoea is not a feature of bovine fasciolosis unless it is complicated by the presence of *Ostertagia* spp. Combined infection with these two parasites has been referred to as the fasciolosis/ostertagiosis complex.

Diagnosis: This is based primarily on clinical signs, seasonal occurrence, prevailing weather patterns, and a previous history of fasciolosis on the farm or the identification of snail habitats. While diagnosis of ovine fasciolosis should present few problems, especially when a postmortem examination is possible, diagnosis of bovine fasciolosis can sometimes prove difficult. In this context, routine haematological tests and examination of faeces for fluke eggs (note: eggs of *Fasciola* are browny yellow and eggs of Paramphistomidae are colourless) are useful and may be supplemented by two other laboratory tests.

The first is the estimation of plasma levels of enzymes released by damaged liver cells. Two enzymes are usually measured. Glutamate dehydrogenase (GLDH) is released when parenchymal cells are damaged and levels become elevated within the first few weeks of infection. The other, gamma glutamyl transpeptidase (GGT) indicates damage to the epithelial cells lining the bile ducts; elevation of this enzyme takes place mainly after the flukes reach the bile ducts and raised levels are maintained for a longer period. The second test is the detection of antibodies against components of flukes in serum or milk samples, the ELISA and the passive haemagglutination test being the most reliable.

Pathology: In cattle, the pathogenesis is similar to that seen in sheep with the added features of calcification of the bile ducts and enlargement of the gallbladder. The calcified bile ducts often protrude from the liver surface, giving rise to the term 'pipe-stem liver' (Fig. 2.25). Aberrant migration of the flukes is more common in cattle and encapsulated parasites are often seen in the lungs.

Epidemiology: For a more detailed description, see entry under sheep.

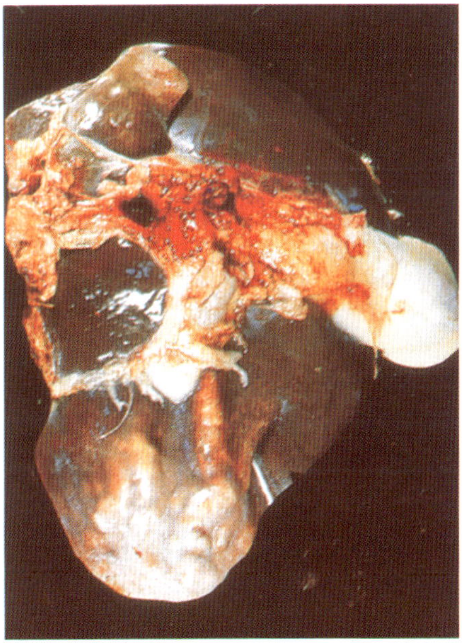

Fig. 2.25 Gross appearance of the liver in bovine fasciolosis.

Treatment: The older drugs such as carbon tetrachloride, hexachlorethane and hexachlorophene may still be used in some countries, but these have been largely replaced by more efficient and less toxic compounds and only the latter will be discussed.

At present there is only one drug, triclabendazole, which will remove the early immature (around 2 weeks of age in cattle) parenchymal stages. Apart from triclabendazole, the two drugs most commonly used for subacute or chronic fasciolosis are nitroxynil and oxyclozanide, and several others, such as clorsulon and niclofolan, are also marketed in some countries. Albendazole, ricobendazole and netobimin are also effective against adult fluke at an increased dosage rate. In lactating cows, where the milk is used for human consumption, the above drugs are either banned or have extended withdrawal periods. An exception is oxyclozanide, which is licensed for use in lactating animals in many countries and has a milk-withholding time of up to 3 days. Resistance to flukicides is not a problem in cattle.

Control: Control of fasciolosis may be approached in two ways: by reducing populations of the intermediate snail host or by using anthelmintics (for a more detailed description see entry under sheep). The timing of treatments will depend on the spectrum of activity of the flukicide. A typical treatment schedule in the northern hemisphere in an average rainfall season would be:

- Dose cattle in autumn with a flukicide, which is effective against young immature fluke to reduce liver damage from fluke migration. This is irrespective of whether cattle will be housed or outwintered.
- Dose grazing cattle in winter with a flukicide, which is effective against adult fluke and immature stages. In-wintered cattle need to be treated after housing (timing of the dose varies with the flukicide used).
- Dose out-wintered cattle in spring with a flukicide, which is effective against adult stages. This will remove fluke burdens and reduce contamination of pastures with fluke eggs and thus reduce the summer infection of snails.

Dairy cows can be treated at drying-off. It is important to monitor the need for treatment. The use of meteorological forecasting of fasciolosis is described in detail under sheep.

Fasciola gigantica

Common name: Tropical large liver fluke

Predilection site: Liver

Parasite class: Trematoda

Family: Fasciolidae

Description, gross: The adult fluke is larger than *F. hepatica*, the body is more transparent, and can reach 7.5 cm in length and 1.5 cm in breadth. The shape is more leaf-like, the conical anterior end is very short and the shoulders, characteristic of *F. hepatica*, are barely perceptible (Fig. 2.23b).

Description, microscopic: The eggs are larger than those of *F. hepatica*, measuring 170–190 × 90–100 μm.

Final hosts: Cattle, buffalo, sheep, goat, pig, camel, deer, man

Intermediate hosts: Snails of the genus *Lymnaea* (syn. *Galba*); in southern Europe it is *L. auricularia*, which is also the important species in the southern USA, the Middle East and the Pacific Islands. Other important *Lymnaea* vectors of *F. gigantica* are:

L. natalensis	Africa
L. rufescens	Indian subcontinent
L. acuminata	Indian subcontinent
L. rubiginosa	Southeast Asia
L. viridis	China and Japan

All these snails are primarily aquatic snails and are found in streams, irrigation channels and marshy swamps.

Life cycle: This is similar to *F. hepatica*, the main differences being in the timescale of the cycle. The immature stages migrate through the liver parenchyma, the adults reaching the bile ducts about 12 weeks after infection. Most parasitic phases are longer and the prepatent period is 13–16 weeks.

Geographical distribution: Africa, Asia, Europe, USA

Clinical signs: Clinical signs are similar to those of *F. hepatica*.

Diagnosis: This is based primarily on clinical signs, seasonal occurrence, prevailing weather patterns and a previous history of fasciolosis on the farm or the identification of snail habitats. Diagnosis can be confirmed by the identification of the typical operculate eggs in faeces samples.

Pathogenesis: Acute and chronic infection occurs in sheep but only the chronic form predominates in cattle. Like *F. hepatica*, *F. gigantica* is capable of infecting man.

Pathology: The pathology is similar to that described for *F. hepatica*. In cattle, the pathology is similar to that seen in sheep with the added features of calcification of the bile ducts and enlargement of the gallbladder. The calcified bile ducts often protrude from the liver surface giving rise to the term 'pipe-stem liver'.

Epidemiology: The snails, which carry the larval stages of *F. gigantica*, are primarily aquatic and as a result the disease is associated with animals grazing on naturally or artificially flooded areas or around permanent water channels or dams. In subtropical or tropical countries with distinct wet and dry seasons, it appears that optimal development of eggs to miracidia occurs at the start of the wet season and development within the snail is complete by the end of the rains. Shedding of cercariae then commences at the start of the dry season when the water level is still high and continues as the water level drops. Under laboratory conditions, a large number of metacercariae simply encyst on the surface of the water rather than on herbage, and under natural conditions this could have a very significant effect on the dissemination of infection. Metacercariae are acquired by animals utilising such areas during the dry season and clinical problems, depending on the rate of infection, occur at the end of that season or at the beginning of the next wet season. Metacercariae encyst on plants under water, such as rice plants, and can survive for up to 4 months on stored plants, such as rice straw.

Treatment: The drugs and dose rates given for the treatment of *F. hepatica* are also generally applicable for the treatment of *F. gigantica*. Only triclabendazole and clorsulon are effective against both mature and immature stages of *F. gigantica* in cattle.

Control: The principles are the same as for the control of *F. hepatica* and are based on the routine use of anthelmintics together with measures to reduce populations of the snail intermediate host. There is, however, the important difference that the latter are water snails whose control depends on a different approach from that for the mud snail, *L. truncatula*.

Routine anthelmintic treatment of animals at seasons when heavy infections of adult flukes accumulate in the host is recommended using a drug effective against adult and immature flukes. This should prevent serious losses in production, but for optimal benefit should be accompanied by snail control.

When watering of stock is from a reservoir or stream, complete control can be achieved by fencing the water source and leading a pipe to troughs. To do this effectively from streams, the water may require to be pumped and in remote areas simple water-driven pumps whose power source depends on the water flow have been found useful. It is important that the water troughs be cleaned out regularly since they can become colonised by snails.

When grazing depends on the dry season use of marshy areas around receding lakebeds, snail control is difficult. Molluscicides are usually impractical because of the large body of water involved and their possible effect on fish, which may form an important part of the local food supply. Apart from repeated anthelmintic treatment to prevent patency of acquired infections of *F. gigantica*, there is often little one can do. Ideally, such areas are often best suited to irrigation and the growing of cash crops, the profit from which can be used to improve the dry season food and water supply to cattle.

Fascioloides magna

Common name: Large American liver fluke

Predilection site: Liver and bile ducts

Parasite class: Trematoda

Family: Fasciolidae

Description, gross: Flukes are large and thick and measure up to 10 × 2.5 cm. The flukes are oval, with a rounded posterior end. They possess no anterior cone and when fresh are flesh-coloured.

Description, microscopic: Eggs are large, operculate, measure 109–168 × 75–96 μm and have a protoplasmic appendage at the pole opposite the operculum.

Final hosts: Deer, cattle, sheep, goat, pig, horse

Intermediate hosts: A variety of freshwater snails, *Fossaria* spp, *Lymnaea* spp, *Stagnicola* spp

Geographical distribution: Mainly occurs in North America, central, eastern and southwestern Europe, South Africa and Mexico.

Pathogenesis: In deer and cattle, the flukes are frequently encapsulated in thin-walled fibrous cysts in the liver parenchyma and this restricted migration results in low pathogenicity. In cattle and in pigs the flukes may become entrapped in a thick-walled fibrous capsule and there is no connection to the bile ducts and consequently it is rare to find fluke eggs in faeces in these livestock. Sometimes flukes can also be found in calcified cysts. Although haemorrhage and fibrosis may be present in the liver there is often no obvious clinical sign of infection.

Clinical signs: In deer and cattle the parasites can cause hepatic damage on reaching the liver but the flukes rapidly become encapsulated by the host reaction and clinical signs are minimal.

Diagnosis: This is based primarily on clinical signs, and history of contact with grazing deer in known endemic areas. Cysts and the large flukes are usually seen on postmortem examination. Faecal examination for the presence of fluke eggs is a useful aid to diagnosis.

Pathology: In cattle and pigs, thick-walled cysts with fibrous capsules or calcified cysts may be present in the liver.

Epidemiology: The various snail intermediate hosts tend to occur in stagnant semi-permanent water that contains large amounts of dead or dying vegetation, swamp areas, or pools and streams. *F. magna* is indigenous to North America and is common in Canada and the Great Lake areas where the white-tailed deer and the elk are commonly infected. Domestic cattle and sheep become infected when they graze pasture where parasitised deer occur.

Treatment: For cattle and sheep the commonly used flukicides, such as triclabendazole, closantel, clorsulon and albendazole, are effective. Mature *F. magna* are susceptible to oxyclosanide.

Control: Avoid grazing sheep or cattle on areas which are frequented by deer. Elimination of the snail intermediate hosts is difficult due to their varied habitats. Similarly, removal of Cervidae may not be practical. Because of these factors sheep rearing, particularly, is difficult in areas where the parasite is prevalent.

Notes: *F. magna* is primarily a parasite of deer (Cervidae) and is commonly found in white-tailed deer, elk and moose. For more details see Chapter 8: Ungulates (Deer).

Dicrocoelium dendriticum

Synonym: *Dicrocoelium lanceolatum*

Common name: Small lanceolate fluke

Predilection site: Liver

Parasite class: Trematoda

Family: Dicrocoeliidae

For more details see Chapter 3 (Sheep and goats).

Dicrocoelium hospes

Predilection site: Liver

Parasite class: Trematoda

Family: Dicrocoeliidae

Hosts: Cattle

Geographical distribution: Parts of Africa

Details are essentially similar to *D. dendriticum*.

Echinococcus granulosus

Subspecies: *granulosus*

Common Name: Dwarf dog tapeworm, hydatidosis

Predilection site: Mainly liver and lungs (intermediate hosts); small intestine (definitive hosts)

Parasite class: Cestoda

Family: Taeniidae

Description, gross: Hydatid cysts are large fluid-filled vesicles, 5–10 cm in diameter, with a thick concentrically laminated cuticle and an internal germinal layer.

Description, microscopic: The germinal layer produces numerous small vesicles or brood capsules each containing up to 40 scolices, invaginated into their neck portions and attached to the wall by stalks. Brood capsules may become detached from the wall of the vesicle and float freely in the vesicular fluid and form 'hydatid sand'.

Final hosts: Dog and many wild canids

Intermediate hosts: Domestic and wild ruminants, man and primates, pig and lagomorphs; horses and donkeys are resistant.

For more details see Chapter 3 (Sheep and goats).

Stilesia hepatica

Predilection site: Bile ducts

Parasite class: Cestoda

Family: Thysanosomidae

Definitive hosts: Sheep and other ruminants

Intermediate hosts: The intermediate host is probably an oribatid mite.

Geographical distribution: Africa and Asia

For more details see Chapter 3 (Sheep and goats).

Taenia hydatigena

Synonym: *Taenia marginata, Cysticercus tenuicollis*

Predilection site: Abdominal cavity, liver (intermediate hosts); small intestine (definitive hosts)

Parasite class: Cestoda

Family: Taeniidae

Definitive hosts: Dog, fox, weasel, stoat, polecat, wolf, hyena

Intermediate hosts: Sheep, cattle, deer, pig, horse

Geographical distribution: Worldwide.

Notes: The correct nomenclature for the intermediate host stage is the 'metacestode stage of *Taenia hydatigena*' rather than '*Cysticercus tenuicollis*'. For more details see Chapter 3 (Sheep and goats).

Thysanosoma actinioides

For more details see Parasites of the small intestine.

PARASITES OF THE PANCREAS

Eurytrema coelomaticum

Common name: Pancreatic fluke

Predilection site: Pancreatic ducts, rarely the bile ducts

Parasite class: Trematoda

Family: Dicrocoeliidae

Description, gross: A leaf-shaped reddish brown fluke. Adults measure around 8–12 mm × 6–7 mm.

Description, microscopic: The body is thick and the juvenile flukes are armed with spines. The oral sucker is large, the pharynx and oesophagus short. Eggs measure around 40–50 × 25–35 µm and are similar to those of *Dicrocoelium*.

Final hosts: Cattle, buffalo, sheep, goats, pigs, camels and man

Intermediate hosts: Two are required:

1. Land snails, particularly of the genus *Bradybaena*
2. Grasshoppers of the genus *Conocephalus* or tree crickets (*Oecanthus*)

Life cycle: Eggs passed in faeces are ingested by a snail where two generations of sporocysts occur. Cercariae are released onto the herbage about 5 months after initial infection and these are ingested by grasshoppers. Infective metacercariae are produced in about 3 weeks. The final host becomes infected by accidentally eating the second intermediate host. Metacercariae encyst in the duodenum and migrate to the pancreas via the pancreatic duct and reside in the small ducts of the pancreas. The prepatent period in cattle is 3–4 months.

Geographical distribution: South America, Asia and Europe

Pathogenesis: Low to moderate infections produce little effect on the host. Heavy infections may cause a sporadic wasting syndrome and emaciation.

Clinical signs: No specific signs but a general weight loss may occur in heavy infections.

Diagnosis: Usually reported as an incidental finding at necropsy.

Pathology: Large numbers of flukes can cause dilation and thickening of the pancreatic ducts and extensive fibrosis. Flukes may also be embedded in the pancreatic parenchyma causing chronic interstitial pancreatitis and there is sometimes a granulomatous reaction around fluke eggs that have penetrated the walls of the ducts.

Epidemiology: Infection is influenced by the availability of the invertebrate intermediate hosts. Prevalence rates of *E. coelomaticum* can be as high as 70% in slaughtered cattle in endemic areas.

Treatment: There is no specific treatment for eurytrematosis.

Control: This is not feasible where the intermediate hosts are endemic.

Eurytrema pancreaticum

Common name: Pancreatic fluke

Predilection site: Pancreatic ducts and occasionally the bile ducts and the duodenum.

Parasite class: Trematoda

Family: Dicrocoeliidae

Description: Similar to *E. coelomaticum*. Adults measure around 8–16 × 5–8 mm.

Geographical distribution: Eastern Asia and South America

Details of the life cycle, host range, pathogenesis, clinical, signs, diagnosis, pathology, epidemiology, treatment and control are as for *E. coelomaticum*.

Thysanosoma actinioides

For more details see Parasites of the small intestine.

PARASITES OF THE CIRCULATORY SYSTEM

Schistosoma bovis

Common name: Blood fluke, bilharziosis

Predilection site: Portal and mesenteric veins, urogenital veins

Parasite class: Trematoda

Family: Schistosomatidae

Description, gross: The sexes are separate; the males are 9–22 mm long and 1–2 mm wide, and the female 12–28 mm long. The suckers and the body of the male behind the suckers are armed with minute spines, while the dorsal surface of the male bears small cuticular tubercles. The slender female worm lies permanently in a ventral groove in the broad flat body of the male.

Description, microscopic: The eggs are usually spindle-shaped, but smaller ones may be oval and measure 187 × 60 μm. There is no operculum.

Final hosts: Cattle, sheep, goat, camel

Intermediate hosts: Snails (*Bulinus contortus, B. truncates, Physopsis africana, P. nasuta*)

Life cycle: The ovigerous female penetrates deeply into the small vessels of the mucosa or submucosa of the intestine and inserts her tail into a small venule and since the genital pore is terminal, the eggs are deposited, or even pushed, into the venule. There, aided by their spines and by proteolytic enzymes secreted by the unhatched miracidia, they penetrate the endothelium to enter the intestinal submucosa and ultimately the gut lumen; they are then passed out in the faeces. Worms present in the vesical veins penetrate the endothelial lining of the bladder where eggs may be passed in the urine. Some eggs are carried away in the bloodstream and locate in other organs such as the liver. The eggs hatch in water and the miracidia penetrate appropriate snails. Cercariae develop from daughter sporocysts, which replace the redia stage and there is no metacercarial phase; penetration of the final host by the motile cercariae occurs via the skin or by ingestion in drinking water. After penetration or ingestion the cercariae lose their forked tails, transform to schistosomula, or young flukes, and travel via the bloodstream through the heart and lungs to the systemic circulation. In the liver they locate in the portal veins and become sexually mature before migrating to their final site, the mesenteric veins. The prepatent period is 6–7 weeks.

Geographical distribution: Africa, Middle East, southern Asia, southern Europe

Pathogenesis: The young flukes cause some damage during migration but most serious damage is caused by the irritation produced by the parasite eggs in the intestine and the blood-sucking habit of the worms. Acute disease is characterised by diarrhoea and anorexia due to response to the deposition of eggs in the mesenteric veins and their subsequent infiltration in the intestinal mucosa. The presence of the worms in veins of the bladder in cattle may cause damage to the bladder wall and haematuria.

Clinical signs: These are diarrhoea, sometimes blood stained and containing mucus, anorexia, thirst, anaemia and emaciation. In cattle, the presence of the worms in the vesical veins may cause haematuria.

Diagnosis: This is based mainly on the clinicopathological picture of diarrhoea, wasting and anaemia, coupled with a history of access to natural water sources. The relatively persistent diarrhoea, often blood stained and containing mucus, may help to differentiate this syndrome from fasciolosis.

The demonstration of the characteristic eggs in the faeces or in squash preparations of blood and mucus from the faeces is useful in the period following patency but less useful as egg production drops in the later stages of infection.

In general, when schistosomosis is suspected, diagnosis is best confirmed by a detailed postmortem examination which will reveal the lesions and, if the mesentery is stretched, the presence of numerous schistosomes in the veins. In epidemological surveys, serological tests may be of value.

Pathology: At necropsy during the acute phase of the disease there are marked haemorrhagic lesions in the mucosa of the intestine, but as the disease progresses the wall of the intestine appears greyish, thickened and oedematous due to confluence of the egg granulomata and the associated inflammatory changes. The liver may be larger than normal, depending on the stage of the disease, and may be markedly cirrhotic in long-standing infections. On microscopic examination there is pigmentation of the liver and numerous eggs may be found, surrounded by cellular infiltration and fibrous tissue. The spleen may be slightly swollen and lymph glands are usually pigmented.

Epidemiology: The epidemiology is totally dependent upon water as a medium for infection of both the intermediate and final host. Small streams, irrigation canals, wet savannah and marshy or damp areas are the main snail habitats. Eggs, miracidia and cercariae are short-lived with seasonal transmission directly related to rainfall and temperature. The fact that percutaneous infection may occur encourages infection where livestock are obliged to wade in water. In cattle, high prevalence is usually associated with low numbers of worms, although worm burdens increase with age whilst egg excretion declines markedly in animals above 2 years of age due to the development of partial immunity.

Treatment: For economic reasons, chemotherapy is not suitable for the control of schistosomiosis in domestic stock except during severe clinical outbreaks. Care has to be exercised in treating clinical cases of schistosomosis since the dislodgement of the damaged flukes may result in emboli being formed and subsequent occlusion of major mesenteric and portal blood vessels with fatal consequences. Older drugs still used in some areas are the antimonial preparations, tartar emetic, antimosan and stibophen, and niridazole and trichlorphon, all of which have to be given over a period of days at high dosage rates. Fatalities associated with the use of these drugs are not uncommon. Praziquantel, which is the drug of choice for treatment of human schistosomosis, is also effective in ruminants at 15–20 mg/kg per os but may be cost prohibitive.

Control: This is similar to that outlined for *F. gigantica* and *Paramphistomum* infections. Since the prevalence of snail populations varies according to temperature, local efforts should be made to identify the months of maximum snail population, and cattle movements planned to avoid their exposure to dangerous stretches of water at these times.

When watering of stock is from a reservoir or stream, fencing the water source and leading a pipe to troughs can achieve control. To do this effectively from streams, the water may require to be pumped and in remote areas simple water-driven pumps whose power source depends on the water flow have been found useful. It is important that the water troughs be cleaned out regularly since they can become colonised by snails.

When grazing depends on the dry season use of marshy areas around receding lakebeds, snail control is difficult. Molluscicides are usually impractical because of the large body of water involved and their possible effect on fish, which may form an important part of the local food supply. Apart from repeated anthelmintic treatment to prevent patency of acquired infections of *Schistosoma*, there is often little one can do. Ideally, such areas are often best suited to irrigation and the growing of cash crops, the profit from which can be used to improve the dry season food and water supply to cattle.

Schistosoma japonicum

Common name: Blood fluke, bilharziosis

Predilection site: Portal and mesenteric veins

Parasite class: Trematoda

Family: Schistosomatidae

Description, gross: The sexes are separate; the male, which is broad and flat, is 9.5–20 mm long, carrying the female which is 12–26 mm long, in the hollow of its inwardly curved body (Fig. 2.26). The suckers lie close together near the anterior end. The cuticle is spiny on the suckers and in the gynaecophoric canal. This characteristic and the vascular predilection site are sufficient for generic identification.

Description, microscopic: The eggs are short, oval, 70–100 μm long, and may have a small sub-terminal spine. There is no operculum.

Final hosts: Cattle, horse, sheep, goat, dog, cat, rabbit, pig, man

Intermediate hosts: Snails belonging to the genus *Oncomelania*.

Life cycle: This is similar to *S. bovis*. Development to the cercarial stage occurs through two generations of sporocyst without a redial form and there is no metacercarial phase, penetration of the final host by the motile cercariae occurring via the skin. The developmental period in the snail can be as short as 5 weeks. Schistosomula, or young flukes, that reach the abdominal vessels and pass to the portal veins become sexually mature in about 4 weeks.

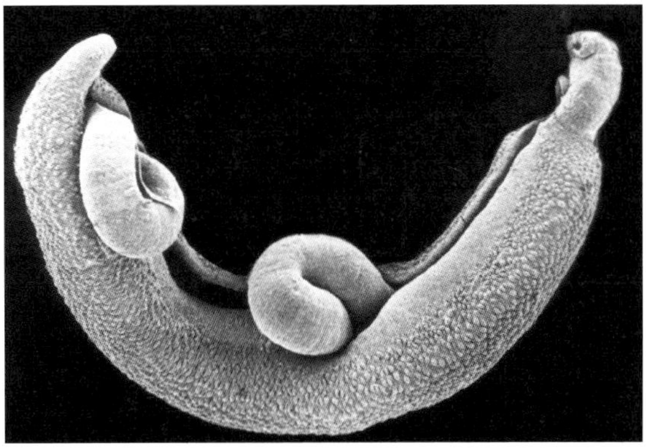

Fig. 2.26 Male and female *Schistosoma* in copula.

Geographical distribution: South and east Asia

Pathogenesis: The penetration of the cercariae through the skin causes dermatitis, which is evident about 24 hours after infection. Passage through the lungs may cause pneumonia in gross infections and abdominal organs such as the liver may become congested during the early stages of the disease due to the arrival of immature worms in the intra-hepatic portal blood vessels. The most serious damage is caused by the adult parasites in the egg-laying stage due to the irritation caused by the eggs lodged in the tissues, which are forced to find their way through small venules to the epithelium and lumen of the gut. The masses of eggs become surrounded by inflamed areas and an infiltration of leucocytes, particularly eosinophils, gives rise to a rather characteristic type of abcess. The abcesses in the intestinal wall usually burst, discharging their contents into the lumen of the gut and eventually heal forming scar tissue. In the liver the abcesses become encapsulated and eventually become calcified, a large number of such foci leading to liver enlargement, cirrhosis and ascites.

Acute disease, characterised by diarrhoea and anorexia, occurs 7–8 weeks after heavy infection and is entirely due to the inflammatory and granulomatous response to the deposition of eggs in the mesenteric veins and their subsequent infiltration in the intestinal mucosa. Following massive infection death can occur rapidly, but more usually the clinical signs abate slowly as the infection progresses. As this occurs, there appears to be a partial shift of worms away from the intestinal mucosa and reactions to these migrating parasites and their eggs can occur in the liver.

Schistosomosis is generally considered to be a much more serious and important infection in sheep than in larger ruminants, and even where a high prevalence of the parasite is detected in slaughtered cattle, clinical signs of the disease are seen only rarely. In sheep, anaemia and hypoalbuminaemia have been shown to be prominent during the clinical phase apparently as a result of mucosal haemorrhage, dyshaemopoeisis and an expansion in plasma volume. The significance of low-level infection is not known, but it has been suggested that this may have a considerable effect on productivity.

There is evidence, experimentally, of acquired resistance to reinfection by homologous species and, from natural infections, that resistance may develop as a result of prior exposure to a heterologous species.

Pathology: This is similar to *S. bovis*. Scar tissue and frequent papillomatous growths may be seen on the intestinal mucosa. On sections of the liver there is also evidence of egg granulomata and of portal fibrosis provoked by eggs, which have, inadvertently, been swept into small portal vessels. The mesentery, mesenteric lymph nodes and spleen are frequently altered due to the presence of abnormal amounts of connective tissue.

Details of the clinical signs, diagnosis, epidemiology, treatment and control are as for *S. bovis*.

Schistosoma nasalis

Synonym: *Schistosoma nasalae*

Common name: Snoring disease

Predilection site: Veins of nasal mucosa

Parasite class: Trematoda

Family: Schistosomatidae

Description, gross: The sexes are separate, the male, which is broad and flat and about 1 cm long, carrying the female in the hollow of its inwardly curved body.

Description, microscopic: The eggs are 336–581 μm long, boomerang shaped, with a terminal spine.

Final hosts: Cattle, goat, sheep, buffalo, horse

Intermediate hosts: Snails (*Lymnaea luteola*, *L. acuminata*, *Indoplanorbis exustus*)

Life cycle: Details of the life cycle are not completely known. The female in the veins of the nasal mucosa lays her eggs, which presumably enter the nasal sinuses and are sneezed out. The eggs hatch in minutes in water and the miracidia penetrate appropriate snails. Development to the cercarial stage occurs without a redial form and there is no metacercarial phase. After penetration or ingestion the cercariae transform to schistosomula, or young flukes, and travel to their final site, the nasal veins.

Geographical distribution: India, Pakistan, SE Asia

Pathogenesis: In heavy infections there is a copious mucopurulent discharge, snoring and dyspnoea. The main pathogenic effects are associated with the eggs, which cause abscess formation in the mucosa. Fibrous granulomatous growths occur which may occlude the nasal passages.

Clinical signs: Coryza, sneezing, dyspnoea and snoring

Diagnosis: Infection is confirmed by the presence of the spindle-shaped eggs in the nasal discharge.

Pathology: The mucosa of the nasal sinuses is studded with small abcesses that contain the eggs of the worms, and later show much fibrous tissue and proliferating epithelium.

Epidemiology: The epidemiology is totally dependent upon water as a medium for infection of both the intermediate and final host.

Treatment and control: As for *S. bovis*

Several other *Schistosoma* species have been reported in cattle. Details on the life cycle, pathogenesis, epidemiology, treatment and control are essentially similar to *S. bovis*.

Schistosoma mattheei

Predilection site: Portal, mesenteric and bladder veins

Parasite class: Trematoda

Family: Schistosomatidae

Description, gross: The sexes are separate; the males are 9–22 mm long and 1–2 mm wide, and the females 12–28 mm long. The suckers and the body of the male behind the suckers are armed with minute spines, while the dorsal surface of the male bears small cuticular tubercles.

Description, microscopic: The eggs are usually spindle-shaped, but smaller ones may be oval and measure 170–280 × 72–84 mm. There is no operculum.

Final hosts: Cattle, sheep, goat, camel, man

Intermediate hosts: Snails (*Bulinus*)

Geographical distribution: South and central Africa, Middle East

Notes: Thought to be synonymous with *S. bovis* but differs on morphological and pathological grounds and is restricted to the alimentary canal.

Schistosoma indicum

Predilection site: Portal, pancreatic, hepatic and mesenteric veins

Parasite class: Trematoda

Family: Schistosomatidae

Description, gross: The sexes are separate; the males are 5–19 mm long, and the females 6–22 mm long.

Description, microscopic: The eggs are oval with a terminal spine and measure 57–140 × 18–72 μm.

Final hosts: Cattle, sheep, goat, horse, donkey, camel

Intermediate hosts: Snails (*Indoplanorbis*)

Geographical distribution: India

Schistosoma spindale

Predilection site: Mesenteric veins

Parasite class: Trematoda

Family: Schistosomatidae

Description, gross: The sexes are separate, the male, which is broad and flat and about 2.0 cm long, carrying the female in the hollow of its inwardly curved body.

Description, microscopic: The eggs are 100–500 μm long, spindle shaped and have a lateral or terminal spine. There is no operculum.

Hosts: Cattle, horse, pig and occasionally dog

Geographical distribution: Parts of Asia and the Far East

Schistosoma turkestanica

Synonym: *Orientobilharzia turkstanicum*

Predilection site: Mesenteric veins and small veins of the pancreas and liver

Parasite class: Trematoda

Family: Schistosomatidae

Description, gross: Small species, the male is 4.2–8 mm and the female 3.4–8 mm.

Description, microscopic: The female uterus contains only one egg at a time, which measures 72–77 × 16–26 μm with a terminal spine and short appendage at the other end.

Hosts: Cattle, sheep, goat, camel, horse, donkey, buffalo

Geographical distribution: Asia

Pathogenesis: Of little significance in cattle but can cause marked debility in sheep and goats, causing liver cirrhosis and nodules in the intestines.

Elaeophora poeli

Common name: Large aortic filariosis

Predilection site: Blood vessels

Parasite class: Nematoda

Superfamily: Filarioidea

Description, gross: Slender worms, males measuring around 4–7 cm and females up to 30 cm.

Description, microscopic: There are no lips and the oesophagus is very long. The tail of the male bears five to seven pairs of papillae, two pairs being pre-cloacal. Microfilariae are 340–360 μm.

Final hosts: Cattle, buffalo, zebu

Intermediate hosts: Not known, possibly Tabanid flies

Life cycle: Indirect life cycle. The microfilariae are ingested by the intermediate host and the L_3, when developed, are released into the wound made when the insect next feeds. The male occurs in nodules in the wall of the aorta, while the female is fixed in nodules by its anterior extremity with the rest of the body free in the lumen of the aorta. Microfilariae occur in the blood and in subcutaneous connective tissue.

Geographical distribution: Parts of Africa, Asia and the Far East

Pathogenesis: In cattle, nodules, from which the female worms protrude, form on the intima of the vessels but in other animals the adults appear to provoke little reaction.

Clinical signs: Infection is usually asymptomatic.

Diagnosis: This is not normally required. Infection is usually diagnosed as an incidental finding on postmortem examination of thickened blood vessels, or those containing nodules.

Pathology: The main affected area is the thoracic region of the aorta. In light infections, the lesions are found chiefly on the dorsal wall of the aorta, near the openings of the intercostal arteries. In heavy infections, the artery becomes swollen, the wall is thickened and the intima contains fibrous tracts. The raised nodules can measure up to 1 cm in diameter.

Epidemiology: Because of the innocuous nature of the infection in cattle, the distribution of the species in these hosts is not completely known.

Treatment: Treatment is not indicated.

Control: Any reduction in vector numbers will reduce transmission.

Onchocerca armillata

Common name: Aortic filariosis

Predilection site: Aorta

Parasite class: Nematoda

Superfamily: Filarioidea

Description, gross: Slender whitish worms. Male worms are about 7 cm and female worms up to 70 cm long.

Description, microscopic: Microfilariae are unsheathed and measure 346–382 μm.

Final hosts: Cattle, rarely camel, sheep, goat

Intermediate hosts: Midges (*Culicoides*), blackflies (*Simulium*)

Life cycle: The life cycle of *Onchocerca armillata* is typically filarioid. The microfilariae are found transiently in the bloodstream and more usually in the skin of the dorsal parts of the body. Biting insects, feeding in this area, ingest microfilariae, which then develop to the infective stage in around 3 weeks. When these infected insects feed on another bovine host, transmission of L_3 occurs.

Geographical distribution: Africa, Middle East, India

Pathogenesis: It is interesting that *O. armillata*, though occurring in a strategically important site in the bovine aorta, is not usually associated with clinical signs. It is usually only discovered at the abattoir, surveys in the Middle East having shown a prevalence as high as 90%.

Clinical signs: Infection is usually inapparent.

Diagnosis: Typical nodular lesions may be found in the wall of the aorta on postmortem examination. Microfilariae may also be found in skin biopsy samples taken from affected areas. The piece of skin is placed in warm saline and teased to allow emergence of the microfilariae, and is then incubated for about 8–12 hours. The microfilariae are readily recognised by their sinuous movements in a centrifuged sample of the saline. Another option is to scarify the skin of a predilection site and examine the fluid exudate for microfilariae.

Pathology: *O. armillata* is found in grossly visible nodules in the intima, media and adventitia of the aorta (Fig. 2.27), and atheromatous plaques are commonly seen on the intima. In chronic infections, the aortic wall is thickened and the intima shows tortuous tunnels with numerous nodules containing yellow caseous fluid and coiled worms. Aortic aneurysms have been noted in about a quarter of infections.

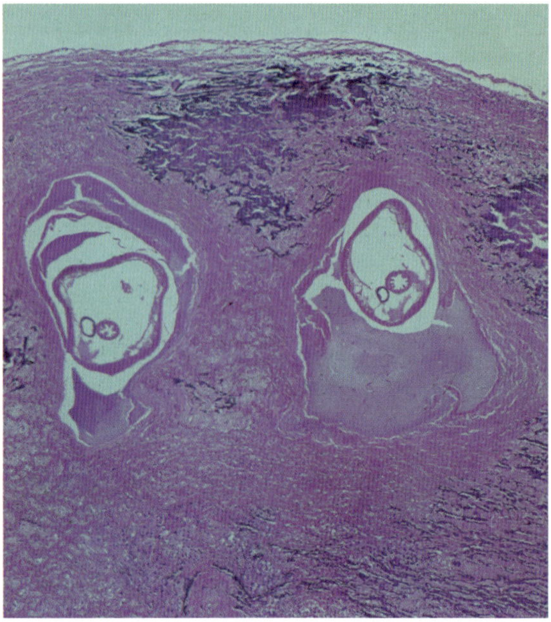

Fig. 2.27 *Onchocerca armillata* within the aorta.

Epidemiology: Prevalence is very high is some regions with 80–90% of animals infected.

Treatment: Rarely indicated. Daily administration of diethylcarbamazine over a period of 21 days acts as a microfilaricide, and a single dose of ivermectin is highly efficient in this respect, although the dying microfilariae may provoke local tissue reactions.

Control: With the ubiquity of the insect vectors there is little possibility of efficient control, though the use of microfilaricides will reduce the numbers of infected flies. In any case, with the relatively innocuous nature of the infection there is unlikely to be any demand for control.

TRYPANOSOMIOSIS

Members of the genus *Trypanosoma* are haemoflagellates of overwhelming importance in cattle in sub-Saharan Africa as a cause of trypanosomiosis. See Chapter 1 (Protozoa – Zoomastigophorasida) for general descriptions.

Salivarian trypanosomes

A number of species of *Trypanosoma*, found in domestic and wild animals, are all transmitted cyclically by

Glossina in much of sub-Saharan Africa. The presence of trypanosomosis precludes the rearing of livestock in many areas while in others, where the vectors are not so numerous, trypanosomosis is often a serious problem, particularly in cattle. The disease, sometimes known as nagana, is characterised by lymphadenopathy and anaemia accompanied by progressive emaciation and, often, death.

Pathogenesis

The signs and effects of the various trypanosomes found in domestic animals are more or less similar. The pathogenesis of trypanosomosis may be considered under three headings:

1. **Lymphoid enlargement** and **splenomegaly** develop associated with plasma cell hyperplasia and hypergammaglobulinaemia, which is primarily due to an increase in IgM. Concurrently there is a variable degree of suppression of immune responses to other antigens such as microbial pathogens or vaccines. Ultimately, in infections of long duration, the lymphoid organs and spleen become shrunken due to exhaustion of their cellular elements.
2. **Anaemia** is a cardinal feature of the disease, particularly in cattle, and initially is proportional to the degree of parasitaemia. Anaemia is caused mainly by extravascular haemolysis through erythrophagocytosis in the mononuclear phagocytic systems of the spleen, liver and lungs, but as the disease becomes chronic there may be decreased haemoglobin synthesis. Leucopenia and thrombocytopenia are caused by mechanisms that predispose leucocytes and platelets to phagocytosis. Immunological mechanisms in the pathogenesis lead to extensive proliferation of activated macrophages, which engulf or destroy erythrocytes, leucocytes, platelets and haematopoietic cells. Later, in infections of several months' duration, when the parasitaemia often becomes low and intermittent, the anaemia may resolve to a variable degree. However, in some chronic cases it may persist despite chemotherapy.
3. **Cell degeneration** and **inflammatory infiltrates** occur in many organs, such as the skeletal muscle and the central nervous system, but perhaps most significantly in the myocardium where there is separation and degeneration of the muscle fibres. The mechanisms underlying these changes are still under study.

Clinical signs

In cattle, the major signs are anaemia, generalised enlargement of the superficial lymph glands, lethargy and progressive loss of bodily condition (Fig. 2.28). Fever and loss of appetite occur intermittently during parasitaemic peaks, the latter becoming marked in the terminal stages of the disease. Typically, the disease is chronic, extending over several months, and usually terminates fatally if untreated. As a herd phenomenon, the growth of young animals is stunted, while adults show decreased fertility, and if pregnant, may abort or give birth to weak offspring. In the terminal stages, animals become extremely weak, the lymph nodes are reduced in size and there is often a jugular pulse. Death is associated with congestive heart failure due to anaemia and myocarditis. Occasionally, the disease is acute, death occurring within 2–3 weeks of infection preceded by fever, anaemia and widespread haemorrhages.

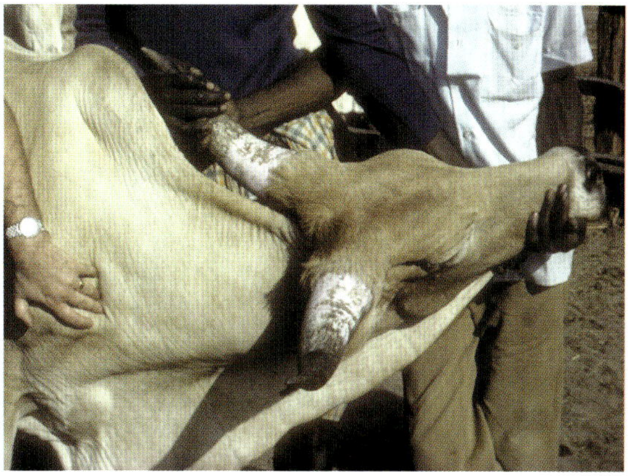

Fig. 2.28 Enlarged prescapular lymph node of Zebu with trypanosomiosis.

Diagnosis

The clinical signs of the disease, although indicative, are not pathognomonic. Confirmation of clinical diagnosis depends on the demonstration of trypanosomes in the blood. If a herd or flock is involved, a representative number of blood samples should be examined, since, in individual animals, the parasitaemia may be in remission or in long-standing cases may be extremely scanty. Occasionally, when the parasitaemia is massive it is possible to detect motile trypanosomes in fresh films of blood. More usually, both thick and thin smears of blood are air-dried and examined later. Thick smears, de-haemoglobinised before staining with Giemsa or Leishman's stain, offer a better chance of finding trypanosomes, while the stained thin smears are used for differentiation of the trypanosome species.

More sensitive techniques utilise centrifugation in a microhaematocrit tube followed by microscopic examination of the interface between the buffy coat and the plasma; alternatively, the tube may be snapped, the buffy coat expressed on to a slide, and the contents examined under dark-ground or phase-contrast microscopy for motile trypanosomes. With these techniques the packed red cell volume is also obtained which is of indirect value in diagnosis if one can eliminate other causes of anaemia, especially helminthosis.

A number of serological tests have been described and include indirect fluorescent antibody test (IFAT) and ELISA and have been partially validated but require further evaluation and standardisation.

Pathology

The carcase is often pale, emaciated and there may be oedematous swellings in the lower part of the abdomen and genital organs with serous atrophy of fat. The liver, lymph nodes and spleen are enlarged and the viscera are congested. Petechiae may appear on lymph nodes, pericardium and intestinal mucosa. The liver is hypertrophic and congested with degeneration and necrosis of the hepatocytes, dilation of blood vessels and parenchymal infiltration of mononuclear cells. A non-suppurative myocarditis, sometimes associated with hydropericarditis, has been reported accompanied by degeneration and necrosis of the myocardial tissue. Other lesions can include glomerulonephritis, renal tubular necrosis, non-suppurative meningio-encephalomyelitis, focal poliomalacia, keratitis, opthalmitis, orchitis, interstitial pneumonia and bone marrow atrophy. Splenic and lymph node hypertrophy occur during the acute phase but the lymphoid tissues are usually exhausted and fibrotic in the chronic stage.

Epidemiology

The vectors are various species of *Glossina* including *G. morsitans*, *G. palpalis*, *G. longipalpis*, *G. pallidipes* and *G. austeni. Typanosoma congolense* can also be transmitted mechanically by other biting flies in tsetse-free areas, although this is uncommon. Since the life cycle of *T. vivax* is short, it is more readily transmitted than other species and mechanical transmission of *T. vivax* by tabanids allows it to spread outside the tsetse belt. The disease can also be transmitted mechanically through contaminated needles and instruments.

The epidemiology depends on three factors: the distribution of the vectors, virulence of the parasite and the response of the host.

- **The vectors**. Of the three groups of tsetse flies (see *Glossina*), the savannah and riverine are the most important since they inhabit areas suitable for grazing and watering. Although the infection rate of *Glossina* with trypanosomes is usually low, ranging from 1–20% of the flies, each is infected for life, and their presence in any number makes the rearing of cattle, pigs and horses extremely difficult. Biting flies may act as mechanical vectors, but their significance in Africa is still undefined.
- **The parasites**. Since parasitaemic animals commonly survive for prolonged periods, there are ample opportunities for fly transmission. Perhaps the most important aspect of trypanosomosis which accounts for the persistent parasitaemia is the way in which the parasite evades the immune response of the host. As noted previously, metacyclic and bloodstream trypanosomes possess a glycoprotein coat which is antigenic and provokes the formation of antibodies which cause opsonisation and lysis of the trypanosomes. Unfortunately, by the time the antibody is produced, a proportion of the trypanosomes have altered the chemical composition of their glycoprotein coat and now, displaying a different antigenic surface, are unaffected by the antibody. Those trypanosomes possessing this new **variant antigen** multiply to produce a second wave of parasitaemia; the host produces a second antibody, but again the glycoprotein coat has altered in a number of trypanosomes so that a third wave of parasitaemia occurs. This process of **antigenic variation** associated with waves and remissions of parasitaemias, often at weekly intervals, may continue for months, usually with a fatal outcome. The repeated switching of the glycoprotein coat is now known to depend on a loosely ordered sequential expression of an undefined number of genes, each coding for a different glycoprotein coat. This, together with the finding that metacyclic trypanosomes may be a mixture of antigenic types, each expressing a different genetic repertoire, explains why domestic animals, even if treated successfully, are often immediately susceptible to reinfection. The complexity of antigens potentially involved has also defeated attempts at vaccination.
- **The hosts**. Trypanosomosis is basically an infection of wildlife in which, by and large, it has achieved a *modus vivendi* in that the animal hosts are parasitaemic for prolonged periods, but generally remain in good health. This situation is known as **trypanotolerance**. In contrast, rearing of domestic livestock in endemic areas has always been associated with excessive morbidity and mortality, although there is evidence that a degree of adaptation or selection has occurred in several breeds. Thus in West Africa small humpless cattle of the *Bos taurus* type, notably the N'Dama, survive and breed in areas of heavy trypanosome challenge despite the absence of control measures (Fig. 2.29). However, their resistance is not absolute and trypanosomosis exacts a heavy toll, particularly in productivity. In other areas of Africa, indigenous breeds of sheep and goats are known to be trypanotolerant, although this may be partly due to their being relatively unattractive hosts for *Glossina*.

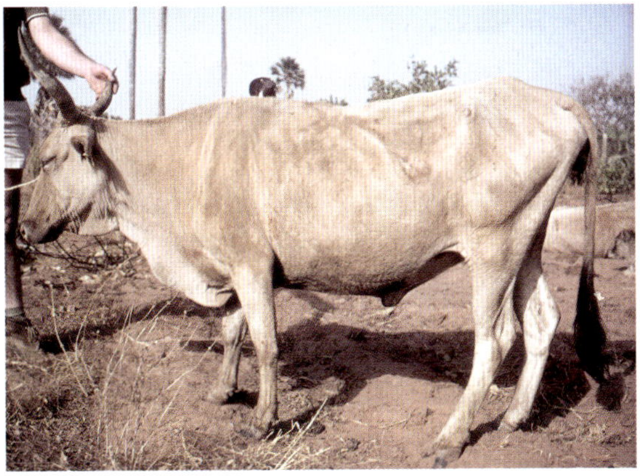

Fig. 2.29 Trypanotolerant N'Dama breed of West Africa.

Precisely how trypanotolerant animals cope with antigenic variation is unknown. It is thought that the control and gradual elimination of their parasitaemias may depend on the possession of a particularly rapid and effective antibody response, although other factors may also be involved.

Trypanosoma brucei brucei

Subgenus: *Trypanozoon*

Common name: Nagana

Predilection site: Blood. *T. brucei brucei* is also found extravascularly in, for example, the myocardium, central nervous system (CNS) and reproductive tract.

Parasite class: Zoomastigophorasida

Family: Trypanosomatidae

Description: *T. brucei brucei* is pleomorphic in form and ranges from long and slender, up to 42 μm (average 29 μm), to short and stumpy, 12–26 μm (mean 18 μm), the two forms often being present in the same blood sample. The undulating membrane is conspicuous, the kinetoplast is small and sub-terminal and the posterior end is pointed. In the slender form the kinetoplast is up to 4 μm from the posterior end, which is usually drawn out, tapering almost to a point, and has a well developed free flagellum; in the stumpy form the flagellum is either short or absent and the posterior end is broad and rounded with the kinetoplast almost terminal. Intermediate forms average 23 μm long and have a blunt posterior end and moderately long flagellum (Fig. 2.30). A fourth form with a posterior nucleus may be seen in laboratory animals. In fresh unfixed blood films, the organism moves rapidly within small areas of the microscope field.

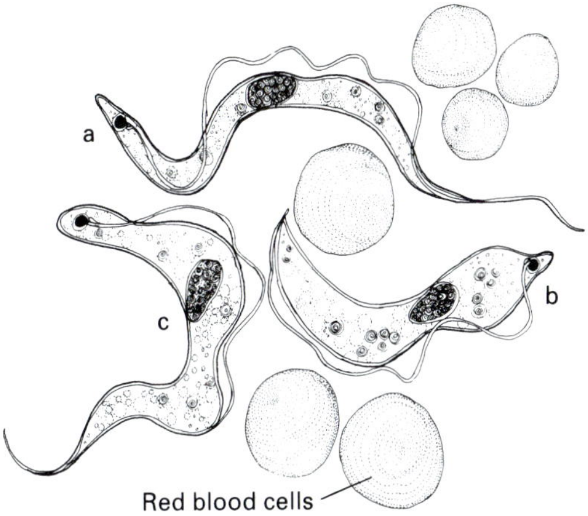

Fig. 2.30 *Trypanosoma brucei* is pleomorphic, showing (a) long slender; (b) short stumpy; and (c) intermediate forms.

Hosts: Cattle, horse, donkey, zebu, sheep, goat, camel, pig, dog, cat, wild game species, particularly antelope

Life cycle: Tsetse flies ingest trypanosomes in the blood or lymph while feeding on an infected host. Thereafter the trypanosomes lose their glycoprotein surface coat, and become elongated and multiply in the midgut before migrating forward to the salivary glands. There they undergo a transformation losing their typical trypanosome, or **trypomastigote**, form and acquire an **epimastigote** form, characterised by the fact that the kinetoplast lies just in front of the nucleus. After further multiplication of the epimastigotes they transform again into small, typically trypomastigote forms with a glycoprotein surface coat. These are the infective forms for the next host and are called **metacyclic** trypanosomes. The entire process takes at least 2–3 weeks and the metacyclic trypanosomes are inoculated into the new host when the tsetse fly feeds.

At the site of inoculation the metacyclic forms multiply locally as the typical blood forms, producing within a few days a raised cutaneous inflammatory swelling called a **chancre**. Thereafter they enter the bloodstream and multiply; a parasitaemia, detectable in the peripheral blood, usually becomes apparent 1–3 weeks later. Subsequently, the parasitaemia may persist for many months although its level may wax and wane due to the immune response of the host.

Geographical distribution: Approximately 10 million square kilometres of sub-Saharan Africa between latitudes 14°N and 29°S.

Pathogenesis: In *T. brucei brucei* infections, the disease is usually more chronic in cattle and animals may survive for several months and may recover.

Treatment: The two drugs in common use are isometamidium and diaminazine aceturate. These are usually successful except where trypanosomes have developed resistance to the drug or in some very chronic cases. Treatment should be followed by surveillance since reinfection, followed by clinical signs and parasitaemia, may occur within a week or two. Alternatively, the animal may relapse after chemotherapy, due to a persisting focus of infection in its tissues or because the trypanosomes are drug resistant.

Notes: Antelope are the natural host species and are reservoirs of infection for domestic animals. Horses, mules and donkeys are very susceptible, and the disease is very severe in sheep, goats, camels and dogs (see respective hosts).

Other subspecies of *T. brucei* – *T.brucei evansi*, *T. brucei equiperdum* – are described separately under their respective subspecies and definitive hosts.

Two other subspecies, *T. brucei gambiense* and *T. brucei rhodesiense*, are important causes of 'sleeping sickness' in humans.

Trypanosoma brucei evansi

Subgenus: *Trypanozoon*

Synonym: *Trypanosoma evansi, T. equinum*

Common name: Surra, el debab, mbori, murrina, mal de Caderas, doukane, dioufar, thaga

Predilection site: Blood

Parasite class: Zoomastigophorasida

Family: Trypanosomatidae

Hosts: Horse, donkey, camel, cattle, zebu, goat, pig, dog, water buffalo, elephant, capybara, tapir, mongoose, ocelot, deer and other wild animals. Many laboratory and wild animals can be infected experimentally.

Geographical distribution: North Africa, Central and South America, central and southern Russia, parts of Asia (India, Burma, Malaysia, southern China, Indonesia, Phillipines)

Pathogenesis: Domestic species such as cattle, buffalo and pigs are commonly infected, but overt disease is uncommon and their main significance is as reservoirs of infection.

Treatment and control: Suramin or quinapyramine (Trypacide) are the drugs of choice for treatment and also confer a short period of prophylaxis. For more prolonged protection a modified quinapyramine known as 'Trypacide Pro-Salt' is also available. Unfortunately, drug resistance, at least to suramin, is not uncommon.

Notes: The original distribution of this parasite coincided with that of the camel, and is often associated with arid desserts and semiarid steppes.

For more details see Chapter 4 (Horses).

Trypanosoma congolense

Subgenus: *Nannomonas*

Common name: Nagana, paranagana, Gambia fever, ghindi, gobial

Predilection site: Blood

Parasite class: Zoomastigophorasida

Family: Trypanosomatidae

Description: *T. congolense* is small, monomorphic in form, 8–20 μm long. The undulating membrane is inconspicuous, the medium-sized kinetoplast is marginal and the posterior end is blunt. There is no free flagellum (Figs 2.31, 2.32). In fresh blood films the organism moves sluggishly, often apparently attached to red cells.

Hosts: Cattle, sheep, goat, horse, camel, dog, pig. Reservoir hosts include antelope, giraffe, zebra, elephant and warthog.

Life cycle: The trypanosomes divide by longitudinal binary fission in the vertebrate host. After ingestion by the tsetse fly they develop in the midgut as long trypomastigotes without a free flagellum. They attach

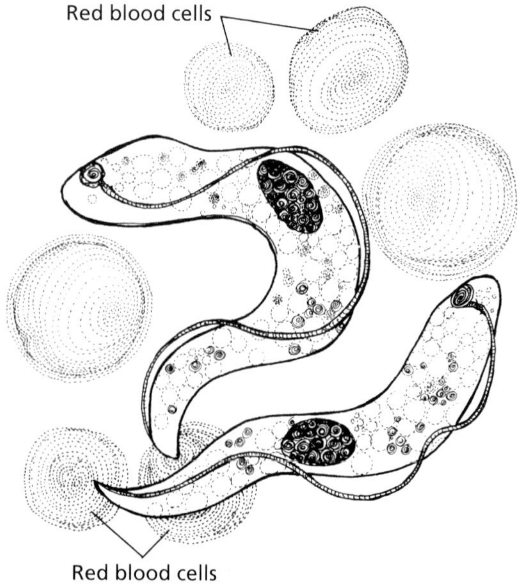

Fig. 2.31 *Trypanosoma congolense* is monomorphic and possesses a marginal kinetoplast.

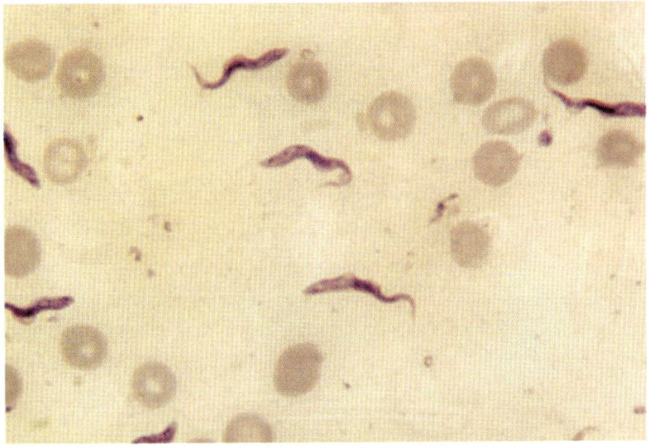

Fig. 2.32 Trypomastigotes of *Trypanosoma congolense*.

first to the wall of the proboscis and multiply there for a time before passing to the hypopharynx where they develop into metacyclic, infective trypomastigotes similar in appearance to the blood forms. These are injected into the vertebrate when the fly bites. Development to the infective stage in *Glossina* takes from 15 to well over 20 days at 23–34°C.

Geographical distribution: Widely distributed in tropical Africa between latitudes 15°N and 25°S.

Pathogenesis: With *T. congolense*, there are many strains which differ markedly in virulence. In cattle, the parasite can cause either an acute fatal disease resulting in death in about 10 weeks, a chronic condition with recovery in about 1 year, or a mild almost asymptomatic condition. The signs caused by this species are similar to those caused by other trypanosomes, but the central nervous system is not affected.

Treatment and control: In infected cattle, the two drugs in common use are diminazene aceturate (Berenil) and homidium salts (Ethidium and Novidium). As with *T. brucei*, these drugs are usually successful except where trypanosomes have developed resistance to the drug or in some very chronic cases.

Additional comments made for treatment and control of *T. brucei* infections equally apply to *T. congolense*.

Notes: *Trypanosoma congolense congolense* is the most important trypanosome of cattle in tropical Africa. The African disease, nagana, is caused by *T. congolense*, often in mixed infection with *T. brucei* and *T. vivax*.

Trypanosoma vivax

Subgenus: *Duttonella*

Common name: Nagana, souma

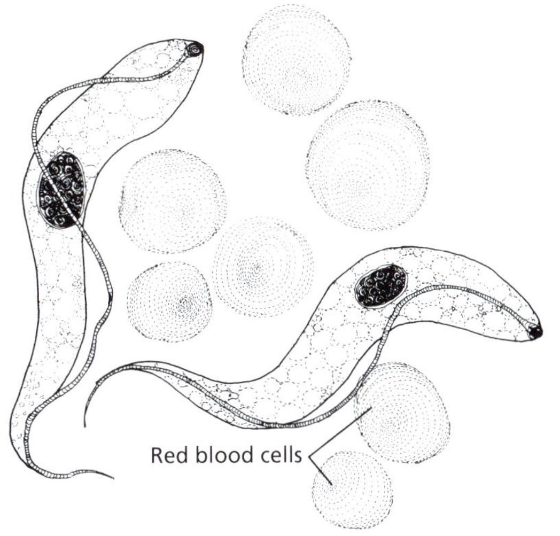

Fig. 2.33 *Trypanosoma vivax* is monomorphic and has a short flagellum and terminal kinetoplast.

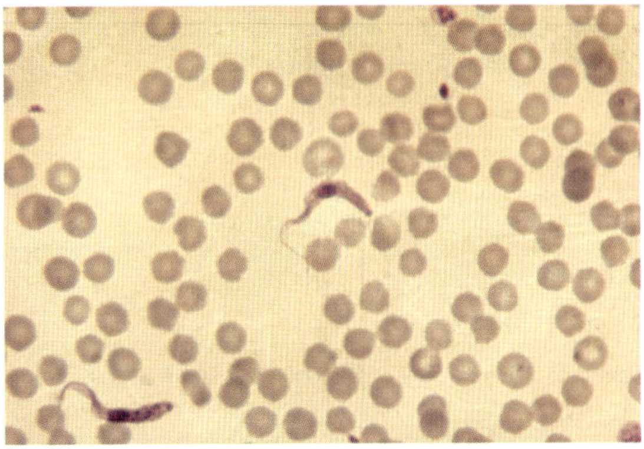

Fig. 2.34 Trypomastigotes of *Trypanosoma vivax*.

Predilection site: Blood

Parasite class: Zoomastigophorasida

Family: Trypanosomatidae

Description: *T. vivax* is monomorphic, ranging from 20–27 μm. The undulating membrane is inconspicuous, the large kinetoplast is terminal and the posterior end is broad and rounded. A short free flagellum is present (Figs 2.33, 2.34). In fresh blood films *T. vivax* moves rapidly across the microscope field.

Hosts: Cattle, sheep, goat, camel, horse; antelope and giraffe are reservoirs.

Life cycle: Development in the insect vector takes place only in the proboscis. The trypanosomes turn first into the epimastigote form, and then the metacyclic, infective trypanosomes that pass to the hypopharynx and infect new hosts when the tsetse flies bite and feed.

Geographical distribution: Africa, Central, West Indies, Central and South America (Brazil, Venezuela, Bolivia, Columbia, Guyana, French Guyana), Mauritius.

Pathogenesis: *T. vivax* is most important in cattle. Generally, strains of *T. vivax* in West Africa are more pathogenic than ones in East Africa, except for one strain in East Africa that causes acute haemorrhagic disease which is very pathogenic.

Treatment: As for *T. congolense*

Notes: There are three subspecies:

- *T. vivax vivax* causes the disease souma in Africa and is found in mixed infections with *T. congolense* and *T. brucei.*
- *T. vivax viennei* occurs in the New World and is transmitted by horseflies. This subspecies occurs in cattle, horses, sheep and goats in northern South America, Central America, West Indies and Mauritius.
- *T. vivax uniforme* is similar to *T. vivax vivax* but is smaller, 12–20 μm long (mean 16 μm). It occurs in cattle, sheep, goats and antelopes in Uganda and Zaire, causing a disease similar to *T. vivax vivax.*

Salivarian trypanosomiosis control

This currently depends on the control of tsetse flies, discussed under Tsetse flies (*Glossina*), and on the use of drugs (Table 2.2).

In cattle, and if necessary in sheep and goats, isometamidium is the drug of choice since it remains in the tissues and has a prophylactic effect for 2–6 months. Otherwise, diminazene may be used as cases arise, these being selected either by clinical examination or on the haematological detection of anaemic animals. To reduce the possible development of drug resistance it may be advisable periodically to change from one trypanocidal drug to another. To further enhance the effective use of trypanocidal drugs, they may be used as 'sanative' pairs and treatment restricted to individual clinically affected animals.

Two important aspects of control are:

- The necessity to protect cattle from a tsetse-free zone while being trekked to market through an area of endemic trypanosomosis.
- An awareness of the dangers of stocking a tsetse-free ranch with cattle from areas where trypanosomosis is present, as mechanical transmission may cause an outbreak of disease.

In both cases treatment with a trypanocidal drug at an appropriate time is advisable.

Table 2.2 Drugs used in the treatment and control of nagana in cattle.

Drug	Recommended dose	Comments
Diminazine aceturate	3–10 mg/kg i.m.	*T. brucei, T. congolense, T. vivax*
Isometamidium	0.25–1 mg/kg i.m.	*T. brucei, T. congolense, T. vivax.* Local reaction
Homidium bromide	1 mg/kg s.c.	*T. congolense, T. vivax*
Homidium chloride		Prophylaxis for 6 weeks
Pyrithidium bromide	2–2.5 mg/kg	*T. congolense, T. vivax* Prophylaxis for 4 months

An alternative approach, using trypanotolerant breeds of ruminants, perhaps combined with judicious drug therapy, may, in the future, offer a realistic solution in many areas where the disease is endemic and this aspect is currently under intensive study.

Stercorarian trypanosomes

These are relatively large trypanosomes found in the blood of cattle, with faecal transmission by tabanid flies (*Tabanus, Haematopota*).

Trypanosoma theileri

Subgenus: *Megatrypanum*

Predilection site: Blood

Parasite class: Zoomastigophorasida

Family: Trypanosomatidae

Description: Large trypanosome, 60–70 μm in length, although may be up to 120 μm with posterior end long and pointed (Figs 2.35, 2.36). There is a medium sized kinetoplast with a prominent undulating membrane and a free flagellum. Both trypomastigote and epimastigote forms may appear in the blood.

Hosts: Cattle

Life cycle: Multiplication occurs in the vertebrate host by longitudinal binary fission of the epimastigote form in the lymph nodes and various tissues. The

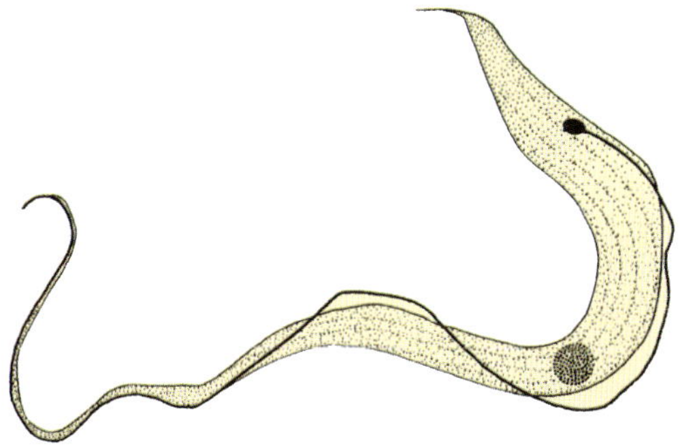

Fig. 2.35 *Trypanosoma theileri.*

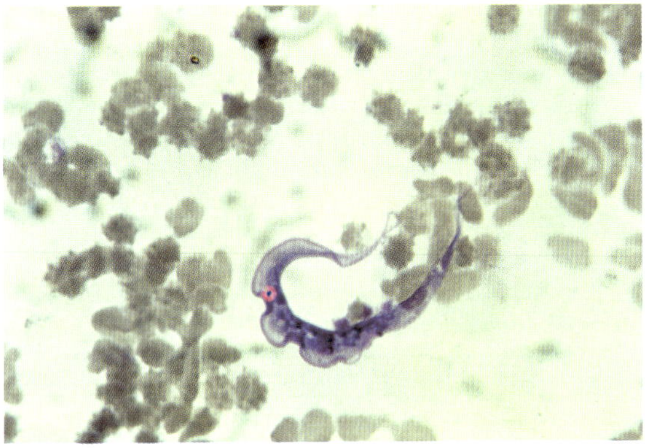

Fig. 2.36 Trypomastigotes of *Trypanosoma theileri.*

trypanosomes develop into small metacyclic tryptomastigotes in the hind gut of tabanid flies (stercorarian development). Transmission back to the vertebrate host occurs through fly faeces, containing the parasite, deposited on mucous membranes.

Geographical distribution: Worldwide

Pathogenesis: Infection produces transient parasitaemias, but is generally considered to be non-pathogenic. Under conditions of stress it may cause abortion and even death.

Clinical signs: Infections are usually asymptomatic

Diagnosis: Can only be usually diagnosed by incubating blood in culture medium suitable for the multiplication of trypanosomes.

Epidemiology: *Trypanosoma theileri* is transmitted by tabanid flies (*Tabanus*, *Haematopota*); the worldwide distribution of the trypanosome corresponds to the range and prevalence of its intermediate hosts. The metacyclic tryptomastigotes, present in the faeces of the vector, gain access to the blood of their mammalian host by penetrating abraded skin, by contamination of mucous membranes, or following ingestion of the vector when the liberated trypanosomes penetrate the mucosa. Intrauterine infection has been reported.

Treatment and control: Not usually required, although general fly control measures may help limit potential transmission from tabanid flies.

Notes: Often referred to as a 'non-pathogenic trypanosome'.

BABESIOSIS

Life cycle

Multiplication of *Babesia* organisms in the vertebrate host occurs in the erythrocytes by binary fission, endodyogeny, endopolyogeny (budding) or merogony to form merozoites. These are liberated from the erythrocyte and invade other cells. The asexual cycle continues indefinitely and the animals may remain infected for life. On ingestion by a tick these forms become vermiform, and enter the body cavity then the ovary and penetrate the eggs where they round up and divide to form small round organisms. When the larval tick moults into the nymph stage, the parasites enter the salivary gland and undergo a series of binary fissions entering the cells of the salivary gland acini. They multiply further until the host cells are filled with thousands of minute parasites. These become vermiform, break out of the host cell and lie in the lumen of the gland and are injected into the mammalian host when the tick sucks blood.

Epidemiology

The epidemiology of the bovine *Babesia* species depends on the interplay of a number of factors and these include:

1. The virulence of the particular species of *Babesia*. *B. bigemina* and *B. bovis* in tropical and subtropical regions are highly pathogenic, *B. divergens* in northern Europe is relatively pathogenic, whilst *B. major* produces only mild and transient anaemia.
2. The age of the host. It is frequently stated that there is an inverse age resistance to *Babesia* infection in that young animals are less susceptible to babesiosis than older animals. The reason for this is not known.
3. The immune status of the host. In endemic areas, the young animal first acquires immunity passively, in the colostrum of the dam and, as a result, often suffers only transient infections with mild clinical signs. However, these infections are apparently sufficient to stimulate active immunity, although recovery is followed by a long period

during which they are carriers when, although showing no clinical signs, their blood remains infective to ticks for many months. It used to be thought that this active immunity was dependent on the persistence of the carrier state and the phenomenon was termed premunity. However, it seems unlikely that this is the case since it is now known that such animals may lose their infection either naturally or by chemotherapy, but still retain a solid immunity.

4. The level of tick challenge. In endemic areas, where there are many infected ticks, the immunity of the host is maintained at a high level through repeated challenge and overt disease is rare. In contrast, where there are few ticks or when they are confined to limited areas, the immune status of the population is low and the young animals receive little, if any, colostral protection. If, in these circumstances, the numbers of ticks suddenly increase due to favourable climatic conditions or to a reduction in dipping frequency, the incidence of clinical cases may rise sharply. This situation is known as enzootic instability.
5. Stress. In endemic areas, the occasional outbreak of clinical disease, particularly in adult animals, is often associated with some form of stress, such as parturition or the presence of another disease, such as tick-borne fever.

Babesia bigemina

Common name: Texas fever

Predilection site: Blood

Parasite class: Sporozoasida

Family: Babesiidae

Description: *B. bigemina* is a large, pleomorphic babesia but characteristically is seen and identified by the pear-shaped bodies joined at an acute angle within the mature erythrocyte. Round forms measure 2 µm and the pear-shaped, elongated ones are 4–5 µm. The erythrocytic stages lack a conoid, micropores and typical mitochondria, but have an anterior and posterior polar ring and typically two rhoptries.

Hosts: Cattle, buffalo

Geographical distribution: Australia, Africa, North, Central and South America, Asia and southern Europe

Pathogenesis: The rapidly dividing parasites in the red cells produce rapid destruction of the erythrocytes with accompanying haemoglobinaemia, haemoglobinuria and fever.

Generally, *B. bigemina* infections are not as virulent as those of *B. bovis*, despite the fact that the parasites may infect 40% of the red cells. Otherwise the disease is typically biphasic, the acute haemolytic crisis, if not fatal, being followed by a prolonged period of recovery.

Clinical signs: Calves are relatively resistant to infection, and do not usually show clinical disease. In older animals, clinical signs can be very severe; however, differences in pathogenicity may occur with various *B. bigemina* isolates associated with different geographical areas. The first sign is usually a high fever with rectal temperatures reaching 41.5°C (106.7°F). There is anorexia and ruminal atony. Often the first visible appearance of infection is that the animal isolates itself from the herd, becomes uneasy, seeks shade and may lie down. Cattle may stand with an arched back, have a roughened hair coat and show evidence of dyspnoea and tachycardia. The mucous membranes are first inflamed and reddened, but as erythrocytic lysis occurs, they become palid and show signs of anaemia. Anaemia is a contributory factor to the weakness and loss of condition seen in cattle that survive the acute phase of the disease. The anaemia may occur very rapidly, with 75% or more of the erythrocytes being destroyed in just a few days. This is usually associated with severe haemoglobinemia and haemoglobinuria. After onset of fever, the crisis will usually pass within a week, and if the animal survives, there is usually severe weight loss, drop in milk production, possible abortion and a protracted recovery. Mortality is extremely variable and may reach 50% or higher, but in the absence of undue stress most animals will survive.

Diagnosis: As for *B. bovis*

Pathology: Acute infections as for *B. bovis*. In cattle that have suffered a more prolonged illness, acute lesions are much less conspicuous. Subepicardial petechial hemorrhages may be present, the carcase is usually emaciated and icteric, the blood is thin and watery, the intermuscular fascia is oedematous, the liver yellowish brown, and the bile may contain flakes of semi-solid material. The kidneys are pale and often oedematous, and the bladder may contain normal urine, depending on how long past the haemolytic crisis the necropsy is performed. Although the spleen is enlarged, the pulp is firmer than in acute babesiosis.

Epidemiology: *Boophilus annulatus*, *B. microplus* and *B. decoloratus* are the principal vectors of *Babesia bigemina*. Mechanical transmission is possible, but it is not efficient enough to maintain infection in the absence of specific tick vectors.

Treatment: As with *B. bovis*, successful treatment of *B. bigemina* depends on early diagnosis and the prompt administration of effective drugs. If medication is administered early, success is the rule, for there are several effective compounds. One of the first successful treatments was trypan blue. This treatment may be used to determine the type of infection present. *B. bigemina* is susceptible to trypan blue treatment, whereas *B. bovis* is not. Generally, the small babesias are more resistant to chemotherapy. The most commonly used compounds for treatment are diminazene diaceturate (3–5 mg/kg), imidocarb (1–3 mg/kg) and amicarbalide (5–10 mg/kg); however, the quinuronium and acridine derivatives are also effective where these are available. Treatment of *B. bigemina* is so effective in some instances that radical cures occur that will eventually leave the animal susceptible to reinfection. For this reason, reduced drug levels are sometimes indicated. Imidocarb has been successfully used as a chemoprophylactic that will prevent clinical infection for as long as 2 months, but allow mild sub-clinical infection to occur as the drug level wanes resulting in premunition and immunity.

Control: Specific control measures are not usually necessary for animals born of mothers in endemic areas, since their colostrum-acquired immunity is gradually reinforced by repeated exposure to infection. Indeed, the veterinary importance of babesiosis is chiefly that it acts as a constraint to the introduction of improved livestock from other areas. Areas of enzootic instability also create problems when tick numbers suddenly increase or animals, for some reason, are forced to use an adjacent tick-infested area.

Immunisation, using blood from carrier animals, has been practised for many years in tropical areas, and more recently in Australia; rapidly passaged strains of *Babesia*, which are relatively non-pathogenic, have been widely utilised in live vaccines. In the near future, these may be superseded by adjuvanted vaccines prepared from several recombinant *Babesia* antigens. Otherwise the control of babesiosis in susceptible animals introduced into endemic areas depends on surveillance for the first few months after their arrival and, if necessary, treatment.

Vaccination of cattle against *B. bigemina* infection is commonly practised in many countries by inoculating blood from donor animals. This is usually obtained from a recently recovered case, any untoward reactions in the 'vaccinates' being controlled by babesicidal drugs. In Australia, the procedure is more sophisticated in that the vaccine is produced from acute infections produced in splenectomised donors. For economy, the blood is collected by exchange transfusion rather than by exsanguination. It is interesting that the rapid passage of the parasite by blood inoculation in splenectomised calves has fortuitously had the very desirable effect of decreasing the virulence of the infection in non-splenectomised calves to the extent that post vaccination surveillance of cattle is frequently not performed. The parasite count of the blood determines the dilution of the latter, which is dispensed in plastic bags, packed in ice and despatched in insulated containers. Each dose of vaccine contains about 10 million parasites. Most of the vaccine is used in cattle under 12 months of age living in conditions of enzootic instability. The degree of protection induced is such that only 1% of vaccinated cattle subsequently develop clinical babesiosis from field challenge, compared to 18% of unvaccinated cattle.

The primary disadvantage of red cell vaccines is their lability and the fact that, unless their preparation is carefully supervised, they may spread diseases such as enzootic bovine leucosis. Obviously there will be no such problem with a vaccine based on recombinant antigens.

A regimen of four injections of long-acting oxytetracycline at weekly intervals, administered to naive cattle during their first month of grazing on tick-infested pastures, has been shown to confer prophylaxis against *B. bigemina* during this period, after which the cattle were immune to subsequent challenge.

Notes: *B. bigemina*, a large *Babesia* is of particular interest historically, since it was the first protozoan infection of man or animals demonstrated to have an arthropod intermediate host; this was shown in 1893 by Smith and Kilborne while investigating the cause of the locally known 'Texas fever' in cattle in the USA. The disease has since been eradicated in that country.

Babesia bovis

Synonym: *Babesia argentina*

Predilection site: Blood

Parasite class: Sporozoasida

Family: Babesiidae

Description: *B. bovis* is a small pleomorphic *babesia*, typically identified as a single body, as small round bodies, or as paired, pear-shaped bodies joined at an obtuse angle within the centre of the mature erythrocyte. The round forms measure 1–1.5 μm, and the pear-shaped bodies 1.5 × 2.4 μm in size. Vacuolated signet ring forms are especially common.

Hosts: Cattle, buffalo, deer

Geographical distribution: Australia, Africa, Central and South America, Asia and southern Europe

Pathogenesis: *B. bovis* is generally regarded as the most pathogenic of the bovine *Babesia*. Although the classical signs of fever, anaemia and haemoglobinuria occur, the degree of anaemia is disproportional to the parasitaemia since haematocrit levels below 20% may be associated with infections of less than 1% of the red cells. The reason for this is unknown. In addition, *B. bovis* infection is associated with sludging of the red cells in the small capillaries. In the cerebrum this causes blockage of the vessels by clumps of infected red cells leading to anoxia and tissue damage. The resulting clinical signs of aggression, incoordination or convulsions and depression are invariably fatal. Finally, recent work has indicated that some of the severity of *B. bovis* infection may be associated with the activation of certain plasma components, leading to circulatory stasis, shock and intravascular coagulation.

Clinical signs: Incoordination, convulsions, depression, death

Diagnosis: The history and clinical signs of fever, anaemia, jaundice, and hemoglobinuria in cattle located in enzootic areas where *Boophilus* ticks occur are usually sufficient to justify a diagnosis of babesiosis. For confirmation, the examination of blood films, stained with Giemsa, will reveal the parasites in the red cells. However, once the acute febrile phase has subsided they are often impossible to find since they are rapidly removed from the circulation. In addition, a technique of brain biopsies has been described that has proven very useful in detecting and diagnosing *Babesia bovis* infections. The characteristic low parasitemias in the circulating blood make this technique very useful in improving the chances of seeing the organism. There is a marked concentration of infected erythrocytes in the capillaries of the brain.

From each animal six blood smears should be made, air-dried and fixed in methanol and/or a sample of whole blood in an anticoagulant and serum should be collected. In cases of chronic infection, diagnosis is usually made using a variety of serological tests for the detection of specific antibodies, since the organism disappears or is present in extremely low numbers soon after the acute infection. Presently, immunofluorescence assay is the test of choice in the serologic diagnosis of *B. bovis*.

Other conditions that should be considered and may resemble babesiosis are anaplasmosis, trypanosomiosis, theileriosis, leptospirosis, bacillary haemoglobinuria, haemobartonellosis and eperythrozoonosis.

Pathology: At necropsy, the carcase is pale and jaundiced and the lungs may be oedematous and congested in cattle that have died early in the course of infection. The pericardial sac may contain serosanguineous fluid and subepicardial and subendocardial petechial haemorrhages. The liver is enlarged and icteric, and the gallbladder, which may have haemorrhage on the mucous surface, is distended with thick, dark green bile. The spleen is markedly enlarged, and has a dark pulpy consistency. The abomasal and intestinal mucosa may be icteric with patches of subserosal haemorrhages (Fig. 2.37). The blood is thin and watery. The urinary bladder is frequently distended, with dark, reddish brown urine. Jaundice is commonly distributed in the connective tissue. The lymph nodes are oedematous and often have petechiation.

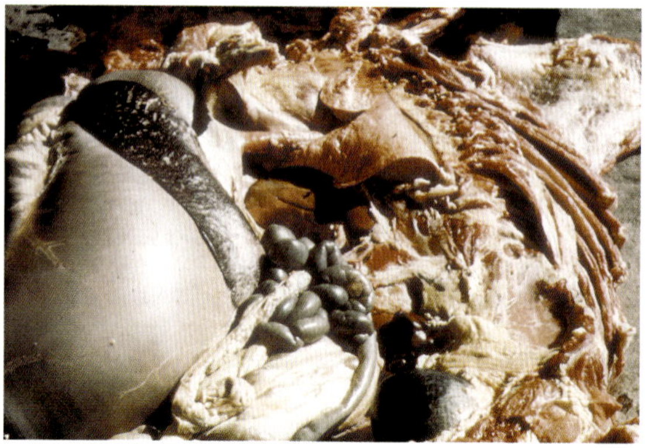

Fig. 2.37 Postmortem findings, *Babesia bovis.*

Epidemiology: *Babesia bovis* is transmitted by the same ticks that transmit *B. bigemina* (*Boophilus annulatus*, *B. microplus*). The tick *Boophilus decoloratus*, which is widely distributed in Africa, does not appear to transmit *Babesia bovis* even though it readily transmits *Babesia bigemina*. There are reports from Europe of *Babesia bovis*, for which the vector is thought to be *Ixodes ricinus*.

Treatment: Successful treatment depends on early diagnosis and the prompt administration of effective drugs. There is less likelihood of success if treatment is delayed until the animal has been weakened by fever and anaemia. Chemotherapy is generally effective, although *B. bovis* is usually somewhat more difficult to treat than other *Babesia* species, and a second treatment, or slightly increased dose rates, may be desirable. The most commonly used compounds for the treatment of babesiosis are diminazene diaceturate (3–5 mg/kg), imidocarb (1–3 mg/kg) and amicarbalide (5–10 mg/kg); however, the quinuronium and acridine derivatives are also effective where these are available. Trypan blue is not effective against *B. bovis*.

Control: The numbers of ticks and therefore the quantum of *Babesia* infection may be reduced by regular spraying or dipping with acaricides. In addition, in cattle, the selection and breeding of cattle which acquire a high degree of resistance to ticks is practised, particularly in Australia. Widespread use of tick vaccines may also have a significant influence on the incidence of infection in cattle (see control of *Babesia bigemina*).

Repeated passage of *B. bovis* in splenectomised calves results in the attenuation of the organism and for many years this attenuated vaccine has been produced and successfully used in Australia for the prevention of *B. bovis*. In some cattle (older, and producing dairy cows), chemotherapy may be indicated, but usually the vaccine may be used without treatment.

The development of in vitro techniques for the cultivation of *B. bovis* on bovine erythrocytes has led to the isolation of soluble antigens, which, when combined with adjuvants, have proven immunogenic. These non-infectious vaccines, although they do not prevent infection, appear to be responsible for moderating the effects of infection. They do not produce as high a level of protection as is seen with premunising vaccines but are safe and do not yield carriers. In some instances, these vaccines, although protective against homologous challenge, may not protect against immunological variants. The continuous in vitro passage of *B. bovis* has been shown to induce a level of attenuation similar to that seen with the passage of the organism in splenectomised calves and infection with this attenuated organism has been reported to prevent clinical infection following a challenge with virulent *B. bovis*. The primary disadvantage of red cell vaccines is their lability and the fact that, unless their preparation is carefully supervised, they may spread diseases such as enzootic bovine leucosis. Obviously there will be no such problem with a vaccine based on recombinant antigens.

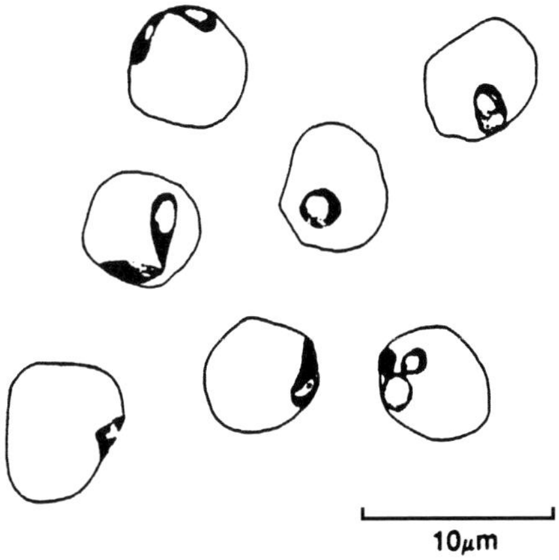

Fig. 2.38 Diverse forms of *Babesia divergens* in bovine red cells.

Babesia divergens

Common name: Redwater fever

Predilection site: Blood

Parasite class: Sporozoasida

Family: Babesiidae

Description: Examination of stained blood films shows the organisms to be within red cells, almost always singly or as pairs, often arranged at a characteristic angle with their narrow ends opposed. Typically, they are pyriform, but may be round, elongated or cigar-shaped. *B. divergens* is a 'small *Babesia*' and in blood films typically appears as paired, widely divergent organisms, 1.5 × 0.4 μm, lying near the edge of the red cell (Fig. 2.38). Other forms may be present measuring 2 × 1 μm, some are circular up to 2 μm in diameter and a few may be vacuolated.

Hosts: Cattle

Geographical distribution: Northern Europe

Pathogenesis: The rapidly dividing parasites in the red cells produce rapid destruction of the erythrocytes with accompanying haemoglobinaemia, haemoglobinuria and fever. This may be so acute as to cause death within a few days, during which the packed red cell volume falls below 20%. The parasitaemia, which is usually detectable once the clinical signs appear, may involve between 0.2% and 45% of the red cells. Milder forms of the disease, associated with relatively resistant hosts, are characterised by fever, anorexia and perhaps slight jaundice for a period of several days.

Clinical signs: Typically the acute disease occurs 1–2 weeks after the tick commences to feed and is characterised by fever and haemoglobinuria ('redwater'). The mucous membranes, at first congested, become jaundiced, the respiratory and pulse rates are increased, the heart beat is usually very audible, and in cattle ruminal movements cease and abortion may occur. If untreated, death commonly occurs in this phase. Otherwise, convalescence is prolonged, there is loss of weight and milk production and diarrhoea followed by constipation is common. In animals previously exposed to infection, clinical signs may be mild or even inapparent.

Diagnosis: The history and clinical signs are usually sufficient to justify a diagnosis of babesiosis. For confirmation, the examination of blood films, stained with Giemsa, will reveal the parasites in the red cells (Fig. 2.39). However, once the acute febrile phase has subsided they are often impossible to find since they are rapidly removed from the circulation.

Pathology: At necropsy, the carcase is pale and jaundiced, the bile is thick and granular and there may be subepicardial and subendocardial haemorrhages.

Epidemiology: *B. divergens* is transmitted by *Ixodes ricinus*, and is widespread and pathogenic, with clinical cases occurring during the periods of tick activity, primarily in the spring and autumn. Infection in

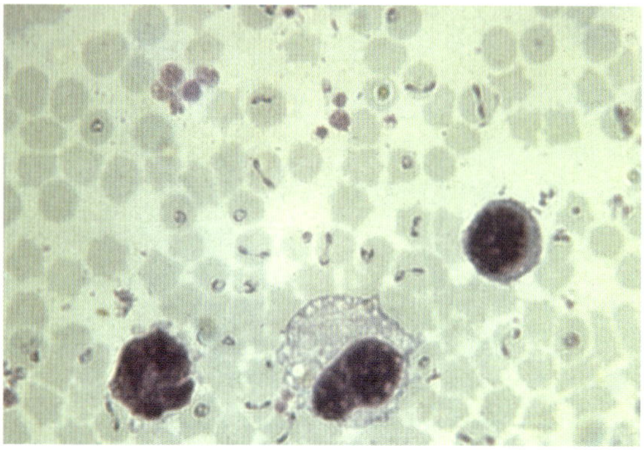

Fig. 2.39 Intraerythrocytic stages of *Babesia divergens*.

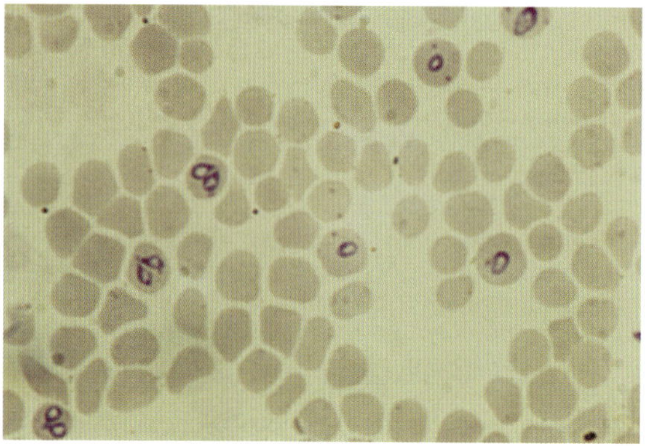

Fig. 2.40 Intraerythrocytic stages of *Babesia major*.

the tick is transovarially transmitted and the larvae, nymphs and adults of the next generation are all able to transmit infection to cattle.

Treatment: Amicarbilide, diminazene aceturate and imidocarb are the most commonly used drugs. Recently, long-acting preparations of oxytetracycline have been shown to have a prophylactic effect against *B. divergens* infection. Imidocarb, due to its persistence in the tissues, has a prophylactic effect for several weeks. During the convalescent phase of the disease, blood transfusions may be valuable as are drugs designed to stimulate food and water intake.

Control: Normally no effort is made to control this infection in endemic areas, although cattle recently introduced require surveillance for some months, since, on average, one in four will develop clinical disease and of these one in six will die if untreated. However, in some parts of mainland Europe, such as the Netherlands, where ticks are confined to rough vegetation on the edges of pastures and on roadsides, it is often possible to take evasive measures. It is thought that the red and roe deer are not important reservoir hosts since only mild infections have been experimentally produced in splenectomised deer.

Notes: Since 1957, several cases of fatal babesiosis due to *B. divergens* infection have occurred in man in Yugoslavia, Russia, Ireland and Scotland. In each case, the individual had been splenectomised sometime previously, or was currently undergoing immunosuppressive treatment.

Babesia major

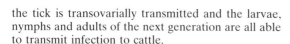

Predilection site: Blood

Parasite class: Sporozoasida

Family: Babesiidae

Description: A 'large *Babesia*', with pyriform bodies 2.6 × 1.5 μm, being characteristically paired at an acute angle less than 90° and found in the centre of the erythrocyte (Fig. 2.40). Round forms about 1.8 μm diameter may form.

Hosts: Cattle

Geographical distribution: Europe, North Africa, South America

Pathogenesis: *Babesia major* is only mildly pathogenic.

Clinical signs: Clinical signs with *B. major* are usually inapparent but where symptoms do occur these are characterised by a haemolytic syndrome with elevated temperature, mild anaemia and haemoglobinuria.

Diagnosis: Examination of blood films, stained with Giemsa, will reveal the parasites in the red cells.

Epidemiology: *B. major* is transmitted by the three-host tick *Haemaphysalis punctata*.

Treatment: Not usually required but amicarbilide, diminazene aceturate and imidocarb are effective.

Control: Specific control measures are not usually necessary for animals born of mothers in endemic areas since, as noted previously, their colostrally acquired immunity is gradually reinforced by repeated exposure to infection. Tick numbers may be reduced by regular spraying or dipping with acaricides. The control of infection in susceptible animals introduced into endemic areas depends on surveillance for the first few months after their arrival and, if necessary, treatment.

THEILERIOSIS

Diseases caused by several species of *Theileria* (theileriosis) are a serious constraint to livestock production in Africa, Asia and the Middle East. The parasites, which are tick transmitted, undergo repeated merogonony in the lymphocytes ultimately releasing small merozoites, which invade the red cells to become piroplasms.

Theileria are widely distributed in cattle and sheep in Africa, Asia, Europe and Australia, have a variety of tick vectors and are associated with infections which range from clinically inapparent to rapidly fatal. Although the speciation of many *Theileria* is still controversial, largely because of their morphological similarity, there are two species of major veterinary importance in cattle. Minor and mildly pathogenic species infecting cattle include *T. velifera* and *T. taurotragi* in Africa, *T. mutans* and the *T. sergenti/orientalis/buffeli* complex.

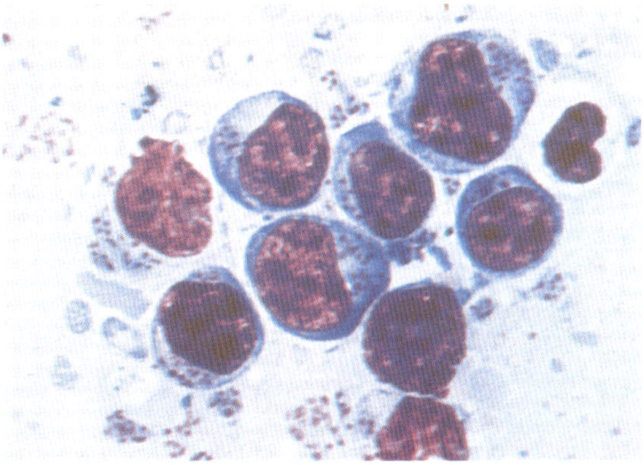

Fig. 2.42 Macroschizonts of *Theileria parva* in a smear of a lymph node.

Theileria parva

Subspecies: *T. parva parva, T. parva lawrencei*

Common name: East coast fever, corridor fever

Predilection site: Blood and lymphatics

Parasite class: Sporozoasida

Family: Theileriidae

Description: Trophozoite forms in the erythrocyte are predominantly rod-shaped (1.5–2.0 × 0.1–1.0 μm), but may also be round, oval and comma-shaped (Fig. 2.41). Koch bodies are in the lymphocytes and endothelial cells of the spleen or lymph nodes where they are very numerous and average 8 μm but can range up to 12 μm or more. Two types have been described; macroschizonts containing chromatin granules 0.4–2.0 μm in diameter (Fig. 2.42); these divide further to become microschizonts that contain chromatin granules 0.3–0.8 μm in diameter and produce merozoites 0.7–1 μm in diameter.

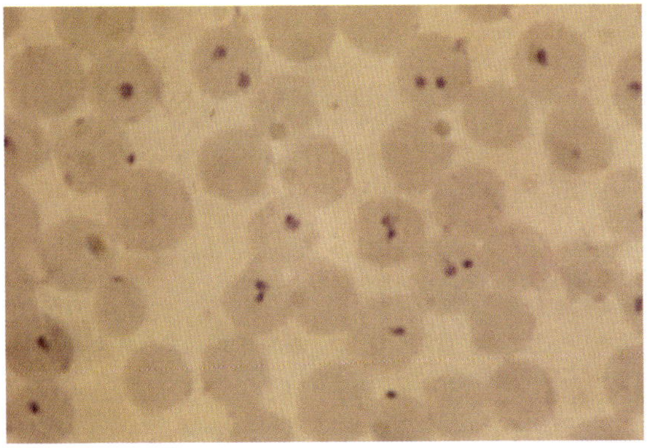

Fig. 2.41 Intraerythrocytic stages of *Theileria parva*.

Hosts: Cattle, African buffalo (*Syncerus caffer*)

Life cycle: Erythrocytic merozoites are ingested by the tick intermediate host, *Rhipicephalus appendiculatus* (the brown ear tick), and develop into macro- and microgamonts to produce zygotes. These develop and enter the haemolymph to become kinetes. These enter the salivary glands to become fission bodies. In adult ticks, the primary fision bodies divide into secondary (primary sporoblasts) and tertiary (secondary sporoblasts) fission bodies and produce sporozoites that are released into the saliva.

Cattle are infected when the ticks suck blood. The sporozoites are inoculated into cattle and quickly enter lymphocytes in an associated lymph gland, usually the parotid. The parasitised lymphocyte transforms to a lymphoblast, which divides rapidly as the macroschizont develops. This division is apparently stimulated by the parasite, which itself divides synchronously with the lymphoblast to produce two infected cells. The rate of proliferation is such that a ten-fold increase of infected cells may occur every 3 days. About 12 days after infection, a proportion of the macroschizonts develop into microschizonts and within a day or so these produce the micromerozoites that enter erythrocytes, which after a few binary fissions produce the varied forms present in the red cells.

For completion of the life cycle, the piroplasms require to be ingested by the larvae or nymphal stages of the three-host vector, *R. appendiculatus*. In these, the sexual phase described above occurs in the tick gut followed by the formation of sporoblasts in the salivary glands. No further development occurs until the next stage of the tick starts to feed when the sporoblasts produce infective sporozoites from about day 4 onwards. Since female ticks feed continuously for about 10 days and males intermittently over a longer period, this allows ample time for infection of the host. Transmission is transtadial, i.e. by the next stage of the tick, and transovarian transmission does not occur. The incubation period following tick transmission is 8–24 days.

Geographical distribution: East and central Africa

Pathogenesis: The sequence of events in a typical acute and fatal infection progresses through three phases, each spanning about 1 week. The first is the incubation period of about 1 week when neither parasite nor lesions can be detected. This is followed during the second week by marked hyperplasia and expansion of the infected lymphoblast population, initially in the regional lymph node draining the site of the tick bite and ultimately throughout the body. During the third week, there is a phase of lymphoid depletion and disorganisation associated with massive lymphocytolysis and depressed leucopoiesis. The cause of the lymphocytolysis is unknown, but is due perhaps to the activation of 'natural killer' cells, like macrophages.

T. parva lawrencei is transmitted from the African buffalo and becomes indistinguishable in its behaviour from *T. parva parva* following several passages in cattle.

Clinical signs: About 1 week after infection, in a fully susceptible animal, the lymph node draining the area of tick bite, usually the parotid, becomes enlarged and the animal becomes pyrexic (40–41.7°C; 104–107°F). Within a few days there is generalised swelling of the superficial lymph nodes, ears, eyes and submandibular regions, the animal becomes anorexic, shows decreased milk production and rapidly loses condition, ceases rumination, becomes weak, with a rapid heartbeat, and petechial haemorrhages may occur under the tongue and on the vulva. Affected animals become emaciated and dyspnoeic and there is terminal diarrhoea, often blood-stained. Recumbency and death almost invariably occur, usually within 3 weeks of infection. Occasionally nervous signs, the so-called 'turning sickness', have been reported and attributed to the presence of meronts in cerebral capillaries.

Milder infections show a mild fever lasting 3–7 days, listlessness and swelling of superficial lymph nodes.

Diagnosis: East coast fever only occurs where *R. appendiculatus* is present, although occasionally outbreaks outwith such areas have been recorded due to the introduction of tick-infected cattle from an enzootic area. In sick animals, macroschizonts are readily detected in biopsy smears of lymph nodes and in dead animals in impression smears of lymph nodes and spleen. In advanced cases, Giemsa-stained blood smears show piroplasms in the red cells, up to 80% of which may be parasitised.

The indirect fluorescent antibody test is of value in detecting cattle, which have recovered from east coast fever.

Pathology: Necropsy during the terminal phase shows lymph nodes are to be swollen with atrophy of the cellular content of the lymph nodes and variable hyperaemia. The spleen is usually enlarged with soft pulp and prominent Malpighian corpuscles. The liver is enlarged, friable, brownish yellow, with parenchymatous degeneration. The kidneys are either congested or pale brown, with variable number of infarcts. The meninges may be slightly congested. The heart is flabby with petechiae on the epicardium and endocardium. The lungs are often congested and oedematous. There may be hydrothorax and hydropericardium, and the kidney capsule may contain a large amount of serous fluid. There may be petechiae in the visceral and parietal pleura, adrenal cortex, urinary bladder and mediastinum. There are characteristic ulcers 2–5 mm or more in diameter in the abomasum, small and large intestines. Peyer's patches are swollen, and the intestinal contents yellowish.

Epidemiology: Since the tick vector, *R. appendiculatus*, is most active following the onset of rain, outbreaks of east coast fever may be seasonal or, where rainfall is relatively constant, may occur at any time. Fortunately, indigenous cattle reared in endemic areas show a high degree of resistance and, although transient mild infection occurs in early life, mortality is negligible. The mechanism of this resistance is unknown. However, such cattle may remain carriers and act as a reservoir of infection for ticks. Susceptible cattle introduced into such areas suffer high mortality, irrespective of age or breed, unless rigid precautions are observed.

In areas where the survival of the tick vector is marginal, challenge is low and indigenous cattle may have little immunity. Such areas, during a prolonged period of rain, may become ecologically suitable for the survival and proliferation of the ticks, ultimately resulting in disastrous outbreaks of east coast fever. In some parts of east and central Africa where populations of cattle and wild African buffalo overlap there is an additional epidemiological complication due to the presence of a strain of *T. parva*, known as *T. parva lawrencei*. This occurs naturally in African buffalo, many of which remain as carriers. The tick vector is also *R. appendiculatus* and, in cattle, the disease causes high mortality. Since infected ticks may survive for nearly 2 years, physical contact between buffalo and cattle need not be close.

Treatment: Although the tetracyclines have a therapeutic effect if given at the time of infection, they are of no value in the treatment of clinical cases.

The drugs of choice in clinical cases of east coast fever are the naphthaquinone compounds parvaquone and buparvaquone and the anti-coccidial drug halofuginone.

Control: Traditionally, the control of east coast fever in areas where improved cattle are raised has relied on legislation to control the movement of cattle, on fencing to prevent access by nomadic cattle and buffalo and on repeated treatment of cattle with acaricides. In areas of high challenge, such treatments may require to be carried out twice weekly in order to kill the tick before the infective sporozoites develop in the salivary glands. This is not only expensive, but creates a population of fully susceptible cattle; if the acaricide fails, through human error or the acquisition of acaricide resistance by the ticks, the consequences can be disastrous.

Great efforts have been made to develop a suitable vaccine, but these have been thwarted by the complex immunological mechanisms involved in immunity to east coast fever and by the discovery of immunologically different strains of *T. parva* in the field. However, an 'infection and treatment' regime which involves the concurrent injection of a virulent stabilate of *T. parva* and long-acting tetracycline has been shown to be successful, although it has not been used on a large scale as yet. Apparently, the tetracycline slows the rate of schizogony, giving the immune response time to develop.

Notes: Because of the wide distribution of its tick vector, *Rhipicephalus*, and the fact that infection in cattle introduced into enzootic areas can be associated with a mortality of 100%, *T. parva* infection is an immense obstacle to livestock improvement.

Theileria annulata

Common name: Mediterranean theileriosis, Mediterranean coast fever

Predilection site: Blood and lymphatics

Parasite class: Sporozoasida

Family: Theileriidae

Description: Trophozoite forms in the erythrocyte are predominently round (0.5–2.7 μm) to oval (2 × 0.6 μm), but may also be rod-shaped or comma-shaped (1.2 × 0.5 μm). Division by binary fission may form two or four daughter cells, the latter in the shape of a cross. Koch bodies are in the lymphocytes of the spleen or lymph nodes or even free in these organs. They average 8 μm but can be up to 27 μm. Two types have been described: macromeronts containing chromatin granules 0.4–1.9 μm in diameter; these divide further to become micromeronts that contain chromatin granules 0.3–0.8 μm in diameter and produce merozoites 0.7–1 μm in diameter.

Hosts: Cattle, domestic buffalo

Life cycle: Erythrocytic merozoites, ingested by the tick intermediate host, develop into macro- and microgamonts to produce zygotes. These develop and enter the haemolymph to become kinetes, which then enter the salivary glands to become fission bodies. In adult ticks, the primary fission bodies divide into secondary (primary sporoblasts) and tertiary (secondary sporoblasts) fission bodies and produce sporozoites that are released into the saliva. Cattle are infected when the ticks suck blood. The sporozoites enter lymphocytes and become meronts, initially macromeronts, and then micromeronts. Micromerozoites enter erythrocytes, and after a few binary fissions produce the varied forms that are taken up by other ticks. The incubation period following tick transmission is 9–25 days (mean 15 days).

Geographical distribution: Mediterranean countries (Portugal and Spain, the Balkans), the Middle East, Indian subcontinent and China

Pathogenesis: The pathogenesis and clinical signs are initially similar to those of east coast fever with pyrexia and lymph node enlargement, but in the late stages there is a haemolytic anaemia and often icterus. Convalescence is protracted in those cases that recover.

Clinical signs: In the acute form there is fever (40–41.7°C; 104–107°F), inappetence, cessation of rumination, rapid heartbeat, weakness, decreased milk production, swelling of superficial lymph nodes and eyelids, diarrhoea (containing blood and mucus), jaundice and petecchial haemorrhages. Affected animals become emaciated and death can occur. In the more chronic form there is intermittent fever, inappetence, emaciation, anaemia and jaundice.

Diagnosis: Diagnosis depends on the detection of meronts in both lymph node biopsy specimens and, unlike *T. parva*, in blood smears. A low-grade piroplasm parasitaemia, in the absence of schizonts, is usually indicative of a recovered carrier animal.

Pathology: The lymph nodes are often but not always swollen; the spleen is often much enlarged and infarcts are usually present in the kidneys. The lungs are usually oedematous; characteristic ulcers are present in the abomasum, small and large intestines.

Epidemiology: *T. annulata* is transmitted transtadially by ticks of the genus *Hyalomma*. *Hyalomma detritum* in north Africa; *H. detritum* and *H. excavatum* in the former Soviet States; *H. truncatum* in parts of Africa; *H. dromedarii* in central Asia; *H. excavatum, H. turanicum* and *H. marginatum* in Asia Minor; *H. marginatum* in India; and *H. longicornis* in Siberia and the Far East. Like east coast fever, indigenous cattle in endemic areas are relatively resistant while improved cattle, particularly European breeds, are highly susceptible. However, unlike east coast fever, the disease in such cattle is not uniformly fatal, although the mortality rate may reach 70%.

Congenital infection can occur occasionally in calves.

Treatment: *See T. parva*

Control: In many areas, the prevention of *T. annulata* infection in imported dairy stock is based on permanent housing. However this is expensive and there is always the possibility that infected ticks may be brought in with the fodder to cause disease and colonise crevices in the cattle accommodation. In some countries immunisation with meronts attenuated by prolonged *in vitro* culture has given excellent results.

Theileria orientalis complex

Synonyms: *Theileria mutans*, *Theileria buffeli*, *Theileria sergenti*

Common name: Benign theileriosis

Predilection site: Blood

Parasite class: Sporozoasida

Family: Theileriidae

Description: Trophozoite forms in erythrocytes are round (1–2 μm diameter), oval (1.5 × 0.6 μm), pyriform, comma-shaped or *Anaplasma*-like (Fig. 2.43). Binary fission produces two or four daughter cells. There are relatively few Koch bodies (8–20 μm) in the lymphocytes of the spleen and lymph nodes, which contain 1–80 chromatin granules (1–2 μm in diameter).

Hosts: Cattle

Life cycle: As for *T. annulata*

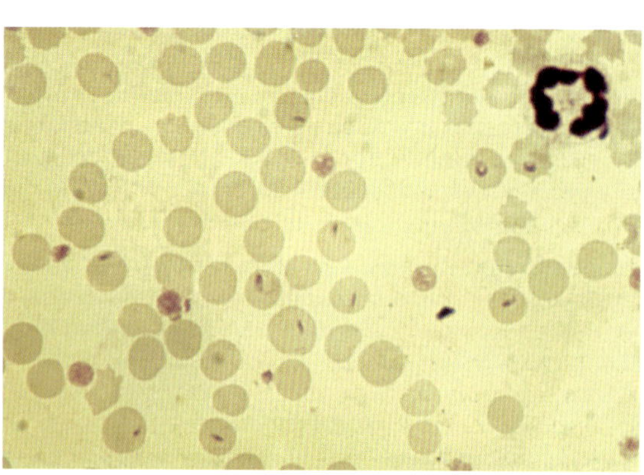

Fig. 2.43 Intraerythrocytic stages of *Theileria mutans.*

Geographical distribution: Southern Europe, Middle East, Asia, Australia

Pathogenesis: Mildly pathogenic

Clinical signs: Similar in appearance to the mild form of *T. annulata* causing anaemia, with jaundice and lymphadenopathy occasionally present.

Diagnosis: Giemsa-stained blood smears may show piroplasms in the red cells, or macroschizonts may be detected in biopsy smears of lymph nodes.

Pathology: In acute cases the spleen and liver are swollen, the lungs may be oedematous and there are characteristic ulcers in the abomasum, and infarcts may be present in the kidneys. Macroschizonts may also be found in impression smears of lymph nodes and spleen taken from dead animals.

Epidemiology: Vectors are *Ambylomma variegatum*, *A. cohaerens*, *A. haebraeum. Haemaphysalis bispinosa* and *H. bancrofti* are the probable vectors in Australia.

Treatment: Little information is available on treatment although the drugs of choice in clinical cases are likely to be parvaquone and buparvaquone.

Control: Tick control methods may be considered including fencing and dipping or cleaning cattle of ticks but these are not usually required.

Notes: The taxonomy of benign theileriosis species is complicated and it is now considered that *T. orientalis* is part of a complex with *T. sergenti*, *T. buffeli* and *T. mutans*.

Theileria taurotragi

Synonym: *Cytauxzoon taurotragi*

Predilection site: Blood

Parasite class: Sporozoasida

Family: Theileriidae

Description: Erythrocytic forms are similar in appearance to *T. parva*. Trophozoite forms in the erythrocyte are predominently round to oval, but may also be rod-shaped or comma-shaped (1.2 × 0.5 μm).

Hosts: Cattle, antelope, particularly the eland (*Taurotragi oryx*)

Life cycle: As for *T. annulata*

Geographical distribution: Africa

Pathogenesis: Mildly pathogenic

Clinical signs: Mild transient fever and anaemia

Diagnosis: Presence of erythrocytic forms in blood smears or meronts in lymph node biopsy specimens.

Morphologically indistinguishable from more pathogenic forms, but generally differentiated on clinical signs and history.

Pathology: Meront stages have been reported in liver, lung and lymph nodes.

Epidemiology: Vectors are *Rhipicephalus appendiculatus* and *R. pulchellus*.

Treatment and control: Not usually required

Theileria velifera

Synonym: *Haematoxenus veliferus*

Predilection site: Blood

Parasite class: Sporozoasida

Family: Theileriidae

Description: Trophozoite forms in erythrocytes are pleomorphic and most often appear as small rods 1–2 μm long. The great majority have a rectangular 'veil' 1–3.5 μm extending out from the side.

Hosts: Cattle, zebu

Life cycle: As for *T. annulata*

Geographical distribution: Africa

Pathogenesis: Non-pathogenic

Clinical signs: Not reported

Diagnosis: Giemsa-stained blood smears may show the characteristic 'veiled' piroplasms in the red cells.

Pathology: No associated pathology

Epidemiology: Known vectors are *Ambylomma variegatum*, *A. lepidu* and *A. haebraeum*.

Treatment and control: Not usually required

RICKETTSIALES

Several rickettsial organisms are of importance in cattle.

Anaplasma marginale

Predilection site: Blood

Order: Rickettsiales

Family: Anaplasmataceae

Description: In Giemsa-stained blood films the organisms of *A. marginale* are seen as small, round, dark red 'inclusion bodies' approximately 0.3–1.0 μm within the red cell (Fig. 2.44). Often there is only one organism in a red cell and characteristically this lies at the outer margin; however these two features are not constant.

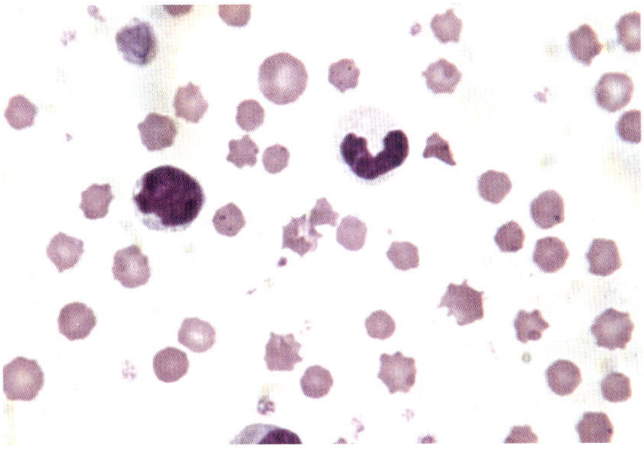

Fig. 2.44 Intraerythrocytic stages of *Anaplasma marginale*.

Hosts: Cattle, sheep, goat, wild ruminants

Life cycle: *Anaplasma* can be transmitted by ticks, and also mechanically by biting flies or contaminated surgical instruments. Once in the blood, the organism enters the red cell by invaginating the cell membrane so that a vacuole is formed; thereafter it divides to form an inclusion body containing up to eight 'initial bodies' packed together. The inclusion bodies are most numerous during the acute phase of the infection, but some persist for years afterwards.

Geographical distribution: Africa, southern Europe, Australia, South America, Asia, former Soviet states and USA

Pathogenesis: Typically, the changes are those of an acute febrile reaction accompanied by a severe haemolytic anaemia. After an incubation period of around 4 weeks, fever and parasitaemia appear, and as the latter develops, the anaemia becomes more severe so that within a week or so up to 70% of the erythrocytes are destroyed. The clinical signs are usually very mild in naive cattle under 1 year old. Thereafter, susceptibility increases so that cattle aged 2–3 years develop typical and often fatal anaplasmosis, while in cattle over 3 years the disease is often peracute and frequently fatal.

Clinical signs: Clinical signs are attributed to severe anaemia and include depression, weakness, fever, laboured breathing, inappetance, dehydration, constipation and jaundice. The acute stage of the disease is characterised by fever (39.4–41.7°C; 103–107°F) that persists for 3–7 days. During the febrile phase there is decreased rumination, dryness of the muzzle, loss of appetite, dullness and depression. Lactating cows show a depression in milk yield and abortion is a common feature in advanced pregnancy. The severity of the disease increases with age, with animals over 3 years of age showing the peracute and possibly fatal disease.

Diagnosis: The clinical signs supplemented, if possible, by a haematocrit estimation and the demonstration of *Anaplasma* inclusions in the red cells, are usually sufficient for diagnosis. For the detection of immune carriers, complement fixation and agglutination tests are available; an indirect fluorescent antibody test and DNA probe have also been developed.

Pathology: Gross pathological lesions are those usually associated with anaemia. Mucous membranes are jaundiced and there is pallor of the tissues. The spleen is often greatly enlarged with enlarged splenic follicles. The liver may be enlarged with rounded borders. The gallbladder is enlarged and obstructed with dark, thick bile. Petechiae may be observed on the epicardium, pericardium, pleura and diaphragm. The lymph glands are enlarged. Microscopically there is hyperplasia of the bone marrow. The spleen shows a decrease of lymphoblasts and increased vacuolation and degeneration of reticular cells and there is reduction of the white pulp and accumulation of pigment resembling haemosiderin.

Epidemiology: The organism is distributed throughout the tropics corresponding to the distribution of the main tick vectors, *Boophilus annulatus, B. decolaratus* and *B. microplus*. In the USA, the main tick vectors are *Dermacentor andersoni, D. occidentalis* and *D. variabilis*. Horse flies (Tabanidae), stable flies (*Stomoxys*), deer flies (*Chrysops*), horn flies and mosquitoes have also been incriminated as potential vectors. Reservoirs of infection are maintained in carrier cattle and in wild ruminants such as deer. Cattle, especially adults, introduced into endemic areas are particularly susceptible, the mortality rate being up to 80%. In contrast, cattle reared in endemic areas are much less susceptible, presumably due to previous exposure when young, although their acquired immunity usually co-exists with a carrier state. This balance may, on occasions, be disturbed and clinical anaplasmosis supervenes when cattle are stressed by other diseases, such as babesiosis.

Treatment: Tetracycline compounds are effective in treatment if given early in the course of the disease and especially before the parasitaemia has reached its peak. More recently, imidocarb has been shown to be effective and may also be used to sterilise carrier animals.

Control: Vaccination of susceptible stock with small quantities of blood containing the mildly pathogenic *A. centrale* or a relatively avirulent strain of *A. marginale* is practised in several countries, any clinical signs in adults being controlled by drugs. In the USA, a killed *A. marginale* vaccine containing erythrocyte stroma is also available. Although all are generally successful in the clinical sense, challenged cattle become carriers and so perpetuate transmission. The killed vaccine has the disadvantage that antibodies produced to the red cell stroma, if transferred in the colostrum, may produce isoerythrolysis in nursing calves. Improved inactivated vaccines are currently under development. Otherwise, control at present depends largely on the reduction of ticks and biting flies.

Anaplasma centrale

Predilection site: Blood

Order: Rickettsiales

Family: Anaplasmataceae

Description: As for *A. marginale*, except that the organisms are commonly found in the centre of the erythrocyte.

Hosts: Cattle, wild ruminants, and perhaps sheep, may act as reservoirs of infection.

Geographical distribution: Worldwide in tropics and subtropics including southern Europe. It is also present in some temperate areas, including parts of the USA.

Pathogenesis: Similar to *A. marginale* but generally considered to be less pathogenic.

Clinical signs: The clinical features include pyrexia, anaemia and often jaundice, anorexia, laboured breathing and in cows, a severe drop in milk yield or abortion. Occasionally peracute cases occur, which usually die within a day of the onset of clinical signs.

Pathology: Necropsy at this time often reveals a jaundiced carcase, a grossly enlarged gallbladder and, on section, a liver suffused with bile. The spleen and lymph nodes are enlarged and congested and there are petechial haemorrhages in the heart muscle. The urine, unlike that in babesiosis, is normal in colour. In survivors, recovery is prolonged.

Epidemiology: Apart from the various modes of transmission described above, little information is available. Reservoirs of infection are maintained in carrier cattle and perhaps in wild ruminants or sheep. Cattle, especially adults, introduced into endemic areas are particularly susceptible, the mortality rate being up to 80%. In contrast, cattle reared in endemic areas are much less susceptible, presumably due to previous exposure when young, although their acquired immunity usually co-exists with a carrier state. This balance may, on occasions be disturbed and clinical anaplasmosis supervenes when cattle are stressed by other diseases, such as babesiosis.

Details on the life cycle, diagnosis, treatment and control are as for *A. marginale.*

Anaplasma phagocytophilum

Synonym: *Anoplasma phagocytophilia, Ehrlichia phagocytophilia, Cytoecetes phagocytophilia*

Common name: Tick-borne fever, pasture fever, canine granulocytic ehrlichiosis, human granulocytic ehrlichiosis, equine granulocytic ehrlichiosis

Predilection site: Blood

Order: Rickettsiales

Family: Rickettsiaceae

For more detailed description see Chapter 3 (Sheep and goats).

Ehrlichia bovis

Predilection site: Blood

Order: Rickettsiales

Family: Rickettsiaceae

Description: Round or irregular-shaped intracytoplasmic organisms (2–10 μm in diameter), present in mononuclear cells, particularly monocytes.

Hosts: Cattle

Life cycle: Infection is transmitted through the bite of an infected tick. Rickettsiae multiply within monocytes forming morulae. The incubation period is reported to be 15–18 days.

Geographical distribution: Africa, Middle East (Turkey, Iran), India, Sri Lanka

Pathogenesis: Has been associated with acute and fatal disease in some regions of Africa.

Clinical signs: Affected animals show anorexia, weakness, muscular trembling, drunken gait and bulging eyes.

Diagnosis: The rickettsiae can be demonstrated by staining blood or organ smears with Giemsa.

Pathology: In fatal cases there is hydropericardium, hydrothorax, splenomegaly and swollen lymph nodes. Monocytosis may occur in terminal infections.

Epidemiology: Transmitted by ticks of the genera *Hyalomma*, *Rhipicephalus* and *Ambylomma*. Known vectors are *Hyalomma anatolicum*, *Rhipicephalus appendiculatus*, *Ambylomma cajennense* and possibly *A. variegatum*.

Treatment: Little information is available although, as with other member of this group, tetracyclines may be effective.

Control: Specific control measures have not been reported but tick control may assist in preventing infection with *E. bovis*.

Ehrlichia ruminantium

Synonym: *Cowdria ruminantum*

Common name: Heartwater, cowdriosis, malkopsiekte (Afrikaans)

Predilection site: Blood

Order: Rickettsiales

Family: Rickettsiaceae

Description: Organisms are seen as close-packed colonies consisting of less than ten to many hundred cocci. The organism varies in size from 0.2 μm to greater than 1.5 μm. The diameter of individual organisms in a given cluster is rather uniform but groups are very pleomorphic. The small granules tend to be coccoid, with larger ones looking like rings, horseshoes, rods and irregular masses.

Hosts: Cattle, sheep, goats and wild ruminants

Life cycle: *Ehrlichia ruminantium* is transmitted by at least five species of *Amblyomma* ticks. In the ruminant host it is first found in reticuloendothelial cells and then parasitises vascular endothelial cells. Division is by binary fission and it produces morula-like colonies in the cytoplasm of infected cells.

Geographical distribution: Africa, south of the Sahara; Caribbean (Guadeloupe, Marie-Galante and Antigua)

Pathogenesis: The pathogenesis of the disease is far from clear. Hydropericardium may lead to cardiac insufficiency and hydrothorax and pulmonary oedema to respiratory difficulties. Oedema is often so pronounced in peracute heartwater that it is responsible for sudden death by asphyxia. The occasional sudden fall in plasma volume preceding death has been associated with the development of the transudates. Brain lesions are not consistent enough to explain the nervous symptoms.

Clinical signs: The average natural incubation period is 2 weeks, but can vary from 10 days to 1 month. In most cases, heartwater is an acute febrile disease, with a sudden rise in body temperature; temperature may exceed 41°C within 1–2 days. It remains high with small fluctuations and drops shortly before death.

A peracute form occurs in exotic breeds introduced into an endemic region. The animal appears clinically normal, but if examined will have a marked pyrexia. It may then suddenly collapse, go into convulsions and die. Thoracic auscultation will often reveal oedema in the lungs and bronchi.

In the acute form, fever is followed by inappetence, sometimes listlessness, diarrhoea, particularly in cattle and dyspnoea indicative of lung oedema. The course of infection is 3–6 days and consists of pyrexia (often over 41°C; 106°F). A mild cough may be heard and, on auscultation, hydrothorax, hydropericardium and lung oedema are noted. A profuse diarrhoea is often present or there may be blood in the faeces. Nervous signs develop gradually. The animal is restless, walks in circles, makes sucking movements and stands rigidly with tremors of the superficial muscles. Cattle may push their head against a wall or present aggressive or anxious behaviour. Finally, the animal falls to the ground, pedalling and exhibiting opisthotonos, nystagmus and chewing movements. The animal usually dies during or following such a nervous attack.

In the subacute form, the signs are like those of the acute form but they are much less severe with a transient fever and sometimes diarrhoea. Disease may last for over a week and the animal usually improves gradually but a few cases progress to collapse and death. This is often the most severe form seen in indigenous cattle, and those previously infected. In these stock symptoms are usually absent.

Diagnosis: There is no specific method for diagnosis in the living animal. A tentative diagnosis of heartwater is based on the presence of *Amblyomma* vectors, of clinical nervous signs, and of transudates in the pericardium and thorax at postmortem examination. Provisional indication can be from the history and clinical signs. Lymph node material can be aspirated to examine for vacuoles containing organisms in the cytoplasm of the reticular cells. Serum can be examined using a capillary flocculation test. A number of serological tests have been described but all suffer from false-positive reactions due to cross-reactions with other *Ehrlichia* species.

Diagnosis is easier at postmortem as the organism can be discerned in brain tissue capillaries that have been fixed in methyl alcohol and stained with Giemsa. Typical colonies of *E. ruminantium* can be observed in brain smears made after death. Slides are examined for the presence of the characteristic colonies. Experience is required to differentiate from other haemoparasites *(Babesia bovis)*, certain blood cells (thrombocytes, granulocytes), normal subcellular structures (mitochondria, mast cell granules), or stain artefacts (stain precipitates), etc. The specificity of the reading can be improved by staining formalin-fixed brain sections using immunoperoxidase techniques. Transmission electron microscopy (TEM) can be used to demonstrate organisms inside a vacuole-like structure, which is surrounded by a membrane in the endothelial cell's cytoplasm.

Differential clinical diagnosis should be made with anthrax, theileriosis, anaplasmosis, botulism, and, in nervous cases rabies, tetanus, strychnine poisoning, cerebral theileriosis, cerebral babesiosis and hypomagnesaemia.

Pathology: The lesions present are very variable and not pathognomonic. In the peracute form there are few gross lesions, but in some there is marked lung oedema with tracheal and bronchial fluids. In the acute form the most common macroscopic lesions are hydropericardium, hydrothorax, pulmonary oedema, intestinal congestion, oedema of the mediastinal and bronchial lymph nodes, petechiae on the epicardium and endocardium, congestion of the brain, and moderate splenomegaly. The liver is often engorged, with the gallbladder distended. The spleen is occasionally enlarged. There may be congestion of the meningeal blood vessels.

Epidemiology: Distribution of heartwater coincides with that of the *Amblyomma* ticks, which require a warm humid climate and bushy grass. A number of African species of the genus *Amblyomma* (*A. haebrum*, *A. variegatum*, *A. pomposum*, *A.gemma*, *A.lepidum*, *A. tholloni*, *A. sparsum*, *A. astrion*, *A. cohaerens*, *A. marmoreum*) and American species (*A. maculatum*, *A. cajennense*, *A. dissimile*) are able to transmit infection. Transmission usually appears to be transtadial although transovarian transmission can occur more rarely. The level of infection is often unknown as indigenous domestic and wild animals often show no signs. It is only when susceptible exotic species are introduced that infection becomes apparent. Besides cattle, sheep, goats, Asian buffalo, antelopes and deer are susceptible to infection and disease. Indigenous cattle undergo inapparent infection. Calves under 3 weeks old, even from susceptible stock, are difficult to infect. Heartwater can occur throughout the year, but incidence declines in the dry season due to reduced tick activity. The incubation period is variable, from 7 to 28 days, with fever starting on average after 18 days. Mortality can be up to 60% in exotic breeds, but less than 5% in local cattle.

Treatment: Therapy is most effective when carried out early in disease. Tetracyclines can be used and do not interfere with development of immunity.

Control: Prevention is aimed at controlling the tick vector by dipping cattle at weekly intervals with reliable acaricides. However, the ticks of the genus *Ambylomma* are less susceptible than those from other genera. As the tick may transmit infection after 24 hours on the host, better control is obtained by applying acaricide by dipping or spraying every

3 days. Resistance to organophosphorus and arsenic has been reported. Care should also be taken not to introduce *Amblyomma* on infected animals or in forage to uninfected cows.

In areas where disease is endemic most cattle are immune. A carrier state develops after infection and remains for several weeks. Non-infected resistance persists a variable time, lasting from a few months to several years. After this time reinfection can occur.

The only method of immunisation is an infection and treatment method using infected blood or homogenised pre-fed infected ticks followed by tetracycline treatment as soon as pyrexia develops.

Notes: Heartwater is one of the main obstacles to the improvement of livestock productivity in sub-Saharan Africa. It was first recognised as a major disease in southern Africa after the introduction of exotic breeds. Its importance depends to a very large extent on the type of livestock present. There are very few reliable figures about its importance in local breeds in endemic areas. However, there is no doubt that in endemic areas indigenous cattle are far more resistant than exotic or crossbred cattle, presumably because of natural selection. In contrast, small ruminants in general, and goats in particular, are not always very resistant.

The name heartwater was used because hydropericardium was regarded as a pathognomonic lesion of the disease. The disease is still also generally known as 'cowdriosis'.

Eperythrozoon wenyonii

Synonym: *Candidatus Mycoplasma wenyonii*

Predilection site: Blood

Order: Rickettsiales

Family: Rickettsiaceae

Description: Coccoid, ring- or rod-shaped structures on the surface of red cells, blue to purple when stained (see diagnosis).

Hosts: Cattle

Geographical distribution: Worldwide

Pathogenesis: Typically, present on red cells, it produces mild and clinically inapparent infections in a variety of domestic animals throughout the world.

Clinical signs: *E. wenyonii* is occasionally responsible for fever, anaemia and loss of weight

Diagnosis: Identification of parasites from staining artefacts requires good blood films and filtered Giemsa stain. They appear as cocci or short rods on the surface of the erythrocytes, often completely surrounding the margin of the red cell. However, the organisms of *Eperythrozoon* are relatively loosely attached to the red cell surface and are often found free in the plasma.

Epidemiology: Vectors are thought to be involved in transmission but precise details are not known.

Treatment: Susceptible to tetracyclines.

Control: Lack of detailed knowledge on the vectors limits any vector control measures.

Notes: The taxonomy of this species is subject to much debate and there is a proposal to re-classify it into the bacterial genus *Mycoplasma* (class Mollicutes) based on 16s rRNA gene sequences and phylogenetic analysis.

Rickettsia conorii

Common name: Boutonneuse fever, Mediterranean spotted fever, Indian tick typhus, east African tick typhus

Predilection site: Blood

Order: Rickettsiales

Family: Rickettsiaceae

For more detailed description see Chapter 6 (Dogs and cats).

PARASITES OF THE NERVOUS SYSTEM

Taenia multiceps

See Chapter 6 (Dogs and cats).

Thelazia rhodesi

Common name: Cattle eyeworm

Predilection site: Eye, conjunctival sac, lachrymal duct

Parasite class: Nematoda

Superfamily: Spiruroidea

Description, gross: Small thin yellowish white worms, 1.0–2.0 cm long. Males are 8–12 mm and females are 12–20 mm.

Description, microscopic: A mouth capsule is present and the cuticle has prominent striations at the anterior end.

Final host: Cattle, buffalo, occasionally sheep, goat

Intermediate host: Muscid flies, particularly *Fannia* spp.

Life cycle: The worms are viviparous. The L_1 passed by the female worm into the lachrymal secretion is ingested by the fly intermediate host as it feeds. Development from L_1 to L_3 occurs in the ovarian follicles of the fly in 15–30 days during the summer months. L_3 migrate to the mouthparts of the fly and are transferred to the final host when the fly feeds. Development in the eye takes place without further migration. The prepatent period is 20–25 days.

Geographical distribution: Worldwide

Pathogenesis: Lesions are caused by the serrated cuticle of the worm and most damage results from movement by the active young adults causing lachrymation, followed by conjunctivitis. In heavy infections the cornea may become cloudy and ulcerated. There is usually complete recovery in about 2 months, although in some cases areas of corneal opacity can persist. Infection may predispose to infectious keratoconjunctivitis ('pink eye') caused by *Moraxella*.

Clinical signs: Lachrymation, conjunctivitis and photophobia. Flies are usually clustered around the eye because of the excessive secretion. In severe cases, the whole cornea can be opaque and without treatment, progressive keratitis and ulceration of the cornea may occur.

Diagnosis: The presence of a conjunctivitis that is coincident with the season of fly activity is an indication of possible infection. In some cases the *Thelazia* worms may be seen on the surface of the conjunctiva or in the conjunctival sac. Sometimes eggs or larvae can be recovered from lachrymal secretions. It may be necessary to instil a few drops of local anaesthetic to facilitate manipulation of the third eyelid.

Pathology: Invasion of the lachrymal gland and ducts may cause inflammation and necrotic exudation leading to occlusion and reduced tear production. Mechanical irritation of the conjunctivitis produces inflammation, whilst damage to the cornea leads to opacity, keratitis and corneal ulceration.

Epidemiology: *Thelazia* infections occur seasonally and are linked to periods of maximum fly activity. The parasite can survive in the eye for several years, but since it is only the young adult which is pathogenic a reservoir of infection may persist in symptomless carrier cattle. Survival of larvae also occurs in the pupal stages of flies during the winter.

Treatment: Treatment was at one time based on manual removal of the worms under a local anaesthetic, but this is now replaced by administering an effective anthelmintic such as levamisole or an avermectin; the former drug may be applied topically as a 1% aqueous solution.

Control: Prevention is difficult because of the ubiquitous nature of the fly vectors. Fly control measures aimed at protecting the face, such as insecticide-impregnated ear tags, aid in the control of eyeworm infection.

Two other species of eyeworm are found in cattle. Details are essentially similar to *T. rhodesi*.

Thelazia gulosa

Synonym: *Thelazia alfortensis*

Common name: Cattle eyeworm

Predilection site: Eye, conjunctival sac and lachrymal duct

Parasite class: Nematoda

Superfamily: Spiruroidea

Geographical distribution: Probably worldwide

Thelazia skrjabini

Common name: Cattle eyeworm

Predilection site: Eye, conjunctival sac and lachrymal duct

Parasite class: Nematoda

Superfamily: Spiruroidea

Geographical distribution: North America, parts of Asia and Europe

Hypoderma bovis

See details under Parasites of the integument.

Toxoplasma gondii

See details and description under Parasites of the locomotory system.

Trypanosoma brucei brucei

See details and description under Parasites of the circulatory system.

PARASITES OF THE REPRODUCTIVE/ UROGENITAL SYSTEM

Stephanurus dentatus

Common name: Pig kidney worm

Predilection site: Kidney, peri-renal fat

Parasite class: Nematoda

Superfamily: Strongyloidea

Hosts: Pig, wild boar, rarely cattle

Pathogenesis: *Stephanurus* may occasionally cause severe liver damage in calves grazing on contaminated ground.

For a more detailed description see Chapter 5 (Pigs).

Tritrichomonas foetus

Synonym: *Trichomonas foetus*

Predilection site: Prepuce, uterus

Parasite class: Zoomastigophorasida

Family: Trichomonadidae

Description: The organism is pear-shaped, approximately 10–25 µm long and 3–15 µm wide and has a single nucleus and four flagella, each arising from a basal body situated at the anterior rounded end. Three of the flagella are free anteriorly, while the fourth extends backwards to form an undulating membrane along the length of the organism and then continues posteriorly as a free flagellum (Figs 2.45, 2.46). The axostyle, a hyaline rod with a skeletal function, extends the length of the cell and usually projects posteriorly. The costa is prominent but there is no pelta.

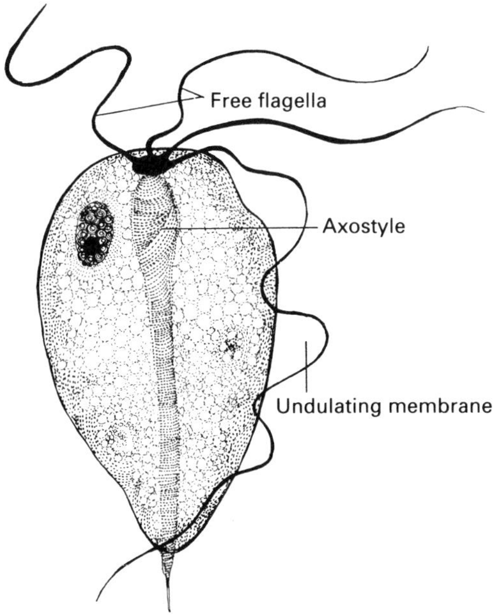

Fig. 2.45 *Tritrichomonas foetus.*

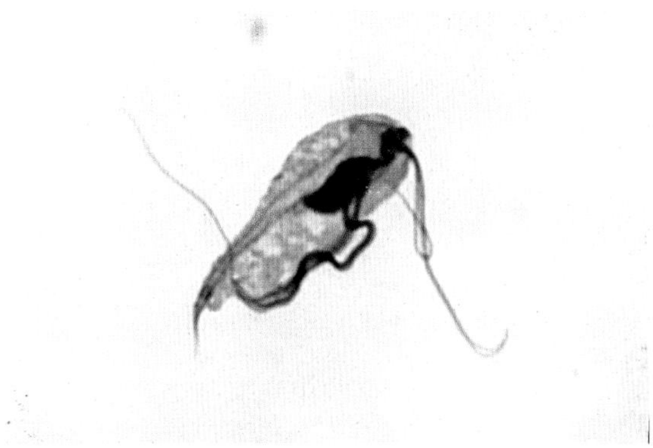

Fig. 2.46 *Tritrichomonas foetus* showing three anterior flagella and trailing posterior flagellum.

In fresh preparations, the organism is motile and progresses by rolling jerky movements, the flickering flagella and the movements of the undulating membrane being readily seen. Occasionally, rounded immobile forms are observed and these are possibly effete.

Hosts: Cattle

Life cycle: The trichomonads reproduce by longitudinal binary fission. No sexual stages are known and there are no cysts. Transmission occurs during coitus.

Geographical distribution: Worldwide. However, the prevalence has now decreased dramatically in areas where artificial insemination is widely practised and in Britain, for example, the disease is now probably extinct.

Pathogenesis: In the bull, a preputial discharge associated with small nodules on the preputial and penile membranes may develop shortly after infection. Organisms are present in small numbers in the preputial cavity of bulls, with some concentration in the fornix and around the glans penis. The chronically infected bull shows no gross lesions.

In the cow, the initial lesion is a vaginitis, which can be followed in animals that become pregnant by invasion of the cervix and uterus. Various sequelae can result, including a placentitis leading to early abortion (1–16 weeks), uterine discharge and pyometra. Abortion before the fourth month of pregnancy is the commonest sequel and this is normally followed by recovery. Occasionally the developing fetal membranes are retained leading to a purulent endometritis, a persistent uterine discharge and anoestrus; infrequently the corpus luteum is retained and the cervical seal remains closed, when a massive pyometra develops which visually simulates the appearance of pregnancy. In some cases, despite infection, pregnancy is not terminated by abortion and a normal, full-term calf is born.

Clinical signs: In the bull, there are no clinical signs once the infection is established. In the cow, early abortion is a characteristic feature although this is often undetected because of the small size of the fetus and the case may present as one of an irregular oestrus cycle. Other clinical signs are those of purulent endometritis or a closed pyrometra and, in these cases, the cow may become permanently sterile. On a herd basis, cows exhibit irregular oestrous cycles, uterine discharge, pyometra and early abortion. The cow usually recovers and generally becomes immune, at least for that breeding season, after infection or abortion.

Diagnosis: A tentative diagnosis of trichomonosis is based on the clinical history, signs of early abortion, repeated returns to service, or irregular oestrous cycles. Confirmation depends on the demonstration of organisms in placental fluid, stomach contents of the aborted fetus, uterine washings, pyometra discharge or vaginal mucus. Apart from a problem of infertility, which usually follows the purchase of a mature bull, confirmation of diagnosis depends on the demonstration of the organism. Vaginal mucus collected from the anterior end of the vagina by suction into a sterile tube, or preputial washings from the bull, may be examined using a warm-stage microscope for the presence of organisms. The number of organisms varies in different situations. They are numerous in the aborted fetus, in the uterus several days after abortion, and, in recently infected cows, they are plentiful in the vaginal mucus 12–20 days after infection. Thereafter the number of organisms varies according to the phase of the oestrous cycle, being highest 3–7 days after ovulation. In the infected bull *T. foetus* organisms are present in highest numbers on the mucosa of the prepuce and penis, apparently not invading the submucosal tissues. It is generally recommended to allow 1 week to pass after the last service before taking a preputial sample. Since the organism is often only present intermittently, the examination may require to be repeated several times. Under phase illumination, the number of flagella observed is an important characteristic as this can help to differentiate *T. foetus* from some bovine flagellates that appear similar. Organisms may be cultured *in vitro,* in Diamond's medium, Clausen's medium or *Trichomonas* medium, which is available commercially. A field culture test that allows for growth of the trichomonads and direct microscopic examination without aspiration of the inoculum has been developed in the USA (InPouch™ TF).

Alternatively, on a herd basis, samples of vaginal mucus may be examined in the laboratory for the presence of specific agglutinins against laboratory cultures of *T. foetus*.

Pathology: Infection in females causes cervicitis and endometritis leading to infertility, abortion or pyometra. The inflammatory changes in the endometrium and cervix are relatively mild and non-specific, although there may be a copious mucopurulent discharge. The exudates may be continuous or intermittent in their discharge, and the number and activity of the trichomonads can vary considerably. Abortions may occur at any time but mainly in the first half of pregnancy. There are no specific fetal lesions, but large numbers of protozoa may be found in the fetal fluids and stomach. The placenta may be covered by white or yellowish flocculent exudates in small amounts, and thickening and haemorrhage without necrosis may be evident on the cotyledons. Pyometra, when it develops, may be copious with watery exudates containing floccules which may be brownish and sticky and contain swarms of trichomonads.

Epidemiology: Bulls, once infected, remain so permanently. The organisms inhabit the preputial cavity and transmission to the cow occurs during coitus. From the vagina, the trichomonads reach the uterus via the cervix to produce a low-grade endometritis. Intermittently, organisms are flushed into the vagina, often 2 or 3 days before oestrus. Infection is usually followed by early abortion, the organisms being found in the amniotic and allantoic fluid. Subsequently cows appear to 'self cure' and, in most cases, appear to develop a sterile immunity.

Treatment: Since the disease is self-limiting in the female only symptomatic treatment and sexual rest for 3 months is normally necessary. In the bull, slaughter is the best policy, although dimetridazole orally or intravenously has been reported to be effective.

Control: Artificial insemination from non-infected donors is the only entirely satisfactory method of control. If a return to natural service is contemplated, recovered cows should be disposed of since some may be carriers.

Notes: Normally one might expect the overall prevalence of trichomonosis to be high, since it is venereally transmitted by bulls, which show no clinical signs. In fact, the advent of supervised schemes of artificial insemination has largely eradicated the disease, and today it is limited to areas where there are many small farms each with their own bulls, or to countries where veterinary supervision is limited.

In a few early studies, three serotypes were recognised based on agglutination: the '*Belfast*' strain, reportedly predominated in Europe, Africa and the USA; the '*Brisbane*' strain in Australia; and the '*Manley*' strain, which has been reported in only a few outbreaks.

Neospora caninum

Synonym: *Histoplasma gondii*

Predilection site: Blood

Order: Sporozoasida

Family: Sarcocystiidae

Description: Tachyzoites measure $6 \times 2\ \mu m$ and are usually located in the cytoplasm of cells. Tissue cysts are oval, 107 μm long, have a thick wall (up to 4 μm) and are found only in neural tissue.

Intermediate hosts: Cattle, sheep, goat

Final host: Dog

Life cycle: The complete life cycle of *Neospora caninum* has only recently been elucidated. It was previously confused with *Toxoplasma gondii* because of the structural similarity of the asexual stages of the two parasites. Similarities between the two organisms suggested that *N. caninum* was a coccidian parasite whose infective stage was an oocyst. The definitive stage has recently been shown to be dogs, which pass small numbers of oocysts in faeces from 8–23 days after infection. Tissue cysts are tachyzoites and can infect a range of animals including cattle, sheep, goats and horses. The dog can also act as an intermediate host.

Geographical distribution: Worldwide

Pathogenesis: *N. caninum* is a major cause of abortion in both dairy and beef cattle. Cows of any age can abort from 3 months of gestation to full term, although most abortions occur at 5–6 months. Fetuses can be born alive or may die *in utero* and be mummified or reabsorbed. Calves that are infected may be born underweight and with neurological symptoms such as ataxia, decreased reflexes and exophthalmia.

Infection is thought to reduce milk production in adult diary cows through its effects on fertility.

Clinical signs: Abortion, mummification, weak calves with ataxia, exophthalmia

Diagnosis: Diagnosis is based on histological examination of freshly aborted fetuses. The lesions in the heart and central nervous system (CNS) are significantly characteristic for diagnosis but can be confirmed by immunocytochemistry. An enzyme-linked immunosorbent assay (ELISA) is commercially available and can be used to test serum samples for *Neospora*-specific antibodies. The ELISA results are expressed as a percentage of a positive control included in each test: per cent positivity (PP) values. Results are negative if less than 20 PP; inconclusive if between 20 and 25 PP; and positive if greater than 25 PP.

Pathology: Tachyzoites and tissue cysts are found intracellularly in the CNS and retina of affected cattle. Although infection can be found in many organs, the commonest site is the brain. Microscopic lesions of non-suppurative encephalitis and myocarditis in aborted fetuses may be seen in the brain, spinal cord and heart. Hepatitis can also be found in epidemic abortions.

Epidemiology: The dog is the final host, and is also an intermediate host in prenatal infections. In cattle, infection can be both vertically transmitted from dam to calf *in utero* and lactogenically, naturally by ingestion of food and water contaminated with dog faeces containing *Neospora caninum* oocysts, or from cow to cow. The mechanisms of repeat congenital transmission are unknown at present.

In cattle, most abortions occur either sporadically on farms with annual abortion rates less than 3%; or as more frequent abortions on farms with annual abortion rates of 5–10%. Occasionally abortion rates may reach 30%, being more common during late summer. It is possible for cattle that have previously aborted due to *Neospora* infection to have a repeat abortion and infected cows are more likely to abort than non-infected cows. Cows infected with *N. caninum* are also likely to infect more than 95% of their calves by transplacental infection.

Treatment: There is no effective treatment in cattle.

Control: Control of *Neospora*-induced abortion in cattle depends on protecting food and water sources from possible contamination with the faeces of any animal and the disposal of aborted fetuses and placentas by incineration. The lack of complete knowledge of both the life cycle and the range of definitive hosts has limited effective control measures but there is a strong argument for the culling of seropositive animals from a herd. Seropositive animals have been shown to suffer a higher risk of abortion than seronegative animals in the herd. Dogs should not be allowed to eat aborted fetuses or fetal membranes, and their faeces should be prevented from contaminating bovine feedstuffs.

Trypanosoma brucei brucei

See details and description under Parasites of the circulatory system.

PARASITES OF THE LOCOMOTORY SYSTEM

Taenia saginata

Synonym: *Cysticercus bovis*

Common name: Beef tapeworm, 'beef measles'

Predilection site: Small intestine (definitive host); muscle, liver, kidney (intermediate host)

Parasite class: Cestoda

Family: Taeniidae

Description, gross: The adult tapeworm is found only in humans and ranges from 5.0–15.0 m in length. The scolex, exceptional among the species of *Taenia*, has neither rostellum nor hooks.

In the bovine animal the mature cysticercus, *C. bovis*, is greyish white, oval, about 0.5–1.0 × 0.5 cm long, and filled with fluid in which the scolex is usually clearly visible. As in the adult tapeworm, it has neither rostellum nor hooks.

Description, microscopic: The uterus of the gravid proglottid has 15–30 lateral branches on each side of the central stem, in contrast to that of *T. solium* with only 7–12 lateral branches. Gravid proglottids may contain around 100 000–200 000 eggs, each being approximately circular with a smooth thick shell, and measuring 30–50 × 20–30 μm.

A subspecies, *Taenia saginata asiatica*, has a rostellum and posterior protruberances on segments and 11–32 uterine buds. The metacestodes are small, about 2 mm, and have a rostellum and two rows of primitive hooks, those of the outer row being numerous and tiny.

Final host: Man

Intermediate host: Cattle

Life cycle: An infected human may pass millions of eggs daily, either free in the faeces or as intact segments each containing about 250 000 eggs, and these can survive on pasture for several months. After ingestion by a susceptible bovine, the oncosphere travels via the blood to striated muscle. It is first grossly visible about 2 weeks later as a pale, semi-transparent spot about 1.0 mm in diameter, but is not infective to man until about 12 weeks later when it has reached its full size of 1.0 cm. By then it is enclosed by the host in a thin fibrous capsule but despite this the scolex can usually still be seen. The longevity of the cysts ranges from weeks to years. When they die they are usually replaced by a caseous, crumbly mass, which may become calcified. Both living and dead cysts are frequently present in the same carcase. Humans become infected by ingesting raw, or inadequately cooked meat. Development to patency takes 2–3 months.

Geographical distribution: Worldwide. Particularly important in Africa and South America.

Pathogenesis: Although *C. bovis* may occur anywhere in the striated muscles the predilection sites, at least from the viewpoint of routine meat inspection, are the heart, the tongue and the masseter and intercostal muscles (Fig. 2.47). Under natural conditions the presence of cysticerci in the muscles of cattle is not associated with clinical signs although, experimentally, calves given massive infections of *T. saginata* eggs have developed severe myocarditis and heart failure associated with developing cysticerci in the heart.

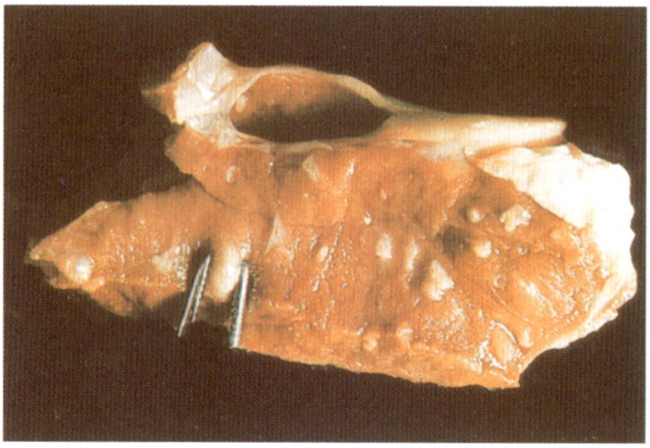

Fig. 2.47 *Cysticercus bovis* in skeletal muscle.

Clinical signs: In humans, the adult tapeworm may produce diarrhoea and hunger pains, but the infection is usually asymptomatic and is mainly objectionable on aesthetic grounds.

Diagnosis: Individual countries have different regulations regarding the inspection of carcases, but invariably the masseter muscle, tongue and heart are incised and examined and the intercostal muscles and diaphragm inspected; the triceps muscle is also incised in many countries. The inspection is inevitably a compromise between detection of cysticerci and the preservation of the economic value of the carcase.

Immunoserology has some usefulness for screening infected herds. In humans, the presence of tapeworms is recognised by the passage of proglottids and/or eggs in faeces.

Pathology: Cysticerci commence to degenerate 4–6 months after infection and by 9 months a substantial number may be dead. With light infections cysticerci may remain viable for 2 years or more.

Epidemiology: There are two quite distinct epidemiological patterns found in developing countries and developed countries respectively.

- Developing countries. In many parts of Africa, Asia and Latin America cattle are reared on an extensive scale, human sanitation is poorly developed and cooking fuel is expensive. In these circumstances the incidence of human infection with *T. saginata* is high, in certain areas being well over 20%. Because of this, calves are usually infected in early life, often within the first few days after birth, from infected stockmen whose hands are contaminated with *Taenia* eggs. Prenatal infection of calves may also occur, but is rare. Of the cysts which develop, a proportion persist for years even though the host has developed an acquired immunity and is completely resistant to further infection. Based on routine carcase inspection, the infection rate is often around 30–60%, although the real prevalence is considerably higher.

- Developed countries. In areas such as Europe, North America, Australia and New Zealand, the standards of sanitation are high and meat is carefully inspected and generally thoroughly cooked before consumption. In such countries, the prevalence of cysticercosis is low, being less than 1% of carcases inspected. Occasionally however, a cysticercosis 'storm', where a high proportion of cattle are infected, has been reported on particular farms. In Britain and in Australia, this has been associated with the use of human sewage on pasture as a fertiliser in the form of sludge, i.e. sedimented or bacterial-digested faeces. Since *T. saginata* eggs may survive for more than 200 days in sludge, the occurrence of these 'storms' is perhaps not surprising. Other causes of a sudden high incidence of infection on particular farms are due to a tapeworm infection in a stockman occurring either as a random event or, as has been reported from feedlots in some of the southern states of the USA, as a result of the use of migrant labour from a country with a high prevalence of infection. As distinct from these 'storms', the cause of the low but persistent prevalence of infection in cattle is obscure, but is thought to be due to the access of cattle to water contaminated with sewage effluents, to the carriage and dispersal of *T. saginata* eggs by birds which frequent sewage works or feed on effluent discharged into rivers or the sea, and to occasional fouling of pasture by itinerant infected individuals. In contrast to the epidemiology in developing countries, cattle of any age are susceptible to infection since they generally possess no acquired immunity. There is also evidence that when cattle are first infected as adults the longevity of the cysticerci is limited, most being dead within 9 months.

Treatment: As yet there is no licensed drug available which will effectively destroy all of the cysticerci in the muscle, although praziquantel has shown efficacy in experimental situations.

Control: In developed countries the control of bovine cysticercosis depends on a high standard of human sanitation, on the general practice of cooking meat thoroughly (the thermal death point of cysticerci is 57°C) and on compulsory meat inspection. Regulations usually require that infected carcases are frozen at –10°C for at least 10 days which is sufficient to kill the cysticerci, although the process reduces the economic value of the meat. Where relatively heavy infections of more than 25 cysticerci are detected, it is usual to destroy the carcase. In agricultural practice the use of human sludge as a fertiliser should be confined to cultivated fields or to those on which cattle will not be grazed for at least 2 years. In developing countries the same measures are necessary, but are not always economically feasible, and at present the most useful step would appear to be the education of communities in both sanitary hygiene and the thorough cooking of meat.

Notes: The intermediate stages of this tapeworm, found in the muscles of cattle, frequently present economic problems to the beef industry and are a public health hazard.

Onchocerca dukei

Predilection site: Muscle connective tissue

Parasite class: Nematoda

Superfamily: Filarioidea

Description, gross: Slender whitish worms; males range from 2–6 cm, females are up to 60 cm long or more.

Description, microscopic: Microfilariae are 250–265 μm long and unsheathed.

Final host: Cattle

Intermediate hosts: Blackflies (*Simulium*)

Life cycle: The life cycle of *Onchocerca* spp is typically filarioid, with the exception that the microfilariae occur in the tissue spaces of the skin, rather than in the peripheral bloodstream. They migrate in subdermal connective tissue in the skin of the back, sometimes ears and neck, where biting blackflies, feeding in this area, ingest microfilariae, which then develop to the infective stage in around 3 weeks. When these infected blackflies feed on another bovine host transmission of L_3 occurs.

Geographical distribution: Africa

Pathogenesis: *O. dukei* is of little clinical or economic importance. Losses may occur by condemnation of localised areas at meat inspection caused by nodular damage.

Clinical signs: Infection in cattle is asymptomatic.

Table 2.3 *Sarcocystis* species found in the muscles of cattle.

Species	Synonym	Definitive host	Pathogenicity (cattle)	Pathogenicity (final host)
S. bovicanis	*S. cruzi, S. fusiformis*	Dog, coyote, wolf	+++	0
S. bovifelis	*S. hirsuta*	Cat	0	0
S. bovihominis	*S. hominis*	Human, primates	0	+

0 = non-pathogenic; + = mildly pathogenic; +++ = severely pathogenic.

Diagnosis: Diagnosis is often made at meat inspection. Nodules are found particularly in the thorax and abdomen and may need to be differentiated from *Cysticercus bovis*. Microfilariae may be identified after soaking skin biopsy specimens in physiological saline for 12 hours and staining with Giemsa.

Epidemiology: The incidence of infection can be very high in endemic areas though the parasite is rarely detected.

Treatment and control: Not required

SARCOCYSTOSIS

The previously complex nomenclature for the large number of *Sarcocystis* spp has largely been discarded by many workers in favour of a new system based on their biology. The new names generally incorporate those of the **intermediate** and **final hosts** in that order. Although unacceptable to systematists, this practice has the virtue of simplicity (Table 2.3).

Life cycle

The life cycle for all species is heteroxenous. Sexual stages occur in the predator and oocysts are passed in the faeces. The intermediate host is infected by ingestion of sporocysts. The final host becomes infected by ingestion of mature sarcocysts containing bradyzoites, usually by eating the prey animal.

Diagnosis

Most cases of *Sarcocystis* infection are only diagnosed at meat inspection when the grossly visible sarcocysts in the muscle are discovered. However, in heavy infections of cattle, diagnosis is based on the clinical signs and on histological demonstration of meronts in the blood vessels of organs, such as kidney or heart, and the presence of cysts in the muscles at necropsy or biopsy. An indirect haemagglutination test, using bradyzoites as antigen, is also a useful aid to diagnosis; however, the presence of a titre need not imply active lesions of *Sarcocystis*. Also, animals may die prior to a detectable humoral response. In cattle, the degenerative muscle changes closely resemble those of vitamin E–selenium deficiency, although the latter lacks an inflammatory cellular response. Examination of faeces from dogs or cats on the farm for the presence of sporocysts may be helpful in the diagnosis.

Epidemiology

Little is known of the epidemiology, but from the high prevalence of symptomless infections observed in abattoirs, it is clear that where dogs or cats are kept in close association with farm animals or their feed, then transmission is likely. Sheepdogs are known to play an important part in the transmission of *S. bovicanis* and farm cats in the transmission of *S. bovifelis* so care should be exercised that only cooked meat is fed to dogs or cats. Acute outbreaks are probably most likely when livestock, which have been reared without dog or cat contact, are subsequently exposed to large numbers of the sporocysts from dog or cat faeces. The longevity of the sporocysts shed in the faeces is not known.

Treatment and control

There is no effective treatment for infection, either in the final or in the intermediate host. Where an outbreak occurs in cattle, it has been suggested that the introduction of amprolium (100 mg/kg, per os, daily over 30 days) into the diet of the animals has a prophylactic effect.

The only control measures possible are those of simple hygiene. Farm dogs and cats should not be housed in, or allowed access to, fodder stores nor should they be allowed to defecate in pens where livestock are housed. It is also important that they are not fed uncooked meat.

Sarcocystis bovicanis

Synonym: *Sarcocystis cruzi, Sarcocystis fusiformis*

Predilection site: Muscle

Order: Sporozoasida

Family: Sarcocystiidae

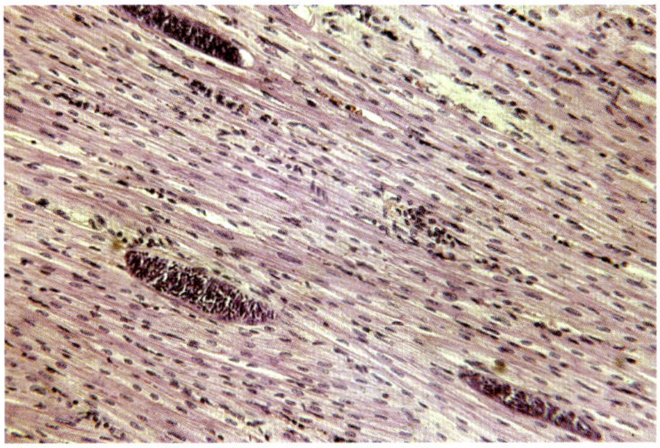

Fig. 2.48 *Sarcocystis bovicanis.*

Description: In cattle, the meronts found in the endothelial cells are quite small, measuring 2–8 μm in diameter. In contrast, the bradyzoite cysts can be very large and visible to the naked eye as whitish streaks running in the direction of the muscle fibres. They have been reported as reaching several centimetres in length, but more commonly they range from 0.5–5.0 mm (Fig. 2.48). The cyst wall is thin and smooth and has a small number of flattened protrusions 0.3–0.6 μm long, without fibrils.

Intermediate hosts: Cattle

Final hosts: Dog, fox, wolf, coyote

Life cycle: The definitive final host is the dog. Infection is by ingestion of the sporocysts and this is followed by at least three asexual generations. In the first, sporozoites, released from the sporocysts, invade the intestinal wall and enter the capillaries where they locate in endothelial cells in the caecum, large intestine, kidney, pancreas and mesenteric lymph node, and undergo two merogonous cycles. A third asexual cycle occurs in the circulating lymphocytes, the resulting merozoites penetrating skeletal and cardiac muscle cells. There they encyst and then divide by a process of budding or endodyogeny giving rise to broad banana-shaped bradyzoites contained within a cyst; this is the mature sarcocyst and is the infective stage for the carnivorous final host.

Geographical distribution: Worldwide

Pathogenesis: Infection in the final host is normally non-pathogenic, although mild diarrhoea has occasionally been reported. The principal pathogenic effect is attributable to the second stage of merogony in the vascular endothelium. Heavy experimental infections of calves with *S. bovicanis* have resulted in mortality 1 month later, with, at necropsy, petechial haemorrhages in almost every organ including the heart, together with generalised lymphadenopathy. Experimental infection of adult cows has resulted in abortion.

A naturally occurring chronic disease of cattle, 'Dalmeny disease', has been recognised in Canada, the USA and Britain. This is characterised by emaciation, submandibular oedema, recumbency and exophthalmia; at postmortem examination, numerous meronts are found in endothelial cells, and developing sarcocysts in areas of degenerative myositis.

Clinical signs: In heavy infections there is anorexia, fever, anaemia, loss of weight, a disinclination to move and sometimes recumbency. In cattle, there is often a marked loss of hair at the end of the tail. These signs may be accompanied by submandibular oedema, exophthalmia and enlargement of lymph nodes. Abortions may occur in breeding stock.

Pathology: Meronts present in endothelial cells of capillaries in various organs lead to endothelial cell destruction. As the organisms enter muscle, a wide range of change may be encountered. Microscopic inspection of *Sarcocystis*-infected muscle often reveals occasional degenerate parasitic cysts surrounded by variable numbers of inflammatory cells (very few of which are eosinophils) or, at a later stage, macrophages and granulation tissue. Usually there is no muscle fibre degeneration, but there may be thin, linear collections of lymphocytes between fibres in the region. The extent of muscle change bears little relationship to the numbers of developing cysts, but generally very low numbers of *Sarcocystis* produce no reaction. As cysts mature, the cyst capsule within the enlarged muscle fibre becomes thicker and more clearly differentiated from the muscle sarcoplasm.

Sarcocystis bovifelis

Synonym: *Sarcocystis hirsuta*

Predilection site: Muscle

Order: Sporozoasida

Family: Sarcocystiidae

Description: The first-generation meronts are 37 × 22 μm and contain more than 100 tachyzoites. Second-generation meronts when mature are 14 × 6.5m and contain up to 35 tachyzoites. Sarcocysts are up to 8 mm long with a striated wall, 7 μm thick, and may be visible to the naked eye as whitish streaks running in the direction of the muscle fibres.

Intermediate hosts: Cattle

Final host: Cat

Life cycle: The definitive final host is the cat. Infection is by ingestion of the sporocysts and this is followed by at least two asexual generations. In the intermediate host, the first-generation meronts are located in mesenteric and intestinal arterioles. Second-generation meronts when mature are found in capillaries of striated muscle and the heart, from which the resulting merozoites penetrate striated muscle cells, most commonly in the oesophageal muscle. There they encyst and metrocytes are formed within the cyst, which divide repeatedly by endodyogeny to form bradyzoites. The mature sarcocyst is the infective stage for the cat, the final host.

Geographical distribution: Worldwide

Pathogenesis: Infections are generally non-pathogenic; and any pathogenic effect is attributable to the second stage of merogony in the vascular endothelium.

Clinical signs: Infections are usually asymptomatic. Heavy infections may occasionally produce anorexia, fever, diarrhoea, anaemia and weight loss.

Pathology: In cattle, the tissue cysts may be visible to the naked eye especially in the oesophagus but are more likely to be detected on histopathology.

Sarcocystis bovihominis

Synonym: *Sarcocystis hominis*

Predilection site: Muscle

Order: Sporozoasida

Family: Sarcocystiidae

Description: In the intermediate host, sarcocysts are compartmented with a radially striated wall of about 6 μm in thickness.

Intermediate hosts: Cattle

Final host: Man, primates

Life cycle: The definitive final host is man. Infection is by ingestion of the sporocysts and this is followed by several generations of merogony, from which the resulting merozoites penetrate striated muscle cells, where they encyst; metrocytes are formed within the cyst, which divide repeatedly by endodyogeny to form elongate bradyzoites. The mature sarcocyst is the infective stage for humans.

Geographical distribution: Worldwide

Pathogenesis: The species is slightly if at all pathogenic for calves.

Clinical signs: Infection is usually asymptomatic in calves.

Pathology: Sarcocysts are present in striated muscle. Usually there is no muscle fibre degeneration, but there may be thin, linear collections of lymphocytes between fibres in the region.

Toxoplasma gondii

Predilection site: Muscle, lung, liver, reproductive system, central nervous system

Order: Sporozoasida

Family: Sarcocystiidae

Intermediate hosts: Any mammal, including man, or birds. Note that the final host, the cat, may also be an intermediate host and harbour extra-intestinal stages.

Final hosts: Cat, other felids

Geographical distribution: Worldwide

Pathogenesis: Most *Toxoplasma* infections in cattle are light and consequently asymptomatic. Infections are usually acquired via the digestive tract, and so organisms are disseminated by the lymphatics and portal system with subsequent invasion of various organs and tissues. Pathogenic effects are always related to the extra-intestinal phase of development. In heavy infections, the multiplying tachyzoites may produce areas of necrosis in vital organs such as the myocardium, lungs, liver and brain, and during this phase the host can become pyrexic and lymphadenopathy occurs. As the disease progresses bradyzoites are formed, this chronic phase being usually asymptomatic.

Clinical signs: There are only a few reports of clinical toxoplasmosis associated with fever, dyspnoea, nervous signs and abortion in cattle.

Pathology: In heavy infections, the multiplying tachyzoites may produce areas of necrosis in vital organs such as the myocardium, lungs, liver and brain.

Epidemiology: The cat plays a central role in the epidemiology of toxoplasmosis and the disease is virtually absent from areas where cats do not occur. Compared with sheep, toxoplasmosis in cattle is relatively uncommon and rarely causes clinical signs.

Treatment: Not indicated

Control: Control on farms is more difficult, but where possible animal feedstuffs should be covered to exclude access by cats.

For more detailed description see Chapter 3 (Sheep and goats).

Trypanosoma brucei brucei

See details and description under Parasites of the circulatory system.

PARASITES OF THE CONNECTIVE TISSUE

Onchocerca gutturosa

Synonym: *Onchocerca lienalis*

Common name: Ligamentary onchocercosis

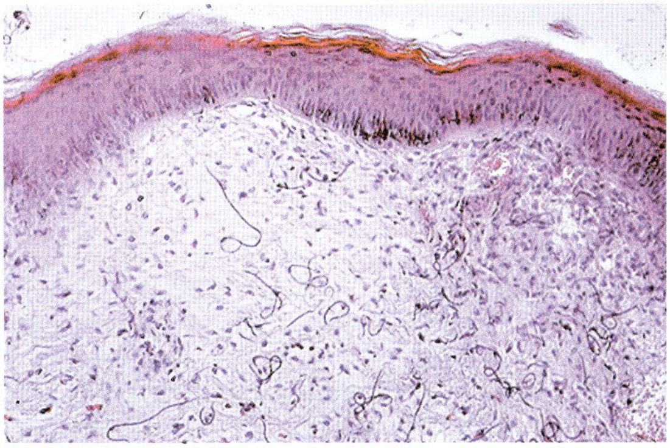

Fig. 2.49 *Onchocerca* spp embedded within connective tissue.

Predilection site: Connective tissue, ligamentum nuchae, gastro-splenic ligament

Parasite class: Nematoda

Superfamily: Filarioidea

Description, gross: Slender whitish worms; males range from 2–6 cm, females are up to 60 cm long or more.

Description, microscopic: Microfilariae are 250–265 μm long and unsheathed.

Final host: Cattle

Intermediate hosts: Blackflies (*Simulium*)

Life cycle: The life cycle of *Onchocerca* spp is typically filarioid, with the exception that the microfilariae occur in the tissue spaces of the skin, rather than in the peripheral bloodstream. They migrate in subdermal connective tissue (Fig. 2.49) in the skin of the back, sometimes ears and neck, where biting blackflies, feeding in this area, ingest microfilariae, which then develop to the infective stage in around 3 weeks. When these infected blackflies feed on another bovine host transmission of L_3 occurs.

Geographical distribution: Worldwide. In Australia and North America the parasite, *O. lienalis* (considered to be synonymous) is found in the gastro-splenic ligament.

Pathogenesis: *O. gutturosa* is of little clinical or economic importance.

Clinical signs: Infection in cattle is asymptomatic.

Diagnosis: Diagnosis is rarely called for and depends on the finding of microfilariae in skin biopsy samples taken from affected areas. The microfilariae are concentrated in the preferred feeding sites of the vectors, which are the back, ears and neck. The piece of skin is placed in warm saline and teased to allow emergence of the microfilariae, and is then incubated for about 8–12 hours. The microfilariae are readily recognised by their sinuous movements in a centrifuged sample of the saline. Another option is to scarify the skin of a predilection site and examine the fluid exudate for microfilariae.

Pathology: Adult worms, which are found in pairs, are most frequently located in the ligamentum nuchae adjacent to the thoracic spines and less frequently in the connective tissue on the scapula, humerus and femur. The worms do not stimulate nodule formation but lie loose in the connective tissue and cause no disease or reaction.

Epidemiology: The incidence of infection can be very high in endemic areas, although the parasite is rarely detected.

Treatment: Not required.

Control: With the ubiquity of the insect vectors there is little possibility of efficient control, though the use of microfilaricides will reduce the numbers of infected flies. In any case, with the relatively innocuous nature of the infection there is unlikely to be any demand for control.

Notes: Some consider this parasite to be synonymous with *O. lienalis.*

Onchocerca gibsoni

Predilection site: Connective tissue

Parasite class: Nematoda

Superfamily: Filarioidea

Description, gross: The slender worms range from 2 to over 20 cm in length and lie tightly coiled in tissue nodules. Males are 3–5 cm and females 14–20 cm, although there have been reports of worms up to 50 cm in length.

Description, microscopic: The tail of the male is curved and bears lateral alae and six to nine papillae at either side. The spicules are unequal in size. Microfilariae are not sheathed and are 240–280 μm long.

Final host: Cattle

Intermediate host: Midges (*Culicoides*)

Life cycle: As for *O. gutturosa*

Geographical distribution: Africa, Asia and Australasia

Pathogenesis: Worms occur in groups 'worm nests', and provoke a fibrous reaction around the coiled-up worms in muscle tissue (nodules can measure up to 5 cm in diameter). The nodules are often in the brisket and can be responsible for economic loss due to carcase trimming.

Clinical signs: Affected animals are not clinically ill and show no presenting signs other than subcutaneous nodules at the predilections sites.

Diagnosis: In active lesions, the presence of worms is readily established on section of the subcutaneous nodules. Microfilariae may also be found in skin biopsy samples taken from affected areas with subcutaneous lymph spaces. The microfilariae are concentrated in the preferred feeding sites of the vectors, which for *Culicoides* spp are usually the shaded lower parts of the trunk, and it is usually recommended that samples should be taken from the region of the linea alba. The piece of skin is placed in warm saline and teased to allow emergence of the microfilariae, and is then incubated for about 8–12 hours. The microfilariae are readily recognised by their sinuous movements in a centrifuged sample of the saline. Another option is to scarify the skin of a predilection site and examine the fluid exudate for microfilariae.

Pathology: A nodule forms around the worms with the head becoming fixed and surrounded by fibroblasts. Successive portions of the worm are drawn into the nodule, where they eventually lie coiled up and surrounded by a fibrous tissue capsule, which increases in thickness as the lesion grows older. In older nodules, degeneration of the tissues and calcification of the worms frequently takes place. The capsule consists of dense fibrous tissue containing blood vessels, leucocytes and lymph spaces. Microfilariae are common and wander in the lymph spaces. Their presence may lead to thickening of the dermis.

Epidemiology: The incidence of infection can be very high in endemic areas.

Treatment: In the past this has consisted of daily administration of diethylcarbamazine over a period as a microfilaricide, but it now appears that a single dose of ivermectin is highly efficient in this respect, although the dying microfilariae may provoke local tissue reactions. Affected carcases must be trimmed to remove the nodules.

Control: With the ubiquity of the insect vectors, there is little possibility of efficient control, though insect repellents will help reduce insect attack. In any case, with the relatively innocuous nature of the infection there is unlikely to be any demand for control.

Onchocerca ochengi

Synonym: *Onchocerca dermata*

Predilection site: Connective tissue, scrotum and udder

Parasite class: Nematoda

Superfamily: Filarioidea

Description: The slender worms range from 2.0–6.0 cm in length and lie tightly coiled in tissue nodules. In active lesions the presence of worms is readily established on section of these nodules.

Final host: Cattle

Intermediate hosts: Unknown

Life cycle: As for *O. gibsoni* although the intermediate host in not known

Geographical distribution: Parts of east and west Africa

Table 2.4 Bovine onchocercosis.

Species	Site	Distribution	Vector	Significance
O. gutturosa	Ligamentum nuchae and other parts of the body	Most parts of the world	*Simulium* spp	No economic significance
(synonym *O. lienalis*)	Gastro-splenic ligaments	Many parts of the world	*Simulium* spp	No economic significance
O. gibsoni	Subcutaneous and intermuscular nodules	Africa, Asia, Australasia	*Culicoides* spp	Carcase trimming
O. armillata	Wall of thoracic aorta	Middle East, Africa, India	*Culicoides* spp *Simulium* spp	No economic significance
O. dukei	Abdomen, thorax, thighs	West Africa	Unknown	Confused with *Cysticercus bovis* at meat inspection
O. cebei	Abdomen, thorax, thighs	Far East	Unknown	No economic significance
O. ochengi	Scrotum, udder	East and West Africa	Unknown	Blemished hides
O. sweetae	Intradermal tissue	Australia	Unknown	Blemished hides

Pathogenesis: *O. ochengi* in the skin causes some economic loss from blemished hides.

Clinical signs: Affected animals are not clinically ill and show no presenting signs other than subcutaneous nodules at the predilection sites.

Diagnosis: As for *O. gibsoni*

Pathology: Not reported

Epidemiology: The incidence of infection can be very high in endemic areas.

Treatment and control: As for *O. gibsoni*

Parafilaria bovicola

Common name: Summer 'bleeding disease', verminous nodules

Predilection site: Subcutaneous and intermuscular connective tissue

Parasite class: Nematoda

Superfamily: Filarioidea

Description, gross: Slender white worms 3.0–6.0 cm in length. Males are 2–3 cm and females 4–5 cm.

Description, microscopic: Anteriorly, there are numerous papillae and circular ridges in the cuticle. In the female the vulva is situated anteriorly near the simple mouth opening.

Small embryonated eggs, 45 × 30 μm, that have a thin flexible shell are laid on the skin surface where they hatch to release the microfilariae or L_1, which are about 200 μm in length.

Final hosts: Cattle, buffalo

Intermediate hosts: Muscid flies; *Musca autumnalis* in Europe

Life cycle: Eggs or free L_1 larvae present in exudates from bleeding points in the skin surface are ingested by muscid flies (e.g. *M. autumnalis* in Europe; and *M. lusoria* and *M. xanthomelas* in Africa), in which they develop to L_3 within several weeks to months, depending on air temperature. Transmission occurs when infected flies feed on lachrymal secretions or skin wounds in other cattle and the L_3 deposited then migrate in the subcutaneous tissue and develop to the adult stage under the skin in 5–7 months. Bleeding points develop 7–9 months after infection, which is about the same duration as patency.

Geographical distribution: Africa, Asia, southern Europe and Sweden

Pathogenesis: Adult worms in the subcutaneous connective tissue induce small inflammatory lesions and haemorrhagic nodules, usually in the upper body regions. When the gravid female punctures the skin to lay her eggs there is a haemorrhagic exudate or 'bleeding point' which streaks and mats the surrounding hairs and attracts flies. Individual lesions only bleed for a short time and healing is rapid. There is some evidence that exposure to sunlight is required to initiate bleeding of the nodules.

At the sites of infection, which are predominantly on the shoulders, withers and thoracic areas, there is inflammation and oedema which, at meat inspection, resemble subcutaneous bruising in early lesions and have a gelatinous greenish yellow appearance with a metallic odour in longer-standing cases. Sometimes the lesions extend into the intermuscular fascia. The affected areas have to be trimmed at marketing and further economic loss is incurred by rejection or downgrading of the hides.

Clinical signs: The signs of parafilarioidosis, such as 'bleeding points' during the warmer seasons, are pathognomonic. Active bleeding lesions are seen most commonly in warm weather, an apparent adaptation to coincide with the presence of the fly intermediate host. The haemorrhagic exudate often streaks the hair and may lead to focal matting.

Diagnosis: This is normally based on clinical signs, but if laboratory confirmation is required, the small embryonated eggs or microfilariae may be found on examination of fresh exudate from bleeding points. The demonstration of eosinophils in smears taken from lesions is also considered a constant diagnostic feature. Serodiagnosis, using an ELISA technique has been developed.

Pathology: Nodules formed in the cutaneous and intermuscular connective tissue are 1–2 cm in diameter, enlarge in the summer months, burst open and haemorrhage and heal with scarring.

Epidemiology: In Europe, bovine parafilarioidosis occurs in spring and summer, disappearing in winter, whereas in tropical areas it is seen mainly after the rainy season. A high prevalence of 36% in cattle has been reported from some endemic areas in South Africa and the disease is now present in Sweden, an area previously free from infection. *Parafilaria* infection may be introduced by the importation of cattle from endemic areas, but its spread will depend on the presence of specific fly vectors. It has been estimated in Sweden that one 'bleeding' cow will act as a source of infection for three other animals.

Treatment: Patent infections in beef and non-lactating dairy cattle may be treated with ivermectin, moxidectin or nitroxynil. The former two drugs are given parenterally as a single dose whereas two doses of nitroxynil are required at an interval of 3 days. None of these drugs is licensed for use in lactating cattle when the less effective levamisole may be tried.

These drugs produce a marked reduction in bleeding points and, due to resolution of the muscle lesions, a significant reduction in meat condemnation if slaughter is delayed for 70 days after treatment.

Control: This is difficult, because of the long prepatent period during which drugs are thought not to be effective. In Sweden, dairy cattle and particularly heifers at pasture, are the main source of infection for *M. autumnalis*, which is an outdoor fly, active in spring and summer. However, infections in young beef cattle are the chief cause of economic loss through carcase damage.

Since neither ivermectin nor nitroxynil is effective against immature worms, treatment is only useful for patent infections recognisable by the clinical signs. However, because of restrictions on the use of ivermectin and nitroxynil in lactating cows, these are rarely treated and instead are kept indoors during the period of fly activity.

In endemic areas, young beef cattle may be treated with an anthelmintic some time before slaughter as described above. In Sweden the use of insecticide-impregnated ear tags has been recommended for vector control.

Notes: The adults of this genus of primitive filarioids live under the skin where they produce inflammatory lesions or nodules and, during egg laying, haemorrhagic exudates or 'bleeding points' on the skin surface.

Setaria labiato-papillosa

Synonym: *Setaria cervi*

Common name: Bovine abdominal filariosis

Predilection site: Peritoneum, pleural cavity

Parasite class: Nematoda

Superfamily: Filarioidea

Description, gross: Long slender whitish worms, up to 12.0 cm in length, and in which the posterior end is spirally coiled. The site and gross appearance are sufficient for generic identification (Fig. 2.50). Males are 40–60 mm and females 60–120 mm in length.

Description, microscopic: The tail of the female ends in a marked button, which is divided into a number of papillae. Microfilariae are sheathed and measure 240–260 μm.

Final hosts: Cattle, buffalo, bison, yak, and various deer, rarely sheep

Intermediate hosts: Mosquitoes (*Aedes*, *Culex*)

Life cycle: Larvae produced by adult worms in the body cavity circulate in the blood and are taken up by culicine mosquitoes, including *Aedes* and *Culex* species.

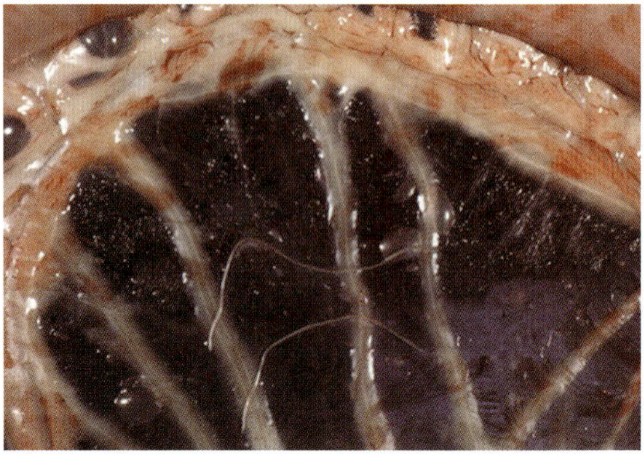

Fig. 2.50 Worms of *Setaria* spp in the mesentery.

Infective larvae develop in the mosquito muscles in 12–16 days, and are re-injected into the final host when the mosquitoes feed. The prepatent period is 8–10 months.

Geographical distribution: Worldwide

Pathogenesis: The worms in their normal site are usually harmless, occasionally inducing a mild fibrinous peritonitis and are only discovered at necropsy. *S. labiato-papillosa* may have an erratic migration in sheep and goats and enter the spinal canal causing cerebrospinal setariosis, 'lumbar paralysis', which is irreversible and often fatal; the condition has only been reported in the Middle and Far East.

Clinical signs: There are no clinical signs when the worms are in their normal site, but when nervous tissue is involved there is locomotor disturbance, usually of the hind limbs, and if the parasites are high in the spinal canal there may be paraplegia.

Diagnosis: Infection with the adult worms is only accidentally discovered in the living animal by the finding of microfilariae in routine blood smears. In cases of cerebrospinal nematodosis, confirmatory diagnosis is only possible by microscopic examination of the spinal cord, since the parasites exist only as larval forms in their aberrant site.

Pathology: A mild, fibrinous peritonitis may be found on postmortem. Migrating larvae affecting the CNS may cause areas of damage seen as brown foci or streaks grossly. The lesions show microcavitation and variable haemorrhage. There is loss of myelin and fragmentation of axons locally with eosinophils, neutrophils and macrophages present along with a mild meningitis and vascular cuffing.

Epidemiology: Since the worms are usually innocuous, their epidemiology has received little study. The prevalence is higher in warmer countries, where there is longer seasonal activity of the mosquito vectors.

Treatment: There is no treatment for setarial paralysis.

Control: This would depend on control of the mosquito vectors, which is unlikely to be applied specifically for this parasite.

Notes: *S. labiato-papillosa* has often been referred to as *S. cervi*, although the latter species is considered a parasite of Axis deer (*Cervus axis*). The parasite is also considered to be identical to *S. digitata*, although some consider the latter to be a valid and distinct species.

Setaria digitatus

Common name: Kumri

Predilection site: Peritoneum, pleural cavity

Parasite class: Nematoda

Superfamily: Filarioidea

Description, gross: As for *S. labiato-papillosa*. The male is 40–50 mm and the female 60–80 mm in length

Description, microscopic: The tail of the female ends in a simple button.

Final hosts: Cattle, buffalo

Intermediate hosts: Mosquitoes (*Armigeres*, *Aedes*, *Anopholes*, *Culex*)

Geographical distribution: Asia

Pathogenesis: The parasites inhabit the thoracic peritoneal cavities and cause little harm. Immature forms have been reported in the CNS of sheep, goats and horses causing epizootic cerebrospinal nematodiosis. Affected animals suffer from acute focal encephalomyelomalacia, which causes acute or subacute tetraplegia or paraplegia of the hindlimbs.

Pathology: Migrating larvae in abherent hosts affecting the CNS may cause areas of damage seen as brown foci or streaks grossly. Acute malacia occurs in the track of the worm such that the lesions show microcavitation and variable haemorrhage. There is loss of myelin and fragmentation of axons locally with eosinophils, neutrophils and macrophages present along with a mild meningitis and vascular cuffing.

Details on the life cycle, epidemiology, treatment and control are as for *S. labiato-papillosa*.

PARASITES OF THE INTEGUMENT

Stephanofilaria stilesi

Predilection site: Skin

Parasite class: Nematoda

Superfamily: Filarioidea

Description, gross: Small nematodes; males are 2.6–3.7 mm and females 3.7–6.9 mm in length.

Description, microscopic: There are four to five cephalic spines and 18–19 peribuccal spines. The male spicules are unequal and the female worms have no anus. The thin-shelled eggs are 58–72 × 42–55 μm in size. Microfilariae are 45–60 μm in length and are characterised by a peribuccal elevation with a single spine and a short and rounded tail.

Final host: Cattle

Intermediate hosts: The horn fly (*Haematobia irritians*, *H. titillans*)

Life cycle: The fly vectors are attracted to the open lesions in the skin caused by the adult parasites, and ingest the microfilariae in the exudate. Development to L_3 takes about 3 weeks, and the final host is infected when the flies deposit larvae on normal skin.

Geographical distribution: USA, Japan, Commonwealth of Independent States (CIS)

Pathogenesis: Lesions begin to appear within 2 weeks of infection. In this species, the lesions are usually localised to the preferred biting areas of the vectors on the lower abdomen, commonly along the midventral line between the brisket and navel, but also on the udder, scrotum, flanks and ears. The flies feed predominantly along the midventral line of the host and their bites create lesions that permit microfilariae to invade the skin. These lesions are attractive to both species of hornflies as well as non-biting muscids. Adult nematodes occur in the dermis and microfilariae in the dermal papillae of lesions but not in adjacent healthy tissue.

Clinical signs: In endemic regions, granulomatous and ulcerative lesions may be seen on the skin, particularly in the midventral line between the brisket and navel. The dermatitis can be exudative and haemorrhagic.

Diagnosis: Though adult worms and microfilariae are present in the lesions they are often scarce and many scrapings prove negative. Diagnosis is therefore usually presumptive in endemic areas, and is based on the appearance and site of the lesions. Deep skin scrapings macerated in saline will release microfilariae and adult worms. Biopsy sections readily reveal microfilariae and adults.

Pathology: The skin is at first nodular, but later there is papular eruption with an exudate of blood and pus. In the centre of the lesion there may be sloughing of the skin, but at the margin there is often hyperkeratosis and alopecia. The condition is essentially an exudative, often haemorrhagic, dermatitis that attracts the fly vectors. Sometimes the lesions are exacerbated by secondary bacterial infection.

Epidemiology: In endemic areas the incidence of infection may be as high as 90% and the occurrence is to a great extent influenced by the type of herbage. Succulent grazing produces soft, moist faeces, which are more suitable breeding sites for the flies than the hard crumbly faeces deposited on sparse dry grazing. Hence, irrigation of pasture may result in an increase of stephanofilariosis. Though the lesions subside in cooler weather, the damage to the hide is permanent and may result in considerable economic loss. Milk yield may be severely diminished from the pain of the lesions and the irritation of cattle by the flies.

Treatment: Organophosphorus compounds, such as trichlorophon, applied topically as an ointment have proved effective. Levamisole at 9–12 mg/kg by injection followed by daily application of zinc oxide ointment has also been reported as effective. Avermectins have reported activity against larval stages but have no appreciable effect against adult stages.

Control: Control of hornflies is feasible by the proper handling of manure and the use of insecticides. Macrocyclic lactones applied topically give reported protection against hornflies for period of up to 5 weeks.

Other filarial species have been reported in cattle and buffalo in India and parts of Asia. The identification of individual species is beyond the scope of this book and interested readers will need to consult a relevant taxonomic specialist.

Stephanofilaria assamensis

Predilection site: Skin

Parasite class: Nematoda

Superfamily: Filarioidea

Geographical distribution: India

Stephanofilaria zaheeri

Predilection site: Skin

Parasite class: Nematoda

Superfamily: Filarioidea

Geographical distribution: India

Clinical signs: With *S. zaheeri*, lesions occur mainly on the head, legs and teats of cattle and buffalo.

Stephanofilaria kaeli

Predilection site: Skin

Parasite class: Nematoda

Superfamily: Filarioidea

Geographical distribution: India

Stephanofilaria dedoesi

Predilection site: Skin

Parasite class: Nematoda

Superfamily: Filarioidea

Description, gross: Small nematodes; males are 2.3–3.2 mm and females 6.1–8.5 mm in length.

Description, microscopic: The oral aperture is surrounded by a protruding cuticular rim with a denticulate edge. The anterior extremity has a circular thickening, which bears a number of small cuticular spines. The male spicules are unequal and the female worms have no anus.

Geographical distribution: Indonesia

Clinical signs: With *S. dedoesi*, lesions occur mainly on the head, legs and teats of cattle. The dermatitis can be exudative and haemorrhagic.

Stephanofilaria okinawaensis

Predilection site: Skin

Parasite class: Nematoda

Superfamily: Filarioidea

Description, gross: The parasites are small, rounded, whitish and slender bodied. Females are 7.0–8.5 mm, and males 2.7–3.5 mm in length

Parafilaria bovicola

See under Parasites of connective tissue.

Dracunculus medinensis

Common name: Guinea worm or Medina worm

Predilection site: Subcutaneous connective tissue

Parasite class: Nematoda

Family: Dracunculidae

Description, gross: Males measure about 2–3 cm and females up to around 100 cm in length.

Description, microscopic: The female worm has no vulva.

Final host: Man and occasionally cattle, horse dog, cat and other mammals

Intermediate hosts: Copepod crustaceans (*Cyclops* spp)

Life cycle: This is indirect. Adult worms mature in deep connective tissue and then migrate to peripheral subcutaneous tissue about 9 months after initial infection. A cutaneous blister develops around the head end of the worm and when this makes contact with water the uterus of the worm ruptures, and liberates large numbers of L_1 larvae. Release of larvae can continue over several weeks if the lesion is repeatedly immersed in water. These larvae develop to the infective stage in a species of *Cyclops*. Infection of the final host is through ingestion of infected copepods with drinking water. The prepatent period is around 12 months.

Geographical distribution: Africa, the Middle East and parts of Asia

Pathogenesis: Following initial infection there are virtually no signs of disease until the gravid adult female emerges in the subcutaneous tissues of the extremities. Pathogenesis is associated with the cutaneous ulcer formation.

Clinical signs: The migration of the worm to the suface of the skin may induce pruritis and urticaria and a blister on an extremity.

Diagnosis: Symptoms of dracunculosis are pathognomonic.

Pathology: Secondary bacterial infection of the ulcer lesion or degeneration of worms can cause marked abscessation.

Epidemiology: A major global eradication programme has reduced the incidence and importance of *D. medinensis*.

Treatment: The worm may be gradually removed through the lesion by winding it round a small stick at a rate of about 2 cm each day or alternatively it may be surgically excised. Treatment with thiabendazole or niridazole, administered over several days might be effective. Ivermectin or albendazole may be useful but efficacy data are lacking.

Control: This is best achieved through the provision of clean drinking water or water that has been adequately sieved to remove any copepods.

Besnoitia besnoiti

Predilection site: Skin, conjunctiva

Order: Sporozoasida

Family: Sarcocystiidae

Description: The pseudocysts are non-septate and about 100–600 μm in diameter, with a thick wall containing thousands of merozoites but no metrocytes.

Intermediate hosts: Cattle, goats, wild ruminants (wildebeest, impala, kudu)

Final host: Cat, wild cats (lion, cheetah, leopard)

Life cycle: The ruminant intermediate hosts are infected by the ingestion of oocysts shed into the environment by infected cats. First generation meronts are present in the endothelial cells of blood cells. Released merozoites then enter cells of the cutis, subcutis, scleral conjunctiva, connective tissue and serosae of the nasal mucosa, larynx, trachea and other tissues of the intermediate host forming pseudocysts.

Geographical distribution: Worldwide, although important tropical and subtropical countries, especially in Africa

Pathogenesis: Following infection in cattle there is a systemic phase accompanied by lymphadenopathy and oedematous swellings in dependent parts of the body. Subsequently bradyzoites develop in fibroblasts in the dermis, subcutaneous tissues and fascia and in the nasal and laryngeal mucosa. The developing cysts in the skin result in a severe condition characterised by painful subcutaneous swellings and thickenings of the skin, loss of hair and necrosis. Apart from the clinical manifestations, which in severe cases can result in death, there can be considerable economic losses due to condemnation of hides at slaughter.

Clinical signs: Affected animals show skin thickening, swelling, hair loss and skin necrosis. Photophobia, excessive lachrymation and hyperaemia of the sclera are present, and the cornea is studded with whitish, elevated specks (pseudocysts).

Diagnosis: Besnoitiosis can be diagnosed by biopsy examination of skin. The spherical, encapsulated cysts are pathognomonic. The best method is examination of the scleral conjunctiva where the pseudocysts can be seen macroscopically.

Pathology: This genus differs from other members of the Sarcocystiidae in that the cysts containing bradyzoites are found mainly in fibroblasts in or under the skin. The host cell enlarges and becomes multinucleate as the *Besnoitia* cyst grows within a parasitophorous vacuole, eventually reaching up to 0.6 mm in diameter.

Epidemiology: Although infection of cattle is thought to be mainly by ingestion of sporulated oocysts from cat faeces, there is a suggestion that mechanical spread by biting flies feeding on skin lesions of cattle may be another route of transmission.

Treatment: There is no known treatment.

Control: Limiting contact of domestic cattle with cats can help reduce the incidence of infection. In countries where the disease is endemic in wildlife populations control is difficult or impossible to achieve and may be limited to the elimination of infected animals.

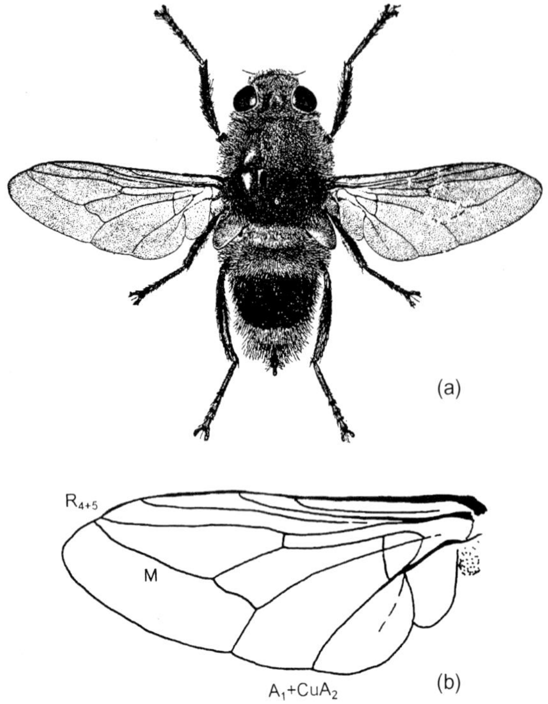

Fig. 2.51 (a) Adult female of *Hypoderma bovis* (reproduced from Castellani and Chalmers, 1910). (b) wing venation typical of *Hypoderma* showing the strongly bent vein M not joining R_{4+5} before the wing margin and vein A_1+CuA_2 reaching the wing margin.

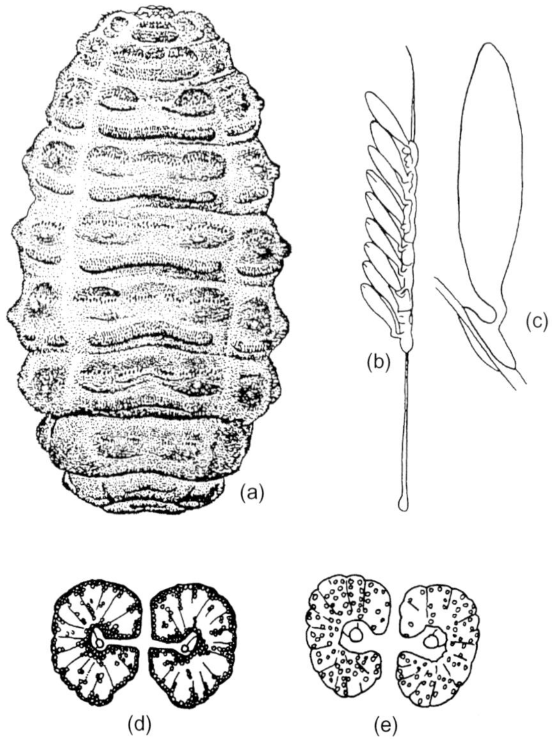

Fig. 2.52 (a) Third stage larva of *Hypoderma bovis*. Eggs of (b) *H. lineatum* and (c) *H. bovis*. Posterior spiracles of third stage larvae of (d) *H. bovis* and (e) *H. lineatum* (reproduced from Zumpt, 1965).

Hypoderma spp

Parasite class: Insecta

Family: Oestridae

Description, adults: The adults are large and the abdomen is covered with yellow-orange hairs giving them a bee-like appearance (Fig. 2.51). The adults have no functioning mouthparts.

Description, larvae: The mature larvae are thick and somewhat barrel-shaped, tapering anteriorly. When mature they are 25–30 mm long, and most segments bear short spines. The colour is dirty white when newly emerged from the host, but rapidly turns to dark brown; the pupa is almost black. The third-stage larvae of the two species of *Hypoderma* that commonly parasitise cattle (*H. bovis* and *H. lineatum*) may be distinguished from other species of *Hypoderma* by examination of the posterior spiracular plate, which is completely surrounded by small spines. The two *Hypoderma* species in cattle may be distinguished from each other by the fact that in *H. bovis* the posterior spiracular plate surrounding the button has a narrow funnel-like channel, whereas in *H. lineatum* it has a broad channel (Fig. 2.52).

Hosts: Cattle; the larvae occur erratically in other animals including equines, sheep and, very rarely, humans.

Life cycle: The adult flies are active only in warm weather, and in the northern hemisphere the peak period is usually in June and July. The females attach their eggs to hairs on the lower parts of the body and on the legs above the hocks. The eggs are 1.0 mm long and are fixed to the hairs using small terminal clasps (Fig. 2.52). One female may lay 100 or more eggs on an individual host. There is no fly activity below approximately 18°C.

The first-stage larvae, which are less than 1.0 mm long, hatch in a few days and crawl down the hairs, penetrate the hair follicles and migrate in the body, following species-specific pathways (see below). The use of paired mouth hooks and the secretion of proteolytic enzymes aid migration. The larvae feed as they travel to the species-specific resting sites, which are reached in late autumn, where they spend the winter.

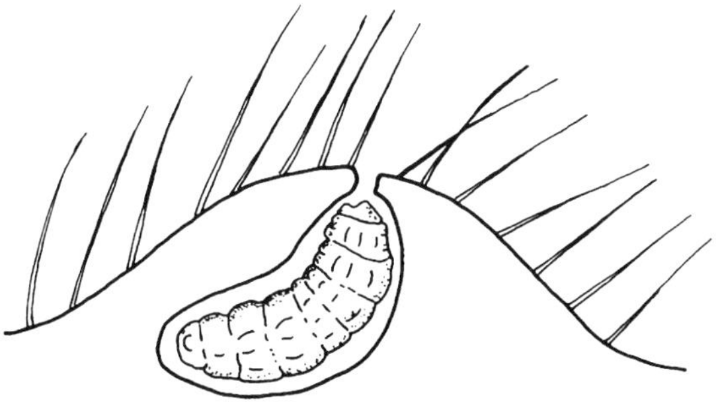

Fig. 2.53 Third stage *Hypoderma* larva in warble on the back of a cow.

The moult to the second stage occurs at this resting site. During this stage they grow to 12–16 mm. In February and March migration is resumed and the L_2 arrive under the skin of the back. Here they moult to the L_3 stage, which can be palpated as distinct swellings ('warbles'). The L_3 makes a cutaneous perforation and the larvae breathe by applying their spiracles to the aperture (Fig. 2.53). A fully grown third-stage larva measures 27–28 mm in length. After about 4–6 weeks in this site they emerge in May–June and fall to the ground, where they pupate under leaves and loose vegetation for about 5 weeks. The adults then emerge, copulate, the females lay their eggs and die, all within 1–2 weeks. Oviposition can take place as soon as 24 hours after emergence from the puparium. The precise timings and duration of events in the life cycle will vary depending on latitude and ambient temperature.

Geographical distribution: Northern hemisphere. However, *Hypoderma* is absent from extreme northern latitudes, including Scandinavia, and it has occasionally been found sparsely south of the equator in Argentina, Chile, Peru and southern Africa, following accidental introduction in imported cattle.

Pathogenesis: By far the most important feature of this genus is the economic loss caused by downgrading and condemnation of hides perforated by larvae. The L_3 under the skin damage the adjacent flesh and this necessitates trimming from the carcase the greenish, gelatinous tissue called 'butcher's jelly', also seen in the infested oesophageal submucosal tissues. In addition the adult flies themselves are responsible for some loss. When they approach animals to lay their eggs, their characteristic buzzing noise, which appears to be instantly recognisable, causes the animals to panic or 'gad', sometimes injuring themselves on posts, barbed wire and other obstacles. Dairy cows show reduced milk yield, and beef animals have reduced weight gains as a result of interrupted feeding. This species will pursue animals for some distance making repeated attacks.

Clinical signs: Except for poor growth and decreased milk yield in bad cases the host animals show no appreciable signs until the larvae appear along the back. The presence of L_3 causes characteristic fluid-filled swellings ('warbles') in the dermis of the back, which can be seen and felt.

Diagnosis: The presence of the larvae under the skin of the back allows diagnosis of warble flies. The eggs may also be found on the hairs of the animals in the summer. Immunodiagnostic tests may be used to detect animals infected with migrating larvae and hence those needing treatment.

Pathology: Warble larvae induce a pronounced tissue inflammation. The cellular reacton is predominantly eosinophilic and lymphocytic. The presence of the larvae also induces the production of a thickened connective tissue lined cavity, surrounding the larva, filled with with inflammatory cells, particularly eosinophils. If larvae die in the spinal canal, the release of a highly toxic proteolysin may cause paraplegia. Larval death in other regions may, in very rare cases, lead to anaphylaxis in sensitised animals.

Treatment: *Hypoderma* is highly susceptible to systemically active organophosphorus insecticides and to the macrocyclic lactones abamectin, ivermectin, doramectin, eprinomectin and moxidectin. The organophosphorus preparations are applied as 'pour-ons' to the backs of cattle and are absorbed systemically from there; macrocyclic lactones can be given by subcutaneous injection or pour-on.

Control: In control schemes in Europe, a single annual treatment is usually recommended, preferably in September, October or November. This is before the larvae of *H. bovis* have reached the spinal canal, so that there is no risk of spinal damage from disintegration of dead larvae. Treatment in the spring when the larvae have left their resting sites and arrived under the skin of the back, although effective in control, is less desirable since the breathing L_3 has then perforated the hide. However, in some countries such as the United Kingdom, such treatment is mandatory if warbles are present on the backs of cattle.

Successful eradication schemes supported by legislation, such as restriction of cattle movement on infected farms and compulsory treatment in the autumn, have been undertaken on islands such as the United Kingdom and Eire. For example, in the UK the prevalence of infected cattle was reduced from around 40% in the 1970s to virtually zero in the 1990s. However, evidence of infection is still encountered occasionally in animals imported into the UK. Other areas that have had successful eradication

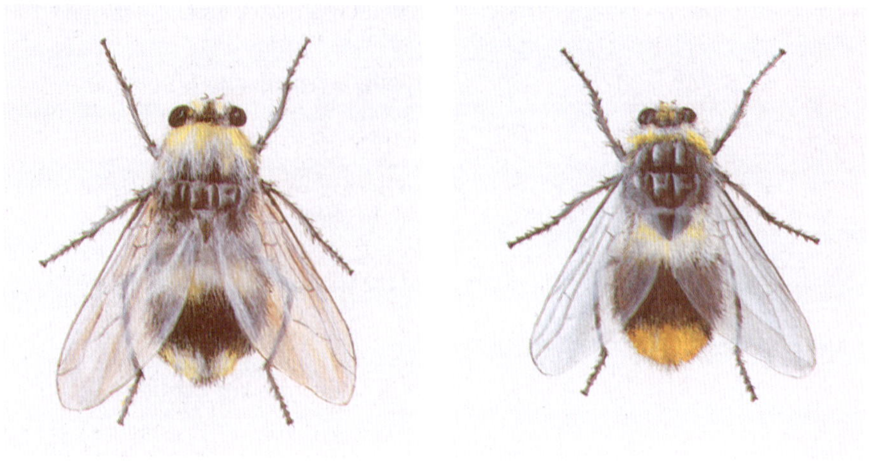
(a) (b)

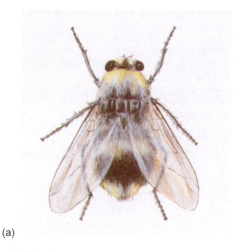

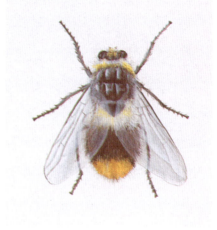

Fig. 2.54 (a) *Hypoderma bovis*. (b) *Hypoderma lineatum*.

such as Denmark and the Netherlands are clearly at greater risk of reintroduction.

Epidemiology: The flies occur in the summer, particularly from mid-June to early September. They are most active on warm days when they lay their eggs on cattle. The flies are limited in dispersal ability and can travel for more than 5 km.

Hypoderma bovis

Common name: Warble fly, northern cattle grub

Predilection site: Subcutaneous tissues, spinal canal

Description: Adult female *Hypoderma bovis* are about 15 mm in length and bee-like in appearance; the abdomen is covered with yellow–orange hairs with a broad band of black hairs around the middle (Fig. 2.54a). The hairs on the head and the anterior part of the thorax are greenish yellow.

Life cycle: Characteristic features of the life cycle of *H. bovis* are that it attaches its eggs singly to hairs on the lower parts of the body (Fig. 2.52c). Following penetration through the skin the larvae migrate along nerves until they reach the epidural fat of the spine in the region of the thoracic and lumber vertebrae, where they overwinter.

Summary of differences between the *Hypoderma* species which parasitise cattle

Feature	*Hypoderma bovis*	*Hypoderma lineatum*
Adult length	15 mm	13 mm
Eggs laid	Singly	In batches
Larval morphology	Posterior spiracular plate surrounding the button has a narrow funnel-like channel	Posterior spiracular plate surrounding the button has a broad channel
Migration path	Along nerves	Between the fascial planes of muscles and along connective tissue
Overwintering site	Epidural fat of the spinal cord	Submucosa of the oesophagus

Hypoderma lineatum

Common name: Warble fly, common cattle grub, heel fly

Predilection site: Subcutaneous tissues, oesophagus

Parasite class: Insecta

Family: Oestridae

Description: Adult female *Hypoderma lineatum* are about 13 mm in length and bee-like in appearance; the abdomen is covered with yellow–orange hairs with a broad band of black hairs around the middle. The hairs on the head and the anterior part of the thorax are yellowish white (Fig. 2.54b).

Life cycle: Characteristic features of the life cycle of *H. lineatum* are that it attaches its eggs in rows of six or more on individual hairs below the hocks (Fig. 2.52b). Following penetration of the skin, the larvae migrate between the fascial planes of muscles and along connective tissue, towards the region of the diaphragm. Eventually they reach the submucosa of the oesophagus where they spend the winter. Adult *H. lineatum* also usually emerge about 1 month before *H. bovis*.

Pathogenesis: The panic reaction provoked by the approach of adult warble flies is less pronounced with *H. lineatum* than *H. bovis*, since it reaches the animals by a series of hops along the ground and remains on the lower limb for a time while it lays its row of eggs, so that the animal may be unaware of its presence. Consequently, in parts of the USA this species is appropriately termed the 'heel fly'. If larvae of *H. lineatum* die in the oesophageal wall they may cause bloat through oesophageal stricture and faulty regurgitation. Larval death in other regions may, in very rare cases, lead to anaphylaxis in sensitised animals.

ECTOPARASITES

FLIES

The larval stages, 'maggots', of a number of species of fly (Diptera) are found in skin wounds on cattle and are listed in the host–parasite checklist at the end of this chapter. More detailed descriptions of these parasites are found in Chapter 11 (Facultative ectoparasites and arthropod vectors).

LICE

Heavy louse infestation is known as pediculosis. Blood-sucking lice have been implicated in the transmission of disease such as those that transmit rickettsial anaplasmosis; however, lice are predominantly of importance because of the direct damage they cause. This effect is usually a function of their density. A small number of lice may be very common and present no problem. However, louse populations can increase dramatically reaching high densities. Transfer of lice from animal to animal or from herd to herd is usually by direct physical contact. Because lice do not survive for long off their host, the potential for animals to pick up infestations from dirty housing is limited, although it cannot be ignored. Occasionally, lice also may be transferred between animals by attachment to flies (phoresy).

Description: Lice have a segmented body divided into a head, thorax and abdomen. They have three pairs of jointed legs and a pair of short antennae. All lice are dorsoventrally flattened and wingless. The sensory organs are poorly developed; the eyes are vestigial or absent.

Geographical distribution: Worldwide, primarily in cooler areas

Pathogenesis: Light infestations are usually only discovered accidentally and should not be considered of any pathogenic importance, lice being almost normal inhabitants of the dermis and coat of many cattle, especially in winter. Moderate infestations are associated only with a mild chronic dermatitis, and are well tolerated. In heavier infestations there is pruritus, with rubbing and licking, but if sucking lice are present in large numbers there may be anaemia and weakness.

Clinical signs: Light infestations are usually only discovered accidentally. In these infections the lice and eggs are easily found by parting the hair, especially along the back, the lice being next to the skin and the eggs scattered like coarse powder throughout the hair. It is important to remember that a heavy louse infestation may itself be merely a symptom of some other underlying condition such as malnutrition or chronic disease, since debilitated animals do not groom themselves and leave the lice undisturbed. In such animals the shedding of the winter coat may be delayed for many weeks, retaining large numbers of lice.

Diagnosis: The lice may be seen on the skin. Removal and examination under a light microscope will allow species identification. The eggs are also visible and appear as white specks attached to the hairs.

Epidemiology: In warm countries there is no marked seasonality of bovine pediculosis, but in cold and temperate regions the heaviest infestations are in late winter and early spring, when the coat is at its thickest, giving a sheltered, bulky and humid habitat for optimal multiplication. The most rapid annual increase in louse populations is seen when cattle are winter-housed, and lice can build up in numbers very quickly. In late spring, there is usually an abrupt fall in the numbers of lice, most of the parasites and eggs being shed with the winter coat. Numbers generally remain low throughout the summer, partly because the thinness of the coat provides a restricted habitat, but partly also because high skin surface temperatures and direct sunlight limit multiplication and may even be lethal.

Treatment: The organophosphorus insecticides (for example, chlorfenvinphos, coumaphos, chlorpyrifos, crotoxyphos, trichlorfon, phosmet and propetamphos), usually applied as pour-on or spot-on applications, are effective in killing all lice. However, most insecticides registered for use on cattle are not very active against louse eggs. This means that after treatment eggs can still hatch and continue the infestation. A second treatment is therefore recommended 2 weeks later to kill newly emerged lice. Pour-on or spot-on synthetic pyrethroids, such as cypermethrin or permethrin, or pour-on avermectins may also be used, although the latter have only limited activity against chewing lice.

Control: The timing and frequency of treatments depends very much on individual circumstances. In many cases treatment in late autumn or early winter will give adequate control of cattle lice. In Europe, louse control is usually undertaken when cattle are housed for the winter. Because a wide variety of chemical classes are effective, louse control is not difficult to achieve. Nevertheless, in an attempt to reduce the risk of selection for resistance, rotation of chemical classes may be advantageous. Treatment of all stock on farm and subsequent initial quarantine and treatment of all newly introduced animals will allow a good degree of louse control to be maintained.

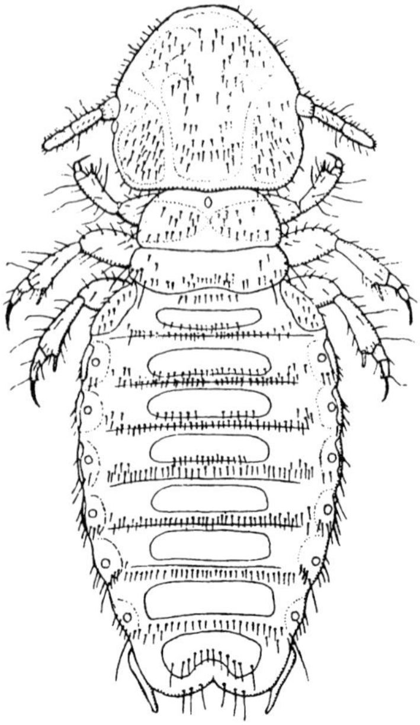

Fig. 2.55 Dorsal view of adult female *Bovicola* (reproduced from Séguy, 1944).

Bovicola bovis

Synonym: *Damalinia bovis*

Common name: Red louse, cattle chewing louse

Predilection site: Favours the top of the head, especially the curly hair of the poll and forehead, the neck, shoulders, back, and rump, and occasionally the tail switch.

Parasite class: Insecta

Parasite order: Phthiraptera

Parasite suborder: Ischnocera

Family: Trichodectidae

Description: *B. bovis* are a reddish brown in colour with dark transverse bands on the abdomen. Adults measure up to 2 mm in length and 0.35–0.55 mm in width. The head is relatively large, as wide as the body and is rounded anteriorly (Fig. 2.55). The mouthparts are ventral and are adapted for chewing. The legs are slender and are adapted for moving amongst the hair. The claws, on each leg, are small.

Hosts: Cattle

Life cycle: During a life span of about a month the female lays an egg every 2 days on average. These eggs are usually whitish, and are glued singly to the hair shaft where they may be seen with the naked eye. The eggs hatch after 7–10 days and each nymphal instar lasts 5–6 days. The nymphs have lighter sclerotisation and less distinct banding than adult lice. The nymph is similar in appearance though much smaller than the adult. After three nymphal stages, the nymph moults again to become an adult. The whole cycle from egg to adult takes 2–3 weeks. Adults may live for up to 10 weeks. *Bovicola* are believed to be capable of increasing their rate of population growth by changing from sexual to asexual reproduction via parthenogenesis. As a result, highly female biased sex ratios may be commonly found in a growing population.

Pathogenesis: The mouthparts of *B. bovis* are equipped for biting and chewing, and these lice feed on the outer layers of the hair shafts, dermal scales and blood scabs. If infestations increase, the lice may spread down the sides and may cover the rest of the body. This louse feeds by scraping away scurf and skin debris from the base of the hairs, causing considerable irritation to the host animal. The skin reaction can cause the hair to loosen and the cattle react to the irritation by rubbing or scratching, which will result in patches of hair being pulled or rubbed off. Scratching may produce wounds or bruises and a roughness to the skin. This may lead to secondary skin infections and skin trauma such as spot and fleck grain loss in the hide, reducing its value.

Epidemiology: *Bovicola bovis* is one of the commonest cattle parasites in Europe and it is the only chewing louse found on cattle in the USA. Though it causes less individual damage than sucking lice, it is present in larger numbers and so can be extremely damaging. Infested cattle may show disrupted feeding patterns.

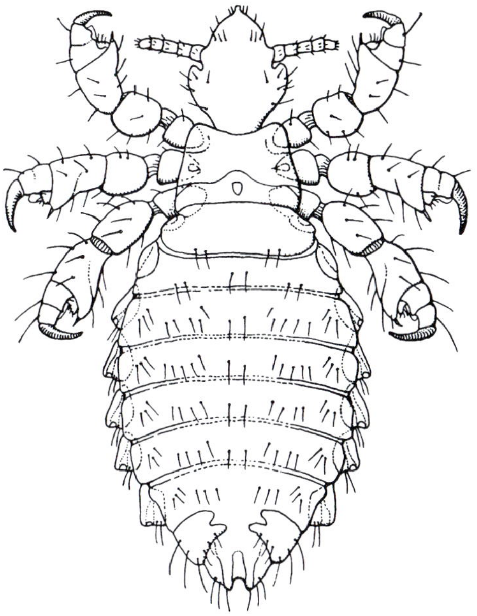

Fig. 2.56 Dorsal view of adult *Haematopinus* (reproduced from Séguy, 1944).

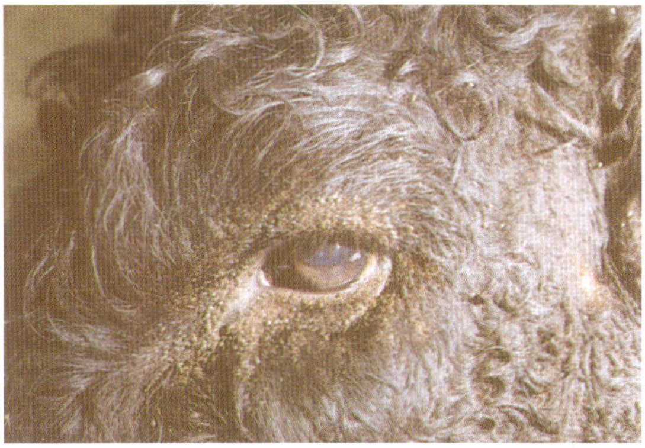

Fig. 2.57 Severe bovine pediculosis due to *Haematopinus eurysternus*.

Pathogenesis: In severe infestations, the entire region from the base of the horns, over the face (Fig. 2.57) to the base of the tail can be infested.

Notes: This species is more commonly found infesting mature cattle than young animals. In North America *Haematopinus eurysternus* is more prevalent in the Great Plains and Rocky Mountain regions.

Haematopinus eurysternus

Common name: The short-nosed louse

Predilection site: Skin, poll and at the base of the horns, in the ears, and around the eyes and nostrils and even in mild infestations it is found in the tail switch.

Parasite class: Insecta

Parasite order: Phthiraptera

Parasite suborder: Anoplura

Family: Haematopinidae

Description: *Haematopinus eurysternus* is one of the largest lice of domestic mammals, measuring 3.4–4.8 mm in length. The louse is broad in shape with a short, pointed head (Fig. 2.56). The head and thorax are yellow or greyish brown, and the abdomen blue-grey with a dark stripe on each side. The hard-shelled eggs are opaque and white and are pointed at their base.

Hosts: Cattle

Life cycle: Adult lice live for 10–15 days and, when mature, females lay one egg per day for approximately 2 weeks. The eggs are glued to the hairs or bristles of the host and hatch in 1–2 weeks. The emerging nymphs resemble the adult louse except in size. Nymphs moult to become adults about 14 days after hatching. The female lice begin to lay eggs after feeding and mating.

Haematopinus quadripertusus

Common name: Tail louse

Predilection site: Tail and perineum

Parasite class: Insecta

Parasite order: Phthiraptera

Parasite suborder: Anoplura

Family: Haematopinidae

Description: *Haematopinus quadripertusus* is a large, eyeless louse about 4–5 mm in length. It has a dark, well developed thoracic sternal plate. Behind the antennae are prominent angular processes, known as ocular points or temporal angles. The legs are of similar sizes, each terminating in a single large claw that opposes the tibial spur. Distinct sclerotised paratergal plates are visible on abdominal segments 2 or 3 to 8.

Hosts: Cattle, commonly zebu cattle (*Bos indicus*)

Life cycle: During a lifespan of about a month the female lays 50–100 operculate eggs ('nits') at a rate of one to six eggs per day. These are usually whitish, and are glued to the hair or feathers where they may be seen with the naked eye. The eggs of this louse are usually deposited on the tail hairs, which become matted with eggs in severe infestations. In very severe cases the tail head may be shed. The eggs hatch after 9–25 days depending on the climatic conditions.

Nymphs disperse over the entire body surface of the host, but adults are most commonly found on the tail head. After three nymphal moults, over a period of about 12 days, the fully mature reproductive adult is present. Within 4 days, after feeding and mating, the adult female begins to lay eggs. The whole cycle from egg to adult takes 2–3 weeks. This species is most commonly found among the long tail hairs at the base of the tail.

Pathogenesis: *Haematopinus quadripertusus* feeds on host blood using its piercing mouthparts. In severe infestations, the entire region from the base of the horns to the base of the tail can be infested.

Epidemiology: Unlike other cattle lice, *Haematopinus quadripertusus* is most abundant during the summer and in warmer climates. The lice are transmitted through direct contact between hosts.

Linognathus vituli

Common name: 'Long-nosed' cattle louse

Predilection site: Skin, preferring the head, neck and dewlap

Parasite class: Insecta

Parasite order: Phthiraptera

Parasite suborder: Anoplura

Family: Linognathidae

Description: Bluish black medium-sized louse with an elongated, pointed head and body, approximately 2.5 mm in length (Fig. 2.58). There are no eyes or ocular points. Forelegs are small. Mid- and hindlegs are larger with a large claw and tibial spur. There are two rows of setae on each segment. The thoracic sternal plate is weakly developed or absent. The eggs may be dark in colour, and are less easy to see on hair. These lice are gregarious in habit, forming dense, isolated clusters. While feeding they extend their bodies in an upright position.

Hosts: Cattle

Life cycle: During a lifespan of about a month the female lays a number of operculate eggs at a rate of about one egg per day. These are glued to the hair where they may be seen with the naked eye. The eggs hatch within 10–15 days. The nymph is similar in appearance to the adult though much smaller. The nymph increases in size as it moults through three instars, to eventually become an adult. The whole cycle from egg to adult takes 2–3 weeks.

Pathogenesis: This species is capable of transmitting bovine anaplasmosis, dermatomycosis (ringworm) and theileriosis.

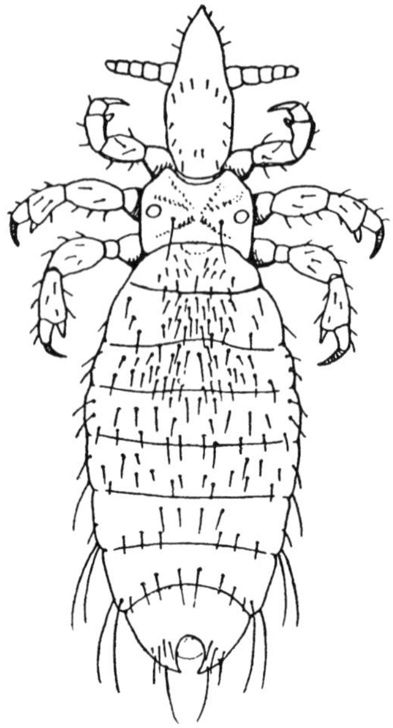

Fig. 2.58 Dorsal view of adult female *Linognathus* (reproduced from Séguy, 1944).

Epidemiology: Heaviest infestation occurs in late winter and early spring.

Solenopotes capillatus

Common name: Little blue cattle louse

Predilection site: Skin of neck, head, shoulders, dewlap, back and tail

Parasite class: Insecta

Parasite order: Phthiraptera

Parasite suborder: Anoplura

Family: Linognathidae

Description: Small bluish lice which tend to occur in clusters on the neck, head, shoulders, dewlap, back and tail. These lice may be distinguished from the genus *Linognathus* by the presence of abdominal spiracles set on slightly sclerotised tubercles, which project slightly from each abdominal segment (Fig. 2.59). At 1.2–1.5 mm in length *Solenopotes capillatus* is the smallest of the anopluran lice found on cattle. Eyes and ocular points are absent, and the louse has a short rostrum. There are no paratergal plates on the abdomen. The second and third pairs of legs are larger than the first pair and end in stout claws. In contrast to species of *Linognathus*, the thoracic sternal plate

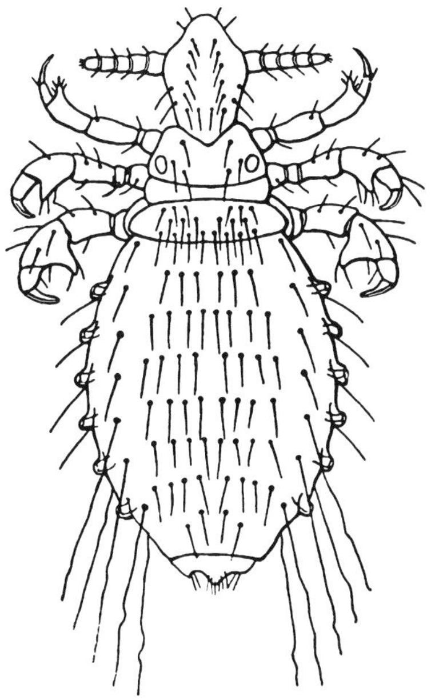

Fig. 2.59 Dorsal view of adult female *Solenopotes* (reproduced from Séguy, 1944).

is distinct. The eggs of this louse species are small, short and dark blue.

Hosts: Cattle

Life cycle: Females lay 1–2 eggs per day, and oviposition usually causes the hairs on which eggs are laid to bend. Eggs hatch after about 10 days and lice moult three times before reaching adulthood 11 days later. The egg-to-adult life cycle requires about 5 weeks.

Haematopinus tuberculatus

Common name: Buffalo louse

Parasite class: Insecta

Parasite order: Phthiraptera

Parasite suborder: Anoplura

Family: Haematopinidae

Description: A large louse measuring about 5.5 mm in length, with prominent ocular points but without eyes.

Hosts: Cattle, buffalo

Pathogenesis: Populations build up during the winter when the animal's coat is longer and thicker but it is not generally considered of any great clinical importance.

Notes: Known originally to infest buffalo but now found to infest cattle in Africa.

MITES

The ectoparasitic mites of cattle feed on blood, lymph, skin debris or sebaceous secretions, which they ingest by puncturing the skin, scavenge from the skin surface or imbibe from epidermal lesions. Most ectoparasitic mites spend their entire lives in intimate contact with their host, so that transmission from host to host is primarily by physical contact. Infestation by mites is called acariasis and can result in severe dermatitis, known as mange, which may cause significant welfare problems and economic losses.

Demodex bovis

Predilection site: Hair follicles and sebaceous glands

Parasite class: Arachnida

Sub-class: Acari

Order: Acariformes

Sub-order: Trombidiformes (Prostigmata)

Family: Demodicidae

Description: Species of *Demodex* have an elongate tapering body, up to 0.1–0.4 mm in length, with four pairs of stumpy legs ending in small blunt claws in the adult (see Fig. 6.32). Setae are absent from the legs and body. The legs are located at the front of the body, and as such the striated opisthosoma forms at least half the body length.

Hosts: Cattle

Life cycle: *Demodex* spp usually live as commensals in the skin, and are highly site-specific, occupying the hair follicles and sebaceous glands. Females lay 20–24 spindle-shaped eggs in the hair follicle that give rise to hexapod larvae, in which each short leg ends in a single, three-pronged claw. Unusually, a second hexapod larval stage follows, in which each leg ends in a pair of three-pronged claws. Octopod protonymph, tritonymph and adult stages then follow. Immature stages and these migrate more deeply into the dermis. One follicle may harbour all life cycle stages concurrently. The life cycle is completed in 18–24 days. In each follicle or gland the mites may occur in large numbers, located in a characteristic head-downward posture. In the newborn and very young these sites are simple in structure, but later they become compounded by outgrowths. The presence of *Demodex* mites much deeper in the dermis than sarcoptids means that they are much less accessible to surface-acting acaricides. Species of *Demodex* are unable to survive off their host.

Geographical distribution: Worldwide

Pathogenesis: The most important effect of bovine demodicosis is the formation of many pea-sized nodules, each containing caseous material and several thousand mites, which cause hide damage and economic loss. Though these nodules can be easily seen in smooth-coated animals, they are often undetected in rough-coated cattle until the hide has been dressed. Problems caused by demodecosis in cattle are primarily a result of the damage caused to the hides. In some rare cases demodecosis may become generalised and fatal.

Clinical signs: Pea-sized nodules containing caseous material and mites, particularly on the withers, lateral neck, back and flanks. Concurrent pyoderma may occur, leading to furunculosis with ulceration and crust formation.

Diagnosis: For confirmatory diagnosis, deep scrapings are necessary to reach the mites deep in the follicles and glands. This is best achieved by taking a fold of skin, applying a drop of liquid paraffin, and scraping until capillary blood appears.

Pathology: In cattle cutaneous nodules consist of follicular cysts lined with squamous epithelium and filled with waxy keratin squames and mites. Eruption of the cysts on to the skin may form a thick crust; rupture within the dermis may form an abcess or granulomatous reaction.

Epidemiology: Probably because of its location deep in the dermis, it is almost impossible to transmit *Demodex* between animals unless there is prolonged contact. Such contact usually only occurs during suckling, and as such it is thought that most infections are acquired in the early weeks of life. The muzzle, neck, withers and back are common sites of infestation.

Treatment: In many cases demodecosis spontaneously resolves and treatment is unnecessary. The organophosphate trichlophon, used on three occasions 2 days apart, and systemic macrocyclic lactones may be effective.

Control: Control is rarely applied since there is little incentive for farmers to treat their animals, as the cost of damage is borne by the hide merchant.

Notes: Species of the genus *Demodex* are highly specialised mites that live in the hair follicles and sebaceous glands of a wide range of wild and domestic animals, including humans. They are believed to form a group of closely related sibling species, which are highly specific to particular hosts: *Demodex phylloides* (pig), *Demodex canis* (dog), *Demodex bovis* (cattle), *Demodex equi* (horse), *Demodex musculi* (mouse), *Demodex ratti* (rat), *Demodex caviae* (guinea-pig), *Demodex cati* (cat) and *Demodex folliculorum* and *Demodex brevis* on humans.

In some parts of Australia 95% of hides are damaged, and surveys in the USA have shown a quarter of the hides to be affected. In Britain 17% of hides have been found to have *Demodex* nodules.

Psorergates bovis

Synonym: *Psorergates bos*

Common name: Cattle itch mite

Predilection site: Skin, all over the body

Parasite class: Arachnida

Sub-class: Acari

Order: Acariformes

Sub-order: Trombidiformes (Prostigmata)

Family: Psorergatidae

Description: *Psorergates bovis* is a small mite, roughly circular in form and less than 0.2 mm in diameter. The legs are arranged more or less equidistantly around the body circumference, giving the mite a crude star shape. Larvae of *P. ovis* have short, stubby legs. The legs become progressively longer during the nymphal stages until, in the adult, the legs are well developed and the mites become mobile. Adults are about 190 μm long and 160 μm wide. The tarsal claws are simple and the empodium is pad-like. The femur of each leg bears a large, inwardly directed curved spine. In the adult female, two pairs of long, whip-like setae are present posteriorly; in the male there is only a single pair.

Hosts: Cattle

Life cycle: The life cycle is typical: egg, hexapod larva, followed by octopod protonymph, tritonymph and adult. All developmental stages occur on the host. The egg-to-adult life cycle requires approximately 35 days.

Geographical distribution: Australia, New Zealand, southern Africa, North and South America. It has not been reported in Europe.

Pathogenesis: Little or no pathogenic effect.

Clinical signs: There are few clinical signs associated with infestations of this mite. Mites may occur on apparently normal skin without causing itching of the host animal.

Diagnosis: To obtain mites it is necessary, having clipped away a patch of hair, to apply a drop of mineral oil and scrape the skin down to the blood capillary level. The mites themselves are easily identified.

Pathology: Rarely the mite may cause alopecia and desquamation, but in the majority of cases there appears to be no recognisable lesion associated with the infection.

Epidemiology: This mite is not normally considered to be of clinical significance.

Treatment: *Psorergates* is relatively unsusceptible to most acaricides, although the formamidine amitraz has recently been shown to be of considerable value. Otherwise, the older arsenic–sulphur preparations may be used. Macrocyclic lactones may be effective.

Control: Regular checks of livestock and treatments will keep infection rate under control.

Psoroptes ovis

Synonyms: *Psoroptes communis* var *ovis*, *Psoroptes cuniculi*, *Psoroptes cervinus*, *Psoroptes bovis*, *Psoroptes equi*

Predilection site: Skin; particularly the legs, feet, base of tail and upper rear surface of the udder

Parasite class: Arachnida

Sub-class: Acari

Order: Acariformes

Sub-order: Sarcoptiformes (Astigmata)

Family: Psoroptidae

Pathogenesis: In cattle these mites cause intense pruritus, papules, crusts, excoriation and lichenification. Lesions may cover almost the entire body; secondary bacterial infections are common in severe cases. Death in untreated calves, weight loss, decreased milk production and increased susceptibility to other diseases can occur.

Treatment: In cattle dipping and topical application of nonsystemic acaricides, such as the organophosphates (diazinon, coumaphos or phosmet), amitraz or a lime–sulphur dip, may be effective. Dippings should be repeated at 2-week intervals. The topical application of flumethrin is also used in some parts of the world. Most treatments are not licensed for use in dairy cattle. Injectable formulations of avermectins (ivermectin and doramectin) and milbemycins (moxidectin) may be effective, though the isolation of treated animals for 2–3 weeks after treatment is required to pevent reinfestation. Eprinomectin is available as a pour-on formulation, and is the only macrocyclic lactone that may be used in dairy cattle.

Following diagnosis, the treatment of all animals on infected premises and subsequent treatment of all incoming stock is recommended.

For more detailed description see Chapter 3 (Sheep and goats).

Psoroptes natalensis

Predilection site: Skin; particularly the legs, feet, base of tail and upper rear surface of the udder

Parasite class: Arachnida

Sub-class: Acari

Order: Acariformes

Sub-order: Sarcoptiformes (Astigmata)

Family: Psoroptidae

Description: Very similar to *P. ovis* but it is believed that *P. natalensis* can be distinguished morphologically by the length and spatulate shape of the fourth outer opisthosomal seta of the male. However, the precise species status of *P. natalensis* has yet to be confirmed.

Hosts: Primarily buffalo but it has been reported on cattle.

For treatment and pathogenesis see *P. ovis*

Chorioptes bovis

Synonym: *Chorioptes ovis*, *Chorioptes equi*, *Chorioptes caprae*, *Chorioptes cuniculi*

Predilection site: Skin, particularly the legs, feet, base of tail and upper rear surface of the udder

Parasite class: Arachnida

Sub-class: Acari

Order: Acariformes

Sub-order: Sarcoptiformes (Astigmata)

Family: Psoroptidae

Description: Adult female *Chorioptes bovis* are about 300 μm in length (Fig. 2.60), considerably smaller than *Psoroptes ovis. Chorioptes* do not have jointed pretarsi; their pretarsi are shorter than in *Psoroptes* and the sucker-like pulvillus is more cup-shaped, as opposed to trumpet-shaped in *Psoroptes*. In the adult female, tarsi I, II and IV have short-stalked pretarsi and tarsi III have a pair of long, terminal, whip-like setae. The first and second pairs of legs are stronger than the others and the fourth pair has long, slender tarsi. In the male, all legs possess short-stalked pretarsi and pulvilli. However, the fourth pair is extremely short, not extending beyond the body margin. Male *C. bovis* have two broad, flat setae and three normal setae on well developed posterior lobes. The mouthparts are distinctly rounder, and the abdominal tubercles of the male are noticeably more truncate than those of *Psoroptes* (see Fig. 3.44).

Hosts: Cattle, sheep, horse, goat, rabbit

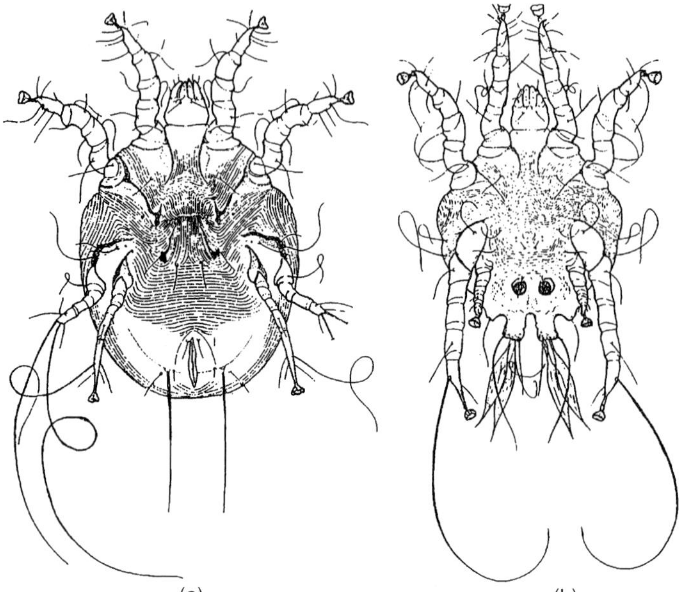

Fig. 2.60 Adult *Chorioptes bovis,* ventral views. (a) Female. (b) Male (reproduced from Baker *et al.*, 1956).

Life cycle: The life cycle is typical: egg, hexapod larva, followed by octopod protonymph, tritonymph and adult. All developmental stages occur on the host. The complete egg-to-adult life cycle takes about 3 weeks. Eggs are deposited at a rate of one per day and are attached to the host skin. Adult females produce 15–20 eggs and live for 2–3 weeks. *Chorioptes bovis* has mouthparts which are adapted for chewing skin debris. Mites may survive for up to 3 weeks off the host, allowing transmission from housing and bedding as well as by direct contact.

Geographical distribution: Worldwide

Pathogenesis: In cattle, chorioptic mange occurs most often in housed animals, particularly dairy animals, affecting mainly the neck, tail-head, udder and legs. Usually only a few animals in a group are clinically affected. The mites are found more commonly on the hindleg than on the foreleg. It is a mild condition, and lesions tend to remain localised, with slow spread. Its importance is economic; the pruritus caused by the mites resulting in rubbing and scratching, with damage to the hide. High infestations have been associated with decreased milk production. The treatment is the same as for sarcoptic mange in cattle.

Clinical signs: Hosts can be asymptomatic with low densities of mites present and thus act as carriers that transfer the mite to other animals. Host reactions are normally only induced when numbers increase to thousands of mites per host. Scabs or scales develop on the skin of the lower parts of the body. There is some exudation and crust formation on the legs and lower body, but this does not spread over a wide area. Infected animals may stamp and scratch infected areas. The majority of the mites are likely to be found on the lower leg, particularly the pastern and foot.

Diagnosis: Skin scrapings from the suspect lesions should be taken for microscopic examination.

Pathology: The pathology is highly variable depending on the intensity and duration of infection; subclinical infections are common. Clinically affected animals may have pustular, crusted, scaly and lichinified lesions and alopecia.

Epidemiology: Mite populations are highest in the winter and may regress over summer. It is the most common type of mange in cattle in the USA.

Treatment: The dips used for psoroptic mange in cattle are also effective against *Chorioptes.* They should be repeated at 2-week intervals. Ivermectin, doramectin, eprinomectin and moxidectin applied topically as a pour-on are also effective against chorioptic mange.

Control: Regular checks of livestock and quarantining of infected animals will help to control the frequency and extent of infestations.

Notes: The names *Chorioptes ovis*, *Chorioptes equi*, *Chorioptes caprae* and *Chorioptes cuniculi* used to describe the chorioptic mites found on sheep, horses, goats and rabbits respectively, are now all thought to be synonyms of *Chorioptes bovis*

Sarcoptes scabiei

Common name: Scabies

Predilection site: Skin

Parasite class: Arachnida

Sub-class: Acari

Order: Acariformes

Sub-order: Sarcoptiformes (Astigmata)

Family: Sarcoptidae

Pathogenesis: Sarcoptic mange is potentially the most severe of the cattle manges, although many cases are mild. Nevertheless, it is being increasingly diagnosed in Britain and in some areas, including Canada and parts of the USA, the disease is notifiable and the entry of cattle carrying *Sarcoptes*, whether clinically affected or not, is not permitted. The mite has partial site preferences, which have given it, in the USA, the common name of 'neck and tail mange', but it may occur on any part of the body. Mild infections merely show scaly skin with little hair loss, but in severe cases the skin becomes thickened, there is marked loss of hair and crusts form on the less well haired parts of the body (Fig. 2.61), such as the escutcheon of cows. There is intense pruritus leading to loss of meat and milk production and to hides being downgraded because of damage by scratching and rubbing.

Treatment and control: Treatment has largely depended on the use of repeated washes or sprays usually organochlorine insecticides such as gamma HCH (hexachlorocyclohexane). However, organochlorine insecticides are not now available in most countries. Systemic macrocyclic lactones may give good results. Alternatively, the application of a pour-on organophosphate such as phosmet, on two occasions at an interval of 14 days, is also effective. Neither macrocyclic lactones nor phosmet are licensed for use in lactating animals whose milk is used for human consumption. The amidine, amitraz, is effective against sarcoptic mange in cattle and has withdrawal periods of 24 and 48 hours respectively for meat and milk.

For further details see Chapter 5 (Pigs).

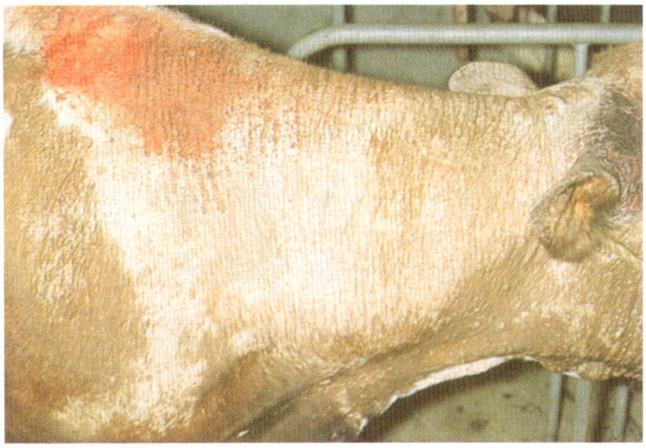

Fig. 2.61 Characteristic lesions of bovine sarcoptic mange.

A number of non-obligate ectoparasites are found on cattle and are listed in the host–parasite checklist at the end of this chapter. More detailed descriptions of these parasites are found in Chapter 11 (Facultative ectoparasites and arthropod vectors).

In the following checklists, the codes listed below apply:

Helminth classes:
N = Nematoda; T = Trematoda; C = Cestoda.

Arthropod classes:
I = Insecta; A = Arachnida.

Protozoal classes:
M = Mastigophora; S = Sarcodina; A = Apicomplexa; R = Rickettsia.

Cattle parasite checklist.

Section/host system	Helminths		Arthropods		Protozoa	
	Parasite	(Super)family	Parasite	Family	Parasite	Family
Digestive						
Oesophagus	*Gongylonema pulchrum*	Spiruroidea (N)	*Hypoderma bovis*	Oestridae (I)		
			Hypoderma lineatum	Oestridae (I)		
Rumen/reticulum	*Gongylonema verrucosum*	Spiruroidea (N)			*Monocercomonas ruminantium*	Monocercomonadidae (M)
	Paramphistomum cervi	Paramphistomatidae (T)			*Entamoeba bovis*	Endamobidae (S)
	Paramphistomum microbothrium	Paramphistomatidae (T)				
	Ceylonocotyle streptocoelium	Paramphistomatidae (T)				
	Cotylophoron cotylophorum	Paramphistomatidae (T)				
Abomasum	*Ostertagia ostertagi*	Trichostrongyloidea (N)			*Cryptosporidium andersoni*	Cryptosporidiidae (A)
	Ostertagia leptospicularis	Trichostrongyloidea (N)				
	Haemonchus contortus	Trichostrongyloidea (N)				
	Haemonchus similis	Trichostrongyloidea (N)				
	Trichostrongylus axei	Trichostrongyloidea (N)				
	Mecistocirrus digitatus	Trichostrongyloidea (N)				
	Parabronema skrjabini	Spiruroidea (N)				
Small intestine	*Trichostrongylus colubriformis*	Trichostrongyloidea (N)			*Eimeria zuernii*	Eimeriidae (A)
	Trichostrongylus longispicularis	Trichostrongyloidea (N)			*Eimeria bovis*	Eimeriidae (A)
	Cooperia oncophora	Trichostrongyloidea (N)			*Eimeria alabamensis*	Eimeriidae (A)
	Cooperia punctata	Trichostrongyloidea (N)			*Eimeria aubernensis*	Eimeriidae (A)
	Cooperia pectinata	Trichostrongyloidea (N)			*Eimeria brasiliensis*	Eimeriidae (A)
	Cooperia surnabada	Trichostrongyloidea (N)			*Eimeria bukidnonensis*	Eimeriidae (A)
	Nematodirus helvetianus	Trichostrongyloidea (N)			*Eimeria canadensis*	Eimeriidae (A)
	Nematodirus battus	Trichostrongyloidea (N)			*Eimeria cylindrica*	Eimeriidae (A)
	Nematodirus spathiger	Trichostrongyloidea (N)			*Eimeria ellipsoidalis*	Eimeriidae (A)
	Bunostomum phlebotomum	Ancylostomatoidea (N)			*Eimeria pellita*	Eimeriidae (A)
	Agriostomum vryburgi	Ancylostomatoidea (N)			*Eimeria subspherica*	Eimeriidae (A)
	Strongyloides papillosus	Rhabditoidea (N)			*Eimeria wyomingensis*	Eimeriidae (A)
	Toxocara (Neoascaris) vitulorum	Ascaridoidea (N)			*Cryptosporidium parvum*	Cryptosporidiidae (A)
	Capillaria bovis	Trichuroidea (N)			*Giardia intestinalis*	Diplomonadidae (M)
	Moniezia benedeni	Anoplocephalidae (C)				
	Moniezia expansa	Anoplocephalidae (C)				
	Thysaniezia ovilla	Thysanosomidae (C)				
	Avitellina centripunctata	Thysanosomidae (C)				
	Stilesia globipunctata	Thysanosomidae (C)				
	Thysanosoma actinoides	Thysanosomidae (C)				
	Cymbiforma indica	Notocotylidae (T)				

Caecum	*Oesophagostomum radiatum*	Strongyloidea (N)	*Eimeria zuernii*	Eimeriidae (A)
Colon	*Trichuris globulosa*	Trichuroidea (N)	*Eimeria bovis*	Eimeriidae (A)
	Trichuris discolor	Trichuroidea (N)	*Tetratrichomonas buttreyi*	Trichomonadidae (M)
	Homalogaster paloniae	Paramphistomatidae (T)	*Tetratrichomonas pavlovi*	Trichomonadidae (M)
			Tritrichomonas enteris	Trichomonadidae (M)
			Retortamonas ovis	Retortamonadorididae (M)
			Buxtonella sulcata	Pycnotrichidae (C)
Respiratory				
Nasal cavities	*Mammomonogamus laryngeus*	Strongyloidea (N)		
	Mammomonogamus nasicola	Strongyloidea (N)		
Trachea Bronchi	*Dictyocaulus viviparus*	Trichostrongyloidea (N)	*Pneumocystis carinii*	Pneumocystidaceae (fungus)
Lung	*Echinococcus granulosus*	Taeniidae (C)		
Liver				
	Fasciola hepatica	Fasciolidae (T)		
	Fasciola gigantica	Fasciolidae (T)		
	Fascioloides magna	Fasciolidae (T)		
	Dicrocoelium dendriticum	Dicrocoeliidae (T)		
	Dicrocoelium hospes	Dicrocoeliidae (T)		
	Echinococcus granulosus	Taeniidae (C)		
	Stilesia hepatica	Thysanosomidae (C)		
	Cysticercus tenuicollis (Taenia hydatigena)	Taeniidae (C)		
	Thysanosoma actinioides	Thysanosomidae (C)		
Pancreas				
	Eurytrema pancreaticum	Dicrocoeliidae (T)		
	Eurytrema coelomaticum	Dicrocoeliidae (T)		
	Thysanosoma actinioides	Thysanosomidae (C)		
Circulatory				
Blood	*Schistosoma bovis*	Schistosomatidae (T)	*Trypanosoma brucei brucei*	Trypanosomatidae (M)
	Schistosoma japonicum	Schistosomatidae (T)	*Trypanosoma brucei evansi*	Trypanosomatidae (M)
	Schistosoma nasalis	Schistosomatidae (T)	*Trypanosoma congolense*	Trypanosomatidae (M)
	Schistosoma mattheei	Schistosomatidae (T)	*Trypanosoma vivax*	Trypanosomatidae (M)
	Schistosoma indicum	Schistosomatidae (T)	*Trypansoma theileri*	Trypanosomatidae (M)
	Schistosoma spindale	Schistosomatidae (T)	*Babesia bigemina*	Babesiidae (A)
	Schistosoma turkestanica	Schistosomatidae (T)	*Babesia bovis*	Babesiidae (A)
			Babesia divergens	Babesiidae (A)

(*continued*)

Cattle parasite checklist (*continued*).

Section/host system	Helminths		Arthropods		Protozoa	
	Parasite	(Super)family	Parasite	Family	Parasite	Family
Blood vessels	*Elaeophora poeli*	Filarioidea (N)			*Babesia major*	Babesiidae (A)
	Onchocerca armillata	Filarioidea (N)			*Theileria parva*	Theileriidae (A)
					Theileria annulata	Theileriidae (A)
					Theileria orientalis complex	Theileriidae (A)
					Theileria taurotragi	Theileriidae (A)
					Theileria velifera	Theileriidae (A)
					Anaplasma marginale	Anaplasmataceae (R)
					Anaplasma centrale	Anaplasmataceae (R)
					Anaplasma phagocytophilum	Anaplasmataceae (R)
					Ehrlichia bovis	Rickettsiaceae (R)
					Ehrlichia ruminantium	Rickettsiaceae (R)
					Eperythrozoon wenyonii	Rickettsiaceae (R)
					Rickettsia conorii	Rickettsiaceae (R)
Nervous						
CNS	*Coenurus cerebralis (Taenia multiceps)*	Taeniidae (C)	*Hypoderma bovis*	Oestridae (I)	*Toxoplasma gondii*	Sarcocystiidae (A)
					Trypanosoma brucei brucei	Trypanosomatidae (M)
Eye	*Thelazia rhodesi*	Spiruroidea (N)				
	Thelazia gulosa	Spiruroidea (N)				
	Thelazia skrjabini	Spiruroidea (N)				
Reproductive/urogenital						
	Stephanurus dentatus	Strongyloidea (N)			*Tritrichomonas foetus*	Trichomonadidae (M)
					Neospora caninum	Sarcocystiidae (A)
					Trypanosoma brucei brucei	Trypanosomatidae (M)
Locomotory						
Muscle	*Cysticercus bovis (metacestode – Taenia saginata)*	Taeniidae (C)			*Sarcocystis bovicanis*	Sarcocystiidae (A)
					Sarcocystis bovifelis	Sarcocystiidae (A)
	Onchocerca dukei	Filarioidea (N)			*Sarcocystis bovihominis*	Sarcocystiidae (A)
					Toxoplasma gondii	Sarcocystiidae (A)
					Trypanosoma brucei brucei	Trypanosomatidae (M)

Connective tissue						
	Onchocerca gutturosa (lienalis)	Filarioidea (N)				
	Onchocerca gibsoni	Filarioidea (N)				
	Onchocerca ochengi	Filarioidea (N)				
	Parafilaria bovicola	Filarioidea (N)				
	Setaria labiato-papillosa	Filarioidea (N)				
	Setaria digitatus	Filarioidea (N)				
Integument						
Skin			*Bovicola bovis*	Trichodectidae (I)	*Besnoitia besnoiti*	Sarcocystiidae (A)
			Haematopinus eurysternus	Haematopinidae (I)		
	Stephanofilaria stilesi	Filarioidea (N)	*Haematopinus quadripertusus*	Haematopinidae (I)		
	Stephanofilaria assamensis	Filarioidea (N)	*Linognathus vituli*	Linognathidae (I)		
	Stephanofilaria zaherii	Filarioidea (N)	*Solenopotes capillatus*	Linognathidae (I)		
	Stephanofilaria kaeli	Filarioidea (N)	*Demodex bovis*	Demodicidae (A)		
	Stephanofilaria dedoesi	Filarioidea (N)	*Psoroptes ovis*	Psoroptidae (A)		
	Stephanofilaria okinawaensis	Filarioidea (N)	*Chorioptes bovis*	Psoroptidae (A)		
			Sarcoptes scabiei	Sarcoptidae (A)		
Subcutaneous			*Hypoderma bovis*	Oestridae (I)		
	Parafilaria bovicola	Filarioidea (N)	*Hypoderma lineatum*	Oestridae (I)		
	Dracunculus medinensis	Dracunculidae (N)	*Dermatobia hominis*	Oestridae (I)		
			Calliphora albifrontis	Calliphoridae (I)		
			Calliphora nociva	Calliphoridae (I)		
			Calliphora stygia	Calliphoridae (I)		
			Calliphora vicina	Calliphoridae (I)		
			Calliphora vomitoria	Calliphoridae (I)		
			Lucilia sericata	Calliphoridae (I)		
			Lucilia cuprina	Calliphoridae (I)		
			Lucilia illustris	Calliphoridae (I)		
			Protophormia terraenovae	Calliphoridae (I)		
			Phormia regina	Calliphoridae (I)		
			Cordylobia anthropophaga	Calliphoridae (I)		
			Cochliomyia hominivorax	Calliphoridae (I)		
			Cochliomyia macellaria	Calliphoridae (I)		
			Chrysomya bezziana	Calliphoridae (I)		
			Chrysomya megacephala	Calliphoridae (I)		
			Wohlfahrtia magnifica	Sarcophagidae (I)		
			Sarcophaga haemorrhoidalis	Sarcophagidae (I)		

The following species of flies and ticks are found on cattle. More detailed descriptions are found in Chapter 11: Facultative ectoparasites and arthropod vectors.

Flies of veterinary importance on cattle

Group	Genus	Species	Family
Blackflies Buffalo gnats	*Simulium*	spp.	Simuliidae (I)
Blowflies and screwworms	*Calliphora*	*albifrontis* *nociva* *stygia* *vicina* *vomitoria*	Calliphoridae (I)
	Chrysomya	*albiceps* *bezziana* *megacephala*	
	Cochliomyia	*hominivorax* *macellaria*	
	Cordylobia	*anthropophaga*	
	Lucilia	*cuprina* *illustris* *sericata*	
	Phormia	*regina*	
	Protophormia	*terraenovae*	
Bot flies	*Gedoelstia*	*haessleri*	Oestridae (I)
	Hypoderma	*bovis* *lineatum*	
	Dermatobia	*hominis*	
Flesh flies	*Sarcophaga*	*fusicausa* *haemorrhoidalis*	Sarcophagidae (I)
	Wohlfahrtia	*magnifica* *meigeni* *vigil*	
Hippoboscids	*Hippobosca*	*equina* *rufipes* *maculata* *camelina*	Hippoboscidae (I)
Midges	*Culicoides*	spp.	Ceratopogonidae (I)
Mosquitoes	*Aedes*	spp.	Culicidae (I)
	Anopheles	spp.	
	Culex	spp.	
Muscids	*Haematobia*	*irritans* *exigua*	Muscidae (I)
	Musca	*autumnalis* *domestica*	
	Stomoxys	*calcitrans*	
Sandflies	*Phlebotomus*	spp.	Psychodidae (I)
Tabanids	*Chrysops*	spp.	Tabanidae (I)
	Haematopota	spp.	
	Tabanus	spp.	
Tsetse flies	*Glossina*	*fusca* *morsitans* *palpalis*	Glossinidae (I)

Tick species found on cattle

Genus	Species	Common name	Family
Ornithodoros	*moubata*	Eyeless or hut tampan	Argasidae (A)
	savignyi	Eyed or sand tampan	
Otobius	*megnini*	Spinose ear tick	Argasidae (A)
Amblyomma	*americanum*	Lone star tick	Ixodidae (A)
	cajennense	Cayenne tick	
	gemma		
	hebraeum	South African bont tick	
	maculatum	Gulf coast tick	
	pomposum		
	variegatum	Tropical bont tick	
Boophilus	*annulatus*	Texas cattle fever tick	Ixodidae (A)
	decoloratus	Blue tick	
	microplus	Pantropical or southern cattle tick	
Dermacentor	*andersoni*	Rocky Mountain wood tick	Ixodidae (A)
	marginatus		
	nutalli		
	reticulatus	Marsh tick	
	occidentalis	Pacific coast tick	
	silvarium		
	varabilis	American dog tick	
Haemaphysalis	*punctata*		Ixodidae (A)
	concinna		
	bispinosa		
	longicornis		
Hyalomma	*anatolicum*	Bont legged tick	Ixodidae (A)
	detritum		
	dromedarii	Camel *Hyalomma*	
	excavatum	Brown ear tick	
	marginatum	Mediterranean *Hyalomma*	
	truncatum		
Ixodes	*ricinus*	Castor bean or European sheep tick	Ixodidae (A)
	holocyclus	Paralysis tick	
	rubicundus	Karoo paralysis tick	
	scapularis		
Rhipicephalus	*appendiculatus*	Brown ear tick	Ixodidae (A)
	bursa		
	capensis	Cape brown tick	
	evertsi	Red or red-legged tick	
	sanguineus	Brown dog or kennel tick	
	simus	Glossy tick	

3
Parasites of sheep and goats

ENDOPARASITES

PARASITES OF THE DIGESTIVE SYSTEM

OESOPHAGUS

Gongylonema pulchrum

Synonym: *Gongylonema scutatum*

Common name: Gullet worm

Predilection site: Oesophagus, rumen

Parasite class: Nematoda

Superfamily: Spiruroidea

Description, gross: A long, slender whitish worm; the males being about 5.0 cm and the females up to about 14.0 cm in length.

Description, microscopic: Worms are easily distinguished microscopically by the presence of longitudinal rows of cuticular bosses in the anterior region of the body. Asymmetrical cervical alae are prominent. The egg is thin-shelled and possesses two opercula. It contains an L_1 when passed in faeces.

Final host: Sheep, goat, cattle, pig, buffalo, horse, donkey, deer, camel, man

Intermediate host: Coprophagous beetles, cockroaches

Life cycle: The life cycle is typically spiruroid. Eggs are passed in faeces and when eaten by an intermediate host they hatch and develop to the infective stage within about 4 weeks. Infection of the definitive host is through the ingestion of infected coprophagous beetles or cockroaches. The adult worms live spirally (in a zipper fashion) embedded in the oesophageal mucosa or submucosa with their anterior and/or posterior ends protruding into the lumen. The prepatent period is about 8 weeks.

Geographical distribution: Probably worldwide

Pathogenesis: Infection is usually regarded as non-pathogenic, though infection has been associated with a mild chronic oesophagitis in ruminants. *G. pulchrum* in humans presents as a painful tumour-like area in the oral epithelium or subcutaneous tissues that contains coiled worms.

Clinical signs: Usually asymptomatic in ruminants

Diagnosis: Usually an incidental finding on postmortem

Pathology: Adult worms bury in the epithelium of the forestomachs producing white or red, blood-filled zigzag tracts in the mucosa.

Epidemiology: Infection is very much dependent on the presence and abundance of the intermediate hosts, principally coprophagous beetles of the genera *Aphodius*, *Onthophagus*, *Blaps*, *Caccobius*, *Onthophagus*. Man can acquire infection through direct ingestion of the intermediate host. Also water can contain infective larvae that have emerged from infected cockroaches in the water source.

Treatment: Not reported

Control: Control is not practical, nor necessary.

RUMEN/RETICULUM

Gongylonema verrucosum

Common name: Rumen gullet worm

Predilection site: Rumen, reticulum, omasum

Parasite class: Nematoda

Superfamily: Spiruroidea

For more details see Chapter 2 (Cattle).

Gongylonema monnig

Common name: Rumen gullet worm

Predilection site: Rumen, reticulum, omasum

Parasite class: Nematoda

Superfamily: Spiruroidea

Description, gross: A long, slender whitish worm; the males being about 4 cm and the females up to about 11 cm in length.

Description, microscopic: Similar to *G. verrucosum* except the cervical alae are not festooned.

Final host: Sheep, goat

Intermediate host: Coprophagous beetles, cockroaches

Geographical distribution: South Africa

Paramphistomum cervi

Synonym: *Paramphistomum explanatum*

Common name: Rumen fluke

Predilection site: Rumen

Parasite class: Trematoda

Family: Paramphistomatidae

Definitive hosts: Cattle, sheep, goat, deer, buffalo, antelope

Intermediate hosts: Water snails, principally *Planorbis* and *Bulinus*

Notes: There is confusion over the classification of paramphistomes and it is likely that many described species such as those listed below are synonymous.

Paramphistomum microbothrium

Common name: Rumen fluke

Predilection site: Rumen

Parasite class: Trematoda

Family: Paramphistomatidae

Definitive hosts: Cattle, sheep, goat, deer, buffalo, antelope

Geographical distribution: Africa

Ceylonocotyle streptocoelium

Synonym: *Paramphistomum streptocoelium*

Common name: Rumen fluke

Predilection site: Rumen

Parasite class: Trematoda

Superfamily: Paramphistomatidae

Definitive hosts: Cattle, sheep, goat and wild ruminants

Geographical distribution: Africa

Cotylophoron cotylophorum

Synonym: *Paramphistomum cotylophorum*

Common name: Rumen fluke

Predilection site: Rumen, reticulum

Parasite class: Trematoda

Family: Paramphistomatidae

Definitive hosts: Cattle, sheep and wild ruminants

Geographical distribution: India, Australia

ABOMASUM

Teladorsagia circumcincta

Synonym: *Ostertagia circumcincta*

Morph species: *Ostertagia trifurcata*, *Teladorsagia davtiani*

Common name: Brown stomach worm

Predilection site: Abomasum

Parasite class: Nematoda

Superfamily: Trichostrongyloidea

Description, gross: Adults are slender, reddish brown worms with a short buccal cavity. Males measure 6–8 mm and females 8–10 mm.

Description, microscopic:

- *Teladorsagia circumcincta.* The lateral lobes of the bursa are well developed but the dorsal lobe is small; telamon is present in the genital cone; the accessory bursal membrane is small, supported by two divergent rays. Spicules are variable in length but normally long and thin (Fig. 3.1a). The posterior end is split into two branches of equal length. A third short offshoot, not readily seen, arises in front of the bifurcation. The gubernaculum is racket-shaped. The vulva is usually covered with a large flap. The tail tapers gradually and ends in a slender, rounded tip that has four to five transverse striations.
- *Ostertagia trifurcata.* Bursa longer than *T. circumcincta.* The lateral lobes of the bursa are well developed, and the dorsal lobe is small; well developed telamon is present in the genital cone. The accessory bursal membrane is modified to form Sjoberg's organ supported by two rays; spicules are short and broad (Fig. 3.1b); the posterior end is divided into three processes, one long and thick with a truncated end, and two short slender branches each tapering to a point. The gubernaculum is somewhat spindle-shaped.

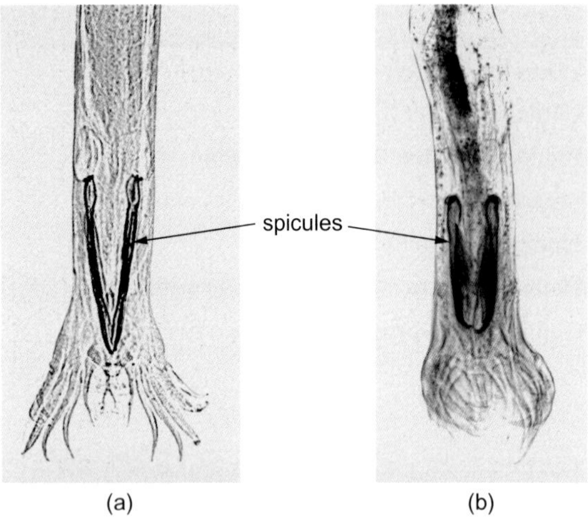

Fig. 3.1 Comparison of spicules of (a) *Teladorsagia circumcincta* and (b) *Ostertagia trifurcata*. Those of *T. circumcincta* are long and thin whereas *O. trifurcata* spicules are short and broad.

- *Teladorsagia davtiani*. Very similar to *O. trifurcata*. The accessory bursal membrane is modified to form Sjoberg's organ and resembles a pair of sessile papillae on the posterior extremity of the genital cone.

Hosts: Sheep, goat

Life cycle: Both the free-living and parasitic phases of the life cycle are similar to those of the bovine species, *O. ostertagi*.

Geographical distribution: Worldwide

Pathogenesis: In clinical infections, this resembles the situation in cattle and similar lesions are present at necropsy, although the morocco leather appearance of the abomasal surface seen in cattle is not common in sheep and goats. In subclinical infections, it has been shown under both experimental and natural conditions that *T. circumcincta* causes a marked depression in appetite and this, together with losses of plasma protein into the gastrointestinal tract and sloughed intestinal epithelium, results in interference with the post-absorptive metabolism of protein. In lambs with moderate infections of *T. circumcincta* carcase evaluation can show poor protein and fat deposition. Skeletal growth can also be impaired.

Clinical signs: The most frequent clinical sign is a marked loss of weight. Diarrhoea is intermittent and although stained hindquarters are common, the fluid faeces, that characterise bovine ostertagiosis, are less frequently seen.

Diagnosis: This is based on clinical signs, seasonality of infection and faecal egg counts and, if possible, post-mortem examination, when the characteristic lesions can be seen in the abomasum. Plasma pepsinogen levels are above the normal of about 0.8 IU tyrosine and usually exceed 2.0 IU in sheep with heavy infections.

Pathology: The pathology is similar to that described for *O. ostertagi* in cattle. The developing parasites cause distension of parasitised gastric glands, leading to a thickened hyperplastic gastric mucosa similar to that seen in cattle (see Fig. 2.5). In heavy infections these nodules coalesce and the abomasal folds are often very oedematous and hyperaemic.

Epidemiology: In sheep, *T. circumcincta* and *O. trifurcata* are responsible for outbreaks of clinical disease, particularly in lambs. In Europe a clinical syndrome analogous to type I bovine ostertagiosis occurs from August to October; thereafter arrested development of many ingested larvae occurs and a type II syndrome has been occasionally reported in late winter and early spring, especially in young adults. In subtropical areas with winter rainfall outbreaks of disease occurs primarily in late winter.

Temperate regions

In Europe, the herbage numbers of *T. circumcincta* L_3 increase markedly from mid-summer onwards and this is when most disease appears. These larvae are derived mainly from eggs passed in the faeces of ewes during the periparturient period, from about 2 weeks prior to lambing until about 6 weeks post-lambing. Eggs passed by lambs, from worm burdens which have accrued from the ingestion of overwintered larvae, also contribute to the pasture contamination. It is these eggs deposited in the first half of the grazing season from April to June which give rise to the potentially dangerous populations of L_3 from July to October. If ingested prior to October, the majority of these larvae mature in 3 weeks; thereafter, many become arrested in development for several months and may precipitate type II disease when they mature.

Immunity is acquired slowly and usually requires exposure over two grazing seasons before a significant resistance to infection develops. Subsequently, adult ewes harbour only very low populations of *Teladorsagia* except during the annual periparturient rise (PPR).

Subtropical regions

The epidemiology in subtropical areas is basically similar to that in temperate zones, except that the seasonal timing of events is different. In many of these areas lambing is geared to an increase in the growth of pasture, which occurs with the onset of rain in late autumn or winter. This coincides with conditions which are favourable to the development of the free-living stages of *Teladorsagia* and so infective larvae accumulate during the winter to cause clinical problems or production loss in the second half of the winter; arrested larval development occurs at the end of the winter or early spring. The sources of pasture contamination are again the ewes during the PPR and the lambs following ingestion of larvae, which have survived the summer. The relative importance of these sources in any country varies according to the conditions during the adverse period for larval survival. Where the summer is very dry and hot, the longevity of L_3 is reduced, except in areas with shade and these can act as reservoirs of infection until the following winter. Although L_3 can persist in sheep faeces during adverse weather conditions the protection is probably less than that afforded by the more abundant bovine faecal pat.

Ostertagia trifurcata

In temperate regions this is similar to *T. circumcincta*. In tropical and subtropical zones where the summer is very dry and hot, the longevity of L_3 is reduced except in areas with shade and these can act as reservoirs of infection until the following winter. Although L_3 can persist in sheep faeces during adverse weather conditions the protection is probably less than that afforded by the more abundant bovine faecal pat. In winter rainfall areas the numbers of *Ostertagia* and *Teladorsagia* larvae on pasture reach a maximum in late winter and decline markedly through spring into summer as the pastures dry out.

Treatment: Ovine teladorsagiosis often responds well to treatment with any of the modern benzimidazoles or pro-benzimidazoles, levamisole, which in sheep is effective against arrested larvae, or the avermectins/milbemycins. However, the widespread prevalence of isolates of *Teladorsagia circumcincta* that are resistant to the benzimidazoles, and increasingly resistant to levamisole and even some macrocyclic lactones, dictates that farmers must monitor the resistance status of their flocks to ensure that an effective anthelmintic is used. Treated lambs should preferably be moved to safe pasture and, if this is not possible, treatment may have to be repeated at 6-weekly intervals until the pasture larval levels decrease in late autumn.

Many of the anthelmintics recommended for sheep are not registered for use in goats. Where goat milk or milk products are used for human consumption, milk-withholding periods for different drugs should be observed. Thiabendazole has anti-fungal properties and should not be used when milk is processed for cheese.

Control: See The treatment and control of parasitic gastroenteritis (PGE) in sheep (below)

Notes: Considered to be a polymorphic species with at least two male morphs, *Teladorsagia circumcincta* and *Ostertagia trifurcata*, and possibly a third, *Teladorsagia davtiani*. The females cannot be differentiated but are distinguishable from other ostertagian females.

The treatment and control of parasitic gastroenteritis (PGE) in sheep

The recommendations outlined below are applicable to temperate areas of the northern hemisphere, but the principles can be adapted to local conditions in other regions.

Treatment

Because of the short period between birth and marketing, the treatment of PGE in lambs is an inferior policy compared with the preventive measures discussed below. However, when necessary, treatment with any of the benzimidazoles, levamisole or an avermectin/milbemycin will remove adult worms and developing stages, unless resistance to these drugs is present in the flock. Following treatment, lambs should be moved to pasture not grazed by sheep that year, otherwise they will immediately become reinfected. The occasional outbreaks of type II teladorsagiosis (ostertagiosis) in young adult sheep in the spring may be treated with the same anthelmintics. Unlike *O. ostertagi* in calves, the arrested stages of the common sheep nematodes are susceptible to the benzimidazoles and levamisole.

Control

Although the control of PGE in sheep is based on the same principles as that described for *O. ostertagi* in cattle, its practice is somewhat different for the following reasons:

1. The PPR (periparturient rise in faecal egg counts) is very marked in ewes and is the most important cause of pasture contamination with nematode eggs in the spring.
2. PGE in sheep is generally associated with a variety of nematode genera with differing epidemiological characteristics.
3. Most sheep graze throughout their lives so that pasture contamination with nematode eggs and the intake of infective larvae is almost continuous and modified only by climatic restrictions.
4. Anthelmintic resistance is now widespread throughout many sheep-rearing areas of the world and therefore strategies are required to manage existing resistance and/or to limit the further development of resistant isolates. Recently, guidelines for the use of anthelmintics in sustainable control strategies for sheep in northern temperate areas have been produced (www.nationalsheep.org) and are outlined below.

Summary of guidelines for the control of gastrointestinal nematodes and use of anthelmintics in sheep and goats

Anthelmintic usage

1. **Use anthelmintics sparingly.** This will reduce the selection pressure for further development of drug resistance. Effective monitoring of faecal egg counts is integral to this approach. This strategy is discussed more fully under treatment of ewes and lambs.
2. **Use anthelmintics effectively.** It is important regularly to check the dosing equipment and to apply correct techniques to maximise the efficacy of the drug. Sheep should be dosed at the rate recommended for the heaviest animal in a subgroup to reduce the likelihood of under-dosing.
3. **Monitor for anthelmintic resistance.** It is essential to ensure that the drug to be administered will be effective. The resistance status of each family of anthelmintic should be assessed on the farm.
4. **Use the appropriate anthelmintic.** In some situations it may be possible to target treatment by using a narrow-spectrum drug, e.g. closantel against a specific infection dominated by *Haemonchus* or a benzimidazole against *Nematodirus*. Avoidance of using a broad-spectrum drug in these circumstances will reduce the selection pressure to this family of anthelmintics. Annual rotation of anthelmintic families can be useful, especially where resistance to the macrocyclic lactones is absent or at a very low level. This strategy will have minimal impact where multiple resistance is firmly established.

Control strategies

1. **Use effective quarantine procedures.** It is essential to treat effectively all sheep and goats imported on to a home farm to prevent the introduction of anthelmintic-resistant worms. This may be difficult on farms with resistance to all three families of drugs, although a narrow-spectrum product may be useful in some circumstances. In many northern temperate areas resistance is mainly to the benzimidazoles with some resistance to levamisole and emerging resistance to the macrocyclic lactones. In these circumstances a quarantine treatment would consist of treatment with a macrocyclic lactone and levamisole administered sequentially, or if available, as a combination product.
2. **Use strategies to conserve susceptible worms.** The aim is to lower the selection pressure for development of resistance which occurs when sheep are treated and moved on to pasture with low contamination or when immune animals are treated. Two approaches are appropriate. Firstly, do not move treated sheep immediately on to low contamination pasture as any worms which survive treatment will not be diluted by large numbers of more susceptible parasites. Instead, delay moving the sheep from contaminated pasture after dosing to allow them to become lightly reinfected and then move them onto the 'cleaner' grazing. Secondly, leave a proportion (about 10%) of the flock untreated so that some animals will shed eggs on to the low-contamination pasture. There is inevitably a trade-off between the potential to reduce selection for resistance versus some loss of productivity.
3. **Use strategies that reduce the reliance on anthelmintics.** Approaches which integrate grazing management will reduce the exposure to infective larvae, and thus reduce the adverse effects of infection on productivity, whilst allowing sufficient exposure to induce a measure of acquired immunity. This strategy is considered in more detail below.

In selecting the best method of prophylaxis much depends on whether the farm consists primarily of permanent pasture or has pastures which are rotated with crops so that new leys or hay and silage aftermaths are available each year.

Prophylaxis on farms consisting of mainly permanent pasture

On such farms control may be obtained either by anthelmintic prophylaxis or by alternate grazing on an annual basis with cattle and sheep. The former is the only feasible method where the farm stock is primarily sheep while the latter can be used where cattle and sheep are both present in reasonable proportions.

Prophylaxis by anthelmintics

Intensive chemoprophylaxis is not a long-term option for the sustainable control of ovine and caprine PGE.

1. **Adult sheep at tupping.** At this time most ewes in good body condition will be carrying low worm burdens as they will have a strong aquired immunity. Treatment at this period can significantly select for anthelmintic resistance. It is therefore recommended that only mature ewes with a low body condition score or immature ewes are dosed around tupping. Use an anthelmintic which is effective against arrested larval stages.
2. **Adult sheep at lambing.** The most important source of infection for the lamb crop is undoubtedly the increase in nematode eggs in ewe faeces during the PPR and prophylaxis will only be efficient if this is kept to a minimum. Effective anthelmintic therapy of ewes during the fourth month of pregnancy should eliminate most of the worm burdens

present at this time, including arrested larval stages and in the case of ewes on extensive grazing, where nutritional status is frequently low, this treatment often results in improved general body condition. Treatment around lambing or turnout, and again 4–5 weeks later will significantly reduce the ewe contribution to pasture contamination, but it may also increase the selection for drug resistance. To reduce the selection pressure it has been suggested that ewes are dosed early in the lactation period to allow them to become reinfected before a high level of immunity is re-established. In addition, leaving a proportion of the ewes untreated will allow the pasture to be contaminated with unselected parasites. Both of these approaches could however increase the risk of disease in the lamb crop later in the season. Where ewes are inwintered or housed for a period before lambing, dose them on entry to the shed. Following turnout on to contaminated pasture they may require further treatment in about 4–5 weeks. An alternative to the gathering of ewes for these treatments is to provide anthelmintic incorporated in a feed or energy block during the periparturient period. The results obtained with the latter system appear to be best when the ewes are contained in small paddocks or fields, as the uptake of drug is less consistent under extensive grazing systems. Rumen boluses designed for the slow release of anthelmintics over a prolonged period are available in some countries for sheep and are recommended for use in ewes during the periparturient period to eliminate worm egg output. Young adults and rams should also be treated at these times.

3. **Lambs.** Treatment for *N. battus* infection is considered separately under the relevant section. In general, lambs should be treated at weaning, and where possible moved to 'safe' pastures, i.e. those not grazed by sheep since the previous year. Where such grazing is not available, prophylactic treatments (using either levamisole, benzimidazoles, pro-benzimidazoles or avermectins/milbemycins) should be repeated until autumn or marketing. The number of treatments will vary depending on the stocking rate, one treatment in September sufficing for lambs under extensive grazing and two between weaning and marketing for those under more intensive conditions. In order to reduce unnecessary dosing of lambs it is recommended that faecal egg counts are monitored to predict the need for treatment. For low level administration, feed blocks have proved useful.

The prophylactic programmes outlined above are relatively costly in terms of drugs and labour but are currently the only practicable options available where the enterprise is heavily dependent on one animal species.

Prophylaxis by alternate grazing of sheep and cattle

On farms where sheep and cattle are both present in significant numbers, effective control is theoretically possible by alternating the grazing of pasture on an annual basis with each host, due to the relative insusceptibility of cattle to sheep nematodes and *vice versa*. However, *Nematodirus battus* can infect young susceptible calves and this may inadvertently contaminate pasture which is being prepared for next season's lambs. In practice, control is best achieved by exchanging, in the spring, pastures grazed by sheep and beef cattle over the previous year, preferably combined with anthelmintic treatment at the time of exchange.

Prophylaxis on farms with alternative grazing

In these mostly intensive farms, rotation of crops and grass is often a feature, and therefore new leys and hay and silage aftermaths are available as safe pastures each year and can be reserved for susceptible stock. In such a situation, control should be based on a combination of grazing management and anthelmintic prophylaxis.

1. **Prophylaxis by grazing management and anthelmintics.** Good control is possible with only one annual anthelmintic treatment of ewes when they leave the lambing field. This will terminate the PPR in faecal egg counts prior to moving the ewes and lambs to a safe pasture. At weaning, the lambs should be moved to another safe pasture and an anthelmintic treatment of the lambs at this time is good policy. A second system has been devised for farms where arable crops, sheep and cattle are major components and involves a 3-year rotation of cattle, sheep and crops. With this system the aftermath grazing available after cropping may be used for weaned calves and weaned lambs. It has been suggested that anthelmintic prophylaxis can be disposed of completely under this system, but clinical PGE has sometimes occurred when treatment has been omitted. As anthelmintics may not remove all the worms present and some cattle nematodes can infect sheep and *vice versa*, and a few infective larvae on the pasture can survive for beyond 2 years, it is advisable to give at least one annual spring treatment to all stock prior to moving to new pastures.
2. **Prophylaxis by grazing management alone.** Systems using strip or creep grazing, which limit the return of sheep to pastures until the contamination has declined to a low level, have been used with some success but are costly in terms of labour

and fencing. A system where sheep are rapidly rotated through a series of paddocks has been used for the control of *Haemonchus* in set tropical areas. Sheep only graze a paddock for 3½ to 4 days and are then moved to the next paddock. A short grazing time is required to prevent autoinfection. Return to the original paddock must not occur at an interval of less than 5 weeks. Under the hot humid environment the infective larvae are very active and die out rapidly on the herbage.

Ostertagia leptospicularis

Synonym: *Ostertagia crimensis, Skrjabinagia kolchida, Grosspiculagia podjapolskyi*

Predilection site: Abomasum

Parasite class: Nematoda

Superfamily: Trichostrongyloidea

Hosts: Deer (roe deer), cattle, sheep, goat, camel

Geographical distribution: Many parts of the world, particularly Europe and New Zealand

For more details see Chapter 2: Cattle

Marshallagia marshalli

Synonym: *Ostertagia marshalli, Ostertagia tricuspis*

Predilection site: Abomasum

Parasite class: Nematoda

Superfamily: Trichostrongyloidea

Description, gross: Similar to *Ostertagia* spp and can be differentiated by its greater length (males 10–13 mm; females 15–20 mm).

Description, microscopic: Males have a long thin dorsal ray, which bifurcates near the posterior extremity. The end of the spicule is divided into three small processes. The ellipsoidal eggs are much larger than *Ostertagia* spp (>150 μm) and resemble those of *Nematodirus battus*.

Hosts: Sheep, goats, deer and wild small ruminants

Life cycle: The life cycle is similar to *Ostertagia* except that L_2 can hatch from the egg. Following ingestion, larvae burrow into the abomasal mucosa and form small greyish white nodules, which may contain several developing parasites. The young L_5 emerge from the nodules around day 16 post-infection and egg laying is usually apparent by 3 weeks. Arrested development of larvae can occur.

Geographical distribution: The tropics and subtropics including southern Europe, USA, South America, India and Russia.

Pathogenesis and clinical signs: Generally *M. marshalli* is not considered to be an important pathogen.

Diagnosis: Adults are readily identified based on the structure of the male spicules. Eggs are recognised in faecal samples by their large size.

Epidemiology: Wild ruminants serve as an important reservoir of infection.

Treatment and control: Anthelminitcs used to treat other gastrointestinal nematodes are likely to be effective.

Notes: Other species include *M. mongolica*, which is found in the abomasum of sheep, goats and camels in parts of Mongolia. *M. schikhobalovi* and *M. dentispicularis* occur in sheep in Russia.

Haemonchus contortus

Synonym: *Haemonchus placei* (see notes)

Common name: Barber's pole worm

Predilection site: Abomasum

Parasite class: Nematoda

Family: Trichostrongyloidea

Description, gross: The adults are easily identified because of their specific location in the abomasum and their large size (2.0–3.0 cm). In fresh specimens, the white ovaries winding spirally around the blood-filled intestine produce a 'barber's pole' appearance (Fig. 3.2).

Description, microscopic: The male has an asymmetrical dorsal lobe and barbed spicules (Fig. 3.3a); the female usually has a vulval flap. In both sexes there are cervical papillae and a tiny lancet inside the buccal capsule (Fig. 3.3b). Infective larvae have 16 gut cells, the head is narrow and rounded and the tail of the

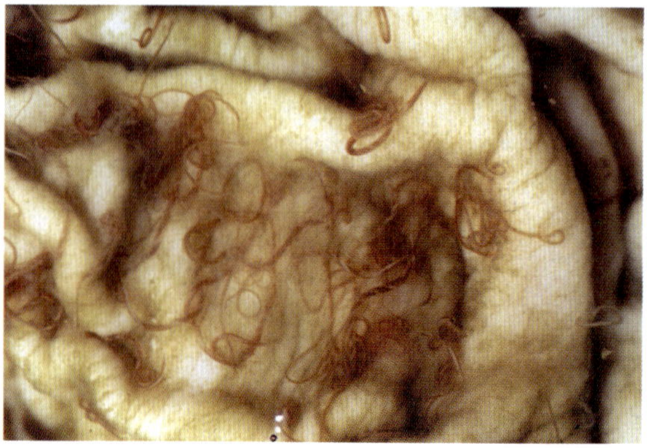

Fig. 3.2 Adult *H. contortus* on the surface of the abomasum.

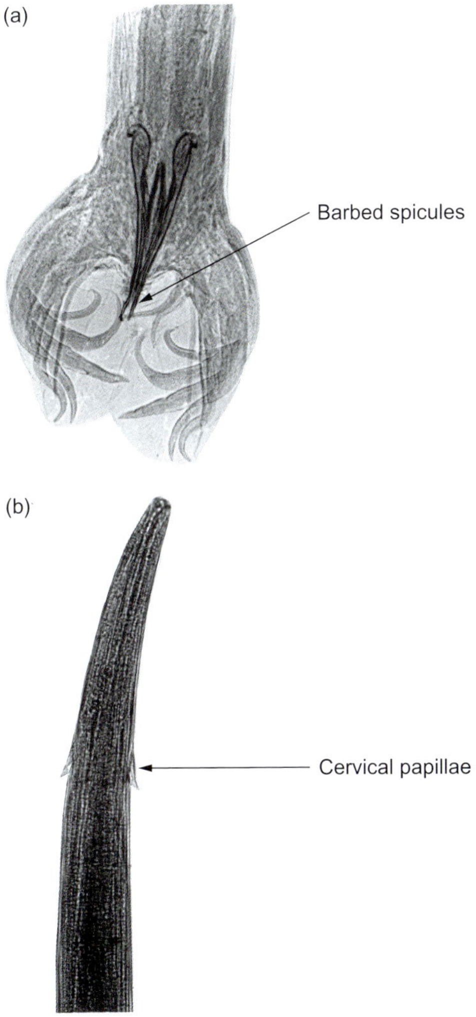

Fig. 3.3 (a) Barbed spicules and bursa of a mature *H. contortus* male worm. (b) Anterior of *Haemonchus contortus* showing the position of the cervical papillae.

sheath is offset. The egg is medium-sized (74 × 44 μm), a regular broad elipse with barrel-shaped sidewalls and numerous blastomeres, which nearly fill the entire egg.

Hosts: Sheep, goat, cattle, deer, camel, llama

Life cycle: This is direct and the preparasitic phase is typically trichostrongyloid. The females are prolific egg layers. The eggs hatch to L_1 on the pasture and may develop to L_3 in as short a period as 5 days but development may be delayed for weeks or months under cool conditions. After ingestion, and exsheathment in the rumen, the larvae moult twice in close apposition to the gastric glands. Just before the final moult they develop the piercing lancet which enables them to obtain blood from the mucosal vessels. As adults they move freely on the surface of the mucosa. The prepatent period is 2–3 weeks in sheep and 4 weeks in cattle.

Geographical distribution: Worldwide. Most important in tropical and subtropical areas.

Pathogenesis: Essentially the pathogenesis of haemonchosis is that of an acute haemorrhagic anaemia due to the blood-sucking habits of the worms. Each worm removes about 0.05 ml of blood per day by ingestion and seepage from the lesions, so that a sheep with 5000 *H. contortus* may lose about 250 ml daily. In acute haemonchosis anaemia becomes apparent about 2 weeks after infection and is characterised by a progressive and dramatic fall in the packed red cell volume. During the subsequent weeks the haematocrit usually stabilises at a low level, but only at the expense of a two- to three-fold compensatory expansion of erythropoiesis. However due to the continual loss of iron and protein into the gastrointestinal tract and increasing inappetence, the marrow eventually becomes exhausted and the haematocrit falls still further before death occurs. When ewes are affected, the consequent agalactia may result in the death of the suckling lambs. Less commonly, in heavier infections of up to 30 000 worms, apparently healthy sheep may die suddenly from severe haemorrhagic gastritis (Fig. 3.4). This is termed hyperacute haemonchosis.

Perhaps as important as acute haemonchosis in tropical areas is the lesser known syndrome of chronic haemonchosis. This develops during a prolonged dry season when reinfection is negligible, but the pasture becomes deficient in nutrients. Over such a period the continual loss of blood from small persisting burdens of several hundred worms is sufficient to produce clinical signs associated primarily with loss of

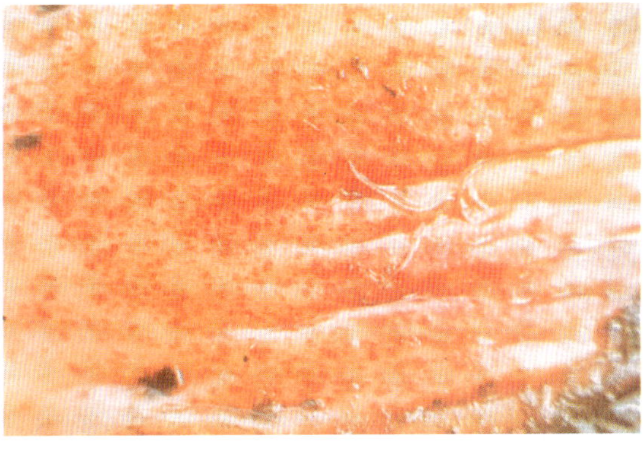

Fig. 3.4 Abomasal haemorrhages in acute haemonchosis.

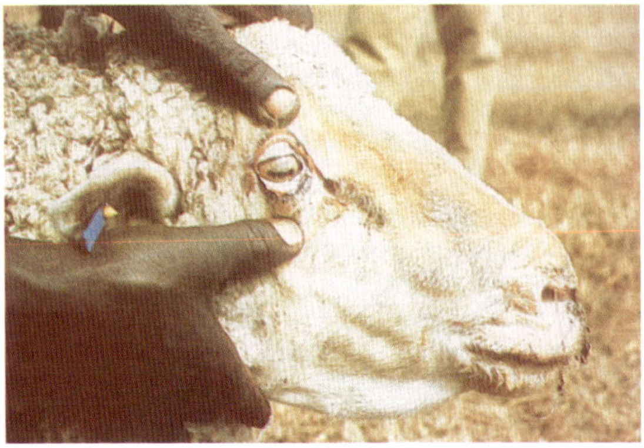

Fig. 3.5 Anaemia and submandibular oedema characteristic of haemonchosis.

weight, weakness and inappetence rather than marked anaemia.

Clinical signs: In hyperacute cases, sheep die suddenly from haemorrhagic gastritis.

Acute haemonchosis is characterised by anaemia, variable degrees of oedema, of which the submandibular form and ascites are most easily recognised, lethargy, dark coloured faeces and falling wool (Fig. 3.5). Diarrhoea is not generally a feature. Chronic haemonchosis is associated with progressive weight loss and weakness, neither severe anaemia nor gross oedema being present.

Diagnosis: The history and clinical signs are often sufficient for the diagnosis of the acute syndrome especially if supported by faecal worm egg counts. Necropsy, paying attention to both the abomasum and the marrow changes in the long bones, is also useful. Changes are usually evident in both, although in sheep, which have just undergone 'self cure' (see below) or are in a terminal stage of the disease, the bulk of the worm burden may have been lost from the abomasum. In hyperacute haemonchosis, only the abomasum may show changes since death may have occurred so rapidly that marrow changes are minimal. The diagnosis of chronic haemonchosis is more difficult because of the concurrent presence of poor nutrition and confirmation may have to depend on the gradual disappearance of the syndrome after anthelmintic treatment.

Pathology: In cases of acute haemonchosis, at necropsy, there may be between 2000 and 20 000 worms present on the abomasal mucosa which shows numerous small haemorrhagic lesions. The abomasal contents are fluid and dark brown due to the presence of altered blood. The carcase is pale and oedematous and the red marrow has expanded from the epiphyses into the medullary cavity.

Epidemiology: The epidemiology of *H. contortus* is best considered separately, depending on whether it occurs in tropical and subtropical or in temperate areas.

Tropical and subtropical areas

Because larval development of *H. contortus* occurs optimally at relatively high temperatures, haemonchosis is primarily a disease of sheep in warm climates. However, since high humidity, at least in the microclimate of the faeces and the herbage, is also essential for larval development and survival, the frequency and severity of outbreaks of disease is largely dependent on the rainfall in any particular area.

Given these climatic conditions, the sudden occurrence of acute clinical haemonchosis appears to depend on two further factors. First, the high faecal worm egg output of between 2000 and 20 000 epg, even in moderate infections, means that massive pasture populations of L_3 may appear very quickly. Second, in contrast to many other helminth infections, there is little evidence that sheep in endemic areas develop an effective acquired immunity to *Haemonchus*, so that there is continuous contamination of the pasture.

In certain areas of the tropics and subtropics, such as Australia, Brazil, the Middle East and Nigeria, the survival of the parasite is also associated with the ability of *H. contortus* larvae to undergo hypobiosis. Although the trigger for this phenomenon is unknown, hypobiosis occurs at the start of a prolonged dry season and permits the parasite to survive in the host as arrested L_4 instead of maturing and producing eggs, which would inevitably fail to develop on the arid pasture. Resumption of development occurs just before the onset of seasonal rains. In other tropical areas such as East Africa, no significant degree of hypobiosis has been observed and this may be due to more frequent rainfall in these areas making such an evolutionary development unnecessary.

The survival of *H. contortus* infection on tropical pastures is variable depending on the climate and degree of shade, but the infective larvae are relatively resistant to desiccation and some may survive for 1–3 months on pasture or in faeces.

In areas of endemic haemonchosis it has often been observed that after the advent of a period of heavy rain the faecal worm egg counts of sheep infected with *H. contortus* drop sharply to near zero levels due to the expulsion of the major part of the adult worm burden. This event is commonly termed the self-cure phenomenon, and has been reproduced experimentally by superimposing an infection of *H. contortus* larvae on an existing adult infection in the abomasum. The expulsion of the adult worm population is considered to be the consequence of an immediate-type hypersensitivity reaction to antigens derived from the developing larvae. It is thought that a similar mechanism operates in the naturally occurring self-cure when large numbers of larvae mature to the infective stage on pasture after rain.

Although this phenomenon has an immunological mechanism it is not necessarily associated with protection against reinfection since the larval challenge often develops to maturity.

Another explanation of the self-cure phenomenon as it occurs in the field is based on the observation that it may happen in lambs and adults contemporaneously and on pasture with insignificant numbers of infective larvae. This suggests that the phenomenon may also be caused, in some non-specific way, by the ingestion of fresh growing grass. Whatever the cause, self-cure is probably of mutual benefit to both host and parasite. The former gains a temporary respite from persistent blood loss while the ageing parasite population is eventually replaced by a vigorous young generation.

Temperate areas

In the British Isles, the Netherlands and presumably in other parts of northern Europe and in Canada, which are among the least favourable areas for the survival of *H. contortus*, the epidemiology is different from that of tropical zones. From the information available, infections seem to develop in two ways. Perhaps most common is the single annual cycle. Infective larvae, which have developed from eggs deposited by ewes in the spring are ingested by ewes and lambs in early summer. The majority of these become arrested in the abomasum as EL_4 and do not complete development until the following spring. During the period of maturation of these hypobiotic larvae, clinical signs of acute haemonchosis may occur and in the ewes this often coincides with lambing. The epidemiology is unknown, but is perhaps associated with pasture contamination by that proportion of ingested larvae, which did not undergo hypobiosis in early summer.

Treatment: When an acute outbreak has occurred the sheep should be treated with one of the benzimidazoles, levamisole, an avermectin/milbemycin or salicylanilide and immediately moved to pasture not recently grazed by sheep. When the original pasture is grazed again, prophylactic measures should be undertaken, as enough larvae may have survived to institute a fresh cycle of infection. Chronic haemonchosis is dealt with in a similar fashion. If possible the new pasture should have a good nutritional value; alternatively some supplementary feeding may be given.

Control: In the tropics and subtropics this varies depending on the duration and number of periods in the year when rainfall and temperature permit high pasture levels of *H. contortus* larvae to develop. At such times it may be necessary to use an anthelmintic at intervals of 2–4 weeks depending on the degree of challenge. Sheep should also be treated at least once at the start of the dry season and preferably also before the start of prolonged rain to remove persisting hypobiotic larvae whose development could pose a future threat. For this purpose, one of the modern benzimidazoles or an avermectin/milbemycin is recommended. In some wool-producing areas where *Haemonchus* is endemic, closantel, which has a residual prophylactic effect, may be used. Because of long withdrawal periods this is of limited use in meat-producing animals.

Apart from anthelmintic prophylaxis, some studies, especially in Kenya, have indicated the potential value of some indigenous breeds of sheep, which seem to be naturally highly resistant to *H. contortus* infection. Presumably such breeds could be of value in developing areas of the world where veterinary surveillance is poor. Rapid rotation through a series of paddocks can be effective in certain wet tropical areas (for details refer to The treatment and control of PGE in sheep – prophylaxis by grazing management alone).

In temperate areas, the measures outlined for the control of parasitic gastroenteritis in sheep are usually sufficient to pre-empt outbreaks of haemonchosis.

Currently trials are in progress to determine the efficacy of a recombinant vaccine based on a membrane glycoprotein of intestinal microvilli of parasitic stages of H. contortus.

Notes: Until recently the sheep species was called *H. contortus* and the cattle species *H. placei*. However there is now increasing evidence that these are the single species *H. contortus* with only strain adaptations for cattle and sheep.

Trichostrongylus axei

Synonym: *Trichostrongylus extenuatus*

Common name: Stomach hairworm

Predilection site: Abomasum or stomach

Parasite class: Nematoda

Superfamily: Trichostrongyloidea

Description, gross: The adults are small, hair-like, light brownish-red and difficult to see with the naked eye. Males measure around 3–6 mm and females 4–8 mm in length.

Description, microscopic: In *T. axei*, the male spicules are dissimilar and unequal in length, the right being shorter than the left (Fig. 3.6a).

Hosts: Cattle, sheep, goat, deer, horse, donkey, pig and occasionally man

Life cycle: This is direct and the preparasitic phase is typically trichostrongyloid. The prepatent period in sheep is about 3 weeks.

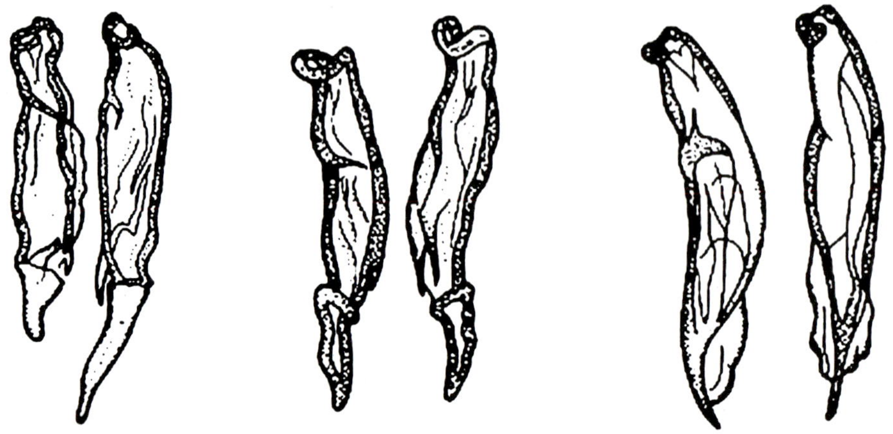

Fig. 3.6 Comparison of spicules of *Trichostrongylus* spp. (a) *T. axei* male showing the dissimilar unequal length spicules. (b) Male *T. colubriformis* showing the characteristic thick spicules of equal length with a barb tip. (c) *T. vitrinus* male showing the thick spicules of equal length which terminate in a point.

Geographical distribution: Worldwide

Pathogenesis: The extent of the lesions in the abomasum or stomach is dependent on the size of the worm population. Small irregular areas, showing diffuse congestion and whitish grey raised flat, circular lesions may be present in the pyloric and fundic regions. These lesions are about 1–2 cm in diameter and have been termed plaques or ringworm lesions (Fig. 3.7). In heavy infections, shallow ulcers may be seen. The changes induced in the gastric mucosa are similar to those of *Ostertagia* with an increase in pH and an increased permeability of the mucosa, leading to an increase in plasma pepsinogen concentration and hypoalbuminaemia.

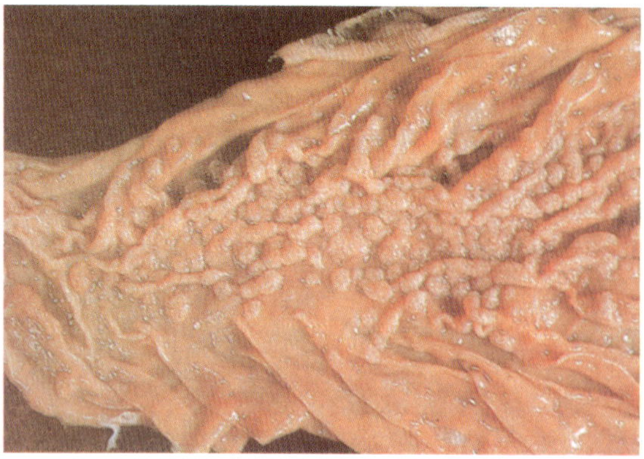

Fig. 3.7 Raised plaques in abomasum due to *Trichostrongylus axei*.

Clinical signs: The principal clinical signs in heavy infections are rapid weight loss and diarrhoea. At lower levels of infection, inappetence and poor growth rates, sometimes accompanied by soft faeces, are the common signs.

Diagnosis: This is based on clinical signs, seasonal occurrence of disease and, if possible, lesions at postmortem examination. Faecal egg counts are a useful aid to diagnosis, although faecal cultures are necessary for generic identification of larvae. At necropsy, *T. axei* is easily identified from washings and digests of the abomasum or stomach.

Pathology: In sheep, there is often extensive desquamation of the superficial epithelium of the mucosa. A mucoid hyperplasia is seen in the plaques and in longer-established infections there may be shallow ulcers in the neck regions of the glands. Cellular infiltration of the lamina propria occurs, particularly an influx of eosinophils and lymphocytes. In most cases there is not a marked reduction in the number of parietal or zymogen cells. Over time, infection can lead to a chronic proliferative inflammation and shallow depressed ulcers may be present.

Epidemiology: The embryonated eggs and infective L_3 of *T. axei* can survive under adverse conditions. Larval numbers increase on pasture in late summer/autumn often giving rise to clinical problems during the winter and early spring. Immunity is slowly acquired and age immunity is not well developed.

Treatment and control: See Treatment and control of parasitic gastroenteritis (PGE) in sheep.

Parabronema skrjabini

Predilection site: Abomasum

Parasite class: Nematoda

Superfamily: Spiruroidea

Description, gross: The white slender adult worms (up to 3.6 cm long) resemble *Haemonchus* spp somewhat in gross form and size, but without the red spiral coloration, while the younger worms are closer to *Ostertagia* in appearance. Males are 15–18 mm with one spicule.

Description, microscopic: The genus is readily distinguished from the other abomasal worms by the presence of large cuticular shields and cordons in the cephalic region. The tail of the male is spiral with four pairs of pre-anal papillae.

Final host: Sheep, goat, cattle, camel

Intermediate host: Muscid flies of the genera *Stomoxys* and *Lyperosia*

Life cycle: Eggs or L_1 are passed in the faeces and the L_1 are ingested by the larval stages of various muscid flies that are often present in faeces. Development to L_3 occurs synchronously with the development to maturity of the fly intermediate host. When the fly feeds around the mouth, lips and nostrils of the host the larvae pass from its mouthparts on to the skin and are swallowed. Alternatively infected flies may be swallowed whole in feed and drinking water. Development to adult takes place in the glandular area of the abomasum.

Geographical distribution: Central and East Africa, Asia, and some Mediterranean countries, notably Cyprus

Pathogenesis: *Parabronema* is usually regarded as non-pathogenic, although it can cause nodular lesions in the abomasal wall.

Clinical signs: Usually inapparent

Diagnosis: Abomasal worms may be found in abomasal scrapings on postmortem.

Pathology: Non-specific. An abomasitis may be found and lesions may become nodular.

Epidemiology: The seasonality of infection is related to the activity of the fly vectors.

Treatment: Treatment is normally not required.

Control: Any measures to reduce fly populations will be beneficial.

Notes: This genus in ruminants is equivalent to *Habronema* in equines.

SMALL INTESTINE

Trichostrongylus

Species of *Trichostrongylus* are small, light brownish red, hair-like worms, and difficult to see with the naked eye. Males measure around 4.0–5.5 mm and females 5.5–7.5 mm in length.

Description, microscopic: The worms have no buccal capsule. A useful generic character is the distinct excretory notch in the oesophageal region. The male bursa has long lateral lobes, while the dorsal lobe is not well defined. Spicules are stout, ridged and pigmented brown, and a gubernaculum is present. Species identification is based on the shape and size of the spicules (Table 3.1; Fig. 3.6). The female tail is bluntly tapered and there is no vulval flap. Eggs are thin-shelled and typically strongyle.

Life cycle: This is direct and the preparasitic phase is typically trichostrongyloid; eggs developing to the infective L_3 in about 7–10 days under optimal conditions. Following ingestion and exsheathment, larvae penetrate the mucosa of the small intestine (Fig. 3.8) and after two moults the fifth-stage worms are present under the intestinal epithelium around 2 weeks after initial infection. The prepatent period is 2–3 weeks.

Diagnosis: This is based on clinical signs, seasonal occurrence of disease and, if possible, lesions at post-mortem examination. Faecal egg counts are a useful aid to diagnosis, although faecal cultures are necessary for generic identification of larvae. At necropsy, the small intestine is often inflamed and the mucosa thickened with an increase in mucus. There may be flattened, red areas that are demarcated from the surrounding mucosa. Digestion of the gut in warm

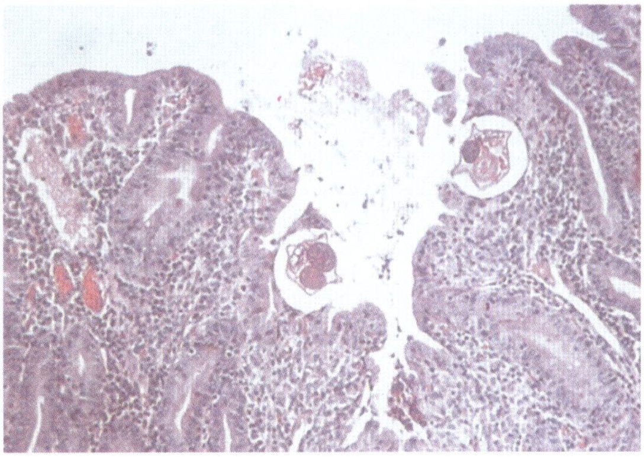

Fig. 3.8 Developing *Trichostrongylus vitrinus* in the small intestinal mucosa.

Table 3.1 Identification of *Trichostrongylus* spp found in sheep and goats based on spicule morphology.

Species	Spicules: description	Spicules: morphology
T. axei	Spicules are dissimilar and unequal in length (the right being shorter than the left)	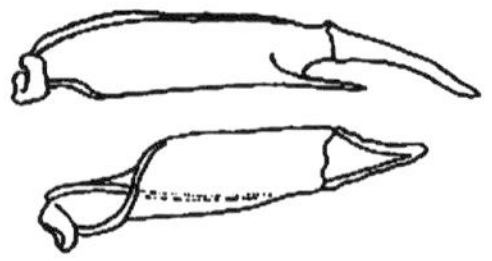
T. colubriformis	Thick, brown, unbranched, of equal length and terminate in a barb-like tip	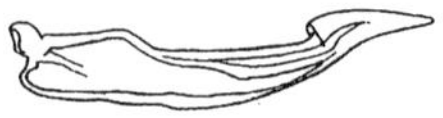
T. vitrinus	Thick, unbranched, of equal length and end in a point	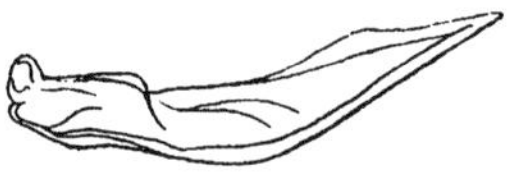
T. longispicularis	The spicules are stout, brown, unbranched, slightly unequal in length and terminate in a tapering blunt tip that has a small semi-transparent protrusion	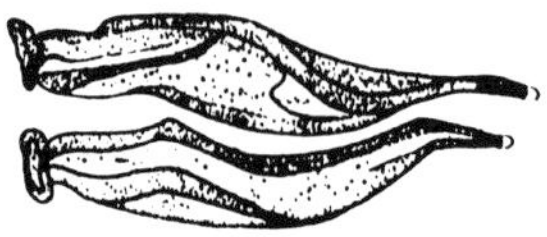
T. rugatus	Spicules are unequal and dissimilar	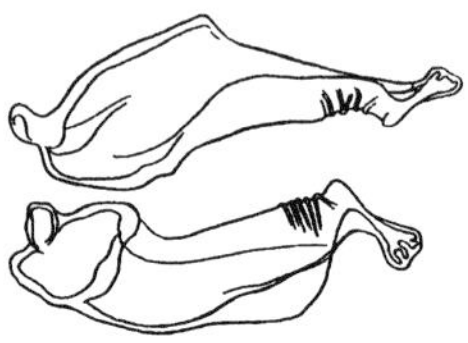
T. falculatus	Spicules sub-equal – 100 μm long	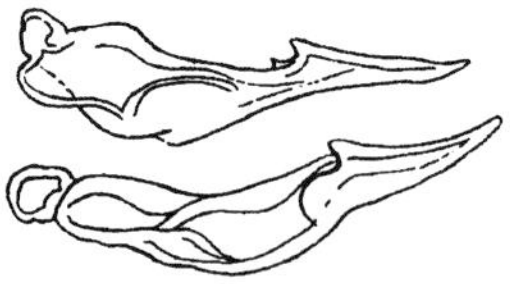
T. capricola	Spicules are equal in length	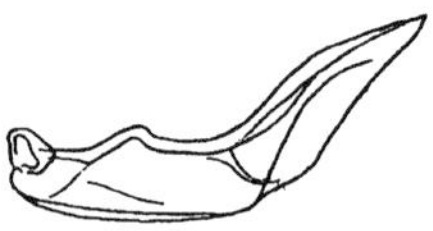
T. retortaeformis	Spicules are stout, unequal in length and terminate in a barb-like tip	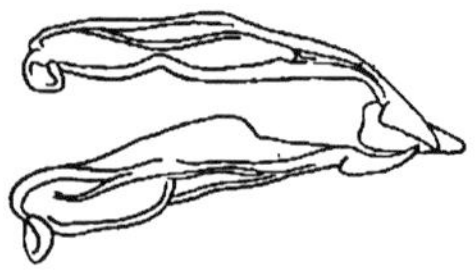

Note: Where spicules are dissimilar, both spicules are illustrated.

physiological saline for 2–3 hours will release the small hair-like worms for examination.

Pathology: Microscopically, there is villous atrophy and fusion of villi with elongation and dilation of the intestinal crypts and an increase in the number of mucus-secreting goblet cells. This is accompanied by marked cellular infiltration of the laminar propria, in particular an increase in eosinophils. Intraepithelial globule leucocytes are numerous, often in the more normal surrounding areas of the mucosa.

Epidemiology: The embryonated eggs and infective L_3 of *Trichostrongylus* can survive under adverse conditions. In temperate areas the L_3 survive the winter, occasionally in sufficient numbers to precipitate clinical disease in the spring, but more commonly, larval numbers increase on pasture in summer and autumn giving rise to clinical problems during these seasons. Hypobiosis plays an important part in the epidemiology, the seasonal occurrence being similar to that of *Ostertagia* spp. In contrast to other trichostrongyles hypobiosis occurs at the L_3 stage although their role in outbreaks of disease has not been fully established.

In the southern hemisphere larvae accumulate in late winter and outbreaks are usually seen in spring. In Australia and Africa, following a period of drought the advent of rain has been shown to rehydrate large numbers of apparently desiccated L_3 (anhydrobiosis) which then become active and rapidly available to grazing animals. *T. colubriformis* also survives adverse environmental conditions as adult parasites within the host and these can persist for many months.

Immunity to *Trichostrongylus*, as in *Ostertagia*, is slowly acquired and in sheep, and probably goats, it wanes during the periparturient period.

Treatment: This is as described for ostertagiosis and parasitic gastroenteritis in sheep.

Control: See Treatment and control of parasitic gastroenteritis (PGE) in sheep

Notes: *Trichostrongylus* is rarely a primary pathogen in temperate areas, but is usually a component of parasitic gastroenteritis in ruminants. By contrast, in the subtropics it is one of the most important causes of parasitic gastroenteritis.

Trichostrongylus colubriformis

Synonym: *Trichostrongylus instabilis*

Common name: Black scour or bankrupt worm

Predilection site: Duodenum and anterior small intestine

Parasite class: Nematoda

Superfamily: Trichostrongyloidea

Description, gross: Males measure around 4.0–5.5 mm and females 5.5–7.5 mm in length.

Description, microscopic: In *T. colubriformis*, the spicules are thick, brown, unbranched, of equal length and terminate in a barb-like tip (Table 3.1; Fig 3.6b).

Hosts: Sheep, goat, cattle, camel and occasionally pig and man

Geographical distribution: Worldwide. Although *T. colubriformis* occurs in temperate regions, it is mainly a parasite of subtropical and tropical zones.

Pathogenesis: Following ingestion, the larvae penetrate the mucosa and developing worms are located in superficial channels sited just beneath the surface epithelium and parallel with the luminal surface, but above the lamina propria. When the sub-epithelial tunnels containing the developing worms rupture to liberate the young worms about 10–12 days after infection, there is considerable haemorrhage and oedema and plasma proteins are lost into the lumen of the gut leading to hypoalbuminaemia and hypoproteinaemia. Grossly there is an enteritis, particularly in the duodenum; the villi become distorted and flattened and the mucosa is inflamed, oedematous and covered in mucus. However many areas may superficially appear normal. Where parasites are congregated within a small area, erosion of the mucosal surface is apparent with severe villous atrophy (Fig. 3.9). In heavy infections diarrhoea occurs, and this, together with the loss of plasma protein into the lumen of the intestine and an increase in turnover of the intestinal epithelium, leads to an impairment in protein metabolism for growth and is reflected as weight loss. Reduced deposition of body protein, calcium and phosphorus and efficiency of food utilisation may occur. Heavy infections can induce osteoporosis and osteomalacia of the skeleton.

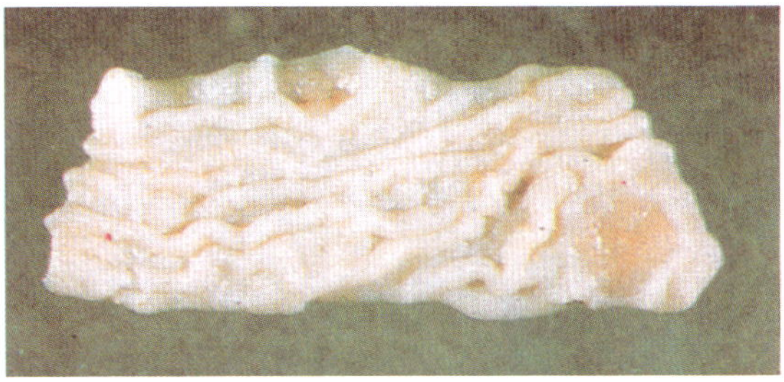

Fig. 3.9 Erosions characteristic of intestinal trichostrongylosis.

Clinical signs: The principal clinical signs in heavy infections are rapid weight loss and diarrhoea, often dark coloured. Deaths can be high, particularly if animals are also malnourished and they receive a high larval challenge over a short period. At lower levels of infection, inappetence and poor growth rates, sometimes accompanied by soft faeces, are the common signs. It is often difficult to distinguish the effects of low infections from malnutrition.

Trichostrongylus vitrinus

Common name: Black scour worm

Predilection site: Duodenum and small intestine

Parasite class: Nematoda

Superfamily: Trichostrongyloidea

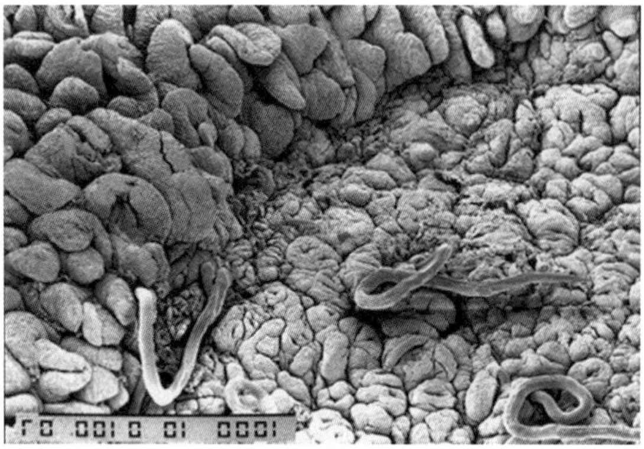

Fig. 3.10 Scanning electron micrograph of small intestine showing villus atrophy in areas where worms are present.

Description, gross: The adults are small, hair-like and light brownish red when fresh. Males measure around 4–6 mm and females 5–8 mm in length.

Description, microscopic: The spicules are thick, unbranched, of equal length and end in a point (Table 3.1; Fig. 3.6c). Eggs are slightly 'brazil nut-shaped' and measure 93–118 × 41–52 µm.

Hosts: Sheep, goat, deer, camel, occasionally pig and man

Geographical distribution: Mainly temperate regions of the world

Pathogenesis: The macroscopic lesions in the intestine are similar to those described for *T. colubriformis*, although they tend not to be as extensive and appear to resolve earlier, possibly being indicative of an earlier expulsion of worms than with *T. colubriformis*. Frequently shallow red depressed areas, demarcated from the more normal coloured surrounding mucosa, are present on the surface of the intestine. These have been termed 'finger print' lesions (Fig. 3.10). These affected areas are devoid of villi, or the villi appear as rounded protruberances, and numerous worms are embedded in the surface mucosa. Infection can induce similar adverse effects on protein and mineral metabolism to those described for *T. colubriformis*.

Clinical signs: The principal clinical signs in heavy infections are weight loss and diarrhoea. At lower levels of infection, inappetence and poor growth rates, sometimes accompanied by soft faeces, are the common signs.

Trichostrongylus longispicularis

Predilection site: Small intestine

Parasite class: Nematoda

Superfamily: Trichostrongyloidea

Description, gross: The adults are similar in size to *T. colubriformis*.

Description, microscopic: The spicules are stout, brown, unbranched, slightly unequal in length and terminate in a tapering blunt tip that has a small semi-transparent protrusion (Table 3.1).

Hosts: Cattle, sheep, goat, deer, camel, llama

Life cycle: This is direct and typically trichostrongyloid. See *T. colubriformis* for details.

Geographical distribution: Ruminants in Australia; and cattle in America and parts of Europe

There are a number of other species of *Trichostrongylus* found in the small intestine of sheep and goats (*T. rugatus*, *T. falculatus*, *T. probolurus*, *T. drepanoformis* and *T. capricola*). These have a more local distribution. The species in rabbits, *T. retortaeformis* and *T. affinus*, have occasionally been recovered from small ruminants.

Cooperia curticei

Predilection site: Small intestine

Parasite class: Nematoda

Superfamily: Trichostrongyloidea

Description, gross: *C. curticei* is moderately small with a large bursa. The most notable feature is the 'watch spring-like' posture. Males measure around 4.5–6.0 mm and females 6.0–8.0 mm in length. When fresh they appear pinkish white.

Description, microscopic: The main generic features are the small cephalic vesicle and the transverse cuticular striations in the oesophageal region. The body possesses longitudinal ridges. The spicules are short and stout and have a distinct wing-like expansion in the middle region, which often bears ridges; there is no gubernaculum. The females have a long tapering tail. Eggs are oval and thin-shelled.

Hosts: Sheep, goat, deer

Life cycle: This is direct and typical of the superfamily. Ingested L_3 exsheath, migrate into the intestinal crypts for two moults and then the adults develop on the surface of the intestinal mucosa. The prepatent period is around 2 weeks. The bionomic requirements of the free-living stages are similar to those of *Teladorsagia*.

Geographical distribution: Worldwide

Pathogenesis: *C. curticei* is generally considered to be a mild pathogen in lambs and kids although in some studies it has been associated with inappetence and poor weight gains. A partial immunity to reinfection develops after about 8–12 months of exposure to infective larvae.

Clinical signs: Low to moderate infections are often asymptomatic but heavy worm burdens can lead to loss of appetite and poor growth rates.

Diagnosis: Eggs of *Cooperia* spp are all very similar morphologically. Faecal culture will allow identification of infective larvae.

Pathology: *Cooperia* do not tunnel into the epithelium but coil among the intestinal villi causing adjacent villous atrophy. In heavy infections there is more widespread villous atrophy in the small intestine leading to loss of brush border enzymes and digestive disturbance.

Epidemiology: In temperate areas, this is similar to that of *Teladorsagia*. Hypobiosis at the EL_4 is a regular feature during late autumn and winter in the northern hemisphere, and spring and summer in the southern hemisphere. Generally, first year grazing animals are most likely to accumulate moderate worm populations. Exposure to infective pasture enables animals to acquire a good level of immunity and as adults they usually show little clinical signs of infection but act as carriers, shedding low numbers of eggs in their faeces. Infective larvae survive well on pasture, being tolerant of cold conditions.

Treatment: The principles are similar to those applied in PGE in sheep. *Cooperia* is one of the dose-limiting species and one should consult the manufacturer's data sheets for efficacy of anthelmintics against adult and L_4 stages.

Control: Similar to that recommended for *Teladorsagia*

Notes: In temperate areas, members of the genus *Cooperia* usually play a secondary role in the pathogenesis of PGE of small ruminants although they may be the most numerous trichostrongyle present.

Cooperia surnabada

Synonym: *Cooperia mcmasteri*

Predilection site: Small intestine

Parasite class: Nematoda

Superfamily: Trichostrongyloidea

Hosts: Cattle, sheep, goat, camel

Geographical distribution: Parts of Europe, North America and Australia

For more details see Chapter 2 (Cattle).

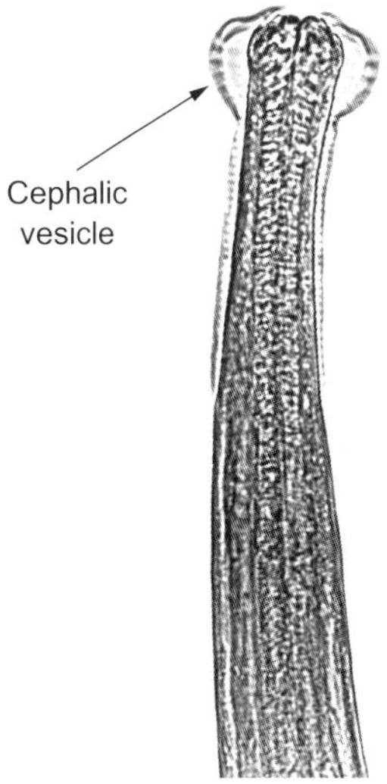

Fig. 3.11 Anterior of *Nematodirus battus* illustrating the small cephalic vesicle.

Nematodirus battus

Common name: Thread-necked worm

Predilection site: Small intestine

Parasite class: Nematoda

Superfamily: Trichostrongyloidea

Description, gross: The adults are slender, the males measuring around 11–16 mm and females 15–25 mm in length. The anterior of the worm is thinner than the posterior region and the cuticle possesses longitudinal ridges.

Microscopic: A small but distinct cephalic vesicle is present (Fig. 3.11). Males are characterised by having only one set of divergent rays in each bursal lobe and the tips of the spicules are fused in a small, flattened oval-shaped projection (Fig. 3.12c). The female worm has a long pointed tail and the large egg is brownish with parallel sides.

Hosts: Sheep, goat and occasionally cattle (calves)

Life cycle: The preparasitic phase is almost unique in the trichostrongylids in that development to the L_3 takes place within the eggshell. Hatching of most eggs requires a prolonged period of chill followed by a mean day/night temperature of more than 10°C, conditions which occur in late spring. Hence most of the eggs from one season's grazing remain unhatched on the ground during the winter and only one generation is possible each year for the bulk of this species. However, some *N. battus* eggs deposited in the spring are capable of hatching in the autumn of the same year resulting in

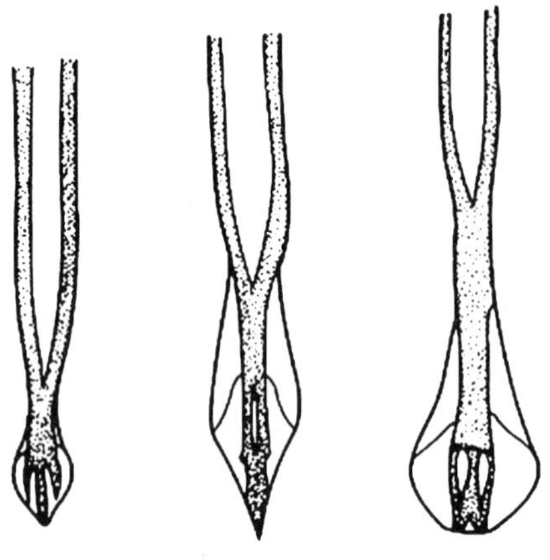

Fig. 3.12 Comparison of spicules of (a) *Nematodirus filicollis*, (b) *N. spathiger* and (c) *N. battus*.

significant numbers of L_3 on the pasture at this time. The ingested L_3 penetrate the mucosa of the small intestine and moult to the L_4 stage around the fourth day. After moulting to the L_5 the parasites inhabit the lumen, sometimes superficially coiled around villi. The prepatent period is 14–16 days.

Geographical distribution: *N. battus* is most important in the British Isles, but also occurs in Norway, Sweden, the Netherlands and parts of Canada.

Pathogenesis: Nematodirosis, due to *N. battus* infection, is an example of a parasitic disease where the principal pathogenic effect is attributable to the larval stages. Following ingestion of large numbers of L_3 there is disruption of the intestinal mucosa, particularly in the ileum, although the majority of developing stages are found on the mucosal surface. Development through L_4 to L_5 is complete by 10–12 days from infection and this coincides with severe damage to the villi and erosion of the mucosa leading to villous atrophy. The ability of the intestine to exchange fluids and nutrients is grossly impaired, and with the onset of diarrhoea the lamb rapidly becomes dehydrated.

Clinical signs: In severe infections, yellowy-green diarrhoea is the most prominent clinical sign and can occur during the prepatent period. As dehydration proceeds, the affected animals become thirsty and in infected flocks the ewes continue to graze, apparently unaffected by the larval challenge, while their inappetent and diarrhoeic lambs congregate round drinking places. At necropsy, the carcase has a dehydrated appearance and there is often an acute enteritis. The intertwining of the thin, twisted worms in the intestine can produce an appearance similar to that of cotton wool. Mortalities can be high in untreated animals. Concurrent infection with pathogenic species of coccidia can exacerbate the severity of disease.

Diagnosis: Because the clinical signs appear during the prepatent period faecal egg counts are of little value in early diagnosis which is best made on grazing history, clinical signs and, if possible, a postmortem examination. Nematodirosis should be differentiated from coccidiosis.

Pathology: Gross pathological changes may be limited to fluid mucoid contents in the upper small intestine with occasional hyperaemia of the mucosa of the duodenum with excess mucus on the surface. Worm counts may reveal tangled, cottony masses of elongate, coiled nematodes. The presence of large numbers of larvae is associated with villous atrophy and fusion, whilst crypts may appear elongate and dilated. Local erosions may occur if villous atrophy is severe and on histopatholgy there is a mixed inflammatory response with large numbers of lymphocytes, plasma cells and eosinophils in the lamina propria.

Epidemiology: The three most important features of the epidemiology of *N. battus* infections are:

1. The capacity of the free-living stages, particularly the egg containing the L_3, to survive on pasture; some for up to 2 years.
2. The critical hatching requirements of most eggs, which ensure the appearance of large numbers of L_3 on the pasture simultaneously, usually in May and June. Though the flush of larvae on the pasture may be an annual event, the appearance of clinical nematodirosis is not; thus if the flush of L_3 is early the suckling lambs may not be consuming sufficient grass to acquire large numbers of L_3, and if it is late the lambs may be old enough to resist the larval challenge. There is some evidence that there is an age resistance to *N. battus*, which commences when lambs are about 3 months old. However, susceptible lambs of 6–7 months can have considerable *N. battus* burdens and it is therefore doubtful if this age immunity is absolute.
3. The negligible role played by the ewe in the annual cycling of *N. battus* which can thus be considered as a lamb-to-lamb disease with usually only one generation of parasites each year in the spring, although in some years an autumn generation of parasites may be seen. Adult sheep often have a few *N. battus* eggs in their faeces, but these are insufficient to precipitate a larval flush, although they are enough to ensure the persistence of infection on the pastures. In management systems that involve both sheep and cattle, young calves can become infected when they graze pasture that carried lambs the previous spring.

Treatment: Several drugs are effective against *Nematodirus* infections: levamisole, an avermectin/milbemycin or one of the modern benzimidazoles. However, *Nematodirus* is one of the dose-limiting species and the manufacturer's data sheets should be consulted as there are differences in efficacy against adults and L_4 stages between oral and parenteral administration for some macrocyclic lactones. The response to treatment is usually rapid and, if diarrhoea persists, coccidiosis should be considered as a complicating factor.

Control: Due to the annual hatching of *N. battus* eggs in spring, the disease can be controlled by avoiding the grazing of successive lamb crops on the same pasture. Where such alternative grazing is not available each year, control can be achieved by anthelmintic prophylaxis, the timing of treatments being based on the knowledge that the peak time for the appearance of *N. battus* L_3 is May to early June. Ideally, dosing should be at 3-week intervals over May and June and it is unwise to await the appearance of clinical signs of diarrhoea before administering the drugs. Forecasting systems are based primarily on soil temperature in the early spring which can predict the likely severity of nematodirosis. In years when the forecast predicts severe disease, three treatments are recommended during May and June; in other years two treatments in May should suffice.

Notes: As anthelmintic resistance is rare in *Nematodirus* species it may be advisable to use a benzimidazole against specific *Nematodirus* infection and in this way reduce the selection pressure on the other families of drugs.

Nematodirus filicollis

Common name: Thread-necked worm

Predilection site: Small intestine

Parasite class: Nematoda

Superfamily: Trichostrongyloidea

Description, gross: The adults are slender worms, males measuring 10–15 mm and females 15–24 mm in length.

Description, microscopic: A small but distinct cephalic vesicle is present. The male has two sets of parallel rays in each of the main bursal lobes. The spicules are long and slender with fused tips and terminate in a narrow pointed swelling (Fig. 3.12a). The female has a truncate blunt tail with a small spine (similar to *N. spathiger*), and the egg is large, ovoid, thin-shelled and colourless and twice the size of the typical trichostrongyle egg.

Hosts: Sheep, goat, occasionally cattle and deer

Life cycle: The preparasitic phase is almost unique in the trichostrongyloids in that development to the L_3 takes place within the egg shell. *N. filicollis* does not have the same critical hatching requirements as *N. battus*. Hatching occurs over a more prolonged period and so larvae often appear on the pasture within 2–3 months of the eggs being excreted in the faeces. The parasitic phase within the host is similar to that of *N. battus*. The prepatent period is 2–3 weeks.

Geographical distribution: Cosmopolitan, but more prevalent in temperate zones

Pathogenesis: Similar to that of *N. battus* but of lesser severity

Clinical signs: Low to moderate infections may produce no obvious clinical manifestations. In severe infections, diarrhoea can occur during the prepatent period and young animals may become dehydrated.

Diagnosis: Examination of faeces will enable the colourless eggs to be differentiated from the brown eggs of *N. battus*. At necropsy the tips of the male spicules will allow diagnosis from other *Nematodirus* species.

Pathology: Third-stage larvae enter the deep layers of the mucosa, penetrating into the crypts. Larvae emerge as fourth- or fifth-stage larvae and coil among the villi with their posterior ends protruding into the lumen. The presence of large numbers of worms leads to the development of villous atrophy, crypt dilation and elongation. If villous atrophy is severe the worms may not be able to maintain their position in the intestine.

Epidemiology: The hatch of L_3 from the eggs occurs over a more prolonged period than with *N. battus*, numbers of larvae accumulate on pasture and often peak in late autumn to early winter. More than one annual generation is possible. Although *N. filicollis* has been associated with outbreaks of nematodirosis in small ruminants it is more common to find it in conjunction with the other trichostrongyles that contribute to ovine PGE.

Treatment: See *Nematodirus battus*.

Control: Disease due to monospecific *Nematodirus filicollis* infections is rarely seen. They are usually part of the worm burden of trichostrongyloid species that are responsible for the syndrome of PGE in sheep and as such may be controlled by the measures outlined elsewhere.

Nematodirus spathiger

Common name: Thread-necked worm

Predilection site: Small intestine

Parasite class: Nematoda

Superfamily: Trichostrongyloidea

Description, gross: The adults are slender worms, males measuring around 10–14 mm and females 15–24 mm in length.

Description, microscopic: A small but distinct cephalic vesicle is present. The male has two sets of parallel rays in each of the main bursal lobes. The spicules are long and slender with fused tips and terminate in a spoon-shaped tip (Fig. 3.12b). The female has a truncate blunt tail with a small spine (similar to *N. filicollis*), and the egg is large, ovoid, thin-shelled and colourless and twice the size of the typical trichostrongyle egg.

Hosts: Sheep, goats, occasionally cattle and other ruminants

Life cycle: The preparasitic phase is almost unique in the trichostrongyloids in that development to the L_3 takes place within the egg shell. *N. spathiger* does not have the same critical hatching requirements as *N. battus*. Larvae can appear on the pasture within 3–4 weeks of eggs being excreted in the faeces; more than one annual generation is therefore possible. The parasitic phase is similar to that of *N. battus*. The prepatent period is 2–3 weeks.

Geographical distribution: Cosmopolitan

Pathogenesis: Similar to that of *N. battus* but of lesser severity

Clinical signs: Low to moderate infections may produce no obvious clinical manifestations. In severe infections, diarrhoea can occur during the prepatent period and young animals may become dehydrated.

Diagnosis: Examination of faeces will enable the colourless eggs to be differentiated from the brown eggs of *N. battus*. At necropsy the tips of the male spicules will allow diagnosis from other *Nematodirus* species.

Pathology: As for *N. filicollis*

Epidemiology: The eggs do not usually exhibit delayed hatching, and the pattern of infection is similar to that of *Trichostrongylus* species.

Treatment and control: See *Nematodirus battus*

Bunostomum trigonocephalum

Synonym: *Monodontus trigonocephalum*

Common name: Hookworm

Predilection site: Small intestine

Parasite class: Nematoda

Superfamily: Ancylostomatoidea

Description, gross: *Bunostomum* is one of the larger nematodes of the small intestine of ruminants, being 1.0–3.0 cm long, stout, greyish white and characteristically hooked at the anterior end with the buccal capsule opening anterodorsally.

Description, microscopic: The large buccal capsule opens anterodorsally and bears on the ventral margin a pair of chitinous cutting plates and internally a large dorsal cone. Dorsal teeth are absent from the buccal capsule but there is a pair of small sub-ventral lancets at its base. In the male the bursa is well developed and has an asymmetrical dorsal lobe. The right externodorsal ray arises higher up on the dorsal stem and is longer than the left. It arises near the bifurcation of the dorsal ray, which divides into two tri-digitate branches. The spicules are slender, twisted and relatively short. In the female the vulva opens a short distance in front of the middle of the body.

The infective larva is small with 16 gut cells and a short filamentous tail. The eggs is medium sized (90×51 µm), irregular broad elipse in shape, with dissimilar sidewalls and 4–8 blastomeres.

Hosts: Sheep, goat, camel, deer

Life cycle: Infection with the L_3 may be percutaneous or oral. After skin penetration, the larvae travel to the lungs and moult to fourth-stage larvae before re-entering the gastrointestinal tract after approximately 11 days. Ingested larvae usually develop without a migration. Further development continues in the gut. The prepatent period is 4–8 weeks.

Geographical distribution: Worldwide

Pathogenesis: The adult worms are blood-suckers and infections of 100–500 worms can produce progressive anaemia, hypoalbuminaemia, loss of weight and occasionally diarrhoea. Worm burdens of around 600 may lead to death in sheep.

Clinical signs: The main clinical signs are progressive anaemia, with associated changes in the blood picture, hydraemia and oedema, which show particularly as submandibular oedema ('bottle jaw'). The animals become weak and emaciated and the appetite usually decreases. The skin is dry and the wool of sheep falls out in irregular patches. Diarrhoea may occur, and the faeces may be dark because of altered blood pigments. Collapse and death may occur.

Diagnosis: The clinical signs of anaemia and perhaps diarrhoea in young sheep are not in themselves pathognomonic of bunostomosis. However, in temperate areas, the epidemiological background may be useful in eliminating the possibility of *Fasciola hepatica* infection. In the tropics, haemonchosis must be considered, possibly originating from hypobiotic larvae. Faecal worm egg counts are useful in that these are lower than in *Haemonchus* infection, while the eggs are more bluntly rounded, with relatively thick sticky shells to which debris is often adherent. For accurate differentiation, larval cultures should be prepared.

Pathology: The carcase is anaemic and cachexic. Oedema and ascites are seen. The liver is light brown and shows fatty changes. The intestinal contents are haemorrhagic and the mucosa is usually swollen, covered with mucus, and shows numerous lesions resulting from the worms feeding. The parasites may be seen still attached to the mucosa or free in the lumen.

Epidemiology: Pathogenic infections are more common in the tropics and subtropics and, in some areas, the highest worm burdens are found at the end of the dry season apparently due to the maturation of hypobiotic larvae. Young animals are most susceptible. In temperate countries, high worm burdens are usually uncommon. The prophylactic dosing regimes, adopted for the control of trichostrongyles, has contributed to the low prevalence of *Bunostomum*.

Treatment: The prophylactic anthelmintic regimes advocated for other gastrointestinal nematodes are usually sufficient.

Control: A combination of strategic dosing with anthelmintics and pasture management as used in the control of ovine PGE is effective. Larvae are susceptible to dessication, and the infection is mainly found on permanently or occasionally moist pastures. Avoiding or draining such pastures is an effective control measure. The ground around water troughs should be kept hard and dry, or treated with liberal applications of salt. Housed sheep and goats should be protected by ensuring the floors and bedding are kept dry and that faeces are removed frequently and are not allowed to contaminate food and water.

Gaigeria pachyscalis

Common name: Hookworm

Predilection site: Duodenum and small intestine

Parasite class: Nematoda

Superfamily: Ancylostomatoidea

Description, gross: Adult males are up to 2 cm; females are up to 3 cm long.

Description, microscopic: The buccal capsule contains a large dorsal cone, but no dorsal tooth, and a pair of sub-ventral lancets, which have several cusps each. The male bursa has small lateral lobes joined together ventrally, and a large dorsal lobe. The antero-lateral ray is short and blunt and is separated widely from other lateral rays. The externo-dorsal rays arise from the main stem of the dorsal ray, which is split for about a quarter of its length, the two short branches ending in very small digitations. The spicules are slender with recurved barb ends.

Hosts: Sheep, goat, wild ruminants

Life cycle: The life cycle is thought to be direct; the main route of infection is percutaneous. Infective L_3 larvae are susceptible to desiccation.

Geographical distribution: South America, South Africa, Indonesia and parts of Asia

Pathogenesis: The parasite is a voracious blood sucker; as few as 100–200 worms are sufficient to produce death in sheep within a few weeks.

Clinical signs: Causes severe anaemia and death.

Diagnosis: Demonstration of the characteristic large eggs in the faeces

Pathology: As for *B. trigonocephalum*

Epidemiology: As for *B. trigonocephalum*

Treatment and control: As for *B. trigonocephalum*

Strongyloides papillosus

Common name: Threadworm

Predilection site: Small intestine

Parasite class: Nematoda

Superfamily: Rhabditoidea

Description, gross: Slender, hair-like worms generally less than 1.0 cm long

Description, microscopic: Only females are parasitic. The long oesophagus may occupy up to one third of the body length and the uterus is intertwined with the intestine giving the appearance of twisted thread. Unlike other intestinal parasites of similar size the tail has a blunt point (Fig. 3.13). Strongyloides eggs are oval, thinshelled and small, being half the size of typical strongyle eggs. In herbivores it is the larvated egg which is passed out in the faeces, but in other animals it is the hatched L_1.

Hosts: Sheep, cattle, other ruminants and rabbits

Life cycle: *Strongyloides* is unique among the nematodes of veterinary importance, being capable of both parasitic and free-living reproductive cycles. The parasitic phase is composed entirely of female worms in the small intestine and these produce larvated eggs by parthenogenesis, i.e. development from an unfertilised egg. After hatching, larvae may develop through four larval stages into free-living adult male

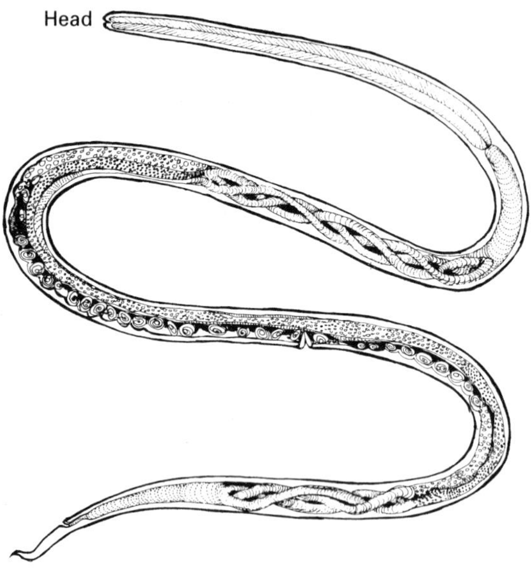

Fig. 3.13 Adult *Strongyloides* female.

and female worms and this can be followed by a succession of free-living generations. However under certain conditions, possibly related to temperature and moisture, the L_3 can become parasitic, infecting the host by skin penetration or ingestion and migrating via the venous system, the lungs and trachea to develop into adult female worms in the small intestine.

Lambs and calves may acquire infection immediately after birth from the mobilisation of arrested larvae in the tissues of the ventral abdominal wall of the dam, which are subsequently excreted in the milk. In addition, prenatal infection has been demonstrated experimentally in cattle. The prepatent period is 8–14 days.

Geographical distribution: Worldwide

Pathogenesis: Skin penetration by infective larvae may cause an erythematous reaction, which in sheep can allow the entry of the causative organisms of foot-rot. Passage of larvae through the lungs has been shown experimentally to result in multiple small haemorrhages visible over most of the lung surfaces. Mature parasites are found in the duodenum and proximal jejunum and if present in large numbers may cause inflammation with oedema and erosion of the epithelium. This results in a catarrhal enteritis with impairment of digestion and absorption.

Clinical signs: The common clinical signs, usually seen only in very young animals, are diarrhoea, anorexia, dullness, loss of weight or reduced growth rate.

Diagnosis: The clinical signs in very young animals, usually within the first few weeks of life, together with the finding of large numbers of the characteristic eggs or larvae in the faeces are suggestive of strongyloidosis. It should be emphasised however that high faecal egg counts may be found in apparently healthy animals.

Pathology: Adult worms establish in tunnels in the epithelium at the base of the villi in the small intestine. In large numbers they may cause villous atrophy, with a mixed mononuclear inflammatory cell infiltration of the lamina propria. Crypt epithelium is hyperplastic and there is villous clubbing.

Epidemiology: *Strongyloides* infective larvae are not ensheathed and are susceptible to extreme climatic conditions. However warmth and moisture favour development and allow the accumulation of large numbers of infective stages. For this reason, it can be a major problem in housed calves up to 6 months of age in some Mediterranean countries. A second major source of infection for the very young animal is the reservoir of larvae in the tissues of their dams and this may lead to clinical strongyloidosis in the first few weeks of life. Successive progeny from the same dam often show heavy infections.

Treatment: Specific control measures for *Strongyloides* infection are rarely called for. The benzimidazoles and the avermectins/milbemycins may be used for the treatment of clinical cases.

Control: Reduction in numbers of free-living larvae by removal of faeces and provision of dry bedding and areas may limit numbers and transmission. Suckling calves should be kept on clean dry areas to prevent infection by skin penetration.

Capillaria longipes

Predilection site: Small intestine

Parasite class: Nematoda

Superfamily: Trichuroidea

Description, gross: These are very fine filamentous worms, the narrow stichosome oesophagus occupying about one third to half the body length. Males measure around 11–13 mm and females up to 20 mm.

Description, microscopic: The males have a long thin single spicule, 1.2 mm long, and often possess a primitive bursa-like structure. The females contain eggs that resemble those of *Trichuris* in possessing bipolar plugs. The eggs are barrel-shaped, 45–50 × 22–25 μm and colourless; they have thick shells that are slightly striated with bipolar plugs.

Hosts: Sheep, goat

Life cycle: The life cycle is direct. The infective L_1 develops within the egg in about 3–4 weeks. Infection of the final host is through ingestion of this embryonated infective stage, development to adult worms occurs without a migration phase. The prepatent period is 3–4 weeks.

Geographical distribution: Worldwide

Pathogenesis: Considered to be of low pathogenicity and of little veterinary significance.

Clinical signs: No clinical signs have been attributed to infection with this parasite.

Diagnosis: Because of the non-specific nature of the clinical signs and the fact that, in heavy infections, these may appear before *Capillaria* eggs are present in the faeces, diagnosis depends on necropsy and careful examination of the small intestine for the presence of the worms. This may be carried out by microscopic examination of mucosal scrapings squeezed between two glass slides; alternatively the contents should be gently washed through a fine sieve and the retained material resuspended in water and examined against a black background.

Pathology: No associated pathology

Epidemiology: Infection is by ingestion of the larvated eggs and is common in sheep though not significant.

Treatment: Not usually required

Control: Not required

Moniezia expansa

Predilection site: Small intestine

Parasite class: Cestoda

Family: Anoplocephalidae

Description, gross: These are long tapeworms, 2 m or more in length, which are unarmed, possessing prominent suckers.

Description, microscopic: Segments are broader than they are long (up to 1.5 cm wide) and contain two sets of genital organs grossly visible along the lateral margin of each segment. There is a row of interproglottidal glands at the posterior border of each segment, which may be used in species differentiation. In *M. expansa* they extend along the full breadth of the segment. The irregularly triangular eggs have a well defined pyriform apparatus and vary from 55–75 μm in diameter.

Final hosts: Sheep, goats, occasionally cattle

Intermediate hosts: Forage mites, mainly of the family Oribatidae

Life cycle: Mature proglottids or eggs are passed in the faeces and on pasture where the oncospheres are ingested by forage mites. The embryos migrate into the body cavity of the mite where they develop to cysticercoids in 1–4 months and infection of the final host is by ingestion of infected mites during grazing. The prepatent period is approximately 6 weeks, but the adult worms appear to be short lived, patent infections persisting for only 3 months.

Geographical distribution: Worldwide

Pathogenesis: Although generally regarded as of little pathogenic significance there are several reports, especially from eastern Europe and New Zealand, of heavy infections causing unthriftiness, diarrhoea and even intestinal obstruction. However, *Moniezia* infections are so obvious, both in life, because of the presence of proglottids in the faeces, and at necropsy, that other causes of ill health may be overlooked. It is interesting that experimental studies have failed to demonstrate substantial clinical effects even with fairly heavy worm burdens.

Clinical signs: While a great variety of clinical signs, including unthriftiness, diarrhoea, respiratory signs and even convulsions, have been attributed to *Moniezia*, infections are generally symptomless. Subclinical effects remain to be established.

Diagnosis: This is based largely on the presence of mature proglottids in the faeces and the characteristic shape of *Moniezia* eggs (triangular, *M. expansa*; quadrangular, *M. benedeni*) that contain the oncosphere. The eggs of *M. benedeni* are slightly larger than those of *M. expansa*.

Pathology: Little pathology is associated with the presence of light infections. Heavy infections may produce a solid mass of tapeworms that may occlude the intestinal lumen.

Epidemiology: Infection is common in lambs, kids and calves during their first year of life and less common in older animals. A seasonal fluctuation in the incidence of *Moniezia* infection can apparently be related to active periods of the forage mite vectors during the summer in temperate areas. The cysticercoids can overwinter in the mites.

Treatment: In many countries several drugs, including niclosamide, praziquantel, bunamidine and a number of broad-spectrum benzimidazole compounds, which have the advantage of also being active against gastrointestinal nematodes, are available for the treatment of *Moniezia* infection. If this is carried out in lambs and calves in late spring, in temperate areas, the numbers of newly infected mites on pasture will be reduced.

Control: Ploughing and reseeding, or avoiding the use of the same pastures for young animals in consecutive years, may prove beneficial.

Notes: This genus of cestodes is common in ruminants and resembles, in most respects, *Anoplocephala* of the horse. *Moniezia* spp are only the tapeworms of ruminants in many countries of western Europe.

Other species of tapeworms are found in the small intestine of sheep and goats. Many of the details are essentially similar to *Moniezia*.

Avitellina centripunctata

Predilection site: Small intestine

Parasite class: Cestoda

Family: Thysanosomidae

Description, gross: This tapeworm resembles *Moniezia* on gross inspection except that the segmentation is so poorly marked that it appears somewhat ribbon-like. It can reach 3 m in length by about 4 mm in width and the posterior end is almost cylindrical in appearance.

Description, microscopic: A single set of genital organs is present with the pores alternating irregularly. Proglottids are short. Eggs lack a pyriform apparatus and measure around 20–45 μm.

Definitive hosts: Sheep, goat, camel and other ruminants

Intermediate hosts: Thought to be oribatid mites or psocid lice

Geographical distribution: Europe, Africa and Asia

Pathogenesis: Of negligible pathogenicity

Clinical signs: Usually asymptomatic

Stilesia globipunctata

Predilection site: Small intestine

Parasite class: Cestoda

Family: Thysanosomidae

Description, gross: Adults measure around 0.5 metres in length by 3–4 mm wide.

Description, microscopic: A single set of genital organs is present.

Definitive hosts: Sheep, cattle and other ruminants

Intermediate hosts: Thought to be oribatid mites and psocid lice

Geographical distribution: Southern Europe, Africa and Asia

Pathogenesis: Generally considered to be of low pathogenicity, although severe infection has been reported to cause death.

Clinical signs: Normally asymptomatic

Pathology: Nodules and desquamation may occur in the jejunum where the scoleces of the immature tapeworms penetrate the epithelium. The scolex and anterior proglottids are embedded within the nodule, the posterior proglottids being free in the lumen of the intestine.

Treatment and control: Treatment is rarely called for, but praziquantel has proved effective.

Thysaniezia ovilla

Synonym: *Thysaniezia giardia*

Predilection site: Small intestine

Parasite class: Cestoda

Family: Thysanosomidae

Description, gross: Adults reach 200 cm in length, varying in width up to 12 mm.

Description, microscopic: The scolex is small, measuring up to 1 mm in diameter. Segments are short, bulge outwards giving the margin of the worm an irregular appearance, and contain a single set of genital organs, rarely two, with genital pores alternating irregularly. Eggs are devoid of a pyriform apparatus and found in groups of 10–15 in elongated paruterine organs (100 μm long), with a thick grey shell and a protruberance at one end.

Final hosts: Cattle, sheep, goat, camel and wild ruminants

Intermediate hosts: Oribatid mites (*Galuma*, *Scheloribates*) and psocids (bark lice, dust lice)

Life cycle: Mature segments are passed in the faeces of the infected host on to pasture, where forage mites ingest the oncospheres. Cysticercoids develop within the orabatid intermediate hosts and infection of the final host is by ingestion of infected mites during grazing.

Geographical distribution: Southern Africa

Pathogenesis: Not considered pathogenic

Diagnosis: The mature segments found in the faeces are readily distinguishable from *Moniezia*.

Epidemiology: Infection is very commonly found in adult cattle in southern Africa.

Treatment and control: As for *Moniezia*

Thysanosoma actinoides

Common name: Fringed tapeworm

Predilection site: Small intestine, bile and pancreatic ducts

Parasite class: Cestoda

Family: Thysanosomidae

Description, gross: Adult tapeworms measure 15–30 cm long by 8 mm wide.

Description, microscopic: The scolex is up to 1.5 mm; segments are short and fringed posteriorly. Each segment contains two sets of genital organs with the testes lying medially. Several paruterine organs are present in each proglottid and the eggs have no pyriform apparatus.

Final hosts: Sheep, cattle, deer

Intermediate hosts: Oribatid mites (*Galuma*, *Scheloribates*) and psocids (bark lice, dust lice)

Life cycle: Mature segments are passed in the faeces of the infected host on to pasture, where forage mites ingest the oncospheres. Cysticercoids develop within the orabatid intermediate hosts and infection of the final host is by ingestion of infected mites during grazing.

Geographical distribution: North and South America

Pathogenesis and clinical signs: Generally not considered pathogenic. Blockage of the bile or pancreatic ducts may occur resulting in digestive disorders and unthriftiness.

Diagnosis: Identification of the mature segments and eggs in the faeces.

Epidemiology: Infection is commonly found in sheep, cattle and deer in the western USA and parts of South America.

Treatment and control: As for *Moniezia*

Cymbiforma indica

Predilection site: Gastrointestinal tract

Parasite class: Trematoda

Family: Notocotylidae

Description, gross: Adult fluke are pear-shaped, concave ventrally and measure 0.8–2.7 cm long by 0.3–0.9 mm wide.

Description, microscopic: There is no ventral sucker and the cuticle is armed with fine spines anteriorly and ventrally. Eggs bear long filaments at both poles and measure 18–37 × 11–13 μm.

Final hosts: Sheep, goat, cattle

Intermediate hosts: Snails

Life cycle: The life cycle has not been described.

Geographical distribution: India

Pathogenesis and clinical signs: Generally not considered pathogenic, despite heavy infections frequently reported.

Diagnosis: Identification of the flukes on postmortem

Treatment and control: Not required

Skrjabinotrema ovis

Predilection site: Small intestine

Parasite class: Trematoda

Family: Brachylaemidae

Description, gross: Adult fluke are small with smooth bodies and measure 1 × 0.3–0.7 mm.

Description, microscopic: Eggs measure 24–32 × 16–20 μm and are slightly flattened on one side with a large operculum at one end and a small appendage at the other.

Final hosts: Sheep

Intermediate hosts: Snails

Life cycle: The life cycle has not been described.

Geographical distribution: China, Russia, eastern CIS

Pathogenesis and clinical signs: Heavy infections may cause catarrhal enteritis.

Diagnosis: Identification of the flukes on postmortem

Sheep coccidia

Eleven species of *Eimeria* have been identified in sheep, distinguished primarily on oocyst morphology (Table 15.6; Fig. 15.20). Each stage of each individual coccidial species has its preferences as to which cells it infects and which parts of the gut it infects. Those infecting the posterior part of the intestine tend to be more harmful.

Although the majority of sheep, particularly those under 1 year old, carry coccidia, only two species (*E. crandallis* and *E. ovinoidalis*) are known to be highly pathogenic. It was thought for many years that the species of *Eimeria* affecting sheep and goats were the same. Cross-transmission studies have shown, however, that although morphologically similar, coccidia in small ruminants are host-specific and cross-infection between sheep and goats does not occur.

The following general descriptions apply to sheep and goat *Eimeria*.

Life cycle: The life cycles of all species are typically coccidian (see Chapter 1: Parasite taxonomy and morphology, Phylum: Apicomplexa). Following ingestion of the sporulated oocyst there are usually two merogony stages, producing initially 'giant' first-generation meronts, in some species, followed by smaller second-generation meronts. During gametogony, fusion of macrogametocytes and microgametocytes leads to zygote formation and the excretion of unsporulated oocysts in the faeces. Sporulation outside the body may be completed in 1–4 days under ideal conditions, but can take several weeks in cold weather. Sporulated oocysts contain four sporocysts each containing two sporozoites. The life cycle takes between 2 and 4 weeks, depending on the species of *Eimeria*.

Pathogenesis: The most pathogenic species of coccidia are those that infect and destroy the crypt cells of the large intestinal mucosa. This is because the ruminant small intestine is very long, providing a large number of host cells and the potential for enormous parasite replication with minimal damage. If the absorption of nutrients is impaired, the large intestine is, to some extent, capable of compensating. Those species that invade the large intestine are more likely to cause pathological changes, particularly if large numbers of oocysts are ingested over a short period of time. Here, the rate of cellular turnover is much lower and there is no compensation effect from other regions of the gut. In lambs or kids that become heavily infected, the mucosa becomes completely denuded resulting in severe haemorrhage and impaired water resorption, leading to diarrhoea, dehydration and death. In lighter infections, the effect on the intestinal mucosa is to impair local absorption. Species that develop more superficially in the small intestine cause a change in villous architecture with a reduction in epithelial cell height and a diminution of the brush border, giving the appearance of a 'flat mucosa'. These changes result in a reduction of the surface area available for absorption and consequently a reduced feed efficiency.

Clinical signs: Clinical signs vary from loss of pellet formation to weight loss, anorexia and diarrhoea (with or without blood) (Fig. 3.14).

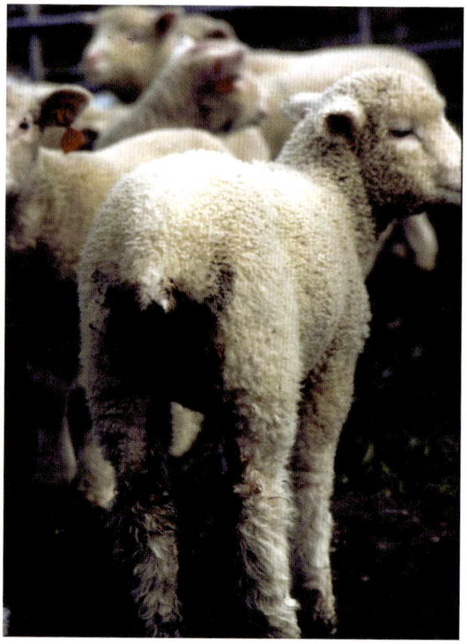

Fig. 3.14 Clinically affected lamb with coccidiosis.

Pathology: On postmortem, there may be little to see beyond thickening and petechiation of the bowel but mucosal scrapings will reveal masses of gamonts and oocysts. Giant meronts may be seen in the mucosa of the small intestine as pin-point white spots (Fig. 3.15), but unless they are in vast numbers they cause little harm. The most pathogenic stages are the gamonts (Fig. 3.16).

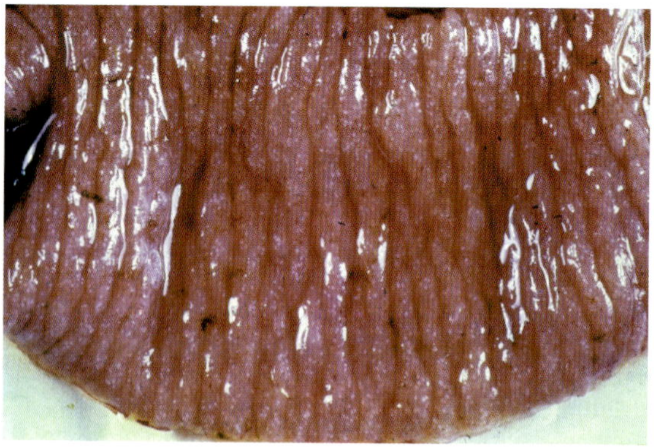

Fig. 3.15 *Eimeria ovinoidalis*. Large intestinal mucosa with 'giant' meronts.

Epidemiology: Coccidia are normally present in animals of all ages and usually cause no clinical signs, as immunity is quickly acquired and maintained by continuous exposure to reinfection. However, intensification may alter the delicate balance between immunity and disease with serious consequences for young animals. Coccidiosis is one of the most important diseases of lambs and kids, particularly in their first few months of life. Whilst coccidial infection is common, the presence of infection does not necessarily lead to the development of clinical signs of disease and, in many situations, low levels of challenge can actually be beneficial by stimulating protective immune responses in the host. Development of disease is dependent on a number of factors, in particular husbandry and management.

Adult animals are highly resistant to the disease, but not totally resistant to infection. As a result, small numbers of parasites manage to complete their life cycle and usually cause no detectable harm. In the wild or under more natural, extensive systems of management,

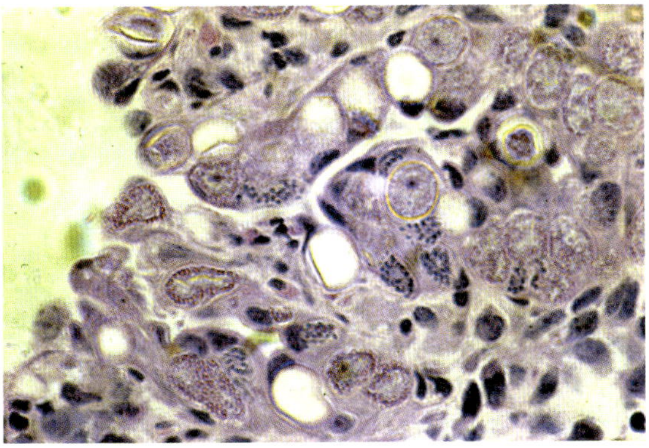

Fig. 3.16 Macrogamonts of *Eimeria ninakohlyakimovae*.

susceptible animals are exposed to only low numbers of oocysts and acquire a protective immunity. Extensive grazing, as occurs under natural conditions in the wild, limits the level of exposure to infective oocysts. Under modern production systems, however, lambs or kids are born into a potentially heavily contaminated environment, and, where the numbers of sporulated oocysts are high, disease often occurs. Three management factors are associated with the development of high levels of infection and the development of disease: pens are not cleaned on a regular basis; overcrowding in the pens; pens are used to house different age groups.

Adult animals, although possibly the original source of infective oocysts in the environment, are not usually responsible for the heavy levels of contamination encountered. The source is often the lambs or kids themselves, which following an initial infection in the first few days of life may produce millions of oocysts within their own environment. Growing animals may then face potentially lethal doses of infective oocysts 3 weeks later when their natural resistance is at its lowest. Later born animals introduced into the same environment are immediately exposed to heavy oocyst challenge. Under unhygienic, overcrowded conditions, the lambs or kids will be exposed to and ingest a large proportion of this infection and will develop severe disease and may even die from the infection. If conditions are less crowded and more hygienic, the infective dose ingested will be lower, they may show moderate, slight or no clinical signs and develop an immunity to reinfection, but they in turn will have multiplied the infection a millionfold. Stress factors, such as poor milk supply, weaning, cold weather and transport, will reduce any acquired resistance and exacerbate the condition. A major problem in milking goatherds is that, in an attempt to ensure a constant year-round milk supply, births often take place over an extended period of time. If the same pens are used constantly for successive batches, or if young kids are added to a pen already housing older animals, then the later born kids are immediately exposed to heavy challenge and can show severe coccidiosis in the first few weeks of life.

Colostrum provides passive immunity to coccidiosis during the first few weeks of life. Thereafter, susceptibility to coccidial infections has been found progressively to increase. Subsequently animals acquire resistance to coccidia as a result of active immunity. While animals of all ages are susceptible to infection, younger animals are generally more susceptible to disease. The majority of lambs or kids will probably become infected during the first few months of life and may or may not show signs of disease. Those that reach adulthood are highly resistant to the pathogenic effects of the parasites but may continue to harbour small numbers throughout their lives.

Occasionally, acute coccidiosis occurs in adult animals with impaired cellular immunity or in those which have been subjected to stress, such as dietary changes, prolonged travel, extremes of temperature and weather conditions, changes in environment or severe concurrent infection. An animal's nutritional status and mineral and vitamin deficiencies can also influence resistance to infection. Suckling animals, in addition to benefiting from colostral intake, may forage less and hence pick up fewer oocysts from pasture. Well nourished animals may simply be able to fight off infection more readily.

Diagnosis: Diagnosis should be based on history, clinical signs (severe diarrhoea in young animals), postmortem findings (inflammation, hyperaemia and thickening of caecum with masses of gamonts and oocysts in scrapings) supported by oocyst counts and speciation to identify pathogenic species. Counts of faecal oocysts identified to species can help to complete the picture, but oocyst numbers may be grossly misleading when considered in isolation. Healthy animals may pass more than a million oocysts per gram of faeces, whereas in animals dying of coccidiosis the count may be less than 10 000. High counts of non-pathogenic species could mask significant numbers of the more pathogenic species, for instance, and give the impression that the abundant species was the cause.

Treatment: Outbreaks of clinical coccidiosis can appear suddenly and may prove troublesome to resolve as they often occur on heavily stocked farms, particularly where good husbandry and management are lacking. If deaths are occurring, early confirmation of the diagnosis is vital and should be based on history, postmortem examination and intestinal smears. Affected animals should be medicated and moved to uncontaminated pens or pasture as soon as possible.

Normally all animals in a group should be treated, as even those showing no symptoms are likely to be infected. Severely infected animals that are diarrhoeic

Table 3.2 Predilection sites and prepatent periods of *Eimeria* species in sheep.

Species	Predilection site	Prepatent period (days)
Eimeria ahsata	Small intestine	18–30
Eimeria bakuensis	Small intestine	18–29
Eimeria crandallis	Small and large intestine	15–20
Eimeria faurei	Small and large intestine	13–15
Eimeria granulosa	Unknown	?
Eimeria intricata	Small and large intestine	23–27
Eimeria marsica	Unknown	14–16
Eimeria ovinoidalis	Small and large intestine	12–15
Eimeria pallida	Unknown	?
Eimeria parva	Small and large intestine	12–14
Eimeria weybridgensis	Small intestine	23–33

and dehydrated may require oral or intravenous rehydration. Where non-specific symptoms of weight loss or ill-thrift are present, it is important to investigate all potential causes and seek laboratory confirmation. If coccidiosis is considered significant, much can be done through advice on management and instigation of preventative measures outlined earlier. Batch rearing of animals of similar ages limits the build-up and spread of oocysts and allows targeting of treatment to susceptible age groups during the danger periods.

Whilst the same compounds used for the treatment and control of coccidiosis in sheep should be effective in goats, little data or information are available on the efficacy of these compounds in goats.

Control: Animals particularly at risk from coccidiosis are those kept indoors on damp bedding, or those on contaminated heavily stocked pastures, particularly in cold wet weather. The incidence of disease can be reduced through avoidance of overcrowding and stress, and attention to hygiene. Raising of food and water troughs, for example, can help avoid contamination by reducing the levels of infection. Young animals should be kept off heavily contaminated pastures when they are most susceptible. Good feeding of dams prior to parturition and creep feeding of their progeny will also help to boost resistance to coccidiosis.

Eimeria crandallis

For details see Large intestine.

Eimeria ovinoidalis

For details see Large intestine.

Eimeria ahsata

Predilection site: Small intestine

Parasite class: Sporozoasida

Family: Eimeriidae

Hosts: Sheep

Description: The oocysts are ellipsoidal to ovoid, yellowish brown, 29–37 × 17–28 μm (mean 33.4 × 22.6 μm) with a micropyle and a micropylar cap and have one or occasionally more polar granules, without a residuum. Sporocysts are 12–22 × 6–10 μm without a Stieda body and with a residuum. The sporozoites are elongate, and lay lengthways head to tail in the sporocysts, and have one to three clear globules each.

First-generation meronts average 184 × 165 μm and may reach 265 × 162 μm by 15 days post infection and contain several thousand merozoites. Second-generation meronts measure 52 × 39 μm and contain approximately 50 merozoites. Intranuclear stages have been observed in small intestinal epithelial cells, 15, 18 and 19 days after experimental infection. The developing parasites are 1.6–5 μm in size and are mostly localised within a tiny cavity of the nucleus. Each intranuclear parasite is surrounded by a halo, and most contain two to four dark-staining and probably dividing nuclei and appear to be second-generation merozoites. The macrogamonts are 35–45 μm in diameter and the microgamonts are 6.5 × 26 μm.

Life cycle: First-generation meronts are localised along the length of the small intestine, but mainly in the jejunum. Second-generation meronts appear in the cytoplasm of epithelial cells 15–20 days after infection. The gamonts appear at 11 days post infection, suggesting that merogony and gametogony run parallel for a time. Most sexual stages develop in epithelial cells of the crypts. The prepatent period is 18–21 days and the patent period is 10–12 days. Sporulation time is 2–3 days.

Geographical distribution: Worldwide

Pathogenesis: Not considered to be pathogenic, although there have been some reports of *E. ahsata* causing diarrhoea, inappetance, weight loss and even death.

Pathology: Thickening of the wall of the ileum, especially anteriorly, with inflammation of Peyer's patches has been reported.

Eimeria bakuensis

Synonym: *Eimeria ovina*

Predilection site: Small intestine

Parasite class: Sporozoasida

Family: Eimeriidae

Hosts: Sheep

Description: Oocysts are ellipsoidal, pale yellowish brown, and are 23–36 × 15–24 µm. There is a micropyle and micropylar cap, one or more polar granules and no residuum. The sporocysts are elongate ovoid, 11–17 × 6–9 µm and contain a residuum and sometimes an inconspicuous Stieda body. Sporozoites are elongate and lie lengthwise head to tail in the sporocysts and have a large clear globule at the broad end and a smaller one at the narrow end. Meronts when mature are 122–146 µm in diameter and contain hundreds of thousands of merozoites (9 × 2 µm).

Life cycle: There appears to be only one asexual generation. The meronts are found in the endothelial cells lining the central lacteals of the small intestine villi and mature 13–21 days after infection. The sexual stages are found in the epithelial cells of the small intestine villi. Synchronous division of the parasites occurs. The microgamonts contain a large residual mass. The sporulation time is 2–4 days. The prepatent period is 19–29 days and the patent period around 10 days.

Geographical distribution: Worldwide

Pathogenesis: Papilloma-like lesions may occur in the small intestine, usually as a sequel to gametocyte formation, but these are not of great pathogenic significance.

Pathology: A few small, slightly haemorrhagic areas are seen scattered throughout the lining of the small intestine and thick, white, opaque patches, made up of groups of heavily parasitised villi, are present leading to the formation of polyps (Fig. 3.17).

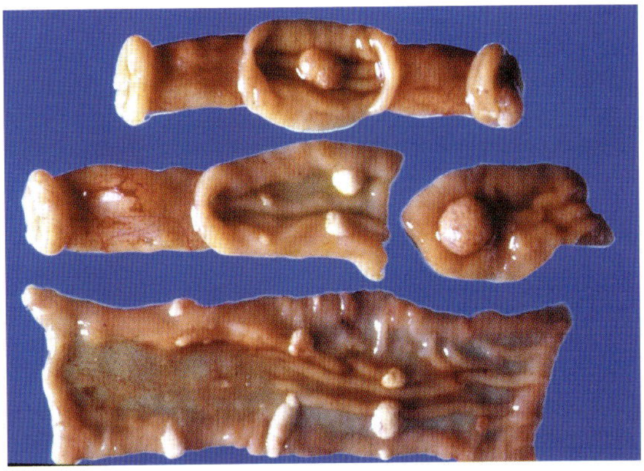

Fig. 3.17 *Eimeria bakuensis* polyps in the small intestine.

Diagnosis: The presence of polyps containing large numbers of gamonts and oocysts is indicative of *E. bakuensis* infection. Oocysts are prevalent in the faeces of sheep of all ages, and coccidiosis cannot be diagnosed solely by finding oocysts. Peak oocyst counts of >1 000 000/g faeces have been reported in clinically healthy lambs.

Eimeria faurei

Predilection site: Small and large intestine

Parasite class: Sporozoasida

Family: Eimeriidae

Hosts: Sheep

Description: The oocyst is ovoid, pale yellow–brown 28–37 × 21–27 µm (32 × 33 µm). There is a conspicuous micropyle 2–3 µm in diameter, without a micropylar cap. There is a polar granule but no oocyst residuum. The sporocysts are ovoid or pyriform, 11–17 × 7–9 µm with a sporocyst residuum. The Stieda body is absent or inconspicuous. The sporozoites are elongate and lie lengthwise head to tail in the sporocysts and have one to two large clear globules each.

Life cycle: Details of the life cycle are not known. The prepatent period is 13–15 days and sporulation time is 1–3 days.

Geographical distribution: Worldwide

Eimeria granulosa

Predilection site: Unknown

Parasite class: Sporozoasida

Family: Eimeriidae

Hosts: Sheep

Description: Oocysts are urn-shaped, 22–35 × 17–25 μm (29.4 × 20.9 μm) with a large micropyle and micropylar cap at the broad end. There is no residuum but polar granules may be present. The sporocysts are ovoid or elongate ovoid, 1–16 × 8–9 μm with a slight Stieda body and a residuum. The sporozoites are elongate, lie lengthwise head to tail in the sporocysts and have one to three clear globules.

Life cycle: Details of the life cycle are not known.

Geographical distribution: Worldwide

Eimeria intricata

Predilection site: Small and large intestine

Parasite class: Sporozoasida

Family: Eimeriidae

Hosts: Sheep

Description: Oocysts are ellipsoidal or slightly ovoid, 40–56 × 30–41 μm (mean 48 × 34 μm), with a thick and striated wall that is granular and transversely striated, brownish yellow to dark brown in colour and 2–3 μm thick. There is a micropyle in the outer wall layer only, and usually a micropylar cap. There are one or more polar granules, but no residuum. The sporocysts are elongate ovoid, 17–22 × 9–14 μm, with a residuum. The Stieda body is very small or absent. Sporozoites are elongate, lie lengthwise head to tail in the sporocysts and have two to three clear globules. Meronts are up to 65 × 45 μm in size and contain large merozoites (19.5 × 4 μm). The mature macrogametes are 32–54 × 25–36 μm, and mature microgamonts are 61–250 × 36–71 μm and contain many slender, flagellated microgametes.

Life cycle: The meronts are mostly in the cells lining the lower small intestine crypts. The gamonts, gametes and oocysts are in the epithelial cells of the crypts of the large and small intestines. The prepatent period is 23–27 days, and sporulation time is 3–7 days.

Geographical distribution: Worldwide

Eimeria marsica

Predilection site: Unknown

Parasite class: Sporozoasida

Family: Eimeriidae

Hosts: Sheep

Description: Oocysts are ellipsoidal 15–22 × 11–14 μm (mean 19 × 13 μm), colourless to slightly greyish or pale yellow, with a micropyle, which may have an inconspicuous micropylar cap. There is no oocyst residuum. The sporocysts are elongate ovoid, 7–11 × 4–7 μm. The Stieda body, if present, is small, and each has a sporocyst residuum. Sporozoites are elongate and lie lengthwise head to tail in the sporocysts and each has a single, small clear globule.

Life cycle: Details of the life cycle are unknown. The prepatent period is 14–16 days and sporulation time is 3 days.

Geographical distribution: Worldwide

Eimeria pallida

Predilection site: Unknown

Parasite class: Sporozoasida

Family: Eimeriidae

Hosts: Sheep

Description: Oocysts are ellipsoidal, colourless to very pale yellow or yellowish green, 12–20 × 8–15 μm (mean 14 × 10 μm) with no micropyle or micropylar cap. A polar granule may be present. There is no oocyst residuum. Sporocysts are elongate ovoid, 6–9 × 4–6 μm. Each has a residuum but no Stieda body. The sporozoites are elongate and usually lie lengthwise, head to tail, although they may lie crosswise in the sporocysts. Each has a single, clear globule.

Life cycle: Details of the life cycle are unknown. The sporulation time is 1–3 days.

Geographical distribution: Worldwide

Eimeria parva

Predilection site: Small and large intestine

Parasite class: Sporozoasida

Family: Eimeriidae

Hosts: Sheep

Description: Oocysts are subspherical, to spherical, smooth, colourless to pale yellow, 13–22 × 11–13 μm (mean 16.5 × 14 μm). There is no micropyle or micropylar cap, but there is a polar granule. There is no oocyst residuum. Sporocysts are ovoid, 6–13 × 5–8 μm. Each has a residuum composed of a few fine granules. The Stieda body is absent or small. The sporozoites each have one clear globule.

Life cycle: The life cycle is typically coccidian with meronts found in the small intestine and the gamonts are found mainly in the caecum and colon, and to a lesser extent in the small intestine. Sporulation time is 3–5 days.

Geographical distribution: Worldwide

Eimeria weybridgensis

Predilection site: Small intestine

Parasite class: Sporozoasida

Family: Eimeriidae

Hosts: Sheep

Description: Oocysts are ellipsoidal to subspherical, colourless or pale yellow, 17–30 × 14–19 μm (mean 24 × 17 μm). There is a micropyle with a micropylar cap and a polar granule is present. There is no oocyst residuum. The sporocysts are elongate ovoid, 13–15 × 6–8 μm and each has a residuum but no Stieda body. The sporozoites are elongate, and lie lengthwise head to tail in the sporocysts. A clear globule is present at each end.

Life cycle: The life cycle is typically coccidian with a prepatent period of 23–33 days and a patent period of 9–12 days. The sporulation time is 1–3 days.

Geographical distribution: Worldwide

Goat coccidia

Nine species of coccidia have been identified in goats based on oocyst morphology and predilection site (Table 15.7; Fig 15.21). *Eimeria ninakohlyakimovae* and *E. caprina* cause widespread denudation of the mucosa in the upper and lower large intestine in young kids. *E. arloingi* is probably the most commonly encountered coccidia causing polyp formation and focal hyperplasia of the mucosa. Other species that are considered pathogenic in goats are *E. christenseni* and *E. hirci*.

Eimeria ninakohlyakimovae

For details see Large intestine.

Eimeria caprina

For details see Large intestine.

Eimeria christenseni

Predilection site: Small intestine

Parasite class: Sporozoasida

Family: Eimeriidae

Hosts: Goat

Description: The oocysts are ovoid or ellipsoidal, 27–44 × 17–31 μm (mean 38 × 25 μm), colourless to pale yellow, with a micropyle and micropylar cap. One or more polar granules are present but there is no oocyst residuum. Sporocysts are broadly ovoid, 12–18 × 8–11 μm. Each has a residuum and the Stieda body is either vestigial or absent. The sporozoites are elongate and lie lengthwise head to tail in the sporocysts. Each has one or more clear globules. First-generation meronts when mature are ellipsoidal, 100–277 × 81–130 μm and contain thousands of straight merozoites about 6–8 × 1–2 μm. Second-generation meronts are 9–20 × 8–12 μm and contain 8–24 merozoites, and sometimes a residuum. Mature macrogametes are 19–35 × 13–25 μm and mature microgamonts are 19–50 × 12–40 μm and contain hundreds of comma-shaped microgametes (3 × 0.5 μm) and a residuum.

Life cycle: First-generation meronts are situated in the endothelial cells of the lacteals of the jejunum and ileum, and in the lamina propria and lymph vessels of the submucosa and mesenteric lymph nodes. Second-generation meronts occur 16 days after infection, mostly in epithelial cells of the crypts, and less often in those of the villi in the small intestine and also in the sinuses of the mesenteric lymph nodes. Gamonts are present in the epithelial cells of the villi and the crypts of the small intestine from 16 days after

Table 3.3 Predilection sites and prepatent periods of *Eimeria* species in goats.

Species	Predilection site	Prepatent period (days)
Eimeria alijevi	Small and large intestine	7–12
Eimeria aspheronica	Unknown	14–17
Eimeria arloingi	Small intestine	14–17
Eimeria caprina	Small and large intestine	17–20
Eimeria caprovina	Unknown	14–20
Eimeria christenseni	Small intestine	14–23
Eimeria hirci	Unknown	13–16
Eimeria jolchijevi	Unknown	14–17
Eimeria ninakohlyakimovae	Small and large intestine	10–13

infection. The prepatent period is 14–23 days and the patent period is 3–30+ days. The sporulation time is 3–6 days.

Geographical distribution: Worldwide

Pathogenesis: This species is one of the more pathogenic in young goats, infection causing desquamation of the mucosa and superficial necrosis.

Pathology: Focal aggregates of coccidia, particularly gamonts and oocysts, occur in the jejunum and ileum and are associated with local infiltration by lymphocytes and plasma cells, epithelial necrosis and submucosal oedema. Superficial desquamation of the mucosa and superficial necrosis are also present. The capillaries are congested and there are petechial haemorrhages. The cellular reaction in the submucosa consists of lymphocytes, macrophages, plasma cells, neutrophils and eosinophils. In the lymph nodes there is oedema and perivascular infiltration by lymphocytes. There are white foci in the intestine consisting essentially of masses of macrogametes, microgamonts and oocysts in the epithelial cells of the tips and sides of the villi and in the crypts.

Eimeria hirci

Predilection site: Unknown

Parasite class: Sporozoasida

Family: Eimeriidae

Hosts: Goat

Description: Oocysts are ellipsoidal, to subspherical, light brown to brownish yellow, 18–23 × 14–19 μm (mean 20.7 × 16.2 μm) with a micropyle and micropylar cap, one or more polar granules, but no oocyst residuum. Sporocysts are ovoid, 8–14 × 4–9 μm with a tiny Stieda body and a residuum. The sporozoites lie lengthwise, at an angle, or even at the ends of the sporocysts and have one to two clear globules.

Life cycle: Details of the life cycle are not known. The prepatent period is 13–16 days and the patent period is 5–14 days. The sporulation time is 1–3 days.

Geographical distribution: Presumed to be worldwide

Pathogenesis: This species is considered pathogenic but lesions and pathology have not been described in detail.

Clinical signs: Clinical signs for *E. christenseni*, *E. hirci*, *E. ninakohlyakimovae* and *E caprina* (see Large intestine) are similar. Infection leads loss of appetite, unthriftiness and profuse diarrhoea, often containing streaks of blood. If left untreated, these animals may continue to scour and eventually die of dehydration.

Diagnosis: Diagnosis is based on history, age, postmortem lesions and faecal examination for oocysts. The latter may be present in very large numbers in both healthy and diseased animals so that postmortem or oocyst differentiation is advisable.

Epidemiology: Managemental factors associated with the development of high levels of infection and the development of disease are overcrowding, dirty conditions and repeat use of rearing pens for different age groups of young goats. If the same pens are used constantly for successive batches, or if young goats are added to a pen already housing older animals, then the later born animals are immediately exposed to heavy challenge and can show severe coccidiosis in the first few weeks of life. On heavily stocked, overgrazed pastures, levels of contamination may be high leading to disease.

Treatment: Few drugs are available for the treatment of coccidiosis in goats but sulphonamides, decoquinate or diclazuril may be effective if disease is suspected.

Control: Good management and hygiene practices, by regular moving of feed and water troughs, avoidance of overcrowding and stress, batch rearing and feeding of dams prior to parturition, can all help to reduce the incidence of infection.

Eimeria alijevi

Predilection site: Small and large intestine

Parasite class: Sporozoasida

Family: Eimeriidae

Hosts: Goat

Description: Oocysts are ovoid or ellipsoidal, pale yellowish to colourless, 15–23 × 12–22 μm (mean 17 × 15 μm) with an inconspicuous micropyle without a micropylar cap or residuum, and one polar granule. Sporocysts are elongate to ovoid, 7–13 × 4–9 μm, with or without a Stieda body, and with a sporocyst residuum. The sporozoites are elongate, and lie at an angle, or lengthwise head to tail in the sporocysts and usually have one to two clear globules. First-generation meronts are 260 × 180 μm and can be seen grossly as whitish bodies. Second-generation meronts are 15–18 × 9–12 μm. The macrogamonts are 14–18 × 9–14 μm, and the microgamonts 22–25 × 15–20 μm.

Life cycle: The life cycle is typically coccidian with first-generation meronts sited in the epithelial cells of the villi in the middle part of the small intestine. Smaller second-generation meronts occur within crypts of the small intestine. Gamonts and oocysts are in the epithelial cells of the colon, caecum and posterior small intestine. The prepatent period is

7–12 days and the patent period, 6–18 days. Sporulation time is 1–5 days.

Geographical distribution: Worldwide

Pathogenesis: Not considered pathogenic although inappetance, weakness and weight loss have been reported.

Eimeria arloingi

Predilection site: Small intestine

Parasite class: Sporozoasida

Family: Eimeriidae

Hosts: Goat

Description: Oocysts are elipsoidal or slightly ovoid, 17–42 × 14–19 μm (mean 27 × 18 μm) with a thick wall and a micropyle and micropylar cap present. There are one or more polar granules but no oocyst residuum. Sporocysts are ovoid, 10–17 × 5–10 μm with a sporocyst residuum, but the Stieda body is either vestigial or not present. The sporozoites are elongate and lie lengthwise head to tail in the sporocysts and usually have a large clear globule at the large end and a small one at the small end. First-generation meronts are 130–350 × 65–240 μm and contain many thousands of merozoites 9–12 × 1–2 μm. Second-generation meronts are 11–44 × 9–20 μm and contain 8–24 merozoites, which are 4–10 μm long. The microgamonts are 19–34 × 13–29 μm and contain a large residuum and several hundred microgametes. The macrogametes are similarly sited and are 19–28 × 14–20 μm.

Life cycle: There are two generations of meronts, with the mature first-generation meronts occuring in the endothelial cells of the lacteals of the villi, in Peyer's patches in the duodenum, jejunum and ileum; and also in the sinuses of the mesenteric lymph nodes draining these regions. These mature 9–12 days after infection. Second-generation meronts lie in the epithelial cells of the villi and the crypts of the small intestine and are mature at about 12 days post infection. Gamonts are found 11–26 days after infection in the epithelial cells lining the crypts and the villi of the jejunum and ileum. The prepatent period is 14–17 days and the patent period 14–15 days. Sporulation time is 1–4 days.

Geographical distribution: Worldwide

Pathogenesis: Papilloma-like lesions or polyps may occur in the small intestine, usually as a sequel to gametocyte formation, but these are not of great pathogenic significance.

Pathology: A few small, slightly haemorrhagic areas are seen scattered throughout the lining of the small intestine and thick, white, opaque patches made up of groups of heavily parasitised villi are present leading to the formation of polyps.

Eimeria aspheronica

Predilection site: Unknown

Parasite class: Sporozoasida

Family: Eimeriidae

Hosts: Goat

Description: Oocysts are ovoid, greenish to yellow-brown, 24–37 × 18–26 μm (mean 31 × 33 μm) with a micropyle but without a micropylar cap. There is a polar granule but no residuum. Sporocysts are piriform or ellipsoidal, 11–17 × 7–11 μm with a sporocyst residuum and a Stieda body that is either vestigial or absent. The sporozoites are elongate and lie lengthwise head to tail in the sporocysts and usually have one to two large clear globules.

Life cycle: Details of the life cycle are not known. The prepatent period is 14–17 days and patent period is 4–9 days. Sporulation time is 1–2 days.

Geographical distribution: Worldwide

Eimeria caprovina

Predilection site: Unknown

Parasite class: Sporozoasida

Family: Eimeriidae

Hosts: Goat

Description: Oocysts are ellipsoidal to subspherical, 26–36 × 21–28 μm (mean 30 × 24 μm), colourless, with a micropyle but without a micropylar cap. One or more polar granules are present. There is no oocyst residuum. Sporocysts are elongate ovoid, 13–17 × 8–9 μm, and each has a Stieda body and a residuum. The sporozoites are elongate, lie lengthwise head to tail in the sporocysts and have a large clear globule at each end.

Life cycle: Details of the life cycle are not known. The prepatent period is 14–20 days and patent period is 4–9 days. Sporulation time is 2–3 days.

Geographical distribution: North America, Europe

Eimeria jolchijevi

Predilection site: Unknown

Parasite class: Sporozoasida

Family: Eimeriidae

Hosts: Goat

Description: Oocysts are ellipsoidal or ovoid, pale yellow, 26–37 × 18–26 μm (mean 31 × 22 μm) with a micropyle at the broad end and a prominent micropylar cap. There is no oocyst residuum. Sporocysts are ovoid, 12–18 × 6–10 μm with a small Stieda body and a residuum. The sporozoites are elongate and lie lengthwise head to tail in the sporocysts and have one or more large clear globules.

Life cycle: Details of the life cycle are not known. The prepatent period is 14–17 days and patent period is 3–10 days. Sporulation time is 2–4 days.

Geographical distribution: Presumed worldwide

Other protozoa

Cryptosporidium parvum

Predilection site: Small intestine

Parasite class: Sporozoasida

Family: Cryptosporidiidae

Hosts: Cattle, sheep, goat, horse, deer, man

Geographical distribution: Worldwide

Epidemiology: A variety of mammals acts as hosts to *C. parvum* but little is known of the importance of their involvement in transmitting infection to, or maintaining infection in, domestic livestock. In young lambs infection appears to be age related with seasonal peaks of disease reported to coincide with birth peaks in spring and autumn. The primary route of infection is mainly by the direct animal-to-animal faecal–oral route. In lambs, chilling due to adverse weather conditions in the neonatal period, intercurrent infections or nutritional or mineral deficiencies could exacerbate or increase the likelihood of disease. Infection in these cases is likely to occur through grooming, nuzzling, coprophagy or by faecal soiling by direct contact with infected animals. Infection may also occur indirectly through consumption of contaminated foods or environmental sources including pasture and water.

For more details see Chapter 2 (Cattle).

Giardia intestinalis

Synonym: *Giardia duodenalis*, *Giardia lamblia*, *Lamblia lamblia*

Predilection site: Small intestine

Parasite class: Zoomastigophorasida

Family: Diplomonadidae

Description: The trophozoite has a pyriform to ellipsoidal, bilaterally symmetrical body; 12–15 μm long by 5–9 μm wide. The dorsal side is convex and there is a large sucking disk on the ventral side. There are two anterior nuclei, two slender axostyles, eight flagellae in four pairs and a pair of darkly staining median bodies. The median bodies are curved bars resembling the claws of a hammer. Cysts are ovoid, 8–12 × 7–10 μm and contain four nuclei.

Hosts: Man, cattle, sheep, goat, pig, horse, alpaca, dog, cat, guinea pig, chinchilla

Geographical distribution: Worldwide

Pathogenesis and clinical signs: Infections in sheep is considered non-pathogenic.

For more details see Chapter 2 (Cattle).

Entamoeba ovis

Synonym: *Entamoeba debliecki*

Predilection site: Small intestine

Parasite class: Sarcodina

Family: Endamoebidae

Description: Trophozoites are 13–14 × 11–12 μm in diameter. The nucleus contains a large pale central endostome composed of several granules, a ring of peripheral chromatin and numerous granules of varying sizes around its periphery. The cysts are 4–13 μm in diameter and each contains a single nucleus when mature, with numerous chromatoid bodies of various sizes and abundance, and a cytoplasmic glycogen granule.

Hosts: Sheep, goat

Life cycle: Trophozoites divide by binary fission. Before encysting, the amoebae round up, become smaller and lay down a cyst wall. Each cyst has one nucleus. Amoebae emerge from the cysts and grow into trophozoites.

Distribution: Worldwide

Pathogenicity: Non-pathogenic

Diagnosis: Identification of trophozoites, or cysts in large intestinal contents of faeces

Treatment and control: Not required

LARGE INTESTINE

Oesophagostomum columbianum

Common name: Nodular worm

Predilection site: Large intestine

Parasite class: Nematoda

Superfamily: Strongyloidea

Description, gross: Adults are slender worms (male 12–17 mm, female 15–22 mm) with large cervical alae, which produce a marked dorsal curvature of the anterior part of the body.

Description, microscopic: The cuticle forms a high mouth-collar shaped like a truncate cone, and separated from the rest of the body by a constriction. The cephalic vesicle is anterior to a cervical groove behind which arise the cervical alae pierced by cervical papillae. External leaf crowns consist of 20–24 elements and the internal has two small elements to each external element. The male bursa is well developed with two equal alate spicules.

The egg is a medium-sized (73–89 × 34–45 μm), regular broad elipse with barrel-shaped walls, and contains 8–16 blastomeres when passed in the faeces. The L_3 have long filamentous tails, 32 gut cells and a rounded head.

Hosts: Sheep, goat, wild ruminants

Life cycle: The preparasitic phase is typically strongyloid and infection is by ingestion of L_3, which enter the mucosa of any part of the small or large intestine becoming enclosed in obvious nodules in which the moult to L_4 takes place. These L_4 then emerge on to the mucosal surface, migrate to the colon and develop to the adult stage. On reinfection with most species the larvae may remain arrested as L_4 in nodules for up to 1 year. The prepatent period is about 45 days.

Geographical distribution: Worldwide; more important in tropical and subtropical areas

Pathogenesis: In the intestine, *O. columbianum* L_3 migrate deep into the mucosa, provoking an inflammatory response with the formation of nodules, which are visible to the naked eye. On reinfection, this response is more marked, the nodules reaching 2.0 cm in diameter and containing greenish eosinophilic pus and an L_4. When the L_4 emerge there may be ulceration of the mucosa. Diarrhoea occurs coincident with emergence about a week after primary infection and from several months to a year after reinfection. In heavy infections, there may be ulcerative colitis and the disease runs a chronic debilitating course with effects on the production of wool and mutton. The nodules in the gut wall also render the intestines useless for processing as sausage skins and surgical suture material.

Clinical signs: In acute infections, severe dark green diarrhoea is the main clinical sign and there is usually a rapid loss of weight, emaciation, prostration and death in young animals. In chronic infections, there is inappetence and emaciation with intermittent diarrhoea and anaemia.

Diagnosis: This is based on clinical signs and postmortem examination. Since the acute disease occurs within the prepatent period, eggs of *Oesophagostomum* spp are not usually present in the faeces. In the chronic disease eggs are present and L_3 can be identified following faecal culture.

Pathology: On postmortem, the carcase is emaciated, the mesenteric lymph nodes are enlarged, and the colonic mucosa is thickened, congested and covered by a layer of mucus in which the worms are scattered. There is hyperplasia of goblet cells, and the lamina propria contains a heavy mixed inflammatory infiltrate with eosinophils, lymphocytes and plasma cells. Nodules caused by histotropic L_4, mainly in the large intestine, are 0.5–3 cm in diameter and comprise a central caseous or mineralised core surrounded by a thin, fibrous, encapsulating stroma. Microscopically, the nematode or its remnants are present among a mass of necrotic debris in which eosinophils are prominent. Giant cells and macophages may surround the necrotic material. Similar nodules may be found in liver, lungs, mesentery and mesenteric lymph nodes. Those in the deeper layers of the gut project from the serosal surface ('pimply gut') and may cause adhesion to adjacent loops of gut or to other organs, and rarely may incite intussusception or peritonitis. In most cases, however, nodules are incidental findings at autopsy. They are probably the response to histotropic L_4 in hosts sensitised by L_3, or the result of prior infection. The nodules caused by the histotropic L_3 consist of small concentrations of suppurative exudate, which resolve as minor foci of granulomatous inflammation after the evacuation of the larvae.

Epidemiology: In tropical and subtropical areas, *O. columbianum* in sheep is especially important. The prolonged survival of the L_4 within the nodules in the gut wall and the lack of an effective immunity made control difficult until the advent of effective anthelmintics.

Treatment: Anthelmintic therapy with broad-spectrum anthelmintics (benzimidazoles, levamisole and avermectins/milbemycins) is highly effective.

Control: A combination of strategic dosing with anthelmintics and pasture management, as used in the control of other nematodes, will also help to control *O. columbianum*.

Notes: The more pathogenic species in sheep occur in the subtropics and tropics and are associated with nodule formation in the intestine.

Oesophagostomum venulosum

Synonym: *Oesophagostomum viginimembrum*

Common name: Large bowel worm

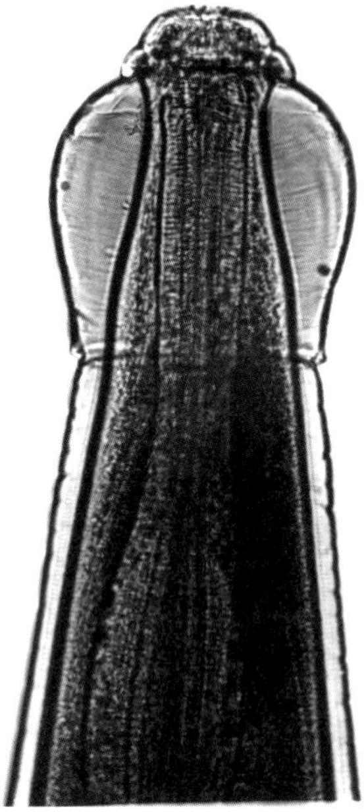

Fig. 3.18 Anterior of *Oesophagostomum venulosum* showing the large inflated cephalic vesicle.

Predilection site: Large intestine

Parasite class: Nematoda

Superfamily: Strongyloidea

Description, gross: Adult worms are slender, with males 11–16 mm, and female 13–24 mm long.

Description, microscopic: The head has a shallow buccal capsule with an external leaf crown of 18 elements. The external crown is compressed so there is only a narrow opening into the buccal capsule. There are no lateral cervical alae and the cervical papillae are posterior to the oesophagus. Around the anterior oesophagus there is an inflated cuticular cephalic vesicle (Fig. 3.18). This terminates in a cervical groove, which is followed in some species by broad cervical alae. In the male the bursa is well developed. The egg is a medium-sized (85 × 51 µm), regular broad elipse with barrel-shaped walls, and contains 16–32 blastomeres when passed in the faeces. The L_3 have long filamentous tails, 32 gut cells and a rounded head.

Hosts: Sheep, goat, deer, camel

Life cycle: The egg hatches on the ground releasing the first-stage larva, which moults to the second stage, and then to the infective third stage. The host is infected by ingestion of the larva with the herbage. There is no migration stage in the body, although there is limited evidence that skin penetration is possible. The larvae moult again and the fourth-stage larvae attach to, or enter, the wall of the intestine. Fourth-stage larvae return to the lumen and pass to the colon. The prepatent period is about 7 weeks.

Geographical distribution: Worldwide

Pathogenesis: Generally considered non-pathogenic

Clinical signs: Not associated with clinical signs

Diagnosis: Diagnosis of gastrointestinal nematodes generally is based on clinical signs, grazing history, postmortem findings and faecal egg counts. Faecal worm egg counts are not that useful, as the eggs of *O. venulosum* are difficult to differentiate from other trichostrongyle eggs. For accurate differentiation, larval cultures should be prepared.

Pathology: *O. venulosum* seldom causes significant nodule formation (c.f. *O. columbianum*) and when it does the nodules are small and mainly confined to the caecum and colon.

Epidemiology: The basic epidemiology of *O. venulosum* is similar to other trichostrongylid infections of sheep and is described in more detail in Chapters 1 and 12. In temperate areas, there is evidence that *O. venulosum* undergoes hypobiosis at the L_4 stage in sheep during autumn and winter, and that this is the principal manner in which this species survives until the next spring. The species is also capable of overwintering on pasture as L_3.

Treatment and control: As for *O. columbianum*

Notes: *Oesophagostomum viginimembrum* is specific to the dromedary camel but is considered to synonymous with *O. venulosum.*

Other species of *Oesophagostomum* have been reported in sheep and goats. Little is known of their pathogenesis and treatment is not usually indicated.

Oesophagostomum multifoliatum

Common name: Nodular worm

Predilection site: Large intestine

Parasite class: Nematoda

Superfamily: Strongyloidea

Hosts: Sheep, goat

Geographical distribution: Eastern Africa

Oesophagostomum asperum

Common name: Nodular worm

Predilection site: Large intestine

Parasite class: Nematoda

Superfamily: Strongyloidea

Hosts: Sheep, goat

Geographical distribution: Asia, Central America

Chabertia ovina

Common name: Large-mouthed bowel worm

Predilection site: Large intestine

Parasite class: Nematoda

Superfamily: Strongyloidea

Description, gross: The adults are 1.5–2.0 cm in length and are the largest nematodes found in the colon of ruminants. They are white, stout with a markedly truncated and enlarged anterior end due to the presence of the very large buccal capsule (Fig. 3.19).

Description, microscopic: The huge buccal capsule, which is bell shaped, has a double row of small papillae around the rim. There are no teeth. There is a shallow ventral cervical groove, and anterior to it a slightly inflated cephalic vesicle. In the male, the bursa is well developed and the spicules are 1.3–1.7 mm long, with a gubernaculum. In the female, the vulva opens about 0.4 mm from the posterior extremity. Infective larvae have a rounded head, 32 gut cells and a long filamentous tail. The egg is a medium-sized (90×50 μm), regular broad elipse, with 16–32 blastomeres.

Hosts: Sheep, goat, occasionally deer, cattle and other ruminants

Life cycle: The life cycle is direct. Eggs are passed in the faeces and hatch on the ground releasing the first-stage larva, which moults to the second stage, and then to the infective third stage. The host is infected by ingestion of the larva with the herbage. In the parasitic phase the L_3 enter the mucosa of the small intestine and occasionally that of the caecum and colon; after a week they moult, the L_4 emerge on to the mucosal surface and migrate to congregate in the caecum where development to the L_5 is completed about 25 days after infection. The young adults then travel to the colon. There is no migration stage in the body. The prepatent period is about 6–7 weeks.

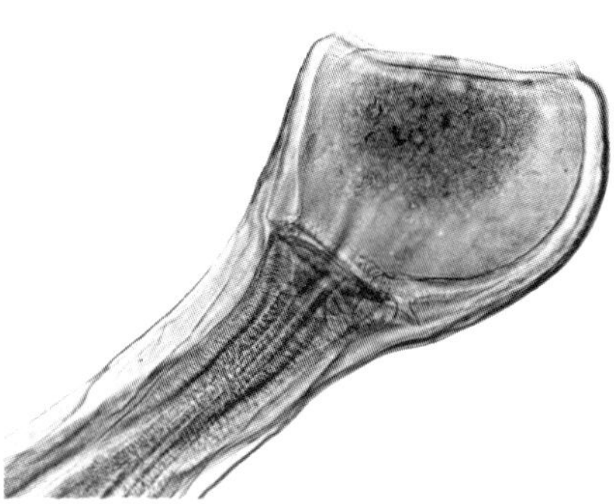

Fig. 3.19 Head of *Chabertia ovina* illustrating the large bell-shaped buccal capsule.

Geographical distribution: Worldwide but more prevalent in temperate regions

Pathogenesis: *Chabertia ovina* is present, usually in low numbers, in the majority of sheep and goats. It contributes to the syndrome of parasitic gastroenteritis and only occasionally occurs in sufficient numbers to cause clinical disease on its own. The major pathogenic effect is caused by the L_5 and by mature adults; these attach to the mucosa of the colon via their buccal capsules and then feed by ingesting large plugs of tissue, resulting in local haemorrhage and loss of protein through the damaged mucosa. A burden of around 300 worms is considered pathogenic and in severe outbreaks the effects become evident during the late prepatent period. The wall of the colon becomes oedematous, congested and thickened with small haemorrhages at the sites of worm attachment.

Clinical signs: Moderate infections are usually asymptomatic. In severe infections, diarrhoea, which may contain blood and mucus and in which worms may be found, is the most common clinical sign. The sheep become anaemic and hypoalbuminaemic and can suffer severe weight loss.

Diagnosis: Since much of the pathogenic effect occurs within the prepatent period, the faecal egg count may be very low. However, during the diarrhoeic phase, the worms may be expelled and they are easily recognised. At necropsy, diagnosis is generally based on the lesions since the worm burden may be negligible following the expulsion of worms in the faeces, although in some cases worms may be observed attached to the mucosa of the colon.

Pathology: There are petechial haemorrhages in the mucosa of colon due to immatures, and immature and adult worms are found in the gut lumen.

Epidemiology: In temperate areas, L_3 are capable of surviving the winter. The parasite may also overwinter in the host as hypobiotic L_4 in the wall of the intestine, emerging in the late winter and early spring. Although outbreaks of chabertiosis have been recorded in goats and sheep in Europe, the disease is more important in the winter rainfall areas of Australasia and South Africa.

Treatment: Anthelmintic therapy with broad-spectrum anthelmintics (benzimidazoles, levamisole and avermectins/milbemycins) is highly effective.

Control: Similar to other strongylid intestinal nematodes.

Skrjabinema ovis

Common name: Pinworms

Predilection site: Caecum, colon

Parasite class: Nematoda

Superfamily: Oxyuroidea

Description, gross: Small worms, up to 7 mm in size; male are 3 mm, and females 6–7 mm. There are three large complicated lips and three small intermediate lips. The oesophagus is cylindrical and terminates in a large spherical bulb.

Description, microscopic: The male worm has a single spicule. The tail is bluntly rounded with a cuticular expansion supported by two pairs of processes. Eggs are asymmetrically flattened, larvated and measure 55–60 × 32–35 μm.

Hosts: Sheep, goat

Life cycle: The life cycle is direct. Embryonated eggs are deposited on the perineal skin by the adult female worms. Infection is by ingestion of the embryonated egg. The prepatent period is about 25 days.

Geographical distribution: Worldwide

Pathogenesis: The pinworms cause negligible pathological disturbance

Clinical signs: These pinworms have rarely been incriminated as a cause of disease and are usually recognised only at necropsy.

Diagnosis: Identification of the worms on post-mortem, or the larvated eggs in faeces

Pathology: No associated pathology

Epidemiology: Infection occurs by ingestion, either through nuzzling or suckling, or through intake of the larvated eggs in grass, hay or bedding.

Treatment: Not usually required

Control: Not required

This genus of small pinworms contains several species parasitic in the caecum and colon, details of which are essentially similar to *Skrjabinema ovis*.

Skrjabinema alata

Common name: Pinworms

Predilection site: Caecum, colon

Parasite class: Nematoda

Superfamily: Oxyuroidea

Hosts: Sheep

Geographical distribution: South Africa

Skrjabinema caprae

Common name: Pinworms

Predilection site: Caecum, colon

Parasite class: Nematoda

Superfamily: Oxyuroidea

Hosts: Goat

Geographical distribution: USA, Mexico

Trichuris ovis

Synonym: *Trichocephalus ovis*

Common name: Whipworms

Predilection site: Large intestine

Parasite class: Nematoda

Superfamily: Trichuroidea

Description, gross: The adults are long white worms about 4–8 cm (male 5–8 cm; females 3.5–7 cm) with a thick broad posterior end tapering rapidly to a long filamentous anterior end that is characteristically embedded in the mucosa.

Description, microscopic: The male tail is coiled and possesses a single spicule in a protrusible sheath. The sheath bears an oblong swelling a short distance from its distal extremity and is covered with minute spines, which decrease in size towards the distal end. The female tail is merely curved. The characteristic eggs are lemon shaped, 75 × 35 μm, with a thick smooth shell and a conspicuous polar plug (operculum) at both ends; in the faeces these eggs appear yellow or brown in colour.

Hosts: Sheep, goats, occasionally cattle and other ruminants

Life cycle: The infective stage is the L_1 within the egg, which develops in 1 or 2 months of being passed in the faeces depending on the temperature. Under optimal conditions, these larvated eggs may subsequently survive and remain viable for several years. After ingestion, the plugs are digested and the released L_1 penetrate the glands of the distal ileum, caecal and colonic mucosa. Subsequently all four moults occur within these glands, the adults emerging to lie on the mucosal surface with their anterior ends embedded in the mucosa. The prepatent period is about 7–10 weeks.

Geographical distribution: Worldwide

Pathogenesis: Most infections are light and asymptomatic. Occasionally when large numbers of worms are present they cause a haemorrhagic colitis and/or a diphtheritic inflammation of the caecal mucosa. This results from the subepithelial location and continuous movement of the anterior end to the whipworm as it searches for blood and fluid.

Clinical signs: Despite the fact that ruminants have a high incidence of light infections, the clinical significance of this genus, especially in ruminants, is generally negligible although isolated outbreaks have been recorded.

Diagnosis: Since the clinical signs are not pathognomonic, diagnosis may depend on finding numbers of lemon-shaped *Trichuris* eggs in the faeces. Egg output is often low in *Trichuris* infections. However, since clinical signs may occur during the prepatent period, diagnosis in food animals may depend on necropsy.

Pathology: In heavy infections there may be a muco-haemorrhagic typhlitis.

Epidemiology: The most important feature is the longevity of the eggs, which may still survive after 3 or 4 years. On pasture, this is less likely since the eggs tend to be washed into the soil.

Treatment: In ruminants, the benzimidazoles, the avermectins/milbemycins or levamisole by injection are very effective against adult *Trichuris*, but less so against larval stages.

Control: Prophylaxis is rarely necessary in ruminants.

Notes: The adults are usually found in the caecum but are only occasionally present in sufficient numbers to be clinically significant.

Other species of *Trichuris* are found less commonly in sheep and goats.

Trichuris skrjabini

Predilection site: Large intestine

Parasite class: Nematoda

Superfamily: Trichuroidea

Geographical distribution: Europe, Asia, USA

Trichuris discolor

Predilection site: Large intestine

Parasite class: Nematoda

Superfamily: Trichuroidea

Geographical distribution: Europe, Asia, USA

For more details see Chapter 2 (Cattle).

Eimeria crandallis

Predilection site: Small and large intestine

Parasite class: Sporozoasida

Family: Eimeriidae

Hosts: Sheep

Description: Oocysts are subspherical to broadly ellipsoidal, 17–23 × 17–22 μm (21.9 × 19.4 μm), with a micropyle, which may be distinct or indistinct, and a micropylar cap. One or more polar granules may be present and there is no residuum. The sporocysts are broadly ovoid, 8–13 × 6–9 μm. There is no Stieda body but a residuum may be present. The sporozoites lie transversely at the ends of the sporocysts and have one to two clear globules. Mature first-generation meronts are 250 μm in diameter, and are visible to the naked eye as pin-point white spots, occurring most frequently in the lower jejunum. They contain an average of 253 000 first-generation merozoites measuring 10 × 1.7 μm.

Life cycle: First-generation meronts appear on day 3 after infection and are mature by day 10. Second-generation meronts appear at day 10–12 after infection in the cytoplasm of epithelial cells of the small intestine and the caecum. Most lie at the base of the crypts and contain five to nine merozoites. Progamonts appear in the nuclei of the epithelial cells in the crypts and villi of the jejunum, ileum and caecum at 11–16 days after infection. The progamonts divide synchronously. By day 16, the progamonts on the villi mature into gamonts, and enlarge and move into the cytoplasm above the nucleus where they differentiate into macro and microgamonts. The progamonts in the crypts mature from day 18. The prepatent period is 13–20 days and sporulation time is 1–3 days.

Geographical distribution: Worldwide

Pathogenesis: The pathogenic lesions are mainly in the caecum and colon where gametogony of *E. crandallis* occurs. The lesions cause local haemorrhage and oedema, and villous atrophy may be a sequel resulting in malabsorption. Infection is particularly a problem in very young lambs, especially if their immune status is poor or they have been colostrum deprived. Light infections produce a very strong immunity.

Pathology: In heavily infected lambs at around 10 days after infection there is whitish discoloration of the mucosa due to masses of first-generation meronts, and this is apparent through the serosa. From the onset of diarrhoea there is hyperaemia and thickening of the wall of the small intestine, increasing in severity towards the caecum. Gamonts were found in scrapings from these areas. In heavy infections, the caecum and colon may be similarly affected. Histologically there is a leucocyte infiltration with loss of villus epithelium associated with first- and second-generation meronts in the small intestine. There is resulting villous atrophy, and the crypt epithelium is also affected resulting in loss of crypts. From day 11 after infection, progamonts can be detected in the small intestine and the large intestine. Infected crypts are hyperplastic with large, basophilic enterocytes and reduced goblet cell numbers.

Eimeria ovinoidalis

Predilection site: Small and large intestine

Parasite class: Sporozoasida

Family: Eimeriidae

Hosts: Sheep

Description: Oocysts are ellipsoidal, colourless or pale yellow, 17–30 × 14–19 μm (mean 19 × 13 μm). There is an inconspicuous micropyle without a micropylar cap. Two or more polar granules are present and there is no residuum. Sporocysts are elongate ovoid, 10–14 × 4–8 μm. Each has a Stieda body and a residuum. The sporozoites are elongate, 11–14 × 2–4 μm and lie lengthwise head to tail in the sporocysts. Each has one large and one small globule. First-generation meronts, at 10 days, average 290 μm in diameter and contain many thousands of merozoites. Second-generation meronts mature at about 10–11 days and have a mean diameter of 12 μm, each containing an average of 24 merozoites. The mature microgamonts average 15 × 12 μm and contain many microgametes arranged peripherally around a central residuum, whilst mature macrogamonts average 16 × 12 μm.

Life cycle: Following ingestion of sporulated oocysts, eight sporozoites emerge from each oocyst into the small intestine and penetrate cells in the intestinal mucosa. The parasites undergo at least one asexual muliplication within the mucosa, giving rise to merozoites within meronts. The first-generation meronts are very large (100–300 μm) and may be visible to the naked eye as pinpoint white spots on the mucosa. These mature in the small intestine lamina propria 9 days after infection, and give rise to a second generation of meronts that are much smaller than the first. Second-generation meronts lie in epithelial cells lining the crypts of the large intestine, maturing 10–11 days after infection. From this last schizont generation, merozoites emerge which give rise to the sexual forms (gamonts), which in turn form oocysts that pass out in the faeces. Once outside, the oocysts sporulate, i.e. they undergo two divisions to produce four sporocysts, each containing two sporozoites. Only the sporulated oocysts are infective. If ingested by a susceptible host, the sporozoites emerge and start the cycle again. The prepatent period is 12–15 days and the patent period is 7–28 days. Sporulation time is 1–3 days.

Geographical distribution: Worldwide

Pathogenesis: The pathogenic lesions are mainly in the caecum and colon where second-stage merogony and gametogony of *E. ovinoidalis* occur. Petechial haemorrhages appear in the small intestine 3–7 days after infection. The small intestine may become thickened and inflamed. The giant first-generation meronts which form in the mucosa of the small intestine 10 days after infection cause leucocyte and macrophage infiltration, crypt hyperplasia and epithelial loss. There is extensive haemorrhage in the posterior small intestine of severely affected lambs by day 15 after infection. The caecum and upper part of the small intestine become thickened and oedematous, and are haemorrhagic by day 19. The gamonts result in loss of crypt and surface epithelium leading to a denuded mucosa. The lesions cause local haemorrhage and oedema, and villous atrophy may be a sequel resulting in malabsorption.

Pathology: On postmortem examination, the caecum is usually inflamed, empty and contracted, with a hyperaemic, oedematous and thickened wall. In some cases the mucosa may be haemorrhagic. Other lesions are more specific but are not usually associated with clinical signs.

Clinical signs: Clinical signs for both *E. crandallis* and *E. ovinoidalis* are similar. The first sign that coccidiosis may be affecting a flock is that lambs may not be thriving as expected. Several lambs may have a tucked-up and open-fleeced appearance with a few showing faecal staining around the hindquarters due to diarrhoea. Lambs eventually lose their appetite and become weak and unthrifty. As the disease progresses, some lambs show profuse watery diarrhoea, often containing streaks of blood. If left untreated, these animals may continue to scour and eventually die of dehydration.

Diagnosis: Diagnosis is based on the management history, the age of the lambs, postmortem lesions and faecal examination for oocysts. The latter may be present in very large numbers in both healthy and diseased lambs so that a necropsy is always advisable.

Epidemiology: In spring-lambing flocks in western Europe, infection of lambs results both from oocysts, which have survived the winter and from those produced by earlier born lambs. Lambs are usually affected between 4 and 8 weeks of age with a peak infection around 6 weeks. The outbreaks reported have occurred where ewes and lambs were housed in unhygienic conditions or grazed intensively. The feeding of concentrates in stationary troughs, around which heavy contamination with oocysts has occurred, can also be a precipitating factor. In the USA, coccidiosis occurs when older lambs are confined in feedlots after weaning.

Treatment and control: Decoquinate and diclazuril are the drugs generally used for the prevention and treatment of these infections. Monensin and amprolium have also been used in some countries for coccidiosis prevention. Several sulphonamides, such as sulphadimidine, sulphamethoxypyridazine, sulphadiazine, sulphadoxine and sulphatroxazole, can also be used for the treatment of infected animals. All animals in a group should be treated and dehydrated animals may require oral or intravenous rehydration. Where non-specific symptoms of weight loss or ill-thrift are present, it is important to investigate all potential causes and seek laboratory confirmation. Good management and hygiene practices, by regular moving of feed and water troughs, avoidance of overcrowding and stress, batch rearing, feeding of dams prior to parturition, and creep feeding, will reduce the incidence of infection.

Eimeria ninakohlyakimovae

Predilection site: Small and large intestine

Parasite class: Sporozoasida

Family: Eimeriidae

Hosts: Goat

Description: Oocysts are ellipsoidal, thin-walled, colourless, 20–22 × 14–16 μm (mean 20.7 × 14.8 μm) without micropyle or micropylar cap and with no oocyst residuum. Sporocysts are ovoid, 9–15 × 4–10 μm, each with a Stieda body and a sporocyst residuum. The sporozoites are elongate, and lie lengthwise head to tail in the sporocysts, each with two clear globules.

Life cycle: The life cycle is typically coccidian. The meronts, gamonts and oocysts are in the epithelial cells of the ileum, caecum and upper large intestine. The prepatent period is 10–13 days. The sporulation time is 1–4 days.

Geographical distribution: Worldwide

Pathogenesis: As for *E. ovinoidalis* in sheep

Eimeria caprina

Predilection site: Small and large intestine

Parasite class: Sporozoasida

Family: Eimeriidae

Hosts: Goat

Description: Oocysts are ellipsoidal or slightly ovoid, dark brown to brownish yellow in colour, 27–40 × 19–26 μm with a smooth wall. There is a micropyle but no micropylar cap or oocyst residuum. One or more polar granules are present. Sporocysts are elongate ovoid, 13–17 × 7–10 μm with a small Stieda body and a residuum. The sporozoites are elongate, lie lengthwise head to tail in the sporocysts and usually have a large clear globule at the large end and a smaller one at the small end.

Life cycle: Details of the life cycle are not known. The prepatent period is 17–20 days and the patent period 3–6 days. Sporulation time is 2–3 days.

Geographical distribution: Worldwide

Pathogenesis: This species is considered pathogenic but lesions and pathology have not been described in detail.

Clinical signs: The clinical signs for *E. ninakohlyakimovae* and *E. caprina* are generally similar. Infection leads loss of appetite, unthriftiness, profuse diarrhoea, often containing streaks of blood. If left untreated, these animals may continue to scour and eventually die of dehydration.

Epidemiology: Management factors associated with the development of high levels of infection and the development of disease are overcrowding, dirty conditions and repeat use of rearing pens for different age groups of young goats. If the same pens are used constantly for successive batches, or if young goats are added to a pen already housing older animals, then the later born animals are immediately exposed to heavy challenge and can show severe coccidiosis in the first few weeks of life. On heavily stocked, overgrazed pastures levels of contamination may be high, leading to disease.

Diagnosis: Diagnosis is based on the management history, postmortem lesions and faecal examination for oocysts.

Treatment and control: Few drugs are available for the treatment of coccidiosis in goats but sulphonamides, decoquinate or diclazuril may be effective if disease is suspected. The incidence of infection can be reduced through avoidance of overcrowding and stress, and attention to hygiene.

Flagellate protozoa

The life cycle of flagellate protozoa is similar for all species found in sheep and goats. The trophozoites reproduce by longitudinal binary fission. No sexual stages are known and there are no cysts. Transmission is thought to occur by ingestion of trophozoites from faeces. All are considered to be non-pathogenic and are generally only identified from smears taken from the large intestine of fresh carcases.

Retortamonas ovis

Predilection site: Large intestine

Parasite class: Zoomastigophorasida

Family: Retortamonadorididae

Description: Trophozoites are pyriform and average 5.2 × 3.4 μm. There is a large cytosome near the anterior end, containing a cytostomal fibril that extends across the anterior end and posteriorly along each side. An anterior flagellum and a posterior trailing flagellum emerge from the cytostomal groove. Cysts are pyriform and ovoid, containing one or two nuclei and retain the cytostomal fibril.

Geographical distribution: Worldwide.

Tetratrichomonas ovis

Synonym: *Trichomonas ovis*, *Ditrichomonas ovis*

Predilection site: Caecum, rumen

Parasite class: Zoomastigophorasida

Family: Trichomonadidae

Description: The body is pyriform, 6–9 × 4–8 μm (mean 7 × 6 μm) and the four anterior flagella are of unequal length. There is a slender, hyaline axostyle which extends approximately 5 μm beyond the body and gradually tapers to a point. There is no chromatic ring at the point at which the axostyle leaves the body. There is an anterior nucleus, and a prominent pelta at the anterior end. There is a prominent undulating membrane which extends 75–100% the length of the body, and which continues as a free posterior flagellum. The costa is prominent and there are several irregular rows of paracostal granules, and an ovoid or club-shaped parabasal body (approximately 2 × 1 μm), containing an intensely chromophilic body and a parabasal filament.

Geographical distribution: Unknown

PARASITES OF THE RESPIRATORY SYSTEM

Mammomonogamus nasicola

Synonym: *Syngamus nasicola*

Predilection site: Nasal cavities

Parasite class: Nematoda

Superfamily: Strongyloidea

Description, gross: The worms are reddish in appearance and about 1–2 cm long. Males are 4–6 mm and females 11–23 mm long and found in permanent copulation. The buccal capsule lacks a cuticular crown.

Description, microscopic: Eggs are ellipsoid, 54–98 μm with no operculum at either end.

Hosts: Sheep, goat, cattle, deer

Life cycle: The life cycle is direct but the mode of transmission is unknown.

Geographical distribution: Central and South America, central Africa, Caribbean islands

Pathogenesis: Heavy infections cause irritation of the nasal mucosa, sneezing and nasal discharges.

Clinical signs: Infections are usually asymptomatic but affected animals may sneeze and have a nasal discharge.

Diagnosis: This is based on clinical signs and the finding of eggs in the faeces or adult worms on postmortem.

Pathology: Not described

Epidemiology: Unknown

Treatment: Successful treatment has not been reported. Benzimidazoles and macrocyclic lactones are likely to be effective.

Control: No preventive or control measures have been described.

Notes: This genus, closely related to *Syngamus*, is parasitic in the respiratory passages of mammals. Infection has been reported in man causing a laryngo-pharyngeal syndrome.

Mammomonogamus laryngeus

Synonym: *Syngamus laryngeus*

Common name: Gapeworm

Predilection site: Larynx

Parasite class: Nematoda

Superfamily: Strongyloidea

Hosts: Cattle, buffalo, goat, sheep, deer, rarely man

For more details of this species see Chapter 2 (Cattle).

Oestrus ovis

Common name: Sheep nasal bot

Predilection site: Nasal passages

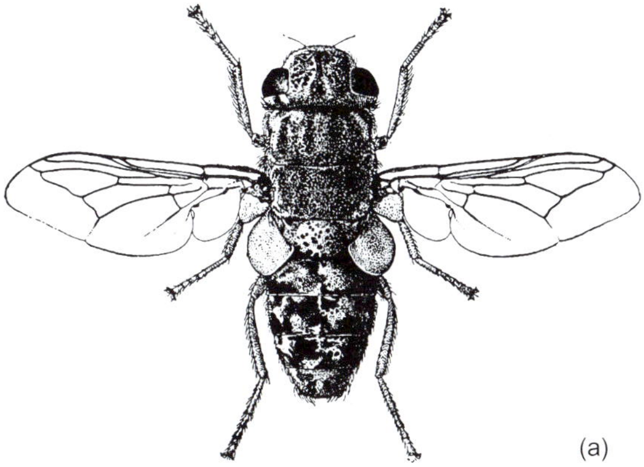

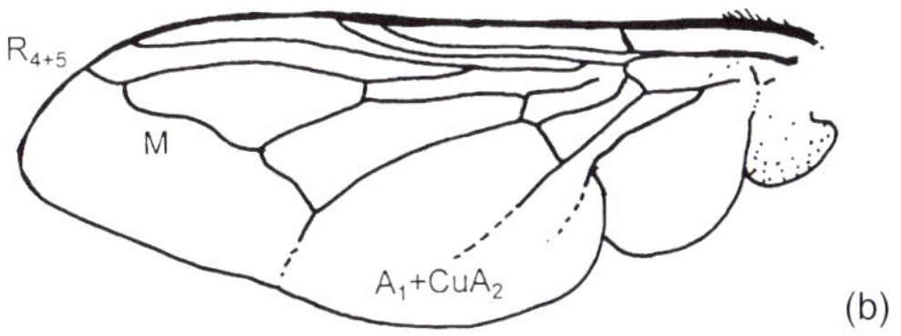

Fig. 3.20 (a) Adult female *Oestrus ovis* and (b) wing venation typical of *Oestrus*, showing the strongly bent vein M joining R_{4+5} before the wing margin (reproduced from Castellani and Chalmers, 1910).

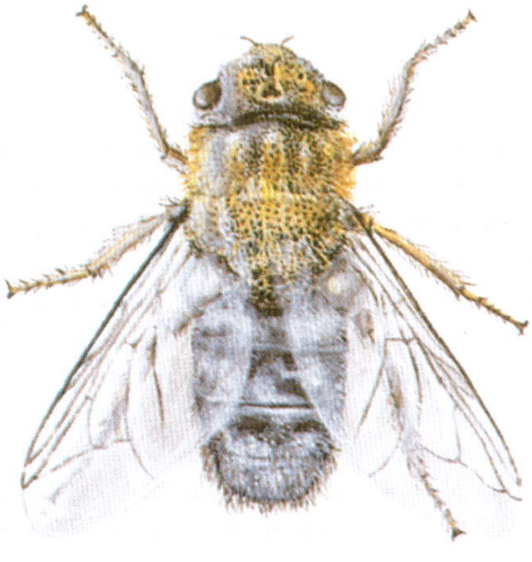

Fig. 3.21 *Oestrus ovis.*

Parasite class: Insecta

Family: Oestridae

Description, adults: Greyish brown flies about 12 mm long, with small black spots on the abdomen and a covering of short brown hairs (Figs 3.20, 3.21). The head is broad, with small eyes, and the frons, scutellum and dorsal thorax bear small wart-like protuberances. The segments of the antennae are small and the arista bare. The mouthparts are reduced to small knobs.

Description, larvae: Mature larvae in the nasal passages are about 30 mm long, yellow–white and tapering anteriorly. Each segment has a dark transverse band dorsally (Fig. 3.22). They have large, black, oral hooks, connected to an internal cephalopharyngeal skeleton. The ventral surface bears rows of small spines.

Hosts: Primarily sheep and goat, but also ibex, camel and, occasionally, humans

Life cycle: The females are viviparous and infect the sheep by squirting a jet of liquid containing larvae at the nostrils during flight, which delivers up to 25 larvae at a time. The newly deposited L_1 are about 1.0 mm long, and migrate through the nasal passages to the frontal sinuses, feeding on the mucus that is secreted in response to the stimulation of larval movement. Larvae attach themselves to the mucous membrane using oral hooks, which cause irritation. The first moult occurs in the nasal passages, and the L_2 crawl into the frontal sinuses where the final moult to L_3 takes place. In the sinuses, the larvae complete their growth and then migrate back to the nostrils, from where they are sneezed to the ground. Larvae pupate in the ground and pupation lasts for between 3–9 weeks. The larvae remain in the nasal passages for a variable period, ranging from 2 weeks in summer to 9 months during colder seasons. Where flies are active throughout the year, two or three generations are possible, but in cool or cold weather the small L_1 and L_2 become dormant and remain in recesses of the nasal passages over winter. They move to the frontal sinuses only in the warmer spring weather, and then complete their development into the L_3, which emerge from the nostrils and pupate on the ground to give a further generation of adults. The females survive only 2 weeks, but during this time each can deposit up to 500 larvae in the nasal passages of sheep.

Geographical distribution: Although originally Palaearctic, it is now found in all sheep-farming areas of the world, having been spread with sheep as they were transported worldwide.

Pathogenesis: Most infections are light, with only an average of 2–20 larvae being present in the frontal sinus of infested animals at any one time. Sheep show nasal discharge and sneezing, and rub their noses on fixed objects. In the rare heavier infections, there is unthriftiness and sheep may circle and show lack of coordination, these signs being termed 'false gid'. If a larva dies in the sinuses, there may be secondary bacterial invasion and cerebral involvement. This

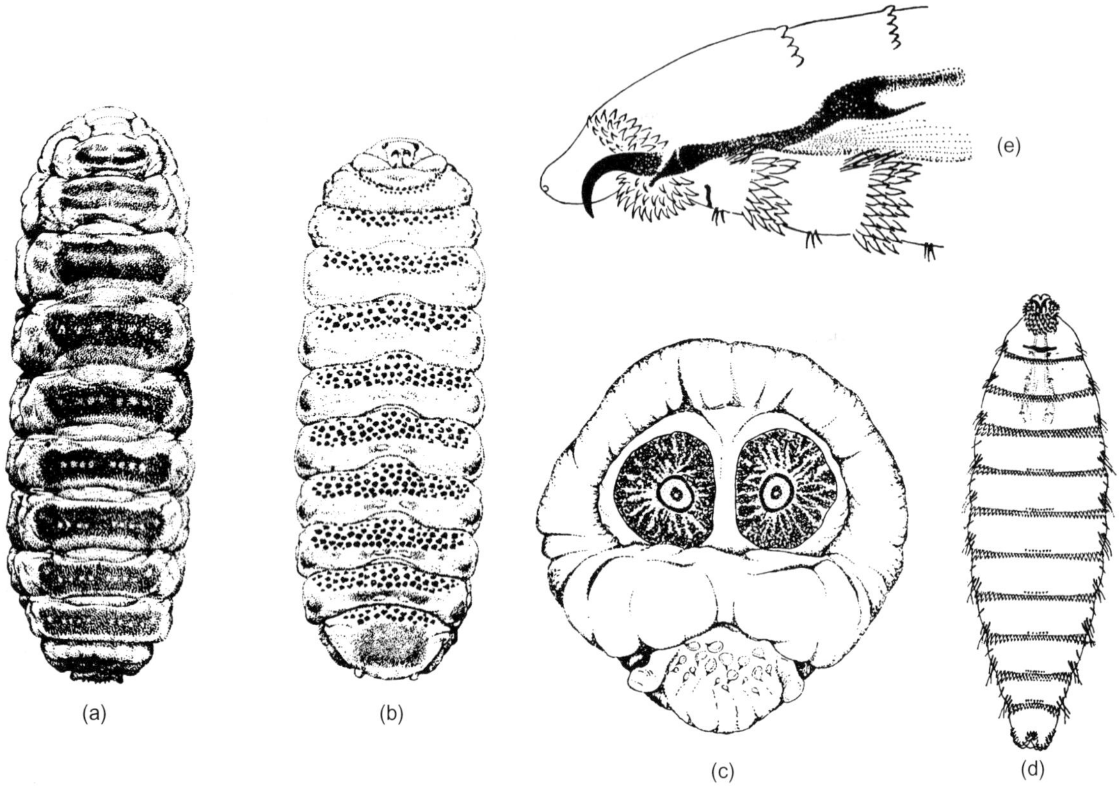

Fig. 3.22 *Oestris ovis*. (a) Dorsal view and (b) ventral view of third-stage larva. (c) Posterior-view of third-stage larva. (d) First-stage larva. (e) Mouthpart of first-stage larva in lateral view (reproduced from Zumpt, 1965).

may occur if larvae crawl into small cavities and are unable to leave when fully grown. Occasionally the larvae may penetrate the bones of the skull and enter the cerebral cavity. The larvae and the thickening of the nasal mucosa may impair respiration. Changes in the nasal tissues of infected sheep include catarrh, infiltration of inflammatory cells and squamous metaplasia, characterised by conversion of secretory epithelium to stratified squamous type. Immune responses by the host to infestation by *O. ovis* have been recorded.

The most important effects, however, are due to the activity of the adult flies. When they approach sheep to deposit larvae the animals panic, stamp their feet, bunch together and press their nostrils into each other's fleeces and against the ground. There may be several attacks each day, so that feeding is interrupted and animals may fail to gain weight.

Oestrus can occasionally also infect humans. Larvae are usually deposited near the eyes, where a catarrhal conjunctivitis may result, or around the lips, leading to a stomatitis. Such larvae never fully develop.

Clinical signs: Nasal discharge, rubbing, sneezing, unthriftiness, circling and lack of coordination. Secondary bacterial infections are common.

Diagnosis: Although the clinical signs may assist in diagnosis, infestations of *Oestrus ovis* must be differentiated from other conditions with similar symptoms. Occasionally a larva may be found on the ground after a severe sneezing attack, but often a positive diagnosis can only be made at necropsy.

Pathology: In addition to mechanical damage to the tissues, infestation induces a marked hypersensitivity reaction where there is an increase in the numbers of serous mast cells and eosinophils and an increased production of IgE. Interstitial pneumonia may develop during the course of ovine oestrosis, marked by increases in the numbers of oesinophils and mast cells in the lung parenchyma, mainly in the peribronchial region. This pathology is probably caused by permanent antigenic stimulation during infection, aspirated larval antigen inducing pulmonary sensitisation.

Epidemiology: The adult flies occur from spring to autumn and are particularly active during the summer months. However in warm climates they may even be active in winter. In southern Europe, three generation peaks in *O. ovis* populations have been recorded in March–April, June–July and September–October. More commonly, however, there are only two generations per year, with adults present in late spring and late summer. Geographically, infestation prevalence tends to be highly localised. The flies hide in warm corners and crevices and in the early morning can be seen sitting on walls and objects in the sun.

Treatment: Where the numbers of larvae are small, it may not be economically viable to treat. However, in heavy infections closantel, nitroxynil, and the endectocides, ivermectin, doramectin and moxidectin, are highly effective, as are the organophosphates trichlorphon and dichlorvos.

Control: Should a control scheme be necessary it has been suggested by South African workers that flock treatment should be given twice a year, the first at the beginning of summer to kill newly acquired larvae, and the second in midwinter to kill any overwintering larvae. Fly repellents may be used but so far these have shown limited success.

Gedoelstia spp

Predilection site: Nasopharynx

Parasite class: Insecta

Family: Oestridae

Description, adults: These are large, robust flies of up to 18 mm in length. The head of the adult is reddish yellow with dark brown spots. The thorax is rusty brown in colour with a pattern of glossy black lines. The abdomen is brown with large black lateral patches and a series of large tubercles with sharply pointed tips.

Description, larvae: The third-stage larvae are ovoid, up to 20 mm in length and may be distinguished from all other oestrids by a vertical slit in the posterior peritremes or a vertical suture if the spiracle is closed.

Hosts: Sheep, occasionally cattle, horses and antelope

Life cycle: The larvae are deposited by the adult flies in the orbit of the natural hosts, which are antelopes, and travel by a vascular route to the nasopharynx where they mature, thus showing some affinity with *Cephenemyia*. Some larvae appear to include the lungs in this migration.

Geographical distribution: Southern Africa

Pathogenesis: In the normal wildlife hosts, larvae appear to cause little pathological damage, although there are reports of loss of coordination. The infection becomes of veterinary importance when domestic ruminants are grazed close to, or among, the wild hosts. In sheep the larvae usually penetrate through the eye or enter via the nose. The larvae then migrate, and arresting eventually in the brain, ocular tissues, nasal cavities or heart. It is in the eye that the signs are most prominent, with glaucoma, extrusion and even rupture of the eyeball.

Clinical signs: In southern Africa this oestrid fly is responsible for an oculo-vascular myiasis, causing extrusion of the eyeball in sheep and, rarely, cattle.

Diagnosis: First-stage larvae may occasionally be observed on the cornea, but often a positive diagnosis can only be made at necropsy.

Pathology: In domestic hosts three main forms of infestation are distinguished: ophthalmic, encephalitic and cardiac, characterised by thrombo-endophlebitis and thrombo-encarditis with encephalomalacia, from vascular thrombosis. Myocardial, pulmonary and renal infarction may also occur.

Epidemiology: Flocks may have a 30% morbidity, of which a third will die, and in some areas sheep farming has had to be abandoned and replaced by cattle farming because of this parasite.

Treatment: Organophosphates such as trichlorphon are effective against the larvae, and flock treatment will reduce the blindness and mortality. Topical application of 0.25% cypermethrin spray to the eye has been used effectively to kill first-stage larvae.

Control: Domestic stock can safely graze with antelope during winter, when the flies are inactive (June–August). They should be removed from such areas in early spring when flies begin to emerge from puparia with the rising temperature.

Dictyocaulus filaria

Common name: Sheep lungworm

Predilection site: Lungs

Parasite class: Nematoda

Superfamily: Trichostrongyloidea

Description, gross: The worms are white with the intestine visible as a dark band. Males measure around 4–8 cm and the females 6–10 cm in length.

Description, microscopic: The L_1 resembles *D. vivivparus* but has a characteristic cuticular knob at the anterior extremity.

Hosts: Sheep, goat and a few wild ruminants

Life cycle: Similar to that of *D. viviparus* in cattle except that the prepatent period is about 4–5 weeks.

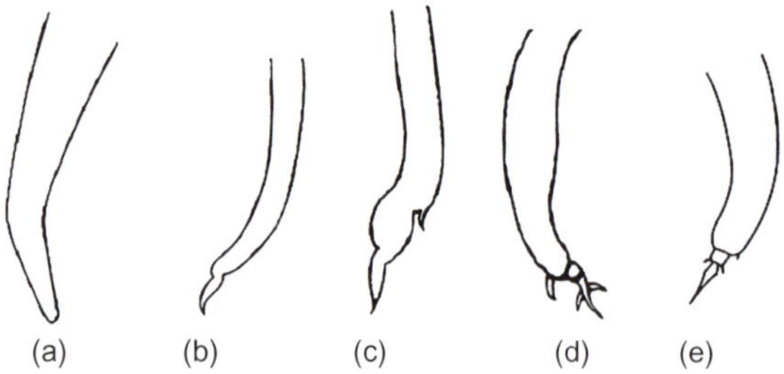

Fig. 3.23 Comparison of the posterior region of the first stage larvae of (a) *Dictyocaulus filaria*, (b) *Protostrongylus rufescens*, (c) *Muellerius capillaris*, (d) *Cystocaulus ocreatus* and (e) *Neostrongylus linearis*.

Eggs contain L_1 when passed from the female. Longevity is variable, and can be up to about 6–9 months.

Geographical distribution: Worldwide

Pathogenesis: Similar to that of *D. viviparus*, infection leading to a catarrhal bronchitis. However, since the number of lungworms in individual animals is generally low (Fig. 3.24), the widespread lesions associated with the bovine infection are not common.

Clinical signs: The most common signs are coughing and unthriftiness which, in endemic areas, is usually confined to young animals. In more severe cases, dyspnoea, tachypnoea and a tenacious nasal discharge are also present. These signs may be accompanied by diarrhoea or anaemia due to concurrent gastrointestinal trichostrongylosis or fasciolosis.

Diagnosis: This is based on history and clinical signs, but should be confirmed by examination of fresh faeces taken from a large proportion of the flock. The L_1 resembles that of *D. viviparus*, but has a characteristic cuticular knob at the anterior extremity and dark granulation of the intestinal cells. It is differentiated from other ovine lungworms by its larger size and blunt-ended tail (Fig. 3.23a).

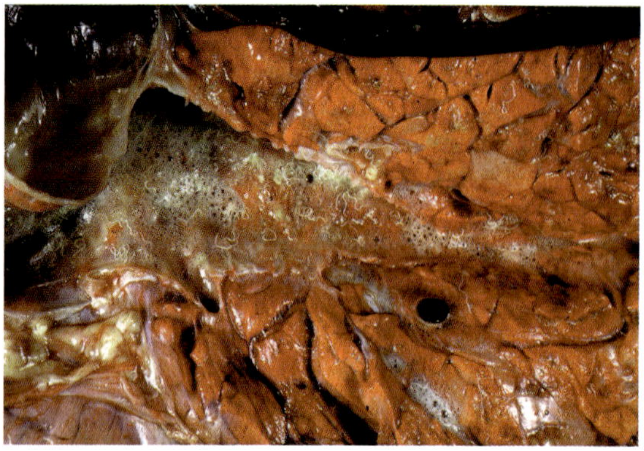

Fig. 3.24 *Dictyocaulus filaria* in the bronchus of an infected sheep.

Pathology: In severe cases, pulmonary oedema and emphysema may occur and the lung surface may be studded with purulent areas of secondary bacterial infection.

Epidemiology: Although this parasite is prevalent worldwide, it is only responsible for sporadic outbreaks of disease in temperate countries such as the UK and North America. It occurs more frequently as a clinical problem in eastern Europe and some Mediterranean countries, the Middle East and India.

In temperate areas the epidemiology is similar to that of *D.viviparus* in that both the survival of overwintered larvae on pasture and the role of the ewe and doe as a carrier are significant factors in the persistence of infection on pasture from year to year in endemic areas. In ewes it is likely that the parasites are present largely as hypobiotic larvae in the lungs during each winter and mature in the spring. Development to the L_3 only occurs during the period from spring to autumn. In lambs and kids, patent infections first occur in early summer, but the heaviest infections are usually seen in autumn. The prevalence of infection is lower in adult animals and their larval output smaller. Infective L_3 can migrate from the faeces without the need for fungal dispersion. It is likely that only two cycles of the parasite occur during each grazing season.

In warmer climates, where conditions are often unsuitable for larval survival, the carrier animal is probably a more important source of pasture contamination and outbreaks of disease in young susceptible animals are most likely to occur after a period of prolonged rain around weaning. Goats are often more susceptible to infection than sheep and can disseminate infection when both are grazed together.

Treatment: Where sporadic outbreaks occur, the affected animals, or preferably the whole flock, should be gathered, treated with a suitable anthelmintic (see *Dictyocaulus viviparus*) and then, if possible, moved to fresh pasture. The prophylactic regimens of control currently recommended for the control of gastrointestinal nematodes in sheep will, in normal years, be effective to a large extent in suppressing *D. filaria* infection.

Control: Where it is necessary to apply specific control measures, it is suggested that the flock should be annually treated with a suitable anthelmintic in late pregnancy. The ewes and lambs should then be grazed on pasture, which, in temperate areas at least, should not have been used by sheep during the previous year.

Notes: This species, the most important lungworm of sheep and goats, is commonly associated with a chronic syndrome of coughing and unthriftiness, which usually affects lambs and kids.

Protostrongylus rufescens

Common name: Red lungworm

Predilection site: Small bronchioles

Parasite class: Nematoda

Superfamily: Metastrongyloidea

Description, gross: Adult worms are slender, reddish worms (male up to 4.5 cm; female up to 6.5 cm).

Description, microscopic: In the male, the bursa is well developed but small. The dorsal ray is globular in shape with six papillae on the ventral side. The spicules are almost straight; the distal ends bear two membraneous alae. The gubernaculum has two boot-shaped prolongations bearing several knobs posteriorly. In the female, the vulva is close to the conoid tail. The first-stage larva has a wavy outline but is devoid of a dorsal spine (Fig. 3.23b).

Definitive hosts: Sheep, goat, deer and wild small ruminants

Intermediate hosts: Snails (*Helicella, Theba, Abida, Zebrina, Arianta*)

Life cycle: The worms are ovo-viviparous, the L_1 being passed in the faeces: these penetrate the foot of the molluscan intermediate host, and develop to L_3 in a minimum period of 2–3 weeks. The final host is infected by ingesting the mollusc. The L_3, freed by digestion, travel to the lungs by the lymphatic–vascular route, the parasitic moults occurring in the mesenteric lymph nodes and lungs. The prepatent period of *Protostrongylus* is 5–6 weeks. The period of patency is very long, exceeding 2 years.

Geographical distribution: Europe, Africa, Australia, North America

Pathogenesis: The worms live in the small bronchioles, where they produce an irritation and local areas of inflammation develop leading to a small foci of lobular pneumonia. The number of nodules on the lung surface may relate to the intensity of infection.

Clinical signs: Pneumonic signs have rarely been observed, and infections are almost always inapparent, being identified only at necropsy.

Diagnosis: The presence of infection is usually noted only during routine faecal examination. The L_1 are first differentiated from those of *Dictyocaulus filaria* by the absence of an anterior protoplasmic knob, and then on the individual characters of the larval tail (Fig. 3.23b).

Pathology: In *Protostrongylus* infection there is a somewhat larger area of lung involvement than with *Muellerius*, the occlusion of small bronchioles by worms, resulting in their lesser branches that occur toward the lung surface being filled with eggs, larvae and cellular debris. The affected alveolar and bronchial epithelium is desquamated, blood vessels are occluded and cellular infiltration and proliferation of connective tissue occurs. This results in a small area of lobular pneumonia and the grey–yellowish lesion has a roughly conical form, with the base on the surface of the lung.

Epidemiology: *Protostrongylus*, whose intermediate host range is restricted to certain species of snail, has a lower prevalence, though its geographic range is just as wide as *Muellerius*. Additional factors which play a part in ensuring the endemicity of these worms are, first, the ability of the L_1 to survive for months in faecal pellets and secondly, the persistence of the L_3 in the intermediate host for the lifetime of the mollusc. Also important in this respect are the long periods of patency and the apparent inability of the final host to develop acquired immunity, so that adult sheep have the heaviest infections and the highest prevalence.

Treatment: The modern benzimidazoles, levamisole and ivermectin have been shown to be effective. However, higher dose rates or repeated treatments may be necessary for high efficacy.

Control: Because of the ubiquity of the molluscan intermediate hosts, and the fact that the L_3 can survive as long as the molluscs, specific control is difficult, but fortunately rarely necessary. In some enterprises it may be practical to reduce snail numbers through the limeing of pastures.

Notes: These worms all inhabit the lungs, but none is a major pathogen and, though common, they are of little economic importance compared with the other helminth parasites of sheep and goats. Although there are several different genera they are sufficiently similar in behaviour to be considered together.

Table 3.4 Other Protostrongylid species.

Species	Distribution
Protostrongylus skrjabini	Eastern Europe and Russia
Protostrongylus stilesi	USA
Protostrongylus rushi	USA
Protostrongylus brevispiculum	USA
Protostrongylus davtiani	USA

Muellerius capillaris

Common name: Nodular lungworms

Predilection site: Lung

Parasite class: Nematoda

Superfamily: Metastrongyloidea

Description, gross: These are grey–reddish, slender hair-like worms about 1.0–3.0 cm long; although large, are often difficult to discern with the naked eye as they are embedded in lung tissue. Males are 12–24 mm and females 19–30 mm.

Description, microscopic: The posterior end of adult male *Muellerius* is spirally coiled and the bursa is very small and folded inwards. The spicules consist of a proximal, alate region and two distal serrated arms. Two sclerotised rods represent the gubernaculum. The first-stage larva has an S-shaped tail, and a small spine adjacent to the tip (Fig. 3.23c).

Definitive hosts: Sheep, goat, deer and wild small ruminants

Intermediate hosts: Snails (*Helix*, *Succinea*) and slugs (*Limax*, *Agriolimax*, *Arion*)

Life cycle: The life cycle is indirect. The worms are ovo-viviparous, the L_1 being passed in the faeces: these penetrate the foot of the molluscan intermediate host, and develop to L_3 in a minimum period of 2–3 weeks. The sheep or goat is infected by ingesting the mollusc. The L_3, freed by digestion, travel to the lungs by the lymphatic–vascular route, the parasitic moults occurring in the mesenteric lymph nodes and lungs. The prepatent period of *Muellerius* is 6–10 weeks. The period of patency is very long, exceeding 2 years.

Geographical distribution: Worldwide except for arctic and subarctic regions

Pathogenesis: Although there can be extensive emphysemic nodules, pneumonic signs have rarely been observed, and infections are usually inapparent, being identified only at necropsy. Sometimes mild infections are accompanied by sporadic coughing. Heavy infections may predispose the lungs to secondary bacterial infection. In goats, heavy infection with *M. capillaris* can induce coughing and dyspnoea and occasionally pneumonia.

Clinical signs: Generally asymptomatic but occasional coughing and dyspnoea in heavy infections

Diagnosis: The presence of infection is usually noted only during routine faecal examination. The L_1 are first differentiated from those of *Dictyocaulus filaria* by the absence of an anterior protoplasmic knob, and then on the individual characters of the larval tail. Frequently several species of small nodular lungworms may be present.

Pathology: *Muellerius* is frequently associated with small, spherical, nodular focal lesions, that occur most commonly near, or on, the lung surface, and on palpation have the feel and size of lead shot. Nodules containing single worms are almost imperceptible, and the visible ones enclose several of the tiny worms as well as eggs and larvae. Occasionally larger greyish nodules, up to 2 cm in diameter, are apparent and sometimes the nodules are calcified. The nodules consist of necrotic masses, resulting from the degeneration of accumulated leucocytes and pulmonary tissue, and they are surrounded by connective tissue and occasional giant cells. Adjoining pulmonary tissue may be hyperaemic and the alveoli become filled with cells and debris.

Epidemiology: *Muellerius* is by far the commonest genus of sheep lungworm, and in many temperate areas such as Britain, the eastern states of the USA and the winter rainfall regions of Australia, almost all sheep carry the infection; the extensive distribution and high prevalence are partly attributable to its wide range of intermediate hosts and the ability of larvae to overwinter in the molluscs. Prevalence of infection tends to increase with age. Additional factors which play a part in ensuring the endemicity of these worms are, first, the ability of the L_1 to survive for months in faecal pellets and secondly, the persistence of the L_3 in the intermediate host for the lifetime of the mollusc. Also important in this respect are the long periods of patency and the apparent inability of the final host to develop acquired immunity, so that adult sheep have the heaviest infections and the highest prevalence. Wild small ruminants are frequently heavily infected and could transmit protostrongylids to grazing sheep and goats under some management systems.

Treatment and control: As for *Protostrongylus rufescens*

The following metastrongylid worms all inhabit the lungs, but none is a major pathogen and, though common, they are of little economic importance compared with the other helminth parasites of sheep and goats. Although there are several different genera they are sufficiently similar in behaviour to be considered together.

Cystocaulus ocreatus

Common name: Small lungworm

Predilection site: Lung

Parasite class: Nematoda

Superfamily: Metastrongyloidea

Description, gross: Adult worms are slender, dark brown worms, up to 9 cm long (males up to 4–5 cm and females up to 9 cm long).

Description, microscopic: In the male, the bursa is small; the spicules consist of a proximal cylindrical region joined distinctly to a distal lance-shaped region. The gubernaculum has a complex structure, with the posterior part consisting of two pointed boot-shaped structures. In the female, the vulva is protected by a bell-shaped expansion of the cuticle. The first-stage larva has a kinked tail and dorsal and ventral spine (Fig. 3.23d).

Definitive hosts: Sheep, goat, deer and wild small ruminants

Intermediate hosts: Snails (*Helicella*, *Helix*, *Theba*, *Cepaea*, *Monacha*)

Life cycle: Similar to *Muellerius*. The prepatent period is 5–6 weeks.

Geographical distribution: Worldwide

Pathogenesis: The worms live in the small bronchioles, where they produce an irritation and local areas of inflammation develop leading to a small foci of lobular pneumonia; the number of nodules on the lung surface may relate to the intensity of infection.

Clinical signs: Pneumonic signs have rarely been observed, and infections are almost always inapparent, being identified only at necropsy.

Diagnosis: The presence of infection is usually noted only during routine faecal examination. The L_1 are first differentiated from those of *Dictyocaulus filaria* by the absence of an anterior protoplasmic knob, and then on the individual characters of the larval tail.

Pathology: In *Cystocaulus* infections, the occlusion of small bronchioles by worms results in their lesser branches that occur toward the lung surface being filled with eggs, larvae and cellular debris. The affected alveolar and bronchial epithelium is desquamated, blood vessels are occluded and cellular infiltration and proliferation of connective tissue occurs. This results in a small area of lobular pneumonia and the dark brown to black lesion has a roughly conical form, with the base on the surface of the lung.

Epidemiology: *Cystocaulus*, whose intermediate host range is restricted to certain species of snail, has a lower prevalence, though its geographic range is just as wide as *Muellerius*. Additional factors which play a part in ensuring the endemicity of these worms are, first, the ability of the L_1 to survive for months in faecal pellets and secondly, the persistence of the L_3 in the intermediate host for the lifetime of the mollusc. Also important in this respect are the long periods of patency and the apparent inability of the final host to develop acquired immunity, so that adult sheep have the heaviest infections and the highest prevalence.

Treatment and control: As for *Protostrongylus rufescens*

Notes: A second species, *C. nigrescens*, is found in eastern Russia and Europe.

The following species are also found in the lungs of sheep and goats. Details are essentially similar to preceeding metastrongylid worms.

Neostrongylus linearis

Common name: Small lungworm

Predilection site: Lung

Parasite class: Nematoda

Superfamily: Metastrongyloidea

Description, gross: Adult worms are slender, small worms (males 5–8 mm and females 13–15 mm long).

Description, microscopic: In the male, the spicules are unequal in size. The first-stage larva has a straight tail with a small dorsal and two small lateral spines (Fig. 3.23e).

Geographical distribution: Central Europe, Middle East

Treatment and control: As for *Protostrongylus rufescens*

Spiculocaulus austriacus

Common name: Small lungworm

Predilection site: Lung

Parasite class: Nematoda

Superfamily: Metastrongyloidea

Description, gross: Adult worms are slender, small worms.

Geographical distribution: Europe

Varestrongylus schulzi

Synonym: *Bicaulus schulzi*

Common name: Small lungworm

Predilection site: Lung

Parasite class: Nematoda

Superfamily: Metastrongyloidea

Description, gross: Adult worms are slender, small worms; males are 12–15 mm and females 22–25 mm.

Geographical distribution: Europe

Echinococcus granulosus

Subspecies: *granulosus*

Common name: Dwarf dog tapeworm, hydatidosis

Predilection site: Mainly liver and lungs (intermediate hosts); small intestine (definitive host)

Parasite class: Cestoda

Family: Taeniidae

Description, gross: 'Hydatid' cysts are large fluid-filled vesicles, 5–10 cm in diameter, with a thick concentrically laminated cuticle and an internal germinal layer.

Description, microscopic: The germinal layer produces numerous small vesicles or brood capsules each containing up to 40 scolices, invaginated into their neck portions and attached to the wall by stalks. Brood capsules may become detached from the wall of the vesicle and float freely in the vesicular fluid and form 'hydatid sand'.

Final hosts: Dog and many wild canids

Intermediate hosts: Domestic and wild ruminants, man and primates, pig and lagomorphs, horses and donkeys are resistant

Life cycle: The prepatent period in the final host is around 40–50 days, after which only one gravid segment is shed per week. The oncospheres are capable of prolonged survival outside the host, being viable on the ground for about 2 years. After ingestion by the intermediate host, the oncosphere penetrates the gut wall and travels in the blood to the liver, or in the lymph to the lungs. These are the two commonest sites for larval development, but occasionally oncospheres escape into the general systemic circulation and develop in other organs and tissues. Growth of the hydatid is slow, maturity being reached in 6–12 months. In the liver and lungs the cyst may have a diameter of up 20 cm, but in the rarer sites, such as the abdominal cavity, where unrestricted growth is possible, it may be very large, and contain several litres of fluid. The cyst capsule consists of an outer membrane and an inner germinal epithelium from which, when cyst growth is almost complete, brood capsules each containing a number of scolices are budded off. Many of these brood capsules become detached and exist free in the hydatid fluid; collectively these and the scolices are often referred to as 'hydatid sand'. Sometimes, complete daughter cysts are formed either inside the mother cyst or externally; in the latter case they may be carried to other parts of the body to form new hydatids.

Geographical distribution: Worldwide

Pathogenesis: In domestic animals the hydatid in the liver or lungs (Figs 3.25, 3.26) is usually tolerated without any clinical signs, and the majority of infections are only revealed at the abattoir. Where oncospheres have been carried in the circulation to other sites, such as the kidney, pancreas, central nervous system (CNS) or marrow cavity of long bones, pressure by the growing cyst may cause a variety of clinical signs.

In contrast, when man is involved as an intermediate host the hydatid in its pulmonary or hepatic site is often of pathogenic significance. One or both lungs may be affected causing respiratory symptoms, and if several hydatids are present in the liver there may be gross abdominal distension. If a cyst should rupture there is a risk of death from anaphylaxis or if the person survives, released daughter cysts may resume development in other regions of the body.

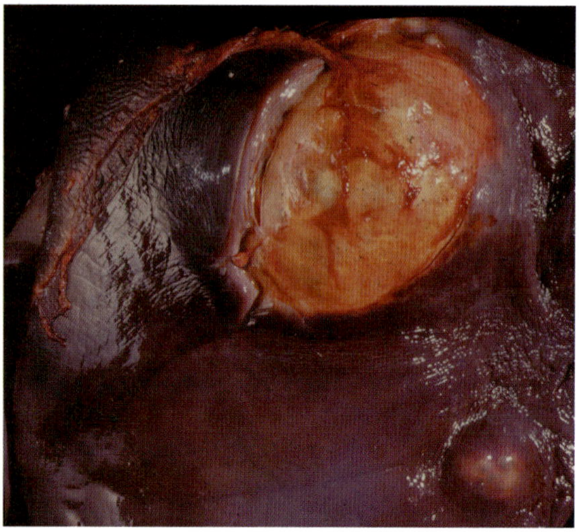

Fig. 3.25 Hydatid cysts of *Echinococcus granulosus* in the lung.

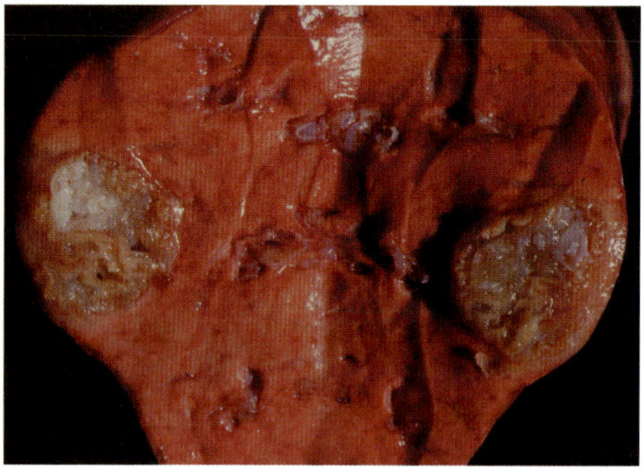

Fig. 3.26 Hydatid cyst of *Echinococcus granulosus* in the liver.

Clinical signs: Infection in cattle or sheep is generally not associated with clinical signs. Human infection can result in respiratory distress or abdominal enlargement depending on whether the lungs or liver are infected.

Diagnosis: The presence of hydatids as a clinical entity is rarely suspected in domestic animals, and specific diagnosis is never called for.

Pathology: In sheep, about 70% of hydatids occur in the lungs, about 25% in the liver, and the remainder in other organs.

Epidemiology: Only a few countries, notably Iceland and Eire, are free from this strain of *E. granulosus*. It is customary to consider the epidemiology as being based on two cycles, pastoral and sylvatic.

In the pastoral cycle the dog is always involved, being infected by the feeding of ruminant offal containing hydatid cysts. The domestic intermediate host will vary according to the local husbandry but the most important is the sheep, which appears to be the natural intermediate host, scolices from these animals being the most highly infective for dogs. In parts of the Middle East the camel is the main reservoir of hydatids, while in northern Europe and northern Russia it is the reindeer. The pastoral cycle is the primary source of hydatidosis in man, infection being by accidental ingestion of oncospheres from the coats of dogs, or from vegetables and other foodstuffs contaminated by dog faeces.

The sylvatic cycle occurs in wild canids and ruminants and is based on predation or carrion feeding. It is less important as a source of human infection, except in hunting communities where the infection may be introduced to domestic dogs by the feeding of viscera of wild ruminants.

Treatment: No treatment in sheep

Control: This is based on the regular treatment of dogs to eliminate the adult tapeworms and on the prevention of infection in dogs by exclusion from their diet of animal material containing hydatids. This is achieved by denying dogs access to abattoirs, and, where possible, by proper disposal of sheep carcases on farms. In some countries these measures have been supported by legislation, with penalties when they are disregarded. In countries where no specific measures for hydatid control exist, it has been found that an incidental benefit from the destruction of stray dogs for rabies control has been a great reduction in the incidence of hydatid infection in humans.

A recombinant DNA vaccine has been developed for *Echinococcus granulosus* but it requires further refinement for practical application and it is currently not available commercially.

Notes: Two biotypes have been described. The 'European' biotype is the most common and involves the dog and a wide variety of domestic livestock intermediate hosts. The dog–sheep cycle is infective to man. Less dominant is the 'northern' biotype that involves the wolf–reindeer or wolf–moose cycles and is not considered a danger to man.

There are two major strains of *E. granulosus* in domestic animals, namely *E. granulosus granulosus* and *E. granulosus equinus* (see Chapter 4: Horses).

PARASITES OF THE LIVER

Fasciola hepatica

Common name: Liver fluke

Predilection site: Liver

Parasite class: Trematoda

Superfamily: Fasciolidae

Description, gross: The young fluke at the time of entry into the liver is 1.0–2.0 mm in length and lancet-like. When it has become fully mature in the bile ducts it is leaf-shaped, grey-brown in colour and is around 2.5–3.5 cm in length and 1.0 cm in width. The anterior end is conical and marked off by distinct shoulders from the body.

Description, microscopic: The tegument is covered with backwardly projecting spines. An oral and ventral sucker may be readily seen. The egg is thin shelled oval, operculate, browny-yellow and large (130–150 × 65–90 μm), and about twice the size of a trichostrongyle egg.

Definitive hosts: Sheep, cattle, goat, horse, deer, man and other mammals

Intermediate hosts: Snails of the genus *Lymnaea*. The most common, *L. truncatula* (syn *Galba*) is an amphibious snail with a wide distribution throughout the world. Other important *Lymnaea* vectors of *F. hepatica* outside Europe are:

L. tomentosa	Australia, New Zealand
L. columella	Central and North America, Australia, New Zealand
L. bulimoides	North and Southern USA and the Caribbean
L. humilis	North America
L. viator	South America
L. diaphena	South America
L. cubensis	South America
L. viridis	China, Papua New Guinea

Life cycle: Adult flukes in the bile ducts shed eggs into the bile, which enter the intestine. Eggs passed in the faeces of the mammalian host develop and hatch, releasing motile ciliated miracidia. This takes 9–10 days at optimal temperatures of 22–26°C and

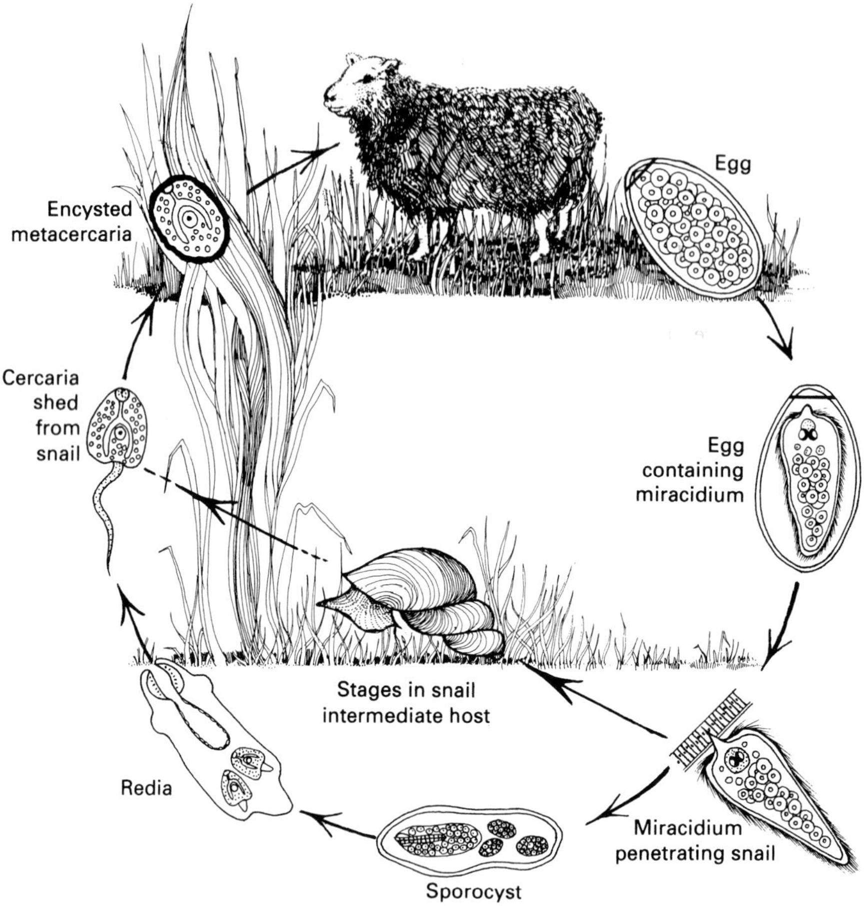

Fig. 3.27 Life cycle of *Fasciola hepatica.*

little development occurs below 10°C. The liberated miracidium has a short lifespan and must locate a suitable snail within about 3 hours if successful penetration of the latter is to occur. In infected snails, development proceeds through the sporocyst and redial stages to the final stage in the intermediate host, the cercaria; these are shed from the snail as motile forms, which attach themselves to firm surfaces, such as grass blades, and encyst there to form the infective metacercariae. It takes a minimum of 6–7 weeks for completion of development from miracidium to metacercaria, although under unfavourable circumstances a period of several months is required. Infection of a snail with one miracidium can produce over 600 metacercariae. Metacercariae ingested by the final host excyst in the small intestine, migrate through the gut wall, cross the peritoneum and penetrate the liver capsule. The young flukes tunnel through the liver parenchyma for 6–8 weeks, then enter the small bile ducts where they migrate to the larger ducts and occasionally the gall bladder and reach sexual maturity. The prepatent period is 10–12 weeks. The minimal period for completion of one entire life cycle of *F. hepatica* is therefore 17–18 weeks (Fig. 3.27). The longevity of *F. hepatica* in untreated sheep may be years; in cattle it is usually less than 1 year.

Geographical distribution: Worldwide

Pathogenesis: This varies according to the number of metacercariae ingested, the phase of parasitic development in the liver and the species of host involved. Essentially the pathogenesis is two-fold. The first phase occurs during migration in the liver parenchyma and is associated with liver damage and haemorrhage. The second occurs when the parasite is in the bile ducts, and results from the haematophagic activity of the adult flukes and from damage to the biliary mucosa by their cuticular spines. Most studies have been in sheep and the disease in this host is discussed in detail. The seasonality of outbreaks is that which occurs in western Europe.

Fasciolosis in sheep may be **acute**, **sub-acute** or **chronic**.

The **acute** disease is the less common type of fasciolosis and occurs 2–6 weeks after the ingestion of large numbers of metacercariae, usually over 2000, and is due to extensive destruction of the liver parenchyma and the severe haemorrhage which results when the young flukes, simultaneously migrating in the liver parenchyma, rupture blood vessels. Damage to the liver parenchyma is also severe. Outbreaks of acute fasciolosis are generally presented as sudden deaths during autumn and early winter. On examination of the remainder of the flock, affected animals are weak, with pale mucous membranes and dyspnoea; in some instances they have palpably enlarged livers associated with abdominal pain and ascites. Sometimes these outbreaks are complicated by concurrent infections with *Clostridium novyi* resulting in clostridial necrotic hepatitis 'black disease', although this is less common nowadays because of widespread vaccination against clostridial diseases.

In the **subacute** disease, metacercariae are ingested over a longer period and while some have reached the bile ducts, where they cause a cholangitis, others are still migrating through the liver parenchyma causing lesions less severe, but similar, to those of the acute disease; thus the liver is enlarged with numerous necrotic or haemorrhagic tracts visible on the surface and in the substance. Subcapsular haemorrhages are usually evident, but rupture of these is rare.

This form of the disease, occurring 6–10 weeks after ingestion of approximately 500–1500 metacercariae, also appears in the late autumn and winter. It is presented as a rapid and severe haemorrhagic anaemia with hypoalbuminaemia, and, if untreated, can result in a high mortality rate. However it is not so rapidly fatal as the acute condition and affected sheep may show clinical signs for 1–2 weeks prior to death; these include a rapid loss of condition, reduced appetite, a marked pallor of the mucous membranes, and an enlarged and palpable liver. Submandibular or facial oedema and ascites may be present.

Chronic fasciolosis, which is seen mainly in late winter/early spring, is the most common form of the disease. It occurs 4–5 months after the ingestion of moderate numbers, 200–500, of metacercariae. The principal pathogenic effects are anaemia and hypoalbuminaemia and more than 0.5 ml blood per fluke can be lost into the bile ducts each day. Additional loss of plasma proteins occurs by leakage through the hyperplastic biliary mucosa and the pathogenic effect is exacerbated if the sheep is on a low plane of nutrition. Clinically, chronic fasciolosis is characterised by a progressive loss of condition, lowered appetite and the development of anaemia and hypoalbuminaemia, which can result in emaciation, an open brittle fleece, pallor of the mucous membranes, submandibular oedema ('bottle-jaw') and ascites. The anaemia is hypochromic and macrocytic with an accompanying eosinophilia. *Fasciola* eggs can be demonstrated in the faeces. In light infections, the clinical effect may not be readily discernible, but the parasites can have a significant effect on production due to an impairment of appetite and to their effect on post-absorptive metabolism of protein, carbohydrates and minerals. There is no evidence for any significant age immunity or acquired resistance to *F. hepatica* infection in sheep.

Clinical signs: Outbreaks of acute fasciolosis in sheep are generally presented as sudden deaths during autumn and early winter. On examination of the remainder of the flock, affected animals are weak, with pale mucous membranes and dyspnoea; in some instances they will have palpably enlarged livers associated with abdominal pain and ascites. Clinically, chronic fasciolosis is characterised by a progressive loss of condition, lowered appetite and the development of anaemia and hypoalbuminaemia which can result in emaciation, an open brittle fleece, pallor of the mucous membranes, submandibular oedema ('bottle-jaw') and ascites. The anaemia is hypochromic and macrocytic with an accompanying eosinophilia. *Fasciola* eggs can be demonstrated in the faeces. In light infections, the clinical effect may not be readily discernible, but the parasites can have a significant effect on production due to an impairment of appetite and to their effect on post-absorptive metabolism of protein, carbohydrates and minerals.

Diagnosis: This is based primarily on clinical signs, seasonal occurrence, prevailing weather patterns, and a previous history of fasciolosis on the farm or the identification of snail habitats. Diagnosis of ovine fasciolosis should present few problems, especially when a postmortem examination is possible. Routine haematological tests and examination of faeces for fluke eggs (note: eggs of *Fasciola* are brown–yellow and eggs of Paramphistomidae are colourless) are useful and may be supplemented by two other laboratory tests.

The first is the estimation of plasma levels of enzymes released by damaged liver cells. Two enzymes are usually measured. Glutamate dehydrogenase (GLDH) is released when parenchymal cells are damaged and levels become elevated within the first few weeks of infection. The other, gamma glutamyl transpeptidase (GGT) indicates damage to the epithelial cells lining the bile ducts; elevation of this enzyme takes place mainly after the flukes reach the bile ducts and raised levels are maintained for a longer period. The second

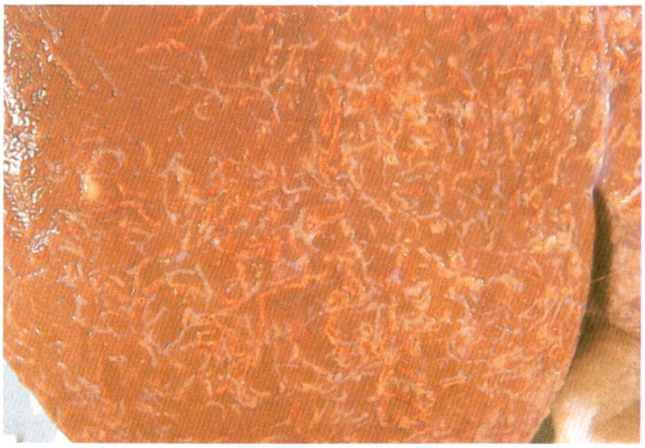

Fig. 3.28 Liver lesions associated with acute ovine fasciolosis.

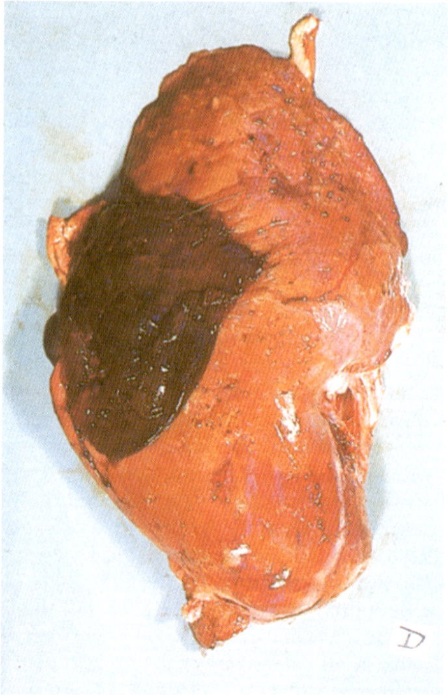

Fig. 3.29 Massive subcapsular haemorrhage frequently seen in acute ovine fasciolosis.

is the detection of antibodies against components of flukes in serum or milk samples, the ELISA and the passive haemagglutination test being the most reliable.

Pathology: In **acute** fluke disease in sheep, at necropsy, the liver is enlarged, friable, haemorrhagic and honeycombed with the tracts of migrating flukes (Fig. 3.28). The surface, particularly over the ventral lobe, is frequently covered with a fibrinous exudate. Subcapsular haemorrhages are common and these may rupture so that a quantity of blood-stained fluid is often present in the abdominal cavity (Fig. 3.29). In the **subacute** form, the liver is enlarged with numerous necrotic or haemorrhagic tracts visible on the surface and in the substance. Subcapsular haemorrhages are usually evident, but rupture of these is rare. In the **chronic** form, the liver has an irregular outline and is pale and firm, the ventral lobe being most affected and reduced in size. The liver pathology is characterised by hepatic fibrosis and hyperplastic cholangitis. Several different types of fibrosis are present. The first to occur is post-necrotic scarring found mainly in the ventral lobe and associated with the healing of fluke tracts. The second, often termed ischaemic fibrosis, is a sequel of infarction caused by damage and thrombosis of large vessels. Thirdly, a peribiliary fibrosis develops when the flukes reach the small bile ducts. Sometimes fluke eggs provoke a granuloma-like reaction, which can result in obliteration of the affected bile ducts. The hyperplastic cholangitis in the larger bile ducts arises from the severe erosion and necrosis of the mucosa caused by the feeding mature flukes.

Epidemiology: There are three main factors influencing the production of the large numbers of metacercariae necessary for outbreaks of fasciolosis.

1. Availability of suitable snail habitats: *L. truncatula* prefers wet mud to free water, and permanent habitats include the banks of ditches or streams and the edges of small ponds. Following heavy rainfall or flooding, temporary habitats may be provided by hoof marks, wheel ruts or rain ponds. Fields with clumps of rushes are often suspect sites. Though a slightly acid pH environment is optimal for *L. truncatula*, excessively acid pH levels are detrimental, such as occur in peat bogs, and areas of sphagnum moss.
2. Temperature: A mean day/night temperature of 10°C or above is necessary both for snails to breed and for the development of *F. hepatica* within the snail, and all activity ceases at 5°C. This is also the minimum range for the development and hatching of *F. hepatica* eggs. However, it is only when temperatures rise to 15°C and are maintained above that level, that a significant multiplication of snails and fluke larval stages ensues.
3. Moisture: The ideal moisture conditions for snail breeding and the development of *F. hepatica* within snails are provided when rainfall exceeds transpiration, and field saturation is attained. Such conditions are also essential for the development of fluke eggs, for miracidia searching for snails and for the dispersal of cercariae being shed from the snails.

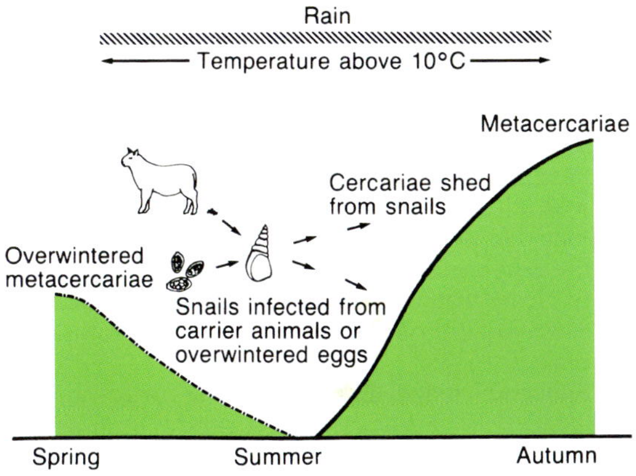

Fig. 3.30 Summer infection of snails.

In temperate countries such as Britain, these factors usually only exist from May to October. A marked increase in numbers of metacercariae on pasture is therefore possible during two periods. First, from what is known as the summer infection of snails, in which metacercariae appear on pasture from August to October (Fig. 3.30). These snail infections arise from miracidia, which have hatched either from eggs excreted in the spring/early summer by infected animals, or from eggs, which have survived the winter in an undeveloped state. Development in the snail occurs during the summer and the cercariae are shed from August until October. Secondly, from the winter infection of snails in which metacercariae appear on the pasture in May to June (Fig. 3.31). These are derived from snails which were infected the previous autumn, and in which larval development had temporarily ceased during the period of winter hibernation of the snail host and had recommenced in the spring. Both *F. hepatica* eggs and metacercariae can

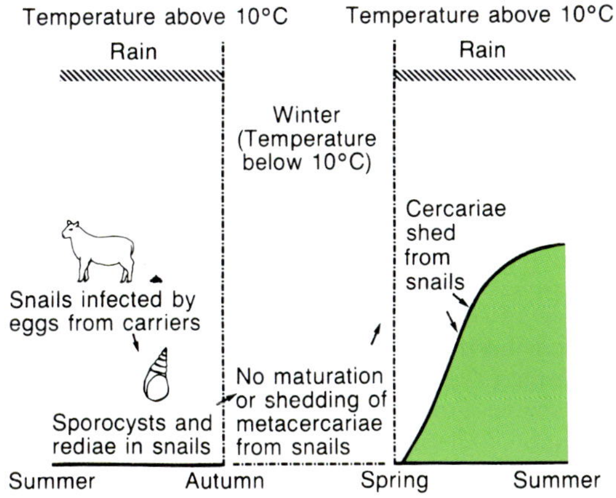

Fig. 3.31 Winter infection of snails.

survive over the winter and play important roles in the epidemiology. The eggs, by hatching into miracidia in late spring, can infect snails. The metacercariae, by infecting stock in early spring, result in eggs being available by mid-summer at the optimal snail breeding season. However, survival of metacercariae is poor under conditions of high temperatures and drought and they rapidly lose their infectivity during processes such as silage making, although they may survive for several months on hay.

In most European countries, the summer infection of snails is the more important and an increase in the numbers of metacercariae occurs annually from August to October. The extent of this increase is highest in years when summer rainfall is heavy. The winter infection of snails is much less important, but occasionally gives rise to large numbers of metacercariae in late spring and early summer, particularly when the preceding months have been unduly wet.

Circulating antibodies to *F. hepatica* are readily detectable in sheep, but there is no evidence that, under field conditions, sheep ever become immune to reinfection with *F. hepatica*, and in the absence of treatment, the flukes will live as long as the sheep. Severe outbreaks of ovine fasciolosis frequently involve adult sheep which have been previously exposed to infection. In contrast, although outbreaks do occur in young cattle, more usually an acquired immunity gradually develops; this limits the lifespan of the primary infection, slows the migration of secondary infection and eventually reduces the numbers of flukes established. Thus, in endemic areas, adult cattle often appear unaffected clinically whereas severe losses from fasciolosis may be occurring in adult sheep. Finally it should be remembered that *F. hepatica* can infect a wide range of mammals, including horses, donkeys, deer, pigs and rabbits, and it is possible that on occasions these hosts may act as reservoirs of infection. Man may also become infected, especially from the consumption of watercress from unfenced beds.

Most of the above comments on the ecology of *L. truncatula* also apply to the other amphibian species of *Lymnaea*, which transmit the parasite. Differentiation of *Lymnaea* species is a specialist task and is usually based on morphological characteristics, although biochemical and immunological methods are now also employed. Note also that taxonomic revisions have resulted in re-classification of many of these species.

In warmer areas, such as the southern USA or Australia, the sequence of events has a different seasonality, but the epidemiological principles are the same. For example, in both Texas and Louisiana snail activity is maximal during the cooler months of autumn with peak numbers of metacercariae appearing in the winter.

The situation differs with *L. tomentosa*, which, although classed as an amphibian snail, is well adapted to aquatic life in swampy areas or irrigation channels, and therefore temperature is the most important controlling biological factor. Thus, in most of eastern Australia, *L. tomentosa* continues to produce egg masses throughout the year, although the rate of reproduction is controlled by temperature and is at its lowest during the winter. The lower winter temperatures also delay hatching of fluke eggs and larval development in the snail so that large numbers of metacercariae first appear in late spring. During the summer and autumn there is a second wave of metacercarial production derived from new generations of snails. *L. tormentosa* can extend its range by floating/drifting on water currents.

There is some evidence that the prevalence of fasciolosis in hot countries is higher after several months of drought, possibly because the animals congregate around areas of water conservation and so the chances of snails becoming infected are increased.

Ecology of *Lymnaea* species in temperate climates

Since *L. truncatula* is the most widespread and important species involved in the transmission of *F. hepatica*, it is discussed in detail. *L. truncatula* is a small snail, the adults being about 1.0 cm in length. The shell is usually dark brown and has a turreted appearance, being coiled in a series of spiral whorls. When held with the turret upright and the aperture facing the observer, the latter is approximately half the length of the snail and is on the right-hand side, and there are 4.5 whorls. The snails are amphibious and although they spend hours in shallow water, they periodically emerge on to surrounding mud. They commonly inhabit drainage ditches and poorly drained land. They are capable of withstanding summer drought or winter freezing for several months by respectively aestivating or hibernating deep in the mud. Optimal conditions include a slightly acid pH environment and a slowly moving water medium to carry away waste products. They feed mostly on algae and the optimum temperature range for development is 15–22°C; below 5°C development ceases. In Britain for example, snails breed continuously from May to October, one snail being capable of producing up to 100 000 descendants over 3 months.

Treatment: The older drugs, such as carbon tetrachloride, hexachlorethane and hexachlorophene, may still be used in some countries, but these have been largely replaced by more efficient and less toxic compounds and only the latter will be discussed.

- **Acute ovine fasciolosis.** Until recently, treatment was not highly successful due to the inefficiency of the older drugs against the early parenchymal stages. However, efficient drugs are now available and the one of choice is triclabendazole, which removes all developing stages over 1 week old. Other drugs are closantel and nitroxynil, which will remove flukes over 4 weeks old. A single dose of triclabendazole accompanied with a move to fluke-free pasture or a well drained, recently cultivated field should be adequate treatment. However with closantel or nitroxynil a second treatment may be necessary 2–3 weeks after moving to fluke-free ground. Where sheep cannot be moved to clean ground, treatment should be repeated at 3-weekly intervals until 6 weeks after deaths have ceased.
- **Subacute ovine fasciolosis.** The drugs recommended for acute fasciolosis can be used against older flukes responsible for subacute fasciolosis. Movement to fluke-free pasture is again advisable following treatment, and where this is not possible treatment should be repeated at 4 and 8 weeks to eliminate maturing flukes. In addition to the above drugs, brotianide (available in some countries) is also effective.
- **Chronic ovine fasciolosis.** Outbreaks of chronic fasciolosis can be successfully treated with a single dose of any of a range of drugs (nitroxynil, brotianide, closantel, oxyclozanide and triclabendazole) and following treatment, the anaemia usually regresses within 2–3 weeks. The roundworm anthelmintics, albendazole, ricobendazole and netobimin are also effective against adult flukes albeit at increased dosage rates.

Frequent treatment with flukicides which belong to the same chemical group, or with the same anthelmintic season after season, could enhance the possibility of development of drug-resistant flukes. It is advisable to plan a control strategy which incorporates a change of flukicides from year to year, although the spectrum of activity of the drugs also needs to be considered.

Control: Control of fasciolosis may be approached in two ways: by reducing populations of the intermediate snail host or by using anthelmintics.

1. **Reduction of snail populations.** Before any scheme of snail control is undertaken a survey of the area for snail habitats should be made to determine whether these are localised or widespread. The best long-term method of reducing mud-snail populations such as *L. truncatula* is drainage, since it ensures permanent destruction of snail habitats. However, farmers are often hesitant to undertake expensive drainage schemes, although in some countries special drainage grants are available. When the snail habitat is limited a simple method of control is to fence off this area or treat annually with a molluscicide. Copper sulphate is the most widely used; although more efficient molluscicides, such

as N-trityl morpholine, have been developed, none are generally available. In Europe, experimental evidence indicates that a molluscicide should be applied either in the spring (May), to kill snail populations prior to the commencement of breeding, or in summer (July/August) to kill infected snails. The spring application should ensure better contact with the snails, because pasture growth is limited, but in practice is often impractical because the saturated nature of the habitat makes vehicular access difficult. In the summer this is less of a problem although molluscicide/snail contact may be reduced because of the increase in herbage growth. The application of a molluscicide should be combined with anthelmintic treatment to remove existing fluke populations and thus the contamination of habitats with eggs. When the intermediate snail host is aquatic, such as *L. tomentosa*, good control is possible by adding a molluscicide, such as N-trityl morpholine or niclosamide, to the water habitat of the snail, but there are many environmental objections to the use of molluscicides in water or irrigation channels and rapid recolonisation of snail habitats can occur.

2. **Use of anthelmintics.** The prophylactic use of fluke anthelmintics is aimed at:

   - Reducing pasture contamination by fluke eggs at a time most suitable for their development, i.e. April to August.
   - Removing fluke populations at a time of heavy burdens or at a period of nutritional and pregnancy stress to the animal. To achieve these objectives, the following control programme for sheep in the British Isles is recommended for years with normal or below average rainfall. Since the timing of treatments is based on the fact that most metacercariae appear in autumn and early winter, it may require modification for use in other areas.

     i. In late April/early May treat all adult sheep with a drug effective against adult stages. At this time, products containing both a fasciolicide and a drug effective against nematodes which contribute to the periparturient rise (PPR) in faecal egg counts in ewes may be used.
     ii. In October, treat the entire flock using a drug effective against parenchymal stages, such as triclabendazole or closantel.
     iii. In January, treat the flock with any drug effective against immature and adult stages.
     iv. In wet years further doses may be nesessary. In June, 4–6 weeks after the April/May dose, all adult sheep should be treated with a drug effective against adult and late immature flukes. In October/November, 4 weeks after the early October dose, treat all sheep with a drug effective against parenchymal stages.
     v. The precise timing of the spring and autumn treatments will depend on lambing and service dates.

3. **Meteorological forecasting of fasciolosis.** The life cycle of the liver fluke and the prevalence of fasciolosis are dependent on climate. This has led to the development of forecasting systems, based on meteorological data, which estimate the likely timing and severity of the disease. In several western European countries, these forecasts are used as the basis for annual control programmes. Two different formulae have been developed:

   i. Estimatation of 'ground surface wetness', which is the critical factor affecting the summer infection of snails. The formula is $M = n(R - P + 5)$ where M is the month, R is the monthly rainfall in inches, P is the evapotranspiration in inches and n is the number of wet days per month. A value of 100 or more per month is optimal for parasite development and therefore values of more than 100 are registered as 100. The formula is applied over the months when temperatures are suitable for snail breeding and parasite development, i.e. May–October in Europe, and the monthly values summated to give a seasonal index or *Mt* value. Since the temperatures are generally lower in May and October, the values for these months are halved prior to summation. Where the *Mt* exceeds 450, the prevalence of fasciolosis is likely to be high. The forecast is used to issue an early warning of disease by calculating data from May to August so that control measures can be introduced prior to shedding of cercariae. The disadvantage of the forecast is that it may overestimate the prevalence where there is an autumn drought or underestimate the likely prevalence where the presence of drainage ditches allows the parasite life cycle to be maintained in dry summers. Although this technique is mainly applied to the summer infection of snails, it is also used for forecasting the winter infection of snails by summating the values for August, September and October; if these exceed 250 and the following May or June has a high rainfall then fasciolosis is forecast for the area.

ii. 'Wet day' forecast. This compares the prevalence of fasciolosis over a number of years with the number of rain-days during the summers of these years. In essence, widespread fasciolosis is associated with 12 wet days (over 1.0 mm of rainfall) per month from June to September where temperatures do not fall below the seasonal normal. Computer-based forecast systems have also been developed.

Fasciola gigantica

Common name: Tropical large liver fluke

Predilection site: Liver

Parasite class: Trematoda

Family: Fasciolidae

Final hosts: Cattle, buffalo, sheep, goat, pig, camel, deer, man

Intermediate hosts: Snails of the genus *Lymnaea*

Geographical distribution: Africa, Asia

Pathology: In acute infections in sheep, the liver is enlarged, friable, haemorrhagic and honeycombed with the tracts of migrating flukes. In the chronic form, the liver has an irregular outline and is pale and firm, the ventral lobe being most affected and reduced in size. The liver pathology is characterised by hepatic fibrosis and hyperplastic cholangitis. The hyperplastic cholangitis in the larger bile ducts arises from the severe erosion and necrosis of the mucosa caused by the feeding mature flukes.

Treatment: For acute fluke infections in sheep, the drug of choice is triclabendazole. Other drugs include closantel and nitroxynil, which will remove flukes over 4 weeks old. Outbreaks of chronic fasciolosis can be successfully treated with a single dose of any of a range of drugs (nitroxynil, brotianide, closantel, oxyclozanide and triclabendazole).

For more details see Chapter 2 (Cattle).

Fascioloides magna

Common name: Large American liver fluke

Predilection site: Liver and bile ducts

Parasite class: Trematoda

Family: Fasciolidae

Final hosts: Deer, cattle, sheep, goat, pig, horse

Intermediate hosts: A variety of freshwater snails, *Fossaria* species, *Lymnaea* species, *Stagnicola* species

Geographical distribution: Mainly occurs in North America, central, eastern and southwest Europe, South Africa and Mexico.

Pathogenesis: In contrast to the situation in deer and cattle, in sheep and goats the host response is negligible and the continual migration of the flukes through the liver parenchyma leads to haemorrhage, hepatitis and fibrosis. Occasionally flukes may be found in the lungs and in the peritoneal cavity. Infection can be fatal in sheep and goats.

Clinical signs: Infection in sheep and goats may cause sudden death.

Diagnosis: This is based primarily on clinical signs, and history of contact with grazing deer in known endemic areas. The presence of cysts and the large flukes are usually seen on postmortem examination. Faecal examination for the presence of fluke eggs is a useful aid to diagnosis.

Pathology: In sheep and goats the presence of migratory flukes in the liver parenchyma leads to haemorrhage, hepatitis and fibrosis. Occasionally flukes may be found in the lungs and in the peritoneal cavity.

Epidemiology: The various snail intermediate hosts tend to occur in stagnant semi-permanent water that contains large amounts of dead or dying vegetation, swamp areas, or pools and streams. *F. magna* is indigenous to North America and is common in Canada and the Great Lake areas where the white-tailed deer and the elk are commonly infected. Domestic cattle and sheep become infected when they graze pasture where parasitised deer occur.

Treatment: For cattle and sheep the commonly used flukicides, such as triclabendazole, closantel, clorsulon and albendazole, are effective. Mature *F. magna* are susceptible to oxyclosanide.

Control: Avoid grazing sheep or cattle on areas which are frequented by deer. Elimination of the snail intermediate hosts is difficult due to their varied habitats. Similarly removal of Cervidae may not be practical. Because of these factors sheep rearing, particularly, is difficult in areas where the parasite is prevalent.

Notes: *F. magna* is primarily a parasite of deer (Cervidae) and is commonly found in white-tailed deer, elk and moose.

For more details see Chapter 8 (Ungulates (deer)).

Dicrocoelium dendriticum

Synonym: *Dicrocoelium lanceolatum*

Common name: Small lanceolate fluke

Predilection site: Liver

Parasite class: Trematoda

Family: Dicrocoeliidae

Description, gross: There is no possibility of confusion with other flukes in the bile ducts of ruminants as *Dicrocoelium* is 6 mm–1.0 cm long and 1.5–2.5 mm wide, distinctly lanceolate and semitransparent. The oral sucker is smaller than the ventral.

Description, microscopic: The gut is simple, consisting of two branches and resembles a tuning fork. Behind the ventral sucker the testes lie in tandem with the ovary immediately posterior. There are no spines on the cuticle (c.f. *Fasciola*). The egg is small, 35–40 μm in length by 29–30 μm in width, dark brown and operculate, usually with a flattened side. It contains a miracidium when passed in the faeces.

Final hosts: Sheep, goats, cattle, deer and rabbits, occasionally horse and pig

Intermediate hosts: Two are required:

1. Land snails of many genera, principally *Cionella lubrica* in N. America and *Zebrina detrita* in Europe. Some 29 other species have been reported to serve as first intermediate hosts, including the genera *Abida*, *Theba*, *Helicella* and *Xerophila*.
2. Brown ants of the genus *Formica*, frequently *F. fusca*

Life cycle: The egg does not hatch until ingested by the first intermediate host, a terrestrial snail, in which two generations of sporocysts develop which then produce cercariae. The latter are extruded in masses cemented together by slime and adhere to vegetation. This phase of development takes at least 3 months. The slime balls of cercariae are ingested by ants in which they develop to metacercariae mainly in the body cavity and occasionally the brain. The presence of a brain lesion in the ant, induced by metacercariae, impels the ant to climb up and remain on the tips of the herbage, thus increasing the chance of ingestion by the final host. This phase in the ant is completed in just over 1 month in summer temperatures. Infection of the final host is by passive ingestion of ants containing metacercariae. The metacercariae hatch in the small intestine and the young flukes migrate up the main bile duct and thence to the smaller ducts in the liver. There is no parenchymal migration and the prepatent period is 10–12 weeks. The total life cycle takes approximately 6 months. The flukes are long-lived and can survive in the final host for several years.

Geographical distribution: Worldwide except for South Africa and Australia. In Europe the prevalence is high but in the British Isles prevalence is low, being confined to small foci throughout the country.

Pathogenesis: Although several thousand *D. dendriticum* are commonly found in the bile ducts, the livers are relatively normal; this is presumably due to the absence of a migratory phase. However, in heavier infections there is fibrosis of the smaller bile ducts and extensive cirrhosis can occur and sometimes the bile ducts become markedly distended. Condemnation of livers at slaughter may cause severe economic losses among cattle herds and sheep flocks.

Clinical signs: In many instances these are absent. Anaemia, oedema, emaciation and reduced wool growth have been reported in severe cases.

Diagnosis: This is entirely based on faecal examination for eggs and necropsy examination of the bile ducts for the presence of flukes.

Pathology: Infected livers are relatively normal; this is presumably due to the absence of a migratory phase. However, in heavier infections there is fibrosis of the smaller bile ducts and extensive cirrhosis can occur and sometimes the bile ducts become markedly distended (Fig. 3.32).

Epidemiology: There are two important features that differentiate the epidemiology of *Dicrocoelium* from that of *Fasciola*:

1. The intermediate hosts are independent of water and are evenly distributed on the terrain.

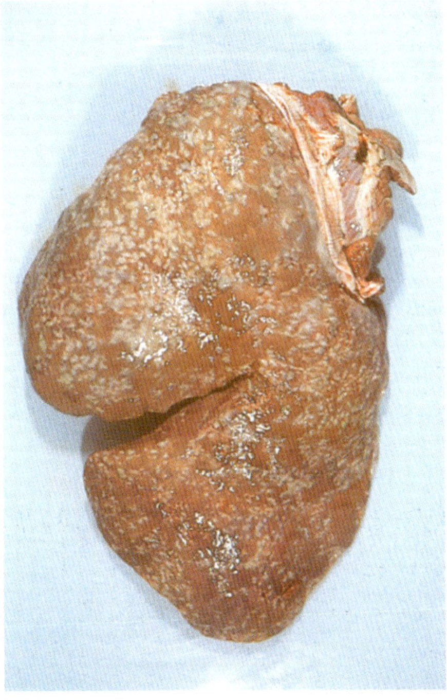

Fig. 3.32 Liver lesions caused by severe *Dicrocoelium dendriticum*.

2. The egg can survive for months on dry pasture, presenting a reservoir additional to that in the intermediate and final hosts.

Treatment: Many flukicides show no activity against *D. dendriticum* when administered at the recommended fluke dose rates. Netobimin has been shown to be highly effective at a dose rate of 20 mg/kg. Albendazole, given at 20 mg/kg, is very effective, as is praziquantel at 50 mg/kg. Other drugs such fenbendazole are also effective, but at very high dose rates (50 mg/kg).

Control: This is difficult because of the longevity of *D. dendriticum* eggs, the wide distribution of the intermediate hosts and the number of reservoir hosts. Control depends almost entirely on regular anthelmintic treatment.

Dicrocoelium hospes

Predilection site: Liver

Parasite class: Trematoda

Family: Dicrocoeliidae

Hosts: Cattle

Geographical distribution: Parts of Africa
Details are essentially similar to *D. dendriticum*

Stilesia hepatica

Predilection site: Bile ducts

Parasite class: Cestoda

Family: Thysanosomidae

Description, gross: The adult tapeworm measures around 0.5 metres in length by 2 mm in width. The neck is broad and the scolex has prominent suckers. The genital organs are single and the opening pores alternate irregularly. The eggs lack a pyriform apparatus.

Final hosts: Sheep and other ruminants

Intermediate hosts: The intermediate host is probably an oribatid mite.

Life cycle: The life cycle is not known but probably involves orabatid mites.

Geographical distribution: Africa and Asia

Clinical signs: Infection is usually asymptomatic.

Diagnosis: Identification of eggs or proglottids in the faeces

Pathogenesis: Generally considered to be of low pathogenicity.

Pathology: No significant lesions are induced despite large numbers of parasites almost occluding the bile ducts.

Epidemiology: *S. hepatica* is very common in sheep and other ruminants.

Treatment and control: Treatment is rarely called for, but praziquantel has proved effective.

Notes: Large numbers of these tapeworms are often found in the bile ducts of sheep at slaughter and although they cause neither clinical signs nor significant hepatic pathology, the liver condemnations are a source of considerable economic loss, on aesthetic grounds.

Thysanosoma actinioides

See under Parasites of the small intestine.

Taenia hydatigena (metacestode)

Synonym: *Taenia marginata*, *Cysticercus tenuicollis*

Predilection site: Abdominal cavity, liver (intermediate hosts); small intestine (definitive hosts)

Parasite class: Cestoda

Family: Taeniidae

Description, gross: The mature metacestode (cysticercus tenuicollis) is about 5–8 cm in diameter and contains a single invaginated scolex (bladderworm) with a long neck.

Final hosts: Dog, fox, weasel, stoat, polecat, wolf, hyena

Intermediate hosts: Sheep, cattle, deer, pig, horse

Life cycle: Dogs and wild canids are infested by consuming the cysticercus in the intermediate host. If untreated, the final host can harbour tapeworms from several months to a year or more. The intermediate host is infected through the ingestion of tapeworm eggs that hatch in the intestine. The oncospheres, infective to sheep, cattle and pigs, are carried in the blood to the liver in which they migrate for about 4 weeks before they emerge on the surface of this organ and attach to the peritoneum. Within a further 4 weeks each develops into the characteristically large metacestode, *Cysticercus tenuicollis*.

Geographical distribution: Worldwide

Pathogenesis: Heavy infections in young lambs can lead to hepatitis and death. Occasionally, also, the developing cysticerci are killed in the liver, presumably in sheep previously exposed to infection; in these cases the subcapsular surface of the liver is

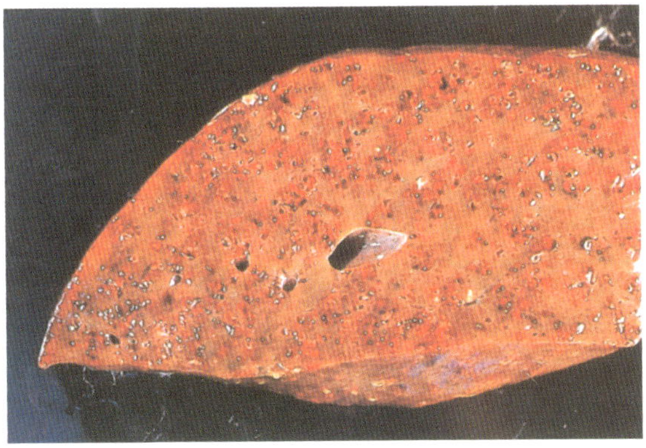

Fig. 3.33 Hepatitis cysticercosa caused by massive infection with *Cysticercus tenuicollis*.

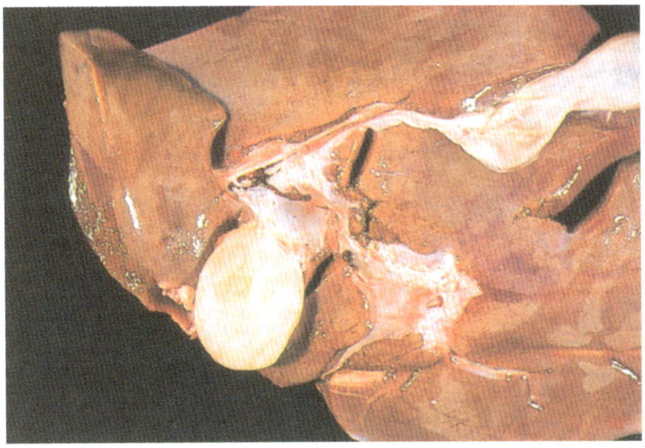

Fig. 3.34 Large fluid-filled *Cysticercus tenuicollis* attached to liver.

studded with greenish nodules of around 1 cm in diameter.

Severe infection of the liver or tissues may result in liver/carcase condemnation at slaughter. The mature cysticerci in the peritoneal cavity are usually benign. Concomitant immunity can occur in the intermediate host allowing metacestodes, acquired from a primary infection, to survive in the host, although the host is resistant to reinfection. Infrequently, large numbers of developing cysticerci migrate contemporaneously in the liver of the sheep or pig producing 'hepatitis cysticercosa', a condition whose gross pathology resembles acute fascioliosis, and which is often fatal (Fig. 3.33).

Clinical signs: Loss of condition, emaciation and ascites may be present.

Diagnosis: Chronic infection in sheep is usually confirmed at meat inspection where the large larval cysts are observed on the mesentery, omentum and abdominal organs. The liver of animals that have died as a result of acute infestation may contain haemorrhagic tracts and developing metacestodes.

Pathology: The main lesions are seen in the liver, which has a number of dark red foci and streaking and young cysticerci may be found in migratory tracts. Metacestode stages are frequently found attached to the omentum, intestinal mesentery and to the serosal surface of abdominal organs, especially the liver in the intermediate ruminant hosts (Fig. 3.34).

Epidemiology: Ruminants are infected by grazing pasture and forages contaminated with dog faeces harbouring eggs of *T. hydatigena*. A wolf and reindeer cycle exists in northern latitudes in which the metacestodes are found in the liver of the intermediate host and dogs can be infected as definitive hosts.

Treatment: No practical treatment is available for the intermediate host.

Control: This is similar to that of other taeniids involving control of infection in the definitive host and through the burial or disposal of ruminant carcases and offal.

Notes: The correct nomenclature for the intermediate host stage is the 'metacestode stage of *Taenia hydatigena*' rather than '*Cysticercus tenuicollis*'.

Echinococcus granulosus

See under Parasites of the respiratory system.

PARASITES OF THE PANCREAS

Eurytrema coelomaticum

Common name: Pancreatic fluke

Predilection site: Pancreatic ducts, rarely the bile ducts

Parasite class: Trematoda

Family: Dicrocoeliidae

Final hosts: Cattle, buffalo, sheep, goats, pigs, camels and man

Intermediate hosts: Two are required:

1. Land snails, particularly of the genus *Bradybaena*
2. Grasshoppers of the genus *Conocephalus* or tree crickets (*Oecanthus*)

Geographical distribution: South America, Asia and Europe

Eurytrema pancreaticum

Common name: Pancreatic fluke

Predilection site: Pancreatic ducts and occasionally the bile ducts and the duodenum

Parasite class: Trematoda

Family: Dicrocoeliidae

Geographical distribution: Eastern Asia and South America

For more details of these species see Chapter 2 (Cattle).

PARASITES OF THE CIRCULATORY SYSTEM

Elaeophora schneideri

Common name: Filarial dermatosis, 'sore head'

Predilection site: Blood vessels

Parasite class: Nematoda

Superfamily: Filarioidea

Description, gross: Slender worms; males are around 5 cm and females up to 12 cm long.

Description, microscopic: Microfilariae are 270 μm, bluntly rounded anteriorly, and tapering posteriorly.

Final hosts: Sheep, goat, deer (elk, moose, mule deer)

Intermediate hosts: Tabanid flies

Life cycle: The life cycle of *E. schneideri* is typically filarioid. The microfilariae are ingested by the intermediate host, when feeding and the L_3, when developed, are released into the wound made when the insect next feeds. Early development appears to be in the meningeal arteries, and the worms migrate to the carotid arteries and are mature and producing microfilariae about 4.5 months after infection. The adult worms are embedded in the arterial intima of the arotid, mesenteric and iliac arteries; occasionally they are found in the digital and tibial arteries with only the anterior part of the female free in the lumen. The prepatent period is around 4–5 months.

Geographical distribution: Western and southern USA

Pathogenesis: In *E. schneideri* infection in sheep, the circulating microfilariae are associated with a facial dermatitis, 'sorehead', in which a granulomatous inflammation of the skin occurs accompanied by intense pruritis. Occasionally the feet are also affected. This appears in the summer months. In severe cases there may be self-injury from rubbing, with abrasion, bleeding and scab formation. Lesions may alternate between periods of activity and inactivity. Lesions ultimately resolve with healing of the skin and regrowth of wool. It is thought that the natural hosts of *E. schneideri* are deer, in which the infection is asymptomatic, and that sheep may be abnormal hosts.

Clinical signs: Only the seasonal facial dermatitis in sheep is recognised as a clinical indication of elaeophorosis.

Diagnosis: Only in sheep is diagnosis required, and though the obvious method is by examination of a skin biopsy, microfilariae are often scarce in samples, and diagnosis is usually presumptive, based on the locality, the facial lesions and the seasonal appearance of the dermatitis.

Pathology: The usual skin lesion seen in sheep is 5–10 cm in diameter, usually on the poll, although lesions may appear on the coronary band. Ischaemic chorioretinitis due to occlusive vasculitis has been reported in elk due to the circulating microfilariae.

Epidemiology: The natural hosts appear to be deer of *Odocoileus* spp (the white-tail and the mule deer), and in these the infection is clinically inapparent. However, in American elk (*Cervus canadensis*) thrombosis due to the worms often results in necrosis of the muzzle, ears and optic nerves, resulting in severe facial damage, blindness and frequently death.

Treatment: No effective treatment reported.

Control: Any reduction in vector numbers will reduce transmission.

Notes: These worms inhabit large blood vessels, but are only of local importance.

Schistosoma bovis

Common name: Blood fluke, bilharziosis

Predilection site: Portal and mesenteric veins, urogenital veins

Parasite class: Trematoda

Family: Schistosomatidae

Final hosts: Cattle, sheep, goat

Intermediate hosts: Snails (*Bulinus contortus*, *B. truncates*, *Physopsis africana*, *P. nasuta*)

Geographical distribution: Africa, Middle East, southern Asia, southern Europe

Schistosoma japonicum

Common name: Blood fluke, bilharziosis

Predilection site: Portal and mesenteric veins

Parasite class: Trematoda

Family: Schistosomatidae

Final hosts: Cattle, horse, sheep, goat, dog, cat, rabbit, pig, man

Intermediate hosts: Snails belonging to the genus *Oncomelania*

Geographical distribution: South and east Asia

Schistosoma mattheei

Predilection site: Portal, mesenteric and bladder veins

Parasite class: Trematoda

Family: Schistosomatidae

Final hosts: Cattle, sheep, goat, man

Intermediate hosts: Snails (*Bulinus*)

Geographical distribution: South and central Africa, Middle East

Notes: Thought to be synonymous with *S. bovis* but differs on morphological and pathological grounds and is restricted to the alimentary canal.

Schistosoma nasalis

Synonym: *Schistosoma nasalae*

Common name: 'Snoring disease'

Predilection site: Veins of nasal mucosa

Parasite class: Trematoda

Family: Schistosomatidae

Final host: Cattle, goat sheep, buffalo, horse

Intermediate hosts: Snails (*Lymnaea luteola, L. acuminata, Indoplanorbis exustus*)

Geographical distribution: India, Pakistan, South East Asia

Schistosoma indicum

Predilection site: Portal, pancreatic, hepatic and mesenteric veins

Parasite class: Trematoda

Family: Schistosomatidae

Final host: Cattle, sheep, goat, horse, donkey, camel

Intermediate hosts: Snails (*Indoplanorbis*)

Geographical distribution: India

Schistosoma turkestanicum

Synonym: *Orientobilharzia turkstanicum*

Predilection site: Mesenteric veins and small veins of the pancreas and liver

Parasite class: Trematoda

Family: Schistosomatidae

Geographical distribution: Asia

More details of these species are in Chapter 2 (Cattle).

Trypanosomes

Members of the genus *Trypanosoma* are haemoflagellates of overwhelming importance in cattle in sub-Saharan Africa but also occur in sheep and goats. See Chapter 1 (Zoomastigophorasida) for general description and Chapter 2 for detailed descriptions of individual species of trypanosomes, and their control.

Trypanosoma brucei brucei

Subgenus: *Trypanozoon*

Common name: Nagana

Predilection site: Blood. *T. brucei bucei* is also found extravascularly in, for example, the myocardium, CNS and reproductive tract.

Parasite class: Zoomastigophorasida

Family: Trypanosomatidae

Hosts: Cattle, horse, donkey, zebu, sheep, goat, camel, pig, dog, cat, wild game species

Distribution: Sub-Saharan Africa

Treatment: The two drugs in common use in cattle are isometamidium and diaminazine aceturate and both should be suitable for use in sheep and goats. These are usually successful except where trypanosomes have developed resistance to the drug or in some very chronic cases. Treatment should be followed by surveillance, since reinfection followed by clinical signs and parasitaemia may occur within a week or two. Alternatively, the animal may relapse after chemotherapy, due to a persisting focus of infection in its tissues or because the trypanosomes are drug-resistant.

Trypanosoma congolense

Subgenus: *nannomonas*

Common name: Nagana, paranagana, Gambia fever, ghindi, gobial

Predilection site: Blood

Parasite class: Zoomastigophorasida

Family: Trypanosomatidae

Hosts: Cattle, sheep, goat, horse, camel, dog, pig. Reservoir hosts include antelope, giraffe, zebra, elephant and warthog.

Distribution: Sub-Saharan Africa

Treatment: In infected cattle, the two drugs in common use are diminazene aceturate (Berenil) and homidium salts (Ethidium and Novidium) and are appropriate for use in sheep and goats infected with *T. congolense*. As with *T. brucei*, these drugs are usually successful except where trypanosomes have developed resistance to the drug or in some very chronic cases.

Trypanosoma vivax

Subspecies: *vivax*

Subgenus: *Duttonella*

Common name: Nagana, souma

Predilection site: Blood

Parasite class: Zoomastigophorasida

Family: Trypanosomatidae

Hosts: Cattle, sheep, goat, camel, horse; antelope and giraffe are reservoirs

Geographical distribution: Africa (central), West Indies, Central and South America (Brazil, Venezuela, Bolivia, Columbia, Guyana, French Guyana), Mauritius

Treatment: As for *T. congolense*

For more details of these species see Chapter 2 (Cattle).

Trypanosoma simiae

Subgenus: *Nannomonas*

Synonym: *Trypanosoma congolense simiae, T. rodhaini, T. porci*

Predilection site: Blood

Parasite class: Zoomastigophorasida

Family: Trypanosomatidae

Hosts: Pig, camel, sheep, goat

Distribution: Central Africa

For more details see Chapter 5 (Pigs).

Trypanosoma melophagium

Subgenus: *Megatrypanum*

Predilection site: Blood

Parasite class: Zoomastigophorasida

Family: Trypanosomatidae

Description: Large trypanosome, 50–60 μm in length with the posterior end long and pointed. There is a prominent undulating membrane and a free flagellum. Tryptomastigote forms are rare in the blood.

Hosts: Sheep, goat

Life cycle: Tryptomastigotes are transmitted by the sheep ked, *Melophagus ovinus*, and epimastigote and amastigote forms in the midgut multiply by binary fission. Epimastigote forms change into small, metacyclic tryptomastigote forms in the hingut. Sheep are infected when they bite into the keds and the tryptomastigotes are released and pass through the intact mucosa. It has been suggested that replication does not occur in the sheep.

Geographical distribution: Worldwide

Pathogenesis: Non-pathogenic

Diagnosis: Infections in the blood are so sparse they can only be detected by culture in selective medium.

Epidemiology: *T. melophagum* is transmitted by the sheep ked *Melophagus ovinus* and infection is linked to the presence and abundance of ked infections.

Treatment and control: Not required although general ectoparasite control strategies effective against keds will also control infection levels of the trypanosome.

Babesiosis

For details on the general life cycle and epidemiology of babesiosis see Chapter 2: Cattle. Control measures are essentially similar and require control of tick vectors. Topical application of acaricides may provide some level of protection but may be difficult in sheep, expensive, and may have a negative cost benefit. Under certain conditions, it may be more beneficial to attain endemic stability, allowing early infection and development of immunity.

Babesia motasi

Predilection site: Blood

Parasite class: Sporozoasida

Family: Babesiidae

Description: *Babesia motasi* is a large species, 2.5–4 × 2 μm, and the parasites are usually piriform. The merozoites occur singly or in pairs and the angle between members of a pair is usually acute.

Hosts: Sheep, goat

Geographical distribution: Southern Europe, the Middle East, the former Soviet Union, southeast Asia and Africa

Pathogenesis: Strains of *B. motasi* from Europe produce a mild clinical response characterised by fever and anaemia but alone is rarely responsible for significant death losses. Strains from the Mediterranean basin may be more pathogenic and some strains are transmissible to goats, but this is not a consistent observation.

Clinical signs: Disease may be acute or chronic. Animals show pyrexia, prostration, marked anaemia and haemoglobinuria in the acute form, and may die. There are no characteristic signs in the chronic disease.

Diagnosis: Examination of blood films, stained with Giemsa, will reveal the parasites in the red cells.

Pathology: In pathogenic infections, the principal lesions include splenomegaly with soft, dark red splenic pulp and prominent splenic corpuscles. The liver is enlarged and yellowish brown and the gall bladder is distended with thick, dark bile. The mucosa of the abomasum and intestine, subcutaneous, subserous and intramuscular connective tissues are oedematous and icteric with patches of haemorrhage. The blood is thin and watery, and the plasma tinged with red.

Epidemiology: Transmitted by ticks of the genus *Haemaphysalis* (*H. punctata*, *H. otophila*), *Dermacentor* (*D. silvarum*) and *Rhipicephalus* (*R. bursa*).

Treatment: Diminazene aceturate is effective against *B. motasi.*

Babesia ovis

Predilection site: Blood

Parasite class: Sporozoasida

Family: Babesiidae

Description: *Babesia ovis* is small species, 1–2.5 μm long, mostly rounded and in the margin of the host erythrocytes, with paired, piriform trophozoites usually lying at an obtuse angle.

Hosts: Sheep, goat

Geographical distribution: Southern Europe, former Soviet States, Middle East, Asia

Pathogenesis: Infections occur as a pathogenic entity in southern Europe and the Middle East but are generally mild in indigenous sheep with severe clinical signs occurring in animals introduced from a non-endemic area. Death, if it occurs, is due to organ failure which, in turn, is due not only to destruction of the erythrocytes with resultant anaemia, oedema and icterus, but also to the clogging of the capillaries of various organs by parasitised cells and free parasites. The stasis from this sludging causes degeneration of the endothelial cells of the small blood vessels, anoxia, accumulation of toxic metabolic products, capillary fragility and eventual perivascular escape of erythrocytes and macroscopic haemorrhage.

Clinical signs: The clinical signs of infection include anaemia, jaundice, oedema and haemoglobinuria. Infections are often mild and often are inapparent.

Diagnosis: Examination of blood films, stained with Giemsa, will reveal the parasites in the red cells. Usually fewer than 0.6% of the erythrocytes are infected.

Pathology: In pathogenic infections, the principal lesions include splenomegaly with soft, dark red splenic pulp and prominent splenic corpuscles. The liver is enlarged and yellowish brown and the gall bladder is distended with thick, dark bile. The mucosa of the abomasum and intestine, subcutaneous, subserous and intramuscular connective tissues are oedematous and icteric with patches of haemorrhage. The blood is thin and watery, and the plasma tinged with red.

Epidemiology: *Rhipicephalus bursa* has been shown to be a vector for this parasite, and *I. ricinus*, *I. persulcatus* and *D. reticulatus* are suspected vectors.

Treatment: Diminazene aceturate is effective against *B. ovis*. Quinuronium sulphate is still used in some countries.

Theileriosis

Theileria spp are widely distributed in cattle and sheep in Africa, Asia, Europe and Australia, have a variety of tick vectors and are associated with infections which range from clinically inapparent to rapidly fatal. Although the speciation of many *Theileria* is still controversial, largely because of their morphological similarity, there are two species of major veterinary importance in sheep.

The life cycle of *Theileria* spp involves erythrocytic merozoites, which are ingested by the tick intermediate host and develop into macro- and microgamonts to produce zygotes. These develop and enter the haemolymph to become kinetes and then the salivary glands to become fission bodies. In adult ticks, the primary fission bodies divide into secondary (primary sporoblasts) and tertiary (secondary sporoblasts) fission bodies and produce sporozoites that are released into the saliva. Animals are infected when the ticks suck blood. The sporozoites enter lymphocytes and become meronts; both macromeronts and micromeronts occur, producing micromerozoites that enter erythrocytes, which after a few binary fissions produce the varied forms that are taken up by other ticks.

Theileria hirci

Synonym: *Theileria lestoquardi*

Common name: Malignant theileriosis of small ruminants

Predilection site: Blood, lymph nodes, spleen

Parasite class: Sporozoasida

Family: Theileriidae

Description: Trophozoites are found in lymphocytes and erythrocytes as round (0.6–2.0 µm in diameter), oval, rod-shaped (1.6 µm long) forms (Fig. 3.35). Binary or quadruple fission takes place in the erythrocytes. Meronts (Koch bodies), averaging 8 µm in diameter (range 10–20 µm) and containing 1–80 granules, are common in the lymphocytes of the spleen and lymph nodes.

Hosts: Sheep, goat

Geographical distribution: Southern Europe, the Middle East, Asia and North and East Africa

Pathogenesis: Highly pathogenic, causing an acute and highly fatal disease in adult sheep and goats with mortalities of 46–100%. The infection is mild in young lambs and kids due to maternal immunity. An acute form is more common, but sabacute and chronic forms have been observed.

Clinical signs: In the acute form there is fever (40–41.7°C; 104–107°F), inappetence, cessation of rumination, rapid heartbeat, weakness, swelling of superficial lymph nodes and eyelids, diarrhoea (containing blood and mucus) and jaundice and haemorrhage in submucous, subserous and subcutaneous tissues may occur. Affected animals become emaciated and death occurs. In chronic infections there is intermittent fever, inappetence, emaciation, anaemia and jaundice.

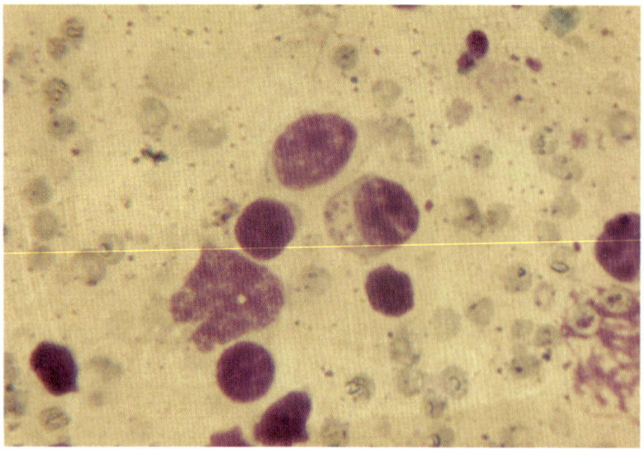

Fig. 3.35 Meront of *Theileria hirci*.

Diagnosis: Diagnosis depends on the detection of meronts in blood smears, lymph node biopsies or lymph node or spleen smears on postmortem.

Pathology: The lymph nodes are always swollen, the liver usually swollen, the spleen markedly enlarged and the lungs oedematous. Infarcts are often present in the kidneys, and there are petechiae on the mucosa of the abomasum and irregularly disseminated red patches on the intestinal mucosa.

Epidemiology: The tick vectors are thought to be *Rhipicephalus bursa* and *Hyalomma anatolicum*.

Treatment: A single injection of parvaquone at a dose rate of 20 mg/kg i.m., or buparvaquone at 2.5 mg/kg given on two occasions are effective. A single dose of halofuginone at 1.2 mg/kg per os is also reported to be effective.

Control: Tick control measures can be considered for controlling disease. Topical application of acaricides may provide some level of protection but may be difficult in sheep, expensive, and may have a negative cost benefit.

Notes: Causes significant losses in small ruminant populations in the Mediterranean and North African regions.

Theileria ovis

Common name: Benign theileriosis of small ruminants

Predilection site: Blood, lymph nodes

Parasite class: Sporozoasida

Family: Theileriidae

Description: Erythrocytic stages are similar in appearance to *T. hirci* and are found in lymphocytes and erythrocytes as round (0.6–2.0 µm in diameter), oval or rod-shaped (1.6 µm long) forms but are much more sparse, with less than 2% of erythrocytes infected.

Hosts: Sheep, goat

Life cycle: Erythrocytic merozoites, ingested by the tick intermediate host, develop into macro- and microgamonts to produce zygotes. These develop and enter the haemolymph to become kinetes and then the salivary glands to become fission bodies. In adult ticks, the primary fission bodies divide into secondary (primary sporoblasts) and tertiary (secondary

Table 3.5 *Theileria* species reported in sheep and goats.

Species	Disease	Tick vectors	Hosts	Distribution
Theileria hirci (Syn: *T. lestoquardi*)	Malignant theileriosis	*Rhipicephalus bursa* *Hyalomma anatolicum*	Sheep, goat	Southern Europe, Middle East, Asia, North and East Africa
Theileria ovis	Benign theieriosis	*Rhipicephalus bursa* in Mediterranean basin *Rhipicephalus evertsi* in Africa	Sheep, goat	Europe, Africa, Asia, India
Theileria recondita	Non-pathogenic	*Haemaphysalis punctata*	Sheep, goat, deer	Western Europe (Germany, UK)
Theileria separata	Non-pathogenic	*Rhipicephalus evertsi*	Sheep, goat	Sub-Saharan Africa
Theileira spp	Pathogenic	*Haemaphysalis* sp.	Sheep	China

sporoblasts) fission bodies and produce sporozoites that are released into the saliva. Animals are infected when the ticks suck blood. The sporozoites enter lymphocytes and become meronts; both macromeronts and micromeronts occur producing micromerozoites that enter erythrocytes, which after a few binary fissions produce the varied forms that are taken up by other ticks.

Geographical distribution: Europe, Africa, Asia, India

Pathogenesis: The pathogenicity and mortality are low although prevalence may be very high in endemic areas

Clinical signs: The infection is usually mild and clinically inapparent.

Diagnosis: Demonstration of the parasites in stained blood or lymph node smears. The organism is indistinguishable from *T. hirci* but the small number of parasites present and the lack of pathogenicity help to differentatiate them.

Pathology: No associated pathology

Epidemiology: The tick vectors are *Rhipicephalus bursa* in the Mediterranean basin and *Rhipicephalus evertsi* in Africa.

Treatment and control: Not usually required

Rickettsiales

Several rickettsial organisms are of significance in sheep and goats.

Anaplasma phagocytophilum

Synonym: *Anoplasma phagocytophilia, Ehrlichia phagocytophilia, Cytoecetes phagocytophilia, Ehrlichia equi, Anaplasma platys*

Common name: Tick-borne fever, pasture fever, canine granulocytic ehrlichiosis, human granulocytic ehrlichiosis, equine granulocyitc erlichiosis

Predilection site: Blood

Order: Rickettsiales

Family: Anaplasmataceae

Description: Blood smears stained with Giemsa or Wright's stains reveal one or more loose aggregates (morulae or inclusion bodies, 1.5–5 μm in diameter) of blue–grey to dark blue coccoid, coccobacillary or pleomorphic organisms within the cytoplasm of neutrophils (Fig. 3.36).

Hosts: Sheep, cattle, dog, horse, deer, rodents

Life cycle: Obligate intracellular organisms infecting ganulocytes, predominantly neutrophils, appearing within the cytoplasm as membrane-bound vacuoles. Multiplication is by binary fission forming large inclusion bodies (morulae). In untreated animals, the

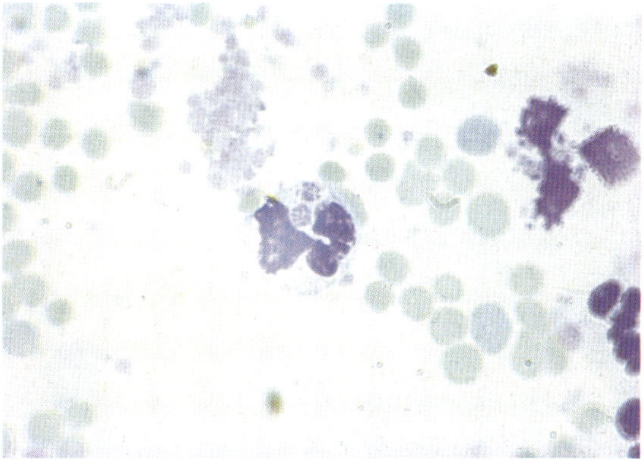

Fig. 3.36 Inclusions of *Anaplasma phagocytophilum*.

cytoplasmic inclusions can be detected in circulating neutrophils for 1–2 weeks. The organisms spend part of their normal life cycle within the tick and are transmitted trans-stadially. As the tick vector feeds on a wide range of vertebrate animals, transmission of the infectious agent may take place to multiple host species.

Geographical distribution: Probably worldwide, Europe (UK, Norway, Finland, the Netherlands and Austria)

Pathogenesis: Organisms enter the dermis via a tick bite and are then spread via the blood and/or the lymph and localise in mature granulocytes, mainly in neutrophils but also in eosinophils, of the peripheral blood. However it is not clear whether they invade mature cells or precursor cells within the myelopoietic system. After endocytosis, multiplication occurs within cytoplasmic phagosomes and the organisms can be found in many organs, e.g. spleen, lungs and liver. The veterinary significance of tick-borne fever in sheep is three-fold. First, although the disease in itself is transient, its occurrence in very young lambs on rough upland pastures may lead to death through inability to maintain contact with the dam. Secondly, the disease, possibly because of the associated leucopenia, predisposes lambs to louping-ill, tick pyaemia (enzootic staphylococcosis) and pasteurellosis. Finally, the occurrence of the disease in adult sheep or cattle newly introduced into an endemic area may cause abortion or temporary sterility in males, possibly as consequences of the pyrexia.

Both animals and humans can be co-infected with various *Anaplasma*, *Ehrlichia*, *Borrelia*, *Bartonella*, *Rickettsia*, *Babesia* and arboviral species. Infection with any of these organisms causes a wide range of clinical and pathological abnormalities, ranging in severity from asymptomatic infection to death. The risk of acquiring one or more tick-bome infections may be dependent on the prevalence of multi-infected vectors. *A. phagocytophilum* and *Borrelia burgdorferi*, for example, share both reservoir hosts and vectors, and in geographical areas where tick-borne fever is endemic, borreliosis is also prevalent.

Clinical signs: In sheep, following an incubation period of 7 days there is fever, dullness and inappetence, which persist for around 10 days. During this time, although leucopenia is marked, the characteristic 'morula' inclusions may be seen in a variable proportion of the polymorphonuclear leucocytes present. Recovery is usually uneventful, although such animals remain carriers for many months.

Diagnosis: Tick-borne fever should be considered when an animal presents with an acute febrile illness in an endemic geographic area. Stained blood smears should be examined and, with Wright's stain, morulae typically appear as dark blue, irregularly stained densities in the cytoplasm of neutrophils. The colour of the morulae is usually darker than that of the cell nucleus. Morulae are often sparse and difficult to detect and a negative blood smear cannot rule out *A. phagocytophilum* infection. Specific diagnostic tests include immunofluorescent antibody test (IFAT), immunoblot analyses, ELISA and polymerase chain reaction (PCR) analyses. The most widely accepted diagnostic criterion is a four-fold change in titre by IFAT. However, cross-reactivity may occur with other members of the genera *Anaplasma* and *Ehrlichia*.

Pathology: The disease is characterised by haematological changes typified by thrombocytopenia and leucopenia. The leucopenia is a result of early lymphopenia later accompanied by neutropenia. Thrombocytopenia is one of the most consistent haematological abnormalities in infected dogs. It may be moderate to severe and persists for a few days before returning to normal. Biochemical abnormalities may include mildly elevated serum alkaline phosphatase and alanine aminotransferase activities.

Epidemiology: Rodents as well as domestic and wild ruminants (sheep and deer), have been reported as reservoir hosts of *A. phagocytophilum* in Europe. The predominant reservoir host varies depending on the local natural and agricultural landscape. The vector of *A. phagocytophilum* in Europe is the common sheep tick, *Ixodes ricinus*. In endemic areas the prevalence of infection in young hill lambs is virtually 100%.

Treatment: Treatment of tick-borne fever in sheep is rarely indicated. When tick pyaemia in lambs is a problem this measure may be supplemented by one or two prophylactic injections of long-acting oxytetracycline, which protects against infection for 2–3 weeks. Doxycycline at 5–10 mg/kg for 3 weeks appears to be most effective regime for treating infections in dogs and cats. Severe disease may require treatment for longer periods. The most common side effects of doxycycline treatment are nausea and vomiting which are avoided by administering the drug with food.

Control: In sheep, prophylaxis depends on tick control by dipping.

Notes: The newly reclassified *Anaplasma phagocytophilum* combo nov. (formerly known as three separate ehrlichiae *E. phagocytophila*, *E. equi*, and *Anaplasma platys* (formerly known as *E. platys*)) causes canine, equine and human granulocytic ehrlichiosis.

Eperythrozoon ovis

Synonym: *Candidatus Mycoplasma ovis*

Predilection site: Blood

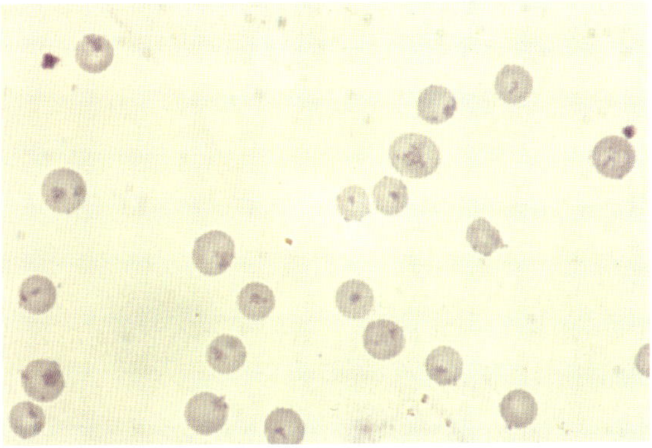

Fig. 3.37 Intraerythrocytic forms of *Eperythrozoon ovis*.

Order: Rickettsiales

Family: Anaplasmataceae

Description: Pleomorphic coccobacilli occurring either as eperythrocytic organisms in depressions on the cell surface, or free in the plasma (Fig. 3.37). Single comma-shaped or ring-form cocci predominate in light to moderate infections but form irregular complex bodies in sever parasitaemias. Cocci appear light blue with Giemsa or Romanowsky's stains.

Hosts: Sheep, goat

Life cycle: Organisms are transmitted by biting insects and ticks. Replication takes place by binary fission or budding.

Geographical distribution: Worldwide

Pathogenesis: Most infections are normally benign, but *E. ovis* is occasionally responsible for fever, anaemia and loss of weight. The onset of clinical signs is insidious. Lambs infected at about 2–3 months of age show growth retardation and are slow to reach sexual maturity.

Clinical signs: Disease in lambs is mild and limited to vague ill-thrift.

Diagnosis: Identification from staining artefacts requires good blood films and filtered Giemsa stain. The organisms appear as cocci or short rods on the surface of the erythrocytes, often completely surrounding the margin of the red cell. However, the organisms of *Eperythrozoon* are relatively loosely attached to the red cell surface and are often found free in the plasma.

Pathology: Initial haematological changes are a fall in packed cell volume, total erythrocytes and haemoglobin and as the parasitaemia drops there is a gradual development of an autoimmune haemolytic anaemia. Platelet counts are reduced and prothrombin times are prolonged

Epidemiology: *E. ovis* is transmitted by stable flies (*Stomoxys calcitrans*) and keds (*Malophagus ovinus*) and in the tropics and subtropics by mosquitoes (*Aedes camptorhynchus*, *Anopheles annulipes*, *Culex annulorostris*) and ticks (*Haemaphysalis plumbeum* and *Rhipicephalus bursa*). Transplacental infection is also thought to occur.

Treatment and control: Tetracyclines should be effective but control is not usually practical or necessary.

Notes: The taxonomy of this species is subject to much debate and there is a proposal to re-classify it into the bacterial genus *Mycoplasma* (class Mollicutes) based on 16s rRNA gene sequences and phylogenetic analysis.

Rickettsia conorii

Common name: Boutonneuse fever, Mediterranean spotted fever, Indian tick typhus, East African tick typhus

Predilection site: Blood

Order: Rickettsiales

Family: Rickettsiaceae

Description: Small pleomorphic Gram-negative, coccoid, obligatory intracellular organisms infecting endothelial cells of smaller blood vessels.

Hosts: Rodents, dog, cattle, sheep, goat, man

Life cycle: Ticks become infected with *R. conorii* by feeding on infected small rodents that are the main reservoir of disease. Immature ticks become infected and infection is transmitted trans-stadially and trans-ovarially to later tick stages, which feed on larger mammals.

Geographical distribution: Southern Europe, Africa, India and the oriental region

Pathogenesis: Infections appear to be non-pathogenic.

Diagnosis: The rickettsiae can be demonstrated by staining blood or organ smears with Giemsa or may be detected serologically.

Epidemiology: The vector of Mediterranean 'boutonneuse' fever is *Rhipicephalus sanguineus.* Apart from dogs, sheep and cattle, other small free-living mammals such as rats, mice and shrews are believed to play an important role in the cycle of infection within tick vectors.

Treatment and control: Not usually required although, if necessary, tetracyclines are usually effective

The following species occur in sheep and goats but are generally of more importance in cattle (see Chapter 2: Cattle for more detailed information).

Anaplasma marginale

Predilection site: Blood

Order: Rickettsiales

Family: Anaplasmataceae

Description: In Giemsa-stained blood films the organisms of *A. marginale* are seen as small, round, dark red 'inclusion bodies' approximately 0.3–1.0 µm within the red cell. Often there is only one organism in a red cell and characteristically this lies at the outer margin; however these two features are not constant.

Hosts: Cattle, sheep, goat, wild ruminants

Geographical distribution: Africa, southern Europe, Australia, South America, Asia, former Soviet states and USA

Anaplasma centrale

Predilection site: Blood

Order: Rickettsiales

Family: Anaplasmataceae

Description: The mildly pathogenic *A. centrale* is similar to *A. marginale*, except that the organisms are commonly found in the centre of the erythrocyte.

Hosts: Cattle, wild ruminants, and perhaps sheep, may act as reservoirs of infection.

Ehrlichia ruminantium

Synonym: *Cowdria ruminantium*

Common name: Heartwater, cowdriosis, malkopsiekte (Afrikaans)

Predilection site: Blood

Order: Rickettsiales

Family: Rickettsiaceae

Description: Organisms are seen as close-packed colonies consisting of less than ten to many hundred cocci. The organism varies in size from 0.2 µm to greater than 1.5 µm. The diameter of individual organisms in a given cluster is rather uniform but groups are very pleomorphic. The small granules tend to be coccoid, with larger ones looking like rings, horseshoes, rods and irregular masses.

Hosts: Cattle, sheep, goats and wild ruminants

PARASITES OF THE NERVOUS SYSTEM

Taenia multiceps

Synonym: *Multiceps multiceps*, *Coenurus cerebralis*

Common name: Gid, sturdy, staggers

Predilection site: Brain and spinal cord (intermediate hosts); small intestine (final hosts)

Parasite class: Cestoda

Family: Taeniidae

Description, gross: When mature the *Coenurus cerebralis* cyst is readily recognised as a large fluid-filled transparent bladder up to 5 cm or more in diameter.

Description, microscopic: The coenurus bears clusters of several hundred protoscolices on its internal wall.

Definitive hosts: Dog, fox, coyote, jackal

Intermediate hosts: Sheep, cattle, deer, pig, horse, man

Life cycle: The intermediate host is infected through the ingestion of *T. multiceps* eggs. Each egg contains an oncosphere that hatches and is activated in the small intestine. The oncosphere then penetrates the intestinal mucosa and is carried via the blood to the brain or spinal cord where each oncosphere develops into the metacestode larval stage (*Coenurus cerebralis*). When mature, this is readily recognised as a large fluid-filled cyst up to 5.0 cm or more in diameter, which bears clusters of scolices on its internal wall. In goats the cysts can also mature in subcutaneous and intramuscular sites. The cysts in sheep and goats often persist throughout the life of the animal. The life cycle is completed when the final host, dog or wild canid, eats an infected sheep brain or spinal cord.

Geographical distribution: Worldwide

Pathogenesis: The *Coenurus* takes about 8 months to mature in the central nervous system and, as it develops, it causes damage to the brain tissue resulting in neurological disturbances. These cysts can cause pressure atrophy, which may lead to perforation of the skull. When cysts locate in the spinal cord the resulting pressure can lead to paresis of the hindlimbs. Although an acute form of coenurosis can occur, chronic disease is more frequently identified. Acute disease is likely to occur when sheep are grazed on pasture heavily contaminated with faeces from untreated dogs. The migration of large numbers of larval stages through the brain can rapidly lead to neurological dysfunction and death. Chronic disease presents as a progressive focal lesion of the brain with signs of neurological dysfunction appearing about 3–6 months from initial infection and is usually seen in sheep of 6–24 months of age. Coenurosis is much less common in cattle.

Clinical signs: Clinical signs depend on the location and size of the cyst or cysts and include circling behaviour, visual defects, peculiarities in gait, stumbling, uncoordinated movements, hyperaesthesia or paraplegia. As the infection progresses animals may become anorexic and lose weight and death may result. The clinical syndrome is often known as 'gid' or 'staggers' in which the animal holds its head to one side and turns in a circle to the affected side.

Diagnosis: It is difficult to diagnose infection in sheep or goats unless obvious neurological signs are apparent. Even then other organisms, such as *Listeria monocytogenes*, *Oestrus ovis* and louping-ill, should be considered in any evaluation of acute coenurosis. Most diagnoses are made at postmortem. Where cysts are located on the surface of the brain it is sometimes possible to palpate the local softening of the frontal bones of the skull.

Pathology: The cyst or cysts are mainly located in one cerebral hemisphere and occur less frequently in the cerebellum and spinal cord (Fig. 3.38). The growth of the cysts within the brain or skull causes pressure atrophy of adjacent cerebral tissue. The migration of large numbers of immature stages in the brain of lambs can lead to acute meningoencephalitis. In acute cases of coenurosis, pale yellow tracts are frequently present on the surface of the brain. They are comprised of necrotic tissue with marked cellular infiltration. In chronic coenurosis there may be compression of brain tissue by the developing cyst and the increased intracranial pressure can result in local softening of the bones of the skull, either above the cyst or in other areas.

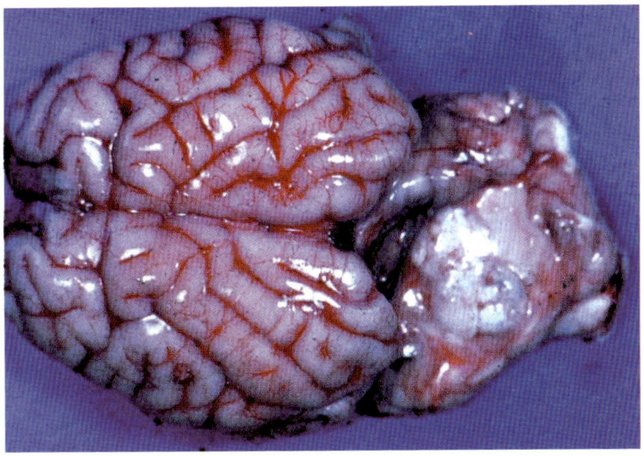

Fig. 3.38 *Coenurus cerebralis* cyst on the surface of the cerebellum from an infected sheep.

Epidemiology: Where livestock, particularly sheep, have access to grazing land that is contaminated with infective dog faeces, then there is a risk of larval migration of the metacestode stage into the central nervous system.

Treatment: Surgical removal is possible if the cyst is situated on the brain surface. This may be detected by local softening of the skull, or by detailed neurological examination. However, for many cases there is no treatment.

Control: This can be achieved through ensuring that dogs, in particular sheep dogs, do not have access to the heads of slaughtered or dead sheep or goats. It is essential that all sheep carcases are buried as soon as possible. In areas where coenurosis is endemic the regular de-worming of dogs with an effective anthelmintic every 6–8 weeks will reduce the contamination into the environment and, by breaking the sheep–dog cycle, may lead to eradication of the disease. Foxes are not thought to be an important final host for *T. multiceps*.

Gedoelstia spp

See details and description under Parasites of the respiratory system.

Toxoplasma gondii

See details and description under Parasites of the reproductive/urogenital system.

PARASITES OF THE REPRODUCTIVE/ UROGENITAL SYSTEM

Toxoplasma gondii

Predilection site: Muscle, lung, liver, reproductive system, central nervous system

Order: Sporozoasida

Family: Sarcocystiidae

Description: Tachyzoites are found developing in vacuoles in many cell types, for example fibroblasts, hepatocytes, reticular cells and myocardial cells. In any one cell there may be 8–16 organisms, each measuring 6.0–8.0 µm. Tissue cysts, measuring up to 100 µm in diameter, are found mainly in the muscle, liver, lung and brain, and may contain several thousand lancet-shaped bradyzoites (Fig. 3.39).

Intermediate hosts: Any mammal, including man, or birds. Note that the final host, the cat, may also be an intermediate host and harbour extra-intestinal stages.

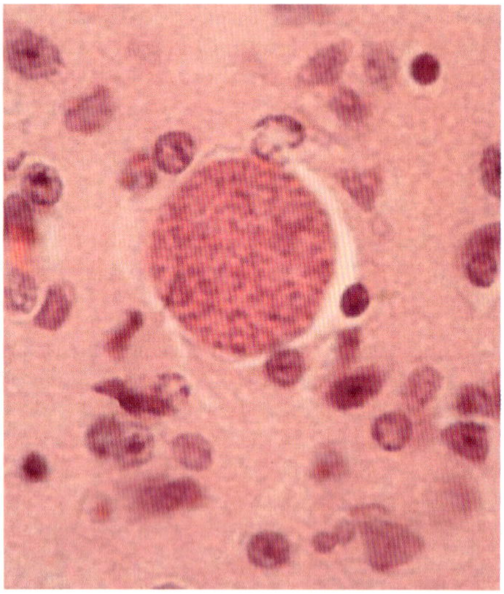

Fig. 3.39 Tissue cyst of *Toxoplasma gondii*.

Final host: Cat, other felids

Life cycle: The final host is the cat, in which gametogony takes place. Sheep and goats act as an intermediate host, in which the cycle is extra-intestinal and results in the formation of tachyzoites and bradyzoites, which are the only forms found in non-feline hosts. Infection usually occurs through the ingestion of sporulated oocysts. The liberated sporozoites rapidly penetrate the intestinal wall and spread by the haematogenous route. This invasive and proliferative stage is called the tachyzoite and, on entering a cell, it multiplies asexually in a vacuole by a process of budding or endodyogeny, in which two individuals are formed within the mother cell, the pellicle of the latter being used by the daughter cells. When 8–16 tachyzoites have accumulated the cell ruptures and new cells are infected. This is the acute phase of toxoplasmosis. In most instances, the host survives and antibody is produced which limits the invasiveness of the tachyzoites and results in the formation of cysts containing thousands of organisms which, because endodyogeny and growth are slow, are termed bradyzoites. The cyst containing the bradyzoites is the latent form, multiplication being held in check by the acquired immunity of the host. If this immunity wanes, the cyst may rupture, releasing the bradyzoites, which become active and resume the invasive characteristics of the tachyzoites.

Geographical distribution: Worldwide

Pathogenesis: Infections are usually acquired via the digestive tract, and so organisms are disseminated by the lymphatics and portal system with subsequent invasion of various organs and tissues. Pathogenic effects are always related to the extra-intestinal phase of development. In heavy infections, the multiplying tachyzoites may produce areas of necrosis in vital organs, such as the myocardium, lungs, liver, and brain; during this phase the host can become pyrexic and lymphadenopathy occurs. As the disease progresses bradyzoites are formed, this chronic phase being usually asymptomatic. In pregnant animals, exposed for the first time to *T. gondii* infection, congenital disease may occur. The predominant lesions are found in the central nervous system, although other tissues may be affected. Thus, retinochoroiditis is a frequent lesion in congenital toxoplasmosis.

Clinical signs: Undoubtedly the most important role of toxoplasmosis, particularly in sheep, is its association with abortion in ewes and perinatal mortality in lambs (Fig. 3.40). If infection of the ewes occurs early in gestation (<55 days), there is death and expulsion of the small fetus, which is seldom observed. If infection occurs in mid-gestation, abortion is more readily detected, the organisms being found in the typical white lesions, 2.0 mm in diameter, in the cotyledons of the placenta and in fetal tissues; alternatively the dead fetus may be retained, mummified and expelled later. If the fetus survives *in utero*, the lamb may be stillborn or, if alive, weak. Ewes that abort due to *T. gondii* in one year, usually lamb normally in subsequent years.

Diagnosis: Tachyzoites of *Toxoplasma gondii* are often difficult to find in tissue sections, but are more likely to be present in sections of brain and placenta. Identification can be confirmed by immunohistochemistry, while the polymerase chain reaction may be used to identify parasite DNA in tissues. Several serological tests have been developed of which the dye test (DT)

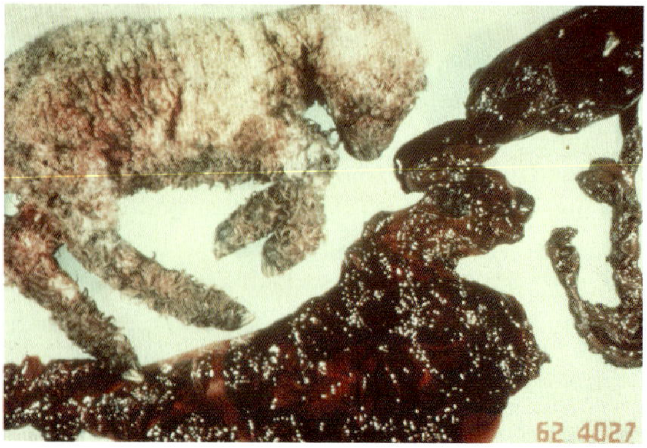

Fig. 3.40 *Toxoplasma gondii*: aborted fetus and necrotic placenta.

is the longest established serological method, and in many ways represents the gold standard, at least in humans. The dye test uses live, virulent *Toxoplasma* tachyzoites, a complement-like 'accessory-factor' and test serum. When specific antibody acts on the tachyzoites, the latter do not stain uniformly with alkaline methylene blue. The test has proven unreliable in some species. The indirect fluorescent antibody test (IFAT) gives titres comparable with the dye test, but is safer as it uses killed tachyzoites and can be used to differentiate IgM and lgG antibodies. Other tests for the detection of *Toxoplasma* antibodies include an direct agglutination test (DAT), a latex agglutination test (LAT) and an enzyme-linked immunosorbent assay (ELISA).

Abortion in sheep and goats due to *T. gondii* must be differentiated from other infectious causes of abortion, including infections with *Chlamydophila abortus* (enzootic abortion), *Coxiella bumetii* (Q fever), *Brucella melitensis*, *Campylobacter fetus fetus*, *Salmonella* spp, border disease, and the viruses that cause bluetongue, Wesselsbron's disease and Akabane disease.

Pathology: In heavy infections, the multiplying tachyzoites may produce areas of necrosis in vital organs such as the myocardium, lungs, liver and brain. In sheep abortions, characteristically the placental intercotyledonary membranes are normal, but white foci of necrosis, approximately 2–3 mm in diameter, may be visible in the cotyledons (Fig. 3.41). Microscopically, these foci appear as areas of coagulative necrosis that are relatively free of inflammation. Inflammation, when present, is non-suppurative. *Toxoplasma* tachyzoites are seen only rarely in association with these foci, usually at the periphery of the lesion. Examination of the brain may reveal focal microgliosis. The lesions often have a small central focus of necrosis that might be mineralised. Focal leucomalacia in cerebral white matter, due to anoxia arising from placental pathology, is often present. Focal microgliosis is more specific, as leucomalacia reflects placental damage, but may occur in other conditions such as border disease or rarely ovine chlamydiosis.

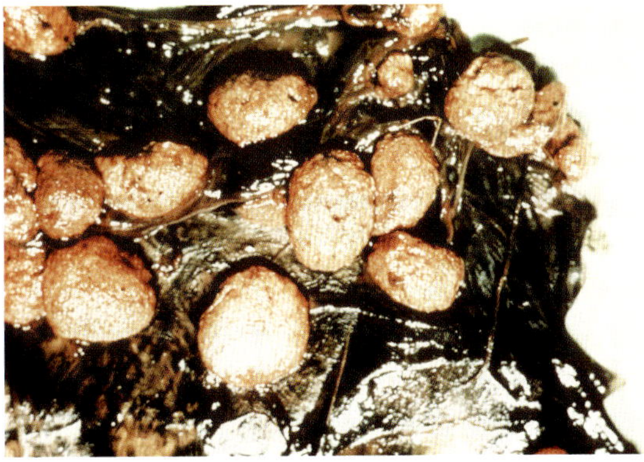

Fig. 3.41 Cotyledons of aborted placenta showing white focal lesions.

Epidemiology: The cat plays a central role in the epidemiology of toxoplasmosis and the disease is virtually absent from areas where cats do not occur. It is difficult to explain the widespread prevalence of toxoplasmosis in ruminants, particularly sheep, in view of the relatively low number of oocysts shed into the environment. It has been suggested that pregnant ewes are most commonly infected during periods of concentrate feeding prior to 'tupping' or lambing, the stored food having been contaminated with cat faeces in which millions of oocysts may be present. Further spread of oocysts may occur via coprophagous insects, which can contaminate vegetables, meat and animal fodder. It has been suggested that venereal transmission can occur in sheep.

Treatment: Not indicated

Control: On farms, control is difficult, but where possible animal feedstuffs should be covered to exclude access by cats and insects. Monensin and decoquinate have also been administered to ewes in mid-pregnancy in attempts to control abortion due to toxoplasmosis. Sheep that abort following toxoplasmosis usually lamb normally in subsequent years. It has often been advised that such sheep should be mixed with replacement stock some weeks before mating in the hope that these will become naturally infected and develop immunity before becoming pregnant. Presumably, the value of this technique depends on the replacements being exposed to circumstances similar to those of the initial outbreak. It is sometimes also advised to mix replacement stock with ewes at the time of the outbreak of abortion in order to facilitate transmission of infection. This is extremely unwise, since other causes of abortion, notably the agent of enzootic abortion of ewes, if also present, may affect the replacement stock and be responsible for abortion in subsequent years. Fortunately, a vaccine is now available for sheep, which is less of a 'hit or miss' than the above techniques. This is a live vaccine consisting of tachyzoites attenuated by repeated passage in mice. The strain used has lost the capacity to form tissue cysts and therefore the potential to form oocysts in cats. It is usually recommended to vaccinate the whole flock initially and thereafter only annual vaccination of replacements. The vaccine consists of 10^4–10^6 tachyzoites and it is given as a single dose intramuscularly at least 3 weeks prior to tupping.

PARASITES OF THE LOCOMOTORY SYSTEM

Taenia ovis

Synonym: *Cysticercus ovis*

Common name: Ovine cysticercosis, 'sheep measles'

Predilection site: Small intestine (final host); muscle (intermediate host)

Parasite class: Cestoda

Family: Taeniidae

Description: Mature cysticerci are ovoid, white and around 3.5–10 mm and contain a single protoscolex, which is invaginated and is armed with hooks and a rostellum.

Definitive hosts: Dog, fox, wild carnivores.

Intermediate hosts: Sheep, goat

Life cycle: Dogs and wild canids are infested by consuming the cysticercus in the intermediate host. The intermediate host is infected through the ingestion of tapeworm eggs that hatch in the intestine. The metacestode stage (*Cysticercus ovis*) infects the musculature and cysts are usually located in the skeletal muscle, heart, diaphragm and intermuscular connective tissue. The cyst becomes infective around 2–3 months after infection of the host. The prepatent period in dogs is around 6–9 weeks.

Geographical distribution: Worldwide.

Pathogenesis: Ovine cysticercosis is primarily important because of aesthetic objections to the appearance of the cysts in sheep meat and, in consequence, it can be a significant cause of economic loss through condemnation at meat inspection.

Clinical signs: Adult tapeworms normally induce only mild symptoms in the host and are considered to be of little pathogenic importance. Infected intermediate hosts do not usually show clinical signs of disease. Sheep can develop a strong acquired immunity to reinfection.

Diagnosis: Diagnosis in sheep and goats is through the identification of cysts at meat inspection.

Pathology: The mature, ovoid white cysticerci are grossly visible in the cardiac and skeletal musculature of sheep and goats. Commonly the cysticerci are degenerate with a green or cream, caseous or calcified centre.

Epidemiology: Ruminants are infected by grazing pasture and forages contaminated with dog or fox faeces harbouring eggs of *T. ovis*.

Treatment: No practical treatment is available for the intermediate host.

Control: Regular treatment of dogs with an effective anthelmintic will reduce contamination of the environment. Dogs should be denied access to raw sheep and goat meat and carcases. A highly protective recombinant vaccine is available in some countries.

Notes: The correct nomenclature for the intermediate host stage is the 'metacestode stage of *Taenia ovis*' rather than '*Cysticercus ovis*'.

Toxoplasma gondii

See details and description under Parasites of the reproductive/urogenital system.

Sarcocystosis

Sarcocystis is one of the most prevalent parasites of livestock. The parasites derive their name from the intramuscular cyst stage (sarcocyst) present in the intermediate (prey) host. The nomenclature used in this book incorporates the names of the **intermediate** and **final hosts** in that order. *Sarcocystis* species affecting sheep and goats are host-specific for their intermediate hosts and family-specific for their final hosts. Further general details on nomenclature, diagnosis and epidemiology are given in Chapter 2: Cattle.

There is no effective treatment for infection, either in the final or in the intermediate host. Where an outbreak occurs in sheep or goats, it has been suggested that the introduction of amprolium into the diet of the animals has a prophylactic effect. Amprolium and halofuginone (0.66 mg/kg, per os on 2 consecutive days) may be used in sheep to avoid clinical disease after infection.

The only control measures possible are those of simple hygiene. Farm dogs should not be housed in, or allowed access to, fodder stores nor should they be allowed to defecate in pens where livestock are housed. It is also important that they are not fed uncooked meat.

Sarcocystis ovicanis

Synonym: *Sarcocystis tenella, Isospora bigemina*

Predilection site: Muscle

Order: Sporozoasida

Family: Sarcocystiidae

Description: In the intermediate host the first-generation meronts found in the endothelial cells are 19–29 × 7.5–24 μm and contain 120–280 merozoites. Tissue cysts are microscopic in size (500 × 60–100 μm)

Table 3.6 *Sarcocystis* species found in the muscles of sheep.

Species	Synonym	Definitive host	Pathogenicity (sheep)	Pathogenicity (final host)
S. ovicanis	*S. tenella*	Dog	+++	0
S. ovifelis	*S. gigantea* *S. medusiformis*	Cat	0	0

0 = non-pathogenic; + = mildly pathogenic; +++ = severely pathogenic.

and are found in skeletal and cardiac muscle. The wall of the cyst appears thick (up to 2.5 μm) and radially striated with long, palisade-like protrusions without fibrils visible on electron microscopy (Fig. 3.42).

Intermediate hosts: Sheep

Final host: Dog

Life cycle: Sheep become infected by ingesting sporocysts, passed in the faeces of the dog. Once ingested there are three asexual generations. In the first, sporozoites, released from the sporocysts, invade the intestinal wall and enter the capillaries where they locate in endothelial cells in many organs and undergo two merogony cycles. A third asexual cycle occurs in the circulating lymphocytes, the resulting merozoites penetrating muscle cells. There they encyst and then divide by a process of budding or endodyogeny giving rise to broad banana-shaped bradyzoites contained within a cyst; this is the mature **sarcocyst** and is the **infective stage** for the dog final host.

Geographical distribution: Worldwide

Pathogenesis: In the sheep intermediate host, the principal pathogenic effect is attributable to the second stage of merogony in the vascular endothelium. *S. ovicanis* is highly pathogenic for lambs reportedly causing severe myositis and encephalomyelitis in lambs in several countries and has been incriminated as the cause of abortion in ewes. Generally, however, clinical signs are rarely observed in *Sarcocystis* infection and the most significant effect is the presence of cysts in the muscles resulting in downgrading or condemnation of carcases. While the dog-borne species were thought to be of primary importance in this context, there is increasing evidence that cat-borne species are also responsible for lesions in meat.

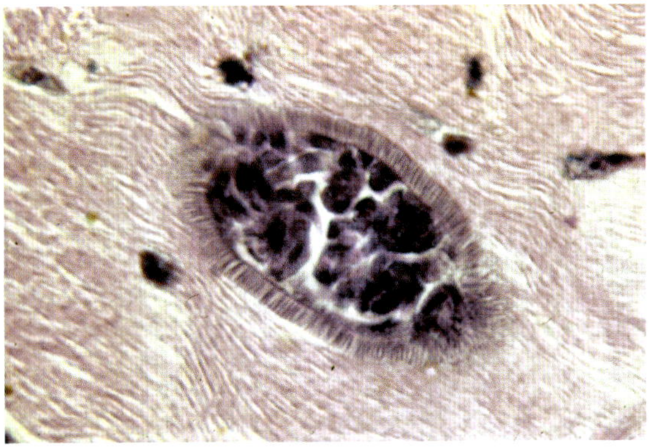

Fig. 3.42 Sarcocyst (*Sarcocystis ovicanis*) in sheep muscle.

Clinical signs: In heavy infections in sheep, there is anorexia, fever, anaemia, loss of weight, a disinclination to move and sometimes recumbency; in lambs a dog-sitting posture has been recorded. Abortions may occur in breeding stock.

Pathology: In sheep, meronts present in endothelial cells of capillaries in various organs lead to endothelial cell destruction. As the organisms enter muscle, a wide range of change may be encountered. Microscopic inspection of *Sarcocystis*-infected muscle often reveals occasional degenerate parasitic cysts surrounded by variable numbers of inflammatory cells (very few of which are eosinophils) or, at a later stage, macrophages and granulation tissue. Usually there is no muscle fibre degeneration, but there may be thin, linear collections of lymphocytes between fibres in the region. The extent of muscle change bears little relationship to the numbers of developing cysts, but generally very low numbers of *Sarcocystis* produce no reaction. As cysts mature, the cyst capsule within the enlarged muscle fibre becomes thicker and more clearly differentiated from the muscle sarcoplasm.

Sarcocystis ovifelis

Synonym: *Sarcocystis gigantea, Sarcocystis medusiformis, Isospora bigemina*

Predilection site: Muscle

Order: Sporozoasida

Family: Sarcocystiidae

Description: In sheep, the meronts found in the endothelial cells are quite small, measuring 2–8 μm in diameter. In contrast, the bradyzoite cysts can be very large and visible to the naked eye as whitish streaks running in the direction of the muscle fibres.

They have been reported as reaching several centimetres in length, but more commonly they range up to 1.5 cm × 0.2–5 mm. The cyst wall has numerous cauliflower-like protrusions 1–4.5 µm long, each containing numerous fibrils. The parasitised host cell is enclosed in connective tissue forming a secondary cyst wall.

Intermediate hosts: Sheep

Final host: Cat

Life cycle: Infection is by ingestion of the sporocysts and this is followed by a single asexual generation in capillaries and arterioles of the lung, kidney and brain, from which the resulting merozoites penetrate muscle cells. There they encyst and then divide by a process of budding or endodyogeny giving rise to broad banana-shaped bradyzoites contained within the sarcocyst. Sarcocysts are found primarily in the muscles of the oesophagus, larynx, tongue and, to a lesser extent, diaphragm and skeletal muscles. Cats are the final host.

Geographical distribution: Worldwide

Pathogenesis: Infection in the final host is normally non-pathogenic, although mild diarrhoea has occasionally been reported. Generally, however, clinical signs are rarely observed in *Sarcocystis* infection and the most significant effect is the presence of cysts in the muscles resulting in downgrading or condemnation of carcases.

Clinical signs: Infection is usually asymptomatic but may occasionally cause a febrile illness.

Pathology: In sheep, the tissue cysts may just be visible to the naked eye, especially in the oesophagus and tongue but are more likely to be detected on histopathology.

Sarcocystis capracanis

Predilection site: Muscle

Order: Sporozoasida

Family: Sarcocystiidae

Description: In goat, the tissue cysts are microscopic in size (130–800 × 50–70 µm) and are found in skeletal and cardiac muscle. The wall of the cyst appears thick (up to 2.6 µm) and radially striated with long, finger-like protrusions.

Intermediate host: Goat

Final host: Dog

Life cycle: As described for sheep species. There are three merogony cycles. Dogs, foxes and wolves are the final host.

Geographical distribution: Worldwide

Pathogenesis: In goats, the merogony stages in the vascular endothelium are pathogenic for the goat and can cause abortion and death. Generally, however, clinical signs are rarely observed in *Sarcocystis* infection and the most significant effect is the presence of cysts in the muscles resulting in downgrading or condemnation of carcases.

Clinical signs: In heavy infections in goats there is anorexia, fever, anaemia, loss of weight, a disinclination to move and sometimes recumbency. Abortions may occur in breeding stock.

Pathology: Similar to that described for *S. ovicanis* in sheep.

Sarcocystis hircicanis

Predilection site: Muscle

Order: Sporozoasida

Family: Sarcocystiidae

Description: In the goat, the tissue cysts are up to 2.5 mm in size and are found in skeletal and cardiac muscle. The wall of the cyst is thin and smooth, striated with long, hair-like protrusions.

Intermediate host: Goat

Final host: Dog

Life cycle: As for *S. capracanis*. The number of merogony stages is unknown. Dogs, foxes and wolves are the final hosts.

Geographical distribution: Europe, Asia

Pathogenesis, clinical signs, pathology: Similar to *S. capracanis*.

Sarcocystis hircifelis

Synonym: *Sarcocystis moulei*

Predilection site: Muscle

Order: Sporozoasida

Family: Sarcocystiidae

Description: The sarcocysts are elongate, compartmented and up to 12 mm in length and have a thick striated wall.

Intermediate host: Goat

Final host: Cat

Life cycle: As described for *S. capracanis*. The number of merogony stages is unknown. Cats are the final host.

Table 3.7 *Sarcocystis* species found in muscles of goats.

Species	Synonym	Definitive host	Pathogenicity (goat)	Pathogenicity (final host)
S. capracanis		Dog, coyote, wolf	+++	0
S. hircicanis		Dog, coyote, wolf	+	0
S. hircifelis	*S. moulei*	Cat	0	0

0 = non-pathogenic; + = mildly pathogenic; +++ = severely pathogenic.

Geographical distribution: Worldwide

Pathogenesis: Non-pathogenic

Clinical signs: Infection is usually asymptomatic.

PARASITES OF THE INTEGUMENT

Besnoitia besnoiti

Predilection site: Skin, conjunctiva

Order: Sporozoasida

Family: Sarcocystiidae

Description: The pseudocysts are non-septate and about 100–600 µm in diameter, with a thick wall containing thousands of merozoites but no metrocytes.

Intermediate hosts: Cattle, goats, wild ruminants (wildebeest, impala, kudu)

Final hosts: Cat, wild cats (lion, cheetah, leopard)

Geographical distribution: Worldwide, although important tropical and subtropical countries, especially in Africa

For further details on pathogenesis, diagnosis, treatment and control, see Chapter 2: Cattle.

Przhevalskiana silenis

Synonym: *Hypoderma ageratum*, *Hypoderma crossi*, *Przhevalskiana ageratum*

Common name: Goat warble

Predilection site: Subcutaneous connective tissue

Parasite class: Insecta

Family: Oestridae

Description, adults: The adult flies are 8–14 mm in length, have large eyes, a grey thorax and grey tesselated abdomen.

Description, larvae: The L_3 larvae are large (up to 25 mm in length), club-shaped, tapering towards the posterior end, with a pair of posterior spiracles. The body is composed of 11 segments with small spines at the conjunction of segments.

Hosts: Domestic goats, less commonly sheep, with gazelles as wild reservoirs over much of its range.

Life cycle: The life cycle of this species is similar in many ways to that of *Hypoderma*, the third-stage larva occurring under the skin of the back. After mating, the adult females lay about 100 black oval eggs that are about 0.8 mm in length. One to four eggs are glued on each hair. The first-stage larvae hatch from the eggs in 5–6 days and penetrate the skin into the subcutaneous tissue. The larvae then migrate in the subcutis directly to the back. However, there is no resting site as seen with *Hypoderma*. Larvae reach the subcutaneous tissue of the host's back and flanks between the end of December and the beginning of February. Here they feed, grow and moult into their second and third stages, causing the characteristic warble swelling at the skin surface. The third-stage larva may be 15–18 mm in length and dark coloured. The L_3 makes a cutaneous perforation, through which the larvae breathe by applying their spiracles to the aperture. When fully mature, in about February to April, the L_3 drops to the ground and pupates. The period required for pupation depends on weather conditions. The adults are active from April to June, lack mouthparts, and survive only 5–10 days on resources accumulated during the larval period.

Geographical distribution: Asia, the Middle East, North Africa and southern Europe

Pathogenesis: Heavy infestations can result in loss of weight, reduction in milk production; however, the chief importance of *Przhevalskiana* is in hide damage.

Clinical signs: Symptoms depend on the intensity of infestation and on the number of larvae in the subcutaneous tissue. Generally hosts are restless, reduce feeding, and significantly infested animals lose condition. Except for poor growth and decreased milk yield in cases of heavy infestation, the host animals show no appreciable signs until the larvae and characteristic 'warbles' appear at the skin surface.

Diagnosis: The presence of the larvae in swellings under the skin, detected by palpaption, allows diagnosis. Respiratory holes at the centre of each swelling, with associated reddish dried exudate may be observed. The eggs may also be found on the hairs of the animals in the summer. Serological diagnosis has been demonstrated to be effective.

Pathology: The pathology is variable and depends on the intensity of infestation. Histologically, a fibrous, thick-walled carivity is formed around the third-stage larva by granulation tissue, surrounded by a hyalinised and eosinophilic cuff. After granulocyte infiltration there may be a second infiltration by lymphocytes, plasma cells, macrophages and giant cells.

Epidemiology: Younger animals appear to be more prone to infestation than older animals. Flock prevalences of between 30 and 90% have been reported in goat herds in southern Italy and Greece, with mean intensities of about five larvae per animal.

Treatment: Organophosphate insecticides, such as trichlorophon, appear to be less effective when used to treat goat warble fly infestation than for bovine hypodermosis. However, the macrocyclic lactones, abamectin, ivermectin, doramectin, eprinomectin and moxidectin, have been shown to be highly effective against *P. silenus* infestation.

Control: A programme of a single annual treatment of macrocyclic lactone should form the basis of effective goat warble fly infestation control in areas where the disease is prevalent.

Notes: Limited geographical distribution, but locally of veterinary importance.

ECTOPARASITES

LICE

Heavy louse infestation is known as pediculosis. Blood-sucking lice have been implicated in the transmission of disease; however, lice are predominantly of importance because of the direct damage they cause. This effect is usually a function of their density. A small number of lice is very common and presents no problem. However, louse populations can increase dramatically reaching high densities. Transfer of lice from animal to animal or from herd to herd is usually by direct physical contact. Because lice do not survive for long off their host, the potential for animals to pick up infestations from dirty housing is limited, although it cannot be ignored. Occasionally, lice also may be transferred between animals by attachment to flies (phoresy).

Description: Lice have a segmented body divided into a head, thorax and abdomen. They have three pairs of jointed legs and a pair of short antennae. All lice are dorsoventrally flattened and wingless. The sensory organs are poorly developed; the eyes are vestigial or absent.

Diagnosis: The lice and their eggs may be seen within the hair and on the skin when the coat is parted. The lice may be removed and identified under a light microscope.

Pathology: The pathology of louse infestation is extremely variable. Infestations may induce alopecia, irritation, papulocrustous dermatitis and self-excoriation. Sucking lice may cause anaemia.

Epidemiology: Generally, for the transfer of louse infestation, close bodily contact is necessary. Transmission occurs when sheep are brought together as in sale yards, and especially when sheep are housed for the winter since the heavy fleece provides a habitat that is readily colonised by lice. Adult lice positioned near to the tip of the wool fibre are passed on to the new host as it brushes past an infested sheep. It takes a single infested sheep just four months to infest the entire flock. Lice populations peak in spring and lambs may be particularly susceptible to infestation.

Treatment: Several topical insecticides, such as amidine, amitraz or organophosphates (for example, chlorfenvinphos, coumaphos, chlorpyrifos, crotoxyphos, trichlorfon, phosmet and propetamphos), applied in dips or spray are effective but are becoming more limited in their availability in some countries due to safety and environmental concerns. Two treatments, 14 days apart, may be required. Topical application of the pour-on pyrethroid, cypermethrin, the spot-on deltamethrin and the insect growth regulator (IGR), triflumuron, have also been shown to be effective. The pyrethroids, which act by diffusion over the body surface in the sebum and give protection for 8–14 weeks, are probably the treatment of choice. Macrocyclic lactones (ivermectin, doramectin and moxidectin) may also be used, although they have only limited activity against chewing lice. The situation for goats is different in that few treatments have been specifically evaluated for use in goats and pour-on treatments may be less effective because of the variability in hair fibres found on different goat breeds.

Control: Louse control in sheep is generally not difficult to achieve due to the wide variety of chemical classes that are effective, although resistance has occurred in some countries. Nevertheless, in an attempt to reduce the risk of selection for resistance, rotation of chemical classes may be advantageous. A good degree of louse control can be achieved by shearing because solar radiation and dehydration reduce the hatch rate of louse eggs. Subsequently, another good management procedure is to treat sheep immediately after shearing, which ensures a greater proportion of lice come into contact with insecticide and reduces the volume of chemical necessary to achieve this. If ewes are dipped during early pregnancy, the risk that they still will be louse infested at lambing is reduced, as is the chance of lambs becoming infested. Then dipping the lambs results in the flock getting as close to louse-free as possible. The ewe lambs, when old enough to be mated, should not then be in a position to so readily infest their progeny. This could lead to a situation where treatment is necessary less frequently, assuming that there is a residual louse population as is commonly the case.

Bovicola ovis

Synonym: *Damalinia ovis*

Predilection site: The upper epidermal layers mainly on the back and upper parts of the body

Parasite class: Insecta

Parasite order: Phthiraptera

Parasite suborder: Ischnocera

Family: Trichodectidae

Description: These chewing lice are up to 3 mm long, reddish brown in colour, with a relatively large head that is as wide as the body and rounded anteriorly. The mouthparts are ventral. *Bovicola* has a three-segmented antenna and a single claw on each tarsus.

Hosts: Sheep

Life cycle: During a lifespan of about 1 month the female lays two to three operculate eggs per day. The eggs are usually whitish, and are glued to the hair where they may be seen with the naked eye. *Bovicola ovis* prefers areas close to the skin such as the back, neck and shoulder, but is highly mobile and severe infestations will spread over the whole body. It is estimated to take about 20 weeks for a population of *B. ovis* on a sheep to increase from 5000 to half a million, under favourable conditions. A nymph hatches from the egg; nymphs are similar to, although much smaller than, the adult. The nymph moults twice, at 5–9-day intervals, until eventually moulting to become an adult. The whole cycle from egg to adult takes 2–3 weeks.

The mouthparts of these lice are adapted for biting and chewing the outer layers of the hair shafts, dermal scales and blood scabs. *Bovicola ovis* is capable of rapid population expansion and this is thought to be aided by their ability to change from sexual to asexual reproduction by parthenogenesis. Hence, highly female-biased sex ratios may be common in a growing population.

Bovicola ovis is very active, roaming in the wool over the entire body. It is susceptible to high temperatures, but it is also intolerant of moisture. In a damp fleece, with a relative humidity of more than 90%, it will die in 6 hours, and when covered by water it will drown in an hour.

Geographical distribution: Worldwide

Pathogenesis: *Bovicola* may cause intense irritation, resulting in rubbing and scratching, with matting and loss of hair, involving almost the whole body in extreme cases. The scratching animal may tear or pull out the fleece and exuded serum from bite wounds may cause wool matting and discoloration. Wounds may attract blowflies. Lice reduce the quality of wool and can reduce wool production if left uncontrolled.

Clinical signs: Restlessness, rubbing and damage to the coat would suggest that lice are present, and when the hair is parted the parasites will be found. Lice appear as small yellowish specks in the hair and the small pale eggs are readily found, scattered throughout the coat.

Bovicola caprae

Synonym: *Damalinia caprae*

Common name: Red louse

Predilection site: Skin

Parasite class: Insecta

Parasite order: Phthiraptera

Parasite suborder: Ischnocera

Family: Trichodectidae

Description: These chewing lice are up to 3 mm long, reddish brown in colour. The head is relatively large, at least as wide as the body, and rounded anteriorly. The mouthparts are ventral. *Bovicola* has a three-segmented antenna and a single claw on each tarsus.

Hosts: Goat

Life cycle: See *B. ovis*.

Geographical distribution: Worldwide

Pathogenesis: See *B. ovis*

Bovicola limbata

Synonym: *Damalinia*

Common name: Red louse

Predilection site: Skin

Parasite class: Insecta

Parasite order: Phthiraptera

Parasite suborder: Ischnocera

Family: Trichodectidae

Description: These chewing lice are up to 3 mm long, reddish brown in colour. The head is relatively large, at least as wide as the body, and rounded anteriorly. The mouthparts are ventral. *Bovicola* has a three-segmented antenna and a single claw on each tarsus.

Hosts: Goat (Angora)

Life cycle: See *B. ovis*

Geographical distribution: Worldwide

Pathogenesis: See *B. ovis*

Linognathus ovillus

Common name: Long-nosed louse, sheep face louse

Predilection site: Skin, found mainly on the face

Parasite class: Insecta

Parasite order: Phthiraptera

Parasite suborder: Anoplura

Family: Linognathidae

Description: This sucking louse is blue–black with a long narrow head and slender body. It measures approximately 2.5 mm in length. Members of this family do not have eyes or ocular points. The second and third pairs of legs are larger than the first pair and end in stout claws. In species of the genus *Linognathus* the thoracic sternal plate is absent or if present is weakly developed. Paratergal plates are absent from the abdomen. The eggs are exceptional in being dark blue, and are less easy to see on hair.

Hosts: Sheep

Life cycle: Adult females lay a single egg per day. Eggs hatch in 10–15 days, giving rise to nymphs that require about 2 weeks to pass through three nymphal stages. The egg-to-adult life cycle requires about 20–40 days.

Geographical distribution: Worldwide, but particularly common in Australia and New Zealand

Pathogenesis: Lice cause sheep to rub and scratch, sometimes to the point of denuding areas of skin. Infestation by *Linognathus* spp results in a chronic dermatitis characterised by constant irritation, rubbing and biting of the fleece. Because they are blood feeders, anaemia is common where high populations of lice exist. Anaemia may predispose animals to respiratory or other diseases. *L. ovillus* is a known vector of *Eperythrozoon ovis* in sheep.

Clinical signs: *Linognathus ovillus* is manly found on the face of sheep but at high densities may spread over the entire body. Infested animals will stamp their feet or bite the infested areas. Sheep infested with lice have a ragged appearance, often with tags of wool hanging from the fleece. Newly infested sheep are very sensitive to lice. Others, which have had lice for long periods, can develop quite severe infestations but show few signs. Often lousy wool has a yellow colour due to a heavy suint and skin secretions.

Linognathus pedalis

Common name: Sheep foot louse

Predilection site: Skin, legs, belly and feet

Parasite class: Insecta

Family: Linognathidae

Description: The foot louse *Linognathus pedalis* is bluish grey, with a long pointed head and can reach up to 2 mm in length when fully engorged. This species does not have eyes or ocular points. The second and third pairs of legs are larger than the first pair and end in stout claws. The thoracic sternal plate is absent or if present is weakly developed. Paratergal plates are absent from the abdomen.

Hosts: Sheep

Life cycle: See *L. ovillus*

Geographical distribution: *L. pedalis* is common in the USA, South America, South Africa and Australasia

Pathogenesis: On the host *L. pedalis* is more sedentary than *L. ovillus* and tends to occur in aggregations in its preferred sites which are the more lightly wooled areas of the body such as the legs, belly and feet. However, at high densities both species may spread over the entire body. Infestation by *Linognathus* results in a chronic dermatitis characterised by constant irritation, rubbing and biting of the fleece. Because they are blood feeders, anaemia may occur where very high populations of lice exist. Anaemia may predispose animals to respiratory or other diseases.

Clinical signs: See *L. ovillus*. In Merinos and other heavily wooled breeds, it is usually first detected at crutching.

Epidemiology: In its normal habitat on the legs, it is exposed to great fluctuations in temperature and, having adapted to survive in these conditions, it is one of the few lice which can live away from the host's body and is viable on pasture for about a week. As a consequence of this, infestations may be picked up off contaminated pasture.

Linognathus stenopsis

Common name: Goat sucking louse

Predilection site: Skin

Parasite class: Insecta

Parasite order: Phthiraptera

Parasite suborder: Anoplura

Family: Linognathidae

Description: *Linognathus stenopsis* is up to 2 mm long when fully fed, with a long pointed head. This species does not have eyes or ocular points. The second and third pairs of legs are larger than the first pair and end in stout claws. The thoracic sternal plate is absent or if present is weakly developed. Paratergal plates are absent from the abdomen.

Hosts: Goat

Life cycle: See *L. ovillus*

Geographical distribution: Worldwide

Pathogenesis: see *L. ovillus*

MITES

The ectoparasitic mites of sheep and goats feed on blood, lymph, skin debris or sebaceous secretions, which they ingest by puncturing the skin, scavenge from the skin surface or imbibe from epidermal lesions. Most ectoparasitic mites spend their entire lives associated their host, so that transmission from host to host is primarily by physical contact. Infestation by mites is called acariasis and can result in severe dermatitis, known as mange, which may cause significant welfare problems and economic losses.

Demodex ovis

Synonym: *Demodex ariae*

Predilection site: Hair follicles and sebaceous glands, most common on the face

Parasite class: Arachnida

Sub-class: Acari

Order: Acariformes

Sub-order: Trombidiformes (Prostigmata)

Family: Demodicidae

Description: Species of *Demodex* have an elongate tapering body, up to 0.1–0.4 mm in length, with four pairs of stumpy legs ending in small blunt claws in the adult (Fig. 6.32). Setae are absent from the legs and body. The legs are located at the front of the body, and as such the striated opisthosoma forms at least half the body length.

Hosts: Sheep

Life cycle: *Demodex* spp usually live as commensals in the skin, and are highly site-specific, occupying the hair follicles and sebaceous glands. Females lay 20–24 spindle-shaped eggs in the hair follicle, and these give rise to hexapod larvae, in which each short leg ends in a single, three-pronged claw. Unusually, a second hexapod larval stage follows, in which each leg ends in a pair of three-pronged claws. Octopod protonymph, tritonymph and adult stages then follow. Immature stages and these migrate more deeply into the dermis. One follicle may harbour all life cycle stages concurrently. The life cycle is completed in 18–24 days. In each follicle or gland the mites may occur in large numbers in a characteristic head-downward posture. In the newborn and very young these sites are simple in structure, but later they become compound by outgrowths. The presence of *Demodex* mites much deeper in the dermis than sarcoptids means that they are much less accessible to surface-acting acaricides. Species of *Demodex* are unable to survive off their host.

Geographical distribution: Worldwide

Pathogenesis: This form of mange is rare in sheep and is of little economic importance, as it is confined to the face region and mild in character. Large numbers of mites may cause hide damage.

Clinical signs: Ovine demodectic mange is uncommon. Clinical signs include alopecia and scaling, especially on the face, neck and shoulders.

Diagnosis: For confirmatory diagnosis, deep scrapings are necessary to reach the mites deep in the follicles and glands. This is best achieved by taking a fold of skin, applying a drop of liquid paraffin, and scraping until capillary blood appears.

Pathology: Lesions may be papular, nodular and, rarely, pustular. The mites in sebaceous glands occasionally induce folliculitis or furunculosis.

Epidemiology: Probably because of its location deep in the dermis, it is very difficult to transmit *Demodex* between animals unless there is prolonged contact. In nature such contact only occurs during suckling, and it is thought that most infections are acquired in the early weeks of life. Transmission appears to occur during the earlier days of suckling.

Treatment: In many cases, demodecosis spontaneously resolves and treatment is unnecessary. Systemic macrocyclic lactones may be effective.

Control: Control is rarely applied.

Notes: Species of the genus *Demodex* are highly specialised mites that live in the hair follicles and sebaceous glands of a wide range of wild and domestic animals, including humans. They are believed to form a group of closely related sibling species, which are highly specific to particular hosts: *Demodex phylloides* (pig), *Demodex canis* (dog), *Demodex bovis* (cattle), *Demodex equi* (horse), *Demodex musculi* (mouse), *Demodex ratti* (rat), *Demodex caviae* (guinea-pig), *Demodex cati* (cat) and *Demodex folliculorum* and *Demodex brevis* on humans. Various morphological variations may be seen on a host, these are sometimes, probably incorrectly, ascribed separate species status.

Demodex caprae

Predilection site: Hair follicles and sebaceous glands

Parasite class: Arachnida

Sub-class: Acari

Order: Acariformes

Sub-order: Trombidiformes (Prostigmata)

Family: Demodicidae

Description: See *D. ovis*

Hosts: Goat

Life cycle: See *D. ovis*

Geographical distribution: Worldwide

Pathogenesis: The disease is similar to that in cattle. The initial lesions on the face and neck extend to the chest and flanks and may eventually involve the whole body, with the formation of cutaneous nodules of up to 20 mm in diameter containing yellowish, caseous material with large numbers of mites. This form of mange is rarely debilitating, and is of greatest importance as a cause of down-grading or condemnation of goat skins.

Clinical signs: Pea-sized nodules containing caseous material and mites, particularly on the withers, lateral neck, back and flanks. Concurrent pyoderma may occur, leading to furunculosis with ulceration and crust formation.

Diagnosis: For confirmatory diagnosis, deep scrapings are necessary to reach the mites deep in the follicles and glands. This is best achieved by taking a fold of skin, applying a drop of liquid paraffin, and scraping until capillary blood appears.

Pathology: Cutaneous nodules consist of follicular cysts lined with squamous epithelium and filled with waxy keratin squames and mites. Eruption of the cysts on to the skin may form a thick cust; rupture within the dermis may form an abcess or granulomatous reaction.

Epidemiology: Probably because of its location deep in the dermis, it is very difficult to transmit *Demodex* between animals unless there is prolonged contact. Such contact usually only occurs during suckling, and as such it is thought that most infections are acquired in the early weeks of life. The muzzle, neck, withers and back are common sites of infestation.

Treatment: In many cases, demodecosis spontaneously resolves and treatment is unnecessary. The organophosphate trichlofon, used on three occasions 2 days apart, and systemic macrocyclic lactones may be effective.

Control: Control is rarely applied.

Psoroptes ovis

Synonym: *Psoroptes communis* var *ovis*, *Psoroptes cuniculi*, *Psoroptes cervinus*, *Psoroptes bovis*, *Psoroptes equi*, *Psoroptes aucheniae*

Common name: Scab mite

Predilection site: Skin

Parasite class: Arachnida

Sub-class: Acari

Order: Acariformes

Sub-order: Sarcoptiformes (Astigmata)

Family: Psoroptidae

Description: Mites of the genus *Psoroptes* are non-burrowing mites, up to 0.75 mm in length and oval in shape (Fig. 3.43). All the legs project beyond the body margin. Its most important recognition features are the pointed mouthparts and the three-jointed pretarsi (pedicels) bearing funnel-shaped suckers (pulvilli) (Fig. 3.44). Adult females have jointed pretarsi and pulvilli on the first, second and fourth pairs of legs and long, whip-like setae on the third pair. In contrast, the smaller adult males, which are recognisable by their copulatory suckers and paired posterior lobes, have pulvilli on the first three pairs of legs and setae on the fourth pair. The legs of adult females are approximately the same length, whereas in males, the fourth pair is extremely short.

Hosts: Sheep, cattle, goat, horse, rabbit, camelids

Life cycle: The eggs of *P. ovis* are relatively large, about 250 μm in length, and oval. The hexapod larva which hatches from the egg is about 330 μm long. The larva moults into a protonymph, the protonymph moults into a tritonymph and the tritonymph moults to become an adult. Egg, larval, protonymph and tritonymph stages and the adult pre-oviposition period each require a minimum of 2 days to be completed, giving a mean egg to adult time of about 10 days.

Adult males attach to female tritonymphs, and occasionally protonymphs, and remain attached until the females moult for the final time, at which point insemination occurs.

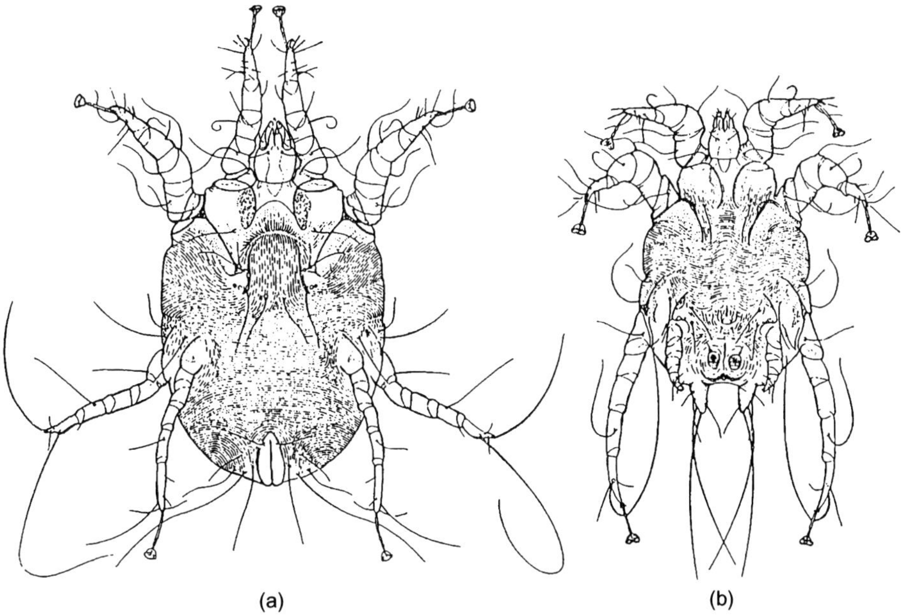

Fig. 3.43 Adult *Psoroptes ovis*, ventral views. (a) Female. (b) Male (reproduced from Baker *et al.*, 1956).

Adult females produce eggs at a rate of about 2–3 per day on average. The median life expectancy for an adult female *P. ovis* is about 16 days, during which it will have laid about 40–50 eggs. Populations of *P. ovis* on a host may therefore grow quickly doubling every 6 days or so.

Geographical distribution: Worldwide; particularly Europe and South America, but not Australia or New Zealand.

Pathogenesis: The mites are non-burrowing and feed superficially on a lipid emulsion of skin cells, bacteria and lymph on the host skin, produced as a result of a hypersensitivity reaction to the presence of antigenic mite faecal material. This hypersensitivity causes inflammation, surface exudation, scale and crust formation, with excoriation (scratching) due to self-trauma. Infestation is described as psoroptic mange or sheep scab (Fig. 3.45). The serous exudate produced in response to the mites dries on the skin to form a dry, yellow crust, surrounded by a border of inflamed skin covered in moist crust. Mites are found on the moist skin at the edge of the lesion, which extends rapidly and may take as little as 6–8 weeks to cover three quarters of the host's skin. Eventually the crust lifts off as the new fleece grows.

Infestation in sheep leads to severe pruritus, wool loss, restlessness, biting and scratching of infested areas, weight loss, reduced weight gain and in some cases, death. When handled, infested sheep may demonstrate a 'nibble reflex', characterised by lip smacking and protrusion of the tongue; others may show epileptiform fits lasting 5–10 minutes. In sheep, lesions may occur on any part of the body, but are particularly obvious on the neck, shoulders, back and flanks. In severe cases the skin may be excoriated, lichenified and secondarily infected, with numerous thick-walled abscesses of between 5 and 20 mm in diameter. Sheep scab can affect sheep of all ages but may be particularly severe in young lambs and sheep in poor condition.

The incidence of the disease varies according to season. In warm weather, mite populations may decline, leaving residual populations in sites such as the axilla, groin, infra-orbital fossa and inner surface of the pinna and auditory canal during spring, summer and early autumn. Populations of *Psoroptes* may also be found localised in the ears of sheep, causing chronic irritation, often associated with haematomas, head shaking and scratching.

Clinical signs: The earliest phase following infection is seen as a zone of inflammation with small vesicles and serous exudate. As the lesion spreads, the centre becomes dry and covered by a yellow crust while the borders, in which the mites are multiplying, are moist. Scab lesions occur most frequently around the shoulders and the back. The first visible sign is usually a patch of lighter wool, but as the area of damage enlarges, the sheep responds to the intense itching associated with mite activity by rubbing and

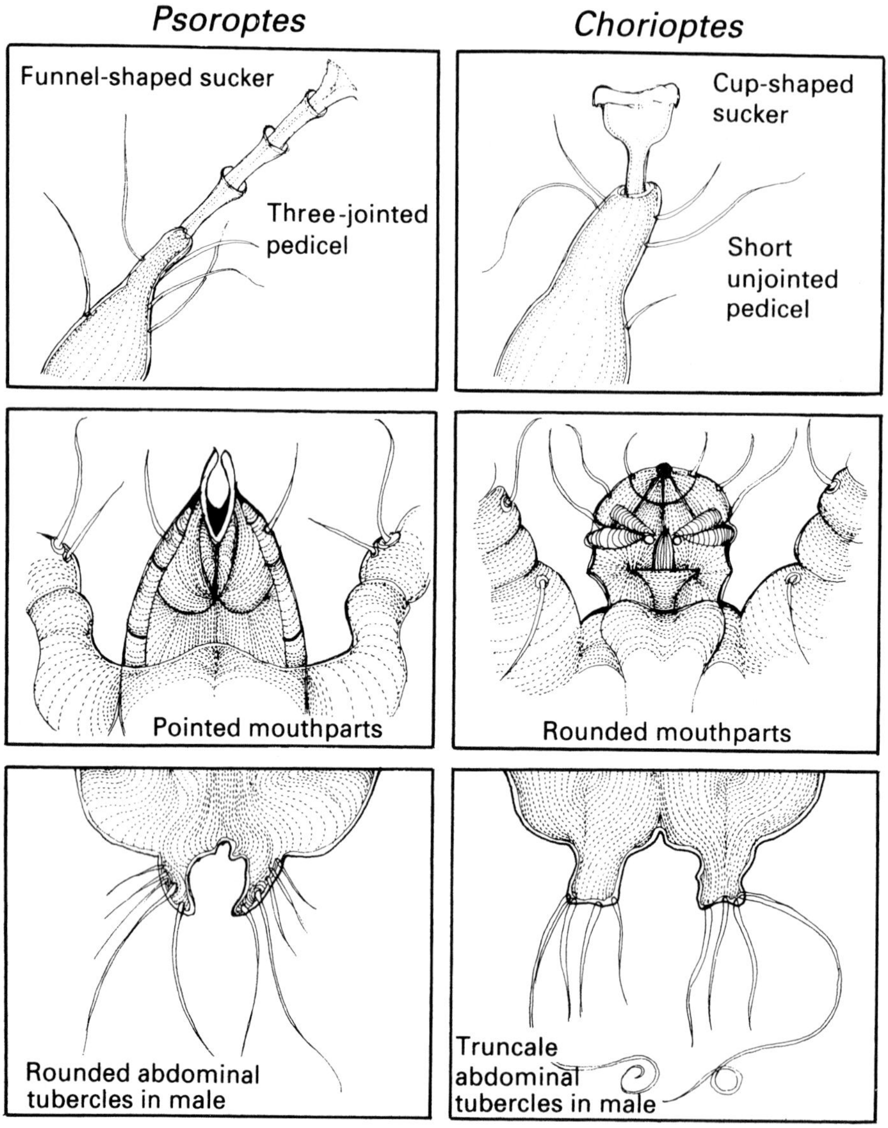

Fig. 3.44 Differential features of *Psoroptes* and *Chorioptes*.

scratching against fence posts and other objects, so that the wool becomes ragged and stained, and is shed from large areas. In addition to wool loss, the sheep may become restless and preoccupied in scratching. As a result, weight gains may be impaired in growing animals, while in adults there may be weight loss.

Diagnosis: Another non-burrowing mite, *Chorioptes*, can be common in sheep, and it is essential that this less pathogenic mite should be differentiated from the pathogenic *Psoroptes*. The important differential features are shown in Fig. 3.44. Although relatively easy to identify the active disease within a flock, the latent lesions make it more difficult to declare a flock free of infection. Particular attention should be paid to the areas in which these lesions are found. A sample may be obtained from skin scrapings taken around the lesion; this can then be examined microscopically.

Pathology: The mite faeces and its flora, shed cuticle and enzymes in the peritrophic membrane which surrounds the faecal pellets, induce a profound inflammatory response by the host. Histopathology includes

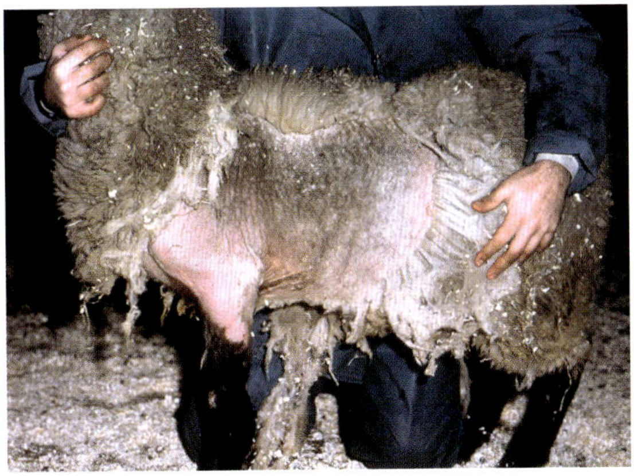

Fig. 3.45 Sheep with psoroptic mange (photograph courtesy of Dr Eduardo Berriatua).

subcorneal oesinophilic pustules, and a dermal infiltrate composed of eosinophils, neutrophils, macrophages and lymphocytes, accompanied by mast cell hyperplasia. There is pronounced dermal oedema.

Epidemiology: Transmission is primarily through physical contact and the majority of sheep become infected while the mites are active and multiplying. However, transmission may also occur via the environment. The length of time a mite can survive off its host is strongly affected by ambient temperature and humidity, but at low temperatures (<15°C) and high humidity (>75% relative humidity), survival may be in excess of 18 days, allowing transmission from housing, bedding or contaminated machinery, such as shearing equipment. Time of year may have an important impact on off-host survival. This has important implications for the potential for transmission from the environment to new hosts, transmission being considerably greater in the winter.

The period when the mite infestation has declined, either as a response to environmental conditions or the host's immune response, is also very significant in the epidemiology of the disease. Sheep that appear to be uninfested but which carry small populations of mites may be introduced to healthy flocks during summer and autumn, and subsequently initiate outbreaks.

Treatment: Although several methods of applying acaricide, such as showering, have been tested, plunge dipping is generally recommended for sheep scab control. Sheep should remain in the bath for at least 1 minute, and the head should be immersed at least twice. They should be held in clean pens before dipping and it is customary to hold them in draining pens for a time afterwards to conserve dip and assist in its proper disposal. Modern acaricides have been developed which have an affinity for wool grease, so that as a succession of sheep go through the bath the acaricide is gradually 'stripped out', and manufacturers give directions for replenishment after a specified number of sheep have been dipped.

In most countries in which control is practised, only specified acaricides are permitted for use in dips. For many years only gamma BHC (gamma hexachlorocyclohexane (HCH)), was used, but this has now been largely replaced by the organophosphates, diazinon and propetamphos, which in addition to giving the required persistence in the fleece, are rapidly detoxified and excreted from tissues. The synthetic pyrethroids, flumethrin and α-cypermethrin, have also been licensed for the control of sheep scab in some countries.

Two treatments with injectable ivermectin at 200 μg/kg and an interval of 7 days have given complete clearance of *Psoroptes ovis*. Additionally, doramectin given at 300 μg/kg or moxidectin at 200 μg/kg give control following a single injection; all are now licensed in several countries for this purpose.

Control: Because of its short population turnover period of 10 days there is very rapid spread, and it is this character which has led to legislative control in many countries since the economic consequences of uncontrolled sheep scab are serious. For example, the disease was presumed to have been eradicated from the United Kingdom in 1952, there having been no notifications of outbreaks for a number of years; it reappeared in 1973, most probably having been introduced as the quiescent phase in imported sheep and very rapidly spread to flocks throughout the UK. It was eradicated from Australia and New Zealand many years ago, but remains notifiable in these countries. Legislation in support of control is based on inspection of flocks, limitation of movement of sheep in, and from, areas in which the infection has been diagnosed, and compulsory treatment of all sheep at prescribed times.

The main source of infection of a flock is through the introduction of new animals. These must be checked over thoroughly and subjected to a quarantine period if possible.

Notes: The taxonomy of the mites in this genus is confused, with mites located in different parts of the body or on different hosts traditionally given different species names; however, little good evidence exists to support this nomenclature.

Psorergates ovis

Synonym: *Psorobia ovis*

Common name: Sheep itch mite

Predilection site: Skin, all over the body

Parasite class: Arachnida

Sub-class: Acari

Order: Acariformes

Sub-order: Trombidiformes (Prostigmata)

Family: Psorergatidae

Description: *Psorergates ovis* is a small mite, roughly circular in form and less than 0.2 mm in diameter (Fig. 3.46). The legs are arranged more or less equidistantly around the body circumference, giving the mite a crude star shape. Larvae of *P. ovis* have short, stubby legs. The legs become progressively longer during the nymphal stages until, in the adult, the legs are well developed and the mites become mobile. Adults are about 190 μm long and 160 μm wide. The tarsal claws are simple and the empodium is pad-like. The femur of each leg bears a large, inwardly directed curved spine. In the adult female, two pairs of long, whip-like setae are present posteriorly; in the male there is only a single pair.

Hosts: Sheep, particularly fine-wooled breeds such as Merino sheep

Life cycle: The life cycle is typical: egg, hexapod larva, followed by octopod protonymph, tritonymph and adult. All developmental stages occur on the host. The egg to adult life cycle requires approximately 35 days.

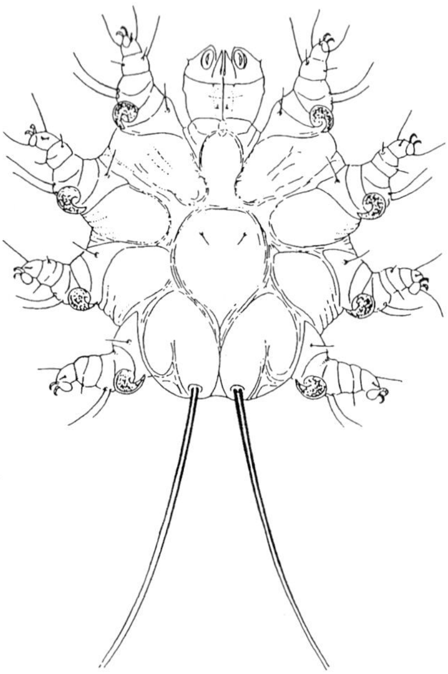

Fig. 3.46 Adult female *Psorergates* (reproduced from Baker *et al.*, 1956).

Geographical distribution: Australia, New Zealand, southern Africa, North and South America. It has not been reported in Europe.

Pathogenesis: Infection is most common in fine-wool breeds such as the Merino and Corriedale and is acquired by contact when the wool is short; as the fleece lengthens, it presents a barrier to the transfer of mites. The spread of the mite population is very slow, and infestation is rarely found in animals less than 6 months old. The animal may be 3 years or more before the whole fleece area is affected.

Though a 'non-burrowing' mite, *Psorergates* attacks the skin itself, living in the superficial layers and causing chronic irritation and skin thickening. The earliest signs are small, pale areas of wool on the shoulders, body and flanks, which gradually extend over the rest of the fleece, with irritation increasing as the mite population grows. Sheep rub, bite and chew their wool, which becomes ragged, with loose strands trailing from the sides of the body. In long-standing cases, large patches of wool may be lost. The fleece itself contains much scurf and has a slightly yellowish hue, while the staple is very dry and easily broken. Microscopically there is a hyperkeratosis and marked desquamation, with the deeper superficial layers showing round-cell infiltration and eosinophilia in the immediate vicinity of the parasite. In severe cases the whole fleece, which is difficult to shear because of its matted consistency, must be discarded. In less severely affected sheep and especially in older animals (which have become tolerant of the itch because of their thickened, damaged skin) fleeces are downgraded.

Clinical signs: These parasites are severely irritating, causing the host animal to rub and bite at their fleece. The fleece may be weakened and the wool may break easily.

Diagnosis: To obtain mites it is necessary, having clipped away a patch of wool, to apply a drop of mineral oil and scrape the skin down to the blood capillary level. The mites themselves are easily identified using a microscope. The absence of mites in a single scraping is not sufficient evidence for a negative diagnosis.

Pathology: Infection induces pruritis; light dry scabs may be present.

Epidemiology: The adult mites are spread by direct contact between hosts and are most often transferred between shorn sheep. Mites are generally found at higher densities in winter and spring. *Psorergates ovis* is very sensitive to desiccation, can only survive for 24–48 hours off the host and only the adults are mobile. As a consequence of these factors, the spread of infestation through a flock is generally slow and is most evident during the winter months.

Treatment: *Psorergates* is relatively unsusceptible to most acaricides, although the formamidine amitraz and lime–sulphur dips have been shown to be of considerable value. Otherwise, the older arsenic–sulphur preparations may be used. Macrocyclic lactones are highly effective against this species, with a single treatment usually killing all the mites.

Control: Sheep should be dipped soon after shearing. Annual dipping after shearing will suppress the mite population, keeping the infestation rate low, but rarely eradicating it completely.

Sarcoptes scabiei

Common name: Scabies

Predilection site: Skin

Parasite class: Arachnida

Sub-class: Acari

Order: Acariformes

Sub-order: Sarcoptiformes (Astigmata)

Family: Sarcoptidae

Pathogenesis, sheep: The mite, unlike the non-burrowing mites of the genus *Psoroptes*, prefers regions without wool, such as the face, ears, axillae and groin, and has a slow spread. Affected areas are at first erythematous and scurfy. The intense pruritus characteristic of sarcoptic mange is present, and sheep scratch and rub the head, body and legs against trees, posts and walls. Because of the itch, sheep are almost continuously restless and are unable to graze, so that there is progressive emaciation. In haired sheep the whole body may be affected. Sarcoptic mange has a wide geographic distribution in many sheep-raising areas of the world, such as the Middle East. In Africa it occurs in the local breeds of haired sheep and, because of hide damage, is of considerable economic importance, more than a million sheepskins being exported from the region annually. Sarcoptic mange of sheep in Britain has not been encountered for more than 30 years.

Pathogenesis, goats: This form of mange in goats is worldwide in distribution, but is of greatest economic importance in areas where the goat is the basic domestic ruminant such as India and West Africa. In goats the condition is often chronic, and may have been present simply as 'skin disease' for many months before definitive diagnosis has been made. As in other sarcoptic infections the main signs are irritation with encrustations, loss of hair and excoriation from rubbing and scratching. In long-standing cases the skin becomes thickened and nodules may develop on the less well haired parts of the skin, including the muzzle, around the eyes, and inside the ears.

Treatment: In sheep, treatment and control are similar to those described for the more common psoroptic mange. In goats, repeated treatment is often necessary, sometimes over several months in long-standing cases. The acaricide which has been most widely used is gamma HCH, and where this is no longer available there may be problems obtaining a suitable drug licensed for use in goats. Although not licensed for the treatment of milking goats, a single injection of systemic macrocyclic lactone may be effective. Corticosteroid therapy has been reported to aid recovery as it suppresses the pruritus.

For further details see Chapter 5 (Pigs).

Chorioptes bovis

Synonym: *Chorioptes ovis*, *Chorioptes equi*, *Chorioptes caprae*, *Chorioptes cuniculi*

Predilection site: Skin, particularly the legs, feet, base of tail and upper rear surface of the udder

Parasite class: Arachnida

Sub-class: Acari

Order: Acariformes

Sub-order: Sarcoptiformes (Astigmata)

Family: Psoroptidae

Hosts: Cattle, sheep, horse, goat, rabbit

Pathogenesis: In sheep, the mites are found mainly on the legs and feet and, though very common, little harm is caused (Fig. 3.44). When clinical cases do occur, they are typically in the form of foot mange, affecting the forefeet. The mites cluster about the accessory digits and along the coronary border of the outer claws, causing crusting below the accessory digits and in the interdigital spaces. Lambs are thought to become infected by contact with the legs of the ewe. In some cases there may be spread from the limbs to the face and other regions and, in occasional severe cases, pustular dermatitis (with wrinkling and thickening of the skin) may occur.

It has been noted in New Zealand that when the mange spreads to the scrotum the thickened and inflamed skin allows the scrotal temperature to remain high with, as a result, testicular atrophy and cessation of spermatogenesis. Infected rams have impaired reproductive ability or sterility, though their general health is not affected. The condition is not irreversible; semen production and fertility return to normal after successful mange treatment. Prevalence of leg and scrotal mange is usually highest in the autumn and winter months, and declines in spring.

In goats, the mites occur mostly on the forefeet around the accessory digits and claws. However, they may also occur higher on the foot and on the pastern. The lesions produced are relatively mild. Infestation rates of *C. bovis* tend to be higher in goats than sheep, with up to 80–90% of goats in individual herds being parasitised.

Treatment: Chorioptic mange in sheep is easily treated by dipping or by local treatment with a suitable acaricide. Macrocyclic lactones are an effective treatment against chorioptic mange. Crotoxyphos (0.25%) applied as a spray can also be used to treat infestations.

In goats, a suitable acaricidal wash, scrubbed on to the lesions on two occasions, 14 days apart, is effective.

Notes: The names *Chorioptes ovis*, *Chorioptes equi*, *Chorioptes caprae* and *Chorioptes cuniculi* used to describe the chorioptic mites found on sheep, horses, goats and rabbits respectively, are now all thought to be synonyms of *Chorioptes bovis*.

For further details see Chapter 2 (Cattle).

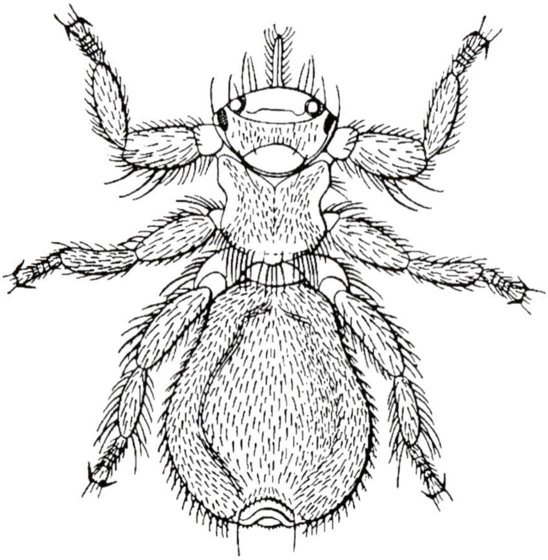

Fig. 3.47 Adult sheep ked, *Melophagus ovinus*.

FLIES

Melophagus ovinus

Common name: Sheep ked

Predilection site: Skin on the neck, shoulders and belly

Parasite class: Insecta

Family: Hippoboscidae

Description, adult: Hairy, brown, wingless, 'degenerate' fly, approximately 5.0–8.0 mm long with a short head and broad, dorsoventrally flattened, brownish thorax and abdomen (Figs 3.47, 3.48). The abdomen is indistinctly segmented and is generally soft and leathery. Both sexes are completely wingless and even the halteres are absent. They have piercing blood-sucking mouthparts and strong legs provided with claws that enable them to cling onto wool and hair.

Hosts: Sheep

Life cycle: Keds are permanent ectoparasites and live for several months feeding on the blood of sheep and sometimes goats. A single egg is ovulated at a time. The egg hatches inside the body of the female and the larva is retained and nourished within the female during its three larval stages, until it is fully developed. The mature larvae produced by the females adhere to the wool. These are immobile and pupate immediately. The 3.0–4.0 mm long brown puparia are easily visible on the fleece. The pupae are fully formed within 12 hours of larviposition and are resistant to treatment. Adult keds emerge in approximately 3 weeks in summer, but this period may be extended considerably during winter. Copulation occurs 3–4 days after emergence, and females are able to produce offspring 14 days after emergence. Although one mating provides sufficient sperm for a lifetime, repeated matings usually occur when multiple males are present. A female produces between 10 and 20 larvae in its lifetime. Ked populations build up slowly since each female produces only one larva every 10–12 days. Adults can only live for short periods off their hosts.

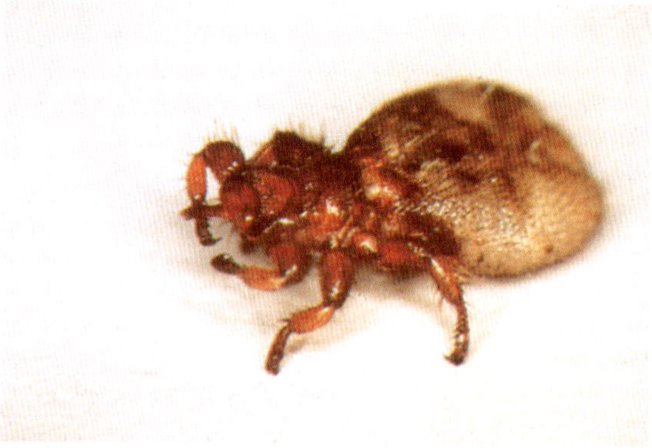

Fig. 3.48 The sheep ked *Melophagus ovinus*.

Geographical distribution: Worldwide, but most common in temperate areas

Pathogenesis: Since keds suck blood, heavy infections may lead to loss of condition and anaemia. Inflammation leads to pruritus, biting, rubbing, wool loss and a vertical ridging of the skin known as 'cockle'. *Melophagus ovinus* is also responsible for an allergic dermatitis in sheep characterised by small nodules on the grain layer of the skin, reduced weight gain and darkened patches at the affected site. They are spread by contact and long-wooled breeds appear to be particularly susceptible.

Melophagus ovinus is the vector of the non-pathogenic *Trypanosoma melophagium*. If the sheep eats a ked the metacyclic stages may penetrate the buccal mucosa.

Clinical signs: Intense irritation from infestation causes sheep to rub, bite and scratch themselves, tearing the fleece. Heavy infestation may cause anaemia. The piercing mouthparts of keds create open wounds susceptible to further bacterial and parasitic infections. The faeces of the keds produce stains in the coat that do not wash out readily.

Diagnosis: Adults and pupae may be seen on the host animal, most frequently around the ribs.

Epidemiology: Keds are permanent ectoparasites. The spread of sheep keds is largely through contact, and the movement of keds from ewes to lambs is an important route of infestation. Within a flock, transfer occurs when sheep keds move to the tips of the fleece in response to increasing air temperature. Air temperature must usually be 21°C or above before many keds are observed on the surface of the fleece. Consequently, transfer between animals is more likely, and occurs more rapidly, in summer than in winter. Sheep with dense, long or clotted fleeces are more likely to spread the infection because the keds come to the surface of such fleeces. Heavy infestations of keds are most commonly seen in autumn and winter. Poorly fed animals or those that are not sufficiently protected against cold weather are most liable to suffer from keds, and the parasites are particularly common towards the end of winter.

Treatment: Organophosphates and pyrethroids applied as dips, sprays or pour-on formulations are highly effective at treating *M. ovinus* infestations. Pupae are resistant to treatment but shearing removes pupae and adults.

Control: Specific measures are rarely undertaken, since the routine use of insecticides for the control of blowflies and ticks usually also results in the efficient control of keds.

Notes: The sheep ked is of considerable economic importance and is generally regarded as one of the most damaging ectoparasites of sheep in North America. The overall losses in the USA due to keds have been estimated to be about US$40 million per year.

FLY STRIKE (MYIASIS)

Myiasis is the infestation of the organs or tissues of host animals by the larval stages of dipterous flies, usually known as maggots or grubs. The fly larvae feed directly on the host's necrotic or living tissue. A small number of species are obligate ectoparasites and must have a living host to complete their development. The majority, however are facultative parasites and these can develop in both living and dead organic matter. The facultative species can be subdivided into primary and secondary facultative species. The primary species usually adopt an ectoparasitic habit and are capable of initiating myiasis, but may occasionally live as saprophages in decaying organic matter and animal carcases. The secondary facultative ectoparasites normally live as saprophages and usually cannot initiate a myiasis; they may secondarily invade pre-existing infestations. The three obligate species of myiasis fly are dealt with in Chapter 11.

Clinical signs: Infestations resulting from small numbers of larvae may be tolerated well by sheep; nothing can be seen until the fleece is parted, revealing the damaged skin and the larvae. Heavily affected sheep are anorexic, appear dull and usually stand away from the main flock. The fleece in the affected area is darker, has a damp appearance and a foul odour.

Diagnosis: This is based on the clinical signs and recognition of maggots in the lesion.

Treatment: Once the problem is diagnosed, all affected sheep should be separated and the area surrounding the lesion clipped. Where possible larvae should be removed and killed; larvare that are more that 24 hours old that are allowed to drop from the lesion will survive and subsequently emerge as adults. The lesion should be dressed with a suitable preparation of dilute insecticide, such as diazinon, cypermethrin or deltamethrin.

Control: This has been based largely on the prophylactic treatment of sheep with insecticides. The problems associated with this are the relatively short period spent by the larvae on the sheep, the repeated infestations (which occur throughout the season) and the rapidity with which severe damage occurs. Any insecticide used must therefore not only kill the larvae, but also persist in the fleece. Organophosphorous and pyrethroids insecticides may give effective protection for up to 10 weeks. Application of these insecticides is made by hand spraying, plunge dipping, in a spray race or by jetting. In the northern hemisphere, two annual treatments, usually in May and August should give protection for the whole of the fly season. The insect growth inhibitors, cyromazine and dicyclanil, give excellent protection for 8 or 12 weeks respectively after a single application. However, these chemicals must be applied as a pour-on before an anticipated challenge.

Other measures that should be taken to aid control are the prevention of diarrhoea by effective worm control and the removal of excess wool from the groin and perineal area to prevent soiling, a technique known as crutching. Shearing reduces strike risk in ewes and the docking of lamb tails will also significantly reduce the risk of breech strike. Appropriate disposal of carcases, which otherwise offer an excellent alternative breeding place for blowflies, is also recommended.

Lucilia

Description, adults: *Lucilia* blowflies measure up to 10 mm in length and are characterised by a metallic greenish to bronze sheen (Fig. 3.49). The adults are characterised by the presence of a bare stem-vein, bare squamae and the presence of three pairs of postsutural, dorso-central bristles on the thorax. The sexes are very similar in appearance, but may be distinguished by the distance between the eyes, which are almost touching anteriorly in males and separated in females.

Adult *Lucilia sericata* and *L. cuprina* may be distinguished from most other species of *Lucilia* by the presence of a pale creamy-white basicostal scale at the base of the wing, three postsutural acrostichal bristles on the thorax and one anterio-dorsal bristle on the tibia of the middle leg. However, definitive identification to species can only be confirmed using a small number of subtle morphological features, such as the colour of the fore femur, the number of paravertical setae present on the back of the head and, most reliably, the shape of the male genitalia.

Larvae: Larvae are smooth, segmented and measure 10–14 mm in length. They possess a pair of oral hooks at the anterior extremity, and, at the posterior, peritremes bearing spiracles (Fig. 3.50).

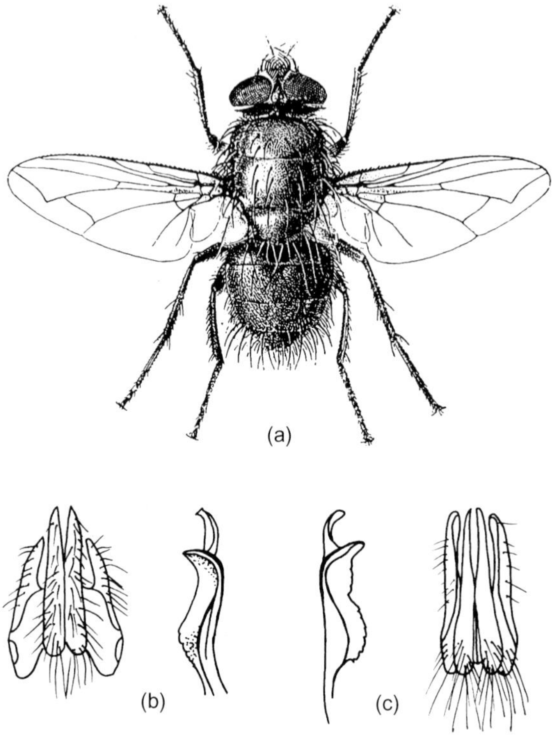

Fig 3.49 (a) Adult *Lucilia sericata* (reproduced from Shtakelbergh, 1956). Male genitalia (aedeagus in lateral view and forceps in dorsal view) of (b) *Lucilia sericata* and (c) *Lucilia cuprina* (reproduced from Aubertin, 1933).

Hosts: Mainly sheep, but a range of other domestic and wild animals may be affected including humans.

Life cycle: *Lucilia* are anautogenous and females must obtain a protein meal before maturing their eggs. When protein is freely available the gravid female blowfly lays clusters of 225–250 yellowish cream eggs on wounds, soiled fleece or dead animals, attracted by the odour of the decomposing matter. The eggs of *Lucilia* hatch into larvae in about 12 hours. The larvae then feed, grow rapidly and moult twice to

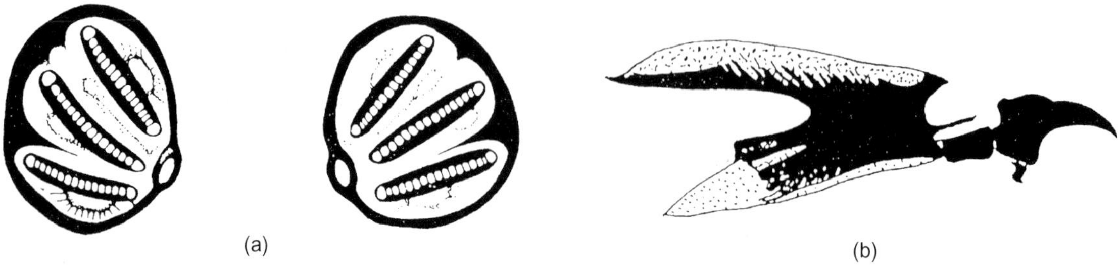

Fig. 3.50 *Lucilia sericata.* (a) Posterior peritremes. (b) Cephalopharyngeal skeleton (reproduced from Zumpt, 1965).

become fully mature maggots in 3 days. The larvae usually feed superficially on the epidermis and lymphatic exudates, or on necrotic tissue. They will only begin to feed on healthy tissue in crowded conditions. The mouth hooks are used to macerate the tissues, and digestion occurs extra-orally by means of amylase in the saliva and proteolytic enzymes in the larval excreta. Mature larvae drop to the ground and pupate. The pupal stage is completed in 3–7 days in summer. Adult flies can live for about 7 days. The time required to complete the life cycle from egg to adult is highly dependent on the ambient temperature but is usually between 2 and 6 weeks.

Pathogenesis: Two species, *L. sericata* and *L. cuprina*, are important primary factulative agents of myiasis. Other species of *Lucilia* may be occasional or secondary invaders of established myiases. After the eggs are deposited on the wool, the larvae emerge and crawl down the wool on to the skin. They secrete proteolytic enzymes, which digest and liquefy the tissues. Second- and third-stage larvae may also abrade the skin with their mouth hooks.

Infestations resulting from a single batch of eggs may be tolerated well by sheep, produce few clinical signs and be difficult to detect without detailed examination. When the larvae cease feeding and leave the host, the lesions created by such small infestations heal well and usually without complications (Fig. 3.51).

However, the odour of an existing infestation may attract more blowflies and induce further oviposition; the high humidity at an active strike lesion may also enhance egg and larval survival. Hence, once infested, sheep become far more likely to receive multiple strikes. At the initial lesion site there may be alopecia and underlying scar tissue formation, while the lesion spreads from its margins as further ovipositions occur and waves of larvae feed under the surrounding wool. The irritation and distress caused by the expanding lesion is extremely debilitating and sheep can rapidly lose condition.

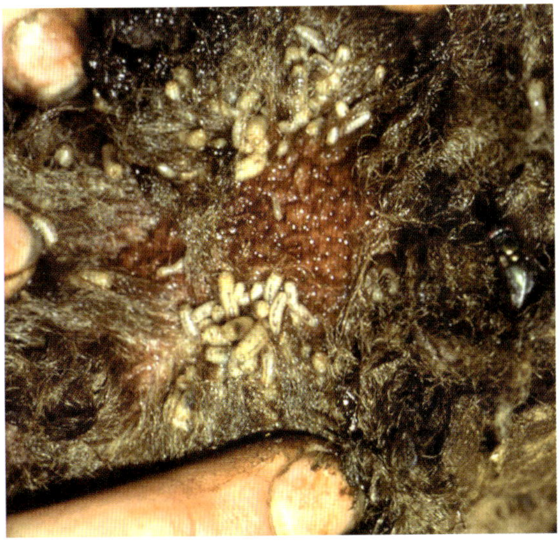

Fig. 3.51 Blowfly strike of sheep by larvae of *Lucilia sericata*.

Pathology: Sheep struck by *Lucilia* show a rapid increase in body temperature and respiratory rate. The animals become anaemic and suffer severe toxaemia, with both kidney and heart tissues affected. The feeding activity of the larvae may cause extensive tissue damage which, in combination with the larval proteases produced, results in the development of inflamed, abraded or undermined areas of skin. Infested animals become lethargic, appear depressed and cease feeeding, resulting in loss of weight and anorexia. If untreated, multiple infestation rapidly leads to death from toxaemia, usually within about 2 weeks of the initial infestation, although the precise time required will depend on the intensity of infestation.

Epidemiology: The epidemiology of cutaneous myiasis in sheep depends on factors that affect the prevalence of blowflies and those which affect host susceptibility. The three principal factors are:

1. Temperature. High ambient temperatures allow elevated levels of fly activity and, provided the relative humidity is also high, favour the creation of suitable areas of microclimate in the fleece that attract the adult flies to lay their eggs. In temperate areas, the rising temperatures of late spring allow overwintering larvae to complete their development and the first wave of adult blowflies to emerge. Ambient temperature then determines the number of generations and, hence, the maximum abundance of flies over the summer.
2. Rainfall. Persistent rain can make the fleece more attractive to the adult female flies, stimulate oviposition and increase the survival of the eggs and first-stage larvae, which require areas of high humidity in the wool to persist.
3. Host susceptibility. This is increased where putrefactive odours, often resulting from the bacterial decomposition of organic matter, develop in the fleece. The commonest causes of this are soiling of the hindquarters due to diarrhoea, bacterial fleece rot and injuries due to fighting, especially on the head in rams. Long fleece, long tails and wrinkled skin folds in some breeds, may also increase host susceptibility. Foot rot, caused by two anaerobic, Gram-negative bacteria, *Bacteroides nodosus* and *Fusobacterium necrophorum*, is also an important predisposing factor leading to foot strike.

Lucilia sericata

Synonym: *Phaenicia sericata*

Common name: Greenbottle, sheep blowfly

Predilection site: Skin, skin wounds

Parasite class: Insecta

Family: Calliphoridae

Geographical distribution: Worldwide. Originally *Lucilia sericata* was probably endemic to the Palaearctic. However, as a result of natural patterns of movement and artificial dispersal by humans and livestock in the past few hundred years the species is now found worldwide. *L. sericata* is more common in cool–temperate habitats, such as Europe, and is often replaced by the closely related *Lucilia cuprina* in warm–temperate and subtropical habitats.

Pathogenesis: Blowfly strike by *L. sericata* occurs most commonly in the perineal and tail head region and is strongly associated with the accumulation of faeces in wool around the anus and tail (Fig. 3.51). There is little recorded involvement of dermatitis in predisposing sheep to strike by *L. sericata* in northern Europe. Following initial strike by *L. sericata* secondary blowfly species may also invade the site of infestation. These secondary invaders include other species of *Lucilia*, *Calliphora* spp and, in some regions, *Chrysomya* spp.

Lucilia sericata adults may act as passive vectors of *Mycobacterium avium* subsp. *avium*, *M. a. paratuberculosis* and *M. a. hominissuis*.

Epidemiology: The risk of myiasis by *L. sericata* has been shown to increase with increasing flock size and stocking density, and to decrease with increasing farm altitude. Initially in spring, unshorn adults may be most at risk. Immediately following shearing the risk of strike in adult sheep is considerably reduced. However, the susceptibility of strike in lambs increases, peaking in late summer as their fleeces grow and as populations of pasture nematodes increase, against which they have no acquired immunity, and lead to diarrhoea and faecal soiling. In temperate areas under summer conditions, up to four generations may develop per year. In these areas, the final generation overwinters in the soil as larvae, to emerge as adults in the following spring. The precise timing of spring emergence and the growth of the population is highly temperature dependent. In warmer climates the number of generations per annum is greater and up to nine or ten have been recorded in southern Africa and Australia. The period of risk is more prolonged in warm, moist weather.

Notes: *Lucilia sericata* is the most important agent of sheep myiasis throughout northern Europe and was first recorded as an ectoparasite in England in the fifteenth century. *Lucilia sericata* arrived in New Zealand over 100 years ago and soon established itself as the primary myiasis fly in the country, occurring in 75% of all cases of sheep strike. However, now *L. cuprina* appears to be displacing *L. sericata* to become the most important primary cause of fly strike in sheep in New Zealand.

Lucilia cuprina

Synonym: *Phaenicia cuprina*, *Phaenicia pallescens*

Common name: Greenbottle, Australian sheep blowfly

Predilection site: Skin wounds

Parasite class: Insecta

Family: Calliphoridae

Geographical distribution: It is thought that the original distribution of *Lucilia cuprina* may have been either Afrotropical or Oriental. However, as a result of natural patterns of movement and artificial dispersal by humans and livestock in the past few hundred years, the species is now found worldwide, although in general *L. cuprina* occurs in warm–temperate and subtropical habitats. There are believed to be two sub-species: *L.c. cuprina* is distributed throughout the Neotropical, Oriental and southern Nearctic regions, while *L.c. dorsalis* is found throughout the sub-Saharan, Afrotropical and Australasian regions. However, the two sub-species interbreed readily in the laboratory and intermediate forms are believed to be common. The simple division into two sub-species is, therefore, certainly an oversimplification of the complex pattern of genetic variation that occurs between populations of *L. cuprina*.

Pathogenesis: In Australia and New Zealand, body strike caused by *L. cuprina* is frequently the main form of myiasis. Body strike occurs most commonly around the shoulders and back region and is frequently associated with the incidence of bacterial dermatophilosis caused by the bacterium *Dermatophilus congolensis*. Body strike in Australasia is also often associated with bacterial fleece rot; a superficial dermatitis induced by moisture and proliferation of the bacteria *Pseudomonas aeruginosa* on the skin, resulting in a matted band of discoloured fleece. It is possible that dermatophilosis and fleece rot act synergistically in attracting blowflies and their subsequent oviposition. However, where the Merino breed is prevalent, breech and tail strike may also be common due to the conformation of this breed and the wrinkled skin in the breech area that favours the accumulation of urine and faeces.

Following initial strike by *Lucilia cuprina* a variety of secondary species may also invade the site of infestation. They frequently extend the injury rendering the strike one of great severity. These secondary invaders include *Calliphora* spp and *Chrysomya* spp.

Lucilia cuprina is suspected of spreading diseases such as gastroenteritis and anthrax among host animals.

Epidemiology: In warmer parts of its range nine or ten generations per year have been recorded and *L. cuprina* may be active all year round in some parts of its range.

Notes: *Lucilia cuprina* is absent from most of Europe, although it has been recorded from southern Spain and north Africa. *Lucilia cuprina* was probably introduced into Australia towards the middle or end of the nineteenth century and it is now the dominant sheep myiasis species for mainland Australia and Tasmania, present in 90–99% of flystrike cases. In the early 1980s *L. cuprina* was discovered in New Zealand and was most probably introduced from Australia. Now, despite its low abundance, in northern areas of New Zealand it appears to be displacing *L. sericata* to become the most important primary cause of flystrike in sheep.

Lucilia cuprina In is also the primary myiasis fly of sheep in southern Africa. Although this species had been known in South Africa since 1830, little sheep strike was recorded until the early decades of the twentieth century, possibly as a result of the introduction of more susceptible Merino breeds or changes in husbandry practices.

In North America, *L. cuprina* (syn. *Phaenicia cuprina*, *Phaenicia pallescens*) is known to be present, although it does not appear to be important in sheep myiasis.

Calliphora

Description: The larvae are smooth, segmented and measure 10–14 mm in length. They possess a pair of oral hooks at the anterior extremity, spiracles on the anterior segment and, posteriorly, spiracular plates. The arrangement of the posterior spiracles on these plates serves to differentiate the species.

Hosts: Mainly sheep, but any other animal may be affected.

Life cycle: Flies oviposit primarily in carrion, but also may act as secondary invaders of myiases on live mammals. The gravid female lays clusters of 100–200 yellowish cream eggs. The eggs hatch into larvae and the larvae then feed, grow rapidly and moult twice to become fully mature maggots. When they have completed feeding, third-stage larvae migrate to the ground and pupate. Following pupation the adult female fly must obtain a protein meal and mate.

Pathogenesis: When involved in myiasis, secondary blowflies are attracted by the odour of the infestation, and their larvae extend and deepen the lesion. The irritation and distress caused by the lesion is extremely debilitating and the host animal can rapidly lose condition. The latter is often the first obvious sign of strike as the lesion occurs at the skin surface and is sometimes observed only on close examination.

Epidemiology: Secondary flies usually follow an initial strike by a primary fly such as *Lucilia cuprina* and invade the site of infestation. They frequently extend the injury rendering the strike one of great severity.

Clinical signs, diagnosis, pathology, epidemiology, treatment and control as for *Lucilia*.

Calliphora augur

Common name: The lesser brown blowfly, blue-bodied blowfly

Predilection site: Skin wounds

Parasite class: Insecta

Family: Calliphoridae

Description: The adult *Calliphora augur* is predominantly brown or brown–yellow in colour with a patch of metallic blue on the medial abdomen. The adult body is approximately 11 mm in length.

Geographical distribution: Australasia; mainly eastern Australia

Pathogenesis: It breeds mostly in carcases but will lay into wounds. As a result *Calliphora augur* is an important native Australasian species found as a secondary or tertiary invader of sheep strikes in the Australasian region.

Calliphora albifrontalis

Synonym: *Calliphora australis*

Common name: Western Australian brown blowfly

Predilection site: Skin wounds

Parasite class: Insecta

Family: Calliphoridae

Description: In the adult *Calliphora albifrontalis* the thorax is non-metallic blue–black in colour but the abdomen is predominantly brown or brown–yellow.

Geographical distribution: Australasia

Pathogenesis: *Calliphora albifrontalis* is an important native Australasian species found as a secondary or tertiary invader of sheep strikes in the Australasian region. In Western Australia *C. albifrontalis* may be responsible for up to 10% of single-species strikes.

Calliphora nociva

Synonym: *Calliphora dubia*

Common name: Lesser brown blowfly

Predilection site: Skin wounds

Parasite class: Insecta

Family: Calliphoridae

Description: The adult *Calliphora nociva* is predominantly brown or brown–yellow in colour and closely resembles *C. augur* except for the colour patch on the abdomen, which is a much brighter blue on *C. nociva* than on *C. augur*. *C. nociva* displaces *C. augur* in Western Australia.

Geographical distribution: Australasia, mainly Western Australia

Pathogenesis: *Calliphora nociva* is an important native Australasian species found as a secondary or tertiary invader of sheep strikes in the Australasian region.

Calliphora stygia

Synonym: *Pollenia stygia, Calliphora laemica*

Common name: Eastern golden haired blowfly

Predilection site: Skin wounds

Parasite class: Insecta

Family: Calliphoridae

Description: The adult *Calliphora stygia* is a large native Australasian blowfly with a grey thorax and yellow–brown mottled abdomen. It is one of the earliest flies to visit a corpse and will also feed on living sheep, causing fly strike.

Geographical distribution: Australasia

Pathogenesis: *Calliphora stygia* is a common secondary invader of ovine myiasis, present in strikes from October to May.

Epidemiology: *Calliphora stygia* is adapted to cooler conditions than other flies and occurs in largest numbers in spring and autumn, but may be found on sunny days in winter as well. This adaptation to the cold gives it an advantage on carrion during the cooler months, and in spring in particular many thousands of these flies can develop from carcases. In summer, high temperatures and competition from species such as *Chrysomya rufifacies* reduce its abundance and *C. stygia* becomes scarce. In Western Australia, *C. stygia* is displaced by the very similar *Calliphora albifrontalis*.

Calliphora vicina

Synonym: *Calliphora erythrocephala*

Common name: Bluebottle

Predilection site: Skin wounds

Parasite class: Insecta

Family: Calliphoridae

Description: Bluebottles are stout and characterised by a metallic blue sheen on the body. The thoracic squamae have long dark hair on the upper surface. *Calliphora vicina* and *C. vomitoria* may be distinguished from each other by the presence of yellow–orange jowls with black hairs in the former and black jowls with predominantly reddish hairs in the latter.

Geographical distribution: Worldwide

Pathogenesis: In addition to acting as a secondary invader of myiases, *C. vicina* has also been recorded laying eggs on living small mammals. Attempts to induce primary sheep strike by *C. vicina* have proved unsuccessful and it has been suggested that this species may be physiologically unable to infest sound sheep, either because the sheep body temperature is fatally high or because larvae are unable to feed on the animal tissues without the prior activity of *Lucilia* larvae.

Calliphora vomitoria

Common name: Bluebottle

Predilection site: Skin wounds

Parasite class: Insecta

Family: Calliphoridae

Description: Bluebottles are stout and characterised by a metallic blue sheen on the body (Fig. 3.52). The thoracic squamae have long dark hair on the upper surface. *Calliphora vicina* and *C. vomitoria* may be distinguished from each other by the presence of yellow–orange jowls with black hairs in the former and black jowls with predominantly reddish hairs in the latter.

Geographical distribution: Worldwide

Phormia regina

Common name: Blackbottle, black blowfly

Predilection site: Skin wounds

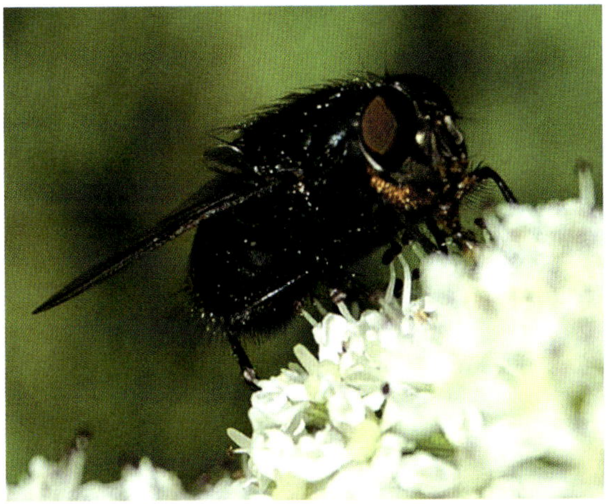

Fig. 3.52 The bluebottle *Calliphora vomitoria*.

Parasite class: Insecta

Family: Calliphoridae

Description, adults: *Phormia regina* is a black-coloured blowfly, with an overlying metallic blue–green coloured sheen. This species is very similar to *Protophormia terraenovae* in appearance. In *P. terraenovae* the anterior thoracic spiracle is black or black–brown and is difficult to distinguish from the general body colour. In contrast, in *Phormia regina* the anterior spiracle is yellow or orange and stands out clearly against the dark background colour of the thorax (Fig. 3.53).

Description, larvae: The third-stage larvae of both *P. terraenovae* and *P. regina* are characterised by strongly developed, fairly pointed tubercles on the posterior face of the last segment. In third-stage larvae of *P. terraenovae* the tubercles on the upper margin of the last segment are longer than those of *P. regina*, being longer than half the width of a posterior spiracle, whereas in *P. regina* they are less than half the width of a posterior spiracle in length. The larvae of *P. terraenovae* also possess dorsal spines on the posterior margins of segment 10, which are absent in larvae of *P. regina*.

Hosts: Mainly sheep, but any other mammals and birds may be affected.

Life cycle: Flies oviposit primarily in carrion, but also may act as secondary invaders of myiases on live mammals. The gravid female lays clusters of 100–200 yellowish cream eggs. The eggs hatch into larvae; the larvae then feed, grow rapidly and moult twice to become fully mature maggots. These then migrate to the ground and pupate. Following pupation the adult female fly must obtain a protein meal and mate. Adult flies can live for approximately 30 days.

Geographical distribution: Northern Canada, USA, Europe, Scandinavia, Russia

Protophormia terraenovae

Synonym: *Phormia terraenovae*

Common name: Blackbottle

Predilection site: Skin wounds

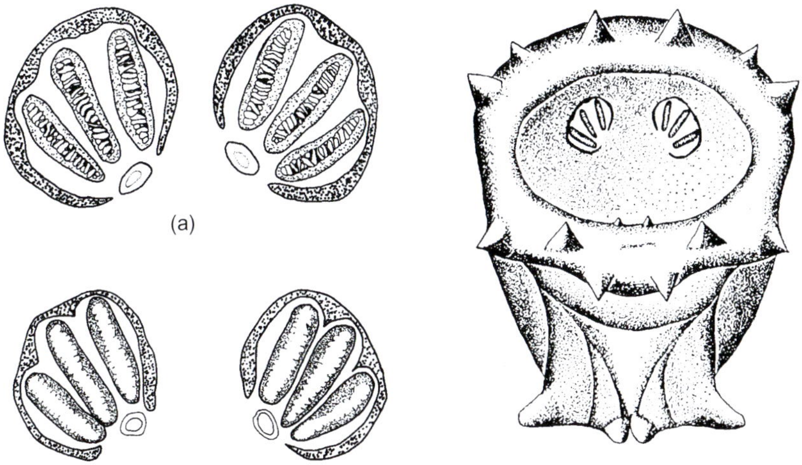

Fig. 3.53 Posterior spiracles of third-stage larvae of (a) *Protophormia terraenovae* and (b) *Phormia regina*. (c) Tubercles on the posterior face of the last segment of third-stage *Protophormia terraenovae* (reproduced from Zumpt, 1965).

Parasite class: Insecta

Family: Calliphoridae

Description, adults: *Protophormia terraenovae* is a black-coloured blowfly with an overlying metallic blue–green coloured sheen. This species is very similar to *Phormia regina* in appearance. In *P. terraenovae* the anterior thoracic spiracle is black or black–brown and is difficult to distinguish from the general body colour. In contrast, in *Phormia regina* the anterior spiracle is yellow or orange and stands out clearly against the dark background colour of the thorax.

Description, larvae: The third-stage larvae of both *P. terraenovae* and *P. regina* are characterised by strongly developed, fairly pointed tubercles on the posterior face of the last segment. In third-stage larvae of *P. terraenovae* the tubercles on the upper margin of the last segment are longer than half the width of a posterior spiracle, whereas in *P. regina* they are less than half the width of a posterior spiracle in length. The larvae of *P. terraenovae* also possess dorsal spines on the posterior margins of segment 10 which are absent in larvae of *P. regina* (Fig. 3.53).

Hosts: Mainly sheep, but may also be a serious pest of cattle and reindeer.

Life cycle: Flies oviposit primarily in carrion but also may act as secondary invaders of myiases on live mammals. The gravid female lays clusters of 100–200 yellowish cream eggs. The eggs hatch into larvae and the larvae then feed, grow rapidly and moult twice to become fully mature maggots. These then migrate to the ground and pupate. Following pupation, the adult female fly must obtain a protein meal and mate. Adult flies can live for about 30 days.

Geographical distribution: Northern Canada, USA, Europe, Scandinavia, Russia

A number of other, more generalist ectoparasites may also be found on sheep and goats and these are listed in the host–parasite checklist at the end of this chapter. More detailed descriptions of these parasites may be found in Chapter 11 (Facultative ectoparasites and arthropod vectors).

In the following checklists, the codes listed below apply:

Helminth classes:
N = Nematoda; T = Trematoda; C = Cestoda.

Arthropod classes:
I = Insecta; A = Arachnida.

Protozoal classes:
M = Mastigophora; S = Sarcodina; A = Apicomplexa; R = Rickettsia.

Sheep parasite checklist.

Section/host system	Helminths		Arthropods		Protozoa	
	Parasite	(Super)family	Parasite	Family	Parasite	Family
Digestive						
Oesophagus	*Gongylonema pulchrum*	Spiruroidea (N)				
Rumen/ reticulum	*Gongylonema verrucosum*	Spiruroidea (N)				
	Gongylonema monnig	Spiruroidea (N)				
	Paramphistomum cervi	Paramphistomatidae (T)				
	Paramphistomum microbothrium	Paramphistomatidae (T)				
	Ceylonocotyle streptocoelium	Paramphistomatidae (T)				
	Cotylophoron cotylophorum	Paramphistomatidae (T)				
Abomasum	*Teladorsagia circumcincta*	Trichostrongyloidea (N)				
	Ostertagia leptospicularis	Trichostrongyloidea (N)				
	Marshallagia marshalli	Trichostrongyloidea (N)				
	Haemonchus contortus	Trichostrongyloidea (N)				
	Trichostrongylus axei	Trichostrongyloidea (N)				
	Parabronema skrjabini	Spiruroidea (N)				
Small intestine	*Trichostrongylus colubriformis*	Trichostrongyloidea (N)			*Eimeria crandallis*	Eimeriidae (A)
	Trichostrongylus vitrinus	Trichostrongyloidea (N)			*Eimeria ovinoidalis*	Eimeriidae (A)
	Trichostrongylus longispicularis	Trichostrongyloidea (N)			*Eimeria ahsata*	Eimeriidae (A)
	Cooperia curticei	Trichostrongyloidea (N)			*Eimeria bakuensis*	Eimeriidae (A)
	Cooperia surnabada	Trichostrongyloidea (N)			*Eimeria faurei*	Eimeriidae (A)
	Nematodirus filicollis	Trichostrongyloidea (N)			*Eimeria granulosa*	Eimeriidae (A)
	Nematodirus battus	Trichostrongyloidea (N)			*Eimeria intricata*	Eimeriidae (A)
	Nematodirus spathiger	Trichostrongyloidea (N)			*Eimeria marsica*	Eimeriidae (A)
	Bunostomum trigonocephalum	Ancylostomatoidea (N)			*Eimeria parva*	Eimeriidae (A)
					Eimeria pallida	Eimeriidae (A)
	Gaigeria pachyscalis	Ancylostomatoidea (N)			*Eimeria weybridgensis*	Eimeriidae (A)
	Strongyloides papillosus	Rhabditoidea (N)			*Cryptosporidium parvum*	Cryptosporidiidae (A)
	Capillaria longipes	Trichuroidea (N)				
	Moniezia expansa	Anoplocephalidae (C)			*Giardia intestinalis*	Diplomonadidae (M)
	Avitellina centripunctata	Thysanosomidae (C)			*Entamoeba ovis*	Endamoebidae (S)
	Stilesia globipunctata	Thysanosomidae (C)				
	Thysaniezia ovilla	Thysanosomidae (C)				
	Thysanosoma actinoides	Thysanosomidae (C)				
	Cymbiforma indica	Notocotylidae (T)				
	Skrjabinotrema ovis	Brachylaemidae (T)				

(*continued*)

Sheep parasite checklist (*continued*).

Section/host system	Helminths		Arthropods		Protozoa	
	Parasite	(Super)family	Parasite	Family	Parasite	Family
Caecum Colon	*Oesophagostomum columbianum*	Strongyloidea (N)			*Eimeria crandallis*	Eimeriidae (A)
	Oesophagostomum venulosum	Strongyloidea (N)			*Eimeria ovinoidalis*	Eimeriidae (A)
	Oesophagostomum multifoliatum	Strongyloidea (N)			*Retortamonas ovis*	Retortamonadorididae (M)
	Oesophagostomum asperum	Strongyloidea (N)			*Tetratrichomonas ovis*	Trichomonadidae (M)
	Chabertia ovina	Strongyloidea (N)				
	Skrjabinema ovis	Oxyuroidea (N)				
	Skrjabinema alata	Oxyuroidea (N)				
	Skrjabinema caprae	Oxyuroidea (N)				
	Trichuris ovis	Trichuroidea (N)				
	Trichuris skrjabini	Trichuroidea (N)				
	Trichuris discolor	Trichuroidea (N)				
	Homologaster palonidae	Paramphistomatidae (T)				
Respiratory						
Nasal cavities	*Mammomonogamus nasicola*	Strongyloidea (N)	*Oestrus ovis*	Oestridae (I)		
	Mammomonogamus laryngeus	Strongyloidea (N)	*Gedoelstia cristata*	Oestridae (I)		
			Gedoelstia haessleri	Oestridae (I)		
Trachea Bronchi	*Dictyocaulus filaria*	Trichostrongyloidea (N)				
	Protostrongylus rufescens	Metastrongyloidea (N)				
Lung	*Muellerius capillaris*	Metastrongyloidea (N)				
	Cystocaulus ocreatus	Metastrongyloidea (N)				
	Neostrongylus linearis	Metastrongyloidea (N)				
	Spiculocaulus austriacus	Metastrongyloidea (N)				
	Varestrongylus schulzi	Metastrongyloidea (N)				
	Echinococcus granulosus	Taeniidae (C)				
Liver						
	Fasciola hepatica	Fasciolidae (T)				
	Fasciola gigantica	Fasciolidae (T)				
	Fascioloides magna	Fasciolidae (T)				
	Dicrocoelium dendriticum	Dicrocoeliidae (T)				
	Dicrocoelium hospes	Dicrocoeliidae (T)				
	Stilesia hepatica	Thysanosomidae (C)				
	Thysanosoma actinioides	Thysanosomidae (C)				
	Cysticercus tenuicollis (metacestode – Taenia hydatigena)	Taeniidae (C)				
	Echinococcus granulosus	Taeniidae (C)				

Pancreas						
	Eurytrema coelomaticum	Dicrocoeliidae (T)				
	Eurytrema pancreaticum	Dicrocoeliidae (T)				
Circulatory					*Trypanosoma brucei brucei*	Trypanosomatidae (M)
Blood	*Schistosoma bovis*	Schistosomatidae (T)				
	Schistosoma japonicum	Schistosomatidae (T)			*Trypanosoma congolense*	Trypanosomatidae (M)
	Schistosoma mattheei	Schistosomatidae (T)				
	Schistosoma nasalis	Schistosomatidae (T)			*Trypansoma simiae*	Trypanosomatidae (M)
	Schistosoma indicum	Schistosomatidae (T)			*Trypanosoma vivax*	Trypanosomatidae (M)
	Schistosoma turkestanicum (Orientobilharzia turkestanicum)	Schistosomatidae (T)			*Trypansoma melophagium*	Trypanosomatidae (M)
					Babesia motasi	Babesiidae (A)
					Babesia ovis	Babesiidae (A)
					Theileria hirci	Theileriidae (A)
					Theileria ovis	Theileriidae (A)
Blood vessels	*Elaeophora schneideri*	Filarioidea (N)			*Anaplasma phagocytophilum*	Anaplasmataceae (R)
					Anaplasma centrale	Anaplasmataceae (R)
					Anaplasma marginale	Anaplasmataceae (R)
					Ehrlichia ruminantium	Rickettsiaceae (R)
					Eperythrozoon ovis	Rickettsiaceae (R)
					Rickettsia conorii	Rickettsiaceae (R)
Nervous						
CNS	*Coenurus cerebralis (metacestode – Taenia multiceps)*	Taeniidae (C)	*Gedoelstia cristata*	Oestridae (I)	*Toxoplasma gondii*	Sarcocystiidae (A)
			Gedoelstia haessleri	Oestridae (I)		
Eye			*Gedoelstia cristata*	Oestridae (I)		
			Gedoelstia haessleri	Oestridae (I)		
Reproductive/ urogenital					*Toxoplasma gondii*	Sarcocystiidae (A)
Locomotory						
Muscle	*Cysticercus ovis (metacestode – Taenia ovis)*	Taeniidae (C)			*Toxoplasma gondii*	Sarcocystiidae (A)
					Sarcocystis ovicanis	Sarcocystiidae (A)
					Sarcocystis ovifelis	Sarcocystiidae (A)

(*continued*)

Sheep parasite checklist (*continued*).

Section/host system	Helminths		Arthropods		Protozoa	
	Parasite	(Super)family	Parasite	Family	Parasite	Family
Connective tissue						
Integument						
Skin			*Linognathus ovillus*	Linognathidae (I)		
			Linognathus pedalis	Linognathidae (I)		
			Bovicola ovis	Trichodectidae (I)		
			Melophagus ovinus	Hippoboscidae (I)		
			Demodex ovis	Demodicidae (A)		
			Demodex ariae	Demodicidae (A)		
			Psoroptes ovis	Psoroptidae (A)		
			Chorioptes bovis	Psoroptidae (A)		
			Psorergates ovis	Psorergatidae (A)		
			Sarcoptes scabiei	Sarcoptidae (A)		
Subcutaneous			*Przhevalskiana silenus*	Oestridae (I)		
			Dermatobia hominis	Oestridae (I)		
			Calliphora augur	Calliphoridae (I)		
			Calliphora albifrontalis	Calliphoridae (I)		
			Calliphora nociva	Calliphoridae (I)		
			Calliphora stygia	Calliphoridae (I)		
			Calliphora vicina	Calliphoridae (I)		
			Calliphora vomitoria	Calliphoridae (I)		
			Lucilia sericata	Calliphoridae (I)		
			Lucilia cuprina	Calliphoridae (I)		
			Protophormia terraenovae	Calliphoridae (I)		
			Phormia regina	Calliphoridae (I)		
			Cordylobia anthrophaga	Calliphoridae (I)		
			Cochliomyia hominivorax	Calliphoridae (I)		
			Cochliomyia macellaria	Calliphoridae (I)		
			Chrysomya bezziana	Calliphoridae (I)		
			Chrysomya megacephala	Calliphoridae (I)		
			Wohlfahrtia magnifica	Sarcophagidae (I)		
			Wohlfahrtia meigeni	Sarcophagidae (I)		
			Wohlfahrtia vigil	Sarcophagidae (I)		

The following species of flies and ticks are found on sheep. More detailed descriptions are found in Chapter 11: Facultative ectoparasites and arthropod vectors.

Flies of veterinary importance on sheep.

Group	Genus	Species	Family
Blackflies Buffalo gnats	*Simulium*	spp	Simuliidae (I)
Blowflies and screwworms	*Calliphora*	*albifrontis* *nociva* *stygia* *vicina* *vomitoria*	Calliphoridae (I)
	Chrysomya	*albiceps* *bezziana* *megacephala*	
	Cochliomyia	*hominivorax* *macellaria*	
	Cordylobia	*anthropophaga*	
	Lucilia	*cuprina* *illustris* *sericata*	
	Phormia	*regina*	
	Protophormia	*terraenovae*	
Bot flies	*Dermatobia*	*hominis*	Oestridae (I)
	Gedoelstia	*haessleri*	
	Oestrus	*ovis*	
	Przhevalskiana	*aegagri* *silenus*	
Flesh flies	*Sarcophaga*	*fusicausa* *haemorrhoidalis*	Sarcophagidae (I)
	Wohlfahrtia	*magnifica* *meigeni* *vigil*	
Hippoboscids	*Hippobosca*	*equina* *rufipes* *maculata*	Hippoboscidae (I)
Midges	*Culicoides*	spp	Ceratopogonidae (I)
Mosquitoes	*Aedes*	spp	Culicidae (I)
	Anopheles	spp	
	Culex	spp	
Muscids	*Hydrotaea*	*irritans*	Muscidae (I)
	Musca	*autumnalis* *domestica*	
	Stomoxys	*calcitrans*	
Sandflies	*Phlebotomus*	spp	Psychodidae (I)
Tabanids	*Chrysops*	spp	Tabanidae (I)
	Haematopota	spp	
	Tabanus	spp	
Tsetse flies	*Glossina*	*fusca* *morsitans* *palpalis*	Glossinidae (I)

Tick species found on sheep.

Genus	Species	Common name	Family
Ornithodoros	*moubata*	Eyeless or hut tampan	Argasidae (A)
	savignyi	Eyed or sand tampan	
Otobius	*megnini*	Spinose ear tick	Argasidae (A)
Amblyomma	*americanum*	Lone star tick	Ixodidae (A)
	cajennense	Cayenne tick	
	gemma		
	hebraeum	South African bont tick	
	maculatum		
	pomposum		
	variegatum	Variegated or tropical bont tick	
Boophilus	*annulatus*	Texas cattle fever tick	Ixodidae (A)
	decoloratus	Blue tick	
	microplus	Pantropical or southern cattle tick	
Dermacentor	*andersoni*	Rocky Mountain wood tick	Ixodidae (A)
	marginatus		
	reticulatus	Marsh tick	
	occidentalis	Pacific coast tick	
	varabilis	American dog tick	
Haemaphysalis	*punctata*		Ixodidae (A)
	concinna		
	bispinosa		
	longicornis		
Hyalomma	*detritum*	Bont leg tick	Ixodidae (A)
	dromedarii	Camel *Hyalomma*	
	marginatum	Mediterranean *Hyalomma*	
	truncatum	Bont leg tick	
Ixodes	*ricinus*	Castor bean or European sheep tick	Ixodidae (A)
	holocyclus		
	rubicundus	Karoo paralysis tick	
	scapularis		
Rhipicephalus	*appendiculatus*	Brown ear tick	Ixodidae (A)
	bursa		
	capensis	Cape brown tick	
	evertsi	Red or red-legged tick	
	sanguineus	Brown dog or kennel tick	
	simus	Glossy tick	

Goat parasite checklist.

Section/host system	Helminths		Arthropods		Protozoa	
	Parasite	(Super)family	Parasite	Family	Parasite	Family
Digestive						
Oesophagus	*Gongylonema pulchrum*	Spiruroidea (N)				
Rumen/ reticulum	*Gongylonema verrucosum*	Spiruroidea (N)				
	Gongylonema monnig	Spiruroidea (N)				
	Paramphistomum cervi	Paramphistomatidae (T)				
	Paramphistomum microbothrium	Paramphistomatidae (T)				
	Ceylonocotyle streptocoelium	Paramphistomatidae (T)				
	Cotylophoron cotylophorum	Paramphistomatidae (T)				
Abomasum	*Teladorsagia circumcincta*	Trichostrongyloidea (N)				
	Ostertagia leptospicularis	Trichostrongyloidea (N)				
	Marshallagia marshalli	Trichostrongyloidea (N)				
	Haemonchus contortus	Trichostrongyloidea (N)				
	Trichostrongylus axei	Trichostrongyloidea (N)				
	Parabronema skrjabini	Spiruriodea (N)				
Small intestine	*Trichostrongylus colubriformis*	Trichostrongyloidea (N)			*Eimeria ninakohlyakimovae*	Eimeriidae (A)
	Trichostrongylus vitrinus	Trichostrongyloidea (N)			*Eimeria alijevi*	Eimeriidae (A)
	Trichostrongylus longispicularis	Trichostrongyloidea (N)			*Eimeria arloingi*	Eimeriidae (A)
	Cooperia curticei	Trichostrongyloidea (N)			*Eimeria aspheronica*	Eimeriidae (A)
	Cooperia surnabada	Trichostrongyloidea (N)			*Eimeria caprina*	Eimeriidae (A)
	Nematodirus filicollis	Trichostrongyloidea (N)			*Eimeria caprovina*	Eimeriidae (A)
	Nematodirus battus	Trichostrongyloidea (N)			*Eimeria christenseni*	Eimeriidae (A)
	Nematodirus spathiger	Trichostrongyloidea (N)			*Eimeria hirci*	Eimeriidae (A)
	Bunostomum trigonocephalum	Ancylostomatoidea (N)			*Eimeria jolchijevi*	Eimeriidae (A)
	Gaigeria pachyscalis	Ancylostomatoidea (N)			*Giardia intestinalis*	Diplomonadidae (M)
	Strongyloides papillosus	Rhabditoidea (N)			*Cryptosporidium parvum*	Cryptosporidiidae (A)
	Capillaria longipes	Trichuroidea (N)				
	Moniezia expansa	Anoplocephalidae (C)				
	Avitellina centripunctata	Thysanosomidae (C)				
	Stilesia globipunctata	Thysanosomidae (C)				
	Thysaniezia ovilla	Thysanosomidae (C)				
	Thysanosoma actinoides	Thysanosomidae (C)				
	Cymbiforma indica	Notocotylidae (T)				

(*continued*)

Goat parasite checklist (*continued*).

Section/host system	Helminths		Arthropods		Protozoa	
	Parasite	(Super)family	Parasite	Family	Parasite	Family
Caecum Colon	*Oesophagostomum columbianum*	Strongyloidea (N)			*Eimeria ninakohlyakimovae*	Eimeriidae (A)
	Oesophagostomum venulosum	Strongyloidea (N)			*Eimeria caprina*	Eimeriidae (A)
					Retortamonas ovis	Retortamonadorididae (M)
	Oesophagostomum multifoliatum	Strongyloidea (N)			*Tetratrichomonas ovis*	Trichomonadidae (M)
	Oesophagostomum asperum	Strongyloidea (N)				
	Chabertia ovina	Strongyloidea (N)				
	Skrjabinema ovis	Oxyuroidea (N)				
	Skrjabinema caprae	Oxyuroidea (N)				
	Trichuris ovis	Trichuroidea (N)				
	Trichuris skrjabini	Trichuroidea (N)				
	Trichuris discolor	Trichuroidea (N)				
	Homologaster palonidae	Paramphistomatidae (T)				
Respiratory						
Nasal cavities	*Mammomonogamus nasicola*	Strongyloidea (N)	*Oestrus ovis*	Oestridae (I)		
			Gedoelstia cristata	Oestridae (I)		
			Gedoelstia haessleri	Oestridae (I)		
Trachea Bronchi	*Dictyocaulus filaria*	Trichostrongyloidea (N)				
	Protostrongylus rufescens	Metastrongyloidea (N)				
Lung	*Muellerius capillaris*	Metastrongyloidea (N)				
	Cystocaulus ocreatus	Metastrongyloidea (N)				
	Neostrongylus linearis	Metastrongyloidea (N)				
	Spiculocaulus austriacus	Metastrongyloidea (N)				
	Varestrongylus schulzi	Metastrongyloidea (N)				
	Echinococcus granulosus	Taeniidae (C)				
Liver						
	Fasciola hepatica	Fasciolidae (T)				
	Fasciola gigantica	Fasciolidae (T)				
	Fascioloides magna	Fasciolidae (T)				
	Dicrocoelium dendriticum	Dicrocoeliidae (T)				
	Dicrocoelium hospes	Dicrocoeliidae (T)				
	Stilesia hepatica	Thysanosomidae (C)				
	Thysanosoma actinoides	Thysanosomidae (C)				
	Cysticercus tenuicollis (metacestode – Taenia hydatigena)	Taeniidae (C)				
	Echinococcus granulosus	Taeniidae (C)				

Pancreas	*Eurytrema coelomaticum*	Dicrocoeliidae				
	Eurytrema pancreaticum	Dicrocoeliidae (T)				
Circulatory						
Blood	*Schistosoma bovis*	Schistosomatidae (T)			*Trypanosoma brucei brucei*	Trypanosomatidae (M)
	Schistosoma japonicum	Schistosomatidae (T)			*Trypanosoma congolense*	Trypanosomatidae (M)
	Schistosoma mattheei	Schistosomatidae (T)			*Trypansoma simiae*	Trypanosomatidae (M)
	Schistosoma nasalis	Schistosomatidae (T)			*Trypansoma vivax*	Trypanosomatidae (M)
	Schistosoma indicum	Schistosomatidae (T)			*Trypansoma melophagium*	Trypanosomatidae (M)
	Schistosoma turkestanicum	Schistosomatidae (T)			*Babesia motasi*	Babesiidae (A)
					Babesia ovis	Babesiidae (A)
					Theileria hirci	Theileriidae (A)
Blood vessels	*Elaeophora schneideri*	Filarioidea (N)			*Theileria ovis*	Theileriidae (A)
					Anaplasma phagocytophilum	Anaplasmataceae (R)
					Anaplasma centrale	Anaplasmataceae (R)
					Anaplasma marginale	Anaplasmataceae (R)
					Ehrlichia ruminantum	Rickettsiaceae (R)
					Eperythrozoon ovis	Rickettsiaceae (R)
					Rickettsia conorii	Rickettsiaceae (R)
Nervous						
CNS	*Coenurus cerebralis (metacestode – Taenia multiceps)*	Taeniidae (C)	*Gedoelstia cristata*	Oestridae (I)	*Toxoplasma gondii*	Sarcocystiidae (A)
			Gedoelstia haessleri	Oestridae (I)		
Eye			*Gedoelstia cristata*	Oestridae (I)		
			Gedoelstia haessleri	Oestridae (I)		
Reproductive/ urogenital					*Toxoplasma gondii*	Sarcocystiidae (A)
Locomotory						
Muscle	*Cysticercus ovis (metacestode – Taenia ovis)*	Taeniidae (C)			*Toxoplasma gondii*	Sarcocystiidae (A)
					Sarcocystis capracanis	Sarcocystiidae (A)
					Sarcocystis hircicanis	Sarcocystiidae (A)
					Sarcocystis hircifelis	Sarcocystiidae (A)
Connective tissue						

(continued)

Goat parasite checklist (*continued*).

Section/host system	Helminths		Arthropods		Protozoa	
	Parasite	(Super)family	Parasite	Family	Parasite	Family
Integument						
Skin			*Bovicola caprae*	Trichodectidae (I)		
			Bovicola limbata	Trichodectidae (I)		
			Linognathus stenopsis	Linognathidae (I)		
			Demodex caprae	Demodicidae (A)		
			Sarcoptes scabiei	Sarcoptidae (A)		
			Psoroptes ovis	Psoroptidae (A)		
			Chorioptes bovis	Psoroptidae (A)		
Subcutaneous			*Przhevalskiana silenus*	Oestridae (I)	*Besnoitia besnoiti*	Sarcocystiidae (A)
			Calliphora augur	Calliphoridae (I)		
			Calliphora albifrontis	Calliphoridae (I)		
			Calliphora nociva	Calliphoridae (I)		
			Calliphora stygia	Calliphoridae (I)		
			Calliphora vicina	Calliphoridae (I)		
			Calliphora vomitoria	Calliphoridae (I)		
			Lucilia cuprina	Calliphoridae (I)		
			Lucilia sericata	Calliphoridae (I)		
			Protophormia terraenovae	Calliphoridae (I)		
			Phormia regina	Calliphoridae (I)		
			Cordylobia anthropophaga	Calliphoridae (I)		
			Cochliomyia hominivorax	Calliphoridae (I)		
			Cochliomyia macellaria	Calliphoridae (I)		
			Chrysomya bezziana	Calliphoridae (I)		
			Chrysomya megacephala	Calliphoridae (I)		
			Wohlfahrtia magnifica	Sarcophagidae (I)		
			Wohlfahrtia meigeni	Sarcophagidae (I)		
			Wohlfahrtia vigil	Sarcophagidae (I)		
			Dermatobia hominis	Oestridae (I)		

The following species of flies and ticks are found on goats. More detailed descriptions are found in Chapter 11: Facultative ectoparasites and arthropod vectors.

Flies of veterinary importance on goats.

Group	Genus	Species	Family
Blackflies Buffalo gnats	*Simulium*	spp	Simuliidae (I)
Blowflies and screwworms	*Calliphora*	*albifrontis* *nociva* *stygia* *vicina* *vomitoria*	Calliphoridae (I)
	Chrysomya	*albiceps* *bezziana* *megacephala*	
	Cochliomyia	*hominivorax* *macellaria*	
	Cordylobia	*anthropophaga*	
	Lucilia	*cuprina* *illustris* *sericata*	
	Phormia	*regina*	
	Protophormia	*terraenovae*	
Bot flies	*Dermatobia*	*hominis*	Oestridae (I)
	Gedoelstia	*haessleri*	
	Oestrus	*ovis*	
	Przhevalskiana	*aegagri* *silenus*	
Flesh flies	*Sarcophaga*	*fusicausa* *haemorrhoidalis*	Sarcophagidae (I)
	Wohlfahrtia	*magnifica* *meigeni* *vigil*	
Hippoboscids	*Hippobosca*	*equina* *rufipes* *maculata*	Hippoboscidae (I)
Midges	*Culicoides*	spp	Ceratopogonidae (I)
Mosquitoes	*Aedes*	spp	Culicidae (I)
	Anopheles	spp	
	Culex	spp	
Muscids	*Hydrotaea*	*irritans*	Muscidae (I)
	Musca	*autumnalis* *domestica*	
	Stomoxys	*calcitrans*	
Sandflies	*Phlebotomus*	spp	Psychodidae (I)
Tabanids	*Chrysops*	spp	Tabanidae (I)
	Haematopota	spp	
	Tabanus	spp	
Tsetse flies	*Glossina*	*fusca* *morsitans* *palpalis*	Glossinidae (I)

Tick species found on goats.

Genus	Species	Common name	Family
Ornithodoros	*moubata*	Eyeless or hut tampan	Argasidae (A)
	savignyi	Eyed or sand tampan	
Otobius	*megnini*	Spinose ear tick	Argasidae (A)
Amblyomma	*americanum*	Lone star tick	Ixodidae (A)
	cajennense	Cayenne tick	
	gemma		
	hebraeum	South African bont tick	
	maculatum		
	pomposum		
	variegatum	Variegated or tropical bont tick	
Boophilus	*annulatus*	Texas cattle fever tick	Ixodidae (A)
	decoloratus	Blue tick	
	microplus	Pantropical or southern cattle tick	
Dermacentor	*andersoni*	Rocky Mountain wood tick	Ixodidae (A)
	marginatus		
	reticulatus	Marsh tick	
	occidentalis	Pacific coast tick	
	varabilis	American dog tick	
Haemaphysalis	*punctata*		Ixodidae (A)
	concinna		
	bispinosa		
	longicornis		
Hyalomma	*detritum*	Bont leg tick	Ixodidae (A)
	dromedarii	Camel *Hyalomma*	
	marginatum	Mediterranean *Hyalomma*	
	truncatum	Bont leg tick	
Ixodes	*ricinus*	Castor bean or European sheep tick	Ixodidae (A)
	holocyclus		
	rubicundus	Karoo paralysis tick	
	scapularis		
Rhipicephalus	*appendiculatus*	Brown ear tick	Ixodidae (A)
	bursa		
	capensis	Cape brown tick	
	evertsi	Red or red-legged tick	
	sanguineus	Brown dog or kennel tick	
	simus	Glossy tick	

4
Parasites of horses

ENDOPARASITES

PARASITES OF THE DIGESTIVE SYSTEM

OESOPHAGUS

No parasites reported.

STOMACH

Members of the genus *Habronema*, and the closely related genus *Draschia*, are parasitic in the stomach of the horse. *Habronema* inhabits the mucus layer of the gastric mucosa and may cause a catarrhal gastritis, but is not considered an important pathogen, while *Draschia* parasitises the fundic region of the stomach wall and provokes the formation of large fibrous nodules that are occasionally significant. The chief importance of these parasites is as a cause of cutaneous habronematidosis or 'summer sores' in warm countries.

Life cycle: The life cycle is similar for all species. Eggs or L_1 are passed in the faeces and the L_1 are ingested by the larval stages of various muscid flies that are often present in faeces. Development to L_3 occurs synchronously with the development to maturity of the fly intermediate host. When the fly feeds around the mouth, lips and nostrils of the horse, the larvae pass from its mouthparts on to the skin and are swallowed. Alternatively infected flies may be swallowed whole in feed and drinking water. Development to adult takes place in the stomach where the larvae burrow into the glandular area of the mucosa and induce the formation of nodules. The worms develop to mature adults within the nodules in about 8 weeks. When *Drachsia* larvae are deposited on a skin wound or around the eyes they can invade the tissues; they do not complete their development but may cause granulomatous skin lesions.

Final hosts: All are parasites of the horse and other equines

Intermediate hosts: Dipteran flies of the genera *Musca*, *Stomoxys* and *Haematobia* (*Lyperosia*)

Epidemiology: The seasonality of cutaneous lesions is related to the activity of the fly vectors.

Treatment: A number of modern broad-spectrum anthelmintics including oxfendazole, oxibendazole and albendazole have been shown to have activity against the adult parasites in the stomach. Cutaneous lesions are best treated with ivermectin. The use of insect repellents has some benefit and radiation therapy and cryosurgery have been used in more chronic cases.

Control: Obviously any measures taken to prevent injuries and to control fly populations will be beneficial. Stacking manure and using insecticides during the day, for example, limit fly populations and attack. Skin wounds should be treated with either fly repellents or a combination of antiseptic and insecticide.

Draschia megastoma

Synonym: *Habronema megastoma*

Predilection site: Stomach

Parasite class: Nematoda

Superfamily: Spiruroidea

Description, gross: Slender white translucent worms 0.7–1.3 cm long; adult male are 7–10 mm and females 10–13 mm. The worms are recognised by their heads, which are slightly constricted from the main body.

Description, microscopic: The pharynx is funnel-shaped. The hind end of the male is usually spirally coiled with four pairs of pre-cloacal papillae. Spicules are uneven in length with the left longer than the right.

Geographical distribution: Worldwide

Pathogenesis: In the stomach the worms live in colonies in the mucosa around which develop large nodular fibrous tumour-like lesions (Fig. 4.1). These occur in the fundus region and seem to be well tolerated unless they protrude into the lumen sufficiently to interfere mechanically with stomach function or,

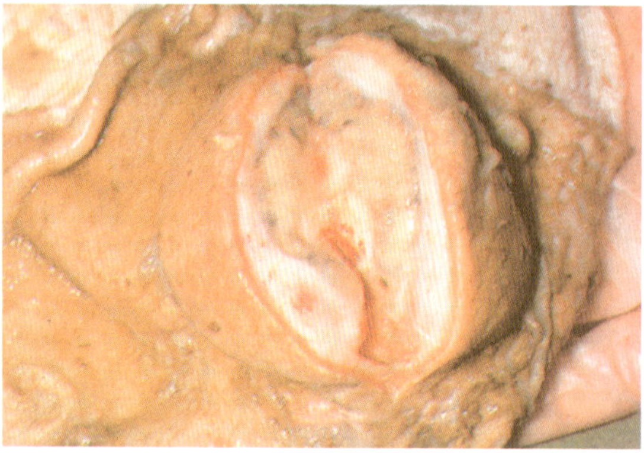

Fig. 4.1 Large nodular tumour-like lesion in the stomach induced by *Draschia megastoma* infection.

more rarely, cause abcessation or perforation when the lesions become secondarily infected with pyogenic bacteria. *D. megastoma* can cause a skin reaction, cutaneous habronematidosis or 'summer sores', when larvae are deposited on broken skin or open wounds by infected flies.

Clinical signs: The presence of adult worms in the stomach causes very little clinical disturbance. Cutaneous habronematidosis presents as intense itching of the affected skin. Non-healing granulomatous lesions, raised above the surface of the skin may be a feature (see *Habronema*).

Diagnosis: Usually only low numbers of eggs or larvae are present in the faeces. Eggs may be demonstrated in gastric lavage taken via a stomach tube. Sometimes larvae can be identified in the small granulomatous skin lesions.

Pathology: Adult worms burrow into the submucosa of the stomach producing large tumour-like nodules causing the mucosa to protrude into the gastric lumen. The worms provoke a surrounding granulomatous reaction, which contains a central core of necrotic and cellular debris and large numbers of eosinophils. Burrowing larvae in the conjunctivae cause an ulcerative, weeping lesion at the medial canthus, which becomes progressively more nodular as the lesion becomes more granulomatous. Mineralised granules, caseous debris and larvae may be found in the lesion. Larvae in the skin cause lesions that are rapidly progressive and proliferative in nature, comprising ulcerated masses of granulation tissue that haemorrhages readily. Lesions may be single or multiple and range in size from 5–15 cm. On section, the lesions are caseous and histologically there are aggregates of eosinophils scattered throughout the connective tissue, which contains a few macrophages and multinucleate giant cells surrounding degenerating larvae. The surface of the lesion is usually covered with a fibronecrotic exudate overlying a highly vascular granulation tissue infiltrated with neutrophils.

Habronema microstoma

Synonym: *Habronema majus*

Predilection site: Stomach

Parasite class: Nematoda

Superfamily: Spiruroidea

Description, gross: Slender white translucent worms 1.5–2.5 cm long; adult males are 16–22 mm and females 15–25 mm. The male has wide caudal alae and the tail has a spiral twist.

Description, microscopic: The pharynx contains a dorsal and ventral tooth in its anterior part. The male has four pairs of pre-cloacal papillae. Spicules are uneven in length with the slender left one longer than the right. The elongated, oval, small eggs are thin-shelled, 45–59 × 16 μm and larvated when shed in faeces.

Geographical distribution: Worldwide

Pathogenesis: The adult *Habronema* in the stomach may cause a mild catarrhal gastritis with excess mucus production. More important are the granulomatous lesions of cutaneous habronematidosis, commonly known as 'summer sores', and the persistent conjunctivitis with nodular thickening and ulceration of the eyelids associated with invasion of the eyes. Larvae have also been found associated with small lung abscesses.

Clinical signs: These are usually absent in gastric habronematidosis. Lesions of cutaneous habronematidosis are most common in areas of the body liable to injury and occur during the fly season in warm humid countries, although it also occurs in temperate regions. During the early stages, there is intense itching of the infected wound or abrasion, which may cause further self-inflicted damage. Subsequently a reddish brown, non-healing cauliflower-like granuloma develops that protrudes above the level of the surrounding skin and may be up to 8.0 cm in diameter. These lesions are known as 'summer sores' in acute cases. Later the lesion may become more chronic, fibrous and inactive, but will not heal until the advent of cooler weather when fly activity ceases (Fig. 4.2). Invasion of the eye produces a persistent conjunctivitis with nodular ulcers, especially at the medial canthus. Sometimes larvae invade the skin of the prepuce and glans penis of stallions.

Diagnosis: This is based on the finding of non-healing, reddish cutaneous granulomas. The larvae,

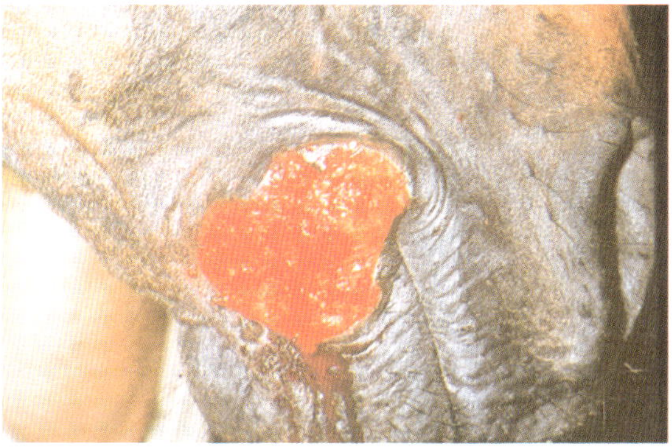

Fig. 4.2 Ulcerated granuloma on commissure of lips of horse due to cutaneous habronematidosis.

recognised by spiny knobs on their tails, may be found in material from these lesions. Gastric infection is not easily diagnosed since *Habronema* eggs and larvae are not readily demonstrable in the faeces by routine techniques.

Pathology: Adult worms in the mucosa of the stomach have been associated with a mild ulceration. Burrowing larvae in the conjunctivae cause an ulcerative, weeping lesion at the medial canthus, which becomes progressively more nodular as the lesion becomes more granulomatous.

Habronema muscae

Predilection site: Stomach

Parasite class: Nematoda

Superfamily: Spiruroidea

Description, gross: Slender white translucent worms, 1.0–2.5 cm long; adult males are 8–14 mm and females 13–22 mm. The male has wide caudal alae and the tail has a spiral twist. It is unlikely to be confused with other nematodes in the stomach since *Draschia* is associated with characteristic lesions and *Trichostrongylus axei* is less than 1.0 cm in length.

Description, microscopic: There are two lateral trilobed lips; the pharynx is cylindrical and has a thick cuticular lining. There are four pairs of pre-cloacal papillae and one or two papillae behind the cloaca. The cloacal region is covered with small cuticlar ridges. Spicules are uneven in length with the slender left one longer than the right. The vulva is situated near the middle of the body and opens dorsolaterally. The elongated, oval, small eggs are thin-shelled, $40–50 \times 10–12\ \mu m$ and larvated when shed in faeces.

Final host: Horse and other equines

Intermediate hosts: Dipteran flies of the genera *Musca*, *Stomoxys* and *Haematobia* (*Lyperosia*)

Geographical distribution: Worldwide

Trichostrongylus axei

Synonym: *Trichostrongylus extenuatus*

Common name: Stomach hairworm

Predilection site: Stomach

Parasite class: Nematoda

Superfamily: Trichostrongyloidea

Description, gross: The adults are small, hair-like, light brownish red and difficult to see with the naked eye. Males measure around 3–6 mm and females 4–8 mm in length.

Description, microscopic: The male spicules are dissimilar and unequal in length (the right being shorter than the left (see Table 3.1, Chapter 3: Sheep and goats).

Hosts: Cattle, sheep, goat, deer, horse, donkey, pig and occasionally man

Life cycle: This is typically trichostrongylid and is described in detail under Sheep and goats in Chapter 3. The prepatent period is about 4 weeks in the horse.

Geographical distribution: Worldwide

Clinical signs: *T. axei* is responsible for gastritis in horses.

Pathology: In the horse, initial lesions are circumscribed areas of hyperaemia in the gastric mucosa, which progresses to catarrhal or lymphocytic inflammation and erosion of the epithelium. This may be associated with necrosis. Over time, infection can lead to a chronic proliferative inflammation and shallow depressed ulcers may be present.

Treatment and control: This is as described under treatment and control of strongylosis in the horse.

Gasterophilus

Species of *Gasterophilus*, known as bots, are obligate parasites of horses, donkeys, mules, zebras, elephants and rhinoceroses. Nine species are recognised in total, six of which are of interest as veterinary parasites of equids.

Description, adults: Bot flies are robust dark flies, 10–15 mm in length (Fig. 4.3). The body is densely covered with yellowish hairs. In the female the ovipositor is strong and protuberant. The wings of adult

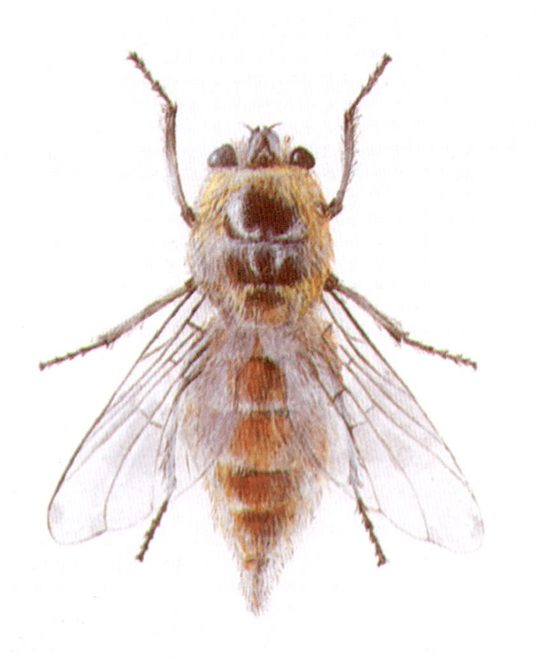

Fig. 4.3 *Gasterophilus* spp.

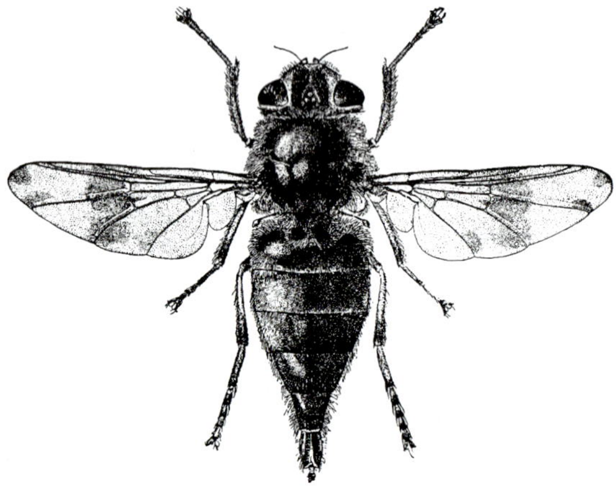

Fig. 4.4 Adult female *Gasterophilus intestinalis* (reproduced from Castellani and Chalmers, 1910).

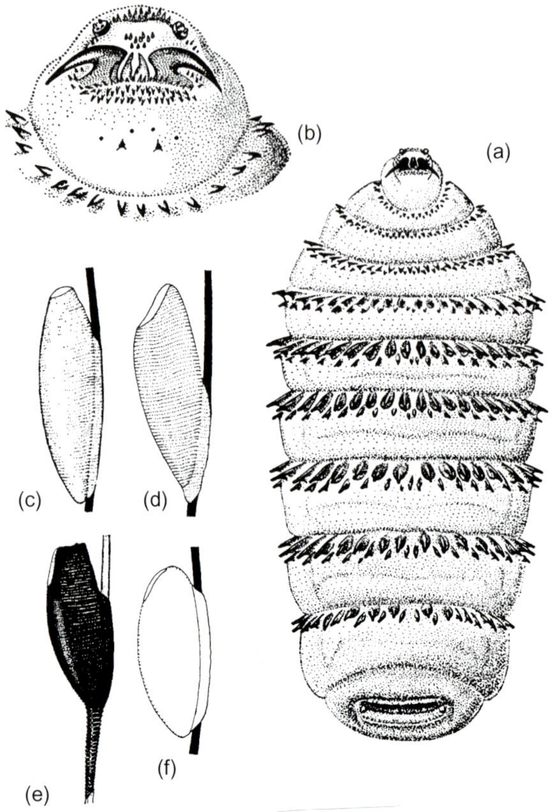

Fig. 4.5 (a) Third-stage larva of *Gasterophilus intestinalis*. (b) Ventral view of pseudocephalon of *G. pecorum*. Eggs of (c) *G. nasalis*; (d) *G. intestinalis*; (e) *G. haemorrhoidalis*; (f) *G. inermis* (reproduced from Zumpt, 1965).

Gasterophilus characteristically have no cross-vein dm-cu (Fig. 4.4).

Description, larvae: When mature and present in the stomach or passed in faeces the larvae are cylindrical, 16–20 mm long and reddish orange with posterior spiracles (Fig. 4.5). Differentiation of mature larvae of the various species can be made on the numbers and distribution of the spines present on various segments (Fig. 4.6).

Life cycle: The life cycles of the various species differ only slightly; key differences will be highlighted below.

Geographical distribution: All species of *Gasterophilus* were originally restricted to the Palaearctic and Afrotropical regions, but three species, *Gasterophilus nasalis*, *G. haemorrhoidalis* and *G. intestinalis*, have been inadvertently introduced into the New World.

Pathogenesis: The presence of larvae in the buccal cavity may lead to stomatitis with ulceration of the tongue. On attachment by their oral hooks to the stomach lining, larvae provoke an inflammatory reaction with the formation of funnel-shaped ulcers surrounded by a rim of hyperplastic epithelium (Fig. 4.7). These are commonly seen at postmortem examination of horses in areas of high fly prevalence and although dramatic in appearance their true pathogenic significance remains obscure.

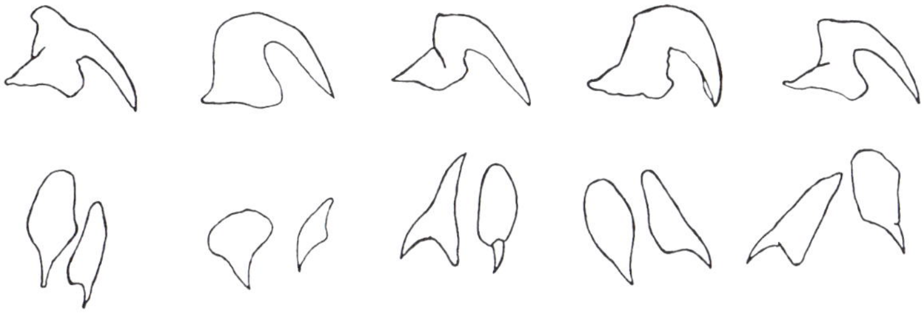

Fig. 4.6 Mouth hooks (top) and ventral spines (bottom) of the fifth segment of (a) *Gasterophilus intestinalis*; (b) *G. inermis*; (c) *G. nasalis*; (d) *G. haemorrhoidalis*; (e) *G. pecorum* (reproduced from Zumpt, 1965).

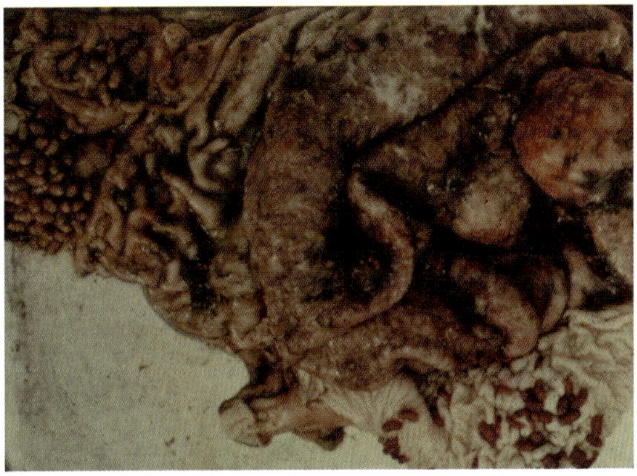

Fig. 4.7 *Gasterophilus* larvae in the stomach of a horse.

Clinical signs: Burrowing of the first-stage larvae in the mouth lining, tongue and gums can produce pus pockets, loosen teeth and cause loss of appetite in the host. Larvae attached to the gastrointestinal mucosa cause inflammation and ulceration. The adult fly can cause irritation and intense avoidance reactions when hovering around the host and laying eggs on the skin. Ovipositing females may be tenacious, laying eggs on mobile as well as stationary animals. Females will pursue galloping horses and immediately resume oviposition when the horse stops.

Diagnosis: The adult flies may be visible and recognisable on and around the host. The eggs are also easily recognisable on the host and may be identified by colour and location. Damage to the mouth and tongue may be detected. The presence of larval parasites in the stomach is difficult to identify except by observation of the larvae in faeces.

Pathology: The burrowing of first- and second-stage *Gasterophilus* larvae in the tissues of the tongue and mouth may result in lesions, the appearance of which is dependent on the degree of burrowing activity. Active tunnelling removes virtually all tissue in the path of the larvae including nerves and capillaries leading to haemorrhage and exocytosis into the tunnels, which fill with erythrocytes mixed with macrophages, lymphocytes and some eosinophils. The tunnels may become infected with bacteria, which result in microabscesses, composed of clotted erythrocytes, bacteria, disintegrating epithelial cells and large numbers of neutrophils. Cells surrounding the tunnel exhibit pyknosis, epithelial hydropic degeneration and became separated from each other.

Interdental gingiva invaded by larvae appear hyperaemic and denuded of epithelia. Recession and ulceration of the gingiva produces periodontal pockets. Extensive invasion by larvae leads to compound periodontal pockets.

The attachment of third-stage larvae results in ulceration at the site of attachment with intense fibrosis below the ulcer. The cephalic portions of embedded larvae become surrounded by a cellular exudate containing erythrocytes and mononuclear cells.

Epidemiology: Adult flies are most active during late summer.

Treatment: The most widely used specific drugs included trichlorphon and dichlorvos, but these have generally been replaced by broad-spectrum macrocyclic lactone compounds, such as ivermectin and moxidectin.

Control: The most effective means of control of this parasite is to remove the eggs from the host's coat. This requires, where possible, daily examination of the animal, paying particular attention to the area around the lips. If eggs are found during the summer and autumn, subsequent infection can be prevented by vigorously sponging with warm water containing an insecticide. The warmth stimulates hatching and the insecticide kills the newly hatched larvae.

From the life cycle it is clear that in temperate areas during the winter almost the entire *Gasterophilus* population will be present as larvae in the stomach, since adult fly activity ceases with the advent of the first frosts in autumn. A single treatment during the winter, therefore, should effectively break the cycle. In certain areas, where adult fly activity is prolonged by mild conditions, additional treatments may be required. Despite the lack of understanding of the pathogenic effect of bots, treatment is usually recommended as owners are concerned when larvae appear in the faeces. Treatment, however, does reduce fly populations and thus the fly worry associated with egg-laying.

Gasterophilus haemorrhoidalis

Common name: Bot flies

Predilection site: Stomach

Parasite class: Insecta

Family: Oestridae

Description: In *G. haemorrhoidalis*, the spines on the ventral surface of the larval segments are arranged in two rows. The head segment has only lateral groups of denticles and the dorsal row of spines on the eighth segment is not broadly interrupted medially. The mouth hooks are uniformly curved dorsally and directed laterally (Fig. 4.6d). The body spines are sharply pointed.

Hosts: Horse, donkey

Life cycle: *G. haemorrhoidalis* lays batches of 150–200 eggs around the lips. The adult flies have a short lifespan and females can deposit all of their eggs within 2–3 hours if the weather is mild and a suitable host is available. The eggs are easily seen: they are 1–2 mm long and usually black in colour. They either hatch spontaneously in about 5 days or are stimulated to do so by warmth, which may be generated during licking and self-grooming. Larvae either crawl into the mouth or are transferred to the tongue during licking. The larvae can burrow into the epidermis of the lips and from there migrate into the mouth. These then penetrate the tongue or buccal mucosa and burrow through in these tissues for several weeks while feeding, before moulting and passing via the pharynx and oesophagus to the stomach where they attach to the gastric epithelium. The larvae remain and develop in the stomach for periods of 10–12 months. When mature in the following spring or early summer, they detach and are passed in the faeces. In this species, the larvae reattach in the rectum for a few days before being passed out. Pupation takes place on the ground, and after 1–2 months the adult flies emerge. These do not feed, and live for only a few days or weeks, during which time they mate and lay eggs. If suitable hosts are unavailable the flies move to high points to aggregate and mate, following which the females initiate a longer-distance search for hosts. There is therefore only one generation of flies per year in temperate areas.

Geographical distribution: Worldwide

Gasterophilus inermis

Common name: Bot flies

Predilection site: Stomach

Parasite class: Insecta

Family: Oestridae

Description: In *G. inermis* the spines on the ventral surface of the larval segments are arranged in two rows. The head segment has only lateral groups of denticles and the dorsal row of spines on the eighth segment are not broadly interrupted medially. The mouth hooks are strongly curved, with their tips directed backwards and approaching the base (Fig. 4.6b). The body spines are sharply pointed. Body segment 3 has three complete rows of spines, and body segment 11 has one row of spines interrupted by a broad median gap.

Hosts: Horse, donkey, zebra

Life cycle: The adult female lays up to 300 eggs on the cheeks and around the mouth of the host animal. These are each attached individually to the base of a hair in these regions. The eggs are easily seen, being 1–2 mm in length and usually creamy white in colour. The eggs either hatch spontaneously in about 5 days or are stimulated to do so by warmth, which may be generated during licking and self-grooming. After hatching, the larvae burrow into the epidermis, and migrate towards the mouth. The migration route of the larvae can be detected by the presence of a track along which the hair has fallen out. The larvae enter at the corner of the mouth and penetrate the mucous membranes of the cheek. The second- and third-stage larvae migrate to the rectum where they reattach. The larvae remain and develop in the host for periods of 10–12 months. When mature in the following spring or early summer, they detach and are passed in the faeces. Pupation takes place on the ground, and after 1–2 months the adult flies emerge. These do not feed and live for only a few days or weeks, during which time they mate and lay eggs. There is therefore only one generation of flies per year in temperate areas.

Geographical distribution: Northern Europe, northern Asia, Africa

Gasterophilus intestinalis

Common name: Bot flies

Predilection site: Stomach

Parasite class: Insecta

Family: Oestridae

Description: In *G. intestinalis*, the mouth hooks are not uniformly curved dorsally and the body spines have blunt tips (Fig. 4.6a).

Hosts: Horse, donkey

Life cycle: Eggs are laid on the hairs of the forelegs and shoulders. Several eggs may be glued to each hair and up to 1000 eggs may be deposited by a female *G. intestinalis* during its lifetime of only a few days. The eggs are easily seen, being 1–2 mm in length and usually creamy white in colour; they either hatch spontaneously in about 7 days or are stimulated to do so by warmth, which may be generated during licking and self-grooming. Larvae either crawl into the mouth or are transferred to the tongue during licking. These then penetrate the tongue or buccal mucosa at the anterior end of the tongue where they excavate galleries in the sub-epithelial layer of the mucous membrane. The larvae wander in these tissues for several weeks before exiting the tongue and moulting. Second-stage larvae attach for a few days to the sides of the pharynx, before moving to the oesophageal portion of the stomach where they cluster at the boundary of glandular and non-glandular epithelium. Larvae remain and develop in this site for periods of 10–12 months. When mature in the following spring or early summer, they detach and are passed in the faeces. Pupation takes place on the ground and after 1–2 months the adult flies emerge. These do not feed and live for only a few days or weeks, during which time they mate and lay eggs. There is therefore only one generation of flies per year in temperate areas.

Geographical distribution: Worldwide

Gasterophilus nasalis

Common name: Throat bot flies

Predilection site: Stomach

Parasite class: Insecta

Family: Oestridae

Description: *G. nasalis* have spines on the ventral surface of the larval segments arranged in a single row. The first three body segments are more or less conical and the third segment has a dorsal row of spines and sometimes ventral spines (Fig. 4.6c).

Hosts: Horse, donkey and zebra

Life cycle: The throat bot fly, *G. nasalis*, lays its eggs in the intermandibular area. Eggs are laid in batches of up to 500, usually with one egg attached per hair. The eggs are easily seen, being 1–2 mm in length and usually creamy white in colour. Eggs either hatch spontaneously in about 7 days or are stimulated to do so by warmth, which may be generated during licking and self-grooming. Larvae either crawl into the mouth or are transferred to the tongue during licking. These then burrow into the spaces around the teeth and between the teeth and gums. This may result in the development of pus sockets and necrosis in the gums. The first larval stage lasts 18–24 days, following which larvae moult and second-stage larvae move via the pharynx and oesophagus to the stomach, where they attach to the gastric epithelium. In the stomach, the yellow *G. nasalis* larvae attach around the pylorus and sometimes the duodenum. Larvae remain and develop in this site for periods of 10–12 months. When mature in the following spring or early summer, they detach and are passed in the faeces. Pupation takes place on the ground, and after 1–2 months the adult flies emerge. These do not feed and live for only a few days or weeks, during which time they mate and lay eggs. There is therefore only one generation of flies per year in temperate areas.

Geographical distribution: Worldwide, particularly the Holarctic

Gasterophilus nigricornis

Common name: Bot flies, broad-bellied horse bot

Predilection site: Stomach

Parasite class: Insecta

Family: Oestridae

Description: In *G. nigricornis* spines on the ventral surface of the larval segments are arranged in a single row. The first three body segments are more or less cylindrical, showing sharp constrictions posteriorly, and the third segment is without spines dorsally or ventrally.

Hosts: Horse, donkey

Life cycle: Female flies alight on the host's cheek to oviposit. The eggs are easily seen; they are 1–2 mm long and usually creamy white in colour. The larvae hatch in 3–9 days and burrow directly into the skin. They then burrow to the corner of the mouth and penetrate the mucous membranes inside the cheek. Once they have reached the central part of the cheek (about 20–30 days after hatching) they moult and leave the mucous membranes. The second-stage larvae are then swallowed, following which they attach themselves to the wall of the duodenum. Larvae remain and develop in this site for periods of 10–12 months, and when mature in the following spring or early summer they detach and are passed in the faeces. Pupation takes place on the ground and after

1–2 months the adult flies emerge. These do not feed and live for only a few days or weeks during which time they mate and lay eggs. There is therefore only one generation of flies per year in temperate areas.

Geographical distribution: Middle East, southern Russia and China

Gasterophilus pecorum

Common name: Bot flies, dark-winged horse bot

Predilection site: Stomach

Parasite class: Insecta

Family: Oestridae

Description: *G. pecorum* has spines on the ventral surface of the larval segments, which are arranged in two rows. The head segment has two lateral groups of denticles and one central group, the latter situated between the antennal lobes and mouth hooks. The dorsal rows of spines are broadly interrupted medially on the 7th and 8th segments. The 10th and 11th segments have no spines.

Hosts: Horse, donkey

Life cycle: Adult *G. pecorum* are most active in late summer and unlike other species, the dark-coloured eggs are laid on pasture and are ingested by horses during grazing. Up to 2000 eggs are laid in batches of 10–115. The eggs are highly resistant and the developed larva may remain viable for months within its egg until ingested by horses. In the mouth, the eggs hatch within 3–5 minutes. First-stage larvae immediately penetrate the mucous membrane of the lips, gums, cheeks, tongue and hard palate and burrow towards the root of the tongue and soft palate, where they may remain for 9–10 months until fully developed. They may also be swallowed and settle in the walls of the pharynx, oesophagus or stomach. When mature in the following spring or early summer, the larvae detach and are passed in the faeces. Pupation takes place on the ground and after 1–2 months the adult flies emerge. These do not feed and live for only a few days or weeks, during which time they mate and lay eggs. There is therefore only one generation of flies per year in temperate areas.

Geographical distribution: Europe, Africa, Asia

Pathogenesis: *Gasterophilus pecorum* is the most pathogenic species in the genus. Large numbers of attached larvae can cause inflammation, hinder swallowing and may eventually lead to death resulting from constriction of the oesophagus.

Clinical signs: Burrowing of the first-stage larvae in the mouth lining, tongue and gums can produce pus pockets, loosen teeth and cause loss of appetite in the host. Large numbers of attached larvae can cause inflammation, choking and hinder swallowing.

Diagnosis: Larvae present in the pharynx can usually be seen on direct inspection. Larvae further down the digestive tract can only be detected by observation of the mature detached larvae in faeces.

SMALL INTESTINE

Strongyloides westeri

Common name: Threadworm

Predilection site: Small intestine

Parasite class: Nematoda

Superfamily: Rhabditoidea

Description, gross: Slender, hair-like worms, 6–9 mm long. Only females are parasitic.

Description, microscopic: The long oesophagus may occupy up to one third of the body length and the uterus is intertwined with the intestine giving the appearance of twisted thread. Unlike other intestinal parasites of similar size the tail has a blunt point. *Strongyloides* eggs are oval, thin-shelled and small, 40–52 × 32–40 μm, being half the size of typical strongyle eggs (Fig. 4.8). The hatched L_1 is passed out in the faeces.

Hosts: Horse, donkey, zebra, rarely pig

Life cycle: *Strongyloides* is unique among the nematodes of veterinary importance, being capable of both parasitic and free-living reproductive cycles. The parasitic phase is composed entirely of female worms in the small intestine and these produce larvated eggs by parthenogenesis, i.e. development from an unfertilised egg. After hatching, larvae may develop through four larval stages into free-living adult male and female worms and this can be followed by a succession of free-living generations. However under certain

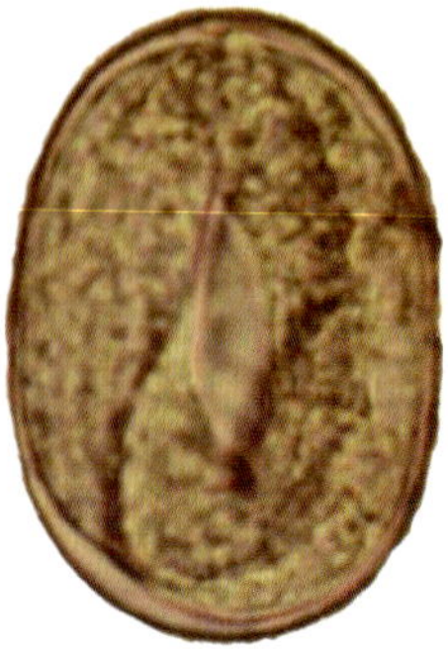

Fig. 4.8 Egg of *Strongyloides westeri*.

conditions, possibly related to temperature and moisture, the L_3 can become parasitic, infecting the host by skin penetration or ingestion and migrating via the venous system, the lungs and trachea to develop into adult female worms in the small intestine.

Foals may acquire infection immediately after birth from the mobilisation of arrested larvae in the tissues of the ventral abdominal wall of the dam, which are subsequently excreted in the milk. The prepatent period is from 8–14 days, depending on the mode of infection.

Geographical distribution: Worldwide

Pathogenesis: Mature parasites are found in the duodenum and proximal jejunum and if present in large numbers may cause inflammation with oedema and erosion of the epithelium. This results in catarrhal enteritis with impairment of digestion and absorption. Migration of larvae through the lungs can cause severe haemorrhage and respiratory distress. Skin penetration may result in irritation and dermatitis.

Clinical signs: Foals with heavy burdens show acute diarrhoea, weakness and emaciation. Older animals may harbour large burdens without showing clinical signs.

Diagnosis: The clinical signs in very young animals, usually within the first few weeks of life, together with the finding of large numbers of the characteristic eggs or larvae in the faeces are suggestive of strongyloidosis. It should be emphasised, however, that high faecal egg counts may be found in apparently healthy animals.

Pathology: Adult worms establish in tunnels in the epithelium at the base of the villi in the small intestine. In large numbers they may cause villous atrophy, with a mixed mononuclear inflammatory cell infiltration of the lamina propria. Crypt epithelium is hyperplastic and there is villous clubbing.

Epidemiology: Infections are very common especially in warm and humid environments. *Strongyloides* infective larvae are not ensheathed and are susceptible to extreme climatic conditions. However, warmth and moisture favour development and allow the accumulation of large numbers of infective stages. A second major source of infection for the very young animal is the reservoir of larvae in the tissues of their dams and this may lead to clinical strongyloidosis in foals in the first few weeks of life. Successive progeny from the same dam often show heavy infections.

Treatment: Specific control measures for infection are rarely called for. Not all anthelmintics show high efficacy, but most of the modern benzimidazoles are effective. Macrocyclic lactones are effective against against adult worms.

Control: Reduction in numbers of free-living larvae by removal of faeces and provision of dry bedding and areas may limit numbers and transmission. On stud farms, foals are often given an anthelmintic treatment at 1–2 weeks of age against *S. westeri*.

Parascaris equorum

Synonym: *Ascaris equorum*, *Ascaris megacephala*

Predilection site: Small intestine

Parasite class: Nematoda

Superfamily: Ascaridoidea

Description, gross: This very large rigid, stout, whitish nematode, up to 40 cm in length, cannot be confused with any other intestinal parasite of equines. Males measure 15–25 cm and females up to 40 cm.

Description, microscopic: The adult parasites have a simple mouth opening surrounded by three large lips and in the male the tail has small caudal alae. The dorsa lip has two double papillae and each ventrolateral lip has one double subventral, and a small lateral papilla. Spicules are long and stout. The egg of *P. equorum* is almost spherical, 50–75 × 40–50 μm, brownish and thick-shelled with an outer, pitted coat.

Hosts: Horse, donkey

Life cycle: The life cycle is direct and migratory involving a hepato-pulmonary route. Eggs produced by the adult female worms are passed in the faeces and can reach the infective stage containing the L_2 in as little as 10–14 days, although development may be delayed at low temperatures. After ingestion and hatching the larvae penetrate the intestinal wall and within 48 hours have reached the liver. By 2 weeks they have arrived in the lungs where they migrate up the bronchi and trachea, are swallowed and return to the small intestine. The site of occurrence and timing of the parasitic larval moults of *P. equorum* are not precisely known, but it would appear that the moult from L_2 to L_3 occurs between the intestinal mucosa and the liver and the two subsequent moults occur in the small intestine. The minimum prepatent period of *P. equorum* is 10 weeks; longevity is up to 2 years. There is no evidence of prenatal infection.

Geographical distribution: Worldwide

Pathogenesis: During the migratory phase of experimental infections, up to 4 weeks following infection, the major signs are frequent coughing, accompanied in some cases by a greyish nasal discharge, although the foals remain bright and alert. Light intestinal infections are well tolerated, but moderate to heavy infections will cause unthriftiness in young animals with poor growth rates, dull coats and lassitude. A wide variety of other clinical signs, including fever, nervous disturbances and colic, has been attributed to field cases of parascariosis, but these have not been observed in experimental studies.

Clinical signs: Adult worms in heavy infections can cause severe enteritis resulting in alternating constipation and foul-smelling diarrhoea. Large numbers of larvae may cause coughing, with fever and anorexia.

Diagnosis: This depends on clinical signs and the presence of spherical, thick, brownish, rough-shelled eggs on faecal examination. Occasionally, atypical thick-walled eggs are seen that lack the dark outer shell. If disease due to prepatent infection is suspected, faecal examination having proved negative, diagnosis may be confirmed by administration of an anthelmintic when large numbers of immature worms may be observed in the faeces.

Pathology: Gross changes are provoked in the liver and lungs by migrating *P. equorum* larvae. In the liver, larvae cause focal haemorrhages and eosinophilic tracts that resolve, leaving whitish areas of fibrosis. Larval migration in the lungs also leads to haemorrhage and infiltration by eosinophils, which are later replaced by accumulations of lymphocytes, while subpleural greyish green lymphocytic nodules develop around dead or dying larvae; these nodules are more numerous following reinfection. These liver and lung lesions are usually of little pathological significance.

Although the presence of worms in the small intestine (Fig. 4.9) is not associated with any specific lesions, heavy infections have occasionally been reported as a cause of impaction and perforation leading to peritonitis. Adult worms may cause catarrhal enteritis and intermittent diarrhoea. However, under experimental conditions, unthriftiness is a major sign and despite maintaining a good appetite infected foals lose weight and may become emaciated. Competition between a large mass of parasites and the host for nutrients may be the underlying cause of this weight loss.

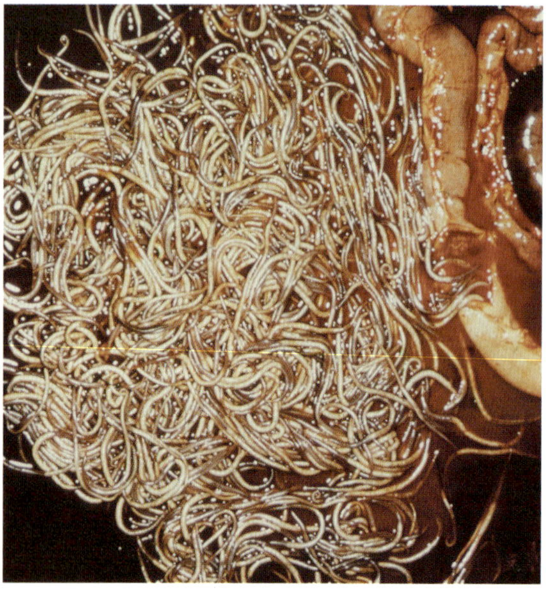

Fig. 4.9 *Parascaris equorum* from the intestine of an infected horse.

Epidemiology: Infection with *Parascaris equorum* is common throughout the world and is a major cause of unthriftiness in young foals. There are two important factors in the epidemiology of infection. First is the high fecundity of the adult female parasite, some infected foals passing millions of eggs in the faeces each day. Secondly, the extreme resistance of the egg in the environment ensures its persistence for several years. The sticky nature of the outer shell may also facilitate passive spread of eggs.

In the northern hemisphere, summer temperatures are such that many eggs become infective at a time when a population of susceptible foals is present. The infections acquired by these result in further contamination of pasture with eggs which may survive during several subsequent grazing seasons. Although mature horses may harbour a few adult worms and act as carriers, heavy burdens are usually confined to yearlings and to foals, which become infected from the first month or so of life; infection is maintained largely by seasonal transmission between these groups of young animals. Exposed foals often develop immunity, resulting in partial or total loss of the worm population.

Treatment: Benzimidazoles (such as fenbendazole, oxfendazole, oxibendazole), pyrantel, ivermectin and moxidectin are all effective against adult and larval stages when given orally.

Control: Since transmission is largely on a foal-to-foal basis it is good policy to avoid using the same paddocks for nursing mares and their foals in successive years. Treatment should start when foals are about 8 weeks old and be repeated at appropriate intervals depending on the anthelmintic used.

Notes: Infection with *Parascaris equorum* is common throughout the world and is a major cause of unthriftiness in young foals.

Tapeworms

Several tapeworm species are found in horses, donkeys and other equines. Intermediate hosts for all species are forage mites of the family Oribatidae, in which the intermediate cysticercoid stages are found.

Life cycle: Mature segments are passed in the faeces and disintegrate, releasing the eggs. These are ingested by forage mites in which they develop to the cysticercoid stage in 2–4 months. The adult tapeworms are found in the intestine of horses 1 or 2 months after the ingestion of infected mites in the herbage.

Diagnosis: Where clinical signs occur they may be difficult to differentiate from more common causes of unthriftiness and digestive upsets. However, it may be possible to confirm the presence of *Anoplocephala* by the demonstration of the typical eggs on faecal examination or on postmortem.

Epidemiology: Horses of all ages may be affected, but clinical cases have been reported mainly in animals up to 3–4 years of age.

Treatment: Specific treatment for *Anoplocephala* infection is rarely called for but a number of compounds have been reported as effective, including pyrantel at increased dosage rates (38 mg/kg). Praziquantel at 1 mg/kg is also effective.

Control: Control is difficult, since forage mites are widespread on pasture. Treatment with an effective anthelmintic before the animals enter new grazing may help to control *Anoplocephala* infections in areas where problems have arisen.

Anoplocephala perfoliata

Predilection site: Terminal ileum, caecum

Parasite class: Cestoda

Family: Anoplocephalidae

Description, gross: *A. perfoliata* is up to 4–8 cm in length by 1.2 cm wide.

Description, microscopic: There is a small, rounded scolex, 2–3 mm in diameter, with a lappet behind each of the four suckers, but there is neither a rostellum nor hooks. It has a very short neck and the strobila widens rapidly, individual proglottids being much wider than they are long. Eggs are irregularly spherical or triangular, 65–80 μm in diameter. The oncosphere is supported by a pair of projections – the **pyriform apparatus**.

Geographical distribution: Worldwide

Pathogenesis: *Anoplocephala perfoliata* has been considered to be relatively non-pathogenic but there is increasing evidence that heavy infections may cause severe clinical signs and may even prove fatal. *A. perfoliata* is usually found around the ileocaecal junction (Fig. 4.10) and causes ulceration of the mucosa at its site of attachment; these lesions have been incriminated as a cause of intussusception. Cases of intestinal obstruction and perforation of the intestinal wall have been recorded associated with massive infections.

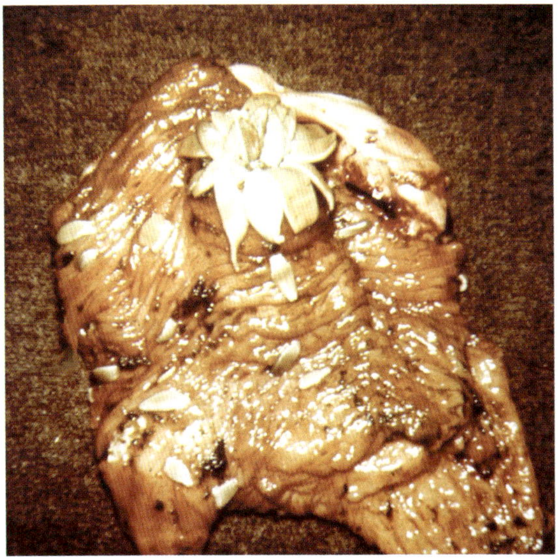

Fig. 4.10 *Anoplocephala perfoliata* tapeworms around the ileocaecal junction.

Clinical signs: In most infections there are no clinical signs. However, when there are significant pathological changes in the intestine there may be unthriftiness, enteritis and colic. Perforation of the intestine will prove rapidly fatal.

Pathology: The mucosa at the site of attachment may be inflamed, thickened and ulcerated, particularly in the areas of the ileocaecal junction where it may lead to partial or fatal occlusion of the ileocaecal orifice.

Anoplocephala magna

Common name: Dwarf equine tapeworm

Predilection site: Small intestine, rarely stomach

Parasite class: Cestoda

Family: Anoplocephalidae

Description, gross: *A. magna* is similar morphologically to *A. perfoliata* but much longer, up to 80.0 cm.

Description, microscopic: The scolex is large, 4–6 mm wide with suckers opening anteriorly, and there are no lappets on the scolex. The neck is short, as are the segments. The genital organs are single and the pores are unilateral. Eggs are similar to *A. perfoliata*.

Geographical distribution: Worldwide

Pathogenesis: Heavy infections of *Anoplocephala magna* may cause catarrhal, haemorrhagic or ulcerative enteritis. Cases of intestinal obstruction, colic and perforation of the intestinal wall have been recorded associated with massive infections.

Clinical signs: Rare, but infection causes diarrhoea and colic.

Pathology: The mucosa at the site of attachment may be inflamed, thickened and ulcerated.

Paranoplocephala mamillana

Synonym: *Anoplocephaloides mamillana*

Predilection site: Small intestine, rarely stomach

Parasite class: Cestoda

Family: Anoplocephalidae

Description, gross: *P. mamillana* is only 6–50 × 4–6 mm in size.

Description, microscopic: There are no lappets on the narrow scolex and the suckers are slit-like. The scolex is large and without rostellum and hooks. The gravid segments are wider than they are long. Eggs are irregularly spherical or triangular, 51 × 37 μm in diameter.

Geographical distribution: Worldwide

Pathogenesis: *Paranoplocephala* is usually considered to be relatively non-pathogenic.

Clinical signs: In most infections there are no clinical signs.

Diagnosis: It may be possible to confirm the presence of *Paranoplocephala* by the demonstration of the typical eggs on faecal examination or on postmortem.

Pathology: Infection is rarely associated with lesions but occasionally the site of attachment is inflamed and slightly ulcerated.

Epidemiology: Horses of all ages may be affected.

Coccidiosis

Several species of coccidia have been reported from horses. Few details are available on the life cycles, pathogenesis and epidemiology and pathogenesis. Similarly, little is also known about treatment and control of equine coccidiosis, but by analogy with other hosts, sulphonamides can be tried. Prevention is based on good management and hygiene. Young animals should be kept off heavily contaminated pastures when they are most susceptible. Good feeding of dams prior to parturition and rearing of animals of similar ages limits the build-up and spread of oocysts.

Eimeria leuckarti

Synonym: *Globidium leuckarti*

Predilection site: Small intestine

Parasite class: Sporozoasida

Family: Eimeriidae

Host: Horse, donkey

Description: Oocysts are ovoid or pyriform, flattened at the small end and very large, measuring 70–90 × 49–69 μm (mean 80 × 60 μm), with a thick dark shell and distinct micropyle. Sporocysts are elongate, 30–43 × 12–15 μm, with a Stieda body and residuum. The sporozoites are up to 35 μm long, lie lengthwise head to tail in the sporocysts and have a clear globule at the broad end.

Life cycle: Complete details of the life cycle are not known and merogony stages have not been described. Early gamonts are in the cells of the intestinal lamina propria of the small intestine. The prepatent period is 15–33 days and sporulation time is 15–41 days.

Geographical distribution: Worldwide

Pathogenesis: Occurs in the small intestine of horses and donkeys and has been incriminated as the cause of an intermittent diarrhoea.

Diagnosis: Diagnosis is difficult, and because of the heavy nature of the oocysts, sedimentation techniques should be employed or, if flotation is used, a concentrated sugar solution is necessary.

Pathology: The pathology includes marked inflammatory changes in the mucosa and a disruption of villous architecture due to the presence of large meront stages (Fig. 4.11).

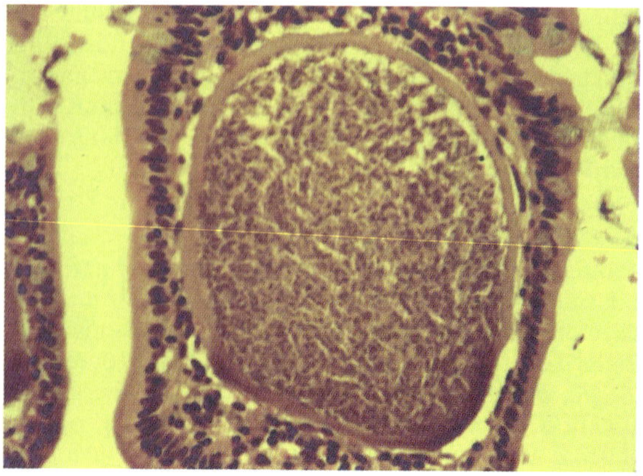

Fig. 4.11 'Giant' meront of *Eimeria leuckarti*.

Eimeria solipedum

Predilection site: Small intestine

Parasite class: Sporozoasida

Family: Eimeriidae

Host: Horse, donkey

Description: Oocysts are spherical, orange to yellowish brown, 15–28 μm in diameter, without an oocyst residuum or micropyle. Sporocysts are ellipsoid to oval, 5 × 3 μm.

Geographical distribution: Russia, CIS

Pathogenesis: Has been reported to cause intermittent diarrhoea.

Diagnosis: Identification of oocysts from faecal samples

Epidemiology: Almost 10% of horses in the former Soviet Union (now Russia and CIS) were found to be infected.

Eimeria uniungulati

Predilection site: Small intestine

Parasite class: Sporozoasida

Family: Eimeriidae

Host: Horse, donkey

Description: Oocysts are oval or ellipsoid, light orange, 15–24 × 12–17 μm, without an oocyst residuum or micropyle. Sporocysts are oval, 6–10.5 × 4–6 μm with a central sporocyst residuum.

Geographical distribution: Russia, CIS

Pathogenesis: Not reported.

Epidemiology: Infection has been reported in 1–10% of horses in the former Soviet Union (now Russia and CIS).

Other protozoa

Cryptosporidium parvum

Predilection site: Small intestine

Parasite class: Sporozoasida

Family: Cryptosporidiidae

Hosts: Cattle, sheep, goat, horse, deer, man

Description: Mature oocysts are ovoidal or spheroidal, 5.0 × 4.5 μm (range 4.6–5.4 × 3.8–4.7 μm) and a length: width ratio of 1.19.

Geographical distribution: Worldwide

Pathogenesis: Cryptosporidiosis has been reported in immunodeficient foals as a cause of diarrhoea.

Clinical signs: Clinically the disease is characterised by anorexia and diarrhoea.

Epidemiology: Several mammals act as hosts to *C. parvum* but little is known of the importance of their involvement in transmitting infection to, or maintaining infection in domestic livestock. In the UK, surveys in horses have shown the presence of *C. parvum* in 28% of thoroughbred foals although there was no association between infection and diarrhoea. Subsequent studies have demonstrated the genotype in horses to be genotype 2.

Treatment: There is no known effective drug therapy, and where cryptosporidiosis is diagnosed, supportive treatment, in the form of antidiarrhoeals and fluids, is usually sufficient.

For more details see Chapter 2 (Cattle).

Giardia intestinalis

Synonym: *Giardia duodenalis*, *Giardia lamblia*, *Lamblia lamblia*

Predilection site: Small intestine

Parasite class: Zoomastigophorasida

Family: Diplomonadidae

Description: The trophozoite has a pyriform to ellipsoidal, bilaterally symmetrical body, 12–15 μm long by 5–9 μm wide. The dorsal side is convex and there is a large sucking disk on the ventral side. There are two anterior nuclei, two slender axostyles, eight flagellae in four pairs and a pair of darkly staining median bodies. The median bodies are curved bars resembling the claws of a hammer. Cysts are ovoid, 8–12 × 7–10 μm and contain four nuclei.

Hosts: Man, cattle, sheep, goat, pig, horse, alpaca, dog, cat, guinea pig, chinchilla

Geographical distribution: Worldwide

Pathogenesis: Infection in horses is considered non-pathogenic.

Clinical signs: No associated clinical signs

Treatment and control: Not required

Notes: There is still controversy over the classification of *Giardia* spp. The current molecular classification places isolates into eight distinct assemblages. Some authors give separate specific names to organisms isolated from different hosts although species specificity of many isolates is unknown. Phylogenetic data suggest that *G. intestinalis* is a species complex composed of several species that are host specific.

For more details see Chapter 2 (Cattle).

LARGE INTESTINE

Cyathostomins ('small strongyles')

The group 'small strongyles' embraces over 40 species, popularly known as trichonemes, cyathostomes or cyathostomins. For many years there has been a great deal of confusion in the classification of this group of parasites and in a new revision it has been proposed that the genus *Trichonema* be discarded and replaced by four main genera, namely *Cyathostomum*, *Cylicocyclus*, *Cylicodontophorus* and *Cylicostephanus*, these being collectively referred to as cyathostomes or more recently, cyathostomins. Other genera of unknown significance included in this group are *Poteriostomum*, *Craterostomum* and *Oesophagodontus*. Since the majority of species involved are similar both morphologically and in behaviour they will be referred to in this text as cyathostomins or small strongyles. Fifteen species of small strongyles are commonly present in large numbers.

The following general descriptions apply to all species of small strongyles.

Pathogenesis and clinical signs: Small strongyles are extremely prevalent, and grazing horses usually carry a mixed burden of large and small strongyles. The major clinical signs associated with heavy infections in animals up to 2–3 years of age are unthriftiness, anaemia and sometimes diarrhoea. Marked clinical signs are less common in older animals, although general performance may be impaired. In temperate countries an acute syndrome of catarrhal and/or haemorrhagic enteritis with severe diarrhoea, leading to emaciation and in some cases death, in horses and ponies in the spring has been reported; this is associated with the simultaneous mass emergence of cyathostome L_4 from the intestinal mucosa and submucosa. This may have aetiological and epidemiological similarities to type II ostertagiosis in young cattle and is often referred to as acute larval cyathostomosis.

Diagnosis: Diagnosis is based on the grazing history and clinical signs of loss of condition and anaemia. Although the finding of typical, oval, thin-shelled strongyle eggs on faecal examination may be a useful aid to diagnosis, it is important to remember that substantial worm burdens may be associated with faecal egg counts of only a few hundred eggs per gram (epg) due either to low fecundity of adult worms, the long prepatent period or to the presence of many immature parasites. On postmortem, it may be possible to visualise the L_4 larvae as tiny grey spots in the intestinal mucosa using the transmural illumination technique. On some occasions when heavy cyathostome infections in the spring cause severe diarrhoea, thousands of bright red cyathostome L_4, apparently unable to establish, may be present in the faeces.

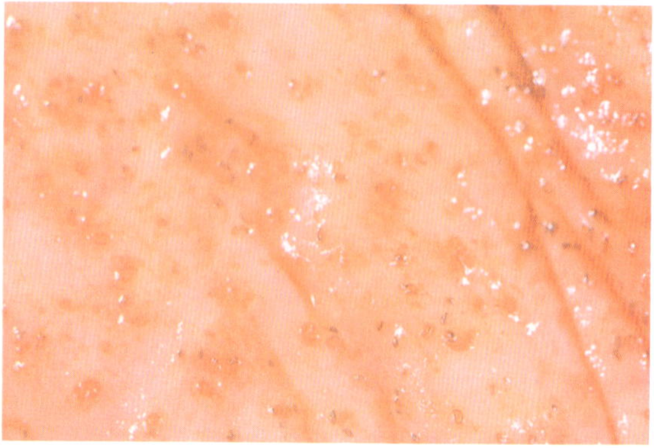

Fig. 4.12 Developing small strongyle larvae in the mucosa of the caecum.

Pathology: Parasitic larval development of most species takes place entirely in the mucosa of the caecum and colon, but a few penetrate the muscularis and develop in the submucosa. The entry of larval cyathostomes (Fig. 4.12) into the lumina of the tubular glands generally provokes an inflammatory response together with marked goblet cell hypertrophy. Emergence of the bright red L_4 into the gut lumen appears to be associated with a massive infiltration of the gut mucosa with eosinophils. Many thousand L_4 may be present, but their pathogenic significance has been little studied. There are, however, reports of heavy natural infections of adult worms and larvae associated with catarrhal and haemorrhagic enteritis, with thickening and oedema of the mucosa, especially in animals of 6 months to 3 years of age.

Mature parasites are frequently present in large numbers in the lumen of the large intestine; during feeding those species with small buccal capsules take in only glandular epithelium, while large species may damage deeper layers of the mucosa. Although the erosions caused by individual parasites may be slight, when large numbers are present a desquamative enteritis may result.

Epidemiology: Strongylosis is most frequently a problem in young horses reared on permanent horse pastures, although cases of severe disease may occur in adult animals kept in suburban paddocks and subjected to overcrowding and poor management. Although the preparasitic larval requirements of the horse strongyles are similar to those of the trichostrongyles of ruminants, adult horses, unlike cattle, may carry substantial worm burdens and therefore have a considerable influence on the epidemiology of infection. Thus there are two sources of infection during the grazing season in temperate areas. First there are infective larvae, which developed during the previous grazing season and have survived on pasture over winter. The second and probably more important source of infective larvae are the eggs passed in the current grazing season by horses, including nursing mares, sharing the same grazing area. Pasture larval levels increase markedly during the summer months when environmental conditions are optimal for rapid development of eggs to L_3 and may lead to the accumulation of large infections in the autumn.

At present there is little evidence for a consistent periparturient rise in faecal egg output in breeding mares due to a relaxation of immunity, since the egg rise in the spring occurs in both breeding and non-breeding animals and is often unrelated to parturition.

There is increasing evidence that many cyathostome L_3 ingested during the autumn show a degree of hypobiosis and remain in the large intestinal mucosa until the following spring. Mass emergence of these larvae results in the severe clinical signs described previously.

Treatment: Treatment for clinical strongylosis should not be necessary if prophylactic measures are adequate. There are several broad-spectrum anthelmintics, including the benzimidazoles, pyrantel and the avermectins/milbemycins (macrocyclic lactones), which are effective in removing lumen-dwelling adult and larval strongyles and these are usually marketed as in-feed or oral preparations. The macrocyclic lactones have the additional advantage of activity against larvae of horse bot flies (*Gasterophilus* spp), which develop in the stomach. Some modern benzimidazoles and macrocyclic lactones are also efficient against both developing cyathostome larvae in the gut wall and some migrating stages of the large strongyles.

Control: Since horses of any age can become infected and excrete eggs, all grazing animals over 2 months of age should be treated every 4–8 weeks with an effective broad-spectrum anthelmintic. This regimen will also control infections with other intestinal parasites such as *Parascaris equorum* and *Oxyuris equi*. Any new animals joining a treated group should receive an anthelmintic and be isolated for 48–72 hours before being introduced. If possible, a paddock rotation system should be adopted so that nursing mares and their foals do not graze the same area in successive years. Avoid overstocking.

If horses are housed in the winter, treatment at that time with an anthelmintic effective against larval cyathostomes will reduce the risk of disease due to their mass emergence in the spring.

There is evidence that some species of cyathostomes are becoming resistant to benzimidazole compounds, pyrantel and piperizine, and to avoid this it is suggested that these should be used strategically alternated with chemically unrelated anthelmintics on an annual or a 6-monthly basis. Faecal samples from groups of horses should be examined at regular intervals to monitor drug efficiency.

The introduction of pasture management techniques may be feasible for some enterprises, such as pasture cleaning twice a week (vacuuming or sweeping) or the alternate grazing of pasture by ruminant livestock.

Cyathostomum spp

Synonym: *Trichonema* spp

Common name: Small strongyles, cyathostomins, cyathostomes, trichonemes

Predilection site: Large intestine

Parasite class: Nematoda

Superfamily: Strongyloidea

Family: Strongylidae

Subfamily: Cyathostominae

Description, gross: Small (5–12 mm in length), bursate nematodes ranging in colour from white to dark red, the majority being visible on close inspection of the large intestinal mucosa or contents (Fig. 4.13).

Description, microscopic: The well developed short buccal capsule is cylindrical, without teeth, and species differentiation is based on characteristics of the buccal capsule, and the internal and external leaf crowns. *Cyathostomum* have a moderately high mouth collar, with cephalic papillae not very prominent. The buccal capsule is broader than deep and has no dorsal gutter. Elements of the external leaf crown are larger, broader and fewer than elements of the internal leaf crown. Inner leaf crown is deep in the buccal capsule and has sclerotised extra-chitinous supports at or near the anterior edge of buccal capsule. The dorsal ray of the male bursa is split to the origin of the externo-dorsal rays

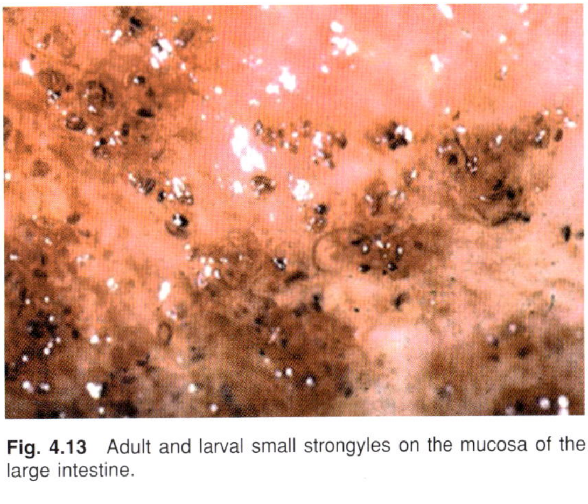

Fig. 4.13 Adult and larval small strongyles on the mucosa of the large intestine.

Table 4.1 *Cyathostomum* species.

Species	Synonyms	Distribution	Description	Comments
C. alveatum	*Cylichnostomum alveatum* *Cylicostomum alveatum* *Trichonema alveatum* *Cylicocercus alveatus*	Africa, Asia, Europe	Walls of buccal capsule uniform thickness posterior to inner leaf crown; which is about one third the depth of buccal capsule	Rare
C. catinatum	*Cylichnostomum catinatum* *Cylicostomum catinatum* *Trichonema catinatum* *Cylicocercus catinatum*	Cosmopolitan	Inner leaf crown more anterior on lateral sides of buccal capsule compared with dorsal and ventral sides, but not in sinous line	Very common
C. coronatum	*Cylichnostomum coronatum* *Cylicostomum coronatum* *Trichonema coronatum* *Cylicostomias coronatum*	Cosmopolitan	Extrachitonous supports prominent and inner leaf crown in even line around buccal cavity, which is as deep as broad and with walls thick and bent inwards	Common
C. labiatum	*Cyathostomum labratum* *Cylichnostomum labiatum* *Cylicostomum labiatum* *Trichonema labiatum* *Cylicostomias labiatum*	Cosmopolitan	Mouth collar notched forming four distinct lips; inner leaf crown elements half length of external leaf crown. Chitinous support spindle-shaped. Excretory pore near junction of mid to posterior third of oesophagus	Common
C. labratum	*Cylichnostomum labratum* *Cylicostomum labratum* *Trichonema labratum* *Cylicostomias labratum*	Cosmopolitan	Mouth collar not notched; inner leaf crown elements more than half length of external leaf crown. Chitinous support pyriform-shaped. Excretory pore near middle of oesophagus	Common
C. montgomeryi	*Cylicostomum montgomeryi* *Trichonema labratum* *Cylicotoichus montgomeryi*	Africa	Similar to *C. labiatum* but without well defined lips. Wall of buccal capsule longer in dorsoventral view	Rare. In zebra, horses and mules
C. pateratum	*Cylicodontophorus pateratum* *Cylicostomum pateratum* *Trichonema pateratum* *Cylicostocercus pateratum*	Cosmopolitan	Inner leaf crown in sinous line deep in buccal cavity (seen in lateral view)	Common
C. saginatum	*Cylicostomum sagittatum* *Trichonema sagittatum* *Cylicostomias sagittatum* *Cylicodontophorus sagittatum*	Europe, Asia	Similar to *C. coronatum* but shallow buccal capsule	Rare
C. tetracanthrum	*Strongylus tetracanthus* *Sclerostomum tetracanthum* *Cylichnostomum tetracanthum* *Cylicostomum tetracanthum* *Trichonema tetracanthum* *Trichonema arcuata* *Trichonema aegypticum* *Cylicostomum aegypticum*	Cosmopolitan	Extrachitonous supports nearly as large as wall of buccal capsule and appear as extensions of buccal capsule wall	Rare

and the spicules are filiform, equal in length with 'pick-shaped' tips. In the female, the vulva is close to the anus. The tail may be straight or bent dorsally with a ventral bulge, anterior to the vulva.

Hosts: Horse, donkey

Life cycle: Hatching of eggs and development to L_3 is complete within 2 weeks during the summer in temperate areas, after which the larvae migrate from the faeces on to the surrounding herbage. After ingestion, the L_3 exsheath and invade the wall of the ileum and large intestine where they develop to L_4 before emerging into the gut lumen and moulting to become young adult worms. The prepatent periods of members of this genus are generally between 2 and 3 months, although this may be extended due to hypobiosis in some species.

Geographical distribution: Worldwide

Cylicocyclus spp

Synonym: *Trichonema* spp

Common name: Small strongyles, cyathostomins, cyathostomes, trichonemes

Predilection site: Large intestine

Parasite class: Nematoda

Superfamily: Strongyloidea

Family: Strongylidae

Subfamily: Cyathostominae

Description, gross: Small to medium size (10–25 mm in length), bursate nematodes ranging in colour from white to dark red, the majority being visible on close inspection of the large intestinal mucosa or contents.

Description, microscopic: The well developed short buccal capsule is cylindrical, without teeth, and species differentiation is based on characteristics of the buccal capsule, and the internal and external leaf crowns. *Cylicocyclus* have a high mouth collar with broad lateral papillae. Elements of the external leaf crown are larger, fewer and broader than those of the inner leaf crown, the latter being short, with thin rods at or near the anterior edge of the buccal capsule. The buccal capsule is short, broader than deep, with thin walls tapering anteriorly, with a hoop-shaped thickening around the posterior margin. In the male the dorsal ray is split to the region of origin of the externodorsal rays and the spicules are filiform, of equal length with pick-shaped tails. In females, the vulva is near the anus and the tail is usually straight but may be bent slightly dorsally.

Hosts: Horse, donkey and other equids

Geographical distribution: Worldwide

Cylicodontophorus spp

Synonym: *Schultzitrichonema*

Common name: Small strongyles, cyathostomins, cyathostomes, trichonemes

Predilection site: Large intestine

Parasite class: Nematoda

Superfamily: Strongyloidea

Family: Strongylidae

Subfamily: Cyathostominae

Description, gross: Small (7–14 mm in length), bursate nematodes ranging in colour from white to dark red, the majority being visible on close inspection of the large intestinal mucosa or contents.

Description, microscopic: The well developed short buccal capsule is cylindrical, without teeth, and species differentiation is based on characteristics of the buccal capsule, and the internal and external leaf crowns. *Cylicodontophorus* have a high mouth collar, with inconspicuous lateral papillae and short and conical submedian papillae. The buccal capsule is short, thick walled, of nearly uniform thickness, and broader than deep. Inner leaf crown elements are longer, broader and less numerous than the external leaf crown elements, and are inserted near the anterior edge of the buccal capsule. The dorsal ray of the male bursa is split only to the proximal branch, and the spicules are filiform, equal in length with 'hook-shaped' tips. In the female, the tail is short with a sharp tip and a prominent ventral bulge may be present anterior to the vulva.

Hosts: Horse, donkey

Geographical distribution: Worldwide

Cylicostephanus spp

Synonym: *Schultzitrichonema, Petrovinema*

Common name: Small strongyles, cyathostomins, cyathostomes

Predilection site: Large intestine

Parasite class: Nematoda

Superfamily: Strongyloidea

Family: Strongylidae

Subfamily: Cyathostominae

Description, gross: Small (4–10 mm in length), bursate nematodes ranging in colour from white to dark red, the majority being visible on close inspection of the large intestinal mucosa or contents.

Table 4.2 Cylicocyclus species.

Species	Synonyms	Distribution	Description	Comments
C. adersi	*Cylicostomum adersi* *Trichonema adersi*	Africa, Asia	Buccal capsule not shallow, walls of uniform thickness; dorsal gutter short but well developed; inner leaf crown elements few and wider than external leaf crown elements and uniform length	Rare
C. auriculatus	*Cylichnostomum auriculatum* *Cylicostomum auriculatum* *Trichonema auriculatum* *Cyathostomum auriculatum*	Africa, Asia, Americas	Buccal capsule not shallow; dorsal gutter absent; lateral papillae long ear-like or horn-like extending much higher than mouth collar; excretory pore and cervical papillae behind oesophago-intestinal junction	Rare
C. brevicapsulatus	*Cylicostomum brevispiculatum* *Cylichobrachytus brevispiculatum* *Trichonema brevispiculatum*	Africa, Asia, Europe, North America	Buccal capsule extremely shallow with delicate inconspicuous walls	Very rare
C. elongatus	*Cyathostomum elongatum* *Cylichnostomum elongatum* *Trichonema elongatum* *Cylicostomum elongatum*	Cosmopoitan	Buccal capsule not shallow; dorsal gutter absent; lateral papillae not long; excretory pore and cervical papillae anterior oesophago-intestinal junction; oesophageal funnel nearly as large as buccal capsule; oesophagus greatly elongated with posterior half enlarged and cylindrical	Common
C. insigne	*Cylichnostomum insigne* *Cylicostomum insigne* *Cylicostomum zebra* *Trichonema insigne*	Cosmopolitan	Buccal capsule not shallow; dorsal gutter absent; lateral papillae not long; excretory pore and cervical papillae anterior to oesophago-intestinal junction; external leaf crown elements narrow; inner leaf crown elements much shorter than external leaf crown elements and uniform length	Very common
C. largocapsulatus	*Trichonema largocapsulatus*	Asia	Oesophago-intestinal valve not elongate; buccal capsule large; elements of external leaf crown almost about half as long as buccal capsule is deep	Very rare
C. leptostomus	*Cylichnostomum leptostomum* *Trichonema leptostomum* *Schultzitrichonema leptostomum* *Cylicotetrapedon leptostomum*	Africa, Asia, Europe, North America	Oesophago-intestinal valve elongate; buccal capsule small; elements of external leaf crown almost as long as buccal capsule is deep	Common
C. maturmurai	*Trichonema maturmurai*	Asia	Buccal capsule not shallow, walls of uniform thickness; inner leaf crown elements more than external leaf crown elements and uniform length	Very rare

(*continued*)

Table 4.2 (*cont'd*)

Species	Synonyms	Distribution	Description	Comments
C. nassatus	*Cyathostomum nassatum* *Cylichnostomum nassatum* *Cylicostomum nassatum* *Trichonema nassatum* *Cylicocyclus bulbiferus*	Cosmopolitan	Buccal capsule not shallow with both lateral papillae and external leaf crown extending beyond mouth collar; dorsal gutter present extending half of depth of buccal capsule; sub-median papillae long extending beyond mouth collar; external leaf crown with 20 elements; buccal capsule with internal shelf-like cuticular projection	Very common
C. radiatus	*Cyathostomum radiatum* *Cylichnostomum radiatum* *Trichonema radiatum* *Cylicostomum prionodes*	Cosmopolitan	Oesophago-intestinal valve not elongate; buccal capsule large; elements of external leaf crown almost about one third as long buccal capsule is deep	Rare
C. triramosus	*Cylicostomum triramosum* *Trichonema triramosum*	Africa, Asia, North America	Buccal capsule not shallow with both lateral papillae and external leaf crown extending beyond mouth collar; dorsal gutter short, button-like; sub-median papillae short and do not extend beyond mouth collar; external leaf crown with 30 elements; buccal capsule without internal projection	Rare
C. ultrajectinus	*Cylicostomum ultrajectinum* *Trichonema ultrajectinum*	Cosmopolitan	Buccal capsule not shallow; dorsal gutter absent; lateral papillae not long; excretory pore and cervical papillae near oesophago-intestinal junction; external leaf crown elements broad; inner leaf crown elements as long or longer than external leaf crown elements	Common

Table 4.3 *Cylicodontophorus* species.

Species	Synonyms	Distribution	Description	Comments
C. bicoronatus	*Cyathostomum bicoronatum* *Cylichnostomum bicoronatum* *Cylicostomum bicoranatum* *Trichonema bicoronatum*	Cosmopolitan	Dorsal gutter well developed; elements of external and internal leaf crowns of nearly equal size	Common
C. euproctus	*Cylichnostomum euproctus* *Cylicostomum euproctus* *Trichonema euproctus*	Cosmopolitan	Dorsal gutter absent; elements of internal leaf crowns twice as long as elements of external leaf crown size; oesophageal funnel not well developed	Rare
C. mettami	*Cylicostoma mettami* *Cylicostomum mettami* *Trichonema mettami* *Cylicocercus mettami* *Cylicostomum ihlei*	Africa, Europe, Asia	Dorsal gutter absent; elements of internal leaf crowns more than twice as long as elements of external leaf crown size; oesophageal funnel well developed	Very rare

Table 4.4 *Cylicostephanus* species.

Species	Synonyms	Distribution	Description	Comments
C. asymetricus	*Cylicostomum asymetricum* *Cylicotrapedon asymetricum* *Schulzitrichonema asymetricum*	Africa, Asia, Europe, North America	Walls of buccal capsule markedly thicker anteriorly; elements of external leaf crown as broad as long, dorsal gutter extends almost to base of inner leaf crown. Buccal capsule asymmetrical in lateral view and walls of capsule concave; teeth in oesophageal funnel not prominent	Very rare
C. bidentatus	*Cylicostomum bidentatum* *Cylicotrapedon bidentatum* *Trichonema bidentatum* *Schulzitrichonema bidentatum*	Europe, North America	Walls of buccal capsule markedly thicker anteriorly; elements of external leaf crown as broad as long, dorsal gutter extends almost to base of inner leaf crown. Buccal capsule symmetrical in lateral view and walls of capsule straight; prominent teeth in oesophageal funnel	Very rare
C. calicatus	*Cyathostomum calicatum* *Cylichnostomum calicatum* *Cylicostomum calicatum* *Trichonema calicatum* *Cylicostomum barbatum* *Trichonema tsengi*	Cosmopolitan	Buccal capsule as broad as deep and wall of uniform thickness. External leaf crowns composed of 8–18 triangular elements; sub-median papillae notched near tips	Very common
C. goldi	*Cylichnostomum goldi* *Cylicostomum goldi* *Trichonema goldi* *Schulzitrichonema goldi* *Cylicostomum tridentatum*	Cosmopolitan	Walls of buccal capsule uniform thick; elements of external leaf crown twice as numerous as elements of inner leaf crown, dorsal gutter button-like. Walls of buccal capsule slight compound curve, slightly thicker posteriorly; female tail bent dorsally; prominent teeth in oesophageal funnel	Common
C. hybridus	*Cylicostomum hybridus* *Trichonema hybridum* *Schulzitrichonema hybridum* *Trichonema parvibursatus*	Asia, Europe	Walls of buccal capsule uniform thick; elements of external leaf crown twice as long as broad, dorsal gutter extends half to base of inner leaf crown. Walls of buccal capsule straight, slightly thicker posteriorly in dorsal view	Rare
C. longibursatus	*Cylicostomum longibursatum* *Trichonema longibursatum* *Cylicostomum nanum* *Cylicostomum calicatiforme*	Cosmopolitan	Walls of buccal capsule uniform thick; elements of external leaf crown twice as long as broad, dorsal gutter button-like. Walls of buccal capsule slight compound curve, slightly thicker posteriorly. Dorsal ray of male bursa very long; female tail straight; teeth in oesophageal funnel not prominent	Very common
C. minutus	*Cylicostomum minutum* *Trichonema minutum*	Cosmopolitan	Buccal capsule as broad as deep and wall of uniform thickness. External leaf crowns composed of 8–18 triangular elements; sub-median papillae notched midway	Very common

(*continued*)

Table 4.4 (*cont'd*)

Species	Synonyms	Distribution	Description	Comments
C. ornatus	*Cylicostomum ornatum* *Trichonema ornatum* *Cylicostomias ornatum* *Cyathostomum ornatum* *Cylicodontophorus ornatum*	Asia, Europe	Walls of buccal capsule markedly thicker anteriorly; elements of external leaf crown as broad as long, dorsal gutter extends almost to base of inner leaf crown. Buccal capsule asymmetrical in lateral view and walls of capsule concave; teeth in oesophageal funnel not prominent. Short, stout bursa	Rare
C. poculatus	*Cyathostomum poculatum* *Cylichnostomum poculatum* *Cylicostomum poculatum* *Trichonema poculatum* *Petrovina poculatum*	Cosmopolitan	Buccal capsule deeper than broader in lateral view and walls much thicker posteriorly. External leaf crown composed of ~36 elements	Rare
C. skrjabini	*Trichonema skrjabini* *Petrovinema skrjabini*	Asia	Buccal capsule deeper than broader in lateral view and walls much thicker posteriorly. External leaf crown composed of ~36 elements. Lacking lateral projection on inner wall of buccal capsule and has rim of dentiform processes at bottom of buccal capsule	Rare

Description, microscopic: The well developed short buccal capsule is cylindrical, without teeth, and species differentiation is based on characteristics of the buccal capsule, and the internal and external leaf crowns. *Cylicostephanus* have a depressed mouth collar, with inconspicuous lateral papillae and prominent submedian papillae. The buccal capsule is slightly narrow anteriorly, with a wall of varying thickness, and with a dorsal gutter. External leaf crown elements are longer, broader and less numerous then the internal leaf crown elements, which are short thin rods inserted near the anterior edge of the buccal capsule. The dorsal ray of the male bursa is split only to the proximal branch, and the spicules are filiform, equal in length with 'pick-shaped' tips. In the female, the vulva is near the anus, and the tail is usually straight.

Hosts: Horse, donkey

Geographical distribution: Worldwide

Poteriostomum imparidentatum

Common name: Non-migratory large strongyles

Predilection site: Large intestine

Parasite class: Nematoda

Superfamily: Strongyloidea

Family: Strongylidae

Subfamily: Cyathostominae

Description, gross: Males are 9–14 mm and females 13–21 mm.

Description, microscopic: This genus is closely related to the genus *Cylicodontophorus*. The two genera are easily separated based on characteristics of the buccal capsule, especially the point of insertion of the internal leaf crown and the character of the dorsal ray. In *P. imparidentatum* six elements of the internal leaf crown are markedly longer than the others.

Hosts: Horse, donkey

Geographical distribution: Worldwide

Poteriostomum ratzii

Common name: Non-migratory large strongyles

Predilection site: Large intestine

Parasite class: Nematoda

Superfamily: Strongyloidea

Family: Strongylidae

Subfamily: Cyathostominae

Description, gross: Males are 9–14 mm and females 13–21 mm.

Description, microscopic: This genus is closely related to the genus *Cylicodontophorus*. The two genera are easily separated based on characteristics of the buccal capsule, especially the point of insertion of the internal leaf crown and the character of the dorsal ray. In *P. ratzii* all elements of the internal leaf crown are of equal length.

Hosts: Horse, donkey

Geographical distribution: Worldwide

Craterostomum acuticaudatum

Synonym: *Cylicostomum acuticaudatum, Cylicostomum mucronatum, Craterostomum mucronatum*

Predilection site: Large intestine

Parasite class: Nematoda

Superfamily: Strongyloidea

Family: Strongylidae

Subfamily: Cyathostominae

Description, gross: Small worms, 6–10 mm long

Description, microscopic: The buccal capsule is of greatest diameter in the middle, the wall is thickened behind the anterior edge. The dorsal gutter is strongly developed. The shallow oesophageal funnel has three small triangular teeth that do not project into the buccal cavity. Elements of the external leaf crown are large and transparent and less numerous than the short, broad elements of the inner leaf crown that ring the anterior ridge of the buccal capsule. Sub-median papillae extend beyond the depressed mouth collar. In the female the tail is long and pointed and the vulva is relatively far from the anus.

Hosts: Horse, donkey

Geographical distribution: Africa, Asia, Europe

Craterostomum tenuicauda

Predilection site: Large intestine

Parasite class: Nematoda

Superfamily: Strongyloidea

Family: Strongylidae

Subfamily: Cyathostominae

Description, gross: Small worms, 6–10 mm long

Description, microscopic: The buccal capsule is of greatest diameter in the middle, the wall is thickened behind the anterior edge. The dorsal gutter is strongly developed. The shallow oesophageal funnel has three small triangular teeth that do not project into the buccal cavity. The elements of the external leaf crown (nine) are large and transparent and less numerous than short, broad elements of the inner leaf crown (18) that ring the anterior ridge of the buccal capsule. Sub-median papillae are unnotched and extend beyond the depressed mouth collar. In the female, the tail is short and pointed and the vulva is relatively far from the anus.

Hosts: Horse, zebra

Geographical distribution: Africa, Asia

Pathogenesis: Not reported

Oesophagodontus robustus

Predilection site: Large intestine

Parasite class: Nematoda

Superfamily: Strongyloidea

Family: Strongylidae

Subfamily: Cyathostominae

Description, gross: Male worms are 15–16 mm and females 19–22 mm. There is a slight constriction between the anterior end and the rest of the body.

Description, microscopic: The buccal capsule is shaped like a funnel with a thickened ring encircling its posterior margin. The oesophageal funnel has three lancet-like teeth that do not project into the buccal capsule. There is no dorsal gutter.

Hosts: Horse, donkey

Geographical distribution: Worldwide

Large strongyles

Members of the genus *Strongylus* live in the large intestine of horses and donkeys and, with *Triodontophorus*, are commonly known as the large strongyles. Since members of these genera form only one component of the total parasitic burdens of the large intestine of the horse, general aspects on their epidemiology, treatment and control have been described under the general introduction to small strongyles.

Diagnosis of these migratory species is difficult during the migratory prepatent phase and is based on grazing history and clinical signs. Due to the long prepatent period, clinically apparent strongylosis may be associated with no, or low, faecal egg counts. Species or generic diagnosis is not usually required but may be undertaken by specialist laboratories based on morphology of larvae or adult worms.

Strongylus edentatus

Synonym: *Alfortia edentatus*

Common name: Large strongyles

Predilection site: Large intestine

Parasite class: Nematoda

Superfamily: Strongyloidea

Family: Strongylidae

Subfamily: Strongylinae

Description, gross: Robust dark red worms which are easily seen against the intestinal mucosa (Fig. 4.14). The well developed buccal capsule of the adult parasite is prominent, as is the bursa of the male. Male are 2.3–2.8 cm in size and females 3.3–4.4 cm. The head end is wider than the rest of the body.

Description, microscopic: Species differentiation is based on size and the presence and shape of the teeth in the base of the buccal capsule. The buccal capsule is wider anteriorly than at the middle and contains no teeth (Fig. 4.15a).

Hosts: Horse, donkey

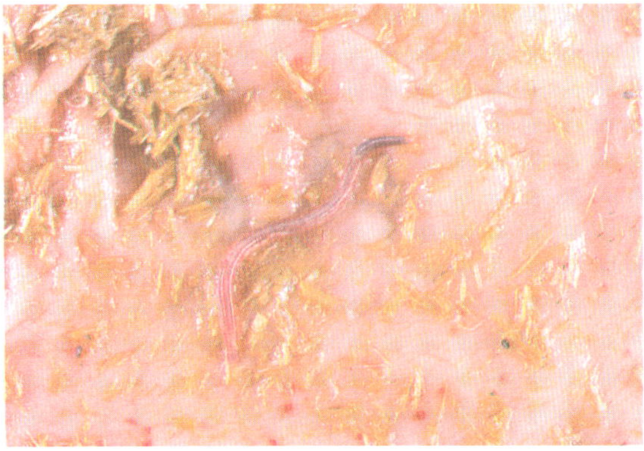

Fig. 4.14 *Strongylus edentatus* feeding on the mucosa of the large intestine.

Life cycle: The adult parasites live in the caecum and colon. Eggs, which resemble those of the trichostrongyles, are passed in the faeces and development from egg to the L_3 under summer conditions in temperate climates requires approximately 2 weeks. Infection is by ingestion of the L_3. Subsequently, parasitic larval development of the three species of *Strongylus* differs and will be dealt with separately.

After penetration of the intestinal mucosa L_3 travel via the portal system, and reach the liver parenchyma

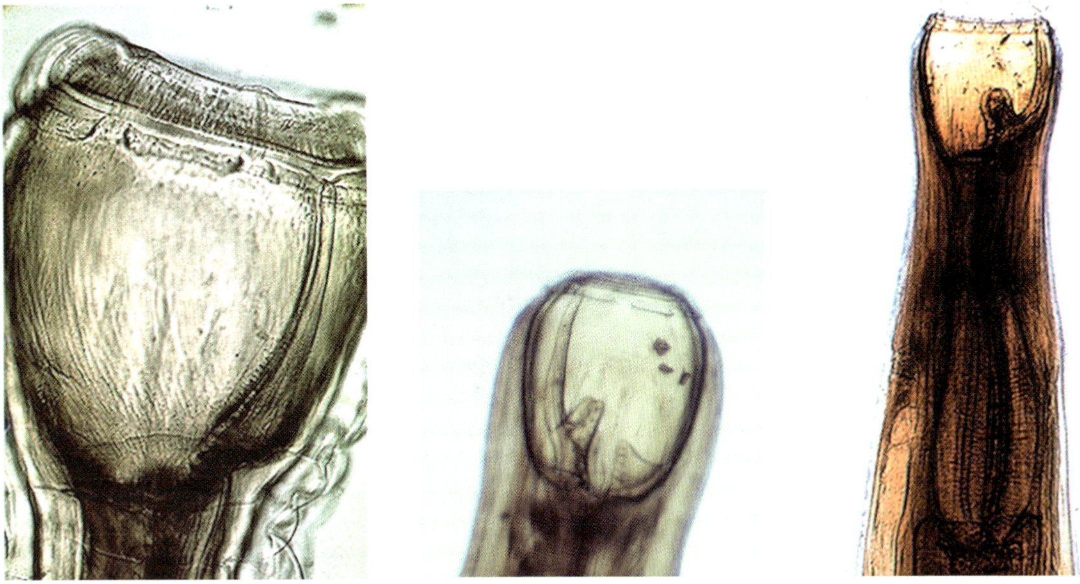

(a) (b) (c)

Fig. 4.15 (a) Anterior of *Strongylus edentatus* showing the cup-shaped buccal capsule, which is devoid of teeth. (b) Anterior of *Strongylus equinus* showing oval buccal capsule with a large dorsal tooth and smaller sub-ventral conical teeth. (c) Anterior of *Strongylus vulgaris* showing ear-shaped rounded teeth at the base of the buccal capsule.

within a few days. About 2 weeks later the moult to L_4 takes place, further migration then occurs in the liver and, by 6–8 weeks post-infection, larvae can be found subperitoneally around the hepatorenal ligament. The larvae then travel under the peritoneum to many sites with a predilection for the flanks and hepatic ligaments. The final moult occurs after 4 months and each L_5 then migrates, still subperitoneally, to the wall of the large intestine where a large purulent nodule is formed, which subsequently ruptures with release of the young adult parasite into the lumen. The prepatent period is 10–12 months.

Geographical distribution: Worldwide

Pathogenesis: In *S. edentatus* infection, there are gross changes in the liver associated with early larval migration, but these rarely result in clinical signs. Similarly, the haemorrhages and fluid-filled nodules, which accompany later larval development in subperitoneal tissues rarely result in clinical signs.

For details of the pathogenesis of infection with adult worms see *S. vulgaris*.

Clinical signs: Diarrhoea, fever, oedema, anorexia, depression and weight loss

Pathology: Haemorrhagic tracts may be produced in the hepatic parenchyma from migrating larvae and parenchymal scars of fibrous tissue on the hepatic capsule are often found on postmortem. Migrating larvae may also elicit subperitoneal haematomas, haemorrhage, peritonitis and omental adhesions. In the gut wall they may form nodules and haemorrhagic foci.

Strongylus equinus

Common name: Large strongyles

Predilection site: Large intestine

Parasite class: Nematoda

Superfamily: Strongyloidea

Family: Strongylidae

Subfamily: Strongylinae

Description, gross: Robust dark red worms which are easily seen against the intestinal mucosa. The well developed buccal capsule of the adult parasite is prominent as is the bursa of the male. Male are 2.6–3.5 cm in size and females 3.8–4.7 cm. The head end is not marked off from the rest of the body.

Description, microscopic: Species differentiation is based on size and the presence and shape of the teeth in the base of the buccal capsule. The buccal capsule is oval in outline and there are external and internal leaf crowns. At the base of the buccal capsule is a large dorsal tooth with a bifid tip and two smaller subventral teeth (Fig. 4.15b). The dorsal oesophageal gland opens into the buccal capsule through a number of pores situated in a thickened ridge, the dorsal gutter, formed by the wall of the buccal capsule. The male has two simple, slender spicules. In the female, the vulva lies 12–14 mm from the posterior extremity. Eggs are oval, 75–92 × 41–54 μm, and thin-shelled.

Hosts: Horse, donkey

Life cycle: The adult parasites live in the caecum and colon. The free-living phase is as described for *S. edentatus*. Of the three *Strongylus* species, least is known of the larval migration of *S. equinus*. It appears that the L_3 lose their sheaths while penetrating the wall of the caecum and ventral colon and within 1 week provoke the formation of nodules in the muscular and subserosal layers of the intestine. The moult to L_4 occurs within these nodules and the larvae then travel across the peritoneal cavity to the liver where they migrate within the parenchyma for 6 weeks or more. After this time, L_4 and L_5 have been found in and around the pancreas before their appearance in the large intestinal lumen. The prepatent period is 8–9 months.

Geographical distribution: Worldwide

Pathogenesis: Despite the invasive behaviour of the parasitic larval stages, little specific pathogenic effect can be attributed to them. There has been little work on the pathogenesis of migrating larvae of *S. equinus*. For details of the pathogenesis of infection with adult worms see *S. vulgaris*.

Clinical signs: Diarrhoea, fever, oedema, anorexia, depression and weight loss

Pathology: Haemorrhagic tracts may be produced in the hepatic parenchyma from migrating larvae and parenchymal scars of fibrous tissue on the hepatic capsule are often found on postmortem. Omental adhesions may also be a sequel to larval migration. In the gut wall they may form nodules and haemorrhagic foci.

Epidemiology: *Strongylus equinus* is relatively less prevalent and abundant than other members of the genus.

Strongylus vulgaris

Common name: Large strongyles

Predilection site: Large intestine

Parasite class: Nematoda

Superfamily: Strongyloidea

Family: Strongylidae

Subfamily: Strongylinae

Description, gross: Robust dark red worms which are easily seen against the intestinal mucosa. The well developed buccal capsule of the adult parasite is prominent as is the bursa of the male. Male are 14–16 mm in size and females 20–24 mm. The head end is not marked off from the rest of the body.

Description, microscopic: Species differentiation is based on size and the presence and shape of the teeth in the base of the buccal capsule. The buccal capsule is oval in outline and contains two ear-shaped teeth at its base (Fig. 4.15c). The elements of the leaf crowns are fringed at their distal extremities. The dorsal oesophageal gland opens into the buccal capsule through a number of pores situated in a thickened ridge, the dorsal gutter, formed by the wall of the buccal capsule. Eggs are oval, 83–93 × 48–52 mm, and thin-shelled.

Hosts: Horse, donkey

Life cycle: The adult parasites live in the caecum and colon. The free-living phase is as described for *S. edentatus*. Following ingestion, the L_3 penetrate the intestinal mucosa and moult to L_4 in the submucosa 7 days later. These then enter small arteries and migrate on the endothelium to their predilection site in the cranial mesenteric artery and its main branches. After a period of development of several months the larvae moult to L_5 and return to the intestinal wall via the arterial lumina. Nodules are formed around the larvae mainly in the wall of the caecum and colon when, due to their size, they can travel no further within the arteries and subsequent rupture of these nodules releases the young adult parasites into the lumen of the intestine. The prepatent period is 6–7 months.

Geographical distribution: Worldwide

Pathogenesis: *Strongylus vulgaris* is less common than it was 20 years ago in many countries, but is still the most significant and pathogenic nematode parasitic in horses. Larval forms cause endoarteritis in the mesenteric circulation, resulting in colic and thromboembolic infarction of the large bowel, while the adults cause anaemia and ill-thrift. Much of the information concerning *S. vulgaris* has been derived from experimental infection of foals. A few weeks after infection with several hundred L_3, a clinical syndrome of fever, inappetence and dullness occurs, sometimes accompanied by colic. At necropsy, these signs are associated with arteritis and thrombosis of intestinal blood vessels, with subsequent infarction and necrosis of areas of bowel. However, a syndrome of this severity is not commonly reported in foals under natural conditions, probably because larval intake is continuous during grazing; it has been shown experimentally that foals may tolerate large numbers of larvae administered in small doses over a long period.

The pathogenesis of infection with adult worms is associated with damage to the large intestinal mucosa due to the feeding habits of the worms and, to some extent, to the disruption caused by emergence of young adults into the intestine following completion of their parasitic larval development. These worms have large buccal capsules and feed by ingestion of plugs of mucosa as they move over the surface of the intestine. Although the worms appear to feed entirely on mucosal material, the incidental damage to blood vessels can cause considerable haemorrhage. Ulcers, which result from these bites, eventually heal, leaving small circular scars. The effects of infection with the adult worms have not been quantified, but the gross damage and subsequent loss of blood and tissue fluids is certainly partly responsible for the unthriftiness and anaemia associated with intestinal helminthosis in the horse.

Clinical signs: Anaemia, poor condition and performance, varying degrees of colic, temporary lameness, intestinal stasis, rarely intestinal rupture and death.

Diagnosis: Colic due to verminous arteritis may be associated with a palpable, painful enlargement at the root of the mesentery.

Pathology: Lesions due to migrating larvae are most common in the cranial mesenteric artery and its main branches (Fig. 4.16), and consist of thrombus formation provoked by larval damage to the endothelium, together with a marked inflammation and thickening of the arterial wall (Fig. 4.17). True aneurysms with dilatation and thinning of the arterial wall, although uncommon, may be found, especially in animals which have experienced repeated infection.

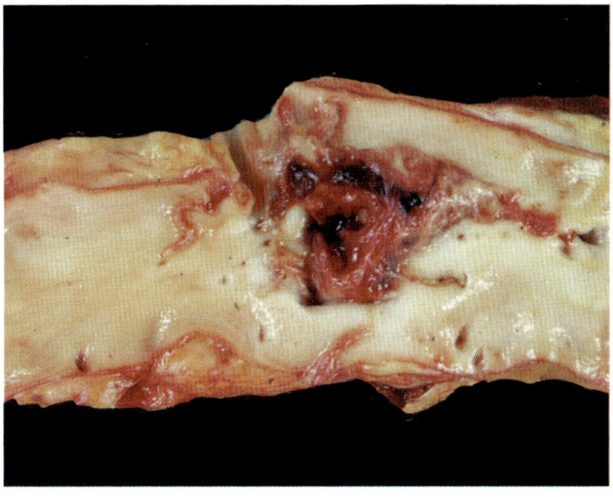

Fig. 4.16 *Strongylus vulgaris* larvae in the cranial mesenteric artery.

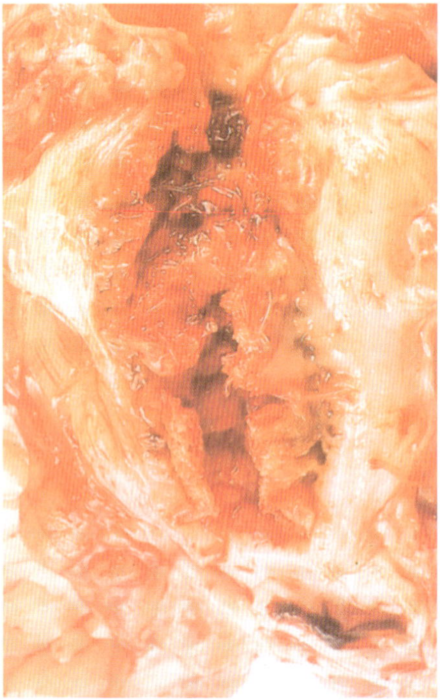

Fig. 4.17 Arteritis and thrombosis of cranial mesenteric artery caused by *Strongylus vulgaris* infection.

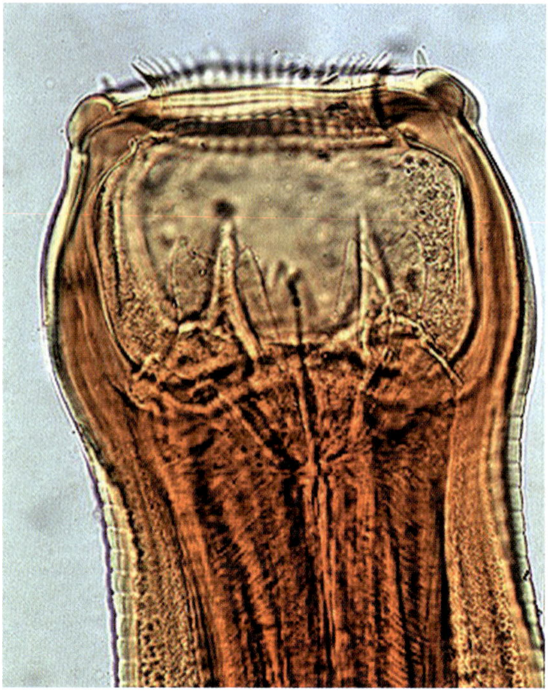

Fig. 4.18 Head of *Triodontophorus* spp, showing the location of teeth at the base of the buccal capsule.

Triodontophorus

Members of the genus *Triodontophorus* are non-migratory, large strongyles frequently found in large numbers in the colon and contribute to the deleterious effects of mixed strongyle infection.

Life cycle: Little information is available on the developmental cycle of this genus, but it is thought to be similar to that of cyathostomes.

Pathogenesis: Like the other horse strongyles, the pathogenic effect of these worms is damage to the large intestinal mucosa from the feeding habits of the adult parasites (Fig. 4.18).

Clinical signs: Loss of condition, anaemia, weakness, diarrhoea

Pathology: Feeding worms lead to the formation of ulcers in the right dorsal colon. The ulcers may be deep and haemorrhagic and bunches of worms may be attached to them (Fig. 4.19).

Triodontophorus brevicauda

Common name: Non-migratory large strongyles

Predilection site: Large intestine

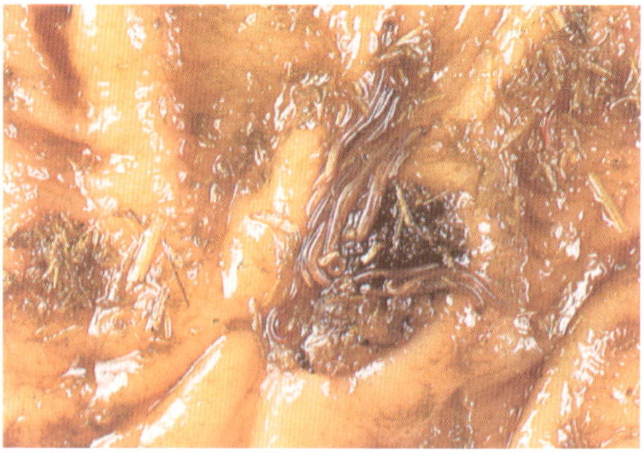

Fig. 4.19 *Triodontophorus tenuicollis* adults feeding around the periphery of an ulcer in the ventral colon.

Parasite class: Nematoda

Superfamily: Strongyloidea

Family: Strongylidae

Subfamily: Strongylinae

Description, gross: Medium-sized worms, varying in size from 9–25 mm

Description, microscopic: The buccal capsule is sub-globular and thick-walled with three large oesophageal teeth composed of two plates, which are smooth except for three elevations on each and protrude into the buccal capsule. The anterior rim of the buccal capsule is thickened anteriorly and surrounded by six plate-like structures. The sub-median papillae are short, broad and conical. The external leaf crown consists of numerous slender elements protruding from the buccal collar, with an equal number of inner leaf crown elements. In the female, the vulva is close to the anus and the tail is very short.

Hosts: Horse, donkey

Geographical distribution: Worldwide

Triodontophorus minor

Common name: Non-migratory large strongyles

Predilection site: Large intestine

Parasite class: Nematoda

Superfamily: Strongyloidea

Family: Strongylidae

Subfamily: Strongylinae

Description, gross: Medium-sized worms, varying in size from 9–25 mm

Description, microscopic: The buccal capsule is sub-globular and thick-walled with three large oesophageal teeth composed of two plates which are strongly denticulated and protrude into the buccal capsule. The anterior rim of the buccal capsule is thickened anteriorly and surrounded by six plate-like structures. The cuticle is strongly serrated in the cervical region. The external leaf crown consists of 44–50 slender elements protruding from the buccal collar, with an equal number of inner leaf crown elements. In the female, the vulva is close to the anus and the tail is short.

Hosts: Horse, donkey

Geographical distribution: Worldwide

Triodontophorus nipponicus

Common name: Non-migratory large strongyles

Predilection site: Large intestine

Parasite class: Nematoda

Superfamily: Strongyloidea

Family: Strongylidae

Subfamily: Strongylinae

Description, gross: Medium-sized worms, varying in size from 9–25 mm

Description, microscopic: The buccal capsule is sub-globular and thick-walled with three large oesophageal teeth, composed of two plates which are strongly denticulated, with three large denticulations, and protrude into the buccal capsule. The anterior rim of the buccal capsule is thickened anteriorly and surrounded by six plate-like structures. The cuticle is strongly serrated in the cervical region. The external leaf crown consists of 56–69 slender elements protruding from the buccal collar, with an equal number of inner leaf crown elements. In the female, the vulva is close to the anus and the tail is short.

Hosts: Horse, donkey

Geographical distribution: Worldwide

Triodontophorus serratus

Common name: Non-migratory large strongyles

Predilection site: Large intestine

Parasite class: Nematoda

Superfamily: Strongyloidea

Family: Strongylidae

Subfamily: Strongylinae

Description, microscopic: The buccal capsule is sub-globular and thick-walled with three large oesophageal teeth composed of two plates that protrude into the buccal capsule. The anterior rim of the buccal capsule is thickened anteriorly and surrounded by six plate-like structures. The mouth collar appears as an inflated round tube around the mouth. The external leaf crown consists of numerous slender elements protruding from the buccal collar, with an equal number of inner leaf crown elements. In the female, the vulva is close to the anus and the tail is long.

Hosts: Horse, donkey

Geographical distribution: Worldwide

Triodontophorus tenuicollis

Common name: Non-migratory large strongyles

Predilection site: Large intestine

Parasite class: Nematoda

Superfamily: Strongyloidea

Family: Strongylidae

Subfamily: Strongylinae

Description, microscopic: The buccal capsule is sub-globular and thick-walled with three large oesophageal teeth composed of two plates which are finely denticulated and protrude into the buccal capsule. The anterior rim of the buccal capsule is thickened anteriorly and surrounded by six plate-like structures. The cuticle is strongly serrated in the cervical region. The external leaf crown consists of numerous slender elements protruding from the buccal collar, with an equal number of inner leaf crown elements. In the female, the vulva is close to the anus.

Hosts: Horse, donkey

Life cycle: As for *T. brevicauda*

Geographical distribution: Worldwide

Oxyuris equi

Common name: Equine pinworm, rat-tail

Predilection site: Caecum, colon and rectum

Parasite class: Nematoda

Superfamily: Oxyuroidea

Description, gross: The mature females are large greyish white, opaque worms with very long tapering tails that may reach 10–15 cm in length, whereas the mature males are generally less than 1.2 cm long (Fig. 4.20). Adult males have one pin-shaped spicule. *O. equi* L_4 are 5–10 mm in length, have tapering tails and are often attached orally to the intestinal mucosa.

Description, microscopic: There is a double oesophageal bulb (Fig. 4.21) and the tiny males have caudal alae and a single spicule. In the female the vulva is situated anteriorly. *O. equi* eggs are ovoid, yellowish, thick-shelled and slightly flattened on one side with a mucoid plug at one end. Eggs contain a morula or larval stage when shed in faeces.

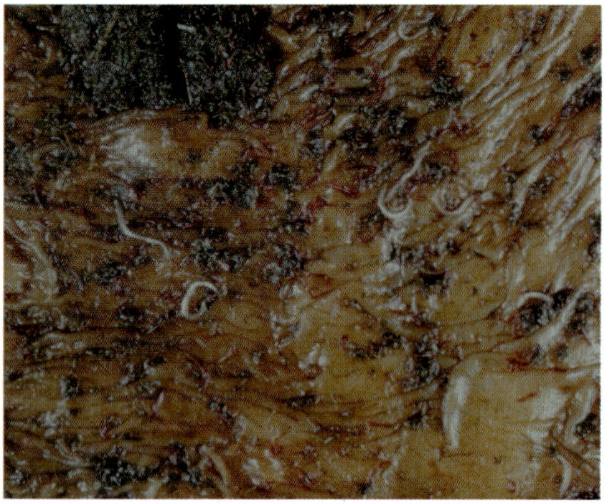

Fig. 4.20 Mixed infection of *Oxyuris equi* adults (white) and small strongyles in the colon.

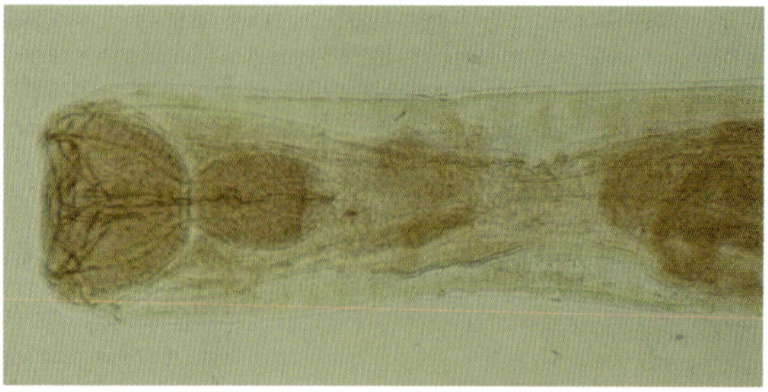

Fig. 4.21 Head of *Oxyuris equi* showing double oesophageal bulb.

Hosts: Horse, donkey

Life cycle: The life cycle is direct. The adult worms are found in the lumen of the caecum and large colon. After fertilisation the gravid female migrates to the anus, extrudes her anterior end and lays her eggs in clumps (up to 50 000 eggs per female), seen grossly as yellowish white gelatinous streaks on the perineal skin or perianal region (Fig. 4.22). Development is rapid, and within 4–5 days the egg contains the infective L_3. Eggs are rubbed off and contaminate the environment. Infection is by ingestion of embryonated eggs on fodder, grass, bedding etc. The larvae are released in the small intestine, move into the large intestine and migrate into the mucosal crypts of the caecum and colon where development to L_4 takes place within 10 days. The L_4 then emerge and feed on the mucosa before maturing to adult stages that inhabit the lumen and feed on intestinal contents. The prepatent period of *O. equi* is 5 months. Longevity of female worms is around 6 months.

Geographical distribution: Worldwide

Pathogenesis: Most of the pathogenic effects of *O. equi* in the intestine are due to the feeding habits of the L_4, which result in small erosions of the mucosa and, in heavy infections, these may be widespread and accompanied by an inflammatory response. Normally, a more important effect is the perineal irritation and anal pruritis caused by the adult females during egg-laying. The resultant dull hair coat and loss of hair is known as 'rat-tail'.

Clinical signs: The presence of parasites in the intestine rarely causes any clinical signs. However, intense pruritis around the anus causes the animal to rub on available solid objects, resulting in broken hairs, bare patches and inflammation and scaling of the skin over the rump and tail head. The intense itching often leads to restlessness and impaired feeding, causing some loss of condition.

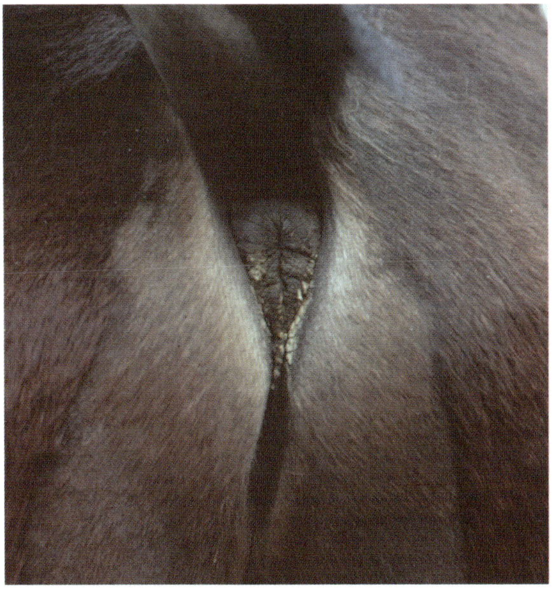

Fig. 4.22 Clumps of *Oxyuris equi eggs* around the rectum of a horse.

Diagnosis: This is based on signs of anal pruritis and tail rubbing and the finding of greyish yellow egg masses on the perineal skin. The large white long-tailed female worms are often seen in the faeces (Fig. 4.23), having been dislodged while laying their eggs. *O. equi* eggs are rarely found on faecal examination of samples taken from the rectum, but may be observed in material from the perineum or in faecal material taken from the ground. The condition needs to be differentiated from mange.

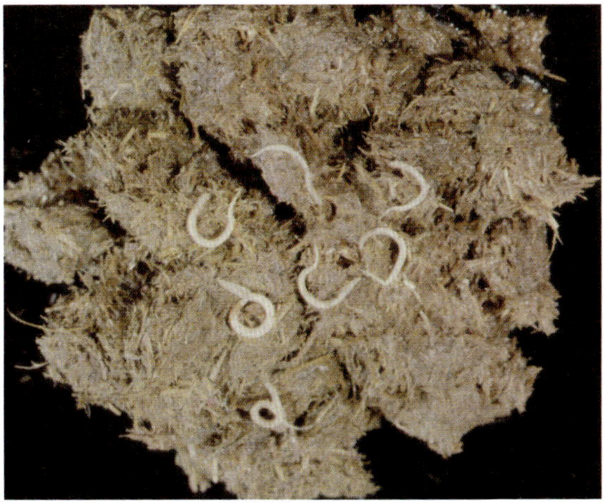

Fig. 4.23 Adult *Oxyuris equi* worms in faeces.

Pathology: Small erosions may occur in the mucosa in heavy infections accompanied by a mixed inflammatory cell response.

Epidemiology: Although the infective stage may be reached on the skin, more often flakes of material containing eggs are dispersed in the environment by the animal rubbing on stable fittings, fencing posts or other solid objects. Heavy burdens may build up in horses in infected stables and there appears to be little immunity to reinfection.

Treatment: *O. equi* is susceptible to many broad-spectrum anthelmintics and should be controlled by routine chemotherapy for the more important horse parasites. Effective anthelmintics include ivermectin, moxidectin, the benzimidazoles (fenbendazole, oxfendazole, oxibendazole) and pyrantel. Newly acquired horses should be treated routinely.

Where animals are showing clinical signs, the perineal skin and underside of the tail should be frequently cleaned (about every 4 days) using a disposable cloth to remove the egg masses prior to their development to L_3 larvae, in addition to anthelmintic treatment.

Control: A high standard of stable hygiene should be observed, such as the frequent removal of bedding and the provision of feeding racks and water troughs than cannot easily be contaminated by bedding.

Notes: Infection with the horse pinworm, *Oxyuris equi*, is extremely common and, although of limited pathogenic significance in the intestine, the female parasites may cause an intense anal pruritis during the process of egg-laying.

Probstmayria vivipara

Common name: Small equine pinworm

Predilection site: Colon

Parasite class: Nematoda

Superfamily: Oxyuroidea

Description, gross: Small slender nematodes, 2.0–3.0 mm, with long filamentous tails

Description, microscopic: The mouth has six small lips and the buccal capsule is cylindrical and long. The oesophagus has an expanded posterior bulb. A large sucker-like excretory pore is present.

Hosts: Horse and various equids

Life cycle: *P. vivipara* is unusual in that it is a perpetual parasite and lives from generation to generation in the equine caecum and colon. The females are viviparous and give birth to larvae almost as large as the adults. Both adults and larvae may be passed in the faeces.

Geographical distribution: Probably worldwide, except some regions of western Europe

Pathogenesis: It is generally considered to be non-pathogenic and although millions of these pinworms may be present they have never given rise to any clinical signs.

Clinical signs: No associated clinical signs

Diagnosis: First-stage larvae may be found in the faeces or larvae and adult worms may be found on necropsy.

Pathology: No associated pathology

Epidemiology: Transmission is probably via coprophagia.

Treatment: The parasite is susceptible to most modern anthelmintics.

Control: Not usually required

Intestinal flukes

Several species of intestinal flukes belonging to the genera *Gastrodiscus* and *Pseudodiscus* are found in the large intestine of horses. Intermediate hosts are snails.

Life cycle: The life cycle of the different species is generally similar. Eggs are passed in the faeces and, following development, release miracidia into water where they enter a species of water snail. Development in the snail proceeds through sporocyst and rediae stages leading to the release of cercariae, which encyst to form metacercariae. Infection of the final host is by ingestion of metacercariae with herbage. Excystation occurs in the intestine where the immature paramphistomes develop to reach maturity.

Pathogenicity: Adult flukes cause little damage to the intestine. Disease is usually caused by large numbers of immature flukes.

Clinical signs: Mild infections are subclinical. Heavy infections are accompanied by diarrhoea, anaemia, oedema, emaciation and marked weakness.

Diagnosis: Diagnosis is based on the presence of eggs in faeces or immature flukes in fluid faeces.

Pathology: Immature flukes are embedded in the mucosa, causing haemorrhage and necrosis. In heavy infections, there may be catarrhal and haemorrhagic enteritis.

Epidemiology: Infection is acquired by ingesting the intermediate hosts with vegetation.

Treatment: Flukicidal drugs, such as nitroxynil, oxyclozanide, closantel, triclabendazole or albendazole and netobimin, are active against the adult flukes; triclabendazole at 10 mg/kg or clasantel at 7 mg/kg are active against immature flukes.

Control: Wet pastures or swamps where the intermediate hosts are found should be avoided.

Gastrodiscus aegyptiacus

Common name: Intestinal fluke

Predilection site: Small and large intestine

Parasite class: Trematoda

Family: Paramphistomatidae

Description, gross: Adult flukes are pink in colour and measure 9–17 × 8–11 mm. The anterior is up to 4 mm and cylindrical, whilst the rest of the body is saucer-shaped, with the margins curved inwards.

Description, microscopic: The ventral surface is covered by a large number of regularly arranged papillae. The oral sucker has two posterolateral pouches; the posterior sucker is small and subterminal. Eggs are oval and measure 131–139 × 78–90 μm.

Final hosts: Horse, pig, warthog

Geographical distribution: Africa, India

Gastrodiscus secundus

Common name: Intestinal fluke

Predilection site: Large intestine

Parasite class: Trematoda

Family: Paramphistomatidae

Final hosts: Horse

Geographical distribution: India

Pseudodiscus collinsi

Common name: Intestinal fluke

Predilection site: Large intestine

Parasite class: Trematoda

Family: Paramphistomatidae

Description, gross: Adult flukes have a conical anterior end widening gradually to an oval leaf-like shape.

Description, microscopic: The conical body has conspicuous serrations along the anterior lateral margins. There is a ventral sucker and the oral sucker has paired pouch-like diverticula.

Final hosts: Horse

Geographical distribution: India

Others

Entamoeba gedoelsti

Predilection site: Large intestine

Parasite subphylum: Sarcodina

Family: Endamoebidae

Hosts: Horse

Description: Trophozoites are 7–13 µm in diameter. The nucleus has an eccentric endostome and a row of relatively coarse chromatin granules around its periphery. Cysts have not been reported.

Life cycle: The life cycle has not been described

Geographical distribution: Worldwide

Pathogenesis: Non-pathogenic

Clinical signs: No associated clinical signs

Diagnosis: Identification of trophozoites in caecal contents or faeces

Epidemiology: Transmission is probably by ingestion of trophozoites. No cyst stage has been described.

Treatment and control: Not required

PARASITES OF THE RESPIRATORY SYSTEM

Rhinoestrus purpureus

Common name: Horse nasal bot fly

Predilection site: Nasal passages

Parasite class: Insecta

Family: Oestridae

Description, adults: A relatively small fly, 8–11 mm in length. The anterior thorax is characterised by a number of glossy black stripes. The head, thorax and abdomen are covered with small wart-like protuberances and a covering of short yellow–brown hairs. The head is broad, with small eyes. The legs are red and yellow–brown. The mouthparts are reduced to small knobs.

Description, larvae: The larvae resemble those of *Oestrus ovis* except that they have strongly recurved mouth hooks and a single row of 8–12 terminal hooklets; there are three larval stages, approximately 1, 3.5 and 20 mm in length respectively.

Hosts: Horse, donkey, occasionally humans

Life cycle: The female fly produces 700 to 800 larvae which are expelled in batches of up to 40 into the nostrils of the hosts. First-stage larvae remain in the nasal cavities, before moving to the pharyngeal area, where they moult to become second- and then third-stage larvae. The rate of development varies considerably depending on location. Third-stage larva are expelled and pupate in the ground.

Geographical distribution: Russia, Ukraine, central Asia

Pathogenesis: This species is a serious veterinary problem in areas such as Russia, and infestation by large numbers of larvae in the throat may result in a high level of mortality.

Clinical signs: Nasal discharge, rubbing, sneezing, unthriftiness, circling and lack of co-ordination. Secondary bacterial infections are common.

Diagnosis: Larvae may be observed in the nasal cavities, throat and base of the tongue.

Pathology: Catarrh, infiltration of inflammatory cells and squamous metaplasia, characterised by conversion of secretory epithelium to stratified squamous type may be observed. Immune responses by the host to infestation may be recorded.

Epidemiology: Adults are on the wing in midsummer. Usually only one generation per year occurs, although a second may be observed in some areas.

Treatment: Where thc numbers of larvae are small, it may not be economically viable to treat. However, in heavy infections closantel, nitroxynil, and the endectocides ivermectin, doramectin and moxidectin are highly effective, as are the organophosphates trichlorfon and dichlorvos.

Control: Area-wide control may be impractical; herd treatment may be given twice a year, the first at the beginning of summer to kill newly acquired larvae, and the second in midwinter to kill any overwintering larvae.

Dictyocaulus arnfieldi

Common name: Equine lungworm

Predilection site: Lungs

Parasite class: Nematoda

Superfamily: Trichostrongyloidea

Description, gross: The adults are slender, thread-like and whitish; the adult males measuring around 3.5 cm and the females 6.5 cm in length. Their location in the trachea and bronchi and their size are diagnostic.

Description, microscopic: Male worms have a small non-lobulated bursa with short rays, with the mediolateral and posteriolateral rays fused for half their

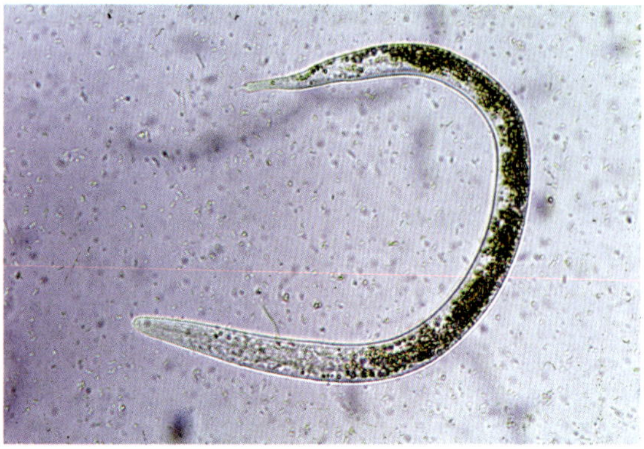

Fig. 4.24 *Dictyocaulus arnfieldi* first-stage larva showing the terminal protuberance.

length. The spicules are short, equal length and slightly curved. Eggs are 80–100 × 50–60 μm and embryonated. First-stage larvae are 290–480 μm with a posterior protuberance (Fig. 4.24).

Hosts: Donkey, other equids and occasionally the horse

Life cycle: The detailed life cycle is not fully known, but is considered to be similar to that of the bovine lungworm, *D. viviparus*, except in the following respects. The adult worms are most often found in the small bronchi and their thin-shelled eggs, containing the first-stage larvae, are coughed up before they are swallowed, passed in the faeces and then hatch soon after being deposited. The prepatent period is around 2–3 months. Patent infections are common in donkeys of all ages, but in horses generally only occur in foals and yearlings. In older horses the adult lungworms rarely attain sexual maturity.

Geographical distribution: Worldwide

Pathogenesis: The characteristic lesion is similar in both horses and donkeys and is somewhat different from bovine parasitic bronchitis.

Clinical signs: Despite the prevalence of patent *D. arnfieldi* infection in donkeys, overt clinical signs are rarely seen; however, on close examination slight hyperpnoea and harsh lung sounds may be detected. This absence of significant clinical abnormality may be partly a reflection of the fact that donkeys are rarely required to perform sustained exercise.

Infection is much less prevalent in horses. However, patent infections may develop in foals and these are not usually associated with clinical signs. In older horses, infections rarely become patent but are often associated with persistent coughing, nasal discharge and an increased respiratory rate.

Diagnosis: In donkeys, patent infections are common and L_1 are readily recovered from fresh faeces. In horses, although a history of donkey contact and clinical signs may be suggestive of *D. arnfieldi* infection, it is often not possible to confirm a diagnosis by demonstrating larvae in the faeces, as many infections do not reach patency. In practice, a presumptive diagnosis of lungworm infection in horses is often only possible in retrospect, when resolution of the clinical signs occurs after treatment.

Pathology: In the caudal lung lobes particularly, there are raised circumscribed areas of over-inflated pulmonary tissue 3.0–5.0 cm in diameter. On section, at the centre of each lesion is a small bronchus containing lungworms and mucopurulent exudate. Microscopically, the epithelium is hyperplastic with an increase in the size and number of mucus-secreting cells while the lamina propria is heavily infiltrated and often surrounded by inflammatory cells, predominantly lymphocytes.

Epidemiology: Donkeys acquire infection as foals and yearlings and tend to remain infected, presumably through re-exposure, all their lives. Horses are thought to acquire infection mainly from pastures contaminated by donkeys during the summer months. Most commonly this occurs when donkeys are grazed as companion animals with horses. However, natural infection in horses can occur in the absence of donkeys. In horses, the prevalence of *D. arnfieldi* is difficult to establish since infections only occasionally achieve patency. *Pilobolus* fungi may play a role in the dissemination of *D. arnfieldi* larvae from faeces, as in *D. viviparus*.

Treatment: Successful treatment of both horses and donkeys has been reported using ivermectin or some benzimidazoles, such as fenbendazole and mebendazole.

Control: Ideally, horses and donkeys should not be grazed together, but if they are, it is advisable to treat the donkeys, preferably in the spring, with a suitable anthelmintic. A similar regimen should be practised in donkey studs and visiting animals should be isolated in separate paddocks.

Echinococcus granulosus

See under Parasites of the liver.

PARASITES OF THE LIVER

Fasciola hepatica

Common name: Liver fluke

Predilection site: Liver

Parasite class: Trematoda

Family: Fasciolidae

For more details see Chapter 3 (Sheep and goats).

Echinococcus granulosus

Subspecies: *equinus*

Common name: Dwarf dog tapeworm, hydatidosis

Predilection site: Mainly liver and lungs (intermediate hosts); small intestine (definitive host)

Parasite class: Cestoda

Family: Taeniidae

Description, gross: Hydatid cysts are large fluid-filled vesicles, 5–10 cm in diameter, with a thick concentrically laminated cuticle and an internal germinal layer.

Description, microscopic: The germinal layer produces numerous small vesicles or brood capsules, each containing up to 40 scolices, invaginated into their neck portions and attached to the wall by stalks. Brood capsules may become detached from the wall of the vesicle and float freely in the vesicular fluid and form 'hydatid sand'.

Final host: Dog, fox

Intermediate hosts: Horse, donkey

Geographical distribution: Mainly Europe

Pathogenesis and clinical signs: Infection in horses is generally not associated with clinical signs.

Epidemiology: Equine hydatidosis is commonest in Europe, and in other parts of the world most cases have been recorded in imported European horses. The strain is highly specific for the horse and the eggs do not develop in the sheep. The domestic dog and the red fox are the final hosts, and the cycle in countries of high prevalence depends on access by dogs to infected equine viscera. On mainland Europe, the most likely source is offal from horse abattoirs and in Britain the viscera of hunting horses, which are fed to foxhounds. The horse strain does not appear to be infective to man.

Treatment: No treatment in horses.

Control: This is based on the regular treatment of dogs to eliminate the adult tapeworms and on the prevention of infection in dogs by exclusion from their diet of animal material containing hydatids. This is achieved by denying dogs access to abattoirs, and, where possible, by proper disposal of equine viscera. In some countries these measures have been supported by legislation, with penalties when they are disregarded.

Notes: There are two major strains of *E. granulosus* in domestic animals, namely *E. granulosus equinus*, which is not infective to man, and *E. granulosus granulosus* (see Chapter 3: Sheep and goats).

PARASITES OF THE CIRCULATORY SYSTEM

Elaeophora bohmi

Predilection site: Blood vessels

Parasite class: Nematoda

Superfamily: Filarioidea

Description, gross: Slender worms, males are 4.5–6 cm and females 4–20 cm long.

Description, microscopic: Microfilariae are 230–290 μm with a long tail.

Final hosts: Horse and other equids

Intermediate hosts: Tabanid and other flies

Life cycle: The microfilariae are ingested by the intermediate host (tabanid flies) when blood feeding and the L_3, when developed, are released into the wound made when the insect next feeds. Microfilariae occur in the blood and in subcutaneous connective tissue.

Geographical distribution: Europe (in particular Austria), Middle East (Iran)

Pathogenesis: Found in the large veins and arteries, often of lower limbs where they usually induce very little pathological reaction.

Clinical signs: Infection is usually asymptomatic.

Diagnosis: This is not normally required. Infection is usually diagnosed as an incidental finding on post-mortem examination of thickened blood vessels, or those containing nodules.

Pathology: Severe infection can cause thickening of the wall of arteries and veins, commonly those in the extremities, and nodules containing calcified worms may be present. The parasites selectively involve the media of the vessels, with the fibrous reaction that develops sometimes causing stenosis of the lumen. The worms are coiled and entwined among the tissue layers, provoking parasitic granulomas with intense eosinophilic and macrophage infiltration. In long-standing infections, the nodular and fibrous thickenings are visible in the vessel walls.

Epidemiology: Because of the innocuous nature of the infection in equines, the distribution of the species in these hosts is not completely known.

Treatment: Treatment is unknown although repeated administration of diethylcarbamazine is effective, but the risk of fatalities from the presence of dead worms in the arteries should be recognised.

Control: Any reduction in vector numbers will reduce transmission.

Notes: These worms inhabit large blood vessels, but are only of local importance.

Schistosoma japonicum

Common name: Blood fluke, bilharziosis

Predilection site: Portal and mesenteric veins

Parasite class: Trematoda

Family: Schistosomatidae

Final hosts: Cattle, horse, sheep, goat, dog, cat, rabbit, pig, man

Intermediate hosts: Snails belonging to the genus *Oncomelania*

Geographical distribution: South and east Asia

For more details see Chapter 2 (Cattle).

Schistosoma nasalis

Synonym: *Schistosoma nasalae*

Common name: Snoring disease

Predilection site: Veins of nasal mucosa

Parasite class: Trematoda

Family: Schistosomatidae

Final host: Cattle, goat sheep, buffalo, horse

Intermediate hosts: Snails (*Lymnaea luteola*, *L. acuminata*, *Indoplanorbis exustus*)

Geographical distribution: India, Pakistan, southeast Asia

For more details see Chapter 2 (Cattle).

Schistosoma indicum

Predilection site: Portal, pancreatic, hepatic and mesenteric veins

Parasite class: Trematoda

Family: Schistosomatidae

Final host: Cattle, sheep, goat, horse, donkey, camel

Intermediate hosts: Snails (*Indoplanorbis*)

Geographical distribution: India

For more details see Chapter 2 (Cattle).

Schistosoma spindale

Predilection site: Mesenteric veins

Parasite class: Trematoda

Family: Schistosomatidae

Hosts: Cattle, horse, pig and occasionally dog

Geographical distribution: Parts of Asia and the Far East

For more details see Chapter 2 (Cattle).

Schistosoma turkestanicum

Synonym: *Orientobilharzia turkstanicum*

Predilection site: Mesenteric veins and small veins of the pancreas and liver

Parasite class: Trematoda

Family: Schistosomatidae

Geographical distribution: Asia

For more details see Chapter 2 (Cattle).

TRYPANOSOMES

See Zoomastigophorasida for general description (Chapter 1: Parasite Morphology and Taxonomy) and Chapter 2: Cattle for detailed descriptions of individual species of trypanosomes and their control.

Trypanosoma brucei brucei

Subgenus: *Trypanozoon*

Common name: Nagana

Predilection site: Blood. *T. brucei bucei* is also found extravascularly in, for example, the myocardium, central nervous sytem (CNS) and reproductive tract.

Parasite class: Zoomastigophorasida

Family: Trypanosomatidae

Description: *T. brucei brucei* is pleomorphic in form and ranges from long and slender up to 42 μm (mean 29 μm), to short and stumpy, 12–26 μm (mean 18 μm), the two forms often being present in the same blood sample. The undulating membrane is conspicuous, the kinetoplast is small and sub-terminal and the posterior end is pointed. In the slender form the kinetoplast is up to 4 μm from the posterior end, which is usually drawn out tapering almost to a point, and has a well-developed free flagellum. In the stumpy form the flagellum is either short or absent and the posterior end is broad and rounded with the kinetoplast almost terminal. Intermediate forms average 23 μm long and have a blunt posterior end and moderately long flagellum. A fourth form with a posterior nucleus may be seen in laboratory animals. In fresh, unfixed blood films, the organism moves rapidly within small areas of the microscope field.

Hosts: Cattle, horse, donkey, zebu, sheep, goat, camel, pig, dog, cat, wild game species

Life cycle: Tsetse flies ingest trypanosomes in the blood or lymph while feeding on an infected host. Thereafter the trypanosomes lose their glycoprotein surface coat, and become elongated and multiply in the midgut before migrating forward to the salivary glands. There they undergo a transformation losing their typical trypanosome, or **trypomastigote**, form and acquire an **epimastigote** form, characterised by the fact that the kinetoplast lies just in front of the nucleus. After further multiplication of the epimastigotes they transform again into small, typically trypomastigote forms with a glycoprotein surface coat. These are the infective forms for the next host and are called **metacyclic** trypanosomes. The entire process takes at least 2–3 weeks and the metacyclic trypanosomes are inoculated into the new host when the tsetse fly feeds.

At the site of inoculation the metacyclic forms multiply locally as the typical blood forms, producing a raised cutaneous inflammatory swelling called a **chancre** within a few days. Thereafter they enter the bloodstream, multiply, and a parasitaemia, detectable in the peripheral blood, usually becomes apparent 1–3 weeks later. Subsequently, the parasitaemia may persist for many months although its level may wax and wane due to the immune response of the host.

Distribution: Sub-Saharan Africa

Pathogenesis: In horses, *T. brucei brucei* infections may be acute or chronic, often accompanied by oedema of the limbs and genitalia.

Treatment: Horses are particularly susceptible to *T. brucei* and suramin and quinapyramine sulphate are the drugs of choice. Diminazene is relatively toxic to horses. Despite treatment, relapse from CNS infection is likely.

Drug	Recommended dose	Comments
Diminazine aceturate	3–10 mg/kg i.m.	Ruminants, pig, horse. Contraindicated in dog and camel
Isometamidium	0.25–1 mg/kg i.m.	Ruminants, horse, dog. Local reaction
Quinapyramine sulphate	3–5 mg/kg i.m.	Horse only. Banned in ruminants
Quinapyramine methylsulphate	5 mg/kg s.c.	Dog
Suramin	7–10 mg/kg i.m. or i.v.	Horse, camel. Local and systemic reactions

Trypanosoma brucei evansi

Subgenus: *Trypanozoon*

Synonym: *Trypanosoma evansi*, *Trypanosoma equinum*

Common name: Surra, el debab, mbori, murrina, mal de caderas, doukane, dioufar, thaga

Predilection site: Blood

Parasite class: Zoomastigophorasida

Family: Trypanosomatidae

Description: *Trypanosoma evansi* is identical to, and structurally indistinguishable in appearance from, the slender forms of *T. brucei brucei*. The mean length varies considerably with typical forms 15–34 μm long (mean 24 μm). Most are slender or intermediate in shape, but stumpy forms occur sporadically. Strains that lack a kinetoplast visible with the light microscope have occasionally arisen spontaneously or can be produced by treatment with certain dyes, drugs or frozen storage.

Hosts: Horse, donkey, camel, cattle, zebu, goat, pig, dog, water buffalo, elephant, capybara, tapir, mongoose, ocelot, deer and other wild animals. Many laboratory and wild animals can be infected experimentally.

Life cycle: Transmission is by biting flies, no cyclical development occurring in the vector, and the trypanosomes remaining in the proboscis.

Geographical distribution: North Africa, Central and South America, central and southern Russia, parts of Asia (India, Burma, Malaysia, southern China, Indonesia, Phillipines)

Pathogenesis: Depending on the virulence of the strain and the susceptibility of the individual host, the disease may be acute in horses, camels and dogs. Other domestic species, such as cattle, buffalo and pigs, are commonly infected, but overt disease is uncommon and their main significance is as reservoirs of infection. The syndrome is similar to that caused by the tsetse-transmitted trypanosomes. Anaemia is caused mainly by extravascular haemolysis through erythrophagocytosis in the mononuclear phagocytic systems of the spleen, liver, and lungs; as the disease becomes chronic there may be decreased haemoglobin synthesis. Leucopenia and thrombocytopenia are caused by mechanisms that predispose leucocytes and platelets to phagocytosis. Immunological mechanisms in the pathogenesis lead to extensive proliferation of activated macrophages, which engulf or destroy erythrocytes, leucocytes, platelets and haematopoietic cells.

Clinical signs: All domestic animals are susceptible but the disease is only fatal in horses, camels and dogs. The disease is manifested by pyrexia, progressive anaemia, loss of condition and depression. Recurrent episodes of fever occur during the course of disease. Oedematous swellings, ranging from cutaneous plaques to frank oedema of the ventral abdomen and genitalia and petechial haemorrhages of the serous membranes are often observed. Abortions have been reported in buffaloes in Asia. Nervous signs may occur and include circling, incoordination, staggering, head pressing, paraplegia, paralysis and prostration.

Diagnosis: The clinical signs of the disease, although indicative, are not pathognomonic. Confirmation of clinical diagnosis depends on the demonstration of trypanosomes in the blood and if a herd or flock is involved a representative number of blood samples should be examined since, in individual animals, the parasitaemia may be in remission or in long-standing cases may be extremely scanty. Occasionally, when the parasitaemia is massive it is possible to detect motile trypanosomes in fresh films of blood. More usually, both thick and thin smears of blood are air dried and examined later. Thick smears, de-haemoglobinised before staining with Giemsa or Leishman's stain, offer a better chance of finding trypanosomes, while the stained thin smears are used for differentiation of the trypanosome species.

More sensitive techniques utilise centrifugation in a microhaematocrit tube followed by microscopic examination of the interface between the buffy coat and the plasma; alternatively, the tube may be snapped, the buffy coat expressed on to a slide, and the contents examined under dark-ground or phase-contrast microscopy for motile trypanosomes. With these techniques the packed red cell volume is also obtained which is of indirect value in diagnosis if one can eliminate other causes of anaemia, especially helminthosis.

A number of serological tests have been described and include IFAT and ELISA and have been partially validated but require further evaluation and standardisation.

Pathology: The carcase is often pale, emaciated and there may be oedematous swellings in the lower part of the abdomen and genital organs with serous atrophy of fat. The liver, lymph nodes and spleen are enlarged and the viscera are congested. Petechiae may appear on lymph nodes, pericardium and intestinal mucosa. The liver is hypertrophic and congested with degeneration and necrosis of the hepatocytes, dilation of blood vessels and parenchymal infiltration of mononuclear cells. A non-suppurative myocarditis, sometimes associated with hydropericarditis, has been reported, accompanied by degeneration and necrosis of the myocardial tissue. Other lesions can include glomerulonephritis, renal tubular necrosis, non-suppurative meningio-encephalomyelitis, focal poliomalacia, keratitis, opthalmitis, orchitis, interstitial pneumonia and bone marrow atrophy. Splenic and lymph node hypertrophy occur during the acute phase but the lymphoid tissues are usually exhausted and fibrotic in the chronic stage.

Epidemiology: This species, although closely related to the salivarian trypanosome *T. brucei brucei*, is mechanically transmitted by biting insects; the usual vectors are horseflies (*Tabanus*) but *Stomoxys*, *Haematopota* and *Lyperosia* can also transmit the infection. In Central and South America the vampire bat is a vector and can transmit the disease (murrina).

Treatment and control: Suramin or quinapyramine (Trypacide) are the drugs of choice for treatment and also confer a short period of prophylaxis. For more prolonged protection a modified quinapyramine known as 'Trypacide Pro-Salt' is also available. Unfortunately, drug resistance, at least to suramin, is not uncommon.

Notes: The original distribution of this parasite coincided with that of the camel, and is often associated with arid desserts and semiarid steppes.

Trypanosoma congolense congolense

Subgenus: *Nannomonas*

Common name: Nagana, paranagana, Gambia fever, ghindi, gobial

Predilection site: Blood

Parasite class: Zoomastigophorasida

Family: Trypanosomatidae

Description: *T. congolense* is small, monomorphic in form, 8–20 μm long. The undulating membrane is inconspicuous, the medium-sized kinetoplast is marginal and the posterior end is blunt. There is no free flagellum. In fresh blood films the organism moves sluggishly, often apparently attached to red cells.

Hosts: Cattle, sheep, goat, horse, camel, dog, pig. Reservoir hosts include antelope, giraffe, zebra, elephant and warthog.

Distribution: Sub-Saharan Africa

Pathogenesis: The signs caused by this species are similar to those caused by other trypanosomes, but the CNS is not affected. Anaemia is caused mainly by extravascular haemolysis through erythrophagocytosis in the mononuclear phagocytic systems of the spleen, liver, and lungs but as the disease becomes chronic there may be decreased haemoglobin synthesis. Leucopenia and thrombocytopenia are caused by mechanisms that predispose leucocytes and platelets to phagocytosis. Immunological mechanisms in the pathogenesis lead to extensive proliferation of activated macrophages, which engulf or destroy erythrocytes, leucocytes, platelets and haematopoietic cells.

Clinical signs: Symptoms include intermittent fever, anaemia, oedema of the limbs and dependent parts, progressive weakness and loss of condition.

Treatment: Homidium salts, isometamidium and pyrithidium can be used for treatment. Diminazene is relatively toxic to horses.

Drug	Recommended dose	Comments
Diminazine aceturate	3–5 mg/kg i.m.	Ruminants, pig, horse. Contraindicated in dog and camel
Homidium bromide	1 mg/kg s.c.	Cattle, sheep, goat and horse
Homidium chloride		Prophylaxis for 6 weeks
Isometamidium	0.25–1 mg/kg i.m.	Ruminants, horse, dog. Local reaction
Pyrithidium bromide	2–2.5 mg/kg i.m.	Cattle, sheep, horse, donkey. Prophylaxis for 4 months

BABESIOSIS/THEILERIOSIS

Two species, the small *Theileria equi* (formerly *Babesia equi*) and the large *B. caballi*, are of importance in horses.

Babesia caballi

Predilection site: Blood

Parasite class: Sporozoasida

Family: Babesiidae

Description: Trophozoites within erythrocytes are pear-shaped, measuring 2–5 μm in length, commonly occurring in pairs joined at the posterior ends with the angle between the organisms acute. Round or oval forms 1.5–3 μm in diameter may also occur.

Hosts: Horse, donkey

Geographical distribution: Europe, Asia, Africa, South and Central America, Southern USA, Australia: related to distribution of ticks.

Pathogenesis: Death, if it occurs, is due to organ failure which, in turn, is due not only to destruction of the erythrocytes with resultant anaemia, oedema and icterus, but also to the clogging of the capillaries of various organs by parasitised cells and free parasites. The stasis from this sludging causes degeneration of the endothelial cells of the small blood vessels, anoxia, and accumulation of toxic metabolic products, capillary fragility and eventual perivascular escape of erythrocytes and macroscopic haemorrhage. The incubation period is 6–10 days.

Clinical signs: The disease may be chronic or acute, and in either case can be mild or fatal. Haemoglobinuria is rare, but fever, anaemia and icterus are present. Gastroenteritis is common. Locomotor signs are usually present, and posterior paralysis may occur.

Diagnosis: Examination of blood films, stained with Romanowsky stains such as Giemsa, will reveal the parasites in the red cells. Species identification is essential with regard to choice of therapeutic drugs. The paired merozoites joined at their posterior ends are considered to be a diagnostic feature of *B. caballi*. Examinations should be made as early as possible, since the parasites begin to disappear from the peripheral blood after the 5th day.

The complement fixation test (CFT) is the primary screening test used for horses travelling between countries. Because the CFT may not identify all infected animals, especially those that have been treated, and because of anti-complementary reactions produced by some sera, the IFAT is used as a supplementary test. Test sera are inactivated for 30 minutes at 60°C and tested in dilutions of 1:5 to 1:5120. A lysis of 50% is recorded as positive, with the titre being the greatest serum dilution giving 50% lysis. A titre of 1:5 is regarded as positive. Anti-complementary samples are examined by the IFAT.

With the indirect fluorescent antibody test (IFAT) the recognition of a strong positive reaction is relatively simple, but any differentiation between weak positive and negative reactions requires considerable experience in interpretation. Each sample of serum is tested against an antigen of *B. caballi*. Test, positive and negative control sera are diluted from 1/80 to 1/1280. Sera diluted 1/80 or more that show a strong fluorescence are usually considered to be positive, although due consideration is also given to the patterns of fluorescence of the positive and negative controls.

Pathology: Principal lesions include splenomegaly with soft, dark red splenic pulp and prominent splenic corpuscles. The liver is enlarged and yellowish brown and the gallbladder is distended with thick, dark bile. The mucosa of the intestine is oedematous and icteric with patches of haemorrhage. Subcutaneous, subserous and intramuscular connective tissues are oedematous and icteric. The blood is thin and watery, and the plasma tinged with red.

Epidemiology: *B. caballi* is transmitted by a variety of tick species, including *Dermacentor*, *Hyalomma* and *Rhipicephalus*. Tick vectors include *Dermacentor reticulatus*, *D. variabilis*, *D. albipictus*, *D. silvarum*, *D. nitens*,

Hyalomma excavatum, *H. scupense*, *Rhipicephalus bursa*, *R. sanguineus* and others according to geographical location. Young animals are less susceptible than old ones. There is cross immunity between *B. caballi* and *Theileria equi*. Recovered horses may remain carriers for 10 months to 4 years.

Treatment: Treatment of equine piroplasmosis is based on a combination of supportive and symptomatic treatment as well as chemotherapy. Supportive treatment is essential in the treatment of acute disease and may include blood transfusion, fluid therapy, vitamins and good nutrition. The chemotherapy of babesiosis in horses is difficult and, due to the toxicity of most effective drugs, care must be taken in the administration of the correct dosage.

The most commonly used drugs for chemotherapy of equine piroplasmosis are:

- Imidocarb diproprionate, given intramuscularly at 2–3 mg/kg body weight in doses 24 hours apart will usually be sufficient for sterilisation of *B. caballi* infections.
- Amicarbalide diisethionate produces clinical recovery at a dose rate of 9–10 mg/kg as a single dose, or as a divided dose over 24 hours. High doses may reportedly cause pronounced side effects.
- Diminazene aceturate given at 5 mg/kg given twice at 24-hour intervals produces clinical recovery.

Control: Immunity in horses after infection lasts for more than 1 year and horses are therefore protected in enzootic areas even with the seasonal fluctuation of the tick population. Tick control is essential. Special attention should be paid to the ears, region under the tail and between the hind legs. Horses introduced into endemic areas are very susceptible and should therefore receive special attention.

Drug	Recommended dose	Frequency	Comments
Imidocarb diproprionate	2–3 mg/kg i.m.	Two doses at 24-hour interval	Pain at injection site
Diminazine aceturate	5 mg/kg i.m.	Two doses at 24-hour interval	Low therapeutic index
Amicarbalide diisethionate	9–10 mg/kg i.m.	Single or repeat 24 hours	Low therapeutic index

Theileria equi

Synonym: *Babesia equi*, *Nuttalia equi*

Predilection site: Blood

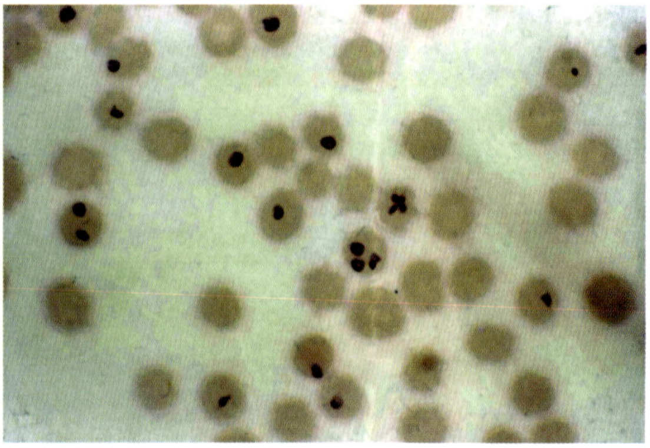

Fig. 4.25 Trophozoites of *Theileria equi*.

Parasite class: Sporozoasida

Family: Theileriidae

Description: The merozoites in the erythrocytes are relatively small, 2–3 µm rounded, amoeboid or most often pyriform, and are readily recognised in blood smears from acute cases. Apart from size, the piroplasms characteristically form a 'Maltese cross' of four organisms (Fig. 4.25).

Hosts: Horse, donkey

Geographical distribution: North, Central, South America, Africa, Asia, mainland Europe

Pathogenesis: Death, if it occurs, is due to organ failure which, in turn, is due not only to destruction of the erythrocytes with resultant anaemia, oedema and icterus, but also to the clogging of the capillaries of various organs by parasitised cells and free parasites. The stasis from this sludging causes degeneration of the endothelial cells of the small blood vessels, anoxia, and accumulation of toxic metabolic products, capillary fragility and eventual perivascular escape of erythrocytes and macroscopic haemorrhage.

Clinical signs: The incubation period following an infective tick bite is 10–21 days. The first sign of disease is a rise in temperature followed by listlessness, depression, marked thirst, inappetence, lachrymation and blepharitis. The most characteristic sign is icterus. There is marked anaemia and more than half the erythrocytes are often destroyed leading to haemoglobinuria. Oedema of the head, legs and ventral part of the body is sometimes present, although posterior paralysis, sometimes seen in *B. caballi* infection, is absent. Affected animals are constipated, and pass small, hard balls of faeces covered with yellow mucus. The animals lose condition fairly rapidly, and may become extremely emaciated. Haemorrhages are present on the mucosa of the nasal passages, vagina and third eyelid. The disease lasts 7–12 days but may be peracute with death occurring in 1–2 days, or may be chronic and last for weeks. Mortality is usually about 10% but may reach 50%. Recovery is slow.

Diagnosis: Examination of blood films, stained with Romanowsky stains such as Giemsa, will reveal the parasites in the red cells. Species identification is essential with regard to choice of therapeutic drugs. The terad or Maltese cross arrangement is a diagnostic feature of *T. equi*. Examinations should be made as early as possible since the parasites begin to disappear from the peripheral blood after the 5th day.

The complement fixation test (CFT) is the primary screening test used for horses travelling between countries. Because the CFT may not identify all infected animals, especially those that have been treated, and because of anti-complementary reactions produced by some sera, the IFAT is used as a supplementary test. Test sera are inactivated for 30 minutes at 60°C and tested in dilutions of 1:5 to 1:5120. A lysis of 50% is recorded as positive, with the titre being the greatest serum dilution giving 50% lysis. A titre of 1:5 is regarded as positive. Anti-complementary samples are examined by the IFAT.

With the indirect fluorescent antibody test (IFAT) the recognition of a strong positive reaction is relatively simple, but any differentiation between weak positive and negative reactions requires considerable experience in interpretation. Each sample of serum is tested against an antigen of *T. equi*. Test, positive and negative control sera are diluted from 1/80 to 1/1280. Sera diluted 1/80 or more that show a strong fluorescence are usually considered to be positive, although due consideration is also given to the patterns of fluorescence of the positive and negative controls.

Pathology: Emaciation, icterus, anaemia and oedema are seen at postmortem examination. There are accumulations of fluid in the pericardial sac and body cavities, and the fat is gelatinous and yellow. The spleen is enlarged, with soft, dark brown pulp. The lymph nodes are swollen and sometimes inflamed. The liver is swollen, engorged and brownish yellow, the hepatic lobules are yellow in the centre and greenish yellow round the edges. The kidneys are pale yellow and may contain petechial haemorrhages. There are petechial or ecchymotic heamorrhages on the mucosa of the intestine and stomach.

Epidemiology: *T. equi* is transmitted by a variety of tick species including *Dermacentor*, *Hyalomma* and *Rhipicephalus*. Vectors are *Dermacentor reticulatus*, *D. albipictus*, *Hyalomma marginatum* (syn. *H. dendritum*), *H. scupense*, *Rhipencephalus bursa* in Russia and former Soviet states; *R. evertsi* in equitorial Africa; *H. anatolicum* and *H. marginatum* in Greece; *H. dromedarii* and *R. sanguineus* in central Asia. The vectors in the USA include *D. variabilis*, *D. albipictus*, *D. (Anocentor) nitens* and *R. sanguineus*; in South America *D. (A.) nitens*.

Treatment: Imidocarb diproprionate given intramuscularly at 2–3 mg/kg body weight in doses 24 hours apart will bring about recovery from *T. equi* infections, but not sterilisation of infection. The use of four doses of 4 mg/kg body weight at 72-hour intervals is reported to sterilise *T. equi* infections, but this high dose rate therapy may cause severe side effects, such as extreme restlessness, sweating and signs of abdominal pain. Treated horses may become seronegative to CFT but remain positive to IFAT and infective to tick vectors. Treatment with amicarbalide diisethionate produces clinical recovery at a dose rate of 9–10 mg/kg as a single dose, or as a divided dose over 24 hours. High doses may reportedly cause pronounced side effects. Diminazene aceturate given at 6–12 mg/kg body weight given twice in a 48-hour period may be required for clinical recovery.

Drug	Recommended dose	Frequency	Comments
Imidocarb diproprionate	2–3 mg/kg i.m. or 4 mg/kg	Two doses at 24-hour interval or four doses at 72-hour interval for sterility	Pain at injection site
Diminazine aceturate	6–12 mg/kg i.m.	Two doses at 48-hour interval	Low therapeutic index
Amicarbalide diisethionate	9–10 mg/kg i.m.	Single or repeat 24 hours	Low therapeutic index

Notes: There is no cross immunity between *T. equi* and *B. caballi*. Young animals are less seriously affected than adults and mixed infections of these parasites can occur.

Neorickettsia risticii

Synonym: *Ehrlichia risticii*

Common name: Equine monocytic ehrlichiosis, Potomac horse fever, ditch fever, Shasta River crud, equine ehrlichial colitis

Predilection site: Reproductive tract

Parasite class: Rickettsiales

Family: Rickettsiaceae

Description: *N. risticii* is a Gram-negative obligate intracellular bacterium, 0.6–1.5 µm in size, with a trophism for monocytes. The organism is not visible in monocytes in blood films from clinical cases.

Hosts: Horse, rarely dog, cat

Life cycle: Details of the life cycle are incomplete but infection to horses appears to involve ingestion of metacercarial stages of trematodes or inadvertent ingestion of aquatic insect stages.

Geographical distribution: USA

Pathogenesis: Potomac horse fever (PHF) is an acute enterocolitis syndrome producing mild colic, fever, and diarrhoea in horses of all ages, as well as abortion in pregnant mares.

Following ingestion within the insect or trematode, the organism is taken up by cells of the monocyte/macrophage series and the organisms accumulate in the reticuloendothelial cells in the wall of the large colon. The infection of enterocytes of the small and large intestine results in acute colitis, which is one of the principal clinical signs. Other signs vary from transient mild fever to severe diarrhoea, which become apparent after 12–18 days. Colic of variable severity and abdominal distension may precede the onset of diarrhoea in about 25% of cases. As well as blood and lymphoid tissue, the organisms have been detected in macrophages, crypt endothelial cells and mast cells in the wall of the colon, caecum and small intestine, where it is thought that a localised endotoxaemia may lead to electrolyte imbalance. A bluish 'toxic ring' surrounding the teeth may be present and affected horses may also exhibit mild to moderate tachypnoea and tachycardia. Mild to severe laminitis has been reported following the onset of diarrhoea. Infection has also been associated with abortion in mares.

Clinical signs: Fever, depression, leucopenia, dehydration, laminitis and diarrhoea

Diagnosis: A provisional diagnosis is often based on the presence of typical clinical signs and the seasonal and geographic occurrence of the disease. Examination of peripheral blood smears is of no value as infected monocytes are present in small numbers in the blood. A definitive diagnosis should be based on isolation or detection of *N. risticii* from the blood or faeces of infected horses. Although serological tests such as IFAT or ELISA exist, serological testing is of limited value as a diagnostic tool, although many infected horses have high antibody titres at the time of infection. Because of the high prevalence of false-positive titres, interpretation of the indirect fluorescent antibody test in individual horses is difficult. Isolation of the agent in cell culture, although possible, is time consuming and not routinely available in many diagnostic laboratories. A recently developed real-time polymerase chain reaction (PCR) assay allows the detection of *N. risticii* DNA within 2 hours, making this a much more feasible test for routine diagnostic examination. To enhance the chances of detection of *N. risticii*, the assay should be performed on a blood as well as a faecal sample, as the presence of the organism in blood and faeces may not necessarily coincide.

Pathology: On postmortem, there are little or no gross pathological changes although histological changes include focal degeneration of endothelial cells in the colon leading to small ulcerative lesions and patchy hyperaemia in the large intestine. There is marked depletion of goblet cells and dilation of intestinal crypts.

Epidemiology: Disease is seen in spring, summer and early autumn and is associated with pastures bordering creeks or rivers. *N. risticii* has been identified in freshwater snails and isolated from trematodes released from the snails. DNA has been detected in 13 species of immature and adult caddisflies (*Trichoptera*), mayflies (*Ephemeroptera*), damselflies (*Odonata, Zygoptera*), dragonflies (*Odonata, Anisoptera*) and stoneflies (*Plecoptera*). Transmission studies using *N. risticii*-infected caddisflies have reproduced the clinical disease. One route of exposure is believed to be inadvertent ingestion of aquatic insects that carry *N. risticii* in the metacercarial stage of a trematode. The incubation period is 10–18 days. Clinically ill horses are not contagious and can be housed with susceptible horses.

Treatment: Oxytetracycline administered at a dose of 6.6 mg/kg i.v. for 5 days is highly effective if given early in the clinical course of the disease. Supportive therapy with fluids, electrolytes, non-steroidal anti-inflammatory drugs (NSAIDs) and antidiarrhoeals may also be indicated in animals exhibiting signs of enterocolitis. Laminitis, if it develops, is usually severe and often refractory to treatment.

Control: Several inactivated, whole-cell vaccines based on the same strain of *N. risticii* are commercially available, although they are only marginally protective in the field. Reduction of snail numbers in rivers and ditches may be attempted to lessen sources of infection.

Notes: The causative agent, formerly known as *Ehrlichia risticii*, has recently been renamed *Neorickettsia risticii* because of its lesser genetic relationships to other *Ehrlichia* groups.

Anaplasma phagocytophilum

Synonym: *Ehrlichia equi*

Common name: Equine granulocytic ehrlichiosis

Predilection site: Blood

Order: Rickettsiales

Family: Anaplasmataceae

Description: Blood smears stained with Giemsa or Wright's stains reveal one or more loose aggregates (morulae or inclusion bodies, 1.5–5 µm in diameter) of blue–grey to dark blue coccoid, coccobacillary or pleomorphic organisms within the cytoplasm of neutrophils.

Hosts: Sheep, cattle, dog, horse, deer, rodents

Life cycle: Obligate intracellular organisms infecting granulocytes, predominantly neutrophils, appearing within the cytoplasm as membrane-bound vacuoles. Multiplication is by binary fission, forming large inclusion bodies (morulae). In untreated animals, the cytoplasmic inclusions can be detected in circulating neutrophils for 1–2 weeks.

Geographical distribution: USA, South America, Europe

Pathogenesis: Equine granulocytic ehrlichiosis is an infectious, non-contagious, seasonal disease. Severity of signs varies with age of the animal and duration of the illness. Signs may be mild. Horses less than 1 year old may have a fever only. Horses 1–3 years old develop fever, depression, mild limb oedema and ataxia. Adults exhibit the characteristic signs of fever, partial anorexia, depression, reluctance to move, limb oedema, petechiation and jaundice. The fever, which is highest during the first 1–3 days (39.5–40°C), persists for 6–12 days. Rarely, myocardial vasculitis may cause transient ventricular arrhythmias. Any concurrent infection can be exacerbated. Cytoplasmic inclusion bodies are few during the first 48 hours and increase to 30–40% of circulating neutrophils at days 3–5 of infection.

Clinical signs: Fever, depression, limb oedema, jaundice and ataxia

Diagnosis: Demonstration of the characteristic cytoplasmic inclusion bodies in blood smears is diagnostic. PCR can detect *A. phagocytophilum* DNA in unclotted blood or buffy coat smears. An IFAT can detect rising antibody body titres to *A. phagocytophilum.*

Pathology: Gross petechiation, ecchymoses and oedema develop in the subcutis and fascia. Vasculitis is regional, with the subcutis and fascia of the legs predominantly affected.

Epidemiology: In endemic areas, the disease is seasonal occurring during periods of peak tick activity. In the USA, transmission to horses is by the tick *Ixodes pacificus* (the western black-legged tick).

Treatment: Oxytetracycline and tetracycline, at 7 mg/kg i.v., for 8 days, has eliminated the infection. Horses with severe ataxia and oedema may benefit from short-term corticosteroid treatment (dexamethasone 20 mg for 2–3 days).

Control: Recovered horses are solidly immune for more than 2 years. There is no vaccine.

Notes: The causal riskettsial agent was initially termed *Ehrlichia equi*, but based on DNA sequence relationships, the organism is now referred to as *Anaplasma phagocytophilum*.

PARASITES OF THE NERVOUS SYSTEM

Thelazia lacrymalis

Common name: Equine eye worm

Predilection site: Eye, conjunctival sac and lachrymal duct

Parasite class: Nematoda

Superfamily: Spiruroidea

Description, gross: Small thin yellowish white worms, 1.0–2.0 cm long. Males are 8–12 mm and females 14–18 mm.

Description, microscopic: A mouth capsule is present and the cuticle has prominent striations at the anterior end. In the male, the tail is blunt and recurved with caudal alae.

Final hosts: Horse and other equids

Intermediate hosts: Muscid flies, particularly *Musca*, *Fannia* and *Morellia*

Life cycle: The worms are viviparous. The L_1 passed by the female worm into the lachrymal secretion is ingested by the fly intermediate host as it feeds. Development from L_1 to L_3 occurs in the ovarian follicles of the fly in 15–30 days during the summer months. L_3 migrate to the mouthparts of the fly and are transferred to the final host when the fly feeds. Development in the eye takes place without further migration and the prepatent period is between about 3–6 weeks.

Geographical distribution: Europe, North and South America and parts of Asia

Pathogenesis: In many hosts, moderate eyeworm infection causes little pathogenic disease. Lesions are caused by the serrated cuticle of the worm and most damage results from movement by the active young adults, causing lachrymation, followed by conjunctivitis. In heavy infections the cornea may become cloudy and ulcerated. There is usually complete recovery in about 2 months, although in some cases areas of corneal opacity can persist. Infection may predispose the host to secondary bacterial infection.

Clinical signs: Often infection can be inapparent but heavy infestations can cause lachrymation, conjunctivitis and photophobia. Flies are usually clustered around the eye because of the excessive secretion. In severe cases the eyes may be swollen, with keratitis, corneal ulceration with a purulent exudate.

Diagnosis: This is based on observation of the parasites in the conjunctival sac. Examination of the lachrymal secretion may reveal first-stage larvae.

Pathology: Invasion of the lachrymal gland and ducts may cause inflammation and necrotic exudation leading to occlusion and reduced tear production. Mechanical irritation of the conjunctiva produces inflammation, whilst damage to the cornea leads to opacity, keratitis and corneal ulceration.

Epidemiology: *Thelazia lacrymalis* is very common in some areas and infestation occurs seasonally, linked to periods of maximum fly activity. The parasite can survive in the eye for several years, but since it is only the young adult that is pathogenic a reservoir of infection may persist in symptomless carrier animals. Only heavy infections cause symptoms. Survival of larvae also occurs in the pupal stages of flies during the winter.

Treatment: Fenbendazole at 10 mg/kg per os for 5 days is effective. Ivermectin given directly into the conjunctival sac may also have some effect, but is not effective when given orally. Mechanical removal with forceps following the application of an ocular local anaesthetic is also useful. In cases of secondary bacterial infection the use of antibiotic eye preparations may be indicated.

Control: Prevention is difficult because of the ubiquitous nature of the fly vectors. Fly control measures aimed at protecting the face, such as headbands, aids in the control of eyeworm infection.

Halicephalobus delitrix

Synonym: *Micronema delatrix*

Parasite class: Nematoda

Superfamily: Rhabditoidea

Pathogenesis: This saprophagous, free-living nematode has been found in the brain and in granulomatous tissues of the nares and maxilla of horses.

Toxoplasma gondii

See details and description under Parasites of the locomotory system.

Sarcocystis neurona

Common name: Equine protozoal myeloencephalitis (EPM)

Predilection site: Brain, spinal cord

Order: Sporozoasida

Family: Sarcocystiidae

Description: Meronts present in the cytoplasm of neural cells, leucocytes and giant cells in the grey and white matter of the brain and spinal cord are 5–35 × 5–20 μm and contain 4–40 merozoites when mature.

Intermediate hosts: Horse

Final host: Opposum (*Dideophis virginiana*). Armadillos, skunks, raccoons, sea otters, seals and domestic cats have all been implicated but their significance is not known.

Life cycle: Details of the life cycle are not completely known. The North American opossum is thought to be one definitive host with transmission to horse via sporocysts in faeces. The life cycle may also involve opposums scavenging on bird carcases containing an identical organism, *Sarcocystis falcatula*, a parasite of several North American bird species. In this respect, horses may be acting as an abnormal, aberrant host.

Geographical distribution: North, Central, South America

Pathogenesis: The organism causes wide-ranging neurological signs associated with infection of any part of the CNS.

Clinical signs: Clinical signs include circling; cranial nerve signs of muscle atrophy, facial paralysis; unilateral vestibular disease; cervical spinal cord disease (wobbler syndrome); monoplegia with muscle atrophy; gait abnormalities, pruritis; cauda equine syndrome.

Diagnosis: Diagnosis is based on clinical signs; analysis of cerebrospinal fluid, response to antiprotozoal therapy and negative response to corticosteroid therapy. Postmortem diagnosis is confirmed by demonstration of the organisms in CNS lesions. A Western blot test for *S. neurona* antibody in CSF has been developed.

Pathology: There is focal discoloration, haemorrhage and malacia of CNS tissue. On histopathology, the parasites are found in association with mixed inflammatory cellular responses, and neuronal degeneration. Meronts in various stages of maturation, or free merozoites, are commonly seen within the cytoplasm of neurons or macrophages, neutrophils, eosinophils, more rarely capillary endothelial cells and myelinated axons.

Epidemiology: The disease is sporadic, although multiple cases have been reported on farms or racing establishments but there is no evidence of horse-to-horse transmission. The disease occurs most frequently in young adult breeding stock.

Treatment: The treatment of choice appears to be trimethoprim/sulphadiazine at 15 mg/kg twice daily combined with 0.25 mg/kg pyrimethamine daily in feed. This may be followed by intermittent therapy with the same drugs at 20 mg/kg and 1 mg/kg respectively once every 1–2 weeks.

Control: The source of the infection is probably opossum faeces so measures to prevent feed contamination should be considered.

PARASITES OF THE REPRODUCTIVE/ UROGENITAL SYSTEM

Trypanosoma equiperdum

Subgenus: *Trypanozoon*

Synonym: *Trypanosoma brucei equiperdum*

Common name: Dourine

Predilection site: Reproductive tract

Parasite class: Zoomastigophorasida

Family: Trypanosomatidae

Description: The organism is identical to, and structurally indistinguishable in appearance from *T. evansi*. The organism is polymorphic, with slender, intermediate and stumpy forms. The mean length varies considerably with typical forms 15–34 µm long (mean 24 µm). The undulating membrane is conspicuous and the kinetoplast small and sub-terminal. Strains that lack a kinetoplast, visible with the light microscope, have occasionally arisen spontaneously or can be produced by treatment with certain dyes, drugs or frozen storage.

Hosts: Horse, donkey

Life cycle: The trypanosome is transmitted at coitus. The organism divides by longitudinal binary fission in various tissue fluids, particularly in subcutaneous urticarial plaques and in the reproductive system.

Geographical distribution: Mediterranean basin, South Africa, Middle East, South America

Pathogenesis: The disease is marked by stages of exacerbation, tolerance or relapse, which vary in duration and which may occur once or several times before death or recovery. The signs most frequently noted are pyrexia, tumefaction and local oedema of the genitalia and mammary glands, oedematous cutaneous eruptions, knuckling of the joints, incoordination, facial paralysis, ocular lesions, anaemia and emaciation. A pathognomonic sign is the oedematous plaque consisting of an elevated lesion in the skin, up to 5–8 cm in diameter and 1 cm thick. The plaques usually appear over the ribs, although they may occur anywhere on the body, and usually persist for between 3 and 7 days. They are not a constant feature. In long-standing cases, the external genitalia may be fibrosed. The incubation period is 2–12 weeks and the disease runs a chronic course over 6 months to 2 years.

Clinical signs: The first sign is oedema of the genitalia and there is slight fever, inappetance and a mucous discharge from the urethra and vagina. Circumscribed areas of the mucosa of the vulva or penis may become depigmented. The second stage of the disease is characterised by urticaria and appears after 4–6 weeks. Circular, sharply circumscribed urticarial plaques about 3 cm in diameter arise on the sides of the body, remain for 3–4 days, and then disappear. The plaques may develop again later. Muscular paralysis develops beginning with the muscles of the nostrils and neck, extending to the hind limbs and finally to the rest of the body. The animal shows incoordination and then complete paralysis. Dourine is usually fatal unless treated, but mild strains of the parasite may occur in some regions.

Diagnosis: Demonstration of the trypanosomes from the urethral or vaginal discharges, the skin plaques or the peripheral blood is generally not possible, although centrifugation of these fluids may help to find the pathogens. The clinical disease is typical in endemic areas to allow diagnosis. Infected animals can be detected with the complement fixation test (CFT) but cross-reaction with *T. evansi* and *T. brucei* are common. An IFAT is used as a confirmatory test for dourine or to resolve inconclusive results obtained by CFT.

Pathology: At postmortem examination, gelatinous exudates are present under the skin. In the stallion, the scrotum, sheath and testicular tunica are thickened and infiltrated. In some cases, the testes are fibrosed and may be unrecognisable. In the mare, the vulva, vaginal mucosa, uterus, bladder and mammary glands may be thickened with gelatinous infiltration. The lymph nodes, particularly in the abdominal cavity, are hypertrophied, softened and, in some cases, haemorrhagic. There is pronounced anaemia and oedematous infiltration of the perineal tissues and ventral abdominal wall and hydrothorax, hydropericardium and ascites are often pronounced. The spinal cord of animals with paraplegia is often soft, pulpy and discoloured, particularly in the lumbar and sacral regions.

Epidemiology: Dourine is the only trypanosome that is not transmitted by an invertebrate vector. Organisms present in the equine reproductive tract are transmitted during coitus and very rarely by biting flies. As trypanosomes are not continually present in the genital tract throughout the course of the disease, transmission of the infection does not necessarily take place at every copulation involving an infected animal. Transmission of infection from mare to foal can occur via the mucosa, such as the conjunctiva. Mares' milk has been shown to be infectious. *T. equiperperdum* occurs in donkeys but the disease is asymptomatic. Oedema on the genitals is not obvious and skin plaques only occur in less than 10% of infected donkeys. Sperm and vaginal discharges contain large numbers of parasites and are therefore a significant reservoir of the pathogen.

Treatment: Quinapyramine sulphate (3–5 mg/kg s.c.) is one of the few compounds effective against *T. equiperdum*. In many countries, chemotherapy is prohibited and strict border controls are required before importation of horses and donkeys.

Control: Strict control of breeding and movements of horses together with quarantine and slaughter in clinical outbreaks has a marked effect on the incidence of disease. Detection and slaughter of carrier equines leads to eventual eradication. In-contact animals are declared free after 3 consecutive monthly negative complement fixation tests.

Notes: *T. equiperdum* causes the most important venereal disease in horses and is responsible for great losses wherever it occurs.

Animals other than equids can be infected experimentally. Rat-adapted strains can be maintained indefinitely; infected rat blood can be satisfactorily cryopreserved. Antigens for serological tests are commonly produced from infected laboratory rats.

Klossiella equi

Predilection site: Kidney

Parasite class: Sporozoasida

Family: Klossiellidae

Description: Meronts in endothelial cells of Bowman's capsule in the kidneys are 8–12 μm in diameter with 20–30 nuclei. Second-generation meronts found in epithelial cells of the proximal convoluted tubules are 15–23 μm in diameter containing 15–20 merozoites. Gamogony and sporogony occur in the epithelial cells of the thick limb of Henle's loop. The microgamonts form 4–10 microgametes. Sporonts, 20–23 μm in diameter, have about 40 buds on their periphery before becoming sporoblasts, 35–45 μm in diameter. Each sporoblast divides by multiple fission, forming 10–15 or more nuclei, which condense and come to lie along the periphery of the sporoblast. The sporocysts each contain 10–15 sporozoites and are themselves contained in a sac formed, by the host cell.

Hosts: Horse, donkey, zebra

Life cycle: The life cycle is not clearly understood. Within epithelial cells of kidney tubules, trophozoites form meronts and merozoites, which in turn form gamonts. Fertilised gametes are believed to develop into sporonts, which bud to form sporoblasts. Each of these sporoblasts undergoes successive divisions to form sporocysts that contain sporozoites. Mature sporocysts are surrounded by a thick wall and pass from the body in the urine. When ingested by another host, the sporozoites are released from the sporocyst, move to the kidney, where they enter epithelial cells and initiate the cycle.

Geographical distribution: Worldwide

Pathogenesis and clinical signs: Non-pathogenic and not usually associated with clinical signs

Diagnosis: Sporocysts may be detected in urine sediments or trophozoite stages may be found on postmortem in the kidney. The site and location are pathognomonic.

Pathology: Only heavily parasitised kidneys have gross lesions, which appear as tiny grey foci on the cortical surface. Microscopically these foci are areas of necrosis, with perivascular infiltration of inflammatory cells, especially lymphocytes, with an increase in interstitial fibroblasts.

Epidemiology: Sporocysts are passed in the urine and infection takes place by the ingestion of the sporulated sporocysts.

Treatment and control: Not required

Notes: This species is apparently quite common throughout the world but seldom seen.

PARASITES OF THE LOCOMOTORY SYSTEM

Trichinella spiralis

Synonym: *Trichina spiralis*

Common name: Muscle worm

Predilection site: Small intestine, muscle

Parasite class: Nematoda

Superfamily: Trichuroidea

For more details see Chapter 5 (Pigs).

Toxoplasma gondii

Predilection site: Muscle, lung, liver, reproductive system, central nervous system

Order: Sporozoasida

Family: Sarcocystiidae

Description: Tachyzoites are found developing in vacuoles in many cell types, for example fibroblasts, hepatocytes, reticular cells and myocardial cells. In any one cell there may be 8–16 organisms, each measuring 6.0–8.0 μm. Tissue cysts, measuring up to 100 μm in diameter, are found mainly in the muscle, liver, lung and brain and may contain several thousand lancet-shaped bradyzoites.

Pathogenesis: *Toxoplasma* has been recorded in horses but there are little, if any, clinical reports of disease.

For more details see Chapter 3 (Sheep and goats).

SARCOCYSTIS

Sarcocystis is one of the most prevalent parasites of grazing animals.

Life cycle: Horses are infected by ingesting sporocysts, passed in the faeces of the dog. In the muscles the parasites divide by a process of budding or endodyogeny, giving rise to broad banana-shaped bradyzoites contained within a cyst; this is the mature sarcocyst and is the infective stage for the carnivorous final host.

Diagnosis: Most cases of *Sarcocystis* infection in horses are only revealed at postmortem, when the grossly visible sarcocysts in the muscle are discovered. Examination of faeces from dogs on the farm for the presence of sporocysts may be helpful in the diagnosis.

Pathology: For the two species reported in horses, microscopic inspection has revealed minimal host reaction in infected tissues.

Epidemiology: Little is known of the epidemiology, but from the high prevalence of symptomless infections observed in abattoirs it is clear that where dogs are kept in close association with horses or their feed, then transmission is likely. Acute outbreaks are probably most likely when horses, which have been reared without dog contact, are subsequently exposed to large numbers of the sporocysts from dog faeces. The longevity of the sporocysts shed in the faeces is not known.

Treatment: There is no effective treatment for *Sarcocystis* infection in horses.

Control: The only control measures possible are those of simple hygiene. Farm dogs should not be housed in, or allowed access to, fodder stores, nor should they be allowed to defecate in pens where horses are housed. It is also important that they are not fed uncooked meat.

Sarcocystis equicanis

Synonym: *Sarcocystis bertrami*

Predilection site: Muscle

Order: Sporozoasida

Family: Sarcocystiidae

Description: Tissue cysts are segmented, up to 10 mm long with a smooth wall less than 1 μm thick with no radial striations. A small number of 0.4–2.0 μm protrusions are evident on electron microscopy.

Intermediate hosts: Horse

Final host: Dog

Geographical distribution: Worldwide

Pathogenesis: The pathogenic effects associated with *S. equicanis* in the horse have not been investigated.

Clinical signs: Infection has not been associated with clinical signs in the final or intermediate host.

Sarcocystis fayeri

Predilection site: Muscle

Order: Sporozoasida

Family: Sarcocystiidae

Description: Tissue cysts are up to 900 × 70 μm. The cyst wall is 1–2 μm thick and radially striated.

Intermediate hosts: Horse

Final host: Dog

Geographical distribution: Worldwide

Pathogenesis: Few pathogenic effects are associated with *S. fayeri* in the horse, although a few cases of severe myositis have been reported

Clinical signs: Occasional myalgia has been reported.

PARASITES OF THE INTEGUMENT

Onchocerca reticulata

Common name: Kasen summer mange, equine dhobie itch

Predilection site: Connective tissue, flexor tendons and suspensory ligament of the fetlock

Parasite class: Nematoda

Superfamily: Filarioidea

Description, gross: Slender whitish worms; males are 15–20 cm and females over 50 cm long

Description, microscopic: Microfilariae are 330–370 μm and possess a long whiplash tail.

Final hosts: Horse, donkey

Intermediate hosts: *Culicoides* spp (biting midges)

Life cycle: The life cycle of *Onchocerca* spp is typically filarioid, with the exception that the microfilariae occur in the tissue spaces of the skin, rather than in the peripheral bloodstream. They migrate in subdermal connective tissue in the ventral midline; biting midges, feeding in this area, ingest microfilariae, which then develop to the infective stage in around 3 weeks. When these infected midges feed on another equine host transmission of L_3 occurs. The prepatent period is around 12–16 months.

Geographical distribution: Worldwide

Pathogenesis: The connective tissue of the flexor tendons and suspensory ligament of the fetlocks is the preferential site. Following inoculation of L_3 by the vector, *Culicoides*, the arrival of the parasites in their final site results in host reaction in the form of a painless, diffuse swelling, which gradually increases in size to become a palpable soft lump, and then regresses to leave a calcified focus, the skin over the area remaining intact. In the lower limbs the reaction to the presence of the parasite leads to the formation of soft painless swellings succeeded by small fibrous nodules.

Clinical signs: Apart from the initial mild reaction, no clinical signs attributable to the adult worms have been demonstrated. The microfilariae are reported to cause a chronic dermatitis of horses, being severe in summer and disappearing during the winter.

Diagnosis: Infection may be confirmed by examination of thick skin sections taken from the predilection sites. The piece of skin is placed in warm saline for about 8–12 hours and teased to allow emergence of the microfilariae. These are readily recognised by their sinuous movements in a centrifuged sample of the saline. Fluid from scarified skin can also be examined for the presence of microfilariae.

Pathology: The ventral skin lesions are indistinguishable from those of *Culicoides* sensitivity. Gross lesions include alopecia, scaling, crusting and leucoderma. Secondary excoriations and ulcerative dermatitis are induced by self-trauma.

Epidemiology: The general prevalence of equine onchocercosis is high, most surveys in the USA having shown rates of more than 50%, though the highest so far recorded in Britain is 23%. The accumulation of microfilariae in the definitive host is highest during the seasons of greatest midge activity.

Treatment: Not usually required. Ivermectin has good activity against the microfilariae stages and will provide relief in cases of onchocercal dermatitis.

Control: Generally not indicated. Insecticidal sprays or repellents may reduce attacks by biting midges.

Notes: Though onchocercosis is an important filarial infection in human medicine, most species in domestic animals are relatively harmless.

Parafilaria multipapillosa

Synonym: *Filaria haemorrhagica*

Common name: Summer bleeding disease, summer sores

Predilection site: Subcutaneous and intermuscular connective tissue

Parasite class: Nematoda

Superfamily: Filarioidea

Description, gross: Slender white worms 3.0–7.0 cm in length. Adult males are 28 mm, females 40–70 mm.

Description, microscopic: Anteriorly, there are numerous papillae and circular ridges in the cuticle. In the female the vulva is situated anteriorly near the simple mouth opening.

Small embryonated eggs, that have a thin flexible shell, are laid on the skin surface where they hatch to release the microfilariae or L_1; these are about 200 μm in length and have a rounded posterior extremity.

Final hosts: Horse, donkey

Intermediate hosts: Horn flies, *Haematobia atripalpis* and other *Haematobia* spp in Europe

Life cycle: Eggs or free L_1 larvae present in exudates from bleeding points in the skin surface are ingested by horn flies (*Haematobia*), in which they develop to L_3 within several weeks to months, depending on air temperature. Transmission occurs when infected flies feed on lachrymal secretions or skin wounds in other horses and the L_3 deposited then migrate in the subcutaneous tissue and develop to the adult stage under the skin in 9–12 months.

Geographical distribution: North Africa, eastern and southern Europe, Asia and South America

Pathogenesis: Infection results in the formation of subcutaneous nodules, which break open and ooze blood (Fig. 4.26). Their distribution in the harness areas may make the animals unsuitable for work.

Clinical signs: Clinically the condition is characterised by matting of the hair due to blood and tissue fluid exudates from ruptured nodules. The lesions are more prominent in the summer and particularly when the animals are hot, so that they appear to be 'sweating blood'. Occasionally, lesions are mistaken for injuries caused by thorns and barbed wire.

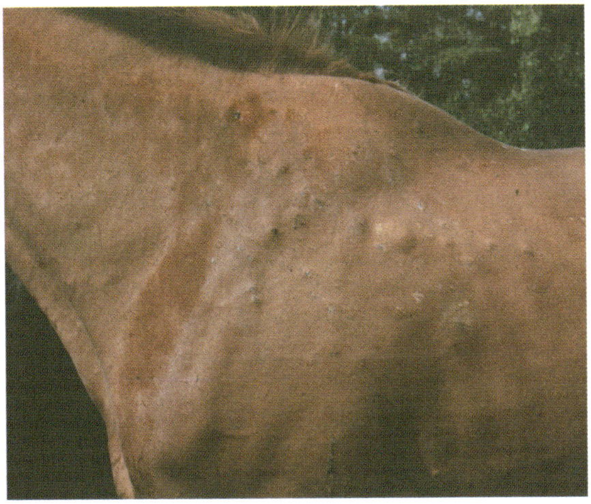

Fig. 4.26 Flank of a horse showing subcutaneous nodules induced by *Parafilaria multipapillosa*.

Diagnosis: The presence of nodules in the skin ('bleeding points') are pathognomonic. Larvated eggs or microfilariae can be demonstrated by microscopic examination of smears taken from the haemorrhagic exudate of fresh lesions. An ELISA is also available in some countries for serodiagnosis.

Pathology: Nodules formed in the cutaneous and intermuscular connective tissue are 1–2 cm in diameter, enlarge in the summer months, burst open and haemorrhage and heal by scarring.

Epidemiology: Disease is usually only apparent in the warmer seasons in temperate regions, whereas in hot tropical areas lesions are often seen after the rainy season. Although the condition tends to disappear in cold weather it will periodically reappear during warmer months for up to 4 years in individual animals.

Treatment: This is difficult, but oral ivermectin or moxidectin may be tried.

Control: Fly control measures will be beneficial.

Setaria equina

Common name: Abdominal worm

Predilection site: Peritoneum, pleural cavity

Parasite class: Nematoda

Superfamily: Filarioidea

Description, gross: The adults are long and slender, reaching 8 cm (males) and 13 cm (females). The posterior end is spirally coiled.

Description, microscopic: The microfilariae present in the blood are about 0.25 mm long.

Final hosts: Horse, donkey

Intermediate host: Mosquitoes

Life cycle: Larvae produced by adult worms in the body cavity circulate in the blood and are taken up by culicine mosquitoes, including *Aedes* and *Culex* species. Infective larvae develop in the mosquito muscles in 2 weeks, and are re-injected into horses when the mosquitoes feed. The prepatent period is 8–10 months.

Geographical distribution: Worldwide

Pathogenesis: The adult worms live in the abdominal body cavity. Occasionally, the adults invade the lungs and eyes. The worms in their normal site are usually harmless and are only discovered at necropsy. Migrating larvae can cause an encephalomyelitis in horses and also can invade the eye and induce blindness.

Clinical signs: There are no clinical signs when the worms are in their normal site, but when nervous tissue is involved there is locomotor disturbance and in severe cases lumbar paralysis.

Diagnosis: Infection with the adult worms is only accidentally discovered in the living animal by the finding of microfilariae in routine blood smears. In cases of cerebrospinal setariosis, confirmatory diagnosis is only possible by microscopic examination of the spinal cord, since the parasites exist only as larval forms in their aberrant site.

Pathology: Migrating larvae affecting the CNS may cause areas of damage seen as brown foci or streaks grossly. The lesions show microcavitation and variable haemorrhage. There is loss of myelin and fragmentation of axons locally with eosinophils, neutrophils and macrophages present along with a mild meningitis and vascular cuffing.

Epidemiology: Since the worms are usually innocuous their epidemiology has received little study. The prevalence is higher in warmer countries, where there is longer seasonal activity of the mosquito vectors.

Treatment: There is no treatment for setarial paralysis. Ivermectin has been reported to be effective against adult *S. equina*.

Control: This would depend on control of the mosquito vectors, which is unlikely to be applied specifically for this parasite.

Notes: The members of this genus are usually harmless inhabitants of the peritoneal and pleural cavities.

Rhabditis spp

Synonym: *Peloderma*

Parasite class: Nematoda

Superfamily: Rhabditoidea

Pathogenesis: Another saprophagous, free-living nematode reported from the skin and gingivae of horses.

ECTOPARASITES

Bovicola equi

Synonym: *Damalinia equi, Trichodectes parumpilosus, Werneckiella equi equi*

Common name: Horse louse

Predilection site: Upper epidermal layers of the neck, flanks and tail base

Parasite class: Insecta

Parasite order: Phthiraptera

Parasite suborder: Ischnocera

Family: Trichodectidae

Description: These lice are up to 1–2 mm long and reddish brown in colour. The relatively large head is as wide as the wingless body, and rounded anteriorly. The mouthparts are ventral. This species has a three-segmented antenna and a single claw on the tarsi.

Hosts: Horse

Life cycle: During a lifespan of about a month females lay one egg approximately every day, glued singly on to a hair shaft. The eggs are usually whitish and may be seen with the naked eye. Females avoid ovipositing on the coarse hairs of the mane and tail, instead preferring finer hairs on the side of the neck, the flanks and the tail base. In severe cases the infestation may cover most of the body. The egg hatches into a nymph that is similar in appearance to the adult, although the nymph is much smaller, with lighter sclerotisation and less distinct banding. The cycle from egg to adult takes 3–4 weeks.

The mouthparts of *Bovicola equi* are adapted for biting and chewing, and allow them to feed on the outer layers of the hair shafts, dermal scales and blood scabs. They also feed on the exudates resulting from their irritant effect. *Bovicola equi* is capable of rapid population expansion.

Geographical distribution: Worldwide

Pathogenesis: *Bovicola equi* may cause intense irritation, resulting in rubbing and scratching, with matting and loss of hair and sometimes self-excoriation, involving almost the entire body in extreme cases. It is possible that heavy louse infestations in equines are themselves symptomatic of some other disorder, such as disease or, more likely, simple neglect. If neglected and left ungroomed, the undisturbed louse population will multiply more rapidly. In addition animals in a debilitated condition will fail to shed their winter coats and hence retain very large numbers of lice.

This species may act as a vector of equine infectious anaemia.

Clinical signs: Restlessness, rubbing and damage to the coat will suggest that lice are present, and when the hair is parted the parasites will be found. *Bovicola equi* appears as small yellowish specks in the hair, and the small pale eggs are readily found scattered throughout the coat. Other symptoms include a rough coat, skin infections, loss of hair and weight loss.

Diagnosis: The lice and their eggs may be seen within the hair and on the skin when the coat is parted. The lice may be removed and identified under a light microscope.

Pathology: The pathology of louse infestation is extremely variable. Infestations may induce alopecia, dermal irritation, papulocrustous dermatitis and self-excoriation.

Epidemiology: Equine pediculosis spreads by contact and via contaminated grooming equipment, blankets, rugs and saddlery. Severe infestations spread over the entire body, and the numbers are greatest in winter and early spring when the winter coat is at its most dense. Longer-haired animals and breeds are more prone to infestation by this species. As in cattle, the shedding of the winter coat is important in ridding animals of the greater part of their louse burden in spring. In hot countries the skin temperature of the animal's back may be high enough to kill lice in the exposed, fine-coated areas.

Treatment: Currently pyrethroid-based insecticides, applied as non-systemic, pour-on formulations are usually used to control lice, as many older drugs are no longer available. All of the horses in the establishment should be treated. Because eggs are relatively resistant to insecticides, treatment should be repeated every 7–14 days to kill newly hatched lice. Systemic treatments, such as the avermectins, are not approved for treatment of lice on horses.

Control: Grooming equipment should be scalded, blankets and rugs thoroughly washed, and saddlery thoroughly cleaned. Ideally, animals should have individual grooming equipment, and saddlery should not be interchanged, but this may not be economically feasible within some establishments. Regular and thorough grooming is, of course, the essence of control.

Haematopinus asini

Common name: Horse sucking louse

Predilection site: Skin of head, neck, back, brisket and between the legs

Parasite class: Insecta

Parasite order: Phthiraptera

Parasite suborder: Anoplura

Family: Haematopinidae

Description: *Haematopinus asini* is 3–3.5 mm long and yellow–brown as an adult. The lice have three pairs of legs and a long, narrow head with piercing mouthparts adapted for sucking blood and tissue fluids. The lice are found only on equines. All the species of *Haematopinus* are large lice, about 4–5 mm in length. They possess prominent angular processes, known as ocular points or temporal angles, behind the antennae. Eyes are absent. The thoracic sternal plate is dark and well developed. The legs are of similar sizes each terminating in a single large claw that opposes the tibial spur. Distinct sclerotised paratergal plates are visible on abdominal segments 2 or 3 to 8.

Hosts: Horse, donkey

Life cycle: During a lifespan of about a month the female lays operculate eggs ('nits') at a rate of one to six eggs per day. These are usually whitish, and are glued to the hair where they may be seen with the naked eye. They hatch in 1–2 weeks. Nymphs grow and moult over a period of about 12 days until the fully grown adult is present. After feeding and mating, the female lice may begin to lay eggs. Adults die after approximately 10–15 days of oviposition, and an average of around 24 eggs are laid per female. The whole cycle from egg to adult takes 3–4 weeks.

Geographical distribution: Worldwide

Pathogenesis: On horses, *Haematopinus asini* is most commonly found on the head, neck, back and inner surface of the upper legs. Symptoms include heavy dandruff and greasy skin and eventually bald spots with raw, red centres. Light infestations may be asymptomatic but, if present in sufficient numbers, they have been known to cause anaemia, weight loss and loss of vitality and appetite. Outbreaks of equine lice tend to be more frequent in the early spring, since the accumulated dirt in the barn and tack room, plus dander from the shedding of winter coats, provides an ideal environment for them. In horses, lice are often associated with poor grooming and management. Thin, aged, stressed or physically compromised horses seem to be more susceptible. Heavy louse infestations may in themselves be symptomatic of some other disorder such as disease or, more likely, simple neglect. Animals in a debilitated condition may harbour very large numbers of lice and the louse population will rapidly multiply on neglected, ungroomed animals.

Clinical signs: *Haematopinus* spp irritate their hosts by taking small but frequent blood meals. Each time they feed, they puncture the skin in a different place. As in other animals, equine lice may cause intense irritation, resulting in rubbing and scratching, with matting and loss of hair and sometimes excoriation, involving almost the whole body in extreme cases. Animals are restless and lose condition and, in heavy *Haematopinus* infestations, there may also be anaemia. Loss of condition and weight may increase the susceptibility of the host animal to other diseases.

Diagnosis: Restlessness, rubbing and damage to the coat would suggest that lice are present, and when the hair is parted the parasites will be found. These lice are large and yellow–brown, and very easily seen, and in temperate countries on warm sunny days will often move on to the surface of the coat.

Pathology: The pathology of louse infestation is extremely variable. Low infestations may induce alopecia, irritation, papulocrustous dermatitis and self-excoriation. The blood-feeding of *Haematopinus* may cause anaemia.

Epidemiology: In normal light infestations, lice occupy sites in the dense hair of the mane, the base of the tail, the submaxillary space, and also on the fetlocks of rough-legged breeds. From these sites spread occurs over the whole body, and the numbers are greatest in winter and early spring when the winter coat is at its most dense. As in cattle, the shedding of the winter coat is important to rid animals of the greater part of their louse burden in spring. In hot conditions the skin temperature of the animal's back may be high enough to kill lice in the exposed, fine-coated areas. Equine pediculosis spreads by contact and via contaminated grooming equipment, blankets, rugs and saddlery.

Treatment: As for *B. equi*

Control: As for *B. equi*

Demodex equi

Predilection site: Hair follicles and sebaceous glands

Parasite class: Arachnida

Sub-class: Acari

Order: Acariformes

Sub-order: Trombidiformes (Prostigmata)

Family: Demodicidae

Description: Species of *Demodex* have an elongate tapering body, up to 0.1–0.4 mm in length, with four pairs of stumpy legs ending in small blunt claws in the adult (Fig. 6.32). Setae are absent from the legs and body. The legs are located at the front of the body, and, as such, the striated opisthosoma forms at least half the body length.

Hosts: Horse

Life cycle: *Demodex* spp usually live as commensals in the skin, and are highly site-specific, occupying the hair follicles and sebaceous glands. Females lay 20–24 spindle-shaped eggs in the hair follicle that give rise to hexapod larvae, in which each short leg ends in a single, three-pronged claw. Unusually, a second hexapod larval stage follows, in which each leg ends in a pair of three-pronged claws. Octopod protonymph, tritonymph and adult stages then follow. Immature stages and these migrate more deeply into the dermis. One follicle may harbour all life cycle stages concurrently. The life cycle is completed in 18–24 days. In each follicle or gland the mites may occur in large numbers, located in a characteristic head-downward posture. In the newborn and very young these sites are simple in structure, but later they become compounded by outgrowths. The presence of *Demodex* mites much deeper in the dermis than sarcoptids means that they are much less accessible to surface-acting acaricides. Species of *Demodex* are unable to survive off their host.

Geographical distribution: Worldwide; but not reported in Australia

Pathogenesis: In the horse demodectic mange is rare, but may occur either as the squamous or the pustular type, affecting initially the muzzle, forehead and peri-ocular area.

Clinical signs: Scaling and alopecia, with or without papules and pustules, largely on the face, shoulders, neck and limbs. Pruritus is absent. Demodecosis in horses has been reported in association with chronic corticosteroid treatment.

Diagnosis: For confirmatory diagnosis, deep scrapings are necessary to reach the mites deep in the follicles and glands. This is best achieved by taking a fold of skin, applying a drop of liquid paraffin, and scraping until capillary blood appears.

Pathology: Lesions in horses, evident as patchy alopecia and scaling or as nodules, usually begin on the head and neck, but may rapidly spread to involve most of the body.

Epidemiology: Probably because of its location deep in the dermis, it is difficult to transmit *Demodex* between animals unless there is prolonged contact. Such contact occurs most commonly at suckling.

Treatment: There is little information regarding the treatment of equine demodecosis. Investigation and treatment of underlying systemic disease should be performed. Amitraz is contraindicated in horses because it can cause severe colic and death.

Control: Not usually required.

Notes: A second species, *D. caballi*, which infests the eyelids and muzzle has been described in horses; whether this is a true species of a morphological variant has not been established.

Sarcoptes scabiei

Common name: Scabies

Predilection site: Skin

Parasite class: Arachnida

Sub-class: Acari

Order: Acariformes

Sub-order: Sarcoptiformes (Astigmata)

Family: Sarcoptidae

Notes: This mange is now uncommon in horses. In Britain, for example, only two cases have been recorded since 1948. In both cases there was strong evidence that the infection had been acquired from other domestic species.

Pathogenesis: When present sacrcoptic mange can be severe. There may be intense pruritus due to hypersensitivity. Early lesions appear on the head, neck and shoulders as small papules and vesicles that later develop into crusts. Alopecia and crusting spread, become lichenified, forming folds. If untreated, lesions may extend over the whole body, leading to emaciation, general weakness and anorexia.

Treatment: If suspected, organophosphate insecticides or lime–sulphur solution can be applied by spray or dipping. Treatment should be repeated at 12- to 14-day intervals at least three to four times. Alternatively, the oral administration of ivermectin or moxidectin at 200 μg/kg can be attempted. Several treatments are required, 2–3 weeks apart, and it is important to treat all contact animals.

More detailed description is found in Chapter 5 (Pig), under Ectoparasites.

Psoroptes equi

Synonym: *Psoroptes cuniculi*, *Psoroptes cervinus*, *Psoroptes bovis*, *Psoroptes ovis*

Common name: Scab mite

Predilection site: Skin

Parasite class: Arachnida

Sub-class: Acari

Order: Acariformes

Sub-order: Sarcoptiformes (Astigmata)

Family: Psoroptidae

Pathogenesis: Infestation is rare in horses. When present, pruritic lesions may be seen on thickly haired regions of the body, such as under the forelock and mane, at the base of the tail, between the hindlegs and in the axillae. Lesions start as papules and alopecia and develop into thick, hemorrhagic crusts.

Treatment: As for sarcoptic mange
More detailed description is found in Chapter 3 under Sheep and Goat Ectoparasites.

Chorioptes bovis

Synonym: *Chorioptes ovis*, *Chorioptes equi*, *Chorioptes caprae*, *Chorioptes cuniculi*

Predilection site: Skin; particularly the legs, feet, base of tail and upper rear surface of the udder.

Parasite class: Arachnida

Sub-class: Acari

Order: Acariformes

Sub-order: Sarcoptiformes (Astigmata)

Family: Psoroptidae

Notes: The names *Chorioptes ovis*, *Chorioptes equi*, *Chorioptes caprae* and *Chorioptes cuniculi* used to describe the chorioptic mites found on sheep, horses, goats and rabbits respectively, are now all thought to be synonyms of *Chorioptes bovis*.

In horses, chorioptic mange due to *C. bovis* is occasionally observed. The mites are restricted to the pastern and occurs as crusty lesions with thickened skin on the legs below the knees and hocks, and is most prevalent in rough-legged animals and in those with heavy feather (Fig. 4.27). Though the mites are active only superficially, their movement causes irritation and restlessness, especially at night when animals are housed and minor injuries may occur in the fetlock region from kicking against walls.

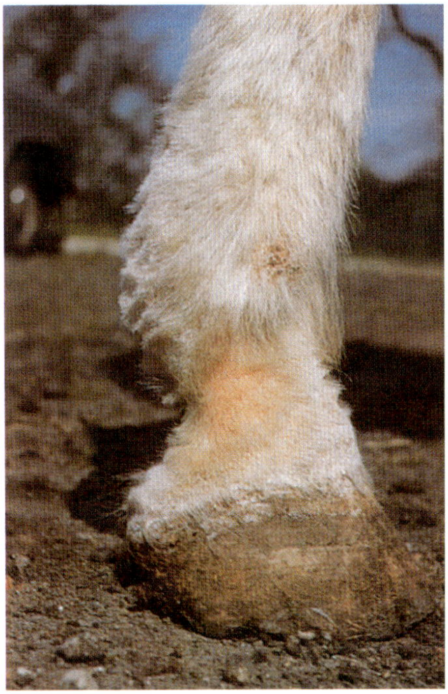

Fig. 4.27 Characteristic leg lesions of chorioptic mange in a horse.

More detailed description is found in Chapter 2 (Cattle) under Ectoparasites.

Several non-obligate ectoparasites are found on horses and are listed in the host–parasite checklist at the end of this chapter. More detailed descriptions of these parasites are found in Chapter 11 (Facultative ectoparasites and arthropod vectors).

In the following checklists, the codes listed below apply:

Helminth classes:
N = Nematoda; T = Trematoda; C = Cestoda.

Arthropod classes:
I = Insecta; A = Arachnida.

Protozoal classes:
M = Mastigophora; S = Sarcodina; A = Apicomplexa; R = Rickettsia.

Horse parasite checklist.

Section/host system	Helminths		Arthropods		Protozoa	
	Parasite	(Super)family	Parasite	Family	Parasite	Family
Digestive						
Oesophagus						
Stomach	*Draschia megastoma*	Spiruroidea (N)	*Gasterophilus haemorrhoidalis*	Oestridae (I)		
	Habronema microstoma	Spiruroidea (N)	*Gasterophilus inermis*	Oestridae (I)		
	Habronema muscae	Spiruroidea (N)	*Gasterophilus intestinalis*	Oestridae (I)		
	Trichostrongylus axei	Trichostrongyloidea (N)	*Gasterophilus nasalis*	Oestridae (I)		
			Gasterophilus nigricornis	Oestridae (I)		
			Gasterophilus pecorum	Oestridae (I)		
Small intestine	*Strongyloides westeri*	Rhabditoidea (N)			*Eimeria leuckarti*	Eimeriidae (A)
	Parascaris equorum	Ascaridoidea (N)			*Eimeria solipedum*	Eimeriidae (A)
	Anoplocephala perfoliata	Anoplocephalidae (C)			*Eimeria uniungulati*	Eimeriidae (A)
	Anoplocephala magna	Anoplocephalidae (C)			*Cryptosporidium parvum*	Cryptosporidiidae (A)
	Paranoplocephala mamillana	Anoplocephalidae (C)			*Giardia intestinalis*	Diplomonadidae (M)
Caecum Colon	*Cyathostomum alveatum*	Strongyloidea (N)			*Entamoeba gedoelsti*	Endamoebidae (S)
	Cyathostomum catinatum	Strongyloidea (N)				
	Cyathostomum coronatum	Strongyloidea (N)				
	Cyathostomum labiatum	Strongyloidea (N)				
	Cyathostomum labratum	Strongyloidea (N)				
	Cyathostomum montgomeryi	Strongyloidea (N)				
	Cyathostomum pateratum	Strongyloidea (N)				
	Cyathostomum saginatum	Strongyloidea (N)				
	Cyathostomum tetracanthrum	Strongyloidea (N)				
	Cylicocyclus adersi	Strongyloidea (N)				
	Cylicocyclus auriculatus	Strongyloidea (N)				
	Cylicocyclus brevicapsulatus	Strongyloidea (N)				
	Cylicocyclus elongatus	Strongyloidea (N)				
	Cylicocyclus insigne	Strongyloidea (N)				
	Cylicocyclus largocapsulatus	Strongyloidea (N)				
	Cylicocyclus leptostomus	Strongyloidea (N)				
	Cylicocyclus maturmurai	Strongyloidea (N)				
	Cylicocyclus nassatus	Strongyloidea (N)				
	Cylicocyclus radiatus	Strongyloidea (N)				

Cylicocyclus triramosus	Strongyloidea (N)
Cylicodontophorus bicoronatus	Strongyloidea (N)
Cylicodontophorus euproctus	Strongyloidea (N)
Cylicodontophorus mettami	Strongyloidea (N)
Cylicostephanus asymetricus	Strongyloidea (N)
Cylicostephanus bidentatus	Strongyloidea (N)
Cylicostephanus calicatus	Strongyloidea (N)
Cylicostephanus goldi	Strongyloidea (N)
Cylicostephanus hybridus	Strongyloidea (N)
Cylicostephanus longibursatus	Strongyloidea (N)
Cylicostephanus minutus	Strongyloidea (N)
Cylicostephanus ornatus	Strongyloidea (N)
Cylicostephanus poculatus	Strongyloidea (N)
Cylicostephanus skrjabini	Strongyloidea (N)
Poteriostomum imparidentatum	Strongyloidea (N)
Poteriostomum ratzii	Strongyloidea (N)
Craterostomum acuticaudatum	Strongyloidea (N)
Craterostomum tenuicauda	Strongyloidea (N)
Oesophagodontus robustus	Strongyloidea (N)
Strongylus edentatus	Strongyloidea (N)
Strongylus equinus	Strongyloidea (N)
Strongylus vulgaris	Strongyloidea (N)
Triodontophorus brevicauda	Strongyloidea (N)
Triodontophorus minor	Strongyloidea (N)
Triodontophorus nipponicus	Strongyloidea (N)
Triodontophorus serratus	Strongyloidea (N)
Triodontophorus tenuicollis	Strongyloidea (N)
Oxyuris equi	Oxyuroidea (N)
Probstmayria vivipara	Oxyuroidea (N)
Gastrodiscus aegyptiacus	Paramphistomatidae (T)
Gastrodiscus secundus	Paramphistomatidae (T)
Pseudodiscus collinsi	Paramphistomatidae (T)
Anoplocephala perfoliata	Anoplocephalidae (C)

(*continued*)

Horse parasite checklist (*continued*).

Section/host system	Helminths		Arthropods		Protozoa	
	Parasite	(Super)family	Parasite	Family	Parasite	Family
Respiratory						
Nose			*Rhinoestrus purpureus*	Oestridae (I)		
Trachea Bronchi	*Dictyocaulus arnfieldi*	Trichostrongyloidea (N)				
Lung	*Echinococcus granulosus*	Taeniidae (C)				
Liver						
	Fasciola hepatica	Fasciolidae (T)				
	Echinococcus granulosus	Taeniidae (C)				
Pancreas						
Circulatory						
Blood	*Schistosoma japonicum*	Schistosomatidae (T)			*Trypanosoma brucei brucei*	Trypanosomatidae (M)
	Schistosoma nasalis	Schistosomatidae (T)			*Trypanosoma brucei evansi*	Trypanosomatidae (M)
	Schistosoma indicum	Schistosomatidae (T)			*Trypanosoma congolense congolense*	Trypanosomatidae (M)
	Schistosoma spindale	Schistosomatidae (T)			*Babesia caballi*	Babesiidae (A)
	Schistosoma turkestanicum	Schistosomatidae (T)			*Theileria equi*	Theileriidae (A)
					Neorickettsia risticii	Rickettsiaceae (R)
					Anaplasma phagocytophilum	Anaplasmataceae (R)
Blood vessels	*Elaeophora bohmi*	Filarioidea (N)				
Nervous						
CNS	*Halicephalobus (Micronema) delitrix*	Rhabditoidea (N)			*Toxoplasma gondii*	Sarcocystiidae (A)
					Sarcocystis neurona	Sarcocystiidae (A)
Eye	*Thelazia lacrymalis*	Spiruroidea (N)				

Reproductive/ urogenital						
					Trypanosoma equiperdum	Trypanosomatidae (M)
Kidneys					*Klossiella equi*	Klossiellidae (A)
Locomotory						
Muscle	*Trichinella spiralis*	Trichuroidea (N)			*Toxoplasma gondii*	Sarcocystiidae (A)
					Sarcocystis equicanis	Sarcocystiidae (A)
					Sarcocystis fayeri	Sarcocystiidae (A)
Connective tissue						
Integument						
Skin	*Rhabditis (Peloderma)* spp.	Rhabditoidea (N)	*Hippobosca equina*	Hippoboscidae (I)		
			Bovicola equi	Trichodectidae (I)		
			Haematopinus asini	Linognathidae (I)		
			Demodex equi	Demodicidae (A)		
			Sarcoptes scabiei	Sarcoptidae (A)		
			Psoroptes ovis	Psoroptidae (A)		
			Chorioptes bovis	Psoroptidae (A)		
Subcutaneous	*Onchocerca reticulata*	Filarioidea (N)	*Cordylobia anthropophaga*	Calliphoridae (I)		
	Parafilaria multipapillosa	Filarioidea (N)	*Cochliomyia hominivorax*	Calliphoridae (I)		
	Setaria equina	Filarioidea (N)	*Cochliomyia macellaria*	Calliphoridae (I)		
	Dracunculus medinensis	Dracunculoidea (N)	*Chrysomya bezziana*	Calliphoridae (I)		
			Chrysomya megacephala	Calliphoridae (I)		
			Wohlfahrtia magnifica	Sarcophagidae (I)		
			Wohlfahrtia meigeni	Sarcophagidae (I)		
			Wohlfahrtia vigil	Sarcophagidae (I)		
			Dermatobia hominis	Oestridae (I)		

The following species of flies and ticks are found on horses. More detailed descriptions are found in Chapter 11: Facultative ectoparasites and arthropod vectors.

Flies of veterinary importance on horses.

Group	Genus	Species	Family
Blackflies Buffalo gnats	*Simulium*	spp	Simuliidae (I)
Bot flies	*Dermatobia*	*hominis*	Oestridae (I)
Flesh flies	*Sarcophaga*	*fusicausa* *haemorrhoidalis*	Sarcophagidae (I)
	Wohlfahrtia	*magnifica* *meigeni* *vigil*	
Midges	*Culicoides*	spp	Ceratopogonidae (I)
Mosquitoes	*Aedes* *Anopheles* *Culex*	spp spp spp	Culicidae (I)
Muscids	*Hydrotaea*	*irritans*	Muscidae (I)
	Musca	*autumnalis* *domestica*	
	Stomoxys	*calcitrans*	
Sandflies	*Phlebotomus*	spp	Psychodidae (I)
Screwworms and blowflies	*Chrysomya*	*albiceps* *bezziana* *megacephala*	Calliphoridae (I)
	Cochliomyia	*hominivorax* *macellaria*	
	Cordylobia	*anthropophaga*	
Tabanids	*Chrysops* *Haematopota* *Tabanus*	spp spp spp	Tabanidae (I)

Tick species found on horses.

Genus	Species	Common name	Family
Ornithodoros	*moubata*	Eyeless or hut tampan	Argasidae (A)
	savignyi	Eyed or sand tampan	
Amblyomma	*cajennense*	Cayenne tick	Ixodidae (A)
	hebraeum	Bont tick	
	maculatum	Gulf coast tick	
	variegatum	Tropical bont tick	
Dermacentor	*albipictus*	Winter or moose tick	Ixodidae (A)
	andersoni	Rocky Mountain wood tick	
	nitens	Tropical horse tick	
	occidentalis	Pacific coast tick	
	reticulatus	Marsh tick	
	silvarum		
Haemaphysalis	*punctata*		Ixodidae (A)
Hyalomma	*anatolicum*	Bont leg tick	Ixodidae (A)
	detritum	Bont leg tick	
	excavatum	Brown ear tick	
	marginatum	Mediterranean *Hyalomma*	
	truncatum	Bont leg tick	
Ixodes	*ricinus*	Castor bean or European sheep tick	Ixodidae (A)
	holocyclus		
	rubicundus	Karoo paralysis tick	
	scapularis	Shoulder tick	
Rhipicephalus	*appendiculatus*	Brown ear tick	Ixodidae (A)
	bursa		
	capensis	Cape brown tick	
	evertsi	Red or red-legged tick	
	sanguineus	Brown dog or kennel tick	

5
Parasites of pigs

ENDOPARASITES

PARASITES OF THE DIGESTIVE SYSTEM

OESOPHAGUS

Gongylonema pulchrum

Synonym: *G. scutatum*

Common name: Gullet worm

Predilection site: Oesophagus, rumen

Parasite class: Nematoda

Superfamily: Spiruroidea

Final host: Sheep, goat, cattle, pig, buffalo, horse, donkey, deer, camel, man

Intermediate host: Coprophagous beetles, cockroaches

For more details see Chapter 3 (Sheep and goats).

STOMACH

Hyostrongylus rubidus

Common name: Red stomach worm

Predilection site: Stomach

Parasite class: Nematoda

Superfamily: Trichostrongyloidea

Description, gross: Slender reddish worms when fresh, males measuring around 5–7 mm and females 6–10 mm in length. The body cuticle is both transversely and longitudinally striated with 40–45 longitudinal striations.

Description, microscopic: A small cephalic vesicle is present and the spicules resemble *Ostertagia* in ruminants, but have only two distal branches. The bursa of the male is well developed and the dorsal lobe small. There is a well developed telamen and short spicules. The vulva of the female opens in the posterior third of the body. Eggs are medium sized, 71–78 × 35–42 μm strongyle-type and are often difficult to differentiate from those of *Oesophagostomum*.

Hosts: Pig, wild boar; occasionally found in rabbits

Life cycle: The free-living and parasitic stages are similar to those of *Ostertagia*; infection is through oral ingestion of L_3. The prepatent period is about 3 weeks. Hypobiosis of L_4 may occur following repeated infection, or be induced by seasonal changes, and is often seen in older animals. In sows these hypobiotic larvae may resume their development during the periparturient relaxation of immunity and/or early lactation, leading to an increase in the faecal egg count.

Geographical distribution: Worldwide

Pathogenesis: Similar to ostertagiosis, with penetration of the gastric glands by the L_3 and replacement of the parietal cells by rapidly dividing undifferentiated cells which proliferate to give rise to nodules on the mucosal surface. The pH becomes elevated in heavy infections and there is an increase in mucus production and a catarrhal gastritis. Sometimes there is ulceration and haemorrhage of the nodular lesions, but more commonly light infections occur and these are associated with decreased appetite and poor feed conversion rates.

Clinical signs: Light infections are often asymptomatic. Heavy infections can lead to inappetence, vomiting, anaemia, loss of condition and bodyweight. Diarrhoea may or may not occur.

Diagnosis: This is based on a history of access to permanent pig pastures and the clinical signs. Confirmatory diagnosis is by examination of faeces for eggs; larval identification following faecal culture may be necessary, particularly to differentiate *Hyostrongylus* from *Oesophagostomum*. At necropsy, the small reddish worms can be seen in the mucous exudates on the

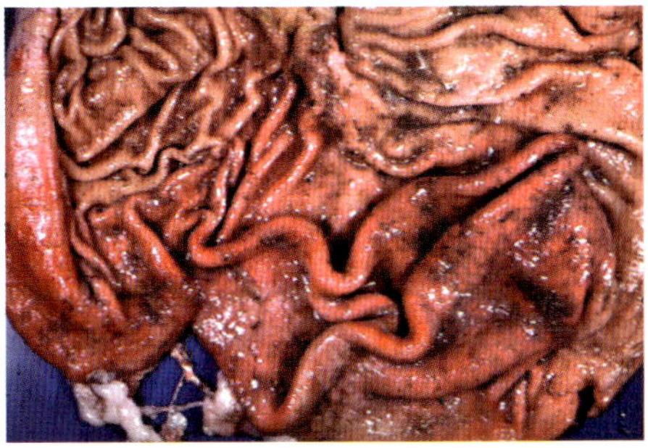

Fig. 5.1 *Hyostrongylus rubidus* on the mucosa of an infected stomach.

gastric mucosa. Other stomach worms, the spiruroid nematodes, are larger: >13 mm.

Pathology: During the course of larval development there is dilation of infected gastric glands and hyperplasia of the glandular epithelium of both infected and neighbouring glands. The lamina propria is oedematous with infiltration by lymphocytes, plasma cells and eosinophils. Larvae are found in the gastric glands with adults mainly on the surface (Fig. 5.1). During the course of development the hyperplasia causes the formation of pale nodules, which may become confluent in heavy infections, leading to the formation of a thickened, convoluted mucosa. There may be focal or diffusely eroded areas and occasionally ulceration of the glandular mucosa.

Epidemiology: Because of the preparasitic larval requirements, infection is confined to pigs with access to pasture or those kept in straw yards. It is therefore more common in breeding stock, particularly gilts. The free-living larvae are particularly sensitive to desiccation and low temperatures. The epidemiology, at least in temperate zones, is similar to that of *Ostertagia* in ruminants with seasonal hypobiosis a feature. Adult pigs often act as a reservoir of infection.

Treatment: When *Hyostrongylus* infection is diagnosed, particularly in breeding stock, it is important to use a drug such as a modern benzimidazole or a macrocyclic lactone, which will remove hypobiotic larvae.

Control: The same principles apply as for the control of parasitic gastroenteritis in ruminants. For example, in temperate areas there should be an annual rotation of pasture with other livestock or crops. The timing of the move to other pastures may be dependent on other farming activities; if it can be delayed until October or later and accompanied by an anthelmintic treatment, then eggs from any worms which survive the treatment are unlikely to develop due to the unfavourable winter temperatures. A second treatment, again using a modern benzimidazole or a macrocyclic lactone is recommended 3–4 weeks later to remove any residual infection. It may be advantageous to treat pregnant pigs before farrowing.

Notes: This parasite is responsible for a chronic gastritis in pigs, particularly gilts and sows.

Ollulanus tricuspis

Predilection site: Stomach

Parasite class: Nematoda

Superfamily: Trichostrongyloidea

Description, gross: This is a very small trichostrongyle (0.7–1.0 mm long). Males are 0.7–0.8 mm, and females 0.8–1 mm long.

Description, microscopic: It is identified microscopically by the spiral coil of the head. The male bursa is well developed and the spicules are stout and each is split into two for a considerable distance. The female has a tail with three or four short cusps. The vulva is in the posterior part of the body and there is only one uterus and ovary.

Hosts: Cats, wild felids; occasionally found in pigs, foxes and domestic dogs

Life cycle: The worms are viviparous, the larvae developing to the L_3 stage in the uterus of the females. Autoinfection can occur, the shed L_3 developing into adult worms on the gastric mucosa in around 4–5 weeks. The whole life cycle may be completed endogenously and transmission, at least in the cat, is thought to be via ingestion of vomit containing the L_3. The worms live under a layer of mucus in the stomach wall and the anterior end of the worm is often located within the gastric crypts.

Geographical distribution: Mainly occurs in Europe, North and South America, Australasia and the Middle East.

Pathogenesis: A chronic gastritis has been reported in the pig.

Clinical signs: Occasional vomiting and emaciation

Diagnosis: Diagnosis of ollulanosis is seldom made because of their small size and lack of eggs and larvae in the faeces. Examination of vomit, following an emetic, for the presence of worms is a useful approach. At necropsy, recovery and identification of the very small worms from the gastric mucosa should lead to a diagnosis.

Pathology: The worms lie beneath the mucus on the surface of the stomach, or partly in the gastric glands, and their presence may lead to mucosal lymphoid hyperplasia and elevated numbers of globule leucocytes in the gastric epithelium. Heavy infections result in hyperplasia of the gastric glands causing the stomach mucosa to become convoluted and thrown into folds.

Epidemiology: The parasite is common in some parts of the world, particularly in cat colonies and cats that roam. The parasite can replicate in the stomach without any need for external egg or larval phases and can spread via vomit. The disease spreads mainly among starving stray cats and from them to other hosts.

Treatment: Not reported in the pig, although benzimidazoles or ivermectin should be effective.

Control: This is mainly achieved through the implementation of good hygiene procedures and prevention of contact with cats.

Ascarops strongylina

Synonym: *Arduenna strongylina*

Predilection site: Stomach

Parasite class: Nematoda

Superfamily: Spiruroidea

Description, gross: Small, slender worms, the males measuring up to 15 mm and the reddish females 22 mm long. They live on the stomach wall under a layer of mucus.

Description, microscopic: A cervical ala is located only on the left side of the body. The wall of the pharynx contains several spiral supports. Eggs are thick-shelled, $34–49 \times 20\,\mu m$, and are embryonated when passed.

Final hosts: Pig, wild boar

Intermediate hosts: Coprophagous beetles (*Aphodius*, *Onthophagus*, *Gymnopleurus*)

Life cycle: The life cycle of *A. strongylina* is typically spiruroid. Eggs passed in the faeces of the infected host develop into infective larvae, if ingested by coprophagous beetles. The life cycle is completed when pigs ingest the beetles. The prepatent period is about 4 weeks.

Geographical distribution: Worldwide

Pathogenesis: *A. strongylina* is not severely pathogenic; the main effect being a catarrhal gastritis, particularly in young animals.

Clinical signs: Clinical signs are usually absent, although, in heavy infections, softening of faeces and inappetence may occur.

Diagnosis: Diagnosis of a particular genus is difficult by faecal examination, but the presence of the small elongate eggs in the faeces of animals showing signs of gastritis will give a tentative indication of spiruroidosis.

Pathology: On postmortem, the gastric mucosa is sometimes reddened and oedematous.

Epidemiology: The epidemiology depends on the presence and abundance of the intermediate beetle hosts. Infection is more prevalent in outdoor pigs at pasture.

Treatment: Treatment has not been considered with this genus.

Control: Not usually required.

Ascarops dentata

Synonym: *Arduenna dentata*

Predilection site: Stomach

Parasite class: Nematoda

Superfamily: Spiruroidea

Geographical distribution: Malaysia, S.E. Asia.

All other details are essentially similar to *A. strongylina*

Gnathostoma hispidum

Predilection site: Stomach

Parasite class: Nematoda

Superfamily: Spiruroidea

Description, gross: Thick-bodied worms; the males are 1.5–2.5 cm and the females 2.0–4.5 cm long. The presence of the worms in gastric nodules is sufficient for generic diagnosis.

Description, microscopic: The whole body is covered with spines. The left spicule is longer than the right. Eggs are oval, $72–74 \times 39–42\,\mu m$ with a thin cap at one pole.

Final host: Pig, rarely man

Intermediate hosts: *Cyclops* spp and related freshwater crustacea

Life cycle: The young worms migrate in the abdominal organs of the host, particularly the liver. Adult worms live in tunnels in the gastric nodules, and the eggs pass from there into the lumen and are dropped into the water in the faeces where they develop to L_2 before hatching after several days. Crustaceans ingest L_2 and development to L_3 takes place within about 10 days. The final host is infected by ingestion of the crustacea and further development occurs in the stomach wall, where the deeply embedded worms provoke the growth of fibrous lesions. A second intermediate host is not required with *G. hispidum*.

Geographical distribution: Europe, Asia, Africa

Pathogenesis: The most obvious effect of gnathostomosis is the presence of fibrous growths on the stomach wall. Ulceration and necrosis of the stomach wall are often present. In some cases a number of larvae will migrate from the stomach to other organs, most commonly the liver, in which they burrow, leaving necrotic tracks in the parenchyma. It occurs erratically in man as a cause of visceral larva migrans.

Clinical signs: *Gnathostoma* infection is usually inapparent. Severe infections may produce a marked gastritis leading to inappetence and weight loss.

Diagnosis: The infection in the living animal can only be diagnosed by the finding of the greenish, oval eggs, which have a thin cap at one pole, in the faeces. Often, however, eggs are not present in faeces.

Pathology: Fibrous growths are of variable size, the largest being 3–4 cm in diameter, and are cavitated, amounting to thick-walled cysts containing several worms and fluid.

Epidemiology: It should be noted that the final hosts are also eligible second intermediate hosts, so that, for example, the pig may harbour L_3 in its liver and muscles as well as adult worms in its stomach.

Treatment: Treatment has not been fully investigated.

Control: With ubiquity of the first and second intermediate hosts, complete control cannot be achieved, but partial limitation is possible by thorough cooking of all food.

Gnathostoma doloresi

Predilection site: Stomach

Parasite class: Nematoda

Superfamily: Spiruroidea

Geographical distribution: Asia

All other details are essentially similar to G. *hispidum*

Physocephalus sexalatus

Predilection site: Stomach

Parasite class: Nematoda

Superfamily: Spiruroidea

Description, gross: Small, slender worms; the males measuring about 10–12 mm and the females up to 22 mm long.

Description, microscopic: The wall of the pharynx contains a single spiral support. The cervical papillae are asymmetrically located. Eggs are thick-shelled and are embryonated when passed.

Final hosts: Pig; occasionally rabbit, hare

Intermediate hosts: Coprophagous beetles

Life cycle: The life cycle is typically spiruroid and the prepatent period is about 6 weeks.

Geographical distribution: Widely distributed in many parts of the world

Pathogenesis: The parasites lie on the surface of the stomach wall under a layer of mucus. *P. sexalatus* is not severely pathogenic, the main effect being a catarrhal gastritis, particularly in young piglets.

Clinical signs: In many infections, obvious clinical signs are absent; in heavy infections, softening of faeces and inappetance may occur.

Diagnosis: As for other spiruroid parasites

Pathology: At necropsy, the gastric mucosa is sometimes reddened and oedematous. The tiny worms can be seen in the mucus covering the gastric mucosa.

Epidemiology: Infection occurs where the intermediate hosts are plentiful. Transmission may also occur through paratenic hosts, such as amphibians or birds.

Treatment: Not reported

Control: Measures that restrict dung beetle populations feeding on pig faeces will be beneficial.

Notes: *P. sexalatus* is not considered to be of great economic or pathogenic importance.

Simondsia paradoxa

Predilection site: Stomach

Parasite class: Nematoda

Superfamily: Spiruroidea

Description, gross: Small slender worms. The females measure up to about 20 mm in length, and males are 12–15 mm long.

Description, microscopic: Females have large lateral alae and a large ventral and dorsal tooth. The gravid female has a characteristic form, the posterior end of the body being a rounded sac filled with eggs. The male has a spirally coiled tail. Eggs are oval or ellipsoid, 20–29 μm.

Final host: Pig

Intermediate hosts: Beetles

Life cycle: The life cycle is indirect. Eggs are passed in the faeces and ingested by beetles in which they hatch and develop to infective larvae. The parasites continue development when the intermediate host is ingested by a pig. Male worms live on the surface of the gastric mucosa, but the females are found in small cysts in the mucosal crypts with their anterior ends protruding.

Geographical distribution: Predominantly a parasite of tropical and subtropical regions; also occurs in parts of Europe.

Pathogenesis: *Simondsia paradoxa* is not severely pathogenic, the main effect being a catarrhal gastritis. In addition, there can be some fibrous reaction around the nodules in the stomach wall.

Clinical signs: Infections are usually asymptomatic.

Diagnosis: Diagnosis of a particular genus is difficult by faecal examination, but the presence of the small elongate eggs in the faeces of animals showing signs of gastritis will give a tentative indication of spiruroidosis.

Pathology: Females are present in nodules 6–8 mm in diameter.

Epidemiology: Infection is likely to be more common in outdoor pigs where the intermediate hosts are more abundant.

Treatment: Treatment is generally not considered.

Control: Attempts to control these spiruroids are unlikely to be successful because of the ready availability of the intermediate hosts.

Trichostrongylus axei

Synonym: *Trichostrongylus extenuatus*

Common name: Stomach hairworm

Predilection site: Stomach

Parasite class: Nematoda

Superfamily: Trichostrongyloidea

Description, gross: The adults are small, hair-like, light brownish red and difficult to see with the naked eye. Males measure around 3–6 mm and females 4–8 mm in length.

Hosts: Cattle, sheep, goat, deer, horse, donkey, pig and occasionally man

Life cycle: This is typically trichostronylid and is described in detail in Chapter 3 (Sheep and goats).

Geographical distribution: Worldwide

Pathogenesis: *T. axei* may occasionally be found in the stomach of pigs, but is considered to be of minor importance.

SMALL INTESTINE

Globocephalus urosubulatus

Synonym: *Globocephalus longemucronatus*

Common name: Pig hookworm

Predilection site: Small intestine

Parasite class: Nematoda

Superfamily: Strongyloidea

Description, gross: A very small, stout whitish worm, 0.4–0.8 cm long

Description, microscopic: The mouth opens subdorsally and the buccal capsule is globular but with an absence of chitinous structures in the buccal capsule. The male bursa is well developed and the spicules are slender.

Hosts: Pig, wild boar

Life cycle: The life cycle is direct, either by oral ingestion of L_3 larvae or by percutaneous penetration. Larval migration through the heart, lungs, trachea, oesophagus and stomach occurs.

Geographical distribution: North and South America, Europe, Africa and Asia

Pathogenesis: Not known but thought to be generally of little pathological significance, although heavy infections may affect piglets severely.

Clinical signs: Generally asymptomatic, although heavily infected piglets may be anaemic and show weight loss and emaciation.

Diagnosis: Identification of eggs in the faeces, or adult worms found in the small intestine on postmortem.

Pathology: Not described

Epidemiology: Not reported

Treatment: Most modern benzimidazoles and macrocyclic lactones are likely to be effective.

Control: Frequent removal of faeces and bedding on dry straw or concrete will help reduce the risk of infection.

Ascaris suum

Common name: Large roundworm, white spot

Predilection site: Small intestine

Parasite class: Nematoda

Superfamily: Ascaridoidea

Description, gross: *A. suum* is by far the largest nematode of the pig; the white, rigid females are up

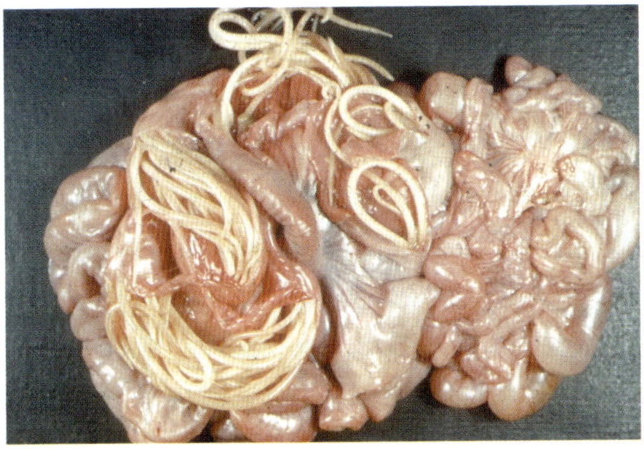

Fig. 5.2 A knot of *Ascaris suum* recovered from the small intestine of an infected pig.

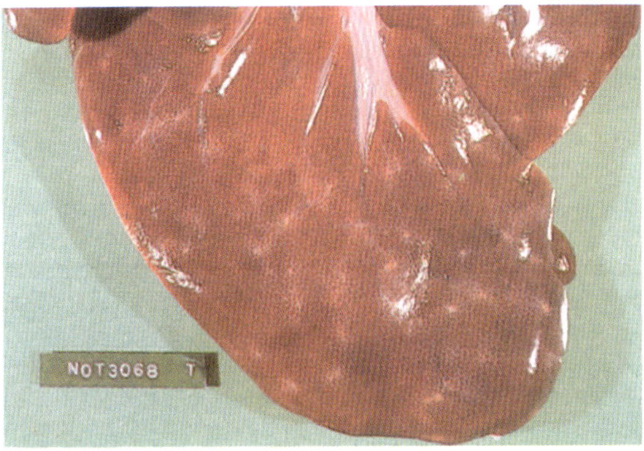

Fig. 5.3 Milk spot lesions in the liver associated with *Ascaris suum*.

to 40.0 cm long and the males up to 25 cm in length, and could only be confused with *Macracanthorhyncus* where this occurs (Fig. 5.2).

Description, microscopic: The egg is ovoid and yellowish brown, with a thick shell, the outer layer of which is irregularly mamillated. The egg is larvated when passed in the faeces and the thick multilayered eggshell enables the egg to survive desiccation and freezing in the environment for several years.

Hosts: Pig, wild boar, rarely sheep, cattle, man

Life cycle: The life cycle is direct. Though the preparasitic moults occur by about 3 weeks after the egg is passed, a period of maturation is necessary, and the egg is not usually infective until a minimum of four weeks after being passed, even in the optimal temperature range of 22–26°C. The egg is very resistant to temperature extremes, and is viable for more than 4 years. After ingestion, the larvated egg hatches in the small intestine, the L_3 larva penetrates the intestinal mucosa and then travels to the liver. The larva then passes in the bloodstream to the lungs and thence to the small intestine via the bronchi, trachea and pharynx. In the intestine the final moult occurs and the young adult worms inhabit the lumen of the small intestine. If the eggs are ingested by an earthworm or dung beetle they will hatch, and the L_3 travel to the tissues of these paratenic hosts, where they can remain, fully infective for pigs, for a long period. The prepatent period is between 7 and 9 weeks, and each female worm is capable of producing more than 200 000 eggs per day. Longevity is around 6–9 months.

Geographical distribution: Worldwide

Pathogenesis: The migrating larval stages in large numbers may cause numerous small haemorrhages, emphysema and a transient pneumonia, but it is now recognised that many cases of so-called '*Ascaris* pneumonia' may be attributable to other infections, or to piglet anaemia. In the liver, the migrating larvae can cause 'milk spot' or 'white spot' which appears as cloudy whitish spots of up to 1.0 cm in diameter on the surface of the liver, and represents the fibrous repair of inflammatory reactions to the passage of larvae in the livers of previously sensitised pigs (Fig. 5.3). Livers showing 'milk spot' lesions may be condemned at meat inspection. The adult worms in the intestine cause little apparent damage to the mucosa, but occasionally, if large numbers are present, there may be obstruction, and rarely a worm may migrate into the bile duct, causing obstructive jaundice and carcase condemnation. Experimental infections have shown that in young pigs the important effect of alimentary ascariosis is economic, with poor feed conversion and slower weight gains, leading to an extension of the fattening period by 6–8 weeks.

Clinical signs: The main effect of the adult worms in pigs is to cause production loss in terms of diminished weight gain. Otherwise, clinical signs are absent except in the occasional case of intestinal or biliary obstruction. Heavy infections may increase the susceptibility of young pigs to other bacterial and viral pathogens. In piglets under 4 months old, larval activity during the pulmonary phase of migration may cause a clinically evident pneumonia, which is usually transient and rapidly resolving. In sheep and cattle exposed to contaminated grazing, there may be acute dyspnoea, tachypnoea and coughing following acute challenge with migrating larvae in the lungs.

Diagnosis: Diagnosis is based on clinical signs, history of disease, and, in infections with the adult worm, on the presence in faeces of the yellow–brown ovoid eggs, with thick mamillated shells. Being dense, the eggs float more readily in saturated solutions of zinc sulphate or magnesium sulphate than in the saturated sodium chloride solution, which is used in most faecal examination techniques. Low counts of *A. suum* eggs in faeces (<200 epg) may represent false-positives due to the coprophagic activity of pigs. At necropsy, the large worms in the small intestine are easy to recognise.

Pathology: Larval migration induces lesions in the liver and lungs. In the lungs, gross lesions are limited largely to numerous focal haemorrhages scattered over and through the pulmonary parenchyma. There may be some oedema, congestion and alveolar emphysema. Microscopically, there is an eosinophilic bronchiolitis. Bronchioles are surrounded by macrophages and eosinophils, and the bronchiolar wall is infiltrated by eosinophils, which are also present, with necrotic debris, in the lumen. Larvae are usually readily found in tissue sections and may be present in alveoli, alveolar ducts, bronchioles or bronchi, and in more chronic cases, are found within eosinophilic granulomas. Lesions in the liver result in considerable economic loss from condemnation at meat inspection. Haemorrhagic tracks are present near portal areas and throughout lobules, visible through the capsule as pinpoint red areas, sometimes slightly depressed and surrounded by a narrow pale zone. These lesions collapse, healing by fibrosis, which extends around portal tracts and extends out more diffusely emphasising lobular outlines. Granulomatous foci containing giant cells, macrophages and eosinophils may centre on the remnants of larvae trapped and destroyed in the liver. The inflammatory infiltrates in livers of animals exposed to larval ascarids may become severe and diffuse, and this is reflected in the gross appearance of the liver, which has extensive 'milk spots' and prominent definition of lobules. The liver is firm, and heavy scars may become confluent, obliterating some lobules and extending out to exaggerate interlobular septa throughout the liver.

The pathogenicity of adult ascarids in the intestine is poorly defined. Heavy infections may obstruct the gut, being visible as rope-like masses through the intestinal wall. Ascarids may occasionally pass to the stomach and be vomited or migrate up the pancreatic or bile ducts. Sometimes biliary obstruction and icterus, or purulent cholangitis, may ensue. Rarely, intestinal perforation occurs. On histology, there may be substantial hypertrophy of the muscularis externa and elongation of the crypts of Lieberkühn, though height of villi is not significantly reduced. Hypertrophy and exhaustion of the goblet-cell population and increased infiltrates of eosinophils and mast cells are also observed in infected intestines.

In sheep, and occasionally cattle, migrating ascarids can cause eosinophilic granulomas and interstitial hepatitis and fibrosis with heavy eosinophilic infiltrates in the livers of sheep grazing contaminated areas. In heavy infections where death ensues, the lungs are moderately consolidated, with alveolar and interstitial emphysema and interlobular oedema. Microscopically, there is thickening of the alveolar septae, and effusion of fluid and macrophages into the alveoli. Larvae present within alveoli and bronchioles provoke an acute bronchiolitis.

Epidemiology: Young suckling piglets can become infected early after birth through the ingestion of embryonated eggs that are attached to the underbelly of the sow. Prevalence of infection is usually highest in pigs of around 3–6 months of age. A partial age immunity operates in pigs from about 4 months of age onwards, and this, coupled with the fact that the worms themselves have a limited life-span of several months, would suggest that the main source of infection is the highly resistant egg on the ground, a common characteristic of the ascaridoids. Hence 'milk spot', which is economically very important, since it is a cause of much liver condemnation, presents a continuous problem in some pig establishments. This condition has been widely noted to have a distinct seasonality of occurrence, appearing in greatest incidence in temperate areas during the warm summer months, and almost disappearing when the temperatures of autumn, winter and spring are too low to allow development of eggs to the infective stage. Also earthworms are generally more active and available during the summer months. Sows and boars act as reservoirs of light infection. *A. suum* may occasionally infect cattle, causing an acute, atypical, interstitial pneumonia, which may prove fatal. In most cases reported the cattle have had access to housing previously occupied by pigs, sometimes several years before, or to land fertilised with pig manure. In lambs, *A. suum* may also be a cause of clinical pneumonia as well as 'milk spot' lesions, resulting in condemnation of livers. In most cases lambs have been grazed on land fertilised with pig manure or slurry, such pasture remaining infective for lambs even after ploughing and cropping. Young adults of *A. suum* are occasionally found in the small intestine of sheep. There are a few recorded cases of patent *A. suum* infection in man but cross-infection is not of epidemiological significance.

Treatment: The intestinal stages are susceptible to most of the anthelmintics in current use in pigs, and the majority of these, such as the benzimidazoles, are given in the feed over several days. In cases of suspected *Ascaris* pneumonia, injectable levamisole and ivermectin may be more convenient. For 3–4 days post-treatment the faeces should be removed from the pens and destroyed, as they often will contain large numbers of eggs and expelled/disintegrating worms.

Control: In the past, elaborate control systems have been designed for ascariosis in pigs, but with the appearance of highly effective anthelmintics these labour-intensive systems are rarely used. The chief problem in control is the great survival capacity of the eggs, but in housed pigs, strict hygiene in feeding and bedding, with frequent hosing/steam cleaning of walls, floors and feeding troughs will limit the risk of infection. Some disinfectants and chemical solutions will limit infectivity. In pigs on free range the problem is greater, and where there is serious ascariosis it may be necessary to discontinue the use of paddocks for several years, since the eggs can survive cultivation. It is good practice to treat in-pig sows at entry to the farrowing pen, and young pigs should receive anthelmintic treatment when purchased or on entry to the finishing house and 8 weeks later; boars should be treated every 3–6 months. Washing of the skin of sows prior to their removal to the farrowing pen should reduce contamination with embryonated eggs.

Notes: The type species, *Ascaris lumbricoides*, occurs in man, and at one time it was not differentiated from *A. suum*, so that the pig was thought to present a zoonotic risk for man. With species distinction now possible, *A. lumbricoides* is accepted as specific for man, and is irrelevant to veterinary medicine.

Strongyloides ransomi

Common name: Threadworm

Predilection site: Small intestine

Parasite class: Nematoda

Superfamily: Rhabditoidea

Description, gross: Slender, hair-like worms 3.4–4.5 mm long. Only females are parasitic.

Description, microscopic: The long oesophagus may occupy up to one third of the body length and the uterus is intertwined with the intestine giving the appearance of twisted thread. Unlike other intestinal parasites of similar size the tail has a blunt point. *Strongyloides* eggs are oval, thin-shelled and small, 45–55 × 26–35 μm.

Hosts: Pig

Life cycle: *Strongyloides* is unique among the nematodes of veterinary importance, being capable of both parasitic and free-living reproductive cycles. The parasitic phase is composed entirely of female worms in the small intestine and these produce larvated eggs by parthenogenesis, i.e. development from an unfertilised egg. After hatching, larvae may develop through four larval stages into free-living adult male and female worms and this can be followed by a succession of free-living generations. However, under certain conditions, possibly related to temperature and moisture, the L_3 can become parasitic, infecting the host by skin penetration or ingestion and migrating via the venous system, the lungs and trachea to develop into adult female worms in the small intestine.

Piglets may acquire infection immediately after birth from the mobilisation of arrested larvae in the tissues of the ventral abdominal wall of the dam, which are subsequently excreted in the milk. In addition, prenatal infection has been demonstrated experimentally in pigs. The prepatent period is 6–9 days.

Geographical distribution: Worldwide

Pathogenesis: Skin penetration by infective larvae may cause an erythematous reaction. Mature parasites are found in the duodenum and proximal jejunum and if present in large numbers may cause inflammation with oedema and erosion of the epithelium. This results in catarrhal enteritis with impairment of digestion and absorption.

Clinical signs: In light infections, animals show no clinical signs. In heavy infections, there is bloody diarrhoea, anaemia and emaciation, and sudden death may occur. During the migratory phase there may be coughing, abdominal pain and vomiting.

Diagnosis: Demonstration of larvated eggs in faeces or the adults in scrapings from the intestine on postmortem is diagnostic.

Pathology: The adult female worms burrow into the intestinal wall and establish in tunnels in the epithelium at the base of the villi in the small intestine, causing an inflammatory response. In large numbers they may cause villous atrophy, with a mixed mononuclear inflammatory cell infiltration of the lamina propria. Crypt epithelium is hyperplastic and there is villous clubbing.

Epidemiology: *Strongyloides* infective larvae are not ensheathed and are susceptible to extreme climatic conditions. However warmth and moisture favour development and allow the accumulation of large numbers of infective stages. Adult breeding stock may be infected with dormant larvae in their subcutaneous fat. Pregnancy and farrowing appear to stimulate the re-emergence of these larvae, which then may infect piglets via the colostrum. This appears to be the major route of infection in young piglets and, in only 7 days after birth, piglets may be passing eggs in their faeces.

Treatment: Specific control measures for *Strongyloides* infection are rarely called for. The benzimidazoles and the macrocyclic lactones may be used for the treatment of clinical cases and a single dose of ivermectin 4–16 days prior to farrowing has been shown to suppress larval excretion in the milk of sows.

Control: Strict hygiene and cleaning of pens before farrowing helps limit levels of infection. Treating the sows before farrowing can also help reduce infections in piglets.

Trichinella spiralis

Synonym: *Trichina spiralis*

Common name: Muscle worm

Predilection site: Small intestine, muscle

Parasite class: Nematoda

Superfamily: Trichuroidea

Description, gross: Because of their short lifespan, the adult worms are rarely found in natural infections. The male is about 1.5 mm and the female 3.5–4.0 mm long.

Description, microscopic: The oesophagus is at least one third of the total body length and the tail in the male has two small cloacal flaps, but no copulatory spicule nor a spicule sheath. In the female, the uterus contains developing larvae. *Trichinella* infection is most easily identified by the presence of coiled larvae in striated muscle (Fig. 5.4). The cysts are lemon-shaped, 0.3–0.8 × 0.2–0.4 mm in size and often transparent.

Hosts: Pig, rat, man, and most mammals

Life cycle: The life cycle is indirect. The adult parasites and infective larvae (muscle trichinae) are unusual in being present within a single host (i.e. development from larva to adult to larva in a single host). *Trichinella* does not have a free-living stage. The developing adults lie between the villi of the small intestine. After fertilisation, the males die while the females burrow deeper into the intestinal mucosa. About a week later, they produce L_1 which enter the lymphatic vessels and travel via the bloodstream to the skeletal muscles. There, still as L_1, they penetrate striated muscle cells where they are encapsulated by the host, grow and assume a characteristic coiled position; the parasitised muscle cell is transformed by microvascularisation into a 'nurse cell'. This process is complete within about 3–4 weeks, by which time the larvae are infective and may remain so for many years. Development is resumed when muscle, containing the encysted trichinae, is ingested by another host, usually as a result of predation or carrion feeding. The L_1 is liberated in the stomach and in the intestine undergoes four moults to become sexually mature within about a week. Patent infections persist for only a few weeks at the most.

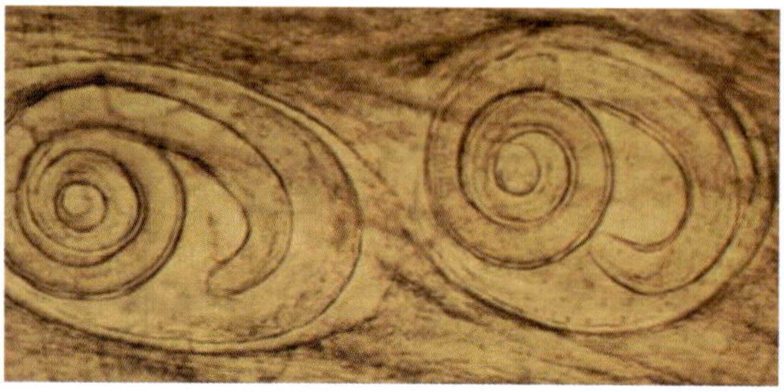

Fig. 5.4 Coiled infective larvae of *Trichinella spiralis* in striated muscle.

Geographical distribution: Worldwide, with the apparent exceptions of Australia, Denmark and Great Britain

Pathogenesis: The adults occur in the glandular crypts of the proximal small intestine and their larvae in the striated muscles; the diaphragmatic, intercostal and masseter muscles and the tongue are considered to be the main predilection sites. Infection in domestic animals is invariably light, and clinical signs do not occur. However, when hundreds of larvae are ingested, as occasionally happens in man and presumably also in predatory animals in the wild, including cats and dogs, the intestinal infection is often associated with catarrhal enteritis and diarrhoea, and 1–2 weeks later the massive larval invasion of the muscles causes acute myositis, fever, eosinophilia and myocarditis. Periorbital oedema and ascites are also common in man, sometimes accompanied by vomiting, diarrhoea, fever and myocarditis. Unless treated with an anthelmintic and anti-inflammatory drugs, such infections may frequently be fatal as a consequence of paralysis of respiratory muscles, but in persons who survive this phase the clinical signs start to abate after 2–3 weeks.

Clinical signs: These are variable and depend on the host and the level of infection. Signs are usually non-specific and resemble those of other diseases, such as diarrhoea, fever, muscular pain, dyspnoea and peripheral eosinophilia. *T. spiralis* infection in young pigs can induce inappetance, weakness and diarrhoea. Older pigs are generally more tolerant of infection.

Diagnosis: This is not relevant in live domestic animals. At meat inspection, heavy larval infections may occasionally be just seen with the naked eye as tiny greyish white spots. For routine purposes small samples of pig muscle (taken from the preferential predilection sites) of about 1 g are squeezed between glass plates, the apparatus being called a compressorium, and examined for the presence of larvae by direct low-power microscopic examination or projection onto a screen using a trichinoscope. Alternatively, small portions of diaphragm tissue may be digested in pepsin/HCl and the sediment examined microscopically for the presence of larvae. The digestion method is now the preferred approach in most countries as it is less expensive and labour intensive to perform. For mass screening purposes, designed to determine the incidence of trichinellosis in pigs within regions or for some high-volume slaughterhouses, immunodiagnostic tests have been used. Of these, the antibody-detection ELISA or EIA appears to be the test of choice.

Pathology: The adults occur in the glandular crypts of the proximal small intestine where there is little associated pathology. Larvae are found in the striated muscles with the diaphragmatic, intercostals, masseter muscles and the tongue considered to be the main predilection sites. On microscpic examination, the larvae lie in a bulging clear segment of muscle fibre, which may be loosely encircled by eosinophils, lymphocytes, plasma cells and macrophages. In a heavy infection, a large proportion of the muscle fibres in the predilection muscles may be infected with larvae and surrounded by reactive zones. As the cellular reaction subsides, muscle fibres surrounded by the larvae have the appearance of a fibrous capsule. Once larvae become encysted, there is muscle fibre degeneration and mineralisation, which doesn't appear to affect larval viability, as larvae can survive for up to 20 years.

Epidemiology: It is important to realise that trichinellosis is basically an infection of animals in the wild and that the involvement of man in these circumstances is accidental. The epidemiology of trichinellosis depends on two factors. First, animals may become infected from a wide variety of sources, predation and cannibalism being perhaps the most common. Others include feeding on carrion, since the encapsulated larvae are capable of surviving for several months in decomposing flesh, and the ingestion of fresh faeces from animals with a patent infection. It is also thought that transport hosts, such as crustaceans and fish, feeding on drowned terrestrial animals, may account for infection in some aquatic mammals such as seals.

The second factor is the wide host range of the parasite, infecting various carnivores and omnivorous mammals. In temperate areas rodents, brown bear, badger and wild pig are most commonly involved; in the arctic, polar bear, wolf and fox; in the tropics, lion, leopard, bushpig, hyena, jackal and warthog. In these sylvatic or feral cycles, man and his animals are only occasionally involved. For example, the consumption of polar bear meat may cause infection in Inuit and sledge-dogs, while in Europe the hunting and subsequent ingestion of wild pigs may also produce disease in man and his companion animals.

The domestic or synanthropic cycle in man and the pig is an 'artificial' zoonosis largely created by feeding pigs on food waste containing the flesh of infected pigs; more recently, tail biting in pigs has been shown to be a mode of transmission. Rats in piggeries also maintain a secondary cycle, which may on occasions pass to pigs or vice versa from the ingestion of infected flesh or faeces. Infection in man is acquired from the ingestion of raw or inadequately cooked pork or its by-products, such as sausages, ham and salami. It is also important to realise that smoking, drying or curing pork does not necessarily kill larvae in pork products. Horsemeat has increasingly been implicated in the transmission of *Trichinella* to man.

In areas such as Poland, Germany and the USA, human trichinosis acquired from pork has, until recently, been an important zoonosis. Over the past few decades, prohibition of feeding uncooked food waste to pigs, improved meat inspection and public awareness have greatly diminished the significance of the problem. In Britain, and other countries in Europe, and in the USA the numbers of outbreaks are few and sporadic.

The decreasing prevalence is also reflected in the fact that inapparent infection in man, as shown by the presence of *T. spiralis* larvae in muscle samples at necropsy, has decreased from 10% to not recorded in Britain, and from 20% to under 5% in the USA over the past 50 years.

Treatment: Although rarely called for in animals, the adult worms and the larvae in muscles are susceptible to several of the benzimidazole anthelmintics, such as in-feed treatment with flubendazole in pigs.

Control: Probably the most important factor in the control of trichinellosis is a legal requirement that swill or waste human food intended for consumption by pigs must be boiled (100°C for 30 minutes). In fact, this practice is mandatory in many countries to limit the potential spread of other diseases, such as foot and mouth disease and swine fever.

Other essential steps include:

1. Meat inspection, which plays an essential role in monitoring the detection of infected carcases. Such carcases must be condemned.
2. Measures to eliminate rodents and other wild animals from piggeries and slaughterhouses.
3. Prevention of exposure of pigs to dead animal carcasses, particularly of rats and pigs.
4. Regulations to ensure that larvae in pork are destroyed by cooking or freezing. In the USA, for example, any pork or pork products, other than fresh pork, must be treated by heating or freezing before marketing and it is likely also that irradiation might soon be introduced as a further method of control.
5. Consumer education, and particularly the recognition that pork or pork products or the flesh of carnivorous game should be thoroughly cooked before consumption. It is worth noting that the larvae of *Trichinella nativa* that occurs in wild carnivores and seals in some arctic and subarctic regions is very resistant to freezing.

Table 5.1 Species of *Trichinella*.

Species	Distribution	Principal hosts	Resistance to freezing
Capsule forming			
T. spiralis	Cosmopolitan	Mammals, pig, rat, man	No
T. nativa	Arctic and subarctic zones: North America, Finland, Sweden	Wild carnivores, seal, polar bear, walrus	High
T. nelsoni	Tropical Africa	Wild carnivores and omnivores	No
T. britovi	Temperate zone of Palaearctic region	Wild carnivores, fox, wild boar, horse, man	Low
T. murrelli	North America	Wildlife, horse, man	No
Non-capsule forming			
T. pseudospiralis	Cosmopolitan	Mammals, birds	No
T. papuae	Papua New Guinea	Wild pig, man	No
T. zimbabwensis	Zimbabwe	Crocodiles	No

Notes: The taxonomy of the genus has been controversial until very recently. It is composed of several sibling species, which cannot be differentiated morphologically but molecular typing, and other criteria, have now identified eight species of *Trichinella* (Table 5.1).

Macracanthorhynchus hirudinaceus

Common name: Thorny-headed worm

Predilection site: Duodenum and proximal small intestine

Parasite class: Acanthocephala

Family: Oligacanthorhynchidae

Description, gross: Adults resemble *Ascaris suum*, but taper posteriorly. The anterior of the worm possesses a retractable proboscis, which is covered with recurved hooks (Fig. 5.5). The males are up to 10 cm and the females around 60 cm in length and slightly pinkish in colour when fresh. The worms are thick (5–10 mm in width) and the cuticle is transversely wrinkled.

Description, microscopic: There is no alimentary canal. The egg is oval with a thick greyish brown pitted shell and contains the acanthor larva when laid. This larva has a small circle of minute hooks at the anterior.

Definitive hosts: Pig, wild boar, occasionally dog, wild carnivores and man

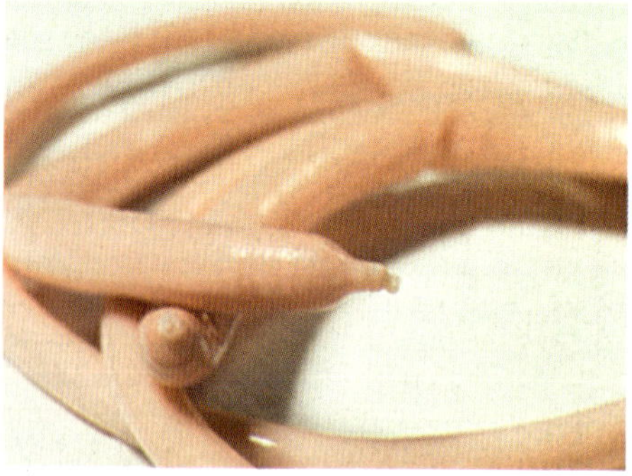

Fig. 5.5 Head of *Macracanthorhynchus hirudinaceus* showing the retractible proboscis.

Intermediate hosts: Various dung beetles and water beetles

Life cycle: Adults, attached to the small intestinal mucosa, lay eggs which are passed in the faeces. These are produced in large numbers, are very resistant to extremes of climate and can survive for years in the environment. After ingestion by dung or water beetle larvae, the acanthor develops to the infective cystacanth stage in approximately 3 months. Infection of pigs occurs after ingestion of either infected beetle grubs or adult beetles. The prepatent period is 2–3 months and longevity can be around 1 year.

Geographical distribution: Worldwide, but absent from certain areas, for example parts of western Europe

Pathogenesis: Mild infections are not very pathogenic, but heavy infections may retard growth rates and cause emaciation.

Clinical signs: Low-level infections are usually asymptomatic. Heavy infections may cause inappetence and weight loss.

Diagnosis: This is based on finding the typical eggs in the faeces. At necropsy the worms superficially appear similar to *Ascaris suum*, but when placed in water the spiny proboscis is protruded, thus aiding differentiation.

Pathology: *M. hirudinaceus* penetrates deep into the intestinal wall with its proboscis and produces inflammation and may provoke granuloma formation at the site of attachment in the wall of the duodenum and the small intestine. Heavy infections may induce a catarrhal enteritis and, rarely, penetration of the intestinal wall, which can result in a fatal peritonitis.

Epidemiology: Infection is seasonal, being partly dependent on the availability of the intermediate hosts. The eggs are able to remain viable in the environment for several years. Infection tends to be more prevalent in pigs of around 1–2 years of age.

Treatment: Although there is little information on treatment, levamisole and ivermectin are reported to be effective.

Control: Pigs should be prevented from access to the intermediate hosts. In modern management systems this may be easily achieved, but where pigs are kept in small sties the faeces should be regularly removed to reduce the prevalence of the dung beetle intermediate hosts.

Fasciolopsis buski

Predilection site: Small intestine

Parasite class: Trematoda

Family: Fasciolidae

Description, gross: Large, thick, elongate-oval fluke without shoulders, broader posteriorly, and variable in size but usually measuring 30–75 × 8–20 mm. The ventral sucker is situated near the anterior extremity and is much larger than the oral sucker. The cuticle bears spines that are frequently lost.

Description, microscopic: Eggs are brown, thin shelled with an operculum, and measure 125–140 × 70–90 μm.

Final hosts: Pig, dog and man

Intermediate hosts: Flat, spiral-shelled freshwater snails of *Planorbis* and *Segmentina* species

Life cycle: The life cycle is similar to *F. hepatica*. The final host is infected through ingestion of metacercariae that encyst on aquatic plants. The prepatent period is 9–13 weeks.

Geographical distribution: India, Pakistan, southeast Asia and China.

Pathogenesis: The parasite is mainly of importance as a cause of disease in humans. It is located in the small intestine where it can cause severe ulceration of the intestinal mucosa in heavy infections in man. Lesions are less severe in the pig and dog.

Clinical signs: Infection causes abdominal pain, diarrhoea, oedema, ascites and occasionally intestinal obstruction leading to malnutrition and death in humans. Symptoms are less severe in pigs and dogs.

Diagnosis: Diagnosis is confirmed by identification of the eggs in faeces that have to be differentiated from eggs of *Fasciola* spp.

Pathology: Heavier infections produce ulceration of the intestinal mucosa.

Epidemiology: The intermediate snail hosts feed on certain plants, water calthrop (*Trapa natans*) and water chestnut (*Eliocharis tuberosa*), which are cultivated for food and usually fertilised with human faeces. The cercariae encyst on the tubers or nuts of these plants, and cause infection if eaten raw. Pigs also become infected through eating these plants.

Treatment: Albendazole (10 mg/kg) and praziquantel (15 mg/kg) are both effective.

Control: The disease is easily preventable by avoiding raw or uncooked aquatic plants in endemic areas. The introduction of good sanitation facilities limits contamination of local watercourses and ponds.

Notes: *F. buski* is primarily a parasite of man, but can occur in the pig and dog, which may act as reservoir hosts.

Coccidiosis

Although some ten species of coccidia have been described from pigs, their importance is not clear. *Isospora suis* is a cause of a naturally occurring severe enteritis in young piglets aged 1–2 weeks. *Eimeria debliecki* has been described as causing clinical disease and severe pathology; *E. polita*, *E. scabra* and *E. spinosa* cause moderate to mild diarrhoea in piglets.

The source of infection appears to be oocysts produced by the sow during the periparturient period, the piglets becoming initially infected by coprophagia; the second phase of diarrhoea is initiated by reinvasion from tissue stages. Diagnosis of the condition is difficult unless postmortem material is available since clinical signs occur prior to the shedding of oocysts and

Table 5.2 Predilection sites and prepatent periods of *Eimeria* species in pigs.

Species	Predilection site	Prepatent period (days)
Isospora suis	Small intestine	5
Eimeria deblieki	Small intestine	6–7
E. polita	Small intestine	7–8
E. scabra	Small and large intestine	7–11
E. spinosa	Small intestine	7
E. porci	Small intestine	5–7
E. neodebliecki	Unknown	10
E. perminuta	Unknown	?
E. suis	Unknown	10

are very similar to those caused by other pathogens such as rotavirus.

Diagnosis of coccidial infections is based on history and clinical signs, and in patent infections, on the presence of oocysts of the pathogenic species in the faeces. Oocysts may not be shed during the diarrhoeal phase so faecal counts are not always of value.

Treatment for all species of *Eimeria* has generally relied on the use of a sulphonamide/trimethoprim product combined with electrolyte and fluid therapy. Treatment with several anticcocidial drugs, such as halofuginone, salinomycin and diclazuril given orally to affected animals, has been reported to be effective, although such treatments may not be licensed or approved in many countries. Control of coccidiosis is based on reducing environmental contamination by improved hygiene. Pens should be kept clean and dry. Ammonia-based disinfectants can be used after thoroughly cleaning farrowing pens by high-pressure hosing or steam disinfection. Overcrowding of piglets and faecal contamination of food and water should be avoided. Prevention can be achieved by the in-feed administration of amprolium to sows during the periparturient period, from 1 week prior to farrowing until 3 weeks post farrowing, where such treatments are licensed or approved.

Isospora suis

Predilection site: Small intestine

Parasite class: Sporozoasida

Family: Eimeriidae

Description: Oocysts are spherical to subspherical, 17–25 × 16–22 µm (mean 20.6 × 18.1 µm) and the wall

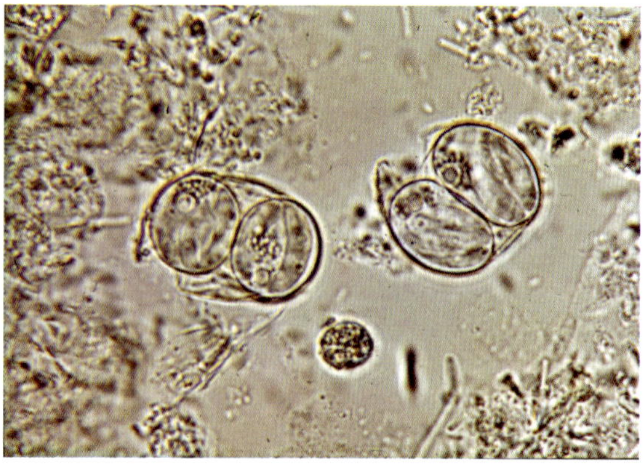

Fig. 5.6 Oocysts of *Isospora suis*.

is colourless and thin. There is no micropyle or residuum and when sporulated the oocysts contain two sporocysts each with four sporozoites characteristic of *Isospora*. The two sporocysts are ellipsoidal, 13–14 × 8–11 µm without a Stieda body but with a sporocyst residuum. The four sporozoites in each sporocyst are sausage-shaped with one pointed end (Fig. 5.6).

Hosts: Pig

Life cycle: Meronts are in the epithelial cells of the villi of the small intestine usually in the distal third and below the host cell nucleus. First-generation meronts are present 2–3 days post infection. Second-generation meronts are present 4 days, and mature gamonts present 5 days post infection. The prepatent period is 4–6 days and the period of patency 3–13 days.

Geographical distribution: Worldwide

Pathogenesis: Infection can occur in all types of farrowing facilities and under all types of management systems. Piglets with clinical infection develop a characteristic non-haemorrhagic disease that is unresponsive to routine antibiotic therapy. Scours tend to occur in individuals from about 6 days of age, but most of the litter scours at 8–10 days of age. The diarrhoea ranges from white to pasty cream faeces through to a watery diarrhoea. Affected piglets tend to be stunted and hairy. Severely affected piglets become dehydrated, continue to suckle but weight gains are reduced. Mortality is generally low to moderate. *I. suis* can cause infection on its own or in combination with other enteropathogens, such as enterotoxigenic *Escherichia coli*, rotavirus and transmissible gastroenteritis virus.

Clinical signs: The main clinical signs are diarrhoea, often biphasic, which varies in its severity from white to pasty cream faeces through to a watery diarrhoea.

Diagnosis: Diagnosis of the condition is difficult unless postmortem material is available, since clinical signs

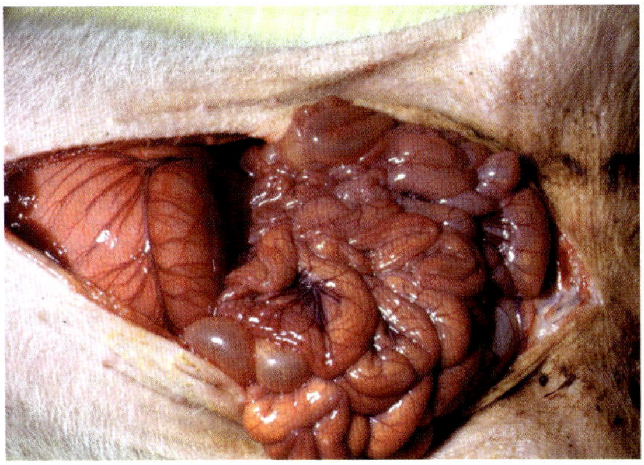

Fig. 5.7 *Isospora suis* infection in a piglet.

occur prior to the shedding of oocysts and are very similar to those caused by other pathogens such as rotavirus.

Pathology: Lesions caused by *I. suis* in young piglets are present in the jejunum and ileum and are associated with the development stages of the parasite. The affected intestine is inflamed and reddened (Fig. 5.7). Microscopic changes include villous atrophy, villous fusion, crypt hyperplasia and necrotic enteritis.

Treatment: Treatment with toltrazuril (1 ml of 5% suspension) given orally to affected piglets at 4 days of age has proved effective.

Eimeria debliecki

Predilection site: Small intestine

Parasite class: Sporozoasida

Family: Eimeriidae

Description: Oocysts are ellipsoid or ovoid, 15–23 × 11–18 μm (mean 18.8 × 14.3 μm), with a smooth and colourless wall. There is a polar granule but no micropyle or oocyst residuum. Sporocysts are elongate ovoid, 13–20 × 5–7 μm with a large Stieda body and a large sporocyst residuum. The sporozoites are vermiform, and each contains two large clear globules.

Hosts: Pig

Life cycle: The endogenous stages are located in the distal part of the columnar epithelial cells of the tips of the villi in the small intestine posterior to the bile duct. First-generation meronts mature at 2 days and second-generation meronts at 4 days; gamonts mature about 5 days after infection. The prepatent period is 6–7 days, and the patent period approximately 5 days. Oocyst sporulation time is 5–7 days.

Geographical distribution: Worldwide

Pathogenesis: *E. debliecki* has been described as causing clinical disease and severe pathology in young piglets. Older animals are seldom if ever affected.

Clinical signs: Diarrhoea, inappetence, emaciation, depressed growth and occasional mortality in young piglets.

Pathology: Catarrhal inflammation of the jejunum is seen. On postmortem there may be enteritis and large numbers of meronts and gamonts may be found in mucosal scrapings. On histopathology, there may be villous atrophy, villous fusion and crypt hyperplasia.

Eimeria polita

Predilection site: Small intestine

Parasite class: Sporozoasida

Family: Eimeriidae

Description: Oocysts are ellipsoidal or broad ovoid, 20–33 × 14–22 μm (mean 25.9 × 18.1 μm) with a slightly rough yellowish brown wall. There is no micropyle or oocyst residuum, although a polar granule may be present. Sporocysts are ellipsoidal to ovoid, 13–19 × 5–9 μm, each has a Stieda body and a residuum. The sporozoites are elongate with one or two clear globules, and lie lengthwise head to tail in the sporocysts. The mature meronts are about 14–24 × 11–23 μm and contain 15–30 merozoites. Macrogametes are 16–29 × 15–25 μm and microgamonts 16–29 × 13–29 μm and possess a residuum.

Hosts: Pig

Life cycle: The endogenous stages occur in the epithelium at the tips of the villi in the jejunum and ileum. There are thought to be two generations of meronts. Gamonts and gametes are found in the same area of the intestine and mature 8–9 days post infection.

The prepatent period is 7–8 days and the patent period is 6–8 days.

Geographical distribution: Worldwide

Pathogenesis: *E. polita* is thought to be moderately pathogenic. Mixed infections are common and several coccidia species may be involved in causing diarrhoea in young piglets.

Clinical signs: Heavy infections may cause diarrhoea, inappetance, weight loss, unthriftiness, dehydration and death

Pathology: On postmortem there may be enteritis and large numbers of meronts and gamonts may be found in mucosal scrapings. On histopathology, there may be villous atrophy, villous fusion and crypt hyperplasia

Eimeria scabra

Predilection site: Small and large intestine

Parasite class: Sporozoasida

Family: Eimeriidae

Description: Oocysts are ovoid or ellipsoidal, 24–42 × 20–24 μm (mean 31.9 × 22.5 μm), with a thick rough, striated wall, yellow brown in colour. There is a micropyle and polar granule, but no oocyst residuum. Sporocysts are ovoid, 14–18 × 7–9 μm, each with a prominent Stieda body and sporocyst residuum. The sporozoites are elongate with two clear globules and lie lengthwise head to tail in the sporocysts. First-generation meronts are 16 × 13 μm in size at 3 days post infection and contain 16–24 merozoites. Second-generation meronts are 16 × 12 μm (5 days), containing 14–22 merozoites; third-generation meronts are 21 × 16 μm in size (7 days) and contain 14–28 merozoites. The macrogametes are 18 × 12 μm and the microgamonts 17 × 13 μm.

Hosts: Pig

Life cycle: The endogenous stages are found in the epithelial cells of the villi, and the necks of the crypts in the posterior small intestine, and also in the caecum and colon. There are three generations of meronts. The first-generation meronts mature at 3 days, second-generation meronts mature at 5 days and a third generation of meronts matures 7 days after infection.

The prepatent period is 7–11 days and the patent period is 4–8 days. Sporulation time is 9–12 days.

Geographical distribution: Worldwide

Pathogenesis: Not generally considered pathogenic, but it may cause mild diarrhoea in piglets.

Clinical signs: Occasional diarrhoea

Pathology: On postmortem there may be enteritis and large numbers of meronts and gamonts may be found in mucosal scrapings. On histopathology, there may be villous atrophy, villous fusion and crypt hyperplasia.

Eimeria spinosa

Predilection site: Small intestine

Parasite class: Sporozoasida

Family: Eimeriidae

Description: Oocysts are ovoid, 17–24 × 12–19 μm (mean 20.6 × 16.2 μm) with a thick, rough, brown wall with long spines. There is a polar granule but no micropyle or oocyst residuum. Sporocysts are elongate ovoid, 10–14 × 5–7 μm, each with a prominent Stieda body and residuum. The sporozoites are elongate, and lie lengthwise head to tail in the sporocysts and each has a clear globule at the large end.

Hosts: Pig

Life cycle: All the endogenous stages are found in the villar epithelial cells of the jejunum and ileum. The number of meront generations is not known. The prepatent period is 7 days.

The sporulation time is 9–10 days.

Geographical distribution: Worldwide

Pathogenesis: *E. spinosa* has been described as causing clinical disease in young piglets. Older animals are generally not affected

Clinical signs: Diarrhoea, inappetence, emaciation, depressed growth and occasional mortality in young piglets

Pathology: Similar to *E. scabra*

The following species of *Eimeria* found in pigs are considered non-pathogenic

Eimeria porci

Predilection site: Small intestine

Parasite class: Sporozoasida

Family: Eimeriidae

Description: Oocysts are ovoid, colourless to yellowish brown, 18–27 × 13–18 μm (mean 21.6 × 15.5 μm) with an indistinct micropyle, a polar granule but no oocyst residuum. Sporocysts are ovoid, 8–12 × 6–8 μm. Each has a Stieda body and a sporocyst residuum. The sporozoites are elongate and either lie at either end of the sporocysts, or lie lengthwise head to tail. Each has an indistinct clear globule.

Hosts: Pig

Life cycle: The endogenous stages occur in the epithelial cells of the lower jejunum and ileum below the host cell nucleus. There are two meront generations. The first occurs 1–3 days, and the second 3–6 days after infection. Young gamonts can be recognised 5 days after infection. The prepatent period is 5–7 days and the patent period is 6 days. Sporulation time is 9 days.

Geographical distribution: Worldwide

Eimeria neodebliecki

Predilection site: Unknown

Parasite class: Sporozoasida

Family: Eimeriidae

Description: Oocysts are ellipsoid; the wall is smooth and colourless 17–26 × 13–20 μm (mean 21.2 × 15.8 μm), with no micropyle or oocyst residuum but there is a polar granule. Sporocysts are elongate or broadly ovoid (9–14 × 5–8 μm); each has a Stieda body and a sporocyst residuum. The sporozoites are vermiform and lie lengthwise head to tail in the sporocysts and each has two clear globules.

Hosts: Pig

Life cycle: Details of the life cycle are unknown. The prepatent period is 10 days and the patent period is 6 days. The sporulation time is 13 days.

Geographical distribution: Worldwide

Eimeria perminuta

Predilection site: Unknown

Parasite class: Sporozoasida

Family: Eimeriidae

Description: Oocysts are ovoid to subspherical, yellow in colour, 12–15 × 10–13 μm (mean 13.3 × 11.7 μm) and the wall has a rough surface. A polar granule is present but no micropyle or oocyst residuum. Sporocysts are ellipsoidal to broadly ovoid, 6–8 × 4–6 μm, each with a Stieda body and residuum. Sporozoites are elongate with two clear globules and lie lengthwise head to tail in the sporocysts.

Hosts: Pig

Life cycle: Details of the lifecycle are unknown. The sporulation time is 10–12 days.

Geographical distribution: Worldwide

Eimeria suis

Predilection site: Unknown

Parasite class: Sporozoasida

Family: Eimeriidae

Description: Oocysts are ellipsoidal, 15–23 × 12–18 μm (mean 18.2 × 14.0 μm) with a smooth and colourless wall. There is a polar granule but no micropyle or oocyst residuum. Sporocysts are elongate ovoid, 8–12 × 4–6 μm, each with a prominent Stieda body and a sporocyst residuum. The sporozoites are elongate and lie lengthwise head to tail in the sporocysts and each has a clear globule at the broad end.

Hosts: Pig

Life cycle: Details of the life cycle are not known. The prepatent period is 10 days and the patent period is 6 days. The sporulation time is 5–6 days.

Geographical distribution: Worldwide

Cryptosporidium parvum

Predilection site: Small intestine

Parasite class: Sporozoasida

Family: Cryptosporidiidae

Host: Cattle, sheep, goat, horse, deer, pig, man

Description: Mature oocysts are ovoidal or spheroidal, 5.0 × 4.5 μm (range 4.6–5.4 × 3.8–4.7 μm) and a length: width ratio of 1.19.

Geographical distribution: Worldwide

Pathogenesis: Most pig cryptosporidial infections are asymptomatic with the majority of infections occurring in 6–12-week-old pigs.

Clinical signs: Clinically the disease is characterised by anorexia and diarrhoea, often intermittent, which may result in poor growth rates. Vomiting and diarrhoea have been reported in young piglets with combined rotavirus and *Cryptosporidium* infections.

Pathology: The meronts and gamonts develop in a parasitophorous envelope apparently derived from the microvilli and so the cell disruption seen in other coccidia does not apparently occur. However, mucosal changes are obvious in the ileum where there is stunting, swelling and eventually fusion of the villi. This has a marked effect on the activity of some of the membrane-bound enzymes.

Epidemiology: The epidemiology of infection has not been studied although it is likely to be similar to *C. parvum* infection in other hosts. Piglets are likely to become infected without showing clinical signs but become sources of infection for other piglets that follow. The primary route of infection is by the direct animal-to-animal faecal–oral route.

Notes: Recent molecular characterisations have shown that there is extensive host adaptation in *Cryptosporidium* evolution, and many mammals or groups of mammals have host-adapted *Cryptosporidium* genotypes, which differ from each other in both DNA sequences and infectivity. Genetic and biological characterisation studies have identified two distinct host adapted strains of *Cryptosporidium* in pigs. Pig genotype I is now considered to be *Cryptosporidium suis*.

Further details of *C. parvum* are given in Chapter 2 (Cattle).

Other protozoa

Cryptosporidium suis

Predilection site: Small and large intestine

Parasite class: Sporozoasida

Family: Cryptosporidiidae

Host: Cattle, sheep, goat, horse, deer, man

Description: Oocysts, passed fully sporulated, are ellipsoid, 4.4–4.9 × 4.0–4.3 μm (mean 4.6 × 4.2 μm), with a length:width ratio of 1.35.

Giardia intestinalis

Synonym: *Giardia duodenalis*, *Giardia lamblia*, *Lamblia lamblia*

Predilection site: Small intestine

Parasite class: Zoomastigophorasida

Family: Diplomonadidae

Hosts: Man, cattle, sheep, goat, pig, alpaca, dog, cat, guinea pig, chinchilla

Geographical distribution: Worldwide

Pathogenesis: Infection in pigs is considered non-pathogenic.

Notes: The current molecular classification places isolates into eight distinct assemblages. Some authors give separate specific names to organisms isolated from different hosts although species specificity of many isolates is unknown. Phylogenetic data suggest that *G. intestinalis* is a species complex composed of several species that are host specific.

Further details of this species are given in Chapter 2 (Cattle).

LARGE INTESTINE

Oesophagostomum

Six species of *Oesophagostomum* have been described from pigs. The identification of individual species is beyond the scope of this book and interested readers will need to consult a relevant taxonomic specialist.

Life cycle: The preparasitic phase is typically strongyloid and infection is by ingestion of L_3, although there is limited evidence that skin penetration is possible in pigs. The L_3 enter the mucosa of any part of the small or large intestine then emerge on to the mucosal surface, migrate to the colon and develop to the adult stage.

Pathogenesis: *Oesophagostomum* infections in the pig are not often associated with clinical disease. Occasional diarrhoea, depression in weight gain and poor food conversion may occur, especially during the period of emergence of larvae and maturation of worms in the lumen of the large intestine. Burdens of about 3000 to 20 000 adult worms are associated with subclinical disease experimentally. Occasionally, infection with *Oesophagostomum*, particularly mucosal damage precipitated by larval encystment, may predispose to necrotic enteritis in association with anaerobic flora and perhaps *Balantidium*.

Clinical signs: Pregnant sows show inappetence, become very thin, and following farrowing, milk production is reduced with effects on litter performance.

Diagnosis: Diagnosis is based on postmortem findings and faecal egg counts. Mixed infections with nodular worms and *Hyostrongylus* occur frequently in pigs at pasture and their eggs are difficult to distinguish, requiring faecal culture to distinguish L_3.

Epidemiology: Infection is more prevalent in older pigs, which are generally less susceptible to the pathogenic effects compared with younger pigs. Survival of free-living L_3 on the pasture and hypobiotic L_4 in the host occur during autumn and winter; the hypobiotic larvae complete their development in the spring often coincident with farrowing. Transmission may also occur by flies, which can carry L_3 on their legs.

Treatment: Adult worms are susceptible to benzimidazoles, levamisole and macrocyclic lactones. Anthelmintic treatment does not always affect the larvae within the nodules and repeat treatments several weeks apart are required to reduce the worm population.

Control: Infections with *Oesophagostomum* are more likely to occur in outdoor pigs kept on pasture. Good management practices, such as provision of clean pastures, rotation, mixed or alternate grazing and strategic dosing regimes should be considered.

Oesophagostomum dentatum

Common name: Nodular worm

Predilection site: Large intestine

Parasite class: Nematoda

Superfamily: Strongyloidea

Description, gross: Adult worms are white in colour 8–14 mm long. Males are 8–10 mm and females 11–14 mm.

Description, microscopic: The cephalic vesicle is prominent, but cervical alae are practically absent. The nine elements of the leaf crown project forward and the internal leaf crown has 18 elements. The buccal capsule is shallow with parallel sides and the oesophagus is club-shaped with a narrow anterior end. In the female, the tail is relatively short. L_3 are less than 600 μm with a tail less than 60 μm.

Hosts: Pig

Geographical distribution: Worldwide

Pathology: In heavy infections there is thickening of the large intestinal wall with catarrhal enteritis. Nodule formation with *O. dentatum* is small compared with other species.

Oesophagostomum quadrispinulatum

Common name: Nodular worm

Predilection site: Large intestine

Parasite class: Nematoda

Superfamily: Strongyloidea

Hosts: Pig, wild boar

Geographical distribution: Worldwide

Oesophagostomum brevicaudum

Common name: Nodular worm

Predilection site: Large intestine

Parasite class: Nematoda

Superfamily: Strongyloidea

Hosts: Pig

Geographical distribution: North America

Oesophagostomum longicaudatum

Common name: Nodular worm

Predilection site: Large intestine

Parasite class: Nematoda

Superfamily: Strongyloidea

Hosts: Pig

Geographical distribution: Europe

Oesophagostomum georgianum

Common name: Nodular worm

Predilection site: Large intestine

Parasite class: Nematoda

Superfamily: Strongyloidea

Geographical distribution: North America

Oesophagostomum granatensis

Common name: Nodular worm

Predilection site: Large intestine

Parasite class: Nematoda

Superfamily: Strongyloidea

Hosts: Pig

Geographical distribution: Europe

Intestinal flukes

Several species of intestinal flukes belonging to the genera, *Gastrodiscus* and *Gastrodiscoides* have been reported in pigs. Further details on the life cycle, epidemiology, treatment and control of intestinal flukes are provided in Chapter 4 (Horses).

Gastrodiscus aegyptiacus

Common name: Intestinal fluke

Predilection site: Small and large intestine

Parasite class: Trematoda

Family: Paramphistomatidae

Description, gross: Adult flukes are pink in colour and measure 9–17 × 8–11 mm. The anterior is up to 4 mm and cylindrical, whilst the rest of the body is saucer-shaped, with the margins curved inwards.

Description, microscopic: The ventral surface is covered by a large number of regularly arranged papillae. The oral sucker has two postero-lateral pouches; the posterior sucker is small and subterminal. Eggs are oval and measure 131–139 × 78–90 μm.

Final hosts: Horse, pig, warthog

Intermediate hosts: Snails of the genus *Bulinus* and *Cleopatra*

Geographical distribution: Africa, India

Gastrodiscoides hominis

Synonym: *Gastrodiscus hominis*

Common name: Intestinal fluke

Predilection site: Large intestine

Parasite class: Trematoda

Family: Paramphistomatidae

Final hosts: Pig, man

Geographical distribution: Asia

Whipworms

Trichuris suis

Synonym: Trichocephalus suis

Common name: Whipworms

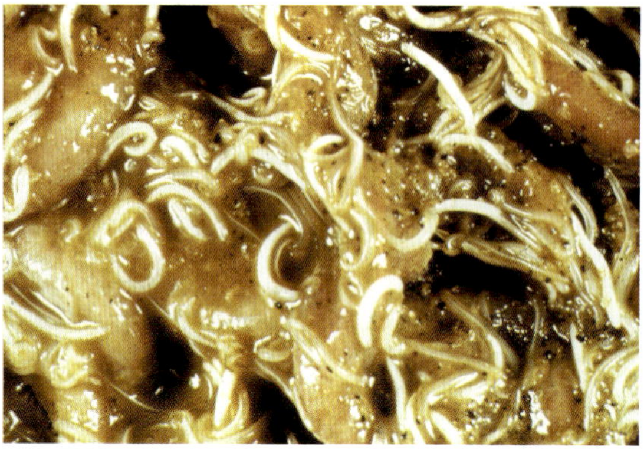

Fig. 5.8 *Trichuris suis* on the surface of the large intestine.

Predilection site: Large intestine

Parasite class: Nematoda

Superfamily: Trichuroidea

Description, gross: The adults are whitish and about 3–5 cm long with a thick broad posterior end tapering rapidly to a long filamentous anterior end that is characteristically embedded in the mucosa (Fig. 5.8).

Description, microscopic: The male tail is coiled and possesses a single spicule in a protrusible sheath. The sheath is variable in shape and in the extent of its spinous armature. The female tail is curved. The characteristic eggs are lemon shaped, 60×25 μm, with a thick smooth shell and a conspicuous polar plug at both ends; in the faeces these eggs appear yellow or brown in colour.

Hosts: Pig, wild boar

Life cycle: The infective stage is the L_1 within the egg, which develops in 1 or 2 months of being passed in the faeces depending on the temperature. Under optimal conditions these may subsequently survive and remain viable for several years. After ingestion, the plugs are digested and the released L_1 penetrate the glands of the distal ileum, caecal and colonic mucosa. Subsequently, all four moults occur within these glands, the adults emerging to lie on the mucosal surface with their anterior ends embedded in the mucosa. The prepatent period is 6–8 weeks. Longevity is 4–5 months.

Geographical distribution: Worldwide

Pathogenesis: Most infections are light and asymptomatic. Occasionally, when large numbers of worms are present, they cause a haemorrhagic colitis and/or a diphtheritic inflammation of the caecal mucosa. This results from the subepithelial location and continuous movement of the anterior end to the whipworm as it searches for blood and fluid. In pigs, heavy infections are thought to facilitate the invasion of potentially pathogenic spirochaetes.

Clinical signs: Despite the fact that pigs have a high incidence of light infections, the clinical significance of this genus is generally negligible, although isolated outbreaks have been recorded. Sporadic disease due to heavy infection is occasionally seen and is associated with an acute or chronic inflammation of the caecal mucosa with watery diarrhoea that often contains blood. Anaemia may be present.

Diagnosis: Since the clinical signs are not pathognomonic, diagnosis may depend on finding numbers of lemon-shaped *Trichuris* eggs in the faeces. However, since clinical signs may occur during the prepatent period, diagnosis in food animals may depend on necropsy.

Pathology: In severe cases, the mucosa of the large intestine is inflamed, haemorrhagic with ulceration and formation of diptheritic membranes.

Epidemiology: The most important feature is the longevity of the eggs, which may still survive after 3 or 4 years as a reservoir of infection in piggeries. Generally pigs of around 2–4 months of age are the most heavily infected.

Treatment: The benzimidazoles or levamisole by injection are effective against adult *Trichuris*, but less so against the larval stage. Some benzimidazoles need to be administered over several days. Doramectin is effective.

Control: Prophylaxis is rarely necessary. Attention should be given to areas where eggs might continue to survive for long periods. Such areas should be thoroughly cleaned and disinfected or sterilised by wet or dry heat.

Notes: The adults are usually found in the caecum but are only occasionally present in sufficient numbers to be clinically significant.

Trichuriosis in man: *Trichuris trichiura*, the whipworm of man and simian primates, is morphologically indistinguishable from *T. suis*. However, it is generally considered that these two parasites are strictly host specific. Worldwide the number of cases in man is several hundred million, with around 10 000 deaths per year attributed to trichuriosis. It is more common in children.

Flagellate protozoa

The life cycle of flagellate protozoa is similar for all species found in pigs. The trichomonads reproduce by longitudinal binary fission. No sexual stages are known and there are no cysts. Transmission is thought to occur by ingestion of trophozoites from faeces. All are considered to be non-pathogenic and are generally only identified from smears taken from the large intestine of fresh carcases.

Tritrichomonas suis

Synonym: *Trichomonas suis*

Predilection site: Nasal passages, stomach, caecum, colon

Parasite class: Zoomastigophorasida

Family: Trichomonadidae

Description: The body is characteristically elongate or spindle-shaped, but may occasionally be piriform or rotund, 9–16 × 2–6 µm (mean 11 × 3 µm), with three anterior flagella, which are approximately equal in length and each ending in a round or spatulate knob (Fig. 5.9). The undulating membrane runs the full length of the body and has four to six folds and its marginal filament continues as a posterior free flagellum. An accessory filament is present. The costa runs the full length of the body, and fine subcostal granules are present. The axostyle is a hyaline rod with a bulbous capitulum and extends beyond the body as a cone-shaped projection narrowing abruptly to a short tip. There is a chromatic ring around its point of exit. The parabasal body is usually a single, slender, tube-like structure, and the nucleus is ovoid or elongated, and has a large, conspicuous endosome surrounded by a relatively clear halo.

Hosts: Pig

Geographical distribution: Worldwide

Pathogenesis: Occurs commonly and is considered non-pathogenic. The organism can cause abortion in sows when experimentally introduced into the reproductive tract.

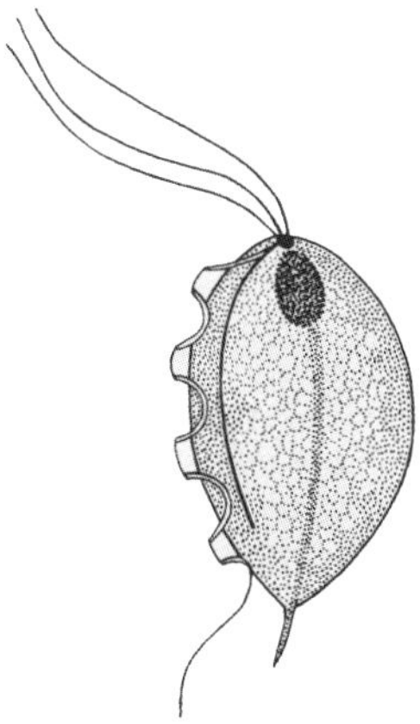

Fig. 5.9 *Tritrichomonas suis*

Tetratrichomonas buttreyi

Synonym: *Trichomonas buttreyi*

Predilection site: Caecum, colon

Parasite class: Zoomastigophorasida

Family: Trichomonadidae

Description: The body is ovoid or ellipsoidal, 4–7 × 2–5 µm (mean 6 × 3 µm). Cytoplasmic inclusions are frequently present. There are three or four anterior flagella, which vary in length from a short stub to more than twice the length of the body; and each ends in a knob or spatulate structure. The undulating membrane runs the full length of the body and has three to five undulations ending in a posterior free flagellum. The accessory filament is prominent, and the costa relatively delicate. The axostyle is relatively narrow, has a spatulate capitulum and extends 3–6 µm beyond the body. There is no chromatic ring at its point of exit. A pelta is present. The nucleus is frequently ovoid (2–3 × 1–2 µm) but is variable in shape and has a small endosome.

Hosts: Cattle, pig

Geographical distribution: Worldwide

Trichomitus rotunda

Synonym: *Trichomonas buttreyi*

Predilection site: Caecum, colon

Parasite class: Zoomastigophorasida

Family: Trichomonadidae

Description: The body is typically broadly piriform, but may occasionally be ovoid or ellipsoidal. It is 7–11 × 5–7 µm (mean 9 × 6 µm). Cytoplasmic inclusions are frequently present. The three anterior flagella are approximately equal in length and each terminates in a knob or spatulate structure. The blepharoplast appears to consist of a single granule. The undulating membrane together with the costa, extends about 50–75% the length of the body, and its undulation pattern varies from smooth to tightly telescoped or coiled waves. The posterior free flagellum is generally shorter than the body. The axostyle is a narrow, straight, non-hyaline rod with a crescent or sickle-shaped capitulum extending about 4 µm beyond the body. The nucleus is practically spherical, 2–3 µm in diameter, with an endosome surrounded by a clear halo. The parabasal body is 2–3 × 0.4–1.3 µm and is composed of two rami forming a 'V'. Each ramus has a parabasal filament.

Hosts: Pig

Geographical distribution: Worldwide

Other intestinal protozoa

Entamoeba suis

Predilection site: Large intestine

Parasite subphylum: Sarcodina

Family: Endamoebidae

Description: Trophozoites are 5–25 μm in diameter. The nucleus varies in appearance. The endostome is central and usually quite large and sometimes fills the nucleus but may be small with a homogeneous ring of peripheral chromatin. The cytoplasm is granular and vacuolated. The cysts are 4–17 μm in diameter and contain a single nucleus and chromatin granules of varying shape and size.

Hosts: Pig

Life cycle: Trophozoites divide by binary fission. Before encysting the amoebae round up, become smaller and lay down a cyst wall. Each cyst has one nucleus. Amoebae emerge from the cysts and grow into trophozoites

Geographical distribution: Worldwide

Pathogenesis: Non-pathogenic

Diagnosis: Identification of trophozoites, or cysts in large intestinal contents or faeces

Treatment and control: Not required

Balantidium coli

Predilection site: Large intestine

Parasite subphylum: Ciliophora

Family: Balantidiidae

Description: An actively motile organism, up to 300 μm, whose pellicle possesses rows of longitudinally arranged cilia (Fig. 5.10). At the anterior end there is a funnel-shaped depression, the peristome, which leads to the cytostome or mouth; from this, food particles are passed to vacuoles in the cytoplasm and digested. Internally there are two nuclei, a reniform macronucleus and adjacent micronucleus, and two contractile vacuoles, which regulate osmotic pressure. Cysts are spherical to ovoid, 40–60 μm in diameter.

Hosts: Pig, man, camel, monkey, dog (rarely), rat

Life cycle: Reproduction is by binary fission. Conjugation, a temporary attachment of two individuals during which nuclear material is exchanged, also occurs, after which both cells separate. Eventually cysts are formed which are passed in the faeces; these have a thick, yellowish wall, through which the parasite may be seen and are viable for 2 weeks at room temperature. Infection of a new host is by ingestion of the cysts.

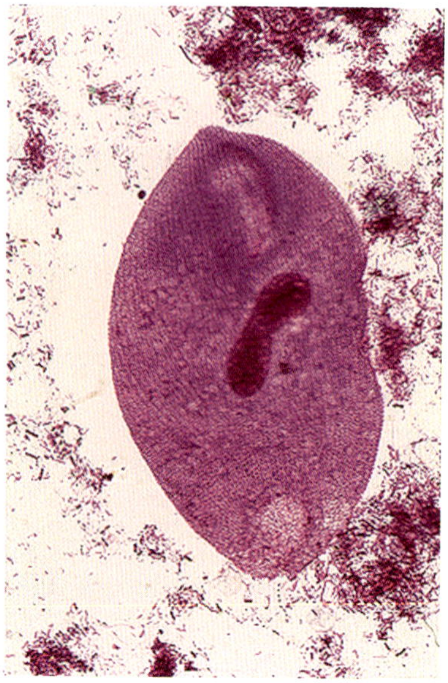

Fig. 5.10 *Balantidium coli.*

Geographical distribution: Worldwide

Pathogenesis: Normally non-pathogenic, these protozoa may, for reasons unknown, occasionally cause ulceration of the mucosa and accompanying dysentery in the pig. *Balantidium* may be a secondary invader within lesions of the large intestine.

Clinical signs: Occasionally causes diarrhoea or dysentery

Diagnosis: *Balantidium* is easily recognised by microscopic examination of intestinal contents or by histological examination of intestinal lesions.

Pathology: The organisms are found in enormous numbers in the lumen of the large intestine with normal caecal mucosa. The organism may, however, be found within mucosal ulcers initiated by other infections. It produces hyaluronidase, which might help to enlarge the lesions by attacking the intercellular ground substance

Epdemiology: *Balantidium coli* probably exists as a commensal in the large intestine of most pigs. Man may occasionally become clinically affected through contamination of foodstuffs or hands with pig faeces. Transmission occurs by ingestion of cysts or trophozoites. The cysts are resistant to environmental conditions and can survive for weeks in pig faeces. The pig is the usual source of infection for man and dogs.

Treatment: Tetracyclines are effective.

Control: Routine hygiene measures to prevent ingestion of cysts or faeces should prevent infection.

PARASITES OF THE RESPIRATORY SYSTEM

NASAL PASSAGES

Ttritrichomonas suis

See details and description under Large intestine.

LUNGS

Metastrongylus

Description, gross: Slender white worms, up to 6.0 cm in length; the host, site and long slender form are sufficient for generic identification. Individual species are differentiated on the size and shape of the male spicules.

Description, microscopic: The elipsoid eggs have rough, thick shells, are 45–57 × 38–41 μm in size and are larvated when laid.

Pathogenesis: The adult worms are found in the lumen of small bronchi and bronchioles, especially those of the posterior lobes of the lungs and provoke a chronic catarrhal and eosinophilic brochiolitis and bronchitis. Purulent staphylococcal infection in the lungs has been noted in many cases of metastrongylosis. The worms are also believed to be responsible for the occasional transmission of swine influenza virus.

Clinical signs: Most infections are light and asymptomatic, particularly in older pigs. However, in heavy infections in young animals, coughing can be marked, and is accompanied by dyspnoea and nasal discharge. Secondary bacterial infection may complicate the signs, inducing inappetance and loss of weight.

Diagnosis: For faecal examination saturated magnesium sulphate should be used as the flotation solution because of the heavy density of the eggs. The small rough-shelled larvated eggs are characteristic, but it should be noted that *Metastrongylus* is often present in normal pigs, and pulmonary signs may be referable to microbial infection rather than lungworms. Egg output may be sporadic in older pigs. The disease is most often encountered in pigs on pasture, though an occasional outbreak has occurred in yarded pigs. Disease history and clinical signs are also an aid to diagnosis.

Pathology: During the prepatent period areas of pulmonary consolidation, bronchial muscular hypertrophy and peribronchial lymphoid hyperplasia develop, often accompanied by areas of over-inflation. When the worms are mature, and eggs are aspirated into the smaller air passages and parenchyma, consolidation increases and emphysema is more marked. Hypersecretion of bronchiolar mucus also occurs during this stage. About 6 weeks after infection, chronic bronchitis and emphysema are established and small greyish nodules may be found in the posterior part of the diaphragmatic lobes; these may aggregate to form larger areas and are slow to resolve.

Epidemiology: Metastrongylosis shows a characteristic age distribution, being most prevalent in pigs of 4–7 months old. It can be of high prevalence in wild boar. The parasite is common in most countries, although outbreaks of disease do not often occur, probably due to the fact that most systems of pig husbandry do not allow ready access to earthworms by pigs. Though it is often suggested that *Metastrongylus* may transmit some of the porcine viruses, and may enhance the effect of pathogens already present in the lungs, the role of the worm is not conclusively proven.

Treatment: Many anthelmintics, including the modern benzimidazoles, levamisole and the macrocyclic lactones, are highly effective.

Control: When pig husbandry is based on pasture, control is extremely difficult because of the ubiquity and longevity of the earthworm intermediate host. On farms where severe outbreaks have occurred, pigs should be housed, dosed and the infected pasture cultivated or grazed with other livestock.

Metastrongylus apri

Synonym: *Metastrongylus elongatus*

Common name: Pig lungworm

Predilection site: Lung

Parasite class: Nematoda

Superfamily: Metastrongyloidea

Description, gross: The adult male is up to 25 mm and the female up to 58 mm.

Description, microscopic: The male bursa is relatively small and the spicules are filiform and each end in a single hook. The vulva of the female is near the anus. The posterior is curved ventrad.

Final hosts: Pig and wild boar; has been recorded in sheep, deer and in other ruminants

Intermediate hosts: Earthworms: *Lumbricus terrestris*, *Lumbricus rubellus*, *Diplocardia* spp, *Eisenia austriaca*, *Dendrobaena rubida*, *Helodrilus foetidus*, *H. caliginosus*

Life cycle: In cold temperatures the eggs are very resistant and can survive for over a year in soil. Normally, however, they hatch almost immediately, the intermediate host ingesting the L_1. In the earthworm, development to L_3 takes about 10 days at optimal temperatures of 22–26°C. The longevity of the L_3 in the earthworm is similar to that of the intermediate host itself and may be up to 7 years. The pig is infected by ingestion of earthworms and the L_3, released by digestion, travel to the mesenteric lymph nodes and moult. The L_4 then reach the lungs by the lymphatic–vascular route, the final moult occurring after arrival in the air passages. The prepatent period is about 24 days.

Geographical distribution: Worldwide

Metastrongylus pudendotectus

Synonym: *Metastrongylus brevivaginatus*

Common name: Pig lungworm

Predilection site: Lung

Parasite class: Nematoda

Superfamily: Metastrongyloidea

Description, microscopic: Differs from *M. apri* in having a larger bursa, and smaller spicules with double hooks in the male. The female tail is straight.

Definitive hosts: Pig and wild boar

Intermediate hosts: Earthworms: *Lumbricus terrestris*, *Lumbricus rubellus*

Life cycle: As for *M. apri*. The prepatent period is about 4 weeks.

Geographical distribution: Worldwide

Metastrongylus salmi

Common name: Pig lungworm

Predilection site: Lung

Parasite class: Nematoda

Superfamily: Metastrongyloidea

Description, microscopic: Differs from the other two species in the length and shape of the male spicules.

Geographical distribution: Parts of Africa, Indo-China, USA

Echinococcus granulosus

See under Parasites of the liver.

PARASITES OF THE LIVER

Ascaris suum

For more details on 'milk spot' liver caused by migrating larvae see under Small intestine.

Fasciola hepatica

Common name: Liver fluke

Predilection site: Liver

Parasite class: Trematoda

Family: Fasciolidae

Definitive hosts: Sheep, cattle, goat, horse, pig, deer, man and other mammals

Geographical distribution: Worldwide

For more details see Chapter 3 (Sheep and goats).

Fasciola gigantica

Common name: Tropical large liver fluke

Predilection site: Liver

Parasite class: Trematoda

Family: Fasciolidae

Final hosts: Cattle, buffalo, sheep, goat, pig, camel, deer, man

Intermediate hosts: Snails of the genus *Lymnaea*

Geographical distribution: Africa, Asia

For more details see Chapter 3 (Sheep and goats).

Echinococcus granulosus

Subspecies: *granulosus*

Common name: Dwarf dog tapeworm, hydatidosis

Predilection site: Mainly liver and lungs (intermediate hosts); small intestine (definitive host)

Parasite class: Cestoda

Family: Taeniidae

Final hosts: Dog and many wild canids

Intermediate hosts: Domestic and wild ruminants, man and primates, pig and lagomorphs

Geographical distribution: Worldwide

Pathogenesis: Hydatid cysts generally cause no clinical signs in pigs. Pressure atrophy of the liver and ascites may be found in heavy infections. Dyspnoea and coughing may be observed in heavily infected lungs.

For more details see Chapter 3 (Sheep and goats).

Taenia hydatigena (metacestode)

Synonym: *Taenia marginata, Cysticercus tenuicollis*

Predilection site: Abdominal cavity, liver (intermediate hosts); small intestine (definitive hosts)

Parasite class: Cestoda

Family: Taeniidae

Gross: The mature metacestode (*Cysticercus tenuicollis*) is about 5–8 cm in diameter and contains a single invaginated scolex (bladderworm) with a long neck.

Definitive hosts: Dog, fox, weasel, stoat, polecat, wolf, hyena

Intermediate hosts: Sheep, cattle, deer, pig, horse

Geographical distribution: Worldwide

Notes: The correct nomenclature for the intermediate host stage is the 'metacestode stage of *Taenia hydatigena*' rather than '*Cysticercus tenuicollis*'.

For more details see Chapter 3 (Sheep and goats).

PARASITES OF THE PANCREAS

Eurytrema pancreaticum

Common name: Pancreatic fluke

Predilection site: Pancreatic ducts and occasionally the bile ducts and the duodenum

Parasite class: Trematoda

Family: Dicrocoeliidae

Description: Similar to *E. coelomaticum*. Adults measure around 8–16 mm × 5–8 mm.

Geographical distribution: Eastern Asia and South America

PARASITES OF THE CIRCULATORY SYSTEM

Schistosoma suis

Common name: Blood fluke, bilharziosis

Synonym: *Schistosoma incognitum*

Predilection site: Mesenteric veins

Parasite class: Trematoda

Family: Schistosomatidae

Description, microscopic: The eggs are 90 × 41 μm, yellowish brown, sub-oval with one side flattened, with a small stout spine inclining towards the flattened side.

Definitive hosts: Pig, dog

Geographical distribution: India

Schistosoma spindale

Common name: Blood fluke, bilharziosis

Predilection site: Mesenteric veins

Parasite class: Trematoda

Family: Schistosomatidae

Hosts: Cattle, horse, pig and occasionally dog

Geographical distribution: Parts of Asia and the Far East

Schistosoma japonicum

Common name: Blood fluke, bilharziosis

Predilection site: Portal and mesenteric veins

Parasite class: Trematoda

Family: Schistosomatidae

Final hosts: Cattle, horse, sheep, goat, dog, cat, rabbit, pig, man

Intermediate hosts: Snails belonging to the genus *Oncomelania*

Geographical distribution: South and East Asia

For more general details of *Schistosoma* species see Chapter 2 (Cattle).

TRYPANOSOMES

See Chapter 1: Parasite taxonomy and morphology (Zoomastigophorasida) for general description and Chapter 2: Cattle for detailed descriptions of individual species of trypanosomes, and their control.

Trypanosoma brucei brucei

Subgenus: *Trypanozoon*

Common name: Nagana

Predilection site: Blood. *T. brucei bucei* is also found extravascularly in, for example, the myocardium, central nervous system (CNS) and reproductive tract.

Parasite class: Zoomastigophorasida

Family: Trypanosomatidae

Hosts: Cattle, horse, donkey, zebu, sheep, goat, camel, pig, dog, cat, wild game species

Distribution: Sub-Saharan Africa

Treatment: The two drugs in common use in cattle are isometamidium and diaminazine aceturate and both should be suitable for use in pigs. These are usually successful except where trypanosomes have developed resistance to the drug or in some very chronic cases. Treatment should be followed by surveillance, since reinfection, followed by clinical signs and parasitaemia, may occur within a week or two. Alternatively, the animal may relapse after chemotherapy, due to a persisting focus of infection in its tissues or because the trypanosomes are drug-resistant.

Trypanosoma congolense congolense

Subgenus: *Nannomonas*

Common name: Nagana, paranagana, Gambia fever, ghindi, gobial

Predilection site: Blood

Parasite class: Zoomastigophorasida

Family: Trypanosomatidae

Distribution: Sub-Saharan Africa

Treatment: In infected cattle, the two drugs in common use are diminazene aceturate (Berenil) and homidium salts (Ethidium and Novidium) and are appropriate for use in pigs infected with *T. congolense*. As with *T. brucei*, these drugs are usually successful except where trypanosomes have developed resistance to the drug or in some very chronic cases.

Trypanosoma simiae

Subgenus: *Nannomonas*

Synonym: *Trypanosoma congolense simiae*, *T. rodhaini*, *T. porci*

Predilection site: Blood

Parasite class: Zoomastigophorasida

Family: Trypanosomatidae

Description: Tryptomastigotes are polymorphic, 12–24 μm long. Around 90% of the forms are long and stout with a conspicuous undulating membrane; around 7% are long and slender with an inconspicuous undulating membrane; and around 3% are short with an inconspicuous undulating membrane. A free flagellum is usually absent.

Hosts: Pig, camel, sheep, goat

Distribution: Central Africa

Life cycle: *T. simiae* is mainly a parasite of warthogs transmitted by tsetse flies, in which the parasites develop in the midgut and proboscis. Tsetse flies also transmit the parasite to pigs, but transmission between pigs is usually mechanically by biting flies. The trypanosome multiplies in the vertebrate host by longitudinal binary fission.

Treatment: In pigs, *T. simiae* is the most important trypanosome pathogen and the rapid onset of death again gives little chance of treatment. Isomethamidium chloride at increased dose rates of 12.5–35 mg/kg i.m. or a combination of quinapyramine (7.5 mg/kg s.c.) and diaminazene aceturate (5 mg/kg i.m.) can be used. A suramin-quinapyramine complex (4 ml/5 kg) has shown some success in prophylaxis in young piglets for a period of 3 months, and in adults for 5 months.

Trypanosoma suis

Subgenus: *Pycnomonas*

Predilection site: Blood

Parasite class: Zoomastigophorasida

Family: Trypanosomatidae

Description: Tryptomastigotes are monomorphic, stout, 14–19 μm long with a small, marginal kinetoplast and a short free flagellum.

Hosts: Pig

Distribution: Central Africa

Treatment: As for *T. simiae*

BABESIA

Two species of *Babesia* are found in pigs. *Babesia perroncitoi* is a small *Babesia*; *B. trautmanni* is a large *Babesia*. Infection is transmitted to pigs via tick vectors.

Life cycle: Multiplication of *Babesia* organisms in the vertebrate host occurs in the erythrocytes by binary fission, endodyogeny, endopolyogeny (budding) or merogony to form merozoites. These are liberated from the erythrocyte and invade other cells. The asexual cycle continues indefinitely and the animals may remain infected for life. The piroplasms are transmitted by ticks but may also be transmitted by mechanical means to another animal. On ingestion by the tick these forms become vermiform and enter the body cavity then the ovary and penetrate the eggs where they round up and divide to form small round organisms. When the larval tick moults into the nymph stage, the parasites enter the salivary gland and undergo a series of binary fissions entering the cells of the salivary gland acini. They multiply further until the host cells are filled with thousands of minute parasites. These become vermiform, break out of the host cell and lie in the lumen of the gland and are injected into the mammalian host when the tick sucks blood.

Pathogenesis: The rapidly dividing parasites in the red cells produce destruction of the erythrocytes with accompanying haemoglobinaemia, haemoglobinuria and fever.

Diagnosis: The history and clinical signs of fever, anaemia, jaundice and haemoglobinuria in pigs located in enzootic areas where ticks occur are usually sufficient to justify a diagnosis of babesiosis. For confirmation, the examination of blood films, stained with Giemsa, will reveal the parasites in the red cells.

Pathology: The spleen is enlarged and there are pulmonary, renal and gastrointestinal hyperaemia and oedema. Subepicardial and subendocardial haemorrhages are present with with petechiation present on the serous membranes.

Treatment: Diminazene aceturate at 3.5 mg/kg i.m. is effective.

Control: Tick control measures can be considered for controlling disease. Topical application of acaricides may provide some level of protection but may be difficult in pigs, be expensive and may have a negative cost-benefit. Under certain conditions, it may be more beneficial to attain endemic stability allowing early infection and development of immunity.

Babesia perroncitoi

Predilection site: Blood

Parasite class: Sporozoasida

Family: Babesiidae

Description: A 'small' *Babesia* occurring most commonly as annular forms measuring 0.7–2 μm, although oval to pyriform forms, 1–3 μm × 1–2 μm in size, may also occur. Merozoites usually occur singly in erythrocytes, but sometimes two or more may be present.

Hosts: Pig

Geographical distribution: Southern Europe, West and Central Africa, Vietnam

Clinical signs: Clinical signs include fever, anaemia, haemoglobinuria, jaundice, oedema and incoordination. Abortion may occur in pregnant sows.

Epidemiology: Wild pigs may act as reservoirs of infection and the tick vectors include *Rhipicephalus* (*R. appendiculatus, R. sanguineus*) and *Dermacentor* (*D. reticulatus*).

Babesia trautmanni

Predilection site: Blood

Parasite class: Sporozoasida

Family: Babesiidae

Description: A 'large' *Babesia* occurring as oval, pyriform and less commonly round forms. Merozoites measure 2.5–4 × 1.5–2 μm, and usually occur in pairs within erythrocytes, but sometimes four or more may be present.

Hosts: Pig

Life cycle: As for *B. perroncitoi*

Geographical distribution: Southern Europe, Africa and parts of Asia

Clinical signs: Clinical signs include fever, anaemia, haemoglobinuria, jaundice, oedema and incoordination. Abortion may occur in pregnant sows. Mortality may reach 50% and pigs of all ages are affected.

Epidemiology: Infection and disease is seasonal according to the activity of the tick vector. Wild boar and warthogs may act as reservoirs of infection and the tick vectors include *Rhipicephalus* (*R. appendiculatus, R. sanguineus*), *Dermacentor* (*D. reticulatus*) and *Boophilus* (*B. decloratus*). Transovarian transmission has been reported in *R. sanguineus*.

Eperythrozoon suis

Synonym: *Candidatus mycoplasma haemosuis*

Predilection site: Blood

Order: Rickettsiales

Family: Anaplasmataceae

Description: Pleomorphic coccobacilli occurring either as eperythrocytic organisms in depressions on the cell surface, or free in the plasma. Single comma-shaped or ring-form cocci predominate in light to moderate infections but irregular complex bodies are formed in severe parasitaemias. Cocci appear light blue with Giemsa or Romanowsky's stains.

Hosts: Pig

Life cycle: Organisms are transmitted by biting insects and possible lice. Replication takes place by binary fission or budding.

Geographical distribution: Worldwide

Pathogenesis: Among the *Eperythrozoon*, *E. suis* is the most pathogenic, and may be very severe and fatal. Pigs are first depressed, inappatent, have high fever and go on to develop anaemia, becoming weaker and constipated, then jaundiced. Infection in sows produces both acute and chronic syndromes. Acute infections often occur postpartum and affected animals are pyrexic, anorexic and may show agalactia, mammary and vulvular oedema. Chronic infections are usually subclinical and often difficult to diagnose. Affected animals are generally in poor condition, pale and jaundiced.

Clinical signs: Jaundice and anaemia in very young pigs

Diagnosis: Identification from staining artefacts requires good blood films and filtered Giemsa stain. They appear as cocci or short rods on the surface of the erythrocytes, often completely surrounding the margin of the red cell. However, the organisms of *Eperythrozoon* are relatively loosely attached to the red cell surface and are often found free in the plasma.

Pathology: The main pathological changes occur in the liver and spleen. In the liver there is fatty degeneration, atrophy and necrosis of central hepatic cells with widespread lymphatic infiltration. Reticulo-endothelial cells in liver, spleen and lymph nodes are hypertrophied and filled with haemosiderin deposits.

Epidemiology: Transmission is seasonal, being more common in summer and autumn when biting flies are active. The pig louse (*Haemotopinus suis*) has also been incriminated in transmission.

Treatment and control: Tetracyclines and the arsenical, roxarsone, are reported to be effective. Control of ectoparasite infections and possibly addition of arsenicals or tetracyclines to the diet have been advocated in countries where the disease is endemic.

Notes: The taxonomy of this species is subject to much debate and there is a proposal to re-classify it into the bacterial genus *Mycoplasma* (class Mollicutes) based on 16s rRNA gene sequences and phylogenetic analysis.

PARASITES OF THE NERVOUS SYSTEM

Toxoplasma gondii

See details and description under Parasites of the locomotory system.

PARASITES OF THE REPRODUCTIVE/UROGENITAL SYSTEM

Stephanurus dentatus

Common name: Pig kidney worm

Predilection site: Kidney, peri-renal fat

Parasite class: Nematoda

Superfamily: Strongyloidea

Description, gross: A large stout worm up to 4.5 cm long, with a prominent buccal capsule and transparent cuticle through which the internal organs may be seen. Males are 2–3 cm, and females 3–4.5 cm long. The colour is usually pinkish. The size and site are diagnostic.

Description, microscopic: The buccal capsule is cup-shaped with small leaf crowns and six external cuticular thickenings (epaulettes) of which the ventral and dorsal are most prominent, and six cusped teeth at the base. The male bursa is short and the two spicules of either equal or unequal length. Eggs are 100×60 µm.

Hosts: Pig, wild boar, rarely cattle

Life cycle: Pre-parasitic development from egg to L_3 is typically strongyloid, though earthworms may intervene as transport hosts. There are three modes of infection: by ingestion of the free L_3, ingestion of earthworms carrying the L_3 and percutaneously. After entering the body, there is an immediate moult, and the L_4 travel to the liver in the bloodstream, either from the intestine by the portal stream, or from the skin by the lungs and systemic circulation. In the liver the final moult takes place, and the young adults wander in the parenchyma for 3 months or more before piercing the capsule and migrating in the peritoneal cavity to the peri-renal region. There they are enclosed in a cyst by the host reaction, and complete their development. The cyst communicates with the ureter either directly or, if it is more distant, by a fine connecting canal, allowing the worm eggs to be excreted in the urine. The prepatent period ranges from 6–19 months and the worms have a longevity of about 2–3 years.

Geographical distribution: Mainly warm to tropical regions of all continents. It does not occur in western Europe.

Pathogenesis: Though the favoured site is in the peri-renal fat, some worms occur in the kidney itself, in the calyces and pelvis (Fig. 5.11). Erratic migration is common in *Stephanurus* infection, and larvae have been found in most organs, including the lungs, spleen, spinal cord, and in muscle. In these sites they are trapped by encapsulation and never reach the perirenal area. Prenatal infection has been reported.

The main pathogenic effect is due to the larvae, which, by the late L_4 stage, have heavily sclerotised buccal capsules capable of tearing tissue and they cause much damage to the liver and occasionally other organs in their wanderings. In heavy infections there may be severe cirrhosis, thrombosis of hepatic vessels and ascites and, in rare cases, liver failure and death. In most infections, however, the effects are

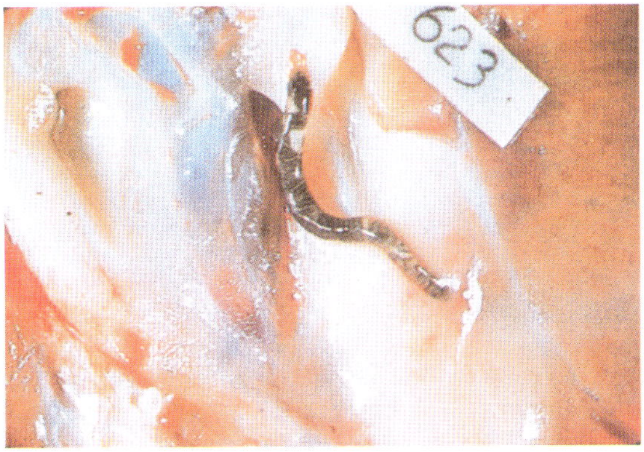

Fig. 5.11 *Stephanurus dentatus* worms in a kidney.

seen only after slaughter as patchy cirrhosis, and the main importance of the worm is economic, from liver condemnation. In general the adult worms are not pathogenic. Usually the adult worms, soon after arrival at the perirenal site, are encapsulated in cysts, which may contain greenish pus. In rare cases the ureters may be thickened and stenosed, with consequent hydronephrosis.

Clinical signs: In most infections the only sign is failure to gain weight or, in more severe cases, weight loss. Where there is more extensive liver damage there may be ascites, but it is only when there is massive invasion, comparable to acute fasciolosis in sheep, that death occurs.

Diagnosis: The clinical signs are likely to be few, and, since most of the damage occurs during the prepatent phase, eggs may not be found in the urine. However, in endemic areas, where pigs are failing to thrive and where local abattoirs record appreciable numbers of cirrhotic livers, a presumptive diagnosis can be made. Worms can be identified at necropsy.

Pathology: Percutaneous infection leads to the formation of nodules in the skin, with oedema and enlargement of the superficial lymph nodes. Migrating larvae produce acute inflammatory lesions especially in the liver. Inflammation may lead to abscess formation and extensive liver cirrhosis. The adult parasite is not markedly pathogenic and is found in cysts, 0.5–4 cm in diameter, each cyst containing a pair of worms. Cysts in the kidney may cause thickening of the ureter, which in chronic cases may be almost occluded.

Epidemiology: Though the adult worms are never numerous, they are very fecund, and an infected pig may pass a million eggs per day. The L_3 is susceptible to desiccation, so that stephanurosis is mainly associated with damp ground. Since it infects readily by skin penetration, the pigs' habit of lying around the feeding area when kept outside presents a risk, as does damp, unhygienic accommodation for housed animals. Such conditions, coupled with prenatal infection and the longevity of the worm, ensure continuity of infection through many generations of pigs. All ages of pigs are susceptible to infection.

Treatment: Levamisole, the modern benzimidazoles and ivermectin are effective.

Control: One approach to control is based on the susceptibility of the L_3 to desiccation and on the fact that a major route of infection is percutaneous. It follows that the provision of impervious surfaces around the feeding areas for outdoor reared pigs, and simple hygiene, ensuring clean dry flooring in pig houses, will help to limit infection. This approach may be supplemented by segregating young pigs from those of more than 9 months of age, which will be excreting eggs.

The 'gilt only' scheme, which was advocated by workers in the United States, consists essentially of using only gilts for breeding. The gilts are reared on land, which is dry and exposed to the sun. A single litter is taken from them, and as soon as the piglets can be weaned the gilts are marketed. The scheme takes advantage of the extremely long prepatent period which allows a single breeding cycle by the gilts to be completed before egg laying begins and so progressively eliminates infection. The boars used in the scheme are housed on concrete.

Regimes incorporating anthelmintic control recommend treatment of sows and gilts 1–2 weeks before putting to the boar, and again 1–2 weeks before farrowing. It should be remembered in designing a control system that the earthworm transport hosts present a continuous reservoir of infection.

PARASITES OF THE LOCOMOTORY SYSTEM

Taenia solium

Synonym: *Cysticercus cellulosae*

Common name: Human pork tapeworm

Predilection site: Small intestine (final host); muscle (intermediate host)

Parasite class: Cestoda

Family: Taeniidae

Description, gross: The adult tapeworm is 3–5 m long with a scolex, typically taeniid, having a rostellum with four suckers and armed with two concentric rows of 22–32 hooks, while the uterus of the gravid segment has 7–13 lateral branches. Adults can survive in humans for many years.

Description, microscopic: Cysts are milky white and have a scolex bearing a rostellum and hooks similar to the adult.

Final host: Man

Intermediate hosts: Pig, wild boar, rarely dog and man

Life cycle: Gravid segments passed in the faeces each contain around 40 000 eggs and because they are non-motile they tend to be concentrated over a small area. Eggs can also resist destruction for a relatively long period of time. After ingestion by a susceptible pig the oncosphere travels via the blood to striated muscle. The principal location is the striated muscles, but cysticerci may also develop in other organs, such as the lungs, liver, kidney and brain. Humans become infected by ingesting raw or inadequately cooked pork containing viable cysticerci. The human final host may also act as an intermediate host and become infected with cysticerci. This is most likely to occur from the accidental ingestion of *T. solium* eggs via unwashed hands or contaminated food. There is also a minor route of autoinfection, apparently, in a person with an adult tapeworm, from the liberation of oncospheres after the digestion of a gravid segment, which has entered the stomach from the duodenum by reverse peristalsis. The prepatent period is 2–3 months.

Geographical distribution: This cestode is most prevalent in South and Central America, India, Africa and parts of the Far East, apart from areas where there are religious sanctions on the eating of pork. It is now uncommon in many developed countries.

Pathogenesis: Clinical signs are inapparent in pigs naturally infected with cysticerci and generally insignificant in humans with adult tapeworms. However, when humans are infected with cysticerci, various clinical signs may occur depending on the location of the cysts in the organs, muscles or subcutaneous tissue. Cysticerci may be found in every organ of the body in humans but are most common in the subcutaneous tissue, eye and brain. Larvae that reach the brain develop in the ventricles and frequently become racemose in character. Most seriously, cysticerci that develop in the central nervous system produce mental disturbances or clinical signs of epilepsy or increased intracranial pressure. They may also develop in the eye with consequent loss of vision. In Latin America alone it is estimated that almost 0.5 million people are affected, either by the nervous or ocular forms of cysticercosis.

Clinical signs: Infected pigs are usually asymptomatic.

Infection is generally insignificant in humans although adult tapeworms can occasionally cause abdominal discomfort and diarrhoea. However when man, acting as the intermediate host, is infected with cysticerci, various clinical signs may occur depending on the location and number of the cysts in the organs, muscles or subcutaneous tissue. CNS signs include mental disturbances or clinical signs of epilepsy and may be fatal. Loss of vision may occur when the eye is involved.

Diagnosis: For all practical purposes, diagnosis in pigs depends on meat inspection procedures but this lacks sensitivity for low infection levels. Individual countries have different regulations regarding the inspection of carcases, but invariably the masseter muscle, tongue and heart are incised and examined and the intercostal muscles and diaphragm inspected. Proglottids can sometimes be seen in faeces. Cysticerci of *T. solium* are larger and more numerous than those of *T. saginata* (see Chapter 2: Cattle). In man the diagnosis of cerebral cysticercosis depends primarily on the detection of cysticerci by CAT (computerised axial tomography) scanning techniques, and on the finding of antibodies to cysticerci in the cerebrospinal fluid.

Pathology: Cysticerci, comprising a single large cyst and inverted scolex, measure 1–2 cm, and are easily visible between muscle fibres. The cysticerci are rapidly ensheathed in connective tissue and create a crescentic zone of degenerative lysis around them, thereby allowing room to grow. Pigs are usually slaughtered at an age when all cysticerci are generally still viable.

Epidemiology: In developing countries this depends primarily on the close association of rural pigs with man, and in particular, their often unrestricted access to human faeces. Indifferent standards of meat inspection and illicit trading in uninspected pork are also major factors in the spread of the infection. Pigs may acquire massive infections because the gravid segments are not active and may remain in faeces. Humans normally become infected when they consume raw or undercooked pork. As noted above, man may become infected with cysticerci and this may occur from the ingestion of eggs on vegetables or other foodstuffs contaminated with human faeces or handled by an infected person.

Treatment: No effective drugs are available to kill cysticerci in the pig although in man praziquantel and albendazole are considered to be of some value as possible alternatives to surgery.

Control: This depends ultimately on the enforcement of meat inspection regulations and deep-freezing procedures. Freezing pork at –10 to –8°C continuously for 4 days kills the cysticerci, but chilling the meat at 0°C is not sufficient and cysts may remain viable in chilled meat for 70 days. The exclusion of pigs from contact with human faeces, the thorough cooking of pork and proper standards of personal hygiene will reduce the prevalence of infection.

Notes: A third form of *Taenia* ('Asian *Taenia*') has been reported throughout eastern Asia and also from parts of East Africa and Poland. The 'Asian *Taenia*' appears to be closely related to *T. saginata* but its molecular profile indicates that it is genetically different. The cysticerci of this tapeworm are located in the liver of the pig and wild boar and occasionally in cattle, goats and monkeys. The 'Asian *Taenia*' is considered not to be an important cause of human cysticercosis.

Trichinella spiralis

See under Small intestine.

Toxoplasma gondii

Predilection site: Muscle, lung, liver, reproductive system, central nervous system

Order: Sporozoasida

Family: Sarcocystiidae

Description: Tachyzoites are found developing in vacuoles in many cell types, for example fibroblasts, hepatocytes, reticular cells and myocardial cells. In any one cell there may be 8–16 organisms, each measuring 6.0–8.0 µm. Tissue cysts, measuring up to 100 µm in diameter, found mainly in the muscle, liver, lung and brain and may contain several thousand lancet-shaped bradyzoites.

Intermediate hosts: Any mammal, including man, or birds. Note that the final host, the cat, may also be an intermediate host and harbour extra-intestinal stages.

Final host: Cat, other felids

Life cycle: The definitive host is the cat in which gametogony takes place (see Chapter 6: Dogs and cats). Pigs act as an intermediate host in which the cycle is extra-intestinal and results in the formation of tachyzoites and bradyzoites, which are the only forms found in non-feline hosts. The liberated sporozoites rapidly penetrate the intestinal wall and spread by the haematogenous route. This invasive and proliferative stage is called the tachyzoite and on entering a cell it multiplies asexually in a vacuole by a process of budding or endodyogeny, in which two individuals are formed within the mother cell, the pellicle of the latter being used by the daughter cells. When 8–16 tachyzoites have accumulated the cell ruptures and new cells are infected. This is the acute phase of toxoplasmosis. In most instances, the host survives and antibody is produced which limits the invasiveness of the tachyzoites and results in the formation of cysts containing thousands of organisms which, because endodyogeny and growth are slow, are termed bradyzoites. The cyst containing the bradyzoites is the latent form, multiplication being held in check by the acquired immunity of the host. If this immunity wanes, the cyst may rupture, releasing the bradyzoites, which become active and resume the invasive characteristics of the tachyzoites.

Geographical distribution: Worldwide

Pathogenesis: Most *Toxoplasma* infections in animals are light and consequently asymptomatic. Toxoplasmosis has been occasionally reported in young pigs and may cause severe fetal losses in pregnant sows, but more usually is mild and unnoticed.

Diagnosis: Tachyzoites of *Toxoplasma gondii* are often difficult to find in tissue sections, but are more likely to be present in sections of brain and placenta. Identification can be confirmed by immunohistochemistry, while the polymerase chain reaction may be used to identify parasite DNA in tissues. A number of serological tests have been developed of which the dye test (DT) is the longest established serological method, and in many ways represents the gold standard. Its reliability for use in pigs is not known.

Pathology: In heavy infections, the multiplying tachyzoites may produce areas of necrosis in vital organs such as the myocardium, lungs, liver and brain. Examination of the brain may reveal focal microgliosis. The lesions often have a small central focus of necrosis that might be mineralised. Focal leucomalacia in cerebral white matter, due to anoxia arising from placental pathology, is often present.

Epidemiology: The cat plays a central role in the epidemiology of toxoplasmosis and infection in pigs may occur through ingestion of feed contaminated with cat faeces or through ingestion of bradyzoites and tachyzoites in the flesh of another intermediate host, such as rats.

Treatment: Not indicated

Control: On farms, control is difficult, but where possible animal feedstuffs should be covered to exclude access by cats and insects. Control of rats and regulation of feeding of swill to pigs are also measures that will limit exposure to infection.

SARCOCYSTIS

Sarcocystis is one of the most prevalent parasites of livestock. Most cases of *Sarcocystis* infection are only revealed at meat inspection when the grossly visible sarcocysts in the muscle are discovered. Little is known of the epidemiology, but from the high prevalence of symptomless infections observed in abattoirs, it is clear that where dogs and cats are kept in close association with farm animals or their feed, then transmission is likely.

The only control measures possible are those of simple hygiene. Farm dogs and cats should not be

Table 5.3 *Sarcocystis* species found in the muscles of pigs.

Species	Synonym	Definitive host	Pathogenicity (pig)	Pathogenicity (final host)
S. suicanis	*S. porcicanis* *S. miescheriana*	Dog, wolf, fox	+++	0
S. porcifelis	*S. suifelis*	Cat	0	0
S. suihominis	*Isospora hominis*	Human	+++	+++

0 = non-pathogenic; + = mildly pathogenic; +++ = severely pathogenic.

housed in, or allowed access to, fodder stores nor should they be allowed to defecate in pens where livestock are housed. It is also important that they are not fed uncooked meat.

Sarcocystis suicanis

Synonym: *Sarcocystis porcicanis*, *Sarcocystis miescheriana*

Predilection site: Muscle

Order: Sporozoasida

Family: Sarcocystiidae

Description: Tissue cysts are compartmented up to 0.5–1.5 mm long × 15–100 μm. The cyst wall has numerous palisade-like processes with randomly arranged filaments seen on electron microscopy.

Intermediate hosts: Pig

Final host: Dog

Life cycle: Infection is by ingestion of the sporocysts and this is followed by three asexual generations. In the first, sporozoites, released from the sporocysts, invade the venules of the liver where they locate in endothelial cells. The second-generation meronts are found in the endothelial cells of capillaries of all organs and the resulting merozoites penetrate muscle cells. There they encyst and then divide by a process of budding or endodyogeny, giving rise to broad banana-shaped bradyzoites contained within a cyst; this is the mature sarcocyst and is the infective stage for the carnivorous final host. Cysts are found in skeletal and cardiac muscle.

Geographical distribution: Worldwide

Pathogenesis: *S. suicanis* is pathogenic to the pig and is known to produce signs of enteritis, myositis and lameness. More generally clinical signs are rarely observed and the most significant effect is the presence of cysts in the muscles of food animals resulting in downgrading or condemnation of carcases.

Clinical signs: In heavy infections of the intermediate hosts there may be anorexia, fever, anaemia, loss of weight, a disinclination to move and sometimes recumbency.

Pathology: In pigs, meronts present in endothelial cells of capillaries in various organs lead to endothelial cell destruction. As the organisms enter muscle, a wide range of change may be encountered. Microscopic inspection of *Sarcocystis*-infected muscle often reveals occasional degenerate parasitic cysts surrounded by variable numbers of inflammatory cells (very few of which are eosinophils) or, at a later stage, macrophages and granulation tissue. Usually there is no muscle fibre degeneration, but there may be thin, linear collections of lymphocytes between fibres in the region. The extent of muscle change bears little relationship to the numbers of developing cysts, but generally very low numbers of *Sarcocystis* produce no reaction. As cysts mature, the cyst capsule within the enlarged muscle fibre becomes thicker and more clearly differentiated from the muscle sarcoplasm.

Sarcocystis porcifelis

Synonym: *Sarcocystis suifelis*

Predilection site: Muscle

Order: Sporozoasida

Family: Sarcocystiidae

Intermediate hosts: Pig

Final host: Cat

Life cycle: As described for *S. suicanis*

Geographical distribution: Unknown

Pathogenesis: Non-pathogenic

Clinical signs: Infection is usually asymptomatic.

Pathology: Cysts are found in oesophageal muscles but their detailed pathology has not been described.

Sarcocystis suihominis

Synonym: *Isospora hominis*

Predilection site: Muscle

Order: Sporozoasida

Family: Sarcocystiidae

Description: In the pig, the mature sarcocysts are thin-walled, compartmented, up to 1.5 mm long, and have protrusions up to 13 μm long, folded closely on the surface.

Intermediate hosts: Pig

Final host: Man, primates

Life cycle: Infection is by ingestion of the sporocysts and this is followed by at least three asexual generations. In the first, sporozoites, released from the sporocysts, invade the intestinal wall and the endothelial cells of blood vessels in the liver, where they undergo two merogony cycles. Sarcocysts can be found in the striated muscles, heart and brain. At first they contain only metrocytes but these divide rapidly to form bradyzoites contained within the thin-walled cyst; this is the mature sarcocyst and is the infective stage for the final host. The prepatent period is about 12–14 days and the patent period lasts at least 18 days.

Geographical distribution: Unknown

Pathogenesis: Infection is not pathogenic for non-human primates but is extremely pathogenic for humans and the pig intermediate host. In the pig, the principal pathogenic effect is attributable to the merogony stages in the vascular endothelium of the liver.

Clinical signs: Acute sarcocystosis in pigs shows a biphasal fever between 5–9 and 11–15 days post infection. During the second phase, there is apathy, dyspnoea, anaemia and cyanosis of the skin, muscle spasms and hyperexcitability and prostration. Abortion may occur in pregnant sows.

Control: The contamination of animal feed and grazing land with human faeces should be avoided. Human infection can be prevented through adequate cooking or freezing of meat.

Notes: In humans, the ingestion of infected pork containing *S. suihominis* produces clinical signs of bloat, nausea, loss of appetite, stomach ache, vomiting, diarrhoea, difficulty breathing and rapid pulse within 6–42 hours. *Sarcocystis* may be responsible for several idiopathic diseases in man, including cardiac diseases such as cardiomyopathy and myocarditis and rheumatic diseases. It has also been suggested that *Sarcocystis* may be associated with muscle aches and fatigue as part of the chronic fatigue syndrome (CFS).

PARASITES OF THE INTEGUMENT

Suifilaria suis

Predilection site: Subcutaneous and connective tissue

Parasite class: Nematoda

Superfamily: Filarioidea

Description, gross: The adult filarioid worms are about 2–4 cm long. Males are 17–25 mm; and females 32–40 mm.

Description, microscopic: The hind end of the male is spirally coiled and the spicules unequal with the left shorter than the right. The tail of the female bears a number of small tubercles on its tip, which ends abruptly. Small embryonated eggs, 51 × 61 μm, that have a thin flexible shell are laid on the skin surface where they hatch to release the microfilariae or L_1, which are about 200 μm in length.

Final host: Pig

Intermediate hosts: Not known

Life cycle: Not known. The females appear to lay their eggs in the skin of the pig.

Geographical distribution: Southern Africa

Pathogenesis: The worms induce small hard whitish nodules in the subcutaneous and intermuscular connective tissues. Infection is generally considered to be non-pathogenic, although erupted skin vesicles may become secondarily infected, forming abscesses.

Clinical signs: Infection is usually asymptomatic causing no effect on productivity.

Diagnosis: This is normally based on clinical signs of small whitish nodules, which eventually burst. Vesicular eruptions contain the eggs.

Pathology: Vesicular nodules may form in the cutaneous and intermuscular connective tissue.

Epidemiology: The epidemiology is unknown.

Treatment: Treatment is seldom required as infection is of little veterinary relevance.

Control: As the intermediate host is unknown control is not feasible or usually required.

ECTOPARASITES

Haematopinus suis

Common name: Hog louse

Predilection site: Skin; most often present on skin folds of the neck and jowl, the flanks and the insides of the legs on thin-coated animals.

Parasite class: Insecta

Parasite order: Phthiraptera

Parasite suborder: Anoplura

Family: Haematopinidae

Description: *Haematopinus suis* is a large, greyish brown louse with brown and black markings, measuring 5–6 mm in length. It is the largest blood-sucking louse found on domestic animals. It has a long narrow head and long mouthparts adapted for sucking blood. It has prominent angular processes, known as ocular points or temporal angles, located behind the antennae. Eyes are absent. The thoracic sternal plate is dark and well developed. The legs are of similar sizes, each terminating in a single large claw that opposes the tibial spur. Distinct sclerotised paratergal plates are visible on abdominal segments 2 or 3 to 8.

Hosts: Pig

Life cycle: During a lifespan of about a month the female lays one to six eggs per day. These are deposited singly, and are glued to the hairs on the lower parts of the body and in skin folds on the neck, and on or in the ears, where they may be seen with the naked eye. The eggs hatch within 13–15 days. The emerging nymphs resemble the adult louse except in size. In about 12 days, the nymphs mature into adults and within 4 days, after feeding and mating, the female lice begin to lay eggs. The entire life cycle, from egg to adult, takes place on the host and is completed in 2–3 weeks. Adults may live for up to 40 days but cannot survive for more than a few days off the host. Between 6 and 15 generations may be completed per year, depending on environmental conditions.

Geographical distribution: Worldwide

Pathogenesis: Infested animals show a reduction in weight gain and are more susceptible to other diseases. In severe infestations piglets may die of anaemia. *Haematopinus suis* is believed to be a vector of African swine fever, *Eperythrozoon suis* and the virus of swine pox.

Clinical signs: This louse is very common, and at low intensities is usually tolerated without any signs apart from occasional mild irritation. It usually occurs in the folds of the neck and jowl, around the ears and on the flanks and backs. The majority of nymphs occur on the head region. However, irritation is caused by the small but frequent blood meals, each of which is taken via a different puncture wound. In heavy infestations, pigs are restless and fail to thrive. Economically, the most important feature of pediculosis in pigs is probably skin damage from scratching, with reduction in hide value. In the most severe cases, pigs may rub most of the hair off their bodies and, if acquired by piglets, *Haematopinus suis* infestation may retard growth. Transfer is usually by contact but *H. suis* may survive for up to 3 days off its host. Hence, transfer can also occur when animals are put into recently vacated dirty accommodation.

Diagnosis: *Haematopinus suis* is the only louse found on pigs. Adults are easily seen on the skin and can be removed and identified under a light microscope.

Pathology: Both epidermis and corium may be affected by inflammatory lesions at the bite puncture sites. Initially neutrophil infiltration with necrosis of epithelial cells prevails. This is followed by capillary proliferation with angioblast and fibroblast multiplication and straggled lymphoid infiltration.

Epidemiology: Infection is primarily by physical contact between pigs, particularly in closely confined fattening animals and in suckling sows penned with their piglets. However, lice may also be acquired when animals are put into recently vacated dirty accommodation.

Treatment: Avermectins given parenterally or the organophosphate phosmet administered as a pour-on have both proved highly effective as a single treatment. Amitraz and deltamethrin are also effective. Once lice have been diagnosed it is essential to treat the entire herd.

Control: Generally, control is based on the application of insecticides or use of a macrocyclic lactone. For herd prophylaxis, gilts and sows should be treated before farrowing to prevent spread of infection to their piglets, and boars treated twice annually.

Sarcoptes scabiei

Common name: Scabies

Predilection site: Skin

Parasite class: Arachnida

Sub-class: Acari

Order: Acariformes

Sub-order: Sarcoptiformes (Astigmata)

Family: Sarcoptidae

Description, adults: The adult of this species has a round, ventrally flattened, dorsally convex body (Fig. 5.12). Adult females are 0.3–0.6 mm long and 0.25–0.4 mm wide, while males are smaller, typically up to 0.3 mm long and 0.1–0.2 mm wide. The posterior two pairs of limbs do not extend beyond the body margin. In both sexes, the pretarsi of the first two pairs of legs bear empodial claws and a sucker-like pulvillus, borne on a long, stalk-like pretarsus. The sucker-like pulvilli help the mite grip the substrate as

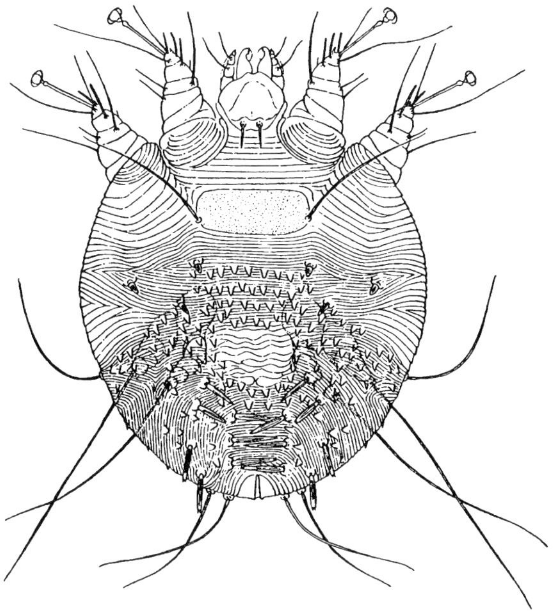

Fig. 5.12 Adult female of *Sarcoptes scabiei* (reproduced from Baker *et al.*, 1956).

it moves. The third and fourth pairs of legs in the female and the third pair of legs in the male end in long setae and lack stalked pulvilli. The mouthparts have a rounded appearance. These mites have no eyes or stigmata. The dorsal surface of the body of *S. scabiei* is covered with transverse ridges, but also bears a central patch of triangular scales. The dorsal setae are strong and spine-like. The anus is terminal and only slightly dorsal. There are several host-adapted varieties of *S. scabiei* that differ subtly in their morphology.

Description, larvae and nymphs: The hexapod larvae and the octopod nymphs resemble the adults in general form.

Hosts: All domestic mammals and humans

Life cycle: The entire life cycle takes place on the host. Mating probably takes place at the skin surface, following which the female creates a permanent winding burrow, parallel to the skin surface, using her chelicerae and the claw-like empodium on the front two pairs of legs. This burrow may be up to 2–3 cm in length and burrowing may proceed at up to 5 mm/day. Each tunnel contains only one female, her eggs and faeces. Maturation of the eggs takes 3 or 4 days, following which the female starts to oviposit one to three eggs per day, over a reproductive life of about 2 months. The eggs, which are oval and about half the length of the adult, are laid singly at the ends of outpockets, which branch off along the length of these tunnels. Three to four days after oviposition, the six-legged larva hatches from the egg. Most larvae will crawl from the burrow towards the skin surface, whilst some remain in the tunnels where they continue their development. Two to three days later the larva moults to become a protonymph. During this time the larva and nymph find shelter and food in the hair follicles. The protonymph moults to become a tritonymph and again a few days later to become an adult.

Both sexes of adult then start to feed and burrow at the skin surface, creating small pockets of up to 1 mm in length in the skin. Mating occurs on the skin. The male dies shortly after copulation. After fertilisation, female mites wander over the pelage to seek a suitable site for a permanent burrow. Despite their short legs, adults are highly mobile, capable of moving at up to 2.5 cm/min. Within an hour of mating the female begins to excavate her burrow. Females burrow without direction, eating the skin and tissue fluids that result from their excavations. Egg laying begins 4–5 days after completion of the initial permanent winding burrow. Female mites rarely leave their burrows and if removed by scratching they will attempt to burrow again.

The total egg to adult life cycle takes between 17 and 21 days, but may be as short as 14 days. During this period, the mortality rate is high, with just 10% of mites that hatch completing their development. During an infection mite numbers increase rapidly, then decline, leaving a relatively stable mite population.

Geographical distribution: Worldwide

Pathogenesis: Host reactions occur primarily in response to the feeding and burrowing activity of the mites and their faecal deposits. This commonly occurs progressively 3 weeks into the initial infection. Lesions can occur anywhere on the body, but are usually found on the head where the hair is relatively thin. The infestation spreads quickly from the initial lesions to cause more generalised mange.

In pigs, the ears are the most common site of infestation, and are usually the primary focus from which the mite population spreads to other areas of the body, especially the back, flanks and abdomen. Many pigs harbour unapparent infections throughout their lives, and the main mode of transmission appears to be between carrier sows and their piglets during suckling. Signs may appear on the face and ears within 3 weeks of birth, later extending to other areas. Transmission may also occur during service, especially from an infected boar to gilts.

Clinical signs: Affected pigs scratch continuously and may lose condition. Common signs are papular eruptions with erythema, pruritus and hair loss. As the infestation progresses the skin becomes thickened, crusted with exudates and secondarily infected due to

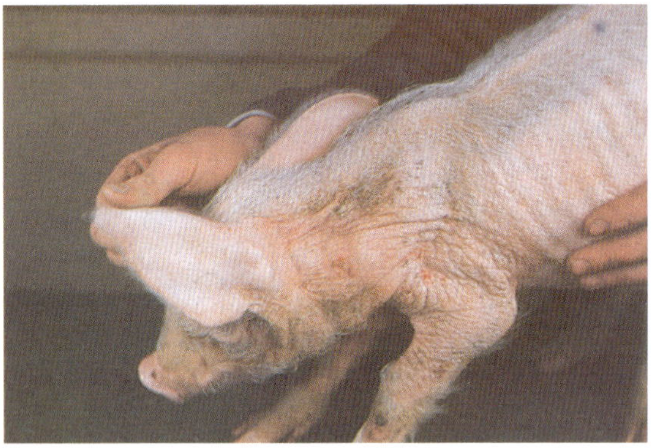

Fig. 5.13 Sarcoptic mange in a pig.

damage caused by the host scratching (Fig. 5.13). Scaly areas around the edge of lesions indicate the spread of mites. Severe cases exhibit loss of appetite and weight, impaired hearing, blindness and exhaustion.

Diagnosis: Useful diagnostic features of porcine sarcoptic mange are:

- The edges of the ears are often first affected, and on rubbing a scratch reflex is readily elicited.
- There is always intense itching, so in cases of dermatitis where there is no itch, sarcoptic mange can be eliminated as a possibility.
- It is a highly contagious condition, and single cases are rarely seen in groups of animals kept in close contact.

Confirmatory diagnosis is by examination of skin scrapings for the presence of mites. However, since these are sometimes difficult to demonstrate, a negative finding should not preclude a tentative diagnosis of mange and initiation of treatment. For confirmatory diagnosis in pigs, a reliable source of material for examination is wax from the ear.

Pathology: The first lesions appear as small red papules or weals and general erythema about the eyes, around the snout, on the concave surface of the external ears, in the axillae and on the front of the hocks where the skin is thin. Scratching results in excoriation of these affected areas and the formation of brownish scabs on the damaged skin. Subsequently, the skin becomes wrinkled, covered with crusty lesions and thickened.

Epidemiology: New hosts are infected by contact with infected individuals, presumably by the transfer of larvae, which are commonly present more superficially on the skin surface. Transmission occurs between mature animals and also from mother to offspring at birth. Transfer of different host-adapted populations of *S. scabiei* between different host species often results in only temporary infestations. Infestation may also occur by indirect transfer, since the mites have been shown to be capable of surviving off the host for short periods. The length of time that *S. scabiei* can survive off the host depends on environmental conditions but may be between 2 and 3 weeks. Consequently, animals' bedding may become contaminated and is a possible source of infestation.

Treatment: In pigs, effective preparations that have been used include amitraz, trichlorphon and bromocyclen. Newer and more convenient products with a better residual effect are the systemic organophosphate pour-on phosmet and the macrocyclic lactones.

Control: In pigs, a common control approach is to treat the sow (the main reservoir of infection) before she goes into the farrowing crate or pen. This procedure will be more successful than having to treat partly grown pigs. The offspring of treated sows show better growth rates and shorter finishing periods than those of untreated sows. It is most important that boars are routinely treated at 6-monthly intervals, and any newly introduced boar is treated and quarantined as they can readily infect sows at service. In the treatment of affected pigs, acaricide may be applied weekly, by wash or by spray, until the signs have regressed. It is recommended that phosmet is applied to the back of the sow 3–7 days before farrowing, pouring a small part of the dose into the ears. As an alternative, systemic macrocyclic lactones may be given.

Demodex phylloides

Predilection site: Hair follicles and sebaceous glands, particularly the eyelids

Parasite class: Arachnida

Sub-class: Acari

Order: Acariformes

Sub-order: Trombidiformes (Prostigmata)

Family: Demodicidae

Description: Species of *Demodex* have an elongate tapering body, up to 0.1–0.4 mm in length, with four pairs of stumpy legs ending in small blunt claws in the adult (Fig. 6.32). Setae are absent from the legs and body. The legs are located at the front of the body, and as such the striated opisthosoma forms at least half the body length.

Hosts: Pig

Life cycle: *Demodex* spp usually live as commensals in the skin, and are highly site-specific, occupying the hair follicles and sebaceous glands. Females lay

20–24 spindle-shaped eggs in the hair follicle that give rise to hexapod larvae, in which each short leg ends in a single, three-pronged claw. Unusually, a second hexapod larval stage follows, in which each leg ends in a pair of three-pronged claws. Octopod protonymph, tritonymph and adult stages then follow. Immature stages and these migrate more deeply into the dermis. One follicle may harbour all life cycle stages concurrently. The life cycle is completed in 18–24 days. In each follicle or gland the mites may occur in large numbers in a characteristic head-downward posture. In the newborn and very young these sites are simple in structure, but later they become compounded by outgrowths. The presence of *Demodex* mites much deeper in the dermis than sarcoptids means that they are much less accessible to surface-acting acaricides. Species of *Demodex* are unable to survive off their host.

Geographical distribution: Worldwide

Pathogenesis: Infestation is usually confined to the head, where there is erythema, papules and thickened skin. If there is secondary bacterial infection or follicular rupture, pustules and nodules may be observed.

Clinical signs: Erythema, papules and thickened skin on the head

Diagnosis: For confirmatory diagnosis, deep scrapings are necessary to reach the mites deep in the follicles and glands. This is best achieved by taking a fold of skin, applying a drop of liquid paraffin, and scraping until capillary blood appears.

Pathology: Lesions typically involve the ventral abdomen, ventral neck, eyelids and snout. They commence as small red macules, developing into cunaneous nodules, covered by surface scale. Excision of the nodules releases thick white caseous debris.

Epidemiology: Probably because of its location deep in the dermis, it is difficult to transmit *Demodex* between animals unless there is prolonged contact. Such contact occurs most commonly at suckling. This mange is rare in pigs, although sporadic incidences of up to 5% have been noted in eastern European countries.

Treatment: In many cases demodecosis spontaneously resolves and treatment is unnecessary. The organophosphates (e.g. malathion, coumaphos, diazinion, fenchlorvos, chlorfenvinphos, phosmet or trichlofon) and systemic macrocyclic lactones may be effective.

Control: Control is rarely applied

Notes: Species of the genus *Demodex* are highly specialised mites that live in the hair follicles and sebaceous glands of a wide range of wild and domestic animals, including humans. They are believed to form a group of closely related sibling species, which are highly specific to particular hosts: *Demodex phylloides* (pig), *Demodex canis* (dog), *Demodex bovis* (cattle), *Demodex equi* (horse), *Demodex musculi* (mouse), *Demodex ratti* (rat), *Demodex caviae* (guinea-pig), *Demodex cati* (cat) and *Demodex folliculorum* and *Demodex brevis* on humans. Various morphological variations may be seen on a host; these are sometimes, probably incorrectly, ascribed separate species status.

A number of non-host-specific ectoparasites are found on pigs and are listed in the host–parasite checklist at the end of this chapter. More detailed descriptions of these parasites are found in Chapter 11 (Facultative ectoparasites and arthropod vectors).

In the following checklists, the codes listed below apply:

Helminth classes:
N = Nematoda; T = Trematoda; C = Cestoda; A = Acanthocephala.

Arthropod classes:
I = Insecta; A = Arachnida.

Protozoal classes:
M = Mastigophora; S = Sarcodina; A = Apicomplexa; R = Rickettsia.

Pig parasite checklist.

Section/host system	Helminths		Arthropods		Protozoa	
	Parasite	(Super)family	Parasite	Family	Parasite	Family
Digestive						
Oesophagus	*Gongylonema pulchrum*	Spiruroidea (N)				
Stomach	*Hyostrongylus rubidus*	Trichostrongyloidea (N)				
	Ollulanus tricuspis	Trichostrongyloidea (N)				
	Ascarops strongylina	Spiruroidea (N)				
	Ascarops dentata	Spiruroidea (N)				
	Gnathostoma hispidum	Spiruroidea (N)				
	Gnathostoma doloresi	Spiruroidea (N)				
	Physocephalus sexalatus	Spiruroidea (N)				
	Simondsia paradoxa	Spiruroidea (N)				
	Trichostrongylus axei	Trichostrongyloidea (N)				
Small intestine	*Globocephalus urosubulatus*	Strongyloidea (N)			*Isospora suis*	Eimeriidae (A)
	Ascaris suum	Ascaridoidea (N)			*Eimeria debliecki*	Eimeriidae (A)
	Strongyloides ransomi	Rhabditoidea (N)			*Eimeria polita*	Eimeriidae (A)
	Trichinella spiralis	Trichuroidea (N)			*Eimeria scabra*	Eimeriidae (A)
	Macracanthorhynchus hirudinaceus	Oligacanthorhynchidae (A)			*Eimeria spinosa*	Eimeriidae (A)
	Fasciolopsis buski	Fasciolidae (T)			*Eimeria porci*	Eimeriidae (A)
					Eimeria neodebliecki	Eimeriidae (A)
					Eimeria perminuta	Eimeriidae (A)
					Eimeria suis	Eimeriidae (A)
					Cryptosporidium parvum	Cryptosporidiidae (A)
					Cryptosporidium suis	Cryptosporidiidae (A)
					Giardia intestinalis	Diplomonadidae (M)
Caecum	*Oesophagostomum dentatum*	Strongyloidea (N)			*Tritrichomonas suis*	Trichomonadidae (M)
Colon	*Oesophagostomum quadrispinulatum*	Strongyloidea (N)			*Tetratrichomonas buttreyi*	Trichomonadidae (M)
	Oesophagostomum brevicaudum	Strongyloidea (N)			*Trichomitus rotunda*	Trichomonadidae (M)
	Oesophagostomum longicaudatum	Strongyloidea (N)			*Entamoeba suis*	Endamoebidae (S)
	Oesophagostomum georgianum	Strongyloidea (N)			*Balantidium coli*	Balantidiidae (C)
	Oesophagostomum granatensis	Strongyloidea (N)				
	Trichuris suis	Trichuroidea (N)				
	Gastrodiscus aegyptiacus	Paramphistomatidae (T)				
	Gastrodiscoides hominis	Paramphistomatidae (T)				

Respiratory				
Nose			*Tritrichomonas suis*	Trichomonadidae (M)
Trachea Bronchi				
Lung	*Metastrongylus apri*	Metastrongyloidea (N)		
	Metastrongylus pudendotectus	Metastrongyloidea (N)		
	Metastrongylus salmi	Metastrongyloidea (N)		
	Echinococcus granulosus	Taeniidae (C)		
Liver				
	Ascaris suum	Ascaridoidea (N)		
	Fasciola hepatica	Fasciolidae (T)		
	Fasciola gigantica	Fasciolidae (T)		
	Echinococcus granulosus	Taeniidae (C)		
	Cysticercus tenuicollis (metacestode – Taenia hydatigena)	Taeniidae (C)		
Pancreas				
	Eurytrema pancreaticum	Dicrocoeliidae (C)		
Circulatory				
Blood	*Schistosoma suis*	Schistosomatidae (T)	*Trypanosoma brucei brucei*	Trypanosomatidae (M)
	Schistosoma spindale	Schistosomatidae (T)	*Trypanosoma congolense congolense*	Trypanosomatidae (M)
	Schistosoma japonicum	Schistosomatidae (T)	*Trypanosoma suis*	Trypanosomatidae (M)
			Trypanosoma simiae	Trypanosomatidae (M)
			Babesia perroncitoi	Babesiidae (A)
			Babesia trautmanni	Babesiidae (A)
			Eperythrozoon suis	Anaplasmataceae (R)
Blood vessels				
Nervous				
CNS			*Toxoplasma gondii*	Sarcocystiidae (A)
Eye				
Reproductive/ urogenital				
	Stephanurus dentatus	Strongyloidea (N)		

(continued)

Pig parasite checklist (*continued*).

Section/host system	Helminths		Arthropods		Protozoa	
	Parasite	(Super)family	Parasite	Family	Parasite	Family
Kidneys						
	Stephanurus dentatus	Strongyloidea (N)				
Locomotory						
Muscle	*Cysticercus cellulosae (metacestode – Taenia solium)*	Taeniidae (C)			*Toxoplasma gondii*	Sarcocystiidae (A)
					Sarcocystis suicanis	Sarcocystiidae (A)
					Sarcocystis porcifelis	Sarcocystiidae (A)
	Trichinella spiralis	Trichuroidea (N)			*Sarcocystis suihominis*	Sarcocystiidae (A)
Connective tissue						
Integument						
Skin	*Suifilaria suis*	Filarioidea (N)	*Haematopinus suis*	Linognathidae (I)		
			Sarcoptes scabiei	Sarcoptidae (A)		
			Demodex phylloides	Demodicidae (A)		
Subcutaneous			*Cordylobia anthropophaga*	Calliphoridae (I)		
			Cochliomyia hominivorax	Calliphoridae (I)		
			Cochliomyia macellaria	Calliphoridae (I)		
			Chrysomya bezziana	Calliphoridae (I)		
			Chrysomya megacephala	Calliphoridae (I)		
			Wohlfahrtia magnifica	Sarcophagidae (I)		
			Wohlfahrtia meigeni	Sarcophagidae (I)		
			Wohlfahrtia vigil	Sarcophagidae (I)		
			Dermatobia hominis	Oestridae (I)		
			Tunga penetrans	Pulicidae (I)		

The following species of flies and ticks are found on pigs. More detailed descriptions are found in Chapter 11: Facultative ectoparasites and arthropod vectors.

Flies of veterinary importance on pigs.

Group	Genus	Species	Family
Blackflies Buffalo gnats	*Simulium*	spp	Simuliidae (I)
Bot flies	*Dermatobia*	*hominis*	Oestridae (I)
Flesh flies	*Sarcophaga* *Wohlfahrtia*	*fusicausa* *haemorrhoidalis* *magnifica* *meigeni* *vigil*	Sarcophagidae (I)
Midges	*Culicoides*	spp	Ceratopogonidae (I)
Mosquitoes	*Aedes* *Anopheles* *Culex*	spp spp spp	Culicidae (I)
Muscids	*Hydrotaea* *Musca* *Stomoxys*	*irritans* *autumnalis* *domestica* *calcitrans*	Muscidae (I)
Sandflies	*Phlebotomus*	spp	Psychodidae (I)
Screwworms and blowflies	*Chrysomya* *Cochliomyia* *Cordylobia*	*albiceps* *bezziana* *megacephala* *hominivorax* *macellaria* *anthropophaga*	Calliphoridae (I)
Tabanids	*Chrysops* *Haematopota* *Tabanus*	spp spp spp	Tabanidae (I)
Tsetse flies	*Glossina*	*fusca* *morsitans* *palpalis*	Glossinidae (I)

Tick species found on pigs.

Genus	Species	Common name	Family
Ornithodoros	*moubata* *savignyi*	Eyeless or hut tampan Eyed or sand tampan	Argasidae (A)
Dermacentor	*reticulatus*	Marsh tick	Ixodidae (A)
Hyalomma	*detritum* *marginatum* *truncatum*	 Mediterranean Hyalomma	Ixodidae (A)
Ixodes	*ricinus* *holocyclus* *rubicundus* *scapularis*	Castor bean or European sheep tick Karoo paralysis tick Shoulder tick	Ixodidae (A)
Rhipicephalus	*evertsi* *sanguineus*	Red or red-legged tick Brown dog or kennel tick	Ixodidae (A)

6
Parasites of dogs and cats

ENDOPARASITES

PARASITES OF THE DIGESTIVE SYSTEM

MOUTH

Tetratrichomonas canistomae

Synonym: *Trichomonas canistomae*

Predilection site: Mouth

Parasite class: Zoomastigophorasida

Family: Trichomonadidae

Description: The body is piriform, 7–12 × 3–4 μm. The four anterior flagella are about as long as the body and arise in pairs from a large blepharoplast (Fig. 6.1). The undulating membrane extends almost the length of the body, and terminates in a free posterior flagellum, which is about half the length of the body. The axostyle is threadlike, stains black with haematoxylin and extends a considerable length beyond the body. The costa is slender and there are no subcostal granules.

Hosts: Dog

Life cycle: The trichomonads reproduce by longitudinal binary fission. No sexual stages are known and there are no cysts.

Geographical distribution: Unknown

Pathogenesis: Considered non-pathogenic

Diagnosis: Morphological identification of the organisms from fresh and stained mouth swab preparations. The organisms can also be cultured in a range of media used for trichomonads.

Epidemiology: Transmission presumably occurs by ingestion of trophozoites from saliva during licking and grooming.

Treatment and control: Not required

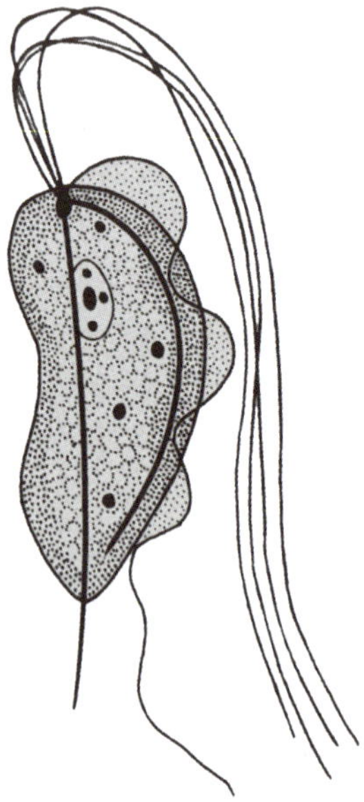

Fig. 6.1 *Tetratrichomonas canistomae.*

Tetratrichomonas felistomae

Predilection site: Mouth

Parasite class: Zoomastigophorasida

Family: Trichomonadidae

Description: The body is piriform, 6–11 × 3–4 μm, (mean 8 × 3 μm). There are four anterior flagella, which are longer than the body. The undulating membrane extends most of the body length and terminates in a free posterior flagellum and the axostyle extends a considerable distance beyond the body.

Hosts: Cat

Notes: The two species may be synonymous. All other details are as for *T. canistomae*

OESOPHAGUS

Spirocerca lupi

Synonym: *Spirocerca sanguinolenta*

Predilection site: Oesophagus, stomach, aorta

Parasite class: Nematoda

Superfamily: Spiruroidea

Description, gross: Adult worms are spirally coiled and have a blood-red colour; males are around 30–55 mm, and females 55–80 mm.

Description, microscopic: The lips are trilobed and the pharynx is short. The male tail bears lateral alae, four pairs and one unpaired median pre-cloacal papillae and two pairs of post-cloacal papillae, with a group of minute papillae near the tail tip. Eggs have thick shells, $30–37 \times 11–15$ μm and are larvated when passed in faeces.

Final hosts: Dog, fox, wild canids and occasionally cat and wild felids

Intermediate hosts: Coprophagous beetles: *Scarabeus sacer*, *Akis*, *Atenchus*, *Gymnopleurus*, *Cauthon* spp. Many vertebrates such as rodents, birds, insectivores and reptiles can act as paratenic hosts.

Life cycle: The thick-shelled elongate egg, containing a larva, is passed in the faeces or vomit and does not hatch until ingested by a dung beetle. In this, the intermediate host, the larva develops to the L_3 and encysts. Paratenic hosts may also be involved if the dung beetle, in turn, is ingested by any of a variety of other animals including the domestic chicken, wild birds and lizards. In these the L_3 becomes encysted in the viscera. On ingestion of the intermediate or paratenic host by the final host the L_3 are liberated, penetrate the stomach wall and migrate via the coeliac artery to the thoracic aorta. About 3 months later the majority of larvae cross to the adjacent oesophagus where they provoke the development of granulomas as they develop to the adult stage in a further 3 months. The prepatent period is therefore about 6 months. Eggs, however, may not be found in the faeces of a proportion of animals with adult infections where the granulomas have no openings into the oesophageal lumen.

Geographical distribution: Tropical and subtropical areas

Pathogenesis: The migrating larvae produce haemorrhages, scarring and/or the formation of fibrotic nodules on the internal wall of the aorta, which, if particularly severe, may cause stenosis or even rupture. The oesophageal granulomas, up to 4.0 cm in size, associated with the adult worms, may be responsible for a variety of clinical signs including dysphagia and vomiting arising from oesophageal obstruction and inflammation.

Two further complications are, first, the development of oesophageal osteosarcoma in a small proportion of infected dogs. These may be highly invasive and produce metastases in the lung and other tissues. Secondly, also relatively rare, is the occurrence of spondylosis of the thoracic vertebrae or of hypertrophic pulmonary osteoarthropathy of the long bones. The aetiology of these lesions is unknown. Occasionally *S. lupi* infection can induce a pyaemic nephritis.

Clinical signs: Despite the potential pathogenicity of this parasite, many infected dogs do not exhibit clinical signs even when extensive aortic lesions and large, often purulent, oesophageal granulomas are present. In some dogs infection will induce persistent vomiting with worms passed in the vomit. In less serious cases there may be difficulty in swallowing or interference with the action of the stomach. Aortic infection is not usually observed until sudden death is caused by rupture.

Diagnosis: The location and appearance of the granulomatous lesions, up to golf-ball size, is usually sufficient for identification. Numerous pink–reddish, stout, spirally coiled worms may be seen on section of the granulomas, but these are difficult to extricate intact since they are coiled and up to 8.0 cm long. Eggs may be found in the faeces or vomit if there are fistulae in the oesophageal granulomas. However, the eggs are similar in appearance to those of other spirurids. Otherwise diagnosis may depend on endoscopy or radiography.

Pathology: The migrating larvae produce characteristic lesions in the wall of the aorta (Fig. 6.2) while the adults are found embedded in granulomatous lesions in the wall of the oesophagus and occasionally the stomach. Aortic lesions include haemorrhage and necrosis with eosinophilic inflammation, intimal roughening with thrombosis, aneurysm with rare aortic rupture, and subintimal and medial mineralisation and heterotopic bone deposition. Spondylosis of the ventral aspects of thoracic vertebrae occurs in some cases with exostoses of the vertebral bodies. Granulomas in the oesophagus contain pleomorphic fibroblasts. In some animals mesencymal neoplasms develop in the wall of the oesophageal granuloma with lesions showing cytological characteristics typical of fibrosarcoma and osteosarcoma, with local tissue invasion and, in many cases, pulmonary metastasis.

Epidemiology: In endemic areas the incidence of infection in dogs is often extremely high, sometimes

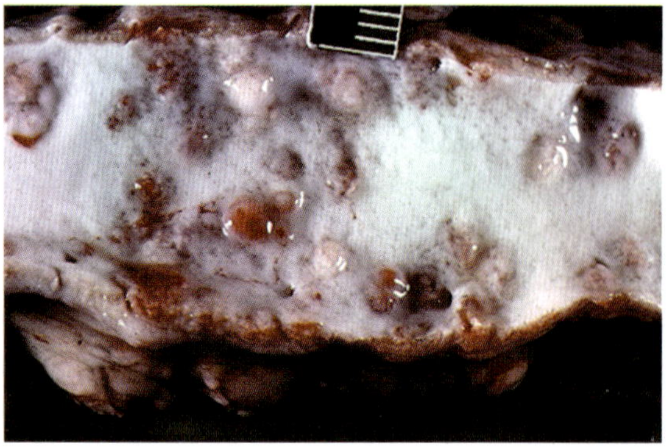

Fig. 6.2 Fibrotic nodules on the internal wall of the aorta from a dog infected with *Spirocerca lupi*.

approaching 100%. Probably this is associated with the many opportunities of acquiring infection from the variety of paratenic hosts.

Treatment: Treatment is rarely practical, but levamisole and albendazole have been reported to be of value. Levamisole is given at 5–10 mg/kg as a single dose. Diethylcarbamazine at oral doses of 10 mg/kg twice daily for 10 days may kill adult worms but not larvae.

Control: This is difficult because of the ubiquity of the intermediate and paratenic hosts. Dogs should not be fed uncooked viscera from wild birds or from free-range domestic chickens.

STOMACH

Ollulanus tricuspis

Predilection site: Stomach

Parasite class: Nematoda

Superfamily: Trichostrongyloidea

Description, gross: This is a very small trichostrongyle. Males are 0.7–0.8 mm, and females 0.8–1 mm long.

Description, microscopic: The worm is identified microscopically by the spiral coil of the head. The male bursa is well developed and the spicules are stout and each is split into two for a considerable distance. The female has a tail with three or four short cusps. The vulva is in the posterior part of the body and there is only one uterus and ovary.

Hosts: Cats, wild felids; occasionally found in pigs, foxes and domestic dogs

Life cycle: The worms are viviparous, the larvae developing to the L_3 stage in the uterus of the females. Autoinfection can occur, the shed L_3 developing into adult worms on the gastric mucosa in around 4–5 weeks. The whole life cycle may be completed endogenously and transmission, at least in the cat, is thought to be via ingestion of vomit containing the L_3. The worms live under a layer of mucus in the stomach wall and the anterior end of the worm is often located within the gastric crypts.

Geographical distribution: Mainly occurs in Europe, North and South America, Australasia and the Middle East.

Pathogenesis: The parasite is considered non-pathogenic in cats. Heavy infections may induce a severe catarrhal gastritis and vomiting. Untreated cats may become emaciated. Little is known of its pathogenicity in other hosts, although a chronic gastritis has been reported in the pig.

Clinical signs: Occasional vomiting and emaciation.

Diagnosis: Diagnosis of ollulanosis is seldom made because of their small size and lack of eggs and larvae in the faeces. Examination of vomit, following an emetic, for the presence of worms is a useful approach. At necropsy, recovery and identification of the very small worms from the gastric mucosa should lead to a diagnosis.

Pathology: The worms lie beneath the mucus on the surface of the stomach, or partly in the gastric glands, and their presence may lead to mucosal lymphoid hyperplasia and elevated numbers of globule leucocytes in the gastric epithelium. Heavy infections cause hyperplasia of the gastric glands causing the stomach mucosa to become convoluted and thrown into folds.

Epidemiology: The parasite is common in some parts of the world, particularly in cat colonies and cats that roam. The parasite can replicate in the stomach without any need for external egg or larval phases and can spread via vomit. The disease spreads mainly among starving stray cats and sometimes stray dogs.

Treatment: Levamisole, ivermectin or repeated doses of oxfendazole at 10 mg/kg twice daily for 5 days are effective.

Control: This is mainly achieved through the implementation of good hygiene procedures.

Spirocerca lupi

See under Oesophagus.

Gnathostoma spinigerum

Predilection site: Stomach

Parasite class: Nematoda

Superfamily: Spiruroidea

Description, gross: Thick-bodied worms, reddish at the front, and greyish posteriorly. The males are 1–2.5 cm and the females up to 3.0 cm long. The presence of the worms in gastric nodules is sufficient for generic diagnosis.

Description, microscopic: Confirmation is easily made with a hand lens when the swollen anterior head bulb covered with transverse rows of 6–11 small hooks will be seen. The head contains four sub-median cavities that each communicate with a cervical sac. The anterior of the body is covered with flat cuticular spines and the ventral caudal region of the male bears small spines and four pairs of large pedunculate papillae as well as several smaller sessile ones. The left spicule is longer than the right. Eggs are oval, greenish, 69×37 µm with a thin cap at one pole.

Final hosts: Cat, dog, man, mink, polecat and several wild carnivores

Intermediate hosts: Host 1: Many species of freshwater crustaceans, copepods. Host 2: Small vertebrates including mammals, birds, reptiles, fish and amphibians

Life cycle: The adult worms live in tunnels in the gastric nodules, and the eggs pass from there into the lumen and are dropped into the water in the faeces where they hatch after several days. The crustaceans (first intermediate hosts) ingest L_1 and development to L_2 takes place. The crustaceans are themselves ingested by vertebrates (second intermediate hosts), such as fish, frogs and reptiles, and development to L_3 occurs and the larvae become encysted. The L_3 can also encyst in many mammals such as mice, rats and dogs. The final host is infected by ingestion of the vertebrate vector and further development occurs in the stomach wall, where the worms provoke the growth of fibrous lesions.

Geographical distribution: Thailand, Japan, South East Asia, China, Mexico

Pathogenesis: *G. spinigerum* is the most pathogenic *Gnathostoma* species, which in cats may cause fatal gastric perforation and peritonitis. In some cases a number of larvae will migrate from the stomach to other organs, most commonly the liver, in which they burrow, leaving necrotic tracks in the parenchyma.

Clinical signs: *Gnathostoma* infection in the cat may cause acute abdominal signs.

Diagnosis: The infection in the living animal can only be diagnosed by the finding of the greenish, oval eggs, which have a thin cap at one pole, in the faeces. Often, however, eggs are not present in faeces.

Pathology: As in many spiruroid infections, the most obvious effect of gnathostomosis is the presence of fibrous growths on the stomach wall. These growths are of variable size, the largest being 3–4 cm in diameter, and are cavitated, amounting to thick-walled cysts containing worms and fluid. Ulceration and necrosis of the stomach wall are often present.

Epidemiology: Dogs, cats and several species of wild mammals are reservoirs of the parasite. These final hosts become infected primarily through eating infected fish or other animals that serve as paratenic hosts. In humans, the ingestion of raw or inadequately cooked fish is the major source of infection. Human infections also are reported from eating raw or poorly cooked catfish, eels, frogs, chickens, ducks and snakes.

Treatment: Treatment has not been fully investigated.

Control: With the ubiquity of the first and second intermediate hosts complete control cannot be achieved. Ensuring only well cooked fish, eels, or other intermediate hosts, such as snakes, frogs, and poultry, are eaten can prevent infections. Potentially copepod infested water should be boiled or treated.

Notes: Like most spiruroids, *Gnathostoma* inhabits the upper alimentary tract, occurring in nodules in the stomach wall of omnivores and carnivores. It is exceptional in requiring two intermediate hosts in most species.

When visceral larva migrans due to *Gnathostoma* occurs in humans, *G. spinigerum* is the species usually involved, and the commonest source of infection is inadequately cooked domestic poultry and fish acting as second intermediate hosts. Infection is particularly common in southeast Asia, Japan and China but occurs in many other countries. The worms never become fully adult, and the immature forms are most commonly found in nodules in subcutaneous tissues and other organs that appear and disappear irregularly as the parasites wander in various parts of the body. In humans, cutaneous gnathostomiosis can result in pruritic swellings and eosinophilia with occasional abscess formation. Ocular gnathostomiosis is characterised by haemorrhage, uveitis and perforation of the iris. A severe form of infection is central nervous system (CNS) gnathostomiosis, leading to haemorrhage and intracranial necrotic tracks that can be fatal.

Physaloptera praeputialis

Predilection site: Stomach

Parasite class: Nematoda

Superfamily: Spiruroidea

Description, gross: Adult worms are larger than most spiruroids, being stout and resembling ascarids. Males measure 1–45 mm and females 1.5–60 mm.

Description, microscopic: The cuticle in both sexes extends posteriorly as a sheath beyond the end of the body. The lips are simple and bear a set of three flattened, internal teeth and a single conical external tooth. The male bears lateral alae, joined anteriorly across the ventral surface. In the female the vulva is slightly anterior to the midbody. The larvated eggs have a thick clear shell and measure 45–58 μm × 30–42 μm.

Final hosts: Cat and wild felids; occasionally the dog

Intermediate hosts: Beetles, cockroaches, crickets and paratenic hosts

Geographical distribution: China, Africa, North and South America

Life cycle: The life cycle is typically spiruroid. Eggs passed in the faeces of the infected host develop into infective larvae if ingested by coprophagous beetles. The life cycle is completed when cats ingest the intermediate hosts. Various transport hosts may also be involved in transmission of infection. The prepatent period is around 8–10 weeks.

Pathogenesis: The adult worms have small teeth on their large triangular lips, and attach strongly to the gastric mucosa, leaving small ulcers when they move to fresh sites. These feeding sites may continue to bleed. They may cause catarrhal gastritis, with emesis, and in heavy infections blood may appear in the faeces.

Clinical signs: In heavy infections there may be vomiting and some degree of anorexia. The faeces may appear dark in colour. Severely affected animals may lose weight.

Diagnosis: Diagnosis is based on clinical signs and by the finding of the elongate eggs, thickened at either pole, in the faeces or vomit.

Pathology: Presence of the adult worms may cause gastric ulceration and haemorrhage.

Epidemiology: The epidemiology depends on the presence and abundance of the intermediate beetle hosts. Infection is more prevalent in outdoor cats that have access to intermediate hosts or paratenic hosts.

Treatment: Treatment with benzimidazoles over a 5-day period has been reported to be effective. Pyrantel is also effective.

Control: The ubiquity of the insect intermediate hosts means that control is not usually feasible.

Physaloptera rara

Predilection site: Stomach

Parasite class: Nematoda

Superfamily: Spiruroidea

Hosts: Cat

Description, gross: Adult male worms are 2.5–3 cm long and females 3–6 cm.

Description, microscopic: This species differs from *P. praeputialis* in that there is no sheath over the posterior portion of the body in both sexes. The female vulva is anterior to the middle of the body. Eggs are thick-shelled and ellipsoid, 42–53 × 29–35 μm.

Geographical distribution: North America

Details of the life cycle, pathogenesis, treatment and control are essentially similar to those of *P. praeputialis*.

Spirura ritypleurites

Predilection site: Stomach, occasionally oesophagus

Parasite class: Nematoda

Superfamily: Spiruroidea

Description, gross: Thick, short white worms with the posterior region thicker than the anterior of the worm and twisted in a spiral.

Description, microscopic: The eggs have a thick shell and are embryonated when passed.

Final hosts: Cat, rarely dog, fox

Intermediate hosts: Coprophagous beetles

Life cycle: The life cycle is typically spiruroid. Eggs develop into infective larvae within an intermediate host. Larvae may then be ingested by paratenic hosts, such as rodents and lizards, in which they become encapsulated. Cats become infected by ingesting the insects or their transport hosts.

Geographical distribution: This worm is endemic in parts of southern Europe, Africa and Asia.

Pathogenesis: *S. ritypleurites* is usually presumed to be non-pathogenic.

Clinical signs: Symptoms of nausea, vomiting and digestive upsets have been reported.

Diagnosis: As for *Physaloptera* spp

Pathology: No associated pathology reported.

Epidemiology: The epidemiology depends on the presence and abundance of the intermediate beetle hosts. Infection is more prevalent in outdoor cats that have access to intermediate hosts or paratenic hosts.

Treatment: Not usually indicated. Treatment with a benzimidazole over an extended period is likely to be effective.

Control: Prevention is difficult because of the large number of intermediate hosts and paratenic hosts.

Capillaria putorii

Synonym: *Aonchotheca putorii*

Predilection site: Stomach, small intestine

Parasite class: Nematoda

Superfamily: Trichuroidea

Description, gross: These are thin, filamentous worms, about 1 cm long; males are 5–8 mm and females 9–15 mm.

Description, microscopic: Eggs have broad flat poles and granular unsegmented contents.

Hosts: Cat, dog, mustelids, hedgehog

Life cycle: Cats are thought to become infected by eating infective eggs from soil contaminated by hedgehog faeces.

Geographical distribution: Europe, New Zealand

Pathogenesis and clinical signs: There are few reports on the clinical signs of infection in cats. Infected cats have reported anorexia and intermittent bloody vomitus.

Diagnosis: Identification of the characteristic eggs in faeces

Pathology: There is reported chronic, hyperplastic pyloric gastritis and ulceration around the pylorus associated with the presence of worms with eggs present in the pyloric mucus and in the lumen of the pyloric glands.

Treatment and control: Levamisole, given as two doses of 7.5 mg/kg at 2-week intervals, and ivermectin, at 300 μg/kg, have been reported to be effective.

SMALL INTESTINE

Toxocara canis

Predilection site: Small intestine

Parasite class: Nematoda

Superfamily: Ascaridoidea

Description, gross: *Toxocara canis* is a large white worm up to about 18.0 cm in length; males are around 10 cm, and females up to 18 cm (Fig. 6.3).

Description, microscopic: The adult head is elliptical due to the presence of large cervical alae. The mouth is surrounded by three large lips. There is no buccal capsule and the oesophagus lacks a bulb. The tail of the male has a terminal narrow appendage and caudal alae. Female genital organs extend anteriorly and posteriorly to the vulval region. The egg is dark brown and subglobular, 90 × 75 μm with a thick, pitted shell.

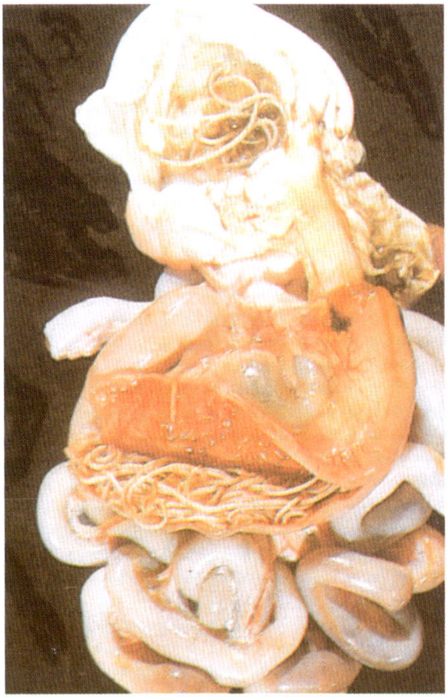

Fig. 6.3 Heavy *Toxocara canis* infection in the small intestine of a pup.

Hosts: Dog, fox

Life cycle: This species has the most complex life cycle in the superfamily, with four possible modes of infection.

The basic form is typically ascaridoid, the egg containing the L_3 being infective, at optimal temperatures, 4 weeks after being passed. After ingestion, and hatching in the small intestine, the larvae travel by the bloodstream via the liver to the lungs, where the second moult occurs, the larvae returning via the trachea to the intestine where the final two moults take place. This form of ascaroid migration occurs regularly only in dogs of up to about 2–3 months old.

In dogs over 3 months of age, the hepatic–tracheal migration occurs less frequently, and at around 4–6 months it has almost ceased and is replaced by somatic migration, followed by hypobiosis. However, some dogs will support hepatic–tracheal migration as adults. Instead of hepatic–tracheal migration, the L_3 travel to a wide range of tissues including the liver, lungs, brain, heart and skeletal muscle, and the walls of the alimentary tract.

In the pregnant bitch, prenatal infection occurs, larvae becoming mobilised at about 3 weeks prior to parturition and migrating to the lungs of the fetus where they moult just before birth. In the newborn pup the cycle is completed when the larvae travel to the intestine via the trachea, and the final moults occur. A bitch, once infected, will usually harbour sufficient larvae to infect all her subsequent litters, even if she never again encounters the infection. A few of these mobilised larvae, instead of going to the uterus, complete the normal migration in the bitch, and the resulting adult worms produce a transient but marked increase in faecal *Toxocara* egg output in the weeks following parturition.

The suckling pup may also be infected by ingestion of L_3 in the milk during the first 3 weeks of lactation. There is no migration in the pup following infection by this route. Paratenic hosts such as rodents or birds may ingest the infective eggs, and the L_3 travel to their tissues where they remain until eaten by a dog when subsequent development is apparently confined to the gastrointestinal tract.

A final complication is recent evidence that bitches may be reinfected during late pregnancy or lactation, leading directly to transmammary infection of the suckling pups and, once patency is established in the bitch, to contamination of the environment with eggs. The bitch may be reinfected via the ingestion of larval stages from the fresh faeces of puppies through her coprophagic activities.

The known minimum prepatent periods are:

- Direct infection following ingestion of eggs or larvae in a paratentic host: 4–5 weeks
- Prenatal infection: 2–3 weeks

Geographical distribution: Worldwide

Pathogenesis: In moderate infections, the larval migratory phase is accomplished without any apparent damage to the tissues, and the adult worms provoke little reaction in the intestine. In heavy infections the pulmonary phase of larval migration is associated with pneumonia, which is sometimes accompanied by pulmonary oedema; the adult worms cause a mucoid enteritis, there may be partial or complete occlusion of the gut and, in rare cases, perforation with peritonitis or in some instances blockage of the bile duct.

Clinical signs: In mild to moderate infections, there are no clinical signs during the pulmonary phase of larval migration. The adults in the intestine may cause tucked-up abdomen or potbelly, with failure to thrive, and occasional vomiting and diarrhoea. Entire worms are sometimes vomited or passed in the faeces. The signs in heavy infections during larval migration result from pulmonary damage and include coughing, increased respiratory rate and a frothy nasal discharge. Most fatalities from *T. canis* infection occur during the pulmonary phase, and pups, which have been heavily infected transplacentally may die within a few days of birth. Nervous convulsions have been attributed by some clinicians to toxocariosis, but there is still some disagreement on whether the parasite can be implicated as a cause of these signs.

Diagnosis: Only a tentative diagnosis is possible during the pulmonary phase of heavy infections when the larvae are migrating, and is based on the simultaneous appearance of pneumonic signs in a litter, often within 2 weeks of birth. The eggs in faeces, subglobular and brown with thick, pitted shells, are species-diagnostic. The egg production of the worms is so high that there is no need to use flotation methods, and they are readily found in simple faecal smears to which a drop of water has been added.

T. canis in the dog can be confused only with *Toxascaris leonina* which is slightly smaller. Differentiation of these two species is difficult, as the only useful character, visible with a hand lens, is the presence of a small finger-like process on the tail of the male *T. canis*.

Pathology: On postmortem, the animal appears poorly grown, potbellied and cachectic. Large numbers of maturing worms are present in the intestines and sometimes the stomach. Focal haemorrhages may be found in the lungs of puppies with migrating *T. canis* larvae. Inflammatory foci are often observed in the kidneys as white, elevated spots 1–2 mm in diameter in the cortex beneath the capsule. In section, they are composed of a small focus of macrophages, lymphocytes, plasma cells and a few eosinophils, possibly containing larvae. Occasionally, granulomas may be found in the eye.

Epidemiology: Surveys of *T. canis* prevalence in dogs have been carried out in most countries and have shown a wide range of infection rates, from 5% to over 80%. The highest rates of prevalence have been recorded in dogs of less than 6 months of age, with the fewest worms in adult animals. Infection induces immunity that results in loss of adult worms.

The widespread distribution and high intensity of infection with *T. canis* depend essentially on three factors. First, the females are extremely fecund, one worm being able to contribute about 700 eggs to each gram of faeces per day, and egg counts of 15 000 epg are not uncommon in pups. Second, the eggs are highly resistant to climatic extremes, and can survive for years on the ground. Third, there is a constant reservoir of infection in the somatic tissues of the bitch, and larvae in these sites are not susceptible to most anthelmintics.

Treatment: The adult worms are easily removed by anthelmintic treatment. The most popular drug used has been piperazine, although this is being superseded by the benzimidazoles (fenbendazole and mebendazole) and by nitroscanate. Pyrantel and the avermectin, selamectin, are also effective. Although several anthelmintics have activity against larval stages and juvenile worms, none are fully effective at their removal.

A simple and frequently recommended regime for control of toxocariosis in young dogs is as follows. All pups should be dosed at 2 weeks of age, and again 2–3 weeks later, to eliminate prenatally acquired infection. It is also recommended that the bitch should be treated at the same time as the pups. A further dose should be given to the pups at 2 months old, to eliminate any infection acquired from the milk of the dam or from any increase in faecal egg output by the dam in the weeks following whelping. Newly purchased pups should be dosed twice at an interval of 14 days.

Since there are likely to be a few worms present, even in adult dogs, in spite of the diversion of the majority of larvae to the somatic tissues, it is recommended that adult dogs should be treated every 3–6 months throughout their lives.

It has been shown that daily administration of high doses of fenbendazole to the bitch from 3 weeks prepartum to 2 days postpartum has largely eliminated transmammary and prenatal infection of the pups, although residual infection in the tissues of the bitch may persist. This regimen may be useful in breeding kennels.

Control: The main aim is to prevent transmammary and intrauterine transmission of infection using the anthelmintic treatment regimens listed above. Hygienic disposal of dog faeces should be encouraged. Where practical, access of rodents to kennels should be prevented.

Notes: Apart from its veterinary importance, this species is responsible for the most widely recognised form of **visceral larva migrans** (VLM) in man. Though this term was originally applied to invasion of the visceral tissues of an animal by parasites whose natural hosts were other animals, it has now, in common usage, come to represent this type of invasion in humans alone and, in particular, by the larvae of *Toxocara canis*, although the larval stages of *T. mystax*, *T. leonina* and *T. vitulorum* (see Chapter 2: Cattle, Small intestine) can be implicated. Its complementary term is cutaneous larva migrans (CLM), for infections by 'foreign' larvae, which are limited to the skin.

The global condition occurs most commonly in children, often under 5 years of age, who have had close contact with household pets, or who have frequented areas such as public parks where there is contamination of the ground by infective dog faeces. Surveys of such areas in many countries have almost invariably shown the presence of viable eggs of *T. canis* in around 10% of soil samples. Despite this high risk of exposure to infection, the reported incidence of clinical cases is small. For example, in 1979 a French survey of the world literature reported that only 430 cases of ocular, and 350 cases of visceral, larva migrans had been recorded. However, it has been suggested that 50–60 clinical cases occur in Britain each year, since many are not recorded.

In many cases, larval invasion is limited to the liver, and may give rise to hepatomegaly and eosinophilia, but on some occasions a larva escapes into the general circulation and arrives in another organ, the most frequently noted being the eye. Here, a granuloma forms around the larva on the retina, often resembling a retinoblastoma. Only in rare cases does the granuloma involve the optic disc, with total loss of vision, and most reports are of partial impairment of vision, with endophthalmitis or granulomatous retinitis. Such cases are currently treated using laser therapy. In a few cases of epilepsy, *T. canis* infection has been identified serologically, but the significance of the association has yet to be established.

Control of visceral larva migrans is based on the anthelmintic regimen described above, on the safe disposal of dog faeces in houses and gardens, and on the limitation of access by dogs to areas where children play, such as public parks and recreation grounds.

Toxocara mystax

Synonym: *Toxocara cati*

Predilection site: Small intestine

Parasite class: Nematoda

Superfamily: Ascaridoidea

Description, gross: Typical of the superfamily, *Toxocara mystax* is a large white worm (up to 10 cm in length), often occurring as a mixed infection with the other ascaridoids of cats, such as *Toxascaris leonina*. Males are 3–6 cm, females 4–10 cm.

Description, microscopic: The tail of the male has a terminal narrow appendage. Differentiation is readily made between *Toxocara mystax* and *Toxascaris leonina* on gross examination or with a hand lens, when the cervical alae of the former are seen to have an arrow-head form, with the posterior margins almost at a right angle to the body, whereas those of *Toxascaris* taper gradually into the body (Fig. 6.4). The male, like that of *Toxocara canis*, has a small finger-like process at the tip of the tail. The egg, subglobular, 65–75 μm with a thick, pitted shell and almost colourless, is characteristic in cat faeces.

Hosts: Cat

Life cycle: The life cycle of *T. mystax* is migratory when infection occurs by ingestion of the L_2 in the egg, and non-migratory after transmammary infection with L_3 or after ingestion of a paratenic host.

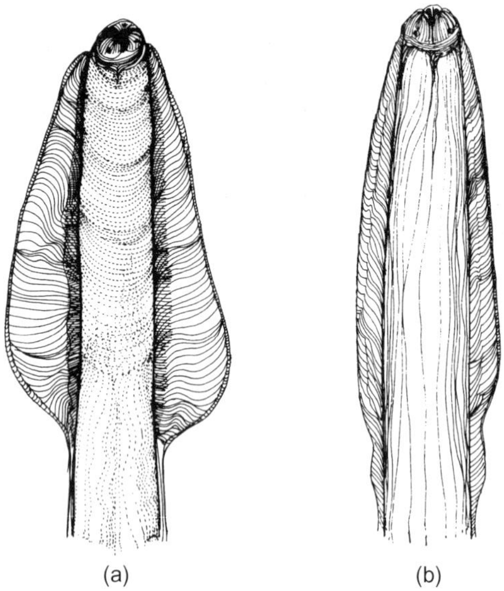

Fig. 6.4 Comparison of the anterior region of (a) *Toxocara mystax* and (b) *Toxascaris leonina*. The cervical alae of *Toxocara mystax* are arrow-shaped whereas those of *Toxascaris leonina* are more slender and less protrusive.

Following ingestion of eggs containing an infective second-stage larva, the larvae enter the stomach wall and then migrate via the liver, lungs and trachea back to the stomach and moult to L_3, while L_4 occur in the stomach contents, the intestinal wall and bowel contents. Rodent infections also play an important part in the life cycle. In these, larvae remain as second-stage forms but when an infected mouse is eaten by a cat the larvae, liberated by digestion, enter the stomach wall of the cat and develop to L_3. As well as mice acting as 'intermediate hosts', L_2 may be found in the tissues of earthworms, cockroaches, chickens, sheep and other animals fed infective eggs.

Transmammary infection is common throughout lactation and the lactogenic route of transmission is the most important. Prenatal infection does not occur. The prepatent period from egg infection is about 8 weeks.

Geographical distribution: Worldwide

Pathogenesis: Because the majority of infections are acquired either in the milk of the dam, or by ingestion of paratenic hosts, there is no migratory phase so any changes are usually confined to the intestine, showing as potbelly, diarrhoea, poor coat and failure to thrive.

Clinical signs: Unthriftiness, potbelly, diarrhoea

Diagnosis: The subglobular eggs, with thick, pitted shells, are easily recognised in faeces.

Pathology: Larvae developing in the mucosa of the stomach may provoke a mild granulomatous reaction comprising lymphocytes and a few macrophages around the coiled larvae.

Epidemiology: The epidemiology of *T. mystax* depends largely on a reservoir of larvae in the tissues of the dam, which are mobilised late in pregnancy and excreted in the milk throughout lactation. The paratenic host is also of considerable significance because of the strong hunting instinct in cats. Exposure to the latter route of infection does not occur until kittens begin to hunt for themselves or to share the prey of their dams.

Treatment: Fenbendazole, mebendazole, piperazine and pyrantel are all effective against adult nematodes. The benzimidazole anthelmintics are more effective against larval ascarids.

Control: Since infection is first acquired during suckling, complete control would be based on removal of kittens from the dam and artificial rearing. Good hygiene is essential in catteries. Young kittens should be wormed regularly with an anthelmintic from 4–6 weeks of age at 3-week intervals until 4 months of age and thereafter at regular intervals.

Notes: *T. mystax* has been reported as a rare cause of visceral larva migrans in man.

Toxocara malayiensis

Predilection site: Small intestine

Parasite class: Nematoda

Superfamily: Ascaridoidea

Description, gross: *Toxocara malayiensis* is a large white worm; males are 5.3–8.5 cm, females 1.1–1.4 cm, morphologically similar to *T. canis* in dogs.

Description, microscopic: There are three well defined lips, each with a deep median notch lined with denticles: a dorsal lip with two large outer papillae, and two subventral lips each with one outer papilla. Cervical alae arise immediately behind the lips, gradually increasing in width to mid-length, then tapering gradually posteriorly

Hosts: Cat

Life cycle: The life cycle has not been fully described.

Geographical distribution: Malaysia

Diagnosis: The subglobular eggs, with thick-pitted shells are similar to those of *T. canis*.

Epidemiology: Not described

Treatment and control: Presumed similar to *T. mystax*.

Details of the pathogenesis, pathology and clinical signs have not been reported.

Toxascaris leonina

Synonym: *Toxascaris limbata*

Predilection site: Small intestine

Parasite class: Nematoda

Superfamily: Ascaridoidea

Description, gross: Males are up to 7 cm long and females up to 10 cm.

Description, microscopic: Adults have an elliptical head due to presence of large cervical alae. Three large lips surround the mouth, there is no buccal capsule and the oesophagus lacks a bulb. The tail of the male is simple. The female genital organs lie behind the level of the vulva. The egg is slightly ovoid, light coloured, 75 × 85 μm with a smooth thick shell, and is characteristic in dog and cat faeces.

Hosts: Dog, cat, fox

Life cycle: The infective stage is the egg containing a second-stage larva or the third-stage larvae present in a mouse intermediate host. Following ingestion and hatching, larvae enter the wall of the intestine and remain for about 2 weeks. No migration of larvae occurs as with other ascarid species. Third-stage larvae appear after about 11 days and moult to L_4 about 3–5 weeks post infection. Adult stages appear from about 6 weeks post infection and lie in the lumen of the intestine. The prepatent period is 10–11 weeks.

Geographical distribution: Worldwide

Pathogenesis: Infection with *Toxascaris* is unlikely to occur in isolation and is more usually accompanied by a *Toxocara* infection. In puppies and young dogs less than 2 months of age the infection is usually absent as there is no prenatal or lactogenic transmission. Damage is caused predominantly by the adult worms and is determined by the number of worms present in the intestine.

Clinical signs: Unthriftiness, potbelly, diarrhoea

Diagnosis: *Toxascaris* is almost indistinguishable grossly from *Toxocara canis*, the only point of difference being the presence of a finger-like process at the tip of the male tail of the latter. In the cat, differentiation from *Toxocara mystax* is based on the shape of the cervical alae, which are lanceolate in *Toxascaris* but arrowhead shaped in *Toxocara mystax*. The characterisitic ovoid, smooth-shelled eggs are easily recognised in the faeces.

Pathology: Pathological effects due to *Toxascaris leonina* are rarely seen. Heavy infections may cause occlusion of the intestinal lumen and are usually associated with the mixed presence of *Toxocara* spp.

Epidemiology: Infection normally occurs through the ingestion of the larvated eggs. Larvae of *Toxascaris leonina* may occur in mice with the third-stage larvae distributed in many tissues. If a dog or cat ingests an infected mouse the larvae are released and develop to maturity in the wall and lumen of the intestine of the final host.

Treatment: Fenbendazole, mebendazole, piperazine and pyrantel are all effective against adult nematodes. The benzimidazole anthelmintics are more effective against larval ascarids.

Control: Ascarid infections in the domestic carnivores invariably include *Toxocara*, such that the measures recommended for control of the latter will also have an effect on *Toxascaris*. Since the two main reservoirs of infection are larvae in the prey or eggs on the ground, control has to be based on treatment of worm infection in the host animals, and on adequate hygiene to limit the possibility of acquisition of infection by ingestion of eggs.

Notes: This genus occurs in domestic carnivores, and though common, is of less significance than *Toxocara* because its parasitic phase is non-migratory.

Ancylostoma caninum

Common name: Canine hookworm

Predilection site: Small intestine

Parasite class: Nematoda

Superfamily: Ancylostomatoidea

Description, gross: The worms are reddish grey in colour, depending on whether the worm has fed, and are readily recognised on the basis of size, and by their characteristic 'hook-like' posture. Males are about 12 mm and females 15–20 mm in length, (much smaller than the common ascarid nematodes, which are also found in the small intestine).

Description, microscopic: The anterior end is bent dorsad and the oral aperture is directed antero-dorsally. The buccal capsule is large with three pairs of marginal teeth and a pair of ventro-lateral teeth and possesses a dorsal gutter (Fig. 6.5). The male bursa is well developed. Eggs are 'strongylate' with dissimilar poles, barrel-shaped sidewalls, 56–75 × 34–47 μm and contain two to eight blastomeres.

Hosts: Dog, fox and occasionally man

Life cycle: The life cycle is direct and, given optimal conditions, the eggs may hatch and develop to L_3 in as little as 5 days. Infection is by skin penetration or

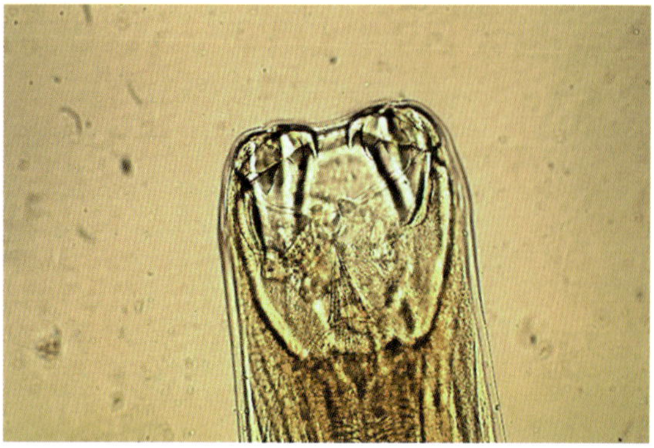

Fig. 6.5 Head of *Ancylostoma caninum* showing the large buccal capsule containing pairs of teeth.

by ingestion, both methods being equally successful. Paratenic hosts can also be important. In percutaneous infection, larvae migrate via the bloodstream to the lungs where they moult to L_4 in the bronchi and trachea, and are then swallowed and pass to the small intestine where the final moult occurs. If infection is by ingestion the larvae may either penetrate the buccal mucosa and undergo the pulmonary migration described above or pass directly to the intestine where the adult worms burrow their buccal capsules into the mucosa. Whichever route is taken, the prepatent period is 14–21 days. The worms are prolific egg layers and an infected dog may pass millions of eggs daily for several weeks.

An important feature of *A. caninum* infection is that, in susceptible bitches, a proportion of the L_3 that reach the lungs migrate to the skeletal muscles where they remain dormant until the bitch is pregnant. They are then reactivated and, still as L_3, are passed in the milk of the bitch for a period of about 3 weeks after whelping. Transplacental transmission does not occur.

Geographical distribution: Worldwide in the tropics and warm temperate areas. In other countries it is sometimes seen in dogs imported from endemic regions.

Pathogenesis: This is essentially that of an acute or chronic haemorrhagic anaemia. The disease is most commonly seen in dogs under 1 year old and young pups, infected by the transmammary route, are particularly susceptible due to their low iron reserves. Transmammary infection is often responsible for severe anaemia in litters of young pups in their second or third week of life. Infection of the bitch on a single occasion has been shown to produce transmammary infections in at least three consecutive litters.

Following infection, blood loss starts about the eighth day of infection when the immature adult has developed the toothed buccal capsule, which enables it to grasp plugs of mucosa containing arterioles. Each worm removes about 0.1 ml of blood daily and in heavy infections of several hundred worms pups quickly become profoundly anaemic. In lighter infections, common in older dogs, the anaemia is not so severe, as the marrow response is able to compensate for a variable period. Ultimately however, the dog may become iron deficient and develop a microcytic hypochromic anaemia. In previously sensitised dogs, skin reactions such as moist eczema and ulceration at the sites of percutaneous infection occur especially affecting the interdigital skin.

It appears that dormant L_3 in the muscles of both bitches and dogs can recommence migration months or years later to mature in the host's intestine. Stress, severe illness or repeated large doses of corticosteroids can all precipitate these apparently new infections in dogs, which may perhaps now be resident in a hookworm-free environment. Experimentally, L_3 of some strains of *A. caninum* exposed to chilling before oral administration have been shown to remain in arrested development in the intestinal mucosa for weeks or months. The significance of this observation is still unknown, but it is thought that such larvae may resume development if the adult hookworm population is removed by an anthelmintic or at times of stress, such as lactation.

Clinical signs: In acute infections, there is anaemia and lassitude and occasionally respiratory embarrassment. In suckled pups the anaemia is often severe and is accompanied by diarrhoea, which may contain blood and mucus. Respiratory signs may be due to larval damage in the lungs or to the anoxic effects of anaemia. In more chronic infections, the animal is usually underweight, the coat is poor, and there is loss of appetite and perhaps pica. Inconsistently there are signs of respiratory embarrassment, skin lesions and lameness. The adverse effects of infection on the coat can have an economic impact where foxes are reared for their fur.

Diagnosis: This depends on the clinical signs and history supplemented by haematological and faecal examination. High faecal worm egg counts are valuable confirmation of diagnosis, but it should be noted that suckled pups may show severe clinical signs before eggs are detected in the faeces. The presence of a few hookworm eggs in the faeces, although giving confirmatory evidence of infection, do not necessarily indicate that an ailing dog is suffering from hookworm disease.

Pathology: Animals dying of ancylostomosis are extremely pale and there is often oedema of subcutaneous tissues and mesenteries, and serous effusion into the body cavities attributable to hypoproteinaemia. In chronic infections, cachexia may be evident. If recent exposure to heavy percutaneous infection has occurred there may be dermatitis and numerous focal haemorrhages in the lung parenchyma. The liver is pale and the intestinal contents are mucoid and red in colour. Worms may be seen attached to the mucosa and pinpoint haemorrhagic sites may be scattered over the intestinal surface.

Epidemiology: In endemic areas the disease is most common in dogs under 1 year old. In older animals, the gradual development of age resistance makes clinical disease less likely, particularly in dogs reared in endemic areas, whose age resistance is reinforced by acquired immunity. The epidemiology is primarily associated with the two main sources of infection, transmammary in suckled pups and percutaneous or oral from the environment. An important aspect of transmammary infection is that disease may occur in suckled pups reared in a clean environment and nursed by a bitch which may have been recently treated with an anthelmintic and has a negative faecal egg count. Contamination of the environment is most likely when dogs are exercised on grass or earth runs that retain moisture and also protect larvae from sunlight. On such surfaces larvae may survive for some weeks. In contrast, dry impervious surfaces, particularly if exposed to sunlight, are lethal to larvae within a day or so. Housing is also important and failure to remove soiled bedding, especially if the kennels are damp or have porous or cracked floors, can lead to a massive build-up of infection.

Treatment: Affected dogs should be treated with an anthelmintic, such as mebendazole, fenbendazole, pyrantel or nitroscanate, all of which will kill both adult and developing intestinal stages; several of the macrocyclic lactones have similar activity. If the disease is severe, it is advisable to give parenteral iron and possibly vitamin B_{12} and to ensure that the dog has a protein-rich diet. Young pups may require a blood transfusion.

Control: A system of regular anthelmintic therapy and hygiene should be adopted. Weaned pups and adult dogs should be treated every 3 months. Pregnant bitches should be dosed at least once during pregnancy with an anthelmintic that has high efficacy against somatic larvae, so as to reduce transmammary infection, and the nursing litters dosed at least twice, at 1–2 weeks of age and again 2 weeks later with a drug specifically recommended for use in pups. This will also help to control ascarid infections. The perinatal transfer of both *Ancylostoma* and *Toxocara* larvae may be reduced by the oral administration of fenbendazole daily from 3 weeks before to 2 days after whelping.

Kennel floors should be free of crevices and dry and the bedding should be disposed of daily. Runs should preferably be of tarmac or concrete and kept as clean and dry as possible; faeces should be removed with a shovel before hosing. If an outbreak has occurred, earth runs may be treated with sodium borate, which is lethal to hookworm larvae, but this also kills grass. A second possibility, which is often used in fox farms, is the provision of wire-mesh flooring in the runs.

Notes: *A. caninum* can occasionally use man as a final host. Although infections do not reach full maturity, they may induce an eosinophilic enteritis.

Ancylostoma braziliense

Common name: Hookworm

Predilection site: Small intestine

Parasite class: Nematoda

Superfamily: Ancylostomatoidea

Description, gross: As for *A. caninum* except it is smaller than either *A. caninum* or *A. tubaeforme*. In the dog, males measure around 7.5 mm and females 9–10 mm in length.

Description, microscopic: The buccal capsule is deep with two pairs of large dorsal and very small ventral teeth. Eggs are similar to *A. caninum*, measuring around 75–95 × 41–45 μm.

Hosts: Dog, cat

Life cycle: Similar in many respects to *A. caninum*, using both oral and percutaneous routes of infection, but transmammary transmission has not been demonstrated. Rodents can act as paratenic hosts. The prepatent period is about 2 weeks in the dog and cat.

Geographical distribution: Tropical and subtropical regions

Pathogenesis: While it may cause a degree of hypoalbuminaemia through an intestinal leak of plasma, it is not a blood sucker and consequently is of little pathogenic significance, causing only mild digestive upsets and occasional diarrhoea. The main importance of *A. braziliense* is that it is regarded as the primary cause of cutaneous larva migrans (CLM) or 'creeping eruption' in man. CLM is characterised by tortuous erythematous inflammatory tracts within the dermis and by severe pruritus, and is caused by infective larvae penetrating the skin and wandering in the dermis. These larvae do not develop, but the skin lesions usually persist for weeks. The severity of the skin lesions relate to the degree of exposure to infective larvae.

Clinical signs: Mild digestive upset and diarrhoea in affected animals. In humans there may be skin erythema and pruritis.

Diagnosis: Worms that have been heat-fixed bend markedly at the position of the vulva. This differs from *A. ceylanicum*.

Pathology: Infected animals may show oedema of subcutaneous tissues and mesenteries, and serous effusion into the body cavities attributable to hypoproteinaemia. If recent exposure to heavy percutaneous infection has occurred there may be dermatitis.

Details of the epidemiology, treatment and control are as for *A. caninum*.

Ancylostoma tubaeforme

Synonym: *Strongylus tubaeformis*

Common name: Feline hookworm

Predilection site: Small intestine

Parasite class: Nematoda

Superfamily: Ancylostomatoidea

Description, gross: Almost identical to *A. caninum*, but slightly smaller, the males measuring around 10 mm and the females 12–15 mm.

Description, microscopic: The buccal capsule is deep with the dorsal gutter ending in a deep notch on the dorsal margin of the buccal capsule, the ventral margin of which bears three teeth on each side. The cuticle is thicker and the deep 'oesophageal' teeth slightly larger than in *A. caninum*. The male bursa is well developed and the spicules are about 50% longer than in *A. caninum*. Eggs are similar to those of *A. caninum* and measure about 56–75 × 34–47 μm.

Hosts: Cat

Life cycle: As for *A. braziliense*. The prepatent period is about 3 weeks.

Geographical distribution: Worldwide

Pathogenesis: *A. tubaeforme* is generally considered to be of low pathogenicity, although heavy infections may lead to a poor coat, anaemia and reduced growth. A strong immunity often develops to infection.

Ancylostoma ceylanicum

Common name: Hookworm

Predilection site: Small intestine

Parasite class: Nematoda

Superfamily: Ancylostomatoidea

Description, gross: Almost identical to *A. braziliense*

Description, microscopic: The cuticular striations are wider than in *A. braziliense*.

Hosts: Dog, cat, wild felids and man.

Life cycle: Similar to *A. braziliense*. The prepatent period is about 2 weeks in the dog.

Geographical distribution: Asia (Malaysia, Sri Lanka)

Pathogenesis: Infections are usually subclinical but heavy infections can induce anaemia and diarrhoea.

Diagnosis: The heat-fixed female worms are not bent as occurs with *A. braziliense*.

Notes: *A. ceylanicum* can complete its life cycle in man and may cause anaemia and abdominal pain and skin penetration by infective larvae may induce cutaneous lesions.

All other details of these two species are in most respects similar to *A. caninum*.

Uncinaria stenocephala

Common name: Northern hookworm

Predilection site: Small intestine

Parasite class: Nematoda

Superfamily: Ancylostomatoidea

Description, gross: A small worm, up to about 1.0 cm long; males are 5–8.5 mm and females 7–12 mm.

Description, microscopic: The adult worms have a large funnel-shaped buccal capsule, which has a pair of chitinous plates, lacks dorsal teeth, but has a pair of sub-ventral teeth at the base (Fig. 6.6). The dorsal cone does not project into the buccal capsule. The male

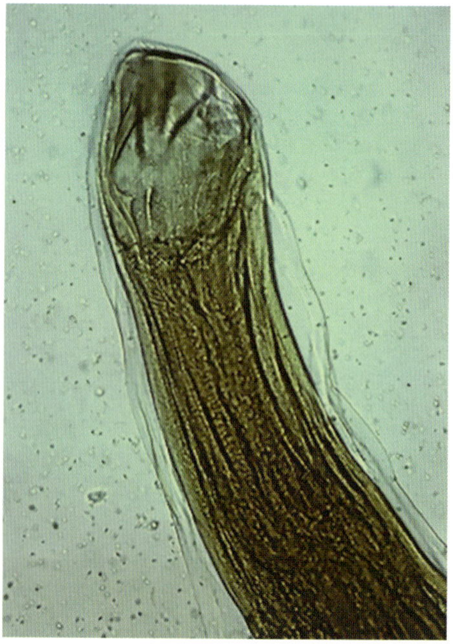

Fig. 6.6 Head of *Uncinaria stenocephala* showing the funnel-shaped buccal capsule and the pair of chitinous plates.

worm has a well developed bursa with a short dorsal lobe and two large and separate lateral lobes and slender spicules. Eggs are ovoidal, $65-80 \times 40-50$ μm.

Hosts: Dog, cat, fox other canids and felids. Various mammals can act as paratenic hosts.

Life cycle: Infection with infective L_3 by oral infection, without pulmonary migration, is the usual route. Although the infective larvae can penetrate the skin, the infection rarely matures and there is no evidence as yet of transmammary or intrauterine transmission. Carnivores may become infected via the consumption of paratenic hosts, such as infected mice. The prepatent period is about 15 days.

Geographical distribution: Temperate and sub-arctic areas, North America and northern Europe

Pathogenesis: The infection is not uncommon in groups of sporting and working dogs. The adult worms attach to the mucosa. They are not voracious blood-suckers like *A. caninum*, but hypoalbuminaemia and low-grade anaemia, accompanied by diarrhoea, anorexia and lethargy, have been recorded in heavily infected pups. Probably the most common lesion in dogs made hypersensitive by previous exposure is pedal dermatitis, affecting particularly the interdigital skin.

Clinical signs: Anaemia, diarrhoea, anorexia, lethargy, interdigital dermatitis

Diagnosis: In areas where *A. caninum* is absent, the clinical signs of the patent infection, together with the demonstration of strongyle eggs in the faeces, is indicative of uncinariosis. Where *Ancylostoma* is also endemic, differential diagnosis may require larval culture, although the treatment is similar.

Pathology: Severe hookworm infections cause villous fusion and atrophy in the small intestine and an inflammatory response in the lamina propria.

Epidemiology: Evidence suggests that in temperate climates like the UK, the seasonal pattern of infective larvae on paddocks used for greyhounds follows that described for gastrointestinal trichostrongyloids in ruminants with a sharp rise in July and a peak in September, suggesting that development to the L_3 is heavily dependent on temperature.

Treatment: Fenbendazole, mebendazole, nitroscanate, piperazine, pyrantel and milbemycin oxime are all active against the northern hookworm.

Control: Regular anthelmintic treatment and good hygiene as outlined for *Ancylostoma* will control *Uncinaria* infection. The combination of ivermectin and pyrantel pamoate or a formulation of chewable ivermectin can give high efficacy. The pedal dermatitis responds poorly to symptomatic treatment, but regresses gradually in the absence of reinfection.

Strongyloides stercoralis

Synonym: *Strongyloides canis, S. intestinalis, Anguillula stercoralis*

Common name: Threadworm

Predilection site: Small intestine

Parasite class: Nematoda

Superfamily: Rhabditoidea

Description, gross: Slender, hair-like worms around 2 mm long. Only females are parasitic.

Description, microscopic: The long oesophagus may occupy up to one third of the body length and the uterus is intertwined with the intestine, giving the appearance of twisted thread. Unlike other intestinal parasites of similar size the tail has a blunt point. *Strongyloides* eggs are oval, thin-shelled and small, $50-58 \times 30-34$ μm. The hatched L_1 is passed out in the faeces.

Hosts: Dog, fox, cat, man

Life cycle: *Strongyloides* is unique among the nematodes of veterinary importance, being capable of both parasitic and free-living reproductive cycles. The parasitic phase is composed entirely of female worms in the small intestine and these produce larvated eggs by parthenogenesis, i.e. development from an unfertilised egg. After hatching, larvae may develop through four larval stages into free-living adult male and female worms and this can be followed by a succession of free-living generations. However under certain conditions, possibly related to temperature and moisture, the L_3 can become parasitic, infecting the host by skin penetration or ingestion and migrating via the venous system, the lungs and trachea to develop into adult female worms in the small intestine. In dogs, autoinfection may occur with L_1 developing rapidly to L_3 in the gut, then penetrating the mucosa of the rectum or perianal skin followed by a pulmonary migration to the gut.

Puppies may acquire infection immediately after birth from the mobilisation of arrested larvae in the tissues of the ventral abdominal wall of the dam, which are subsequently excreted in the milk. The prepatent period is 9 days.

Geographical distribution: Worldwide in warmer climates, Europe (Portugal, France, Poland, Ukraine, Romania, Hungary)

Pathogenesis: Severe infections can occur in dogs, especially in puppies. Mature parasites are found in the duodenum and proximal jejunum and, if present in large numbers, may cause inflammation with oedema and erosion of the epithelium. This results in a catarrhal enteritis with impairment of digestion and absorption.

Table 6.1 *Strongyloides* species reported in cats.

Species	Description	Pathogenicity
S. planiceps	Parasitic females are 2.4–3.3 mm long (mean, 2.8 mm). The tail of the parasitic female narrows abruptly to a blunt tip and the ovaries have a spiral appearance	Non-pathogenic
S. felis (syn *S. cati*)	Similar to *S. planiceps*. Parasitic females of *S. felis* have a long tail narrowing slowly to the tip. Ovaries are straight	Non-pathogenic
S. tumefaciens	Parasitic female is about 5 mm long	Found in tumours in the mucosa of the large intestine

Clinical signs: Bloody diarrhoea, dehydration, sometimes death

Diagnosis: The clinical signs in very young animals, usually within the first few weeks of life, together with the finding of large numbers of the characteristic eggs or larvae in the faeces are suggestive of strongyloidosis.

Pathology: Lesions consist of catarrhal inflammation of the small intestine while in severe infections there may be necrosis and sloughing of the mucosa. Adult worms establish in tunnels in the epithelium at the base of the villi in the small intestine.

Epidemiology: The dog may act as a natural host for this species. Transmission is either by the oral or percutaneous route or by autoinfection. The latter route can lead to cases of persistent strongyloidosis occurring without external reinfection. Unweaned puppies are infected orally from larvae adhering to the teats and with larvae ingested with colostrum. Infection is most commonly seen in the summer when the weather is hot and humid and is frequently a kennel problem.

A strain of *Strongyloides stercoralis* has become adapted to man and usually occurs in warm climates.

Treatment: In dogs, oral fenbendazole at 10–20 mg/kg daily for 3 days is effective. Ivermectin is effective against adult worms.

Control: Disinfection or replacement of kennels and bedding eliminates the sources of infection.

Notes: *S. stercoralis* can cause several forms of disease in man:

1. Penetration and subcutaneous migration of filariform larvae (larval migrans) can cause an itching dermatitis that often resolves spontaneously.
2. Migration in the mucosa of the intestinal tract can cause a chronic intestinal syndrome. Symptoms include sporadic diarrhoea, epigastric abdominal pain, heartburn, bloating and weight loss.
3. A mild transient pulmonary form can occasionally occur that induces mild coughing.
4. Occasionally disseminated infection can induce neurological manifestations, such as Gram-negative polymicrobial meningitis. Less frequently, *S. stercoralis* has been associated with cerebral and cerebellar abscesses.

Three other species of *Strongyloides* are found in cats (see Table 6.1). Details of the life cycle, diagnosis, treatment and control of these species are as for *S. stercoralis*.

Trichinella spiralis

See Chapter 5 (Pigs).

Alaria alata

Common name: Intestinal carnivore fluke

Predilection site: Small intestine

Parasite class: Trematoda

Family: Diplostomatidae

Description, gross: Adult flukes are 2–6 mm in length and the flat expanded anterior part is much longer than the posterior cylindrical part.

Description, microscopic: At the anterior lateral corners of the anterior part there are two tentacle-like processes. The suckers are very small and the adhesive organ consists of two long folds with distinct lateral margins. The eggs are large, 98–134 μm × 62–68 μm, operculate and unembryonated.

Final hosts: Dog, cat, fox, mink, wild carnivores and rarely man

Intermediate hosts: 1. Fresh water snails (*Planorbis* spp). 2. Frogs and toads.

Life cycle: Eggs are passed in the faeces from which miracidia eventually hatch and enter fresh water snails (*Planorbis*). Sporocysts produce cercariae with bifurcated tails. These leave the snail and infect tadpoles or frogs where the cercariae encyst in the muscles forming mesocercariae. If a frog, snake or mouse eats the tadpole, the mesocercariae become encysted, these animals acting as paratenic hosts. Dogs and foxes may be infected by eating rodents infected with mesocercariae. Once infected the mesocercariae migrate extensively, including passage through the lungs and diaphragm, becoming metacercariae before returning to the small intestine and maturing into flukes. The prepatent period is 1–2 weeks.

Geographical distribution: Eastern Europe

Pathogenesis: Adult fluke attach to the mucous membrane of the small intestine (Fig. 6.7) but cause little harm. However the migratory mesocercariae may cause clinical symptoms. Heavy infections may cause a severe duodenitis and pulmonary damage in dogs and cats. A fatal case has been recorded in man through eating inadequately cooked frogs' legs; the principal lesions were in the lungs.

Clinical signs: Infection is not usually associated with clinical signs.

Diagnosis: Diagnosis is by identifying the presence of eggs in the faeces.

Pathology: Effects are generally limited to the attachment of flukes to the intestinal mucosa and may include local irritation, erosion and ulceration and the production of excessive intestinal mucus and, rarely, haemorrhagic enteritis.

Epidemiology: Infection is maintained in endemic areas where intermediate hosts are abundant. Transmammary infection has been reported with some species in cats and rodents.

Treatment: Treatment with praziquantel or niclosamide is recommended.

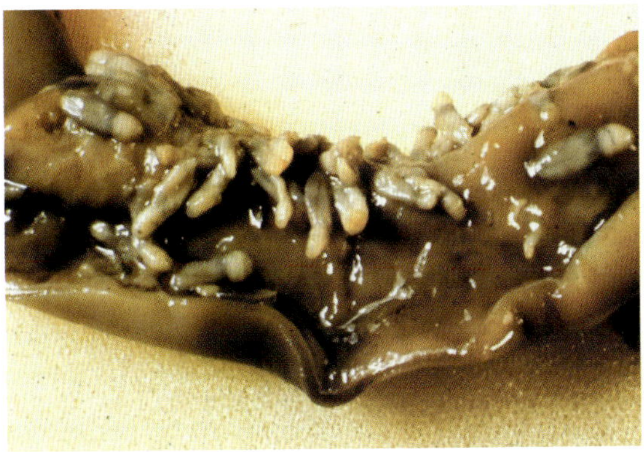

Fig. 6.7 *Alaria* spp attached to the mucosa of the small intestine.

Control: Dogs and cats should be prevented from catching or consuming paratenic hosts such as frogs, rodents and snakes.

Nanophyetus salmincola

Synonym: *Troglotrema salmincola*

Predilection site: Small intestine

Parasite class: Trematoda

Family: Troglotrematidae

Description, gross: The fluke is small, oval, white or cream in colour, about 1–2.5 mm long × 0.3 mm wide.

Description, microscopic: The large testes are oval and situated side by side in the posterior third of the segment. Eggs are yellowish brown in colour, unembryonated and measure about 64–80 × 34–50 μm. They have an indistinct operculum and a small rounded abopercular knob.

Final hosts: Dog, cat, racoon, mink, bear, lynx, other fish-eating mammals and rarely man

Intermediate hosts: 1. Snails (*Oxytrema silicula*, *Goniobasis*, *Semisulcospira* spp). 2. Various salmonid fish

Life cycle: Eggs are passed in the faeces of the host and after hatching, which takes about 3 months, infect the snail first intermediate host. The liberated cercariae swim for a while before penetrating a fish, encysting in the kidneys, muscles and other organs. Infection of the final host occurs when the fish is eaten. The prepatent period is as short as 5 days in the dog.

Geographical distribution: North America (northwest Pacific) and eastern Russia.

Pathogenesis: The trematodes penetrate deeply into the mucosa of the duodenum or attach to the mucosa of other parts of the small or large intestine. In large numbers they produce a superficial enteritis which may lead to haemorrhagic enteritis. The real importance of *N. salmincola* lies in its ability to transmit *Neorickettsia helminthoeca* the agent of 'salmon poisoning', which frequently produces severe and fatal infections in dogs, foxes and other animals.

Clinical signs: The presence of large numbers of flukes may cause diarrhoea. With complicated infections involving *Neorickettsia helminthoeca*, there is a sudden onset of fever and complete loss of appetite. Within a few days there is purulent discharge from the eyes, vomiting and profuse diarrhoea, which may be haemorrhagic. Mortality varies from 50–90% of infected animals.

Diagnosis: Diagnosis is by identifying the presence of eggs in the faeces.

Table 6.2 Intestinal flukes of dogs and cats.

Species	Final hosts	Intermediate hosts	Distribution
Family: Diplostomatidae			
Alaria alata	Dog, cat, fox, mink, wild carnivores, man	1. Snails 2. Frogs and toads	Eastern Europe
Alaria americana	Dog, fox and other canids	1. Snails 2. Frogs and toads	North America
Alaria minnesotae	Cat, skunk	1. Snails 2. Frogs and toads	North America
Alaria canis	Dog, fox	1. Snails 2. Frogs and toads	North America
Alaria michiganensis	Dog, fox	1. Snails 2. Frogs and toads	North America
Alaria marcianae	Cat	1. Snails 2. Frogs and toads	North America
Family: Troglotrematidae			
Nanophyetus salmincola	Dog, cat, racoon, mink, bear, lynx, fish-eating mammals and rarely man	1. Snails 2. Fish	North America, eastern Russia
Family: Heterophyidae			
Heterophyes heterophyes	Dog, cat, fox, man	1. Snails 2. Fish	Egypt, Asia
Heterophyes nocens	Dog, cat, fox, man	1. Snails 2. Fish	Egypt, Asia
Metagonimus yokagawai	Dog, cat, pig, man	1. Snails 2. Fish	Asia, Balkans
Cryptocotyle lingua	Gulls, terns, kittiwake, seal, mink, dog, cat	1. Shellfish 2. Fish	Europe (Germany, Denmark, UK)
Apophallus muhlingi	Gulls, cormorants, dog, cat	1. Unknown 2. Fish	Europe
Apophallus (*Rossicotrema*) *donicum*	Cat, dog, fox, seal	1. Unknown 2. Fish	Europe, North America
Family: Echinosomatidae			
Echinochasmus perfoliatus	Dog, cat, fox, pig	1. Snails 2. Fish	Europe Asia
Euparyphium melis	Cat, fox, polecat, mink, badger, otter, hedgehog	1. Snail 2. Tadpole	Europe
Euparyphium ilocanum	Dog, rat, man	1. Snail 2. Freshwater molluscs	Europe

Pathology: In large numbers, superficial enteritis leading to haemorrhagic enteritis may occur.

Epidemiology: Infection is maintained in endemic areas where intermediate hosts are abundant.

Treatment: Since the rickettsial organisms cause the main pathogenic effects, tetracycline therapy is indicated. High doses of albendazole or fenbendazole over a prolonged period can be effective in treating the fluke infections.

Control: Dogs and cats should not be fed raw fish and should be kept away from salmon rivers and streams.

Notes: *Nanophyetus* can occasionally infect man where it penetrates between the villi and causes inflamation and necrosis of the mucosa.

Several other trematodes parasitise the small intestine of dogs and cats and other definitive hosts, including birds and man, but they are usually of minor veterinary significance and are only briefly summarised in Table 6.2.

Diphyllobothrium latum

Common name: Broad tapeworm

Predilection site: Small intestine

Parasite class: Cestoda

Family: Diphyllobothriidae

Description, gross: A very long, ivory coloured, tapeworm, up to 20 m in length, with several hundred proglottids. The scolex is unarmed with two muscular longitudinal grooves or bothria as organs of attachment.

Description, microscopic: The mature and gravid segments are rectangular-shaped with a central genital pore, being broader than they are long. Eggs are yellow, ovoid, operculate and measure around 70×50 μm.

Final hosts: Man and fish-eating mammals, such as the dog, cat, pig and polar bear

Intermediate hosts: 1. Copepods. 2. Freshwater fish (pike, trout, perch)

Life cycle: Eggs are continuously discharged from the genital pores of the attached gravid segments of the strobila and pass to the exterior in the faeces. They resemble *F. hepatica* eggs being yellow and operculate, but are approximately half the size. The eggs must develop in water and within a few weeks each hatches to liberate a motile ciliated coracidium, which, if ingested by a copepod, develops into the first parasitic larval stage, a procercoid. When the copepod is ingested by a freshwater fish, the procercoid migrates to the muscles or viscera to form the second larval stage, the plerocercoid; this solid larval metacestode is about 5.0 mm long and possesses the characteristic scolex. The life cycle is completed when the infected fish is eaten raw, or insufficiently cooked, by the final host. Development to patency is rapid, occurring within 4 weeks of ingestion of the plerocercoid. However, if the infected fish is eaten by a larger fish, the plerocercoid has the ability to establish itself in its new host.

Geographical distribution: Parts of Scandinavia, Russia, Japan and North America

Pathogenesis and clinical signs: In man, infections are often asymptomatic but there can be fatigue, dyspepsia, vomiting and transient diarrhoea. Infection is usually asymptomatic in animals although occasionally vitamin B_{12} deficiency can occur.

Diagnosis: This depends on the detection of the characteristic eggs in the faeces.

Pathology: Does not induce damage to the intestine.

Epidemiology: *D. latum* is essentially a parasite of man since in other hosts the cestode produces few fertile eggs. The epidemiology is therefore largely centred around two factors, the access of human sewage to freshwater lakes and the ingestion of uncooked fish. Domestic animals, such as dogs or pigs, become infected by eating raw fish or fish offal.

Treatment: Praziquantel and niclosamide are effective against the adult tapeworm.

Control: In areas where infection is common, domestic animals should not be fed fish products unless these have been thoroughly cooked or deep-frozen.

Notes: *Diphyllobothrium latum* is an important cestode parasite of the small intestine of man in northern climates; it may also infect other fish-eating mammals.

Dipylidium caninum

Common name: Double-pored or cucumber seed tapeworm

Predilection site: Small intestine

Parasite class: Cestode

Family: Dilepididae

Description, gross: *Dipylidium* is a much shorter tapeworm than *Taenia*, the maximum length being about 80 cm.

Description, microscopic: The scolex has a protrusible rostellum, which is armed with four or five rows of small rose-thorn shaped hooks (Fig. 6.8). The proglottid is easily recognised, being elongate, like a large rice grain, and has two sets of genital organs, with a pore opening on each margin. Eggs containing a hexacanth embryo are 25–50 μm and are contained in an egg capsule containing up to 30 eggs (Fig. 6.9).

Final hosts: Dog, fox and cat; rarely man

Intermediate hosts: Fleas (*Ctenocephalides* spp, *Pulex irritans*) and lice (*Trichodectes canis*)

Life cycle: The newly passed segments are active, and can crawl about on the tail region of the animal. The oncospheres are contained in egg packets or capsules, each with about 20 eggs, and these are either expelled by the active segment or released by its disintegration.

After ingestion by the intermediate host, the oncospheres travel to the abdominal cavity where they develop into cysticercoids. All stages of the biting

Table 6.3 Tapeworms of dogs and cats.

Genus	Species	Hosts	Intermediate hosts	Infective larva	
				Name	Site
Echinococcus	*granulosus*	Dog (wolf, fox, jackal, dingo, hyena)	Livestock, man	Hydatidosis, hydatid cyst	Liver, lungs, etc.
Echinococcus	*multilocularis*	Fox, dog, cat	Rodents, man, (pig, horse)	Alveolar echinococcus	Liver, lungs, etc.
Echinococcus	*vogeli*	Bush dog, dog, rarely man	Rodents	Hydatid	Liver, lung and other visceral organs
Echinococcus	*oligarthus*	Cougar, jaguar, ocelot and other felids	Rodents	Hydatid	Viscera, musculature and skin
Taenia	*pisiformis*	Dog, fox	Rabbit	*Cysticercus pisiformis*	Abdominal cavity, liver
Taenia	*hydatigena*	Dog, fox	Livestock	*Cysticercus tenuicollis*	Abdominal cavity, liver
Taenia (syn. *Multiceps*)	*multiceps*	Dog	Sheep, cattle, man	*Coenurus cerebralis*	Brain, spinal cord
Taenia (syn. *Multiceps*)	*skrjabini*	Dog, fox	Sheep	*Coenurus skrjabini*	Muscle, subcutis
Taenia	*cervi*	Fox, dog	Deer, roe deer	*Cysticercus cervi*	Muscle
Taenia	*krabbei*	Dog	Reindeer	*Cysticercus tarandi*	Muscle
Taenia	*ovis*	Dog, fox	Sheep, goat	*Cysticercus ovis*	Muscle
Taenia	*crassiceps*	Fox, dog	Small rodents	*Cysticercus longicollis*	Abdominal cavity
Taenia (syn. *Hydatigera*)	*taeniaeformis*	Cat	Small rodents	*Strobilocercus fasciolaris* syn. *crassicollis*	Liver
Taenia	*serialis*	Dog	Rabbit	*Coenurus serialis*	Connective tissue
Taenia	*hyaenae*	Hyena	Camel (dromedary)	*Cysticercus dromedarii*	Muscle, liver
Dipylidium	*caninum*	Dog, cat, fox	Flea, louse	Cysticercoid	Abdominal cavity
Mesocestoides	*lineatus*	Dog, fox, cat	1. Oribatid mite 2. Mammals, reptiles, frogs, birds	Tetrathyridium	Abdominal cavity, liver
Diphyllobothrium	*latum*	Man, dog, pig, cat	1. Copepods 2. Fish	Plerocercoid	Abdominal cavity, Muscle
Spirometra	*mansoni*	Dogs, cat, wild carnivores, and occasionally man	1. Copepods 2. Amphibians, reptiles, birds	Plerocercoid	Muscles, subcutaneous tissues
Spirometra	*mansonoides*	Cat, bobcat and occasionally dog	1. Crustacea 2. Rats, mice, snakes	Plerocercoid	Muscles, subcutaneous tissues
Spirometra	*erinacei*	Cat, fox	1. Crustacea 2. Frogs	Plerocercoid	Muscles, subcutaneous tissues

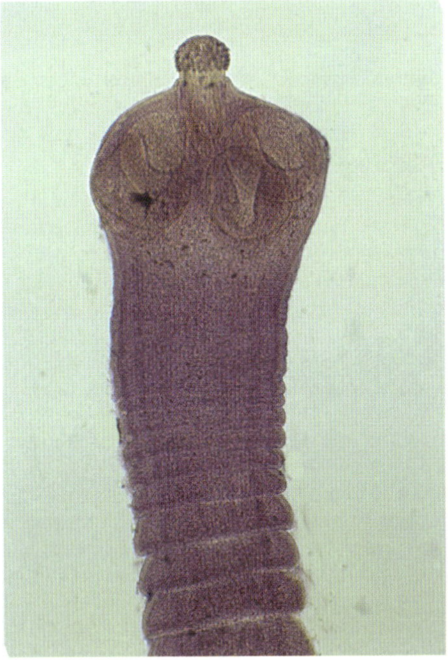

Fig. 6.8 Head of *Dipylidium caninum* showing the protrusible rostellum.

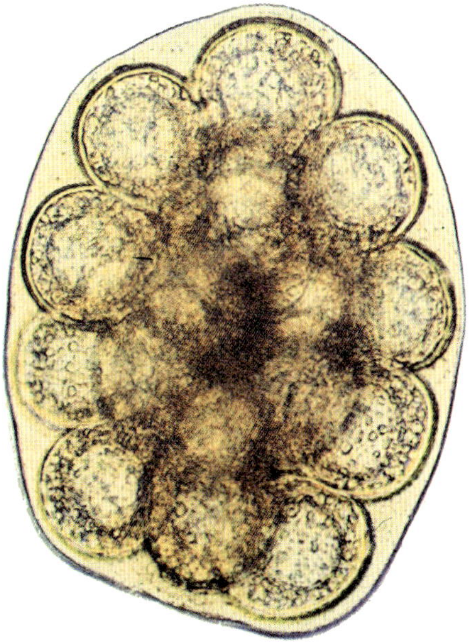

Fig. 6.9 Egg capsule of *Dipylidium caninum*.

louse can ingest oncospheres, but the adult flea, with its mouthparts adapted for piercing, cannot do so, and infection is only acquired during the larval stage, which has chewing mouthparts. Development in the louse, which is permanently parasitic and therefore enjoys a warm habitat, takes about 30 days, but in the flea larva and the developing adult in the cocoon, both of which are on the ground, development may extend over several months. The final host is infected by ingestion of the flea or louse containing the cysticercoids. Development to patency, when the first gravid segments are shed, takes about 3 weeks.

Geographical distribution: Worldwide

Pathogenesis: The adult is non-pathogenic and several hundreds can be tolerated without clinical effect. They shed segments, which, as they crawl actively from the anus, may cause some discomfort, and a useful sign of infection is excessive grooming of the perineum. It has been suggested that infected dogs form the habit of rubbing the anus along the floor, but impacted anal glands are a more common cause of this behaviour.

Clinical signs: Anal discomfort, itching

Diagnosis: Often the first indication of infection is the presence of a segment on the coat around the perineum. If the segment is freshly passed, preliminary identification may be made on the elongate shape, and the double genital organs, which may be seen with a hand lens. If it is dried and distorted it will be necessary to break it up with mounted needles in water, where the egg packets are easily seen under the microscope, thus differentiating the segment from that of *Taenia* spp, which contains only numerous single oncospheres.

Pathology: Adult tapeworms are of little pathogenic significance.

Epidemiology: *Dipylidium* infection is very common and, being dependent on the continuous presence of ectoparasites for its local endemicity, it is more prevalent in neglected animals, though infestations are also seen in well kept dogs and cats.

Treatment and control: In *Dipylidium* infection, treatment and control must be instituted together, for it is clearly of no value to eliminate the adult tapeworm while leaving a reservoir in the animal's ectoparasites. Hence, administration of anthelmintics, such as nitroscanate and praziquantel, should be accompanied by the use of insecticides. It is also imperative that the animal's bedding and customary resting places should receive attention with insecticides to eliminate the immature stages of the flea, which are many times more numerous than the adult parasites feeding on the dog or cat.

Notes: This is the commonest tapeworm genus of the domestic dog and cat

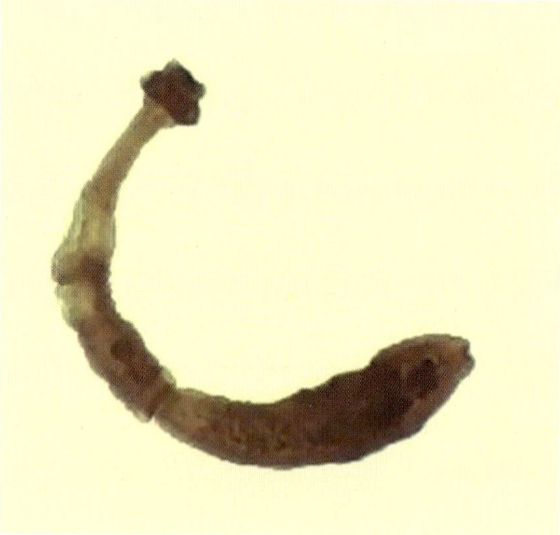

Fig. 6.10 *Echinococcus granulosus* showing the scolex, and the large gravid posterior proglottid.

Echinococcus granulosus

Subspecies: *granulosus*

Subspecies: *equinus*

Common name: Dwarf dog tapeworm, hydatidosis

Predilection site: Anterior small intestine (final host); mainly liver and lungs (intermediate host)

Parasite class: Cestoda

Family: Taeniidae

Description, gross: The entire cestode is only about 6.0 mm long, and is therefore difficult to find in the freshly opened intestine. It consists of a scolex and three or four segments, the terminal gravid one occupying about half the length of the complete tapeworm (Fig. 6.10).

'Hydatid' cysts are large fluid-filled vesicles, 5–10 cm in diameter.

Description, microscopic: The scolex is typically taeniid and the rostellum has two rows of hooks, varying from 30–60 in number. Each segment has a single genital opening, with the penultimate segment sexually mature and the last segment gravid. The genital pores alternate irregularly. For more detailed morphology of hydatid cysts see description of *E. granulosus* in Chapter 3 (Sheep and goats).

The eggs are typically 'taenid' and measure 32–36 × 25–30 μm and the embryophore is radially striated with a six-hooked oncosphere.

Final hosts: *E. granulosus granulosus*: dog and many wild canids; *E. granulosus equinus*: dog and red fox

Intermediate hosts: *E. granulosus granulosus*: domestic and wild ruminants, man and primates, pig and lagomorphs; horses and donkeys are resistant. *E. granulosus equinus*: horse and donkey

Life cycle: The prepatent period in the final host is around 40–50 days, after which only one gravid segment is shed per week. The oncospheres are capable of prolonged survival outside the host, being viable on the ground for about 2 years. After ingestion by the intermediate host, the oncosphere penetrates the gut wall and travels in the blood to the liver, or in the lymph to the lungs. These are the two commonest sites for larval development, but occasionally oncospheres escape into the general systemic circulation and develop in other organs and tissues.

Growth of the hydatid within intermediate hosts is slow, maturity being reached in 6–12 months. In the liver and lungs the cyst may have a diameter of up to 20 cm, but in the rarer sites, such as the abdominal cavity where unrestricted growth is possible, it may be very large, and contain several litres of fluid. The cyst capsule consists of an outer membrane and an inner germinal epithelium from which, when cyst growth is almost complete, brood capsules each containing a number of scolices are budded off. Many of these brood capsules become detached and exist free in the hydatid fluid; collectively these and the scolices are often referred to as 'hydatid sand'.

Sometimes, complete daughter cysts are formed either inside the mother cyst or externally; in the latter case they may be carried to other parts of the body to form new hydatids.

Geographical distribution: *E. granulosus granulosus*: worldwide; *E. granulosus equinus*: mainly Europe

Pathogenesis: The adult tapeworm is not pathogenic, and thousands may be present in a dog without clinical signs. In domestic animals the hydatid in the liver or lungs is usually tolerated without any clinical signs, and the majority of infections are only revealed at the abattoir. Where oncospheres have been carried in the circulation to other sites, such as the kidney, pancreas, CNS or marrow cavity of long bones, pressure by the growing cyst may cause a variety of clinical signs.

In contrast, when man is involved as an intermediate host, the hydatid in its pulmonary or hepatic site is often of pathogenic significance. One or both lungs may be affected causing respiratory symptoms, and if several hydatids are present in the liver there may be gross abdominal distension. If a cyst should rupture there is a risk of death from anaphylaxis or if the person survives, released daughter cysts may resume development in other regions of the body.

Clinical signs: Asymptomatic in the dog and infection in cattle or sheep is also generally not associated with clinical signs. Human infection can result in respiratory distress or abdominal enlargement depending on whether the lungs or liver are infected.

Diagnosis: Diagnosis of infection in dogs with adult tapeworms is difficult, because the segments are small and are only shed sparsely. When found, identification is based on their size (2.0–3.0 mm), ovoid shape and single genital pore.

In some countries control regimes have involved the administration of purgative anthelmintics, such as arecoline hydrochloride, so that the whole tapeworm is expelled in mucus and can be searched for in the faeces. If a necropsy is available the small intestine should be opened and immersed in shallow water, when the attached tapeworms will be seen as small slender papillae. Immunodiagnostic tests have been developed that are based on the faecal antigen detection antibody sandwich ELISA technique.

Pathology: No reported pathology in the final hosts.

Epidemiology:

- *E. granulosus granulosus*. Only a few countries, notably Iceland and Eire, are free from this strain of *E. granulosus*. It is customary to consider the epidemiology as being based on two cycles, pastoral and sylvatic. In the pastoral cycle the dog is always involved, being infected by the feeding of ruminant offal containing hydatid cysts. The domestic intermediate host will vary according to the local husbandry but the most important is the sheep, which appears to be the natural intermediate host, scolices from these animals being the most highly infective for dogs. In parts of the Middle East the camel is the main reservoir of hydatids, while in northern Europe and northern Russia it is the reindeer. The pastoral cycle is the primary source of hydatidosis in man, infection being by accidental ingestion of oncospheres from the coats of dogs, or from vegetables and other foodstuffs contaminated by dog faeces. The sylvatic cycle occurs in wild canids and ruminants and is based on predation or carrion feeding. It is less important as a source of human infection, except in hunting communities where the infection may be introduced to domestic dogs by the feeding of viscera of wild ruminants.
- *E. granulosus equinus*. Equine hydatidosis is commonest in Europe, and in other parts of the world most cases have been recorded in imported European horses. The strain is highly specific for the horse and the eggs do not develop in the sheep. The domestic dog and the red fox are the final hosts, and the cycle in countries of high prevalence depends on access by dogs to infected equine viscera. On mainland Europe, the most likely source is offal from horse abattoirs and in Britain the viscera of hunting horses, which are fed to foxhounds. The horse strain does not appear to be infective to man.

Treatment: *Echinococcus* tapeworms are more difficult to remove than *Taenia*, but several drugs, notably praziquantel, are now available which are highly effective. After treatment it is advisable to confine dogs for 48 hours to facilitate the collection and disposal of infected faeces. In man, hydatid cysts may be excised surgically, although mebendazole, albendazole and praziquantel therapies have been reported to be effective.

Control: This is based on the regular treatment of dogs to eliminate the adult tapeworms and on the prevention of infection in dogs by exclusion from their diet of animal material containing hydatids. This is achieved by denying dogs access to abattoirs, and where possible, by proper disposal of sheep carcases on farms. In some countries these measures have been supported by legislation, with penalties when they are disregarded. In countries where no specific measures for hydatid control exist, it has been found that an incidental benefit from the destruction of stray dogs for rabies control has been a great reduction in the incidence of hydatid infection in humans.

A recombinant DNA vaccine has been developed for *Echinococcus granulosus* but it requires further refinement for practical application and it is currently not available commercially.

Notes: Two biotypes have been described. The 'European' biotype is the most common and involves the dog and a wide variety of domestic livestock intermediate hosts. The dog–sheep cycle is infective to man. Less dominant is the 'Northern' biotype that involves the wolf–reindeer or wolf–moose cycles and is not considered a danger to man.

Echinococcus multilocularis

Common name: Dwarf fox tapeworm, alveolar ecchinococcosis

Predilection site: Lower small intestine (final hosts); liver also lungs, brain, muscles, lymph nodes (intermediate hosts)

Parasite class: Cestoda

Family: Taeniidae

Description, gross: *E. multilocularis* is a very small tapeworm (2–4 mm) and is generally similar to *E. granulosus*, but usually with three to five segments, the terminal one measuring less than half the length of the whole worm.

Description, microscopic: The scolex has four suckers and possesses a double row of large and small hooks. The third segment of the adult tapeworm is sexually mature and the genital pores are in front of the middle of each segment. The uterus is sac-like with no lateral sacculations in the terminal proglottid. Gravid segments contain around 200–300 spherical eggs. Eggs that are shed have a diameter of about 30–40 μm. The structure of the metacestode consists of a germinative gelatinous matrix that forms multiple compartments.

Final hosts: Wild canids (primarily foxes but in some areas coyote, wolf and raccoon dog may be involved), domestic dog and cat, although the cat is a less suitable host than canids.

Intermediate hosts: Mainly microtine rodents, such as voles, muskrats and lemmings, and insectivores; some of the larger mammals, including man, are also susceptible.

Life cycle: *E. multilocularis* is typically maintained in a sylvatic (wildlife) cycle, although in some rural communities a synanthropic cycle occurs with the domestic dog acting as definitive host. The intermediate host is infected by ingestion of the oncosphere and subsequent passage, via the circulatory system, to the liver where it develops into a multilocular or alveolar cyst (metacestode stage). The cycle is completed when the definitive host consumes an infected intermediate host, the mature tapeworm developing in about 5 weeks. Adult tapeworms are relatively short lived, about 6 months.

Geographical distribution: Northern hemisphere, including North America, Greenland, Scandinavia, central Europe, Russia, Middle East; also India, China and Japan

Pathogenesis: The larval metacestode stage develops primarily in the liver as the so-called multilocular or alveolar cyst, a diffuse growth with many compartments containing a gelatinous matrix into which the protoscolices are budded off. Growth of the intermediate stage is invasive, extending locally and capable of systemic metastases to other sites such as lungs, brain, muscles and lymph nodes. These hydatids are the causative agent of alveococcosis or alveolar echinococcosis.

Clinical signs: Usually asymptomatic in the definitive host. In the intermediate host, clinical signs are dependent on the level of infection and the location of the metacestode stages. Infection in man often presents with few signs until the infection has markedly progressed. The slow infiltration of organs may cause symptoms resembling those of a slow-growing carcinoma.

Diagnosis: The sedimentation and counting technique at necropsy is the well established method for the detection of intestinal *E. multilocularis* in the definitive host, although the intestinal scraping technique is also useful. More recent research techniques include the detection of copro-DNA by PCR and the detection of *E. multilocularis* specific copro-antigen in an ELISA based assay.

Serological and PCR-based tests are available for the early detection of infection in man.

Pathology: The adult tapeworm causes little damage in the intestine of the definitive host.

In the liver, invasion by the metacestode stage can result in atrophy of the parenchyma and cause cirrhosis. Expansion of alveolar echinococcus in the liver produces aggregates of small gelatinous cysts that appear similar to malignant neoplasia.

Epidemiology: Though *E. multilocularis* has a wide distribution in the northern hemisphere, it is essentially a parasite of tundra regions with its greatest prevalence in the subarctic regions of Canada, Alaska and Russia. Its basic epidemiological cycle in these regions is in the arctic fox and wolf, and their prey, small rodents and insectivores. In North America, its range is extending south from Canada into the United States where the red fox and coyote act as final hosts. The cycle is therefore sylvatic, and most cases in humans occur in trappers and their families following contact with the contaminated fur of foxes and wolves. However, eating vegetables or fruit contaminated by infected foxes seeking garden voles, may occasionally infect suburban man.

Over the last decade the population of red foxes has expanded in Europe and foxes have also extended their distribution into urban and peri-urban areas. The demonstration of an urban wildlife cycle of *E. multilocularis* in foxes has implications for human health in areas where this parasite is endemic. In addition, the expansion of the synanthropic cycle, involving domestic dogs that prey on metacestode-infected rodents, may lead to an increase in the prevalence of human alveolar echinococcosis. *E. multilocularis* egg contamination has been predicted to be maximal where the urban and rural habitats overlap.

Treatment: Dogs and cats can be treated with praziquantel or epsiprantel. Treatment of domestic intermediate hosts is not advised. The invasive growth in man simulates malignant neoplasia, and because of its infiltrative spread in tissues and its readiness to develop metastatically, surgery is not advisable; instead treatment with mebendazole or praziquantel is recommended.

Control: Because of the large sylvatic reservoir, control of *E. multilocularis* is unlikely ever to be achieved. Precautionary measures include:

(1) The wearing of protective rubber gloves when handling fresh skins/furs of foxes, wolves etc.

(2) The thorough washing of forest fruits and berries prior to consumption in regions where infection is endemic.
(3) The treatment of dogs and cats with an effective cestocidal anthelmintic.

Two further species of *Echinococcus* occur, *E. oligarthrus* and *E. vogeli*. These are briefly summarised below. The metacestode stages can establish and develop in man. Intermediate hosts include rodents such as the paca (*Cuniculus paca*), spiny rat (*Proechimys guyannensis*) and agouti (*Dasyprocta* spp).

Echinococcus vogeli

Predilection site: Small intestine (final hosts); liver, lung and other visceral organs (intermediate hosts)

Parasite class: Cestoda

Family: Taeniidae

Description, gross: *E. vogeli* is a very small tapeworm (4–6 mm) and usually has three segments, the terminal gravid segment being very long in comparison to the rest of the tapeworm.

Description, microscopic: The uterus is sac-like, long and tubular in shape. The metacestode has a polycystic structure.

Final hosts: Bush dog (*Speothos venaticus*) and occasionally domestic dog. Man can be an accidental host.

Geographical distribution: Central and South America

Echinococcus oligarthrus

Predilection site: Small intestine (final hosts); viscera, musculature and skin (intermediate hosts)

Parasite class: Cestoda

Family: Taeniidae

Description, gross: *E. oligarthrus* is an extremely small tapeworm (2.5–3.0 mm) and usually has three segments.

Description, microscopic: The uterus is sac-like in the gravid proglottid. The metacestode is polycystic in form.

Final hosts: Cougar, jaguar, ocelot and other felids; man can be an accidental host.

Geographical distribution: Central and South America

Other details for both species are similar to those for *E. multilocularis*

Spirometra mansoni

Predilection site: Small intestine

Parasite class: Cestoda

Family: Diphyllobothriidae

Description, gross: The adult tapeworms are very similar to *Diphyllobothrium*. The plerocercoids, also called spargana, are white, ribbon-like, crinkled and can measure around 300–400 mm.

Description, microscopic: The tapeworm possesses both a uterine and a vaginal pore and the uterus is spiral in shape. Eggs have pointed ends.

Final hosts: Dogs, cat, wild carnivores and occasionally man

Intermediate hosts: 1. Copepods. 2. Amphibia, reptiles, birds and mammals

Life cycle: The morphology and life cycle of these tapeworms is similar to that of *D. latum*, the procercoids being found in crustaceans, such as Cyclops, and the plerocercoids in a wide variety of hosts. These can also act as paratenic hosts. The plerocercoids can also transfer between intermediate hosts.

Geographical distribution: South America and Asia

Pathogenesis and pathology: The tapeworm usually causes little effect in the intestine of dogs and cats.

Clinical signs: Usually asymptomatic in animals.

Notes: Other details are similar in most respects to *D. latum*. Occasionally, man may become infected with plerocercoids, either through drinking water containing procercoid-infected crustacea or from eating a plerocercoid-infected host such as a pig. This zoonosis, known as sparganosis (*Sparganum* was the old name for these plerocercoids), is characterised by the presence of larvae up to 35 mm long in the muscles and subcutaneous tissues, particularly the periorbital area, causing oedema and inflammation. Occasionally the spargana disintegrates into several pieces (proliferating disease), which develop separately, and this can be fatal.

Other species of *Spirometra* found in dogs and cats are detailed in Table 6.4.

Taenia hydatigena

Synonym: *Taenia marginata*, *Cysticercus tenuicollis*

Predilection site: Small intestine (final hosts); abdominal cavity, liver (intermediate hosts)

Parasite class: Cestoda

Family: Taeniidae

Description, gross: *T. hydatigena* is a large tapeworm measuring up to 5 m in length. The scolex is large and has two rows of 26 and 46 rostellar hooks. Gravid proglottids are 12 × 6 mm and the uterus has five to ten lateral branches.

Description, microscopic: Eggs are oval or elliptical and measure 36–39 × 34–35 μm.

Table 6.4 Species of *Spirometra* found in dogs and cats.

Species	Final hosts	Intermediate hosts	Distribution
Spirometra mansoni	Dogs, cat, wild carnivores, and occasionally man	1. Copepods 2. Amphibia, reptiles, birds	South America and Asia
Spirometra mansonoides	Cat, bobcat and occasionally dog	1. Crustacea 2. Rats, snakes, mice	North America
Spirometra erinacei	Cat, fox	1. Crustacea 2. Frogs	Far East, Australia

Final hosts: Dog, fox, weasel, stoat, polecat, wolf, hyena

Intermediate hosts: Sheep, cattle, deer, pig, horse

Life cycle: Dogs and wild canids are infested by consuming the cysticercus in the intermediate host. The intermediate host is infected through the ingestion of tapeworm eggs that hatch in the intestine. The oncospheres, infective to sheep, cattle and pigs, are carried in the blood to the liver in which they migrate for about 4 weeks before they emerge on the surface of this organ and attach to the peritoneum. Within a further 4 weeks each develops into the characteristically large metacestode, *Cysticercus tenuicollis*.

Geographical distribution: Worldwide

Pathogenesis and clinical signs: Adult tapeworms in dogs are usually asymptomatic. However, in heavy infections there may be gastrointestinal disturbances such as diarrhoea, abdominal pain and anal pruritis that result from the migration of proglottids from the perianal area.

Diagnosis: Often the first signs of tapeworm infection in dogs is the presence of proglottids in the faeces or more frequently the perianal area as a result of the active migration of the segments.

Pathology: Usually causes little damage to the intestine although there have been occasional reports of obstruction when several worm are present.

Epidemiology: If untreated, the final host can harbour tapeworms from several months to a year or more.

Treatment: Tapeworms can be removed from dogs through the administration of an effective cestocidal anthelmintic, such as niclosamide, praziquantel, nitroscanate or multiple doses of mebendazole or fenbendazole (Table 6.5). No practical treatment is available for the intermediate host.

Table 6.5 Tapeworm treatments for dogs and cats.

Anthelmintic	Dose rate (mg/kg)	*Taenia* spp	*Echinococcus* spp	*Dipylidium*	Comments
Praziquantel	5 (oral) 8 (spot on) 3.5–7.5 (inj)	+ + +	+ + +	+ + +	Good activity against *E. multilocularis*
Dichlorophen	200	+		+	
Nitroscanate	50	+	(+)	+	Active against *E. granulosus*. Use in dogs only
Niclosamide	125	+		(+)	
Fenbendazole	100 single dose 50 for 3 days	+			
Mebendazole	Variable (3.5–50) Given for 2–5 days	(+)	(+)		Activity against tapeworms variable. Some activity against *E. granulosus*
Epsiprantel	5.5	+		+	Combined with pyrantel pamoate
Bunamidine	50	+	+	+	No longer available in many countries

+ active; (+) variable activity.

Control: This is similar to that of other taeniids involving control of infection in the final host and through the burial or disposal of ruminant carcasses and offal.

Notes: The correct nomenclature for the intermediate host stage is the 'metacestode stage of *Taenia hydatigena*' rather than '*Cysticercus tenuicollis*'.

Taenia hyaenae

Synonym: *Cysticercus dromedarii*, *Cysticercus cameli*

Common name: Cysticercosis

Predilection site: Muscle, liver and other organs

Parasite class: Cestoda

Family: Taeniidae

Description, gross: Small tapeworms 200–300 cm long.

Description, microscopic: The cysticercus of *T. hyaenae* is 12–18 mm in length and has an armed protoscolex with a double row of hooks.

Final hosts: Hyena

Intermediate hosts: Camel, cattle, goat, rarely sheep and various antelopes

Life cycle: Eggs passed by hyenas are ingested by the intermediate hosts in which the oncospheres migrate to the muscles via the blood before developing to infective cycticerci.

Geographical distribution: Tropical Africa

Pathogenesis and clinical signs: Infection is usually asymptomatic.

Taenia multiceps

Synonym: *Multiceps multiceps*, *Coenurus cerebralis*

Common name: Gid, sturdy, staggers

Predilection site: Small intestine (definitive hosts); brain and spinal cord (intermediate hosts)

Parasite class: Cestoda

Family: Taeniidae

Description, gross: Adult tapeworms are 40–100 cm in length.

Description, microscopic: Adults have a small head about 0.8 mm in diameter with four suckers. There is a double ring of 22–32 rostellar hooks. The gravid segments measure 8–12 × 3–4 mm and the uterus has 18–26 lateral branches which contain taeniid eggs. Eggs are approximately 29–37 μm in diameter.

Final hosts: Dog, fox, coyote, jackal and wolf

Intermediate hosts: Sheep, goat, cattle, deer, pig, horse, man

Life cycle: The intermediate host is infected through the ingestion of *T. multiceps* eggs. Each egg contains an oncosphere that hatches and is activated in the small intestine. The oncosphere then penetrates the intestinal mucosa and is carried via the blood to the brain or spinal cord where each oncosphere develops into the metacestode larval stage (*Coenurus cerebralis*). When mature, this is readily recognised as a large fluid-filled cyst up to 5.0 cm or more in diameter. This bears clusters of up to several hundred scolices on its internal wall. In goats the cysts can also mature in subcutaneous and intramuscular sites. The cysts in sheep and goats often persist throughout the life of the animal. The life cycle is completed when the final host, dog or wild canid, eats an infected sheep brain or spinal cord.

Geographical distribution: Worldwide, but absent from the USA and New Zealand

Pathogenesis and clinical signs: Infection in the intermediate hosts is usually asymptomatic.

Diagnosis: As for *T. hydatigena*

Pathology: No associated pathology

Epidemiology: This is largely influenced by whether sheepdogs and stray dogs have access to the heads or spinal cords of infected intermediate hosts

Treatment: As for other taenid species

Control: This can be achieved through ensuring that dogs, in particular sheep dogs, do not have access to the heads of slaughtered or dead sheep or goats. It is essential that all sheep carcases are buried as soon as possible. In areas where coenurosis is endemic the regular de-worming of dogs with an effective anthelmintic every 6–8 weeks will reduce the contamination into the environment and, by breaking the sheep–dog cycle, may lead to eradication of the disease. Foxes are not thought to be an important final host for *T. multiceps*.

Taenia ovis

Synonym: *Cysticercus ovis*

Common name: Ovine cysticercosis, 'sheep measles'

Predilection site: Small intestine (final host); muscle (intermediate host)

Parasite class: Cestoda

Family: Taeniidae

Description, gross: The adult tapeworm is large, measuring 0.5–1.5 m in length.

Microscopic: The rostellum bears 24–36 hooks. The strobila has a scalloped edge and is often coiled into a spiral. The mature proglottids have a vaginal sphincter and the ovary and vagina cross each other. The uterus of the gravid proglottids has 20–25 lateral branches on either side. The oval egg measures 34 × 24–28 μm.

Final hosts: Dog, fox, wild carnivores

Intermediate hosts: Sheep, goat

Life cycle: Dogs and wild canids are infested by consuming the cysticercus in the intermediate host. The intermediate host is infected through the ingestion of tapeworm eggs that hatch in the intestine. The metacestode stage (*Cysticercus ovis*) infects the musculature and cysts are usually located in the skeletal muscle, heart, diaphragm and intermuscular connective tissue. The cyst becomes infective around 2–3 months after infection of the host. The prepatent period in dogs is around 6–9 weeks.

Geographical distribution: Worldwide

Pathogenesis and clinical signs: Heavy infections in young dogs can sometimes cause diarrhoea and ill-thrift.

Diagnosis: Tapeworm infection in dogs is often recognised through the presence of shed proglottids and/or tapeworm segments in fresh faeces.

Epidemiology: Adult tapeworms shed three segments each containing 78 000–95 000 eggs. The eggs can survive 90–150 days at 16°C but survive for shorter periods at higher temperatures. Ruminants are infected by grazing pasture and forages contaminated with dog or fox faeces harbouring eggs of *T. ovis*.

Treatment: As for other taenid species

Control: Regular treatment of dogs with an effective anthelmintic will reduce contamination of the environment. Dogs should be denied access to raw sheep and goat meat and carcases. A highly protective recombinant vaccine is available in some countries.

Notes: The correct nomenclature for the intermediate host stage is the 'metacestode stage of *Taenia ovis*' rather than '*Cysticercus ovis*'.

Taenia pisiformis

Synonym: *Cysticercus pisiformis*

Predilection site: Small intestine (final host); peritoneum, liver (intermediate host)

Parasite class: Cestoda

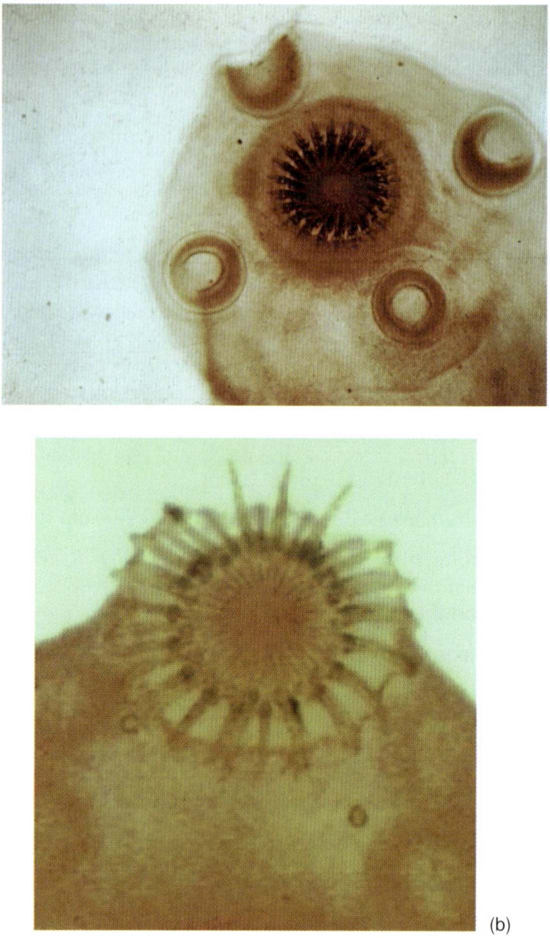

(a)

(b)

Fig. 6.11 (a) Scolex of *Taenia pisiformis* showing the four suckers and armed rostellum. (b) Scolex of *Taenia serialis*.

Family: Taeniidae

Description, gross: The adult tapeworm can measure up to 2 m in length.

Microscopic: The adult tapeworm has a large scolex with narrow strobila and the rostellum has 34–48 hooks (Fig. 6.11a). Gravid segments have a uterus with 8–14 lateral branches on either side. *Cysticercus pisiformis* is a small pea-like transparent cyst. Eggs are oval or elliptical and measure 37 × 32 μm.

Final hosts: Dog, fox

Intermediate hosts: Rabbit, hare

Life cycle: Infection of the intermediate host is through ingestion of tapeworm eggs shed by dogs. Ingested eggs hatch in the small intestine of the intermediate host and penetrate the intestinal wall and pass via the portal system to the liver. Juvenile stages migrate through the liver parenchyma and locate in the abdominal cavity after 2–4 weeks, where they develop into cysts (*Cysticercus pisiformis*) attached to the wall of the mesentery and omentum. Cysts can survive the life of the host. The final host is infected by ingesting the cysticercus. The prepatent period in the dog is around 6–8 weeks.

Geographical distribution: Worldwide

Pathogenesis: Infection is usually asymptomatic in both the final and the intermediate host. However, in heavy infections liver damage can occur in the intermediate host as a result of migration of juvenile worms through the liver parenchyma. This can lead to hepatitis and cirrhosis.

Clinical signs: Infection is usually asymptomatic. In heavy infections the intermediate hosts may show emaciation and jaundice.

Diagnosis: Infection of the intermediate host is detected through the presence of a single cyst or a cluster of several cysts in the abdominal cavity.

Pathology: Pea-like cysts present on the peritoneum, wall of the mesentery and omentum.

Epidemiology: There is a high prevalence in hunting dogs.

Treatment: As for other taenid species

Control: Hunting dogs should be wormed regularly with an effective anthelmintic and should not be fed raw carcases or offal from rabbits and hares.

Notes: The correct nomenclature for the intermediate host stage is the 'metacestode stage of *Taenia pisiformis*' rather than '*Cysticercus pisiformis*'.

Taenia serialis

Synonym: *Coenurus serialis*

Predilection site: small intestine (definitive host); intramuscular and subcutaneous connective tissue (intermediate host)

Parasite class: Cestoda

Family: Taeniidae

Description, gross: The adult tapeworm is of medium length, around 0.5–0.7 m, and bears two rows of hooks (Fig. 6.11b). The metacestode cysts may be 4–6 cm in size.

Microscopic: The numerous scolices in the *Coenurus* are arranged in lines or strands as the name '*serialis*' implies. The gravid uterus has 10–18 lateral branches and the vaginal sphincter is well developed.

Final hosts: Dog, fox and other canids

Intermediate hosts: Rabbit, hare and rarely rodents and man

Life cycle: Infection of the intermediate host is through ingestion of tapeworm eggs shed by dogs. The intermediate stage *Coenurus serialis* is found in the rabbit, usually subcutaneously or in the intermuscular connective tissue. The final host is infected by ingesting the metacestode stage.

Geographical distribution: Worldwide

Pathogenesis: Infection is usually asymptomatic in both the definitive and the intermediate host.

Clinical signs: No clinical signs reported.

Diagnosis: Infection of the intermediate host is detected through the presence of cysts in subcutaneous or intramuscular connective tissue.

Pathology: Pea-like cysts are present in subcutaneous or intramuscular connective tissue.

Epidemiology: There is a high prevalence in hunting dogs.

Treatment: As for other taenid species

Control: Hunting dogs should be wormed regularly with an effective anthelmintic and should not be fed raw carcases or offal from rabbits and hares.

Notes: The correct nomenclature for the intermediate host stage is the 'metacestode stage of *Taenia serialis*' rather than '*Coenurus serialis*'. Another species *Taenia brauni* is very similar to *T. serialis* and is found in parts of Africa. The adult tapeworm occurs in the dog and other wild canids and the metacestode in rodents.

Taenia taeniaeformis

Synonym: *Hydatigera taeniaeformis*, *Taenia crassicollis*, *Cysticercus fasciolaris*, *Strobilocercus fasciolaris*

Predilection site: Small intestine (final host); liver (intermediate host)

Parasite class: Cestoda

Family: Taeniidae

Description, gross: The adult tapeworm is of medium size, up to 70 cm in length.

Description, microscopic: The scolex is large and there is absence of a neck region. The uterus has five to nine lateral branches and the posterior proglottids are bell-shaped. The metacestode stage is a strobilocercus (*Strobilocercus fasciolaris*), which is a small cyst connected with an evaginated scolex by a segmented juvenile strobila.

Final host: Cat, lynx, stoat, fox

Intermediate hosts: Mouse, rat, rabbit, squirrel

Table 6.6 Taenid tapeworms of dogs.

Parasite species	Scolex size, μm (range)	Number of hooks	Length of hooks (μm)		Number of testes (layers)	Genital pores	Number of uterine branches	Notes
			Large hooks	Small hooks				
T. hydatigena	206 (170–220)	28–36 (26–44)	191–218 (170–235)	118–143 (110–168)	600–700 (1)	5–10 prominent	6–10 that re-divide	Lobes of ovary unequal in size. No vaginal sphincter. Testes extend to vitellarium, but not confluent behind
T. ovis	180 (156–188)	30–34 (24–38)	170–191 (131–202)	111–127 (89–157)	350–750 (1)	15–30	11–20 that re-divide	Lobes of ovary unequal in size. Well developed vaginal sphincter. Testes extend to posterior edge of ovary
T. multiceps	(150–170)	22–30 (20–34)	157–177 (120–190)	98–136 (73–160)	284–388 (2)		14–20 that re-divide	Lobes of ovary equal in size. Pad of muscle on anterior wall of vagina. Testes extend to vitellarium, but not confluent behind
T. serialis	160 (135–175)	26–32	137–175	78–120			20–25	
T. pisiformis	250 (225–294)	34–48	225–294	132–177			5–15 barely visible	

Life cycle: The metacestode (*Cysticercus fasciolaris*) develops in the liver of rodents and is infective to cats after about 9 weeks. When a cat ingests the metacestode the scolex attaches to the wall of the intestine. Tapeworms in cats become patent around 6 weeks and eggs are ingested by the intermediate host.

Geographical distribution: Cosmopolitan

Pathogenesis: Adult tapeworms are of minor pathogenic significance and infections are usually subclinical.

Clinical signs: None reported.

Diagnosis: Diagnosis depends on the demonstration of segments or individual taeniid eggs in the faeces. Specific identification of the adult tapeworm is a specialised task.

Epidemiology: Rodents are infected by grazing pasture and forages contaminated with cat faeces harbouring eggs of *T. taeniaeformis*. Two cycles can occur: an urban cycle that involves the domestic cat and house and field rodents; and a sylvatic cycle that in North America uses bobcats and wild rodents.

Treatment: Cats should be treated regularly with an effective cestocidal anthelmintic. For adult tapeworms a number of effective drugs are available, including praziquantel, mebendazole, fenbendazole and dichlorophen.

Control: Control depends on dietary methods that exclude access to the larval stage in the intermediate host. Where practical, cats should be prevented from eating rodents.

Taenia cervi

Synonym: *Cysticercus cervi, Taenia krabbei, Cysticercus tarandi*

Predilection site: Small intestine (definitive host); muscle (intermediate host)

Parasite class: Cestoda

Family: Taeniidae

Description, gross: The adult worm is about 26 cm long.

Description, microscopic: The mature segments are much broader than long and the organs are compressed and transversely elongated. The scolex bears 26–34 hooks.

Final hosts: Wolf, red fox, arctic fox

Intermediate hosts: Red deer (*Cervus elaphus*), roe deer (*Capreolus capreolus*), reindeer (*Rangifer tarandus*)

Life cycle: Wild canids are infested by consuming the cysticercus in the intermediate host. The intermediate host is infected through the ingestion of tapeworm eggs that hatch in the intestine.

Geographical distribution: Worldwide

Pathogenesis: Cysticerci may cause economic loss through condemnation at meat inspection.

Clinical signs: Adult tapeworms are considered to be of little pathogenic importance. Infected intermediate hosts do not usually show clinical signs of disease.

Diagnosis: Diagnosis is through the identification of cysts at postmortem.

Pathology: The mature, ovoid white cysticerci are grossly visible in the muscle, heart, lung, liver and brain.

Epidemiology: Deer are infected by grazing pasture and forages contaminated with carnivore faeces harbouring taenid eggs.

Treatment and control: Control is not practical.

Notes: The correct nomenclature for the intermediate host stage is the 'metacestode stage of *Taenia cervi*' rather than '*Cysticercus cervi*'. It is unclear whether *Taenia krabbei*, found mainly in reindeer, is synonymous with *T. cervi*, which is found mainly in red deer and roe deer, and that they are one and the same species present in different hosts.

Mesocestoides lineatus

Predilection site: Small intestine

Parasite class: Cestoda

Family: Mesocestoididae

Description, gross: The adult tapeworm is 30–250 cm in length and up to 3 mm wide.

Description, microscopic: The scolex is large and the suckers are elongate and oval. Mature segments each contain a sinle set of reproductive organs. The eggs are oval and measure 40–60 × 35–43 μm.

Final host: Dog, cat, fox, mink and wild carnivores

Intermediate hosts: 1. Orabatid mites. 2. Birds, amphibians, reptiles

Life cycle: The life cycle requires two intermediate hosts. A cysticercoid is produced in the first intermediate host, which, when eaten by the second intermediate hosts forms a terathrydium; this may remain as an encapsulated form for some time.

Geographical distribution: Europe, Asia, Africa

Pathogenesis: Adult tapeworms are of minor pathogenic significance and infections are usually subclinical.

Clinical signs: None reported

Macracanthorhynchus hirudinaceus

Common name: Thorny-headed worm

Predilection site: Duodenum and proximal small intestine

Parasite class: Acanthocephala

Family: Oligacanthorhynchidae

Final hosts: Pig, wild boar, occasionally dog, wild carnivores and man

Intermediate hosts: Various dung beetles and water beetles

Geographical distribution: Worldwide, but absent from certain areas, for example parts of western Europe

For more details see Chapter 5 (Pigs).

Coccidiosis

Dogs and cats are infected with coccidian parasites belonging to the genus, *Isospora*. In the dog, the common *Isospora* species are *I. canis* and *I. ohioensis*. In the cat the common species are *I. felis* and *I. rivolta*.

Pathogenesis: There is no real evidence that these species are pathogenic on their own, but infection may be exacerbated by intercurrent viral disease, or other immunosuppressive agents.

Clinical signs: Diarrhoea in young puppies or kittens

Diagnosis: Coccidiosis may be diagnosed on postmortem by finding coccidial stages in the intestines. Affected animals with diarrhoea or dysentery may be shedding oocysts in the faeces. The presence of oocysts is not in itself sufficient for diagnosis but should be considered with presenting signs of sudden onset of enteritis. Oocysts may need to be differentiated from other oocysts of other coccidia genera found in dogs (see Table 6.7) and cats (see Table 6.8 and Fig. 6.12).

Pathology: Coccidial stages are found in the epithelial cells lining the villi of the small intestine. In heavy infections there is villous stunting and reduction in the absorptive area of the lower small intestine leading to diarrhoea.

Epidemiology: Crowding and lack of good sanitation promote spread of coccidiosis. Breeding establishments, kennels and rescue centres are potential sources of infection. Older dogs and cats are generally immune from disease, but may seed the environment with oocysts leading to infection in young puppies and kittens that have no previous exposure.

Treatment: Information on treatment in the dog and cat is scanty, although by analogy with other host

Table 6.7 Coccidian parasites in the faeces of dogs.

Coccidian species	Alternative name	Intermediate host	Oocyst* condition	Oocyst size (μm)	Sporocyst size (μm)
Sarcocystis bovicanis	*S. cruzi, S. fusiformis*	Cattle	S	19–21 × 15–18	**16.3 × 10.8**
Sarcocystis ovicanis	*S. tenella*	Sheep	S		**14.8 × 9.9**
Sarcocystis suicanis	*S. porcicanis* *S. mieschiriana*	Pig	S		**12.7 × 10.1**
Sarcocystis equicanis	*S. bertrami*	Horse	S		**15.2 × 10**
Sarcocystis fayeri		Horse	S		**12.0 × 7.9**
Sarcocystis capracanis		Goat	S		**12–15 × 8–10**
Sarcocystis hircicanis		Goat	S		
Sarcocystis cameli		Camel	S		**12 × 9**
Sarcocystis hovarthi	*S. gallinarum*	Chicken	S		**10–13 × 7–9**
Hammondia heydorni	*Toxoplasma heydorni*	Various	U	**13 × 11**	
Isospora canis	*Cystoisospora canis*	–	U	**38 × 30**	21 × 16
Isospora ohioensis	*Cystoisospora ohioensis*	–	U	**23 × 19**	14.5 × 10

* Sporulated (S) or unsporulated (U) oocysts in faeces; oocysts or sporocysts (**in bold**) generally found free in faeces.

Table 6.8 Coccidian parasites in the faeces of cats.

Coccidian species	Alternative name	Intermediate host	Oocyst condition*	Oocyst size (μm)	Sporocyst size (μm)
Sarcocystis bovifelis	*S. hirsuta*	Cattle	S	12–18 × 11–14	**12.5 × 7.8**
Sarcocystis ovifelis	*S. tenella*	Sheep	S		**12.4 × 8.1**
Sarcocystis hircifelis	*S. moulei*	Goat	S		**12.4 × 9.1**
Sarcocystis porcifelis		Pig	S		**13.5 × 8**
Sarcocystis cuniculi	*S. cuniculorum*	Rabbit	S		**13 × 10**
Sarcocystis muris		Mouse	S		**10.3 × 8.5**
Besnoitia besnoiti	*Sarcocystis besnoiti*	Ruminants	U	**14–16 × 12–14**	
Toxoplasma gondii			U	**13 × 12**	9 × 6.5
Hammondia hammondi	*Toxoplasma hammondi*	Rodents	U	**13.2 × 10.6**	9.8 × 6.5
Isospora felis	*Cystoisospora felis*	–	U	**41.6 × 30.5**	22.6 × 18.4
Isospora rivolta	*Cystoisospora rivolta*	–	U	**25 × 21.1**	15.2 × 11.6

* Sporulated (S) or unsporulated (U) oocysts in faeces; oocysts or sporocysts (**in bold**) generally found free in faeces.

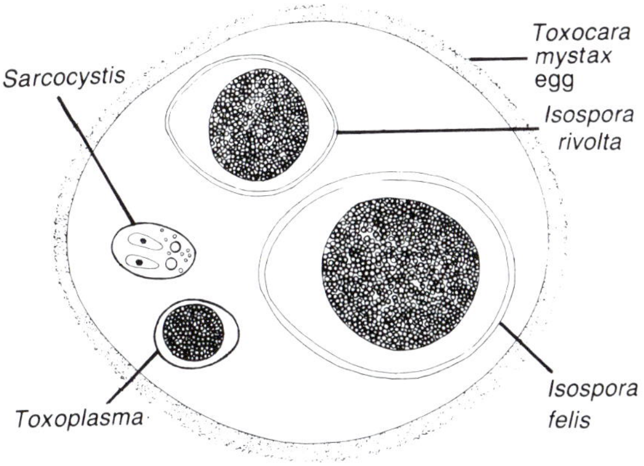

Fig. 6.12 Diagram of cat oocysts relative to ascarid eggs of *Toxocara mystax*.

species, the use of sulphonamides, such as sulphadimidine, should be tried.

Control: Good sanitation and isolation are effective measures in preventing coccidiosis. In kennels or rescue centres, animal accommodation should be cleaned daily. Standard disinfectants are ineffective against coccidial oocysts but ammonia-based products are effective.

Notes: At one time it was thought that species of the genus *Isospora* were freely transmissible between dogs and cats, but it is now established that this is not the case.

Isospora canis

Predilection site: Small intestine

Parasite class: Sporozoasida

Family: Eimeriidae

Description: Oocysts are ellipsoidal to slightly ovoid, 34–42 × 23–36 μm (mean 38 × 30 μm) with a smooth, pale wall without a micropyle, polar granule or residuum but with a tiny blob adherent to the oocyst wall at the broad end. The two sporocysts are ellipsoidal 18–28 × 15–19 μm with a smooth, colourless wall and a prominent residuum. Each sporocyst contains four sausage-shaped sporozoites with clear sub-central globules.

Hosts: Dog

Isospora ohioensis

Predilection site: Small intestine

Parasite class: Sporozoasida

Family: Eimeriidae

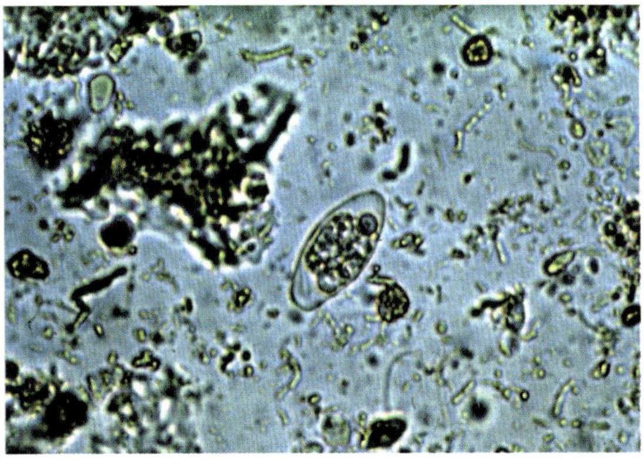

Fig. 6.13 Oocysts of *Isospora felis*.

Description: Oocyst is ellipsoidal to oval, 20–27 × 14–24 μm (mean 23 × 19 μm) with a smooth, colourless to pale yellow wall without a micropyle, polar granule or residuum. The two sporocysts are ellipsoidal, 12–19 × 9–13 μm (mean 14.5 × 10 μm) with a residuum and four sporozoites with one or more, clear globules.

Hosts: Dog

Isospora felis

Predilection site: Small intestine

Parasite class: Sporozoasida

Family: Eimeriidae

Description: Oocyst is ovoid, 32–53 × 26–43 μm (mean 43 × 32 μm) with a smooth, yellowish to pale brown wall without micropyle, polar granule or residuum. Sporulated oocyst contains two sporocysts each with four sporozoites (Fig. 6.13). The two sporocysts are ellipsoidal 20–27 × 17–22 μm with a smooth colourless wall and a prominent residuum. Each sporocyst contains four sausage-shaped sporozoites with clear sub-central globules.

Hosts: Cat

Isospora rivolta

Predilection site: Small intestine

Parasite class: Sporozoasida

Family: Eimeriidae

Description: Oocysts are ellipsoidal to ovoid 21–29 × 18–26 μm (mean 25 × 21 μm) with a smooth, colourless to pale brown wall without a micropyle, polar granule or residuum. The two sporocysts are ellipsoidal 14–16 × 10–13 μm with a residuum and four sporozoites each with clear sub-central globules.

Hosts: Cat

Life cycle: Rodents may ingest sporulated oocysts and become infected with asexual stages, thereby acting as reservoirs of infection. A number of rodent species can act as transport hosts. The life cycle is normally direct, although there is some evidence that a predator–prey relationship may be involved and that dogs and cats can acquire infection from the tissues of rodents.

Geographical distribution: Worldwide

Pathogenesis: The pathogenicity of *I. rivolta* is generally thought to be low, although severe diarrhoea in young kittens has been associated with high oocyst counts.

Hammondia heydorni

Predilection site: Small intestine

Parasite class: Sporozoasida

Family: Sarcocystiidae

Description: Oocysts are 13 × 11 μm without a micropyle or residuum and appear dumb-bell shaped after sporulation. The sporocysts have no Stieda body but have a residuum.

Final hosts: Dog

Intermediate hosts: Cattle, sheep, goat, rodents, guinea pig

Life cycle: Unsporulated oocysts are produced in the faeces, and following infection of the intermediate hosts, the multiplication of tachyzoites in the lamina propria of the intestinal wall is followed by the production of cysts containing bradyzoites in the skeletal muscle. The prepatent period is 6–7 days. Sporulation time is 3 days.

Geographical distribution: Presumed worldwide

Pathogenesis: Non-pathogenic

Clinical signs: Diarrhoea in young puppies

Diagnosis: Identification of oocysts in dog faeces and differentiation from other coccidia species of dogs (see Table 6.7)

Pathology: Not reported

Epidemiology: The dog is infected following the consumption of zoite-containing tissues of the intermediate host. Direct dog-to-dog transmission does not occur.

Treatment: Not indicated

Control: The only control measures possible are those of simple hygiene. Dogs should also not be fed raw or uncooked meat.

Hammondia hammondi

Synonym: *Isospora hammondi*, *Toxoplasma hammondi*

Predilection site: Small intestine

Parasite class: Sporozoasida

Family: Sarcocystiidae

Description: Unsporulated oocysts are colourless, spherical to subspherical, 11–13 × 10–13 μm without a micropyle or residuum and subspherical to ellipsoidal, 13–14 × 10–11 μm (mean 13 × 11 μm) after sporulation. The sporocysts are ellipsoidal, 8–11 × 6–8 μm (mean 10 × 6.5 μm) and have no Stieda body but have a residuum. The sporozoites are elongate and curved with a nucleus near the centre.

Final hosts: Cat

Intermediate hosts: Rodents (mouse, rat, guinea pig)

Life cycle: The cat is infected by ingesting the infected rodents containing meronts. After ingestion, there is multiplication in the small intestine epithelium followed by gametogony. The prepatent period in the cat is 5–16 days and the patent period can be as long as 136 days.

Geographical distribution: Presumed worldwide

Pathogenesis: Non-pathogenic to either host, but it is important to recognise that the oocysts of *Hammondia* closely resemble those of *Toxoplasma* and that their differentiation in cat faeces is a specialist task.

Clinical signs: No associated clinical signs

Diagnosis: Identification of oocysts in cat faeces and differentiation from other coccidia species of cats (see Table 6.8)

Pathology: Not reported

Epidemiology: The cat is infected following the consumption of zoite-containing tissues of the intermediate host. Direct cat-to-cat transmission does not occur.

Treatment: Not indicated

Control: The only control measures possible are those of simple hygiene. Cats should not be fed raw or uncooked meat.

Sarcocystis

The previously complex nomenclature for the large number of *Sarcocystis* spp has largely been discarded by many workers in favour of a new system based on their biology. The new names generally incorporate those of the **intermediate** and **final hosts** in that order. Although unacceptable to systematists, this practice has the virtue of simplicity.

At present the most important species recognised with the dog as a final host are:

- *Sarcocystis bovicanis* (*Sarcocystis cruzi*)
- *Sarcocystis ovicanis* (*Sarcocystis tenella*)
- *Sarcocystis capricanis*
- *Sarcocystis hircicanis*
- *Sarcocystis suicanis* (*Sarcocystis porcicanis*, *Sarcocystis miescheriana*)
- *Sarcocystis equicanis* (*Sarcocystis bertrami*)
- *Sarcocystis fayeri*
- *Sarcocystis hovarthi*
- *Sarcocystis cameli*

The most important species recognised with the cat as a final host are:

- *Sarcocystis bovifelis* (syn *S. hirsuta*)
- *Sarcocystis ovifelis* (*S. tenella, S. medusiformis*)
- *Sarcocystis porcifelis* (*Sarcocystis suifelis*)

Life cycle: The life cycle for all species is heteroxenous. Sexual stages occur in the predator and oocysts are passed in the faeces. Infection in the dog and cat is by ingestion of bradyzoite cysts in the muscles of infected intermediate hosts. The bradyzoites are liberated in the intestine and the freed zoites pass to the subepithelial lamina propria and differentiate into micro- and macrogametocytes. Following conjugation of gametes, thin-walled oocysts are formed which, unlike those of most other enteric sporozoans, sporulate within the body. Two sporocysts are formed, each containing four sporozoites. Usually the fragile oocyst wall ruptures and free sporocysts are found in the faeces.

Pathogenesis: Infection in the dog and cat is normally non-pathogenic although mild diarrhoea has occasionally been reported with some infections.

Clinical signs: Occasional diarrhoea

Diagnosis: Identification of oocysts in dog or cat faeces and differentiation from other coccidia species of dogs and cats (see Tables 6.7 and 6.8)

Pathology: Infection in the final host is not normally associated with pathological changes. Oocysts may be seen in the lamina propria and within the epithelium at the tips of the villi.

Epidemiology: Little is known of the epidemiology, but from the high prevalence of symptomless infections observed in abattoirs, it is clear that where dogs and cats are kept in close association with farm animals or their feed, then transmission is likely. Sheep dogs and farm cats are known to play an important part in the transmission of *Sarcocystis* and care should be exercised that only cooked meat is fed to dogs and cats. Acute outbreaks of *Sarcocystis* in livestock are probably most likely when livestock, which have been reared without contact with farm dogs particularly, are subsequently exposed to large numbers of the sporocysts from dog faeces. The longevity of the sporocysts shed in the faeces is not known.

Treatment and control: There is no effective treatment for infection in dogs or cats. The only control measures possible are those of simple hygiene. Farm dogs and cats should not be housed in, or allowed access to, fodder stores, nor should they be allowed to defecate in pens where livestock are housed. It is also important that they are not fed uncooked meat.

Sarcocystis bovicanis

Synonym: *Sarcocystis cruzi*, *Sarcocystis fusiformis*

Predilection site: Small intestine

Order: Sporozoasida

Family: Sarcocystiidae

Description: Sporulated oocysts are fully sporulated and dumb-bell shaped when passed in the faeces, 19–21 × 15–18 μm, with a thin oocyst wall sunken between two sporocysts, without a micropyle, polar granule or oocyst residuum (Fig. 6.14). However, it is usually the sporulated sporocyst that is found free in the faeces. Sporocysts are ellipsoidal, 14.3–17.4 × 8.7–13.3 μm (mean 16.3 × 10.8 μm), smooth, colourless without a Stieda body but with a residuum and each has four sporozoites.

Final host: Dog, fox, wolf, coyote

Intermediate hosts: Cattle

Geographical distribution: Worldwide

Sarcocystis ovicanis

Synonym: *Sarcocystis tenella*, *Isospora bigemina*

Predilection site: Small intestine

Order: Sporozoasida

Family: Sarcocystiidae

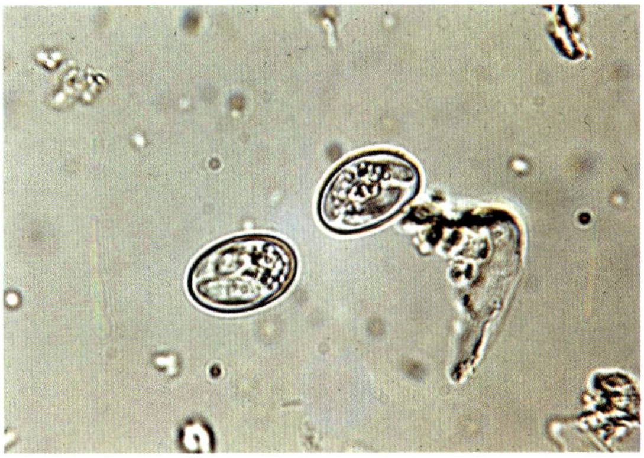

Fig. 6.14 Oocysts of *Sarcocystis bovicanis*.

Description: Oocysts are sporulated when passed in the faeces and contain two sporocysts each with four sporozoites; usually the sporulated sporocyst is found free in the faeces. In *S. ovicanis*, the sporulated sporocysts measure approximately 13.1–16.1 × 8.5–10.8 μm (mean 14.8 × 9.9 μm).

Final host: Dog

Intermediate hosts: Sheep

Geographical distribution: Worldwide

Sarcocystis capracanis

Predilection site: Small intestine

Order: Sporozoasida

Family: Sarcocystiidae

Description: The oocysts have not been described. The sporulated sporocysts are ellipsoidal and measure approximately 12–15 × 8–10 μm

Final host: Dog

Intermediate hosts: Goat

Geographical distribution: Worldwide

Sarcocystis hircicanis

Predilection site: Small intestine

Order: Sporozoasida

Family: Sarcocystiidae

Description: The oocysts have not been described. The sporulated sporocysts are ellipsoidal and measure approximately 15–17.3 × 10.5–11.3 μm.

Final host: Dog

Intermediate hosts: Goat

Geographical distribution: Worldwide

Sarcocystis suicanis

Synonym: *Sarcocystis porcicanis*, *Sarcocystis miescheriana*

Predilection site: Small intestine

Order: Sporozoasida

Family: Sarcocystiidae

Description: Sporulated sporocysts found free in the faeces measure approximately 12.7 × 10.1 μm.

Final host: Dog

Intermediate hosts: Pig

Geographical distribution: Worldwide

Sarcocystis equicanis

Synonym: *Sarcocystis bertrami*

Predilection site: Small intestine

Order: Sporozoasida

Family: Sarcocystiidae

Description: The sporulated sporocysts measure 15–16.3 × 8.8–11.3 μm (mean 15.2–10 μm).

Final host: Dog

Intermediate hosts: Horse

Geographical distribution: Worldwide

Sarcocystis fayeri

Synonym: *Sarcocystis bertrami*

Predilection site: Small intestine

Order: Sporozoasida

Family: Sarcocystiidae

Description: In *S. fayeri*, the sporulated sporocysts measure 11–13 × 7–8.5 μm (mean 12.0 × 7.9 μm).

Final host: Dog

Intermediate hosts: Horse

Geographical distribution: Worldwide

Sarcocystis hovarthi

Synonym: *Sarcocystis gallinarum*

Predilection site: Small intestine

Order: Sporozoasida

Family: Sarcocystiidae

Description: The oocysts have not been described. The sporulated sporocysts are ellipsoidal and measure approximately 10–13 × 7–9 μm.

Final host: Dog

Intermediate hosts: Chicken

Geographical distribution: Presumed worldwide

Sarcocystis cameli

Predilection site: Small intestine

Order: Sporozoasida

Family: Sarcocystiidae

Description: The oocysts have not been described. The sporulated sporocysts are ellipsoidal and measure approximately 12 × 9 μm

Final host: Dog

Intermediate hosts: Camel (Bactrian and dromedary)

Geographical distribution: North Africa (Egypt, Morocco, Sudan)

Sarcocystis bovifelis

Synonym: *Sarcocystis hirsuta*, *Sarcocystis fusiformis*

Predilection site: Small intestine

Order: Sporozoasida

Family: Sarcocystiidae

Description: Oocysts are smooth, colourless, 12–18 × 11–14 µm and contain two sporocysts each with four sporozoites and are dumb-bell-like in appearance, with no micropyle, polar granule or oocyst residuum. Sporocysts are ellipsoidal, 11–14 × 7–9 µm (mean 12.5 × 7.8 µm) without a Stieda body but with a residuum.

Final host: Cat

Intermediate hosts: Cattle

Geographical distribution: Worldwide

Sarcocystis ovifelis

Synonym: *Sarcocystis tenella, Sarcocystis gigantea, Sarcocystis medusiformis, Isospora bigemina*

Predilection site: Small intestine

Order: Sporozoasida

Family: Sarcocystiidae

Description In *S. ovifelis*, the sporulated sporocysts are ellipsoidal and measure 10.8–13.9 × 7.7–9.3 µm (mean 12.4 × 8.1 µm).

Final host: Cat

Intermediate hosts: Sheep

Geographical distribution: Worldwide

Sarcocystis porcifelis

Synonym: *Sarcocystis suifelis*

Predilection site: Small intestine

Order: Sporozoasida

Family: Sarcocystiidae

Description: The sporulated sporocysts are ellipsoidal and measure 13.2–13.5 × 7.2–8 µm, without a Stieda body, but with a residuum

Final host: Cat

Intermediate hosts: Pig

Geographical distribution: Worldwide

Besnoitia besnoiti

Synonym: *Sarcocystis besnoiti*, *Globidium besnoiti*

Predilection site: Small intestine

Order: Sporozoasida

Family: Sarcocystiidae

Description: Oocysts are ovoid, 14–14 × 12–14 µm, unsporulated and without a micropyle when passed in the faeces of cats. After sporulation they contain two sporocysts each with four sporozoites. The prepatent period in cats is 4–25 days and the patent period 3–15 days.

Final host: Cat, wild cats (lion, cheetah, leopard)

Intermediate hosts: Cattle, goats, wild ruminants (wildebeest, impala, kudu)

Life cycle: The ruminant intermediate hosts are infected by the ingestion of oocysts shed into the environment by infected cats. Cats are infected following ingestion of cysts present in the subcutaneous tissues of infected intermediate hosts.

Geographical distribution: Worldwide, although important in tropical and subtropical countries, especially in Africa

Pathogenesis and clinical signs: *Besnoitia besnoiti* is non-pathogenic in the cat final host.

Diagnosis: Identification of oocysts in cat faeces and differentiation from other coccidia species of cats (see Table 6.8).

Epidemiology: The natural mode of transmission is by ingestion of pseudocysts present in the skin of animal carcases.

Treatment: There is no effective treatment for infection in cats.

Control: As for *Sarcocystis* species

Cryptosporidium parvum

Predilection site: Small intestine

Parasite class: Sporozoasida

Family: Cryptosporidiidae

Hosts: Cattle, sheep, goat, horse, deer, dog, cat, man

Description: Mature oocysts are ovoidal or spheroidal, 5.0 × 4.5 μm (range 4.6–5.4 × 3.8–4.7 μm) and have a length:width ratio of 1.19.

Geographical distribution: Worldwide

Cryptosporidium canis

Predilection site: Small intestine

Parasite class: Sporozoasida

Family: Cryptosporidiidae

Hosts: Dog, fox, man

Description: Mature oocysts are colourless, ovoidal or spheroidal, 4.95 × 4.71 μm and have a length:width ratio of 1.05.

Geographical distribution: Thought to be worldwide

Other protozoa

Cryptosporidium felis

Predilection site: Small intestine

Parasite class: Sporozoasida

Family: Cryptosporidiidae

Hosts: Cat, cattle, man

Description: Oocysts are morphologically indistinguishable from those of *C. parvum*.

Geographical distribution: Thought to be worldwide

Life cycle: The life cycle of all *Cryptosporidium* species is basically similar to that of other intestinal coccidia although sporulation takes place within the host. Oocysts, each with four sporozoites, are liberated in the faeces. Following ingestion, the sporozoites invade the microvillous brush border of the enterocytes and the trophozoites rapidly differentiate to form meronts with four to eight merozoites. Gametogony follows, after one to two generations of meronts leading to the production of oocysts.

Pathogenesis: Chronic diarrhoea may occur in dogs that are immunosuppressed because of concurrent illness or toxicity. Puppies with distemper virus, for example, have developed persistent diarrhoea and persistently excreted *Cryptosporidium* oocysts. Infection with *C. felis* in cats is not considered pathogenic.

Clinical signs: Infection with *Cryptosporidium* is generally asymptomatic but may cause acute diarrhoea in neonatal animals or more chronic diarrhoea in young immunosuppressed animals or in animals with intercurrent and debilitating diseases such as distemper in dogs or FeLV/FIV in cats.

Diagnosis: Oocysts may be demonstrated using Ziehl–Nielsen stained faecal smears in which the sporozoites appear as bright red granules. Speciation of *Cryptosporidium* is difficult, if not impossible, using conventional techniques. A range of molecular and immunological techniques has been developed, that include the use of immunofluorescence (IF) or enzyme-linked immunosorbent assays (ELISA). More recently, DNA-based techniques have been used for the molecular characterisations of *Cryptosporidium* species.

Pathology: The meronts and gamonts develop in a parasitophorous envelope apparently derived from the microvilli and so the cell disruption seen in other coccidia does not apparently occur. However, mucosal changes are obvious in the ileum where there is stunting, swelling and eventually fusion of the villi. This has a marked effect on the activity of some of the membrane-bound enzymes.

Epidemiology: A variety of mammals acts as hosts to *C. parvum* but *C. canis* appears to be adapted to dogs and *C. felis* to cats. Transmission appears to be mainly by the faecal–oral route.

Treatment: There is no known treatment. Supportive treatment and therapy of any concurrent illness may be required.

Control: Good hygiene and management are important in preventing disease from cryptosporidiosis.

Notes: Recent molecular characterisations have shown that there is extensive host adaptation in *Cryptosporidium* evolution, and many mammals or groups of mammals have host-adapted *Cryptosporidium* genotypes, which differ from each other in both DNA sequences and infectivity. These genotypes are now delineated as distinct species and include *C. hominis* (previously termed the human genotype or genotype 1), *C. parvum* (also termed the bovine genotype or genotype 2), *C. canis* (the dog genotype). Other genotypes have been associated with mouse, pig, bear, deer, marsupial, monkey, muskrat, skunk, cattle, and ferret. Most of these organisms probably represent individual *Cryptosporidium* species.

Giardia intestinalis

Synonym: *Giardia duodenalis*, *Giardia lamblia*, *Lamblia lamblia*

Predilection site: Small intestine

Parasite class: Zoomastigophorasida

Family: Diplomonadidae

Description: The trophozoite has a pyriform to ellipsoidal, bilaterally symmetrical body, 12–15 × 5–9 μm. The dorsal side is convex and there is a large sucking disk on the ventral side. There are two anterior nuclei, two slender axostyles, eight flagellae in four pairs and a pair of darkly staining median bodies. The median bodies are curved bars resembling the claws of a hammer. Cysts are ovoid, 8–12 × 7–10 µm and contain four nuclei.

Hosts: Man, cattle, sheep, goat, pig, alpaca, dog, cat, guinea pig, chinchilla

Life cycle: The life cycle is simple and direct, the trophozoite stage dividing by binary fission to produce further trophozoites. Intermittently, trophozoites encyst forming resistant cyst stages that pass out in the faeces of the host in the faeces.

Geographical distribution: Worldwide

Pathogenesis: Although *Giardia* cysts are commonly excreted in the faeces of dogs and cats there is no consistent relationship with diarrhoea or other signs of gastrointestinal problems, although they could act as reservoirs of infection for humans.

Clinical signs: When disease does occur, the signs often include chronic, pasty diarrhoea, weight loss, lethargy and failure to thrive.

Diagnosis: *Giardia* cysts can be detected in faeces by a number of methods. Traditional methods of identification involve direct examination of faecal smears, or faecal concentration by formalin-ethyl acetate or zinc sulphate methods and subsequent microscopic examination. It is generally recommended that three consecutive samples be examined as cysts are excreted intermittently.

Pathology: There may be villous atrophy, crypt hypertrophy and an increased number of intraepithelial lymphocytes. Trophozoites may be seen between villi, attached by their concave surface to the brush border of epithelial cells

Epidemiology: Molecular studies have revealed a substantial level of genetic diversity in *G. intestinalis* isolates. Human isolates fall into two major groups (assemblage A and B) with a wide host range in other mammals and it may prove to be the case that separate species names may be applicable. Other assemblages may also represent distinct species. Limited epidemiological studies suggest that in animal isolates, direct animal-to-animal contact and faecal soiling are the most likely methods of transmission, although water contamination can also be considered as a possible route. Zoonotic transmission has been reported from dogs.

Treatment and control: Several benzimidazole anthelmintics (e.g. albendazole, fenbendazole) and nitroimidazole drugs (metronidazole, tinidazole) are effective and may prove to be of benefit in the treatment of *Giardia* infections in animals. As infection is transmitted by the faecal–oral route, good hygiene and prevention of faecal contamination of feed and water are essential.

Notes: The parasite is important because of water-borne outbreaks that have occurred in human populations. There is still controversy over the classification of *Giardia* spp. The current molecular classification places isolates into eight distinct assemblages. Some authors give separate specific names to organisms isolated from different hosts, although species specificity of many isolates is unknown. Phylogenetic data suggest that *G. intestinalis* is a species complex composed of several species that are host specific.

LARGE INTESTINE

Trichuris vulpis

Synonym: *Trichocephalus vulpis*

Common name: Whipworms

Predilection site: Large intestine

Parasite class: Nematoda

Superfamily: Trichuroidea

Description, gross: The adults are whitish and about 4.5–7.5 cm long with a thick broad posterior end tapering rapidly to a long filamentous anterior end that is characteristically embedded in the mucosa (Fig. 6.15).

Description, microscopic: The male tail is coiled and possesses a single spicule in a protrusible sheath. The sheath bears small spines only on its anterior portion. The characteristic eggs are lemon shaped, 85 × 40 µm with a thick smooth shell and conspicuous polar plug at both ends; in the faeces these eggs appear yellow or brown in colour.

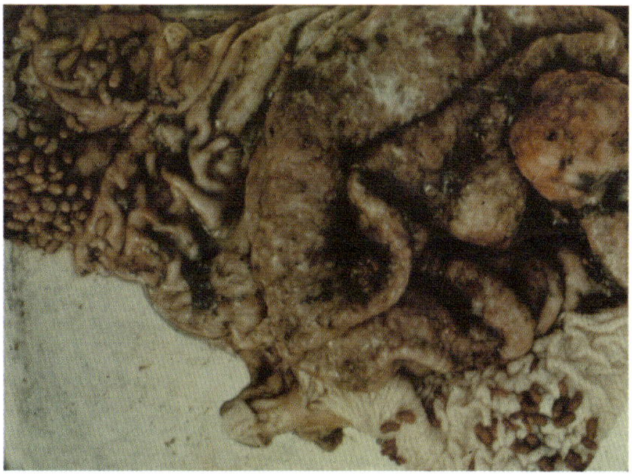

Fig. 6.15 *Trichuris vulpis* adults recovered from an infected intestine.

Hosts: Dog, fox, cat

Life cycle: The infective stage is the L_1 within the egg, which develops in 1 or 2 months of being passed in the faeces depending on the temperature. Under optimal conditions, these may subsequently survive and remain viable for several years. After ingestion, the plugs are digested and the released L_1 penetrate the glands of the distal ileum, caecal and colonic mucosa. Subsequently, all four moults occur within these glands, the adults emerging to lie on the mucosal surface with their anterior ends embedded in the mucosa. The prepatent period is around 3 months.

Geographical distribution: Many parts of the world

Pathogenesis: Most infections are light and asymptomatic. Occasionally, when large numbers of worms are present, they cause a haemorrhagic colitis and/or a diphtheritic inflammation of the caecal mucosa. This results from the subepithelial location and continuous movement of the anterior end to the whipworm as it searches for blood and fluid.

Clinical signs: Sporadic disease due to heavy infection is more common in dogs and is associated with an acute or chronic inflammation of the caecal mucosa with watery diarrhoea that often contains blood. Anaemia may be present and animals can lose weight.

Diagnosis: Since the clinical signs are not pathognomonic, diagnosis may depend on finding numbers of lemon-shaped *Trichuris* eggs in the faeces. Egg output is often low in *Trichuris* infections. However, since clinical signs may occur during the prepatent period, diagnosis may depend on necropsy or a favourable response to anthelmintic treatment. Occasionally expelled adult worms may be present in faeces.

Pathology: In severe cases, the mucosa of the large intestine is inflamed and haemorrhagic with ulceration and formation of diptheritic membranes.

Epidemiology: The most important feature is the longevity of the eggs. Older dogs tend to have higher whipworm burdens than young dogs.

Treatment: The probenzimidazoles and benzimidazoles, administered over several days, are effective against adult *Trichuris*, but less so against the larval stage. Milbemycins are effective.

Control: Prophylaxis is rarely necessary. Attention should be given to areas where eggs might continue to survive for long periods. Such areas should be thoroughly cleaned and disinfected or sterilised by wet or dry heat.

Notes: The adults are usually found in the caecum but are only occasionally present in sufficient numbers to be clinically significant.

Two other species, ***Trichuris serrata*** and ***Trichuris campanula***, are occasionally found in the cat, mainly in North and South America and the Caribbean. Details on the life cycle, pathogenesis, treatment and control are essentially similar to those for *T. vulpis*.

Entamoeba histolytica

Predilection site: Large intestine, liver

Parasite subphylum: Sarcodina

Family: Endamoebidae

Description: Trophozoites of the large form are 20–30 μm in diameter, those of the small form are 12–15 μm. The nucleus, when stained, has a small central endostome with a ring of small peripheral granules. The cysts of both forms are 10–12 μm in size, contain four nuclei when mature and often contain rod-like chromatin bodies with rounded ends.

Hosts: Man, dog, cat, pig, rat, monkey

Life cycle: *E. histolytica* multiplies by binary fission, but eventually encysts and cysts are passed in the faeces. Cysts contain four nuclei and are relatively resistant. When ingested the amoebae emerge from the cyst and both the nuclei and cytoplasm divide resulting in eight small amoebae from each cyst.

Geographical distribution: Worldwide

Pathogenesis: Two forms of the parasite exist. Non-pathogenic forms of the organism normally live in the lumen of the large intestine. Pathogenic forms invade the mucosa causing ulceration and dysentery. From there they may be carried via the portal system to the liver and other organs where large abscesses may form. The amoeba-like trophozoites secrete proteolytic enzymes and produce characteristic flask-shaped ulcers in the mucosa of the large intestine. Their erosion may allow the parasites to enter the bloodstream when the most common sequel is the formation of amoebic abscesses in the liver. The veterinary significance of amoebosis is that natural infections, usually without clinical signs, can occur occasionally in dogs from the human reservoir of active or carrier infections. Kittens are also susceptible to experimental infection, although they do not produce cysts. Monkeys have their own strains of *E. histolytica* and these can be infective to man.

Clinical signs: Infection causes diarrhoea or dysentery.

Diagnosis: Motile organisms and cysts of *E. histolytica* may be detected in smears from faeces. Trophozoites and cysts can be stained with iodine, trichrome or iron haematoxylin. The organisms can also be cultured in a number of media including Boeck and Drbohlav's, Dobell and Laidlaw's, TYI-S-33 and Robinson's medium. Isoenzyme markers can be used to differentiate the two forms seen, but there is some debate as to whether the two types represent different species or if they can change from one type to another under certain circumstances.

A number of serological tests have been evaluated for the diagnosis of *E. histolytica* infections. These include ELISA, latex agglutination, complement fixation and indirect haemagglutination. A number of polymerase chain reactions (PCRs) have also been used to detect *E. histolytica* in clinical samples. The PCRs are based upon the amplification of specific DNA sequences that correlate to the pathogenic/non-pathogenic isoenzyme analysis categorisation and appear to be very sensitive and specific.

Pathology: Pathogenic strains of amoebae penetrate the mucosa of the large intestine and multiply to form small colonies that extend into the submucosa and muscularis. In the absence of bacterial infection there is little reaction, but in complicated infections there is hyperaemia and inflammation with predominantly neutrophils. Amoebae may pass into the lymphatic system and mediastinal lymph nodes and from there migrate in the portal system to the liver where they may cause abcessation. Abcesses may also form in other organs including the lungs and brain.

Epidemiology: *E. histolytica* is primarily a parasite of primates, man is the reservoir for animals. Infection in dogs has only been reported sporadically and often through human contacts.

Treatment: Treatment, if required, relies on the combined use of metronidazole and diiodohydroxyquin.

Control: Dogs are not a significant reservoir of infection for man so that prophylaxis ultimately depends on personal and sanitary hygiene in the human population.

Pentatrichomonas hominis

Synonym: *Pentatrichomonas felis*, *Cercomonas hominis*, *Monocercomonas hominis*, *Trichomonas felis*, *Trichomonas intestinalis*

Predilection site: Large intestine

Parasite subphylum: Sarcodina

Family: Trichomonadidae

Description: The body is pyriform, 8–20 μm long and there are usually five anterior flagella. Four of the anterior flagella are grouped together, and the fifth is separate and directed posteriorly. A sixth flagella runs along the undulating membrane and extends beyond the body as a free trailing flagellum. The undulating membrane extends the length of the body. The axostyle is thick, hyaline with a sharply pointed tip. The pelta is crescent shaped.

Hosts: Man, monkey, dog, cat, rat, mouse, hamster, guinea pig

Life cycle: The trichomonads reproduce by longitudinal binary fission. No sexual stages are known and there are no cysts.

Geographical distribution: Worldwide

Pathogenesis: *P. hominis* is considered non-pathogenic.

Diagnosis: Morphological identification of the organisms from fresh and stained faecal preparations. The organism can also be cultured in trichomonads culture medium.

Treatment and control: Not required

PARASITES OF THE RESPIRATORY SYSTEM

Two species of the genus, *Mammomonogamus*, which is closely related to *Syngamus*, are parasitic in the nasal cavities of cats. Infections are usually asymptomatic but affected animals may sneeze and have a nasal discharge due to irritation of the nasal mucosa. Adult worms are red in colour, 1–2 cm long and permanently joined in copula. Diagnosis is based on clinical signs and the finding of eggs in the faeces or adult worms on postmortem. Details of the life cycle are unknown and there is no known effective treatment.

Mammomonogamus ierei

Predilection site: Nasal cavities

Parasite class: Nematoda

Superfamily: Strongyloidea

Hosts: Cat

Geographical distribution: Caribbean

Mammomonogamus mcgaughei

Predilection site: Frontal sinuses

Parasite class: Nematoda

Superfamily: Strongyloidea

Hosts: Cat

Geographical distribution: Sri Lanka

Capillaria aerophila

Synonym: *Eucoleus aerophila*

Common name: Tracheal worm

Predilection site: Trachea, bronchi, occasionally nasal passages and frontal sinuses

Parasite class: Nematoda

Superfamily: Trichuroidea

Description, gross: These are very fine whitish, filamentous worms, the narrow stichosome oesophagus occupying about one third to half the body length. Males measure around 24 mm and females 32 mm.

Description, microscopic: The males have a long thin single spicule and often possess a primitive bursa-like structure. The females contain eggs that resemble those of *Trichuris* in possessing bipolar plugs. The eggs are barrel-shaped and colourless, 59–80 × 30–40 μm and have thick shells that are slightly striated with bipolar plugs.

Final hosts: Fox, particularly those reared on fur farms, and mustelids; occasionally dogs, cats and man.

Intermediate hosts: Earthworms

Life cycle: The parasite can have both a direct and an indirect life cycle. The females deposit eggs in the lungs and these are coughed up, swallowed and pass out in the faeces onto soil. These eggs take around 5–6 weeks to reach the infective stage and can survive for months in the environment. In the direct cycle, following ingestion of the embryonated eggs, the larvae hatch and penetrate the small intestine and migrate via the lymphatics and bloodstream to the respiratory passages where they invade the mucosa. In the indirect cycle, eggs that are ingested by earthworms hatch and the larvae are infective. The final host is infected following consumption of the earthworm. The prepatent period is around 6 weeks.

Geographical distribution: Worldwide.

Pathogenesis: The nematode causes irritation to the respiratory mucosa with a resultant increase in secretion. There may be some constriction of the lumen of the air passages and some areas may show emphysema. Heavy infections can induce bronchopneumonia with occasional abscess formation in the lung tissue. Secondary bacterial infection can sometimes occur which often is fatal in younger animals.

Clinical signs: Light infections are usually asymptomatic. The clinical signs of moderate to severe infection are those of rhinotracheitis and/or bronchitis and in this respect are similar to those caused by *Oslerus* or *Crenosoma* infection. In such cases, there may be a nasal discharge, a wheezing cough and/or sneezing. Dyspnoea can be observed in heavy infections.

Diagnosis: The presence of eggs in faeces and a nasal discharge are indicative of infection. Note that the eggs are morphologically similar to those of *Capillaria plica* (see under Parasites of the reproductive/urogenital system).

Pathology: The effects depend on the number of worms present. Mild infections cause a mild catarrhal inflammation whilst heavy infections cause more severe irritation and obstruction to the lumen of the airways.

Epidemiology: Although infection can be acquired through the consumption of infective earthworms, the major route of transmission is usually via the ingestion of embryonated infective eggs. *C. aerophila* is particularly a problem in farmed animals reared for their fur. Disease is usually seen in foxes of less than 18 months of age.

Treatment: Modern benzimidazoles or ivermection are effective. Levamisole at 7.5 mg/kg on two consecutive days and repeating 14 days later is also effective.

Control: On fox-rearing farms, care should be taken to ensure that runs are created in areas where the soil is dry and free-draining. Alternatively, the animals should be housed in cages raised above the soil. Breeding pens need to be cleaned thoroughly to reduce the accumulation of infective eggs. Periodic treatment with anthelmintic is essential.

Notes: The taxonomic situation regarding many species of *Capillaria* is complex and recently it has been split into several genera; the old species names are listed with the new proposed generic names.

Crenosoma vulpis

Common name: Fox lungworm

Predilection site: Trachea, bronchi and bronchioles

Parasite class: Nematoda

Superfamily: Metastrongyloidea

Description, gross: Slender white worms, up to 1.5 cm long. Males are 3.5–8 mm with well developed bursae with a large dorsal ray. Females are 12–15 mm. The host and site are sufficient for generic diagnosis.

Description, microscopic: Microscopic confirmation is based on the presence of annular folds of the cuticle, which bear small backwardly directed spines on their margins.

Final hosts: Dog, fox

Intermediate hosts: Slugs, snails (*Helix*, *Cepea*, *Arianta*, *Agriolimax*, *Arion*)

Life cycle: *C. vulpis* is ovo-viviparous and L_1 are passed in the faeces. Larvae penetrate the foot of the intermediate molluscan host and are infective in about 3 weeks. After ingestion of the molluscan host by the final host, the L_3 are released by digestion and travel to the lungs, via the lymphatic glands and hepatic circulation, where both parasitic moults take place. The prepatent period is around 3 weeks.

Geographical distribution: Worldwide

Pathogenesis: The spiny cuticular folds abrade the mucosa of the air passages with resulting bronchopneumonia and occlusion of the smaller bronchi and bronchioles.

Clinical signs: The symptoms are those of a chronic respiratory infection, with coughing, sneezing and nasal discharge associated with tachypnoea. Farmed foxes may become emaciated, with fur of poor quality. In the infrequent acute infections there may be high mortality.

Diagnosis: Examination of faeces by smear, flotation or Baerman technique will reveal the L_1 with a straight tail which differentiates it in fresh canine faeces from those of *Oslerus*, *Filaroides* and *Angiostrongylus*. The L_1 somewhat resembles that of *Strongyloides* spp. Infection should be differentiated from that caused by *Capillaria aerophila* as the two disease entities are similar.

Pathology: The gross lesions usually observed in dogs are greyish consolidations in dorsal regions of the caudal lobes. Histologically, the lesions are catarrhal, eosinophilic bronchitis and bronchiolitis.

Epidemiology: *C. vulpis* is more common in the fox than in the dog, and can be a problem in farmed foxes. The infection has a seasonality corresponding to fluctuations in population of its snail vectors so that, though cubs may begin to acquire L_3 in early summer, the highest incidence of clinical crenosomosis is seen in autumn.

Treatment: Diethylcarbamazine has been reported to be effective but is no longer widely available. Levamisole has reported activity at 8 mg/kg and ivermectin is likely to be active.

Control: The snail vectors may be eliminated by spraying fox runs with molluscicide and painting woodwork with creosote up to 20 cm from the ground. Faeces should be disposed of in a manner that will avoid access by molluscs.

Oslerus osleri

Synonym: *Filaroides osleri*

Common name: Dog lungworm

Predilection site: Bronchii

Parasite class: Nematoda

Superfamily: Metastrongyloidea

Description, gross: Small, pale, slender worms, up to 15 mm long; males are 5 mm, and females 9–15 mm long.

Description, microscopic: The tail of the male is rounded and bears a few papillae; spicules are short and slightly unequal. The larva has a short S-shaped tail.

Hosts: Dog

Life cycle: *Oslerus*, and its closely related genus, *Filaroides*, are exceptional in the superfamily Metastrongyloidea in having direct life cycles. The females are ovo-viviparous, and most eggs hatch in the trachea. Many larvae are coughed up and swallowed, and passed in the faeces and infection may occur by ingestion of these; more commonly, transmission occurs when an infected bitch licks the pup and transfers the newly hatched L_1, which are present in her sputum. After ingestion, the first moult occurs in the small intestine and the L_2 travel to the lungs by the lymphatic–vascular route. Development through to L_5 takes place in the alveoli and bronchi, and the adults migrate to their predilection site, the tracheal bifurcation. The prepatent period varies from 10–18 weeks.

Geographical distribution: Worldwide

Pathogenesis: The worms are embedded in fibrous nodules (2–20 mm) in the trachea at the region of bifurcation, and in the adjacent bronchi (Fig. 6.16). Rarely found deeper in the lungs. The nodules in which the worms live first appear at about two months from infection. They are pinkish-grey granulomas, and the small worms may be seen partly protruding from their surfaces. These nodules are fibrous in character

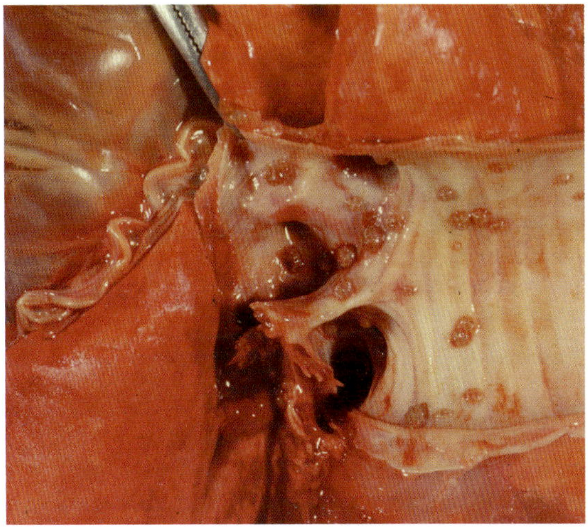

Fig. 6.16 Fibrous nodules in the bronchus caused by infection with *Oslerus osleri*.

and are very firmly applied to the mucosa; they may be up to 2.0 cm in diameter. Though the majority occur near the tracheal bifurcation a few may be found several centimetres from this area. Infection can cause chronic tracheobronchitis.

Clinical signs: Many infections are clinically inapparent, and the characteristic nodules are only discovered incidentally at necropsy. The major signs of *Oslerus* infection are respiratory distress and a dry rasping persistent cough, especially after exercise. The most severe cases have usually been seen in dogs of 6–12 months old, and obviously the infection is of greater importance in working dogs. Heavy chronic infections can impair appetite and lead to emaciation. In household pets, whose exercise is limited, the presence of the tracheal nodules is well tolerated, and animals show little respiratory distress.

Diagnosis: Swabs of pharyngeal mucus give variable results and repeated sampling may be necessary. However, in paroxysmal coughing, large amounts of bronchial mucus are often expelled, containing large numbers of larvae. Less rewarding techniques are those based on faecal examination, either by flotation or by the Baerman method. Although requiring general anaesthesia, bronchoscopy is the most reliable method, as it will indicate not only the presence, size and location of many of the nodules, but will also allow the collection of tracheal mucus for confirmatory examination for eggs and larvae; the latter are invariably coiled, sluggish and have an S-shaped tail. Large nodules may be detected by lateral thoracic radiography.

Pathology: Typical lesions are protruding submucosal nodules, greyish white in colour, in the region of the tracheal bifurcation. Lesions vary in size from barely visible to larger nodules or protruding plaques that project over 1 cm into the lumen of the trachea. Smaller nodules contain immature worms, and the larger ones a mass of tightly coiled adults. The worms lie in tissue spaces between the cartilage rings of the trachea and large bronchii. Live worms provoke formation of a thin capsule and lymphocytic infiltration locally. Superficially the nodules are covered by intact epithelium, except for small pores through which the female worms protrude their tails to lay eggs. Dead worms provoke a foreign body reaction with neutrophils and a few giant cells.

Epidemiology: Transmission occurs when an infected bitch licks the pups and transfers the newly hatched L_1 present in the sputum. Though *Oslerus* has been recorded from many countries there is little data on its local prevalence. In the UK, one survey has given a figure of 6% for all types of dog. In further surveys in the same area, greyhounds have shown a prevalence rate of 18%, but there is no evidence of breed susceptibility. In general the focus of infection appears to be the nursing bitch. Infection rates may be high in kennel-housed dogs.

Treatment: There are reports of amelioration of clinical signs, apparently due to a reduction in the size of the nodules, after prolonged treatment with some benzimidazoles. Fenbendazole and albendazole at increased dosage rates are licensed for the treatment of *Oslerus* infection in dogs.

Control: This is difficult unless infected bitches can be identified and treated before whelping and during lactation. In the past the only certain method of control was the removal of pups from infected dams at birth, and hand rearing or fostering on uninfected bitches.

Notes: This genus was, until recently, part of the larger genus *Filaroides*, but has now been separated on morphological grounds from the other members. Though distinction has been made on morphology it is also useful from the veterinary standpoint, for it separates the single harmful species, *Oslerus osleri*, living in the upper air passages, from the relatively harmless species which are retained in the genus *Filaroides*, and which live in the lung parenchyma.

Filaroides hirthi

Common name: Dog lungworm

Predilection site: Lung

Parasite class: Nematoda

Superfamily: Metastrongyloidea

Description, gross: The worms are very small (0.5–1.0 cm long), slender, hair-like and greyish, and are not only difficult to see with the naked eye in the lung parenchyma but are unlikely to be recovered intact from the tissue. *F. hirthi* is smaller than *F. milksi* (see later).

Description, microscopic: The L_1, present in the faeces and sputum, is coiled, and the tail has a notch, followed by a constriction, and has a terminal lance-like point.

Hosts: Domestic dog, wild carnivores

Life cycle: The life cycle is direct. The worms are ovo-viviparous and the hatched L_1 are passed in faeces or expelled in sputum. Though infection may be acquired by ingestion of faecal larvae, the important route, as in *Oslerus* infection, is thought to be by transfer of L_1 in the bitch's saliva when the pup is licked. The prepatent period of *F. hirthi* is 5 weeks.

Geographical distribution: North America, Europe and Japan

Pathogenesis: Infection is almost invariably asymptomatic, and is discovered only at postmortem examination. However, in the rare heavy infection, hyperpnoea may occur.

Clinical signs: Asymptomatic, rarely hyperpnoea in heavy infections

Diagnosis: A squeeze preparation from a cut surface of the lung will show worm fragments, eggs and larvae, and this, with the host and site, is sufficient for generic diagnosis. Only *F. hirthi* has been diagnosed in the live animal and this was in experimental dogs. The L_1, present in the faeces and sputum, is coiled, and the tail has a notch, followed by a constriction, and has a terminal lance-like point. Zinc sulphate is an effective flotation solution for the detection of larvae.

Pathology: The chief lesions are the small, soft, greyish miliary nodules which are associated with the presence of worms and which are distributed subpleurally and throughout the lung parenchyma; in heavy infections, sometimes observed in experimental dogs subjected to immunosuppressive drugs, the nodules may coalesce into greyish masses.

Epidemiology: Little is known of the epidemiology. *F. hirthi* was first observed in a breeding colony of experimental beagles, and it would be fair to suggest, in view of its mode of transmission, that a high prevalence could be expected in dogs from breeding kennels.

Treatment: Albendazole has been reported to be effective although treatment is rarely called for.

Control: Unlikely to be required.

Filaroides milksi

Common name: Dog lungworm

Predilection site: Lung

Parasite class: Nematoda

Superfamily: Metastrongyloidea

Description: As for *F. hirthi*. *F. milksi* is larger than *F. hirthi*

Hosts: Domestic dog, wild carnivores

Geographical distribution: North America

Anafilaroides rostratus

Predilection site: Lung

Parasite class: Nematoda

Superfamily: Metastrongyloidea

Description: As for *F. hirthi*

Hosts: Cat, rodents

Geographical distribution: North America, Sri Lanka

All other details are as for *F. hirthi*.

Aelurostrongylus abstrusus

Common name: Cat lungworm

Predilection site: Lung parenchyma and small bronchioles

Parasite class: Nematoda

Superfamily: Metastrongyloidea

Description, gross: Aggregations of worms, eggs and larvae are present throughout the lung tissue. The worms, about 0.5–1.0 cm long, are very slender and delicate, and are difficult to recover intact for examination.

Description, microscopic: The male bursa is short and the lobes are indistinct. Eggs measure $80 \times 70\ \mu m$; L_1 in faeces bear a sub-terminal spine on their S-shaped tail.

Final host: Cat

Intermediate hosts: Many terrestrial molluscs, such as snails and slugs; paratenic hosts include rodents, birds, amphibians and reptiles.

Life cycle: The life cycle is indirect. The worms are ovo-viviparous, and the L_1 are passed in the faeces. These penetrate the foot of the molluscan intermediate host and develop to the infective L_3 and during this phase paratenic hosts, such as birds and rodents, may eat the mollusc. The cat is usually infected by ingestion of these paratenic hosts and less frequently by ingestion of the intermediate hosts. The L_3 released in the alimentary tract, travel to the lungs by the lymphatics or bloodstream. After the final moult the adults are located in the alveolar ducts and the terminal bronchioles. The prepatent period is between 4 and 6 weeks, and the duration of patency is about 4 months, though some worms may survive in the lungs for several years despite the absence of larvae in the faeces.

Geographical distribution: Presumed worldwide

Pathogenesis: The worm generally has a low pathogenicity, and the majority of infections are discovered only incidentally at postmortem examination as multiple small, greyish foci or bigger consolidated granulomas in the lungs.

Clinical signs: The clinical effects are slight, and in the resting cat are limited to a chronic mild cough. Following exercise or handling, there may be coughing, sneezing and nasal discharge with slight dyspnoea and production of mucoid sputum. In heavy experimental infections the most severe signs have appeared at

6–12 weeks after infection when egg laying is maximal. Heavy infections may be accompanied by diarrhoea and weight loss.

Diagnosis: Repeated faecal examination by smear, flotation, or Baerman technique may be necessary to find the characteristic L_1, which bears a sub-terminal spine on its S-shaped tail. Examination of pharyngeal swabs may be a useful additional procedure. At necropsy a squeeze preparation from a cut surface of the lung will often show the worm material including the characteristic L_1. Radiography has revealed the increased vascular and focal parenchymal densities, which would be expected from the changes described above.

Pathology: In most cases the lungs show only multiple small raised subpleural foci with greyish centres containing the worms and tissue debris, but in the rare severe infections larger nodules are present, up to 1.0 cm in diameter with caseous centres, projecting from the lung surface; these nodules may coalesce to form areas of consolidation. Microscopically the alveoli may be blocked with worms, eggs, larvae and cellular aggregations, which may progress to granuloma formation. A characteristic change is muscular hypertrophy and hyperplasia, which affects not only the bronchioles and alveolar ducts, but also the media of the pulmonary arteries. In these heavy infections the pleural cavity can be filled with a whitish fluid and occasionally fatalities have been reported. With the exception of the muscular changes, which appear to be irreversible, resolution is rapid and the lungs appear almost completely normal within 6 months of experimental infection, though a few worms may still be present.

Epidemiology: *Aelurostrongylus* infection is widespread, partly because it is almost indiscriminate in its ability to develop in slugs and snails, and partly because of its wide range of paratenic hosts. So far all surveys have shown prevalences greater than 5%.

Treatment: Fenbendazole at 50 mg/kg daily for 3 days has proved effective.

Control: In household pets, and especially those of a nomadic disposition or living in rural locations, access to the intermediate and paratenic hosts is difficult to prevent and control is not often easy or practical.

Notes: Other nematodes can invade the lungs of cats, but generally they are considered to be of low pathogenicity.

Paragonimus westermani

Common name: Oriental lung fluke

Predilection site: Lung

Parasite class: Trematoda

Family: Troglotrematidae

Description, gross: The parasite is rounded and thick, reddish brown in colour 7.5–16 × 4–8 mm, and covered in scale-like spines. The ventral sucker is situated slightly anterior to the middle of the fluke.

Description, microscopic: Species differentiation is based on the shape of the spines. Those in *P. westermani* are large and have bifid points. Eggs are yellowish brown in colour, operculate, 75–118 × 42–67 μm and the shell is thickened at the opposite end to the operculum. Diploid and triploid flukes occur in the Far East.

Hosts: Dog, cat, pig, goat, cattle, fox, other carnivores and man

Life cycle: The life cycle involves an amphibious or water snail, and a crayfish or fresh water crab. Snails of the genera *Melania*, *Ampullaria* or *Pomatiopsis* are infected by miracidia in which further development through sporocyst, redia and cerceria takes place. After escaping the snail, the cercariae swim about and, on contact with a freshwater crab or crayfish, penetrate it and encyst. Crabs and crayfish can also eat cercaria-infected snails. Infection of the final host occurs by ingestion of the metacercariae in the liver or muscles of the crustacean. Infection can also be aquired through consumpion of paratenic hosts which have eaten infected crabs or crayfish. The young flukes migrate to the lungs where they are encapsulated by fibrous cysts connected by fistulae to the bronchioles to facilitate egg excretion. Eggs pass up from the lung in the sputum which the animals usually swallow such that eggs are passed in the faeces. The prepatent period is 5–6 weeks.

Geographical distribution: Asia

Pathogenesis: Parasites in the lungs are not usually of great importance, but some may lodge in the brain or other organs causing more severe damage. Pulmonary signs are comparatively rare in cats or dogs and the veterinary interest is in the potential reservoir of infection for man. Extrapulmonary infections may produce a cutaneous larval migrans and abscess formation in the skin and viscera. Brain and spinal cord involvement may lead to seizures, paraplegia and occasional deaths.

Clinical signs: In lung infections there may be a cough and eggs may be found in the sputum in large numbers.

Diagnosis: Diagnosis is by identifying the presence of eggs in the sputum or faeces.

Pathology: In the lungs the parasitic cyst is surrounded by diffuse connective tissue and the cyst wall becomes infiltrated by leucocytes and giant cells. The cyst usually contains two parasites surrounded by a purulent fluid mixed with blood and eggs. Pleural adhesions sometimes occur and there is usually hyperplasia of the bronchial epithelium and focal areas of inflammation in the lung parenchyma.

Epidemiology: Infection is maintained in endemic areas where intermediate hosts are abundant.

Treatment: High doses of albendazole, fenbendazole or niclofolan over a prolonged period can be effective in control.

Control: The complex life cycle makes control in endemic areas impossible.

Notes: There are over ten species of *Paragonimus* which infect man.

Paragonimus kellicotti

Common name: Lung fluke

Predilection site: Lung

Parasite class: Trematoda

Family: Troglotrematidae

Description, gross: The parasite is rounded, reddish brown in colour, 7.5–16 × 4–8 mm and covered in scale-like spines. The ventral sucker is situated slightly anterior to the middle of the fluke.

Description, microscopic: Species differentiation is based on the shape of the spines. Those in *P. kellicotti* are very large and have a number of points. Eggs are golden-brown in colour, 80–118 × 48–60 μm and have a partly flattened operculum.

Hosts: Cat, pig, dog

Life cycle: As for *P. westermani*

Geographical distribution: North America, South Africa

Pathogenesis: Similar to *P. westermani*

Pneumonyssus caninum

Common name: Nasal mite

Predilection site: Nasal cavity, sinuses

Parasite class: Arachnida

Parasite sub-class: Acari

Family: Halarachnidae

Description: The mites are oval and pale yellow, adults measuring approximately 1–1.5 × 0.6–0.9 mm. They have a smooth cuticle with relatively few setae. The mites have a single irregularly shaped dorsal plate and a small sternal plate. Genital plates are absent in this species and the genital opening is a transverse slit between the coxae of the fourth pair of legs. They have long legs, relative to their body size, which terminate in claws, short pre-tarsi (though these are relatively longer on the first pair of legs) and small suckers.

Hosts: Dog

Life cycle: The details on the life history of these mites is not fully known. There appear to be two main life stages, the adult and a six-legged larval stage. There is no nymphal stage in the life cycle of this parasite. The female is ovo-viviparous and mature females often contain eggs and it is probable that they give birth to larvae.

Geographical distribution: Worldwide; particularly prevalent in Scandanavia

Pathogenesis: *Pneumonyssus caninum* has been associated with head shaking and 'inverted' sneezing, as well as with chronic rhinitis, sinusitis and tonsillitis, although the majority of infections seem to be subclinical. In working and hunting dogs the most obvious result of nasal mite infection is a markedly impaired sense of smell. There is evidence that *P. caninum* can penetrate host tissues and move beyond the respiratory system to cause lesions in the liver and kidney.

Clinical signs: The presence of mites causes excessive nasal secretion and hyperaemia of the nasal mucosa. Extreme infestations may result in listlessness, loss of appetite, irritation and scratching at the eyes, chronic sneezing, bronchial cough and rhinitis or sinusitis.

Diagnosis: The mites can be seen crawling over the tissue surface of the nasal sinuses. Specific diagnosis may be achieved through microscopic examination.

Epidemiology: The infection is probably transmitted by direct nose-to-nose contact between animals. This species appears to be particularly common in Scandinavia; a prevalence of 24% in pet dogs at necropsy has been reported in Sweden.

Treatment and control: Treatment with ivermectin has proved effective.

Linguatula serrata

Common name: Tongue worm

Predilection site: Nasal cavity, sinuses

Parasite class: Pentastomida

Family: Linguatulidae

Description: Males measure up to 20 mm in length while females are 30–130 mm in length. Both sexes are transversely striated, expanded anteriorly and shaped like an elongated tongue (see Fig 1.45). Anteriorly there are five small protuberances, one bearing a small mouth at its extremity, the others bearing tiny claws. The eggs measure about 90 × 70 μm. The larval stage is up to 500 μm in size and devoid of annulations and mouthparts.

Hosts: Principal hosts are tropical reptiles, such as snakes and crocodiles, but some species parasitise mammals and birds. *Linguatula serrata* occurs in dogs, cats and foxes, the adult occurring in the nasal passages and sinuses.

Life cycle: With most pentastomids the life cycle requires an intermediate host. In the case of *Linguatula serrata*, eggs are expelled from the respiratory passage of the host by coughing or sneezing. Eggs are ingested by the herbivorous intermediate host, commonly sheep or cattle or rabbits, and pass into the gut where they hatch. The larva bores through the intestinal wall to the mesenteric glands, liver and lungs. Here, larval development involving a number of moults takes place. The larvae then encyst to develop into the infective nymphal stage. The cysts, about 1.0 mm in diameter, may be visible in cut surfaces of mesenteric glands. The final host is infected by eating uncooked viscera. Following ingestion, the nymph migrates to the nasal passages where the final moult, mating and egg production occur.

Geographical distribution: Worldwide: North America, Europe and Australia

Pathogenesis and clinical signs: Infrequently, heavy infections in dogs may cause sneezing, coughing and a nasal discharge. The parasites live for about 15 months in the host, after which the animal usually recovers.

Diagnosis: Eggs may be found in the faeces or the nasal discharge. Encysted nymphs may be visible in cut surfaces of mesenteric glands.

Treatment and control: There is no specific treatment recommended, although systemic insecticides should be considered. It is possible to remove the parasites surgically. Infection can be avoided by preventing animals from eating potentially infected material.

Pneumocystis carinii

Synonym: *Pneumocystis jiroveci*

Common name: Pneumocystosis

Predilection site: Lung

Parasite class: Archiascomycetes

Family: Pneumocystidaceae

Description: Two major forms of *P. carinii* have been consistently identified from histological and ultrastructural analysis of organisms found in human and rat lung. These are a trophic form and a larger cyst stage containing eight intracystic stages.

Hosts: Man, cattle, rat, ferret, mouse, dog, horse, pig and rabbit

Life cycle: The life cycle of *Pneumocystis* still remains poorly understood. Information is mostly derived from histochemical and ultrastructural analysis of the lung tissue of rodents and infected humans. The presumed life cycle of *Pneumocystis* includes an asexual and a sexual growth phase. Current knowledge suggests that the trophic (trophozoite) forms are produced during asexual development. These forms are usually pleomorphic and found in clusters. They appear capable of replicating asexually by binary fission and also replicate sexually by conjugation, producing a diploid zygote; this undergoes meiosis and subsequent mitosis, resulting in the formation of a precyst initially, and then an early cyst and a mature cyst eventually. During differentiation of the organism from precyst to mature cyst, eight intracystic spores or 'daughter cells' are produced. These intracystic spores are subsequently released, as the mature cyst ruptures, and develop into trophic forms.

Geographical distribution: Worldwide

Pathogenesis: *Pneumocystis* is one of the major causes of opportunistic mycoses in the immunocompromised, including those with congenital immunodeficiencies, retrovirus infections such as AIDS, and cases receiving immunosuppressive therapy.

Clinical signs: Not reported in dogs

Diagnosis: Gomori's methenamine silver (GMS) and Giemsa stain may be used for microscopic visualisation of *Pneumocystis*. Toluidine blue (TBO) is the most effective for cyst stages while Giemsa stains are used to show trophozoites.

Axenic culture methods have been described; however, *in vitro* cultivation, especially from clinical samples, is not always successful. Flourescence antibody staining techniques can be used to detect both cyst and trophozoite stages of *P. carinii*. A number of PCRs have been reported which amplify specific regions of DNA from *P. carinii* and are approximately 100 times more sensitive than conventional staining techniques.

Pathology: The lesion is characterised by a massive plasma cell or histiocyte infiltration of the alveoli in which the organisms may be detected by a silver staining procedure. A foamy eosinophilic material is observed in the lungs during infection. This material is composed of masses of the organism, alveolar macrophages, desquamated epithelial alveolar cells, polymorphonuclear leucocytes and other host cells.

Epidemiology: The organism is apparently quite widely distributed in latent form in healthy individuals and in the dog, as well as a wide variety of other domestic and wild animals. The organism is thought to be transmitted by aerosol, although the natural habitats and modes of transmission of infections in humans are current areas of research. *Pneumocystis* DNA has been detected in air and water suggesting that the free forms of the organism may survive in the environment long enough to infect a susceptible host. However, little information on the means of transmission exists currently. In humans, infections appear to spread between immunosuppressed patients colonised with *Pneumocystis*, and immunocompetent individuals transiently parasitised with the organism. Human and non-human *Pneumocystis* species have been shown to be different and host-specific, suggesting that zoonotic transmission does not occur.

Treatment: Trimethroprim–sulphamethoxazole is the drug of choice for treatment and prophylaxis of *Pneumocystis* infections. Pentamidine and atovaquone are the alternative therapeutic agents in humans.

Control: Control is difficult given that the details of the routes of transmission are unknown. Infection is generally asymptomatic in animals and is only likely to be detected in immunocompromised individuals.

Notes: Initially reported as a morphological form of *Trypanosoma cruzi*, this microorganism later proved to be a separate genus and was named *Pneumocystis carinii* and classified as a protozoan until the late 1980s. Following further taxonomic revision, *Pneumocystis* is now classified as a fungus, not a protozoan. The taxonomy is still complicated in that *Pneumocystis* from humans and other animals are quite different and there appear to be multiple species in this genus. Genetic variations and DNA sequence polymorphisms are often observed, suggesting the existence of numerous strains even within a single species of *Pneumocystis*.

PARASITES OF THE LIVER

Fasciola hepatica

See Chapter 3 (Sheep and goats).

Capillaria hepatica

Synonym: *Callodium hepatica, Hepaticola hepatica*

Predilection site: Liver

Parasite class: Nematoda

Superfamily: Trichuroidea

Description, gross: These are very fine filamentous worms generally measuring between 1 and 5 cm in length.

Description, microscopic: The males have a long thin single spicule and often possess a primitive bursa-like structure. The eggs are barrel-shaped and colourless have thick shells that are slightly striated with bipolar plugs.

Hosts: Rat, mouse, squirrel, rabbit and farmed mustelids; occasionally dog, cat and man

Life cycle: The life cycle is direct and differs from that of other *Capillaria* species. Adult *C. hepatica* worms reproduce in the liver and females lay groups of eggs in the parenchyma where they become encapsulated by the host's reaction. These eggs are therefore not released directly from the host. Infection is acquired by ingestion of either the liver, following predation, cannibalism or carrion feeding, or eggs on the ground that have been freed by decomposition of the host. Eggs in the soil will embryonate and be infective in about 4 weeks. When infective eggs are ingested by the host, they hatch in the intestine and the larvae penetrate the intestinal wall and are carried to the liver via the lymphatics and the bloodstream.

Geographical distribution: Worldwide (in rodents)

Pathogenesis: Adult worms are found in the parenchyma of the liver where they provoke traumatic hepatitis. Eggs are laid in groups in the liver parenchyma from which there is no natural access to the exterior. Granulomas develop around the eggs, accompanied by fibrosis. Heavy infections can cause hepatitis and/or cirrhosis and ascites. The liver may be enlarged and severe infections can be fatal. Heavy infections in man induce similar hepatic lesions to those seen in other mammalian hosts and hepatic capillariosis is usually fatal.

Clinical signs: Mild infections are usually asymptomatic. At autopsy, the liver may have yellowy white streaks on the surface.

Diagnosis: Most infections are discovered at routine autopsy. Granulomatous tissue in the liver parenchyma can be examined for the presence of eggs or worm fragments after squashing between microscope slides.

Pathology: The eggs, which are deposited in clusters, provoke the development of localised granulomas, which are visible through the capsule as yellowish streaks or patches.

Epidemiology: Although the prevalence of *C. hepatica* is high in the liver of rodents it lacks host specificity and occurs in a variety of mammals. Human infection is acquired through ingestion of soil, containing embryonated eggs, or by consuming contaminated food or water.

Treatment: Oral administration of a modern benzimidazole over several days can be effective at preventing egg deposition in the liver tissues. Once egg deposition has occurred, treatment may not be effective.

Control: Destruction of rodents will assist in control.

Notes: The taxonomic situation regarding many species of *Capillaria* is complex and recently it has been split into several genera; the old species names are listed with the new proposed generic names.

Capillariosis in man: three species of *Capillaria* (*C. philippinensis*, *C. hepatica* and *C. aerophila*) can infect man. Man acquires *C. hepatica* infection through ingestion of soil, containing embryonated eggs, or by consuming contaminated food or water. Heavy infections in man induce similar hepatic lesions to those seen in other mammalian hosts and hepatic capillariosis is usually fatal. *C. philippinensis* infects the small intestine and causes a severe enteropathy that can be fatal. It occurs mainly in the Philippines and Thailand with sporadic outbreaks in other parts of southeast Asia, India, the Middle East and southern Europe. Eggs shed into water embryonate and are ingested by freshwater or brackish-water fish and develop to the infective stage in the intestinal mucosa. Infection is acquired through the consumption of raw or undercooked fish. Large infections can accumulate through autoinfection. Fish-eating birds are thought to be the reservoir host. Clinical signs include intermittent diarrhoea, followed by anorexia, abdominal distention and weight loss. There is a protein-losing enteropathy. Human capillariosis resulting from *C. aerophila* is very rare.

Opisthorchis sinensis

Synonym: *Clonorchis sinensis*

Common name: Chinese or oriental liver fluke

Predilection site: Bile ducts, pancreatic ducts and occasionally small intestine

Parasite class: Trematoda

Family: Opisthorchiidae

Description, gross: The adult fluke is flat, transparent pinkish, wide posteriorly and tapering anteriorly and may reach a size of 25 × 5 mm. The cuticle is spiny in the young fluke but smooth in the adult.

Description, microscopic: The testes are multibranched. Eggs have a thick light yellowish brown wall, 27–35 × 12–20 μm in size; they contain a miracidium when they are laid, the internal structure of which is asymmetrical. The convex operculum of the egg fits into a prominent rim of the shell, while the opposite pole frequently bears a small hook-like structure.

Final hosts: Man, dog, cat, pig, mink, badger

Intermediate hosts: Two are required: 1. Operculated snails (*Parafossalurus*, *Bulimus* spp, *Bithynia*, *Melania* and *Vivipara*). 2. Fishes belonging to several genera of the family Cyprinidae (more than 40 have been reported naturally infected)

Life cycle: The eggs normally hatch only after they have been swallowed by the snail first intermediate host. In the snails the miracidium develops into a sporocyst, which produces rediae and these in turn produce cercariae, which have fairly long tails and elongate bodies with pigmented eye-spots. After breaking out of the snail the cercaria swims about, and on meeting a suitable fish it penetrates partly or completely into the tissues of the fish and, losing its tail, becomes encysted in the fish. Infection of the final host occurs through eating raw, infected fish. The metacercariae are liberated in the duodenum of the final host and reach the liver by way of the bile duct. The prepatent period is 16 days.

Geographical distribution: China, Taiwan, Korea, Vietnam, Japan, India and parts of the former Soviet Union

Pathogenesis: The worms live in the narrow proximal parts of the bile ducts. The young flukes, in particular, with their cuticular spines, cause cholangitis, pericholangitis, cholecystitis with desquamation of the epithelium, and may in rare cases bring about bile stasis by blocking up the passages, resulting in jaundice.

Clinical signs: Symptoms are not generally seen except in heavy infections. The symptoms in humans include anaemia, emaciation, ascites, jaundice and diarrhoea.

Diagnosis: Diagnosis is based on the identification of the characteristic eggs in faecal samples, which have to be differentiated from other trematode eggs such as *Heterophyes*, *Metagonimus* and other *Opisthorchis* species. Several serological tests have been developed, but most are non-specific. A reported enzyme-linked immunosorbent assay (ELISA) may be of value.

Pathology: Light infestations may cause little pathology, but in heavier infections there is fibrosis of the smaller bile ducts and cholangiohepatitis and severe biliary fibrosis may develop. Papillomatous or even adenomatous proliferation of the epithelium of the bile ducts takes place, together with cirrhosis of the liver and this frequently leads to the formation of cysts enclosing eggs and flukes.

Epidemiology: Carnivores or humans usually acquire infection by eating raw fish. In some fish, the metacercariae are found only under the scales and animals that are fed with the scales and offal of such fish become infected, while humans who eat the rest of the fish do not. Infection is usually aggregated in a small number of individuals.

Treatment: Praziquantel at 25 mg/kg on 3 consecutive days has been reported to be effective.

Control: Cats and dogs act as reservoirs for human infection. Prevention relies on avoiding feeding or eating of raw, undercooked or improperly pickled, salted, smoked or dried fish. Freezing fish for a week at −10°C may be beneficial, but even frozen fish has been incriminated with outbreaks of infection in non-endemic areas. In endemic areas, treatment of all infected persons and improved sanitation would help control infection. In these areas where fish are raised in ponds, human and animal faeces should be composted or sterilised before being applied as fertiliser to ponds.

Opisthorchis felineus

Synonym: *Opisthorchis tenuicollis*, *Opisthorchis viverrini*

Common name: Cat liver fluke

Predilection site: Bile ducts, pancreatic ducts and occasionally small intestine

Parasite class: Trematoda

Family: Opisthorchiidae

Description, gross: Adult fluke are reddish in colour, with a smooth cuticle and measure 7–12 × 1.5–2.5 mm.

Description, microscopic: The testes are lobed and not branched. Eggs are 26–30 × 11–15 μm in size, and contain a miracidium when they are laid, the internal structure of which is asymmetrical. The operculum of the egg fits into a prominent rim of the shell and may have a tubercular appendage.

Final hosts: Cat, dog, fox, pig, man, cetaceans (seals, porpoises)

Intermediate hosts: Two are required: 1. Operculated snails (*Bithynia*). 2. Freshwater fish belonging to several genera (*Leuciscus*, *Blicca*, *Tinca*, *Barbus*). In Europe, metacercariae are common in freshwater fish such as orfe, bream, tench and barbel.

Life cycle: The prepatent period is 2–3 weeks

Geographical distribution: Southern Asia, Europe, Russia, Canada

Pathogenesis: Most infections are asymptomatic, depending on the level and duration of infection. Adult fluke in the bile ducts, gallbladder and occasionally the pancreatic duct cause thickening of the ducts predisposing to cholangiocarcinoma and hepatocellular carcinoma.

Pathology: Light infestations may cause little pathology, but in heavier infections there is fibrosis of the smaller bile ducts, and cholangiohepatitis and severe biliary fibrosis may develop in advanced cases. Adenocarcinoma of the liver or pancreas in cats and humans has been reported.

Notes: There is some uncertainty regarding the proper classification of opisthorcid flukes and many texts suggest the reported species of *Opisthorchis* are synonymous.

Metorchis albidus

Synonym: *Distoma albicum*, *Opisthorchis albidus*

Common name: Liver fluke

Predilection site: Bile ducts, gallbladder

Parasite class: Trematoda

Family: Opisthorchiidae

Description, gross: The fluke is spatulate, pointed anteriorly, rounded and flat posteriorly, 2.5–3.5 × 1.0–1.6 mm with a spinous cuticle. The genital pore is in front of the ventral sucker.

Description, microscopic: Eggs are small, 24–30 × 13–16 μm.

Definitive hosts: Dog, cat, fox, seal

Intermediate hosts: Two are required: 1. Freshwater snails. 2. Fish, *Blicca bjorkna*

Geographical distribution: Europe, Asia, North America

Several other species of liver flukes of the family Opisthochiidae are found in dogs and cats and are summarised in Table 6.9. Details are essentially similar to those of other opisthorcid flukes.

Platynosomum fastosum

Synonym: *Platynosomum concinnum*

Common name: Cat liver fluke, 'lizard poisoning'

Predilection site: Bile and pancreatic ducts

Parasite class: Trematoda

Family: Dicrocoeliidae

Description, gross: The adult fluke is lanceolate and measures 4–8 × 1.5–2.5 mm.

Description, microscopic: The eggs are brown, oval, thick-shelled and operculate 34–50 × 23–35 μm.

Hosts: Cat

Life cycle: Eggs passed in the faeces develop in a land snail (*Sublima*), and a crustacean (woodlouse).

Table 6.9 Liver flukes of dogs and cats.

Species	Hosts	Intermediate hosts	Distribution
Opisthorcis sinensis	Man, dog, cat, pig, mink, badger	1. Freshwater snails (*Parafossalurus, Bulimus* spp, *Bithynia, Melania* and *Vivipara*) 2. Fish (*Cyprinidae*)	China, Taiwan, Korea, Vietnam, Japan, India and parts of the former Soviet Union
Opisthorcis felineus	Cat, dog, fox, pig, man, cetaceans (seals, porpoises)	1. Freshwater snails (*Bithynia*) 2. Fish (*Leuciscus, Blicca, Tinca, Barbus*)	Southern Asia, Europe, Russia, Canada
Metorchis albidus	Dog, cat, fox, seal	1. Freshwater snails (*Amnicola limosa porosa*) 2. Fish (*Blicca bjorkna*)	Europe, Asia, North America
Metorchis conjunctus	Dog, cat, fox, mink, racoon	1. Freshwater snails (*Amnicola limosa porosa*) 2. Fish (Common sucker, *Catostomus commersoni*)	North America
Platynosomum fastosum	Cat	1. Land snails (*Sublima*) 2. Crustacean (Woodlouse) 3. Lizard (paratenic)	South America, the Caribbean, southern USA, west Africa, Malaysia and the Pacific Islands
Parametorchis complexus	Cat, dog	Not known but probably similar to other liver flukes	North America
Eurytrema procyonis	Cat, fox, racoon	Unknown – thought to be snail (*Mesodon*)	North America
Pseudamphistomum truncatum	Dog, cat, fox, rarely man	1. Snail (unknown) 2. Fish (*Leuciscus, Sardinius, Blicca, Abramis*)	Europe, India

Cercariae encyst when a lizard eats the wood louse. The cat is infected by ingesting an infected lizard, which acts as an obligate paratenic host.

Geographical distribution: South America, the Caribbean, southern USA, west Africa, Malaysia and the Pacific Islands

Pathogenesis: Most infections are well tolerated by the cat causing only a mild inappetence but in heavy infestations, so-called 'lizard poisoning', cirrhosis and jaundice have been reported with diarrhoea and vomiting in terminal cases.

Clinical signs: In mild cases, vague chronic signs of unthriftiness may be observed. Severe infections cause anorexia, vomiting, diarrhoea and jaundice leading to death.

Diagnosis: Based on faecal examination for eggs and necropsy examination of the bile and pancreatic ducts for the presence of flukes.

Pathology: Liver cirrhosis and cholangitis have been reported and the bile ducts are often markedly distended.

Epidemiology: Infection is maintained in endemic areas where intermediate hosts and lizards are abundant.

Treatment: Praziquantel (20 mg/kg) and nitroscanate (100 mg/kg) are reported to be effective treatments.

Control: Preventing cats from hunting lizards can control infection.

Eurytrema procyonis

Predilection site: Bile and pancreatic ducts

Parasite class: Trematoda

Family: Dicrocoeliidae

Description, gross: The body is thick, 8–16 × 5–8.5 mm in size, armed with spines and with large suckers.

Description, microscopic: The eggs are small, 45 × 35 μm, asymmetrical, dark brown with an operculum and a miracidium.

Hosts: Cat, fox, racoon

Life cycle: The life cycle is unknown but is thought to involve snail intermediate hosts of the genus *Mesodon*. Animals are likely to become infected by ingestion of the snail intermediate host.

Geographical distribution: North America

Pathogenesis: Infection is usually well tolerated, and causes no apparent ill-health. Infection in the cat has been reported to cause weight loss and vomiting due to pancreatic fibrosis and atrophy.

Clinical signs: Mild infections are usually asymptomatic.

Diagnosis: Based on faecal examination for eggs and necropsy examination of the bile and pancreatic ducts for the presence of flukes

Pathology: Periductal fibrosis may produce cord-like ducts and there may be atrophy of glandular acini.

Epidemiology: This is a common parasite of the pancreatic ducts of the racoon. Cats presumably become infected by ingestion of the intermediate host.

Treatment: Praziquantel may be effective against these flukes.

Control: This is difficult because of the longevity of the eggs, the wide distribution of the intermediate hosts and the number of reservoir hosts.

Leishmania donovani infantum

Subspecies: *Leishmania infantum* (*Leishmania chagasi*)

Synonym: *Leishmania donovani* complex

Common name: Visceral leishmaniosis, kala-azar, infantile or Mediterranean leishmaniosis (*L. infantum*)

Predilection site: Skin, liver, spleen

Parasite class: Zoomastigophorasida

Family: Trypanosomatidae

Description: *Leishmania* amastigotes are small, round or oval bodies, 1.5–3.0 × 2.5–6.5 μm, located within macrophages and possessing a large nucleus and rod-shaped kinetoplast associated with a rudimentary flagellum, which does not extend beyond the cell margin.

Hosts: Man, dog, fox (*Vulpes vulpes*), black rat (*Rattus rattus*), racoon (*Nyctereutes procyonoides*), jackal (*Canis aureus*), wolf and fennic fox (*Fennecus zerda*), bush dog (*Lycalopex vetulus*)

Life cycle: The leishmanial, or amastigote form, after ingestion by a sandfly, transforms into a promastigote form in the insect gut in which the kinetoplast is situated at the posterior end of the body. These divide repeatedly by binary fission, migrate to the proboscis, and when the insect subsequently feeds, are inoculated into a new host. Once within a macrophage the promastigote reverts to the amastigote form and again starts to divide.

Geographical distribution: Southern France (Cevennes Hills), central and western Mediterranean basin (Europe and Africa), Iran (*L. infantum*), central and southern America (Mexico to northern Argentina) (*L. chagasi*)

Pathogenesis: In dogs, *L. donovani infantum* may cause either visceral or cutaneous lesions, the latter being more common (Fig. 6.17). It may take many months or even years for infected dogs to develop clinical signs, so that the disease may only become apparent long after dogs have left endemic areas. The disease is usually chronic with low mortality, although it can manifest as an acute, rapidly fatal form. Recovery depends on the proper expression of cell-mediated immunity; if this does not occur, the active lesion persists, leading to chronic enlargement of the spleen, liver and lymph nodes and persistent cutaneous lesions.

Clinical signs: In the cutaneous form in the dog, lesions are confined to shallow skin ulcers often on the lip or eyelid, from which recovery is often spontaneous. In the visceral form, which is more common, dogs initially develop 'spectacles' due to depilation of hair around the eyes and this is followed by generalised loss of body hair and eczema, leishmanial organisms

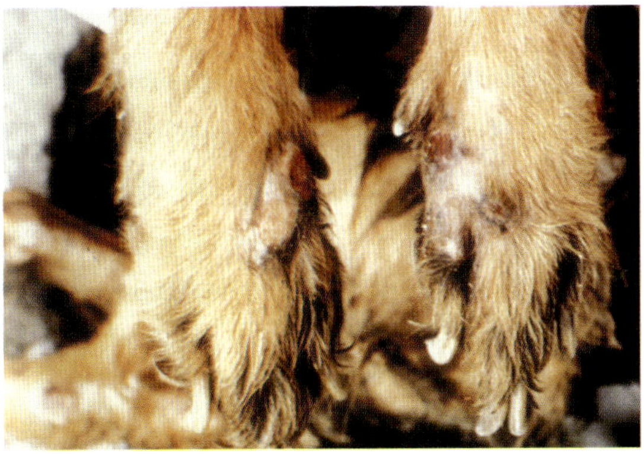

Fig. 6.17 Forelimbs of dog with cutaneous lesions of *Leishmania infantum*.

being present in large numbers in the infected skin. Intermittent fever, anaemia, cachexia and generalised lymphadenopathy are also typical signs. Long periods of remission followed by the reappearance of clinical signs is not uncommon.

Diagnosis: This depends on the demonstration of the amastigote parasites in smears or scrapings from affected skin or from lymph node or marrow biopsies. Confirmation in an individual case may be difficult, particularly if signs are non-specific. Intracellular or extracellular amastigotes can be identified in Giemsa or Leishman's stained aspirates, impression or biopsy samples from lymph node, bone marrow, spleen or skin lesions. PCR and immunocytochemistry methods have been developed for use on these samples offering greater sensitivity. Serological assays using indirect immunofluoresence (IFAT), enzyme linked immunoabsorbent assay (ELISA) and western blot have also been developed. Specialist laboratories can carry out culture and species identification using isoenzyme analysis and RAPD PCR.

Pathology: Visceral leishmaniosis is essentially a reticuloentotheliosis. Reticuloendothelial cells are increased in number and invaded by the parasites. The enormously enlarged spleen is congested with prominent Malpighian corpuscles. The liver is enlarged with fatty infiltration of Kuppfer cells. Macrophages, myelocytes and neutrophils of the bone marrow are filled with parasites. Lymph nodes are usually enlarged and the intestinal mucosa is infiltrated with macrophages filled with parasites.

Epidemiology: Dogs are commonly infected and transmission is by sandflies of the genus *Phlebotomus* (*P. ariasi*, *P. perniciosus*, *P. longcuspis*, *P. chinensis*, *P. mongolensis*, *P. caucasius*) in the Mediterranean area and the genus *Lutzomyia* (*L. longipalpis*, *L. evansi*) in Central and South America. The dog is the principal urban reservoir, with infection rates as high as 20% in some countries, and the most important source of human infection. It is probable that most dogs in endemic areas are exposed to disease and will either develop clinical or subclinical infection or become immune and resistant to infection. Leishmaniosis is diagnosed in dogs in countries where sandfly vectors do not occur, suggesting a currently unknown mechanism of transmission. Vertical transmission from dam to offspring has been reported and transmission by infected blood transfusion has been reported.

Treatment: Several drugs are used for treating canine leishmaniosis (Table 6.10). These include the pentavalent antimonials, of which meglumine antimonate is the main drug, used either alone, or in combination with other drugs, particularly allopurinol. Allopurinol can also be given alone following initial therapy with meglumine antimonite. Other drugs that have been used include Amphotercin B, pentamidine, aminoside and ketoconazole.

Control: From the public health aspect, the destruction of infected dogs, and stray dogs generally, is desirable, although often unacceptable. In some areas, the population of sandflies has been reduced as a result of mosquito control for malaria, and as a result the incidence of leishmaniosis has decreased. Generally though, chemical control of sandfly vectors has had very limited success. A deltamethrin-impregnated collar offers some protection of dogs from sandfly bites and appears to decrease the rate of infection in dogs and people in endemic areas.

Notes: *Leishmania donovani donovani* is a highly fatal infection of man and causes visceral leishmani-

Table 6.10 Drugs used in the treatment of leishmaniosis in dogs.

Drug	Drug group	Dose rate	Notes
Meglumine antimonate	Pentavalent antimonial	100 mg/kg s.c. for 3–4 weeks	Nephrotoxic. May cause pain and muscle fibrosis at injection site
Allopurinol	Pirimidine derivative	20 mg/kg orally daily 20 mg/kg orally daily combined with meglumine antimoniate (100 mg/kg daily s.c. for 20 days) then continue with 20 mg/kg allopurinol indefinitely	
Amphoteracin B	Polyene macrolide	0.5–0.8 mg/kg i.v. or s.c., 2–3 times weekly 1–2.5 mg/kg i.v. in lipid emulsion, twice weekly 3 mg/kg/day i.v. in liposamalised formulation	Nephrotoxic. Administer until cumulative dose of 15 mg/kg is reached Administer until cumulative dose of 10 mg/kg is reached Administer until cumulative dose of 15 mg/kg is reached

osis. In humans the incubation period may be several months with spasmodic fever. Hepatomegaly and splenomegaly follow with mortality of 75–95%.

Hepatozoon canis

Synonym: *Leucocytozoon canis*

Common name: Canine hepatozoonosis

Predilection site: Blood, liver, kidney

Parasite class: Sporozoasida

Family: Hepatozoidae

Description: Gamonts, found in circulating neutrophils are ellipsoidal in shape, about 11 × 4 μm, and are enveloped in a thick membrane (Fig. 6.18). Meronts are usually round to oval, about 30 μm in diameter, and include elongated micromerozoites with defined nuclei, which in cross-section have a 'wheel-spoke' appearance.

Hosts: Dog

Life cycle: The life cycle involves two hosts. The tick is a final host in which syngamy occurs, and the dog is an intermediate host in which asexual reproduction occurs. Nymphal ticks engorge with gamont-infected leucocytes in an infected dog. Following ingestion the gamonts are freed from the leucocytes, associate in pairs and transform into male and female gametes leading to the formation of zygotes and oocysts. Each mature oocyst contains numerous sporocysts each containing 10–26 sporozoites. After the tick moults, oocysts are found in the haemocoele and each tick may carry thousands of infective sporozoites. Since the sporozoites remain in the body cavity, the dog is apparently infected by ingesting the tick. Once ingested the sporozoites are released from the oocysts, penetrate the intestinal wall and are transported to target tissues and organs, in the blood and lymph. They primarily infect the spleen, lymph nodes and bone marrow where merogony occurs in macrophages and endothelial cells. Two forms of meronts are found in infected tissues, one type containing two to four macromerozoites, and a second type containing 20 elongated micromerozoites. When the meront matures and ruptures, merozoites are released and penetrate circulating neutrophils, in which they develop into gamonts that circulate in peripheral blood. The cycle is completed when the tick ingests infected blood. The period of development in the dog from infection to the appearance of gamonts is about 28 days.

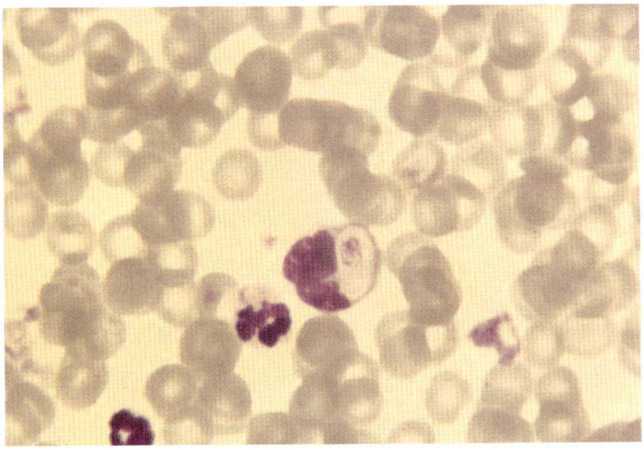

Fig. 6.18 Gamont of *Hepatozoon canis* in circulating neutrophil.

Geographical distribution: Southern Europe, Middle East, Africa, southeast Asia, South America

Pathogenesis: Most dogs infected with *H. canis* appear to undergo a mild infection associated with a limited degree of inflammatory reaction. However, infection may vary from asymptomatic in dogs with a low parasitaemia, to life threatening in animals that present with a high parasitaemia. Symptoms may be exacerbated by the presence of concurrent infections with parvovirus, *Ehrlichia canis*, *Anaplasma platys*, *Toxoplasma gondii*, *Leishmania infantum*, or immune suppression in the young neonate or those with primary or induced immunodeficiency. High parasitaemias can cause direct injury to the affected tissues and affect the immune system, leading to extreme loss of weight and cachexia, although infected dogs may maintain a good appetite.

Clinical signs: Infection with *H. canis* may be subclinical in some animals but produce severe and fatal disease in others. Mild disease is common and is usually associated with low level *H. canis* parasitaemia (1–5%), frequently in association with a concurrent disease. A more severe disease, characterised by lethargy, fever and severe weight loss, is found in dogs with high parasitaemia often approaching 100% of circulating neutrophils. Dogs presenting with both leucocytosis and high parasitaemia may have a massive number of circulating gamonts (>50 000 gamonts/mm^3 blood).

Diagnosis: Diagnosis is usually made on the identification of gamonts in the cytoplasm of neutrophils (more rarely monocytes) in Giemsa or Wright's stained blood smears. Between 0.5% and 5% of neutrophils are commonly infected although this may reach as high as 100% in severe infections. An indirect fluorescent antibody test (IFAT) and western blot have been developed using gamont antigens. Dogs with a high parasitaemia frequently have neutrophilia and a normocytic, normochromic non-regenerative anaemia.

Pathology: Infection may be found as an incidental finding in histopathological specimens in dogs from endemic areas. In dogs with low parasitaemias, few lesions are usually observed. In dogs with high parasitaemias, there may be hepatitis, pneumonia and glomerulonephritis associated with numerous meronts. Meronts and developing gamonts are also found in lymph nodes, spleen and bone marrow.

Epidemiology: The main vector of *H. canis* is the brown dog tick, *Rhipicephalus sanguineus*, which is found in warm and temperate regions all over the world. Infection is transmitted trans-stadially from nymph to adult stages of the tick vectors. Infection appears to be mainly from ingestion of infected ticks. Vertical transmission has been reported.

Treatment: Infection is treated with imidocarb dipropionate at 5–6 mg/kg every 14 days until gamonts are no longer present in blood smears. Oral doxycycline at 10 mg/kg daily for 21 days in combination with imidocarb may also be used. Treatment may take up to 8 weeks to eliminate gamonts from peripheral blood and require regular haematological evaluation. Treatment of all infected dogs is recommended as parasitaemia may increase over time and develop into a severe infection. The prognosis for dogs with a low parasitaemia is generally good, but less favourable for those with a high parasitaemia.

Control: Prophylaxis depends on regular tick control using an effective acaricide and close examination of animals for the presence of ticks. In areas where the disease is endemic, dogs should be prevented from scavenging or eating raw meat or organs from wildlife.

Notes: The closely related *H. americanum* was initially reported to be a strain of *H. canis* but is now considered a separate species, based on clinical disease manifestations, pathology, morphological and genetic differences.

PARASITES OF THE CIRCULATORY SYSTEM

Angiostrongylus vasorum

Synonym: *Haemostrongylus vasorum*

Common name: French heartworm

Predilection site: Right ventricle, pulmonary artery

Parasite class: Nematoda

Superfamily: Metastrongyloidea

Description, gross: Slender worms up to 2.5 cm long. Males are 14–18 mm with a small bursa in which the rays are distinguishable.

Description, microscopic: The ventral rays are fused for most of their length and the dorsal ray is stout with stout terminal branches. Females are 18–25 mm

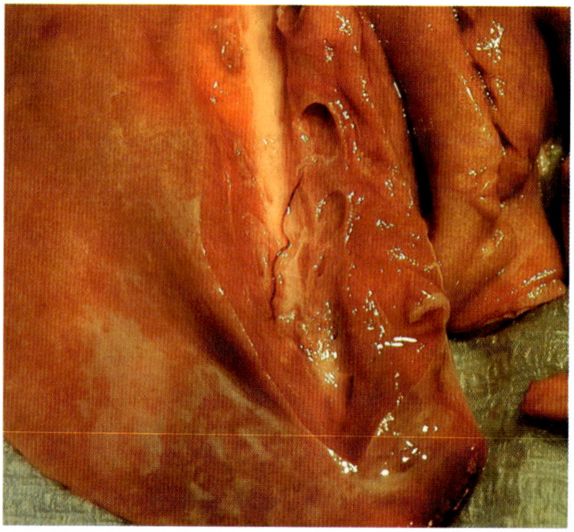

Fig. 6.19 Female *Angiostrongylus vasorum* in the pulmonary artery.

and the white ovaries are coiled round the red intestine (Fig. 6.19) with the vulva in the posterior half of the body.

First-stage larvae are 330 µm in length and have a small cephalic button and a wavy tail with a sub-terminal notch.

Final hosts: Dog, fox and other canids

Intermediate hosts: Terrestrial molluscs, mainly snails and slugs

Life cycle: The genus is ovo-viviparous. The adult worms in the larger pulmonary vessels lay eggs, which are carried to the capillaries, where they hatch. The L_1 break into the alveoli, migrate to the trachea and thence to the alimentary tract to be passed in the faeces. Further development takes place after entry into the intermediate host, the infective stage being reached in 17 days. After the mollusc has been ingested by the dog, the infective L_3, freed by digestion, travel to the lymph nodes adjacent to the alimentary tract, where both parasitic moults take place, and then to the vascular predilection site. L_5 have also been found in the liver. The prepatent period is 7 weeks, and the worms can live in the dog for more than 2 years.

Geographical distribution: Worldwide, except in the Americas. Prevalent in western Europe

Pathogenesis: Canine angiostrongylosis is usually a chronic condition, extending over months or even years. Much of the pathogenic effect is attributable to the presence of the adult worms in the larger vessels and eggs and larvae in the pulmonary arterioles and capillaries. Blockage of these results in circulatory impediment, which may eventually lead to congestive cardiac failure.

Clinical signs: In recently established infections the resting dog usually shows no clinical signs, but if a substantial number of worms is present, the active animal will often show tachycardia, tachypnoea, with a heavy productive cough, the sputum sometimes showing blood. In longer established severe infections signs are present even in the resting dog. There may be recurrent syncope. As a consequence of reduced blood-clotting capacity, slowly developing painless swellings may appear in dependent areas, such as the lower abdomen and intermandibular space, and on the limbs where bruising has occurred. Chronic infections may be accompanied by reduced appetite, anaemia and ascites and deaths can occur. The rare acute infection, normally seen in young animals, shows dyspnoea and violent cough with white–yellow, occasionally bloody, sputum.

Diagnosis: The L_1, which may be present in faeces and sputum, has a small cephalic button, and a wavy tail with a sub-terminal notch, and its presence in association with respiratory and circulatory signs is accepted as confirmatory.

Pathology: The cut surface of the lung is mottled and reddish purple. One reported systemic effect, which is unusual in helminth infections, is interference with the blood-clotting mechanism, so that subcutaneous haematomata may be present. In the larger blood vessels, there is endarteritis and periarteritis which progress to fibrosis, and at necropsy the vessels have a pipe-stem feel on palpation. The vascular change may extend to the right ventricle, with endocarditis involving the tricuspid valve.

Epidemiology: Though worldwide in general distribution, *A. vasorum* is only prevalent in certain localities, and these are invariably rural. In Europe, endemic foci have been recognised in France, Spain, Eire and England.

Treatment: Mebendazole and fenbendazole at increased dose rates and levamisole have proved effective.

Control: Control is impractical in most cases, due to the ubiquity of the molluscan intermediate hosts.

Dirofilaria immitis

Synonym: *Nochtiella immitis*

Common name: Canine heartworm

Predilection site: Cardiovascular system. Adults are in the right ventricle, right atrium, pulmonary artery and posterior vena cava

Parasite class: Nematoda

Superfamily: Filarioidea

Description, gross: Long slender white–grey worms 15–30 cm long. Adult females measure 25–30 cm, with the males about half as long. Many worms are usually found together in a tangled mass. The size and site are diagnostic for *D. immitis*.

Description, microscopic: The male tail has the typical loose spiral common to the filarioids, and the tail bears small lateral alae. There are 4–6 pairs of ovoid papillae. The left spicule is long and pointed; the right spicule is smaller and ends bluntly. In the female the vulva is situated just behind the end of the oesophagus. The microfilariae in the blood are not ensheathed and are 307–332 μm in length by 6.8 μm wide. They have a tapered anterior end and blunt posterior end.

Final hosts: Dog, fox, wild canids; occasionally cat and other wild felids and rarely man

Intermediate hosts: Mosquitoes of the genera *Aedes*, *Anopheles* and *Culex*

Life cycle: The adults live in the heart and adjacent blood vessels and the females release microfilariae directly into the bloodstream. These microfilariae can live for several months in the visceral blood vessels. Microfilariae are ingested by female mosquitoes during feeding. Development to L_3 in the mosquito takes about 2 weeks, by which time the larvae are present in the mouthparts and the final host is infected when the mosquito takes a further blood meal. In the dog the L_3 migrate to the subcutaneous or subserosal tissues and undergo two moults over the next few months; only after the final moult do the young *D. immitis* pass to the heart via the venous circulation. The minimum prepatent period is about 6 months. The adult worms survive for several years and patency has been recorded for over 5 years.

Geographical distribution: Warm–temperate and tropical zones throughout the world including North and South America, southern Europe, India, China, Japan, Australia.

Pathogenesis: This is associated with the adult parasites (Fig. 6.20). Many dogs infected with low numbers of *D. immitis* show no apparent ill effects and it is only in heavy chronic infections that circulatory distress occurs, primarily due to obstruction to normal blood flow leading to chronic congestive right-sided heart failure. The presence of a mass of active worms can cause an endocarditis in the heart valves and a proliferative pulmonary endarteritis, possibly due to a response to parasite excretory products. In addition, dead or dying worms may cause pulmonary embolism. After a period of about 9 months the effect of the developing pulmonary hypertension is compensated for

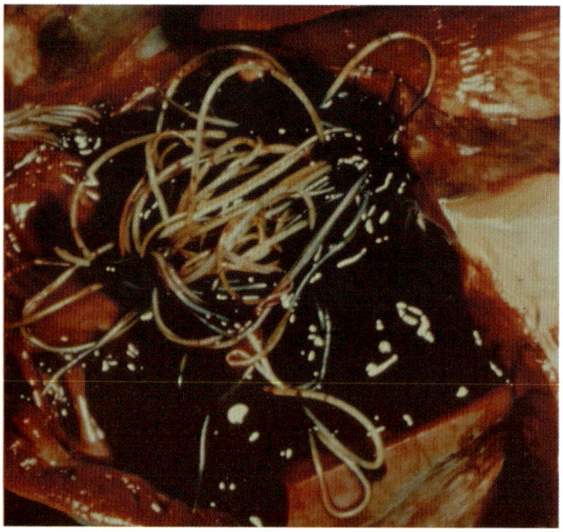

Fig. 6.20 *Dirofilaria immitis* in a section of an infected heart.

by right ventricular hypertrophy, which may lead to congestive heart failure with the usual accompanying signs of oedema and ascites. At this stage the dog is listless and weak.

A mass of worms may lodge in the posterior vena cava and the resulting obstruction leads to an acute, sometimes fatal, syndrome known as the vena caval syndrome. This is characterised by haemolysis, haemoglobinuria, bilirubinaemia, icterus, dyspnoea, anorexia and collapse. Death may occur within 2–3 days. Very occasionally there is blockage of the renal capillaries by microfilariae leading to a glomerulonephritis, possibly related to the deposition of immune complexes.

In cats, pulmonary hypertension, right-sided heart failure and caval syndrome are less common, and more commonly the presence of the parasites in the distal pulmonary arteries may induce a diffuse pulmonary pneumonia. Ectopic infections are more commonly seen in cats with parasites reported in the eye, CNS and subcutaneous tissues.

Clinical signs: Heavily infected dogs are often listless and there is a gradual loss of condition and exercise intolerance. They have a chronic soft cough with haemoptysis and in the later stages of the disease become dyspnoeic and may develop oedema and ascites. The acute vena caval syndrome described above is characterised by haemoglobinuria, icterus and collapse. Lighter infections in working dogs may be responsible for poor performance during periods of sustained exercise. Infected cats may show coughing, tachypnoea and dyspnoea and heavy infections can be fatal.

Diagnosis: This is based on the clinical signs of cardiovascular dysfunction and the demonstration of the appropriate microfilariae in the blood. Non-microfilaraemic dogs may however still harbour adult parasites. Affected dogs are seldom less than 1 year old and most are over 2 years. In suspected cases in which the microfilariae cannot be demonstrated, thoracic radiography may show the thickening of the pulmonary artery, its tortuous course and right ventricular hypertrophy. Angiography may also be used to demonstrate the vascular changes more clearly. At necropsy, adult worms are often present in the right heart chambers and adjacent large blood vessels.

Immunodiagnostic tests are also available commercially to identify cases that do not have a detectable microfilaraemia. For example there are a number of ELISA test kits for the detection of circulating heartworm antigens, or specific antibodies, that will identify most mature infections and which are highly specific.

The identification of the microfilariae in the blood (samples ideally taken in the early evening) is aided by concentrating the parasites following lysis, filtration and then staining with methylene blue or May–Grunwald Giemsa. Commercial kits are available for this technique. Alternatively one part of blood and nine parts of formalin are centrifuged and the sediment mixed with a blue stain and examined as a microscopic smear. The microfilariae have to be differentiated from those of *Dipetalonema reconditum*, a filarial parasite commonly found in the subcutis in dogs. Those of *D. immitis* are more than 300 μm in length and have a tapered head and a straight tail; those of *D. reconditum* are less than 300 μm in length and have a blunt head and a hooked posterior end. More precise differentiation may be achieved by using histochemical stains for acid phosphatase activity. *D. immitis* show distinct red acid-phosphate positive spots at the excretory pore and anus, while *D. reconditum* stains pink overall. Differential diagnosis may be achieved through the application of PCR-based recombinant DNA technology.

Heartworm infection in cats can be difficult to diagnose as a result of low parasite populations.

Pathology: Heartworm disease is primarily a pulmonary vascular disease characterised by endoarteritis with infiltration of leucocytes, mainly eosinophils, followed by myointimal proliferations which produce irregular rugose to villous projections that enmesh the worms. Thrombosis may be associated with either dead or live worms, and thromboembolism and pulmonary infarction following adulticide therapy. Pulmonary changes include haemosiderosis, diffuse interalveolar fibrosis and proliferation of alveolar epithelium. Dead worms commonly result in pulmonary granuloma formation. Additional lesions of heartworm disease include those of right heart failure, such as chronic congestion of the liver and occasionally ascites. Glomerulonephropathy occurs primarily due to glomerular deposition of immune complexes, leading to a mild to moderate proteinuria. Venal caval syndrome causes severe hepatic congestion leading to cavernous enlargement of hepatic venules with phlebosclerosis and thrombosis in the caudal vena cava and hepatic veins.

Epidemiology: Host species vary in their susceptibility to infection, the dog being the most susceptible natural host. Infection commonly occurs in dogs older than 1 year. Intra-uterine infection of puppies can also occur. The important factors in the spread of heartworm disease can be divided into those affecting the host and those affecting the vector.

Host factors include a high density of dogs in areas where the vectors exist, the lengthy patent period of up to 5 years during which time circulating microfilariae are present, and the lack of an effective immune response against established parasites. Also a diurnal periodicity of microfilaraemia ensures that high numbers of microfilariae are circulating in the peripheral blood during the period of mosquito activity.

Vector factors include the ubiquity of the mosquito intermediate hosts, their capacity for rapid population increase and the short development period from microfilariae to L_3 at optimal temperatures. At one point it was considered that the worms do not occur in areas where the temperature falls below 16°C, but more recently spread has occurred to colder zones in Canada and USA.

Treatment: Drug treatment is complex, as the adult heartworms and the microfilariae differ in their susceptibility to anthelmintics. Treatment should not be undertaken without a physical examination of the dog and an assessment of heart, lung, liver and kidney function. Where these functions are grossly abnormal it may be necessary to give prior treatment for cardiac insufficiency. The usual recommendation is that infected dogs are first treated intravenously with thiacetarsamide twice daily over a 2-day period or intramuscularly with melarsamide over 2 days to remove the adult worms; toxic reactions are not uncommon following this treatment due to the dying and disintegrating heartworms and resultant embolism; activity of the dog should be restricted for a period of 2–6 weeks. This drug should be used with extreme care (Table 6.11).

A further treatment with a different drug is then given 6 weeks later to remove the microfilariae that are not susceptible to thiacetarsamide or melarsamide treatment. Several drugs are now available for this purpose; the traditional one was dithiazanine iodide, administered over 7 days, and either this or levamisole given orally over a 10–14-day period has proved effective. The avermectins are also highly efficient against microfilariae, as is milbemycin at the heartworm prophylactic dose of 500 μg/kg. These induce rapid clearance of microfilariae but are not licensed for this purpose because of occasional toxic or microfilaricidal side effects. Veterinarians who choose to use either drug as a microfilaricide should realise that this is an 'extra-label' application and that they take responsibility for administration of the correct dose and provide appropriate monitoring and aftercare.

With all of these drugs there is a risk of adverse reactions to dying microfilariae. In some severe cases, heartworms have been removed surgically rather than risk adverse reactions following drug therapy. Following treatment it is usual to place dogs on a prophylactic programme and this is considered under the next section, on control.

There are currently no licensed anthelmintics for treatment of cats.

Control: Mosquito control is difficult and therefore prophylaxis is based almost entirely on medication (Table 6.12). The drug widely used for this has been diethylcarbamazine, which in endemic areas is given orally to pups daily from 2–3 months of age. This kills developing larvae and so pre-empts the problems of treating patent infections and microfilaraemia. In tropical areas the drug is given all year round, but in more temperate zones, where the mosquito has a limited season, treatment commences 1 month prior to the mosquito season and ceases 2 months after it ends. Where prophylaxis is introduced in older dogs or after treatment of an infected dog, care must be exercised to ensure that the dog is free from microfilarial

Table 6.11 Adulticides for dirofilariosis.

Chemical	Trade name	Dose rate	Comments
Thiacetarsamide sodium	Caparsolate	2.2 mg/kg twice daily for 2 days	Intravenous injection. No longer available
Melarsomine dihydrochloride	Immiticide	2.5 mg/kg i.m. repeated after 24 hours	In severely affected dogs, single injection given followed one month later by two injections 24 hours apart to reduce post-adulticide complications

Table 6.12 Drugs available for heartworm prevention.

Chemical(s)	Host	Recommended dosing interval	Route of administration
Ivermectin	Dog, cat	Monthly	Oral tablet
Ivermectin (+ pyrantel)	Dog	Monthly	Oral tablet
Ivermectin (+ imidacloprid)	Dog	Monthly	Spot-on
Milbemycin oxime	Dog	Monthly	Oral tablet
Milbemycin oxime (+ lufenuron)	Dog	Monthly	Oral tablet
Moxidectin	Dog	Monthly	Oral
Moxidectin microspheres	Dog	6-monthly	Injectable
Selamectin	Dog, cat	Monthly	Spot-on
Diethylcarbamazine citrate (DEC) (+ oxibendazole)	Dog	Daily	Oral

infection as anaphylactoid reactions may occur in infected dogs after diethylcarbamazine treatment. Once prophylaxis is introduced, regular checks for microfilariae should be made every 6 months.

The most up-to-date methods of preventing heartworm infection involve monthly administration, throughout the mosquito season, of ivermectin or milbemycin especially formulated for this use in dogs.

Notes: Of the two species occurring in domestic carnivores, *Dirofilaria immitis* is by far the more important. The adults, which are found in the right side of the heart and adjacent blood vessels of dogs, are responsible for a debilitating condition known as canine heartworm disease. Although primarily a problem of warm countries where the mosquito intermediate host abounds, the disease has become much more widespread in the past decade and the problem in North America is now so extensive that special heartworm clinics have been created.

Dirofilariosis in man: *D. immitis* and *D. repens* can cause aberrant infections in man. *D. immitis* induces pulmonary coin lesions that are normally of little pathological significance. *D. repens* (see parasites of integument) more commonly occurs in subcutaneous nodules, particularly in the ocular area.

Schistosoma spindale

See Chapter 2 (Cattle), Parasites of the circulatory system.

Schistosoma incognitum

See Chapter 5 (Pigs), Parasites of the circulatory system.

TRYPANOSOMES

Members of the genus *Trypanosoma* are haemoflagellates of overwhelming importance in cattle in sub-Saharan Africa but also occur in many other hosts including dogs and cats. See Chapter 1: Parasite taxonomy and morphology (Zoomastigophorasida) for general description and Chapter 2: Cattle for detailed descriptions of individual species of trypanosomes, and their control.

Trypanosoma brucei (brucei)

Subspecies: *brucei*

Subgenus: *Trypanozoon*

Common name: Nagana

Predilection site: Blood. *T. brucei bucei* is also found extravascularly in, for example, the myocardium, CNS and reproductive tract

Parasite class: Zoomastigophorasida

Family: Trypanosomatidae

Description: *T. brucei brucei* is pleomorphic in form and ranges from long and slender, up to 42 μm (average 29 μm), to short and stumpy, 12–26 μm (mean 18 μm), the two forms often being present in the same blood sample. The undulating membrane is conspicuous, the kinetoplast is small and sub-terminal and the posterior end is pointed. In the slender form the kinetoplast is up to 4 μm from the posterior end, which is usually drawn out tapering almost to a point, and has a well developed free flagellum. In the stumpy form the flagellum is either short or absent and the posterior end is broad and rounded with the kinetoplast almost terminal. Intermediate forms average 23 μm long and have a blunt posterior end and moderately long flagellum. A fourth form with a posterior nucleus may be seen in laboratory animals. In fresh unfixed blood films, the organism moves rapidly within small areas of the microscope field.

Hosts: Cattle, horse, donkey, zebu, sheep, goat, camel, pig, dog, cat, wild game species

Distribution: Sub-Saharan Africa

Clinical signs: The dog and cat are susceptible to *T. brucei brucei*. The disease is usually acute, and apart from signs of fever, anaemia and myocarditis, corneal opacity is often a feature. There may also be neurological changes resulting in aggressive signs, ataxia or convulsions.

Treatment: Dogs can be treated with either isometamidium or quinapyramine.

Drug	Recommended dose
Isometamidium	0.25–1 mg/kg i.m.
Quinapyramine dimethylsulphate	5 mg/kg s.c.

Trypanosoma brucei (evansi)

Subspecies: *evansi*

Subgenus: *Trypanozoon*

Synonym: *Trypanosoma evansi*, *T. equinum*

Common name: Surra, el debab, mbori, murrina, mal de Caderas, doukane, dioufar, thaga

Predilection site: Blood

Parasite class: Zoomastigophorasida

Family: Trypanosomatidae

Description: *Trypanosoma evansi* is identical to, and structurally indistinguishable in appearance from, the slender forms of *T. brucei*. The mean length varies considerably, with typical forms 15–34 μm long (mean 24 μm). Most are slender or intermediate in shape, but stumpy forms occur sporadically. Strains that lack a kinetoplast visible with the light microscope have occasionally arisen spontaneously or can be produced by treatment with certain dyes, drugs or frozen storage.

Hosts: Horse, donkey, camel, cattle, zebu, goat, pig, dog, water buffalo, elephant, capybara, tapir, mongoose, ocelot, deer and other wild animals. Many laboratory and wild animals can be infected experimentally.

Life cycle: Transmission is by biting flies, no cyclical development occurring in the vector, and the trypanosomes remaining in the proboscis.

Geographical distribution: North Africa, Central and South America, central and southern Russia, parts of Asia (India, Burma, Malaysia, southern China, Indonesia, Phillipines)

Pathogenesis: Depending on the virulence of the strain and the susceptibility of the individual host, the disease may be acute in horses, camels and dogs. The syndrome is similar to that caused by the tsetse-transmitted trypanosomes. Anaemia is caused mainly by extravascular haemolysis through erythrophagocytosis in the mononuclear phagocytic systems of the spleen, liver and lungs, but as the disease becomes chronic there may be decreased haemoglobin synthesis. Leucopenia and thrombocytopenia are caused by mechanisms that predispose leucocytes and platelets to phagocytosis. Immunological mechanisms in the pathogenesis lead to extensive proliferation of activated macrophages, which engulf or destroy erythrocytes, leucocytes, platelets and haematopoietic cells.

Clinical signs: All domestic animals are susceptible but the disease is only fatal in horses, camels and dogs. The disease is manifested by pyrexia, progressive anaemia, loss of condition and depression. Recurrent episodes of fever occur during the course of disease. Oedematous swellings ranging from cutaneous plaques to frank oedema of the ventral abdomen and genitalia and petechial haemorrhages of the serous membranes are often observed. Nervous signs may occur and include circling, incoordination, staggering, head pressing, paraplegia, paralysis and prostration.

Diagnosis: The clinical signs of the disease, although indicative, are not pathognomonic. Confirmation of clinical diagnosis depends on the demonstration of trypanosomes in the blood. Occasionally, when the parasitaemia is massive it is possible to detect motile trypanosomes in fresh films of blood. More usually, both thick and thin smears of blood are air-dried and examined later. Thick smears, de-haemoglobinised before staining with Giemsa or Leishman's stain, offer a better chance of finding trypanosomes while the stained thin smears are used for differentiation of the trypanosome species.

More sensitive techniques utilise centrifugation in a microhaematocrit tube followed by microscopic examination of the interface between the buffy coat and the plasma; alternatively, the tube may be snapped, the buffy coat expressed on to a slide, and the contents examined under dark-ground or phase-contrast microscopy for motile trypanosomes. With these techniques the packed red cell volume is also obtained which is of indirect value in diagnosis if one can eliminate other causes of anaemia, especially helminthosis.

A number of serological tests have been described and include IFAT and ELISA and have been partially validated but require further evaluation and standardisation.

Pathology: The carcase is often pale, emaciated and there may be oedematous swellings in the lower part of the abdomen and genital organs with serous atrophy of fat. The liver, lymph nodes and spleen are enlarged and the viscera are congested. Petechiae may appear on lymph nodes, pericardium and intestinal mucosa. The liver is hypertrophic and congested with degeneration and necrosis of the hepatocytes, dilation of blood vessels and parenchymal infiltration of mononuclear cells. A non-suppurative myocarditis, sometimes associated with hydropericarditis, has been reported, accompanied by degeneration and necrosis of the myocardial tissue. Other lesions can include glomerulonephritis, renal tubular necrosis, non-suppurative meningio-encephalomyelitis, focal poliomalacia, keratitis, opthalmitis, orchitis, interstitial pneumonia and bone marrow atrophy. Splenic and lymph node hypertrophy occur during the acute phase but the lymphoid tissues are usually exhausted and fibrotic in the chronic stage.

Epidemiology: This species, although closely related to the salivarian trypanosome *T. brucei brucei*, is mechanically transmitted by biting insects; the usual vectors are horseflies (*Tabanus*) but *Stomoxys*, *Haematopota* and *Lyperosia* can also transmit the infection. In Central and South America the vampire bat is a vector and can transmit the disease (murrina).

Treatment: Dogs can be treated with quinapyramine.

Notes: The original distribution of this parasite coincided with that of the camel, and is often associated with arid desserts and semiarid steppes.

Trypanosoma congolense

Subspecies: *congolense*

Subgenus: *Nannomonas*

Common name: Nagana, paranagana, Gambia fever, ghindi, gobial

Predilection site: Blood

Parasite class: Zoomastigophorasida

Family: Trypanosomatidae

Description: *T. congolense* is small, monomorphic in form, 8–20 μm long. The undulating membrane is inconspicuous, the medium-sized kinetoplast is marginal and the posterior end is blunt. There is no free flagellum. In fresh blood films the organism moves sluggishly, often apparently attached to red cells.

Hosts: Cattle, sheep, goat, horse, camel, dog, pig. Reservoir hosts include antelope, giraffe, zebra, elephant and warthog

Distribution: Sub-Saharan Africa

Clinical signs: The dog and cat are susceptible to *T. congolense*. The disease is usually acute, and apart from signs of fever, anaemia and myocarditis, corneal opacity is often a feature. There may also be neurological changes resulting in aggressive signs, ataxia or convulsions.

Treatment: Dogs can be treated with quinapyramine.

Babesia canis

Subspecies: *canis, rossi, vogeli*

Subspecies	Distribution	Vector	Virulence
B. canis canis	Southern and central Europe	*Dermacentor reticulatus*	Moderate–severe
B. canis rossi	Southern Africa	*Haemaphysalis leachi*	Severe
B. canis vogeli	Africa, Asia, North and South America, Australia, Europe	*Rhipicephalus sanguineus*	Mild–moderate

Common name: Canine piroplasmosis

Predilection site: Blood

Parasite class: Sporozoasida

Family: Babesiidae

Description: Large piroplasms, pyriform in shape, 4–5 μm in length, pointed at one end and rounded at the other. Amoeboid forms have been described that are 2–4 μm in diameter and usually contain a vacuole.

Hosts: Dog

Life cycle: Infective sporozoites present in the tick are injected into the dog within saliva when the tick feeds. These organisms then invade, feed and divide by binary fission within erythrocytes, causing the latter to rupture during repeated phase of merogony releasing merozoites that invade other erythrocytes. In chronic infections parasites become sequestered within capillary networks of the spleen, liver and other organs from where they are released periodically into the circulation. On ingestion by the tick these forms become vermiform and enter the body cavity then the ovary and penetrate the eggs where they round up and divide to form small round organisms. When the larval tick moults into the nymph stage, the parasites enter the salivary gland and undergo a series of binary fissions entering the cells of the salivary gland. They multiply further until the host cells are filled with thousands of minute parasites. These become vermiform, break out of the host cell, lie in the lumen of the gland, and are injected into the mammalian host when the tick feeds.

Geographical distribution: Southern Europe, Africa, Asia, USA, Central and South America

Pathogenesis: *Babesia canis* is recognised to represent at least three subspecies, *B. canis canis*, *B. canis rossi* and *B. canis vogeli*, each transmitted by different tick vectors. The severity of infection is determined by the strain of parasite as well as other factors, such as age, immune status and presence of concurrent infections. Haemolytic anaemia is the principal pathogenic mechanism caused by the parasite but other factors, such as immune-mediated destruction of erythrocytes, may occur. Infection may be classified as uncomplicated or complicated. The former is usually associated with mild to moderate anaemia, lethargy, weakness and hepato-splenomegaly. Complicated babesiosis refers to manifestations that cannot be explained by the haemolytic crisis alone and is characterised by severe anaemia and organic dysfunction. Mortality in complicated babesiosis often exceeds 80%.

Clinical signs: The more severe forms of the disease in adult dogs are associated with virulent infections (*B. canis rossi*, *B. canis canis*), whilst pups are more severely affected irrespective of the species of *Babesia*. Peracute infections are a feature of *B. canis rossi* and are characterised by rapid onset collapse, with findings typical of hypotensive shock, pale (sometimes cyanotic) mucous membranes, tachycardia, weak pulse, weakness and depression. Severe intravascular haemolysis produces haemoglobinuria and there may be widespread organ dysfunction associated with hypotension, hypoxaemia leading to coma and death.

In acute cases the first sign is fever, followed by marked anaemia, jaundice, inappetance, marked thirst, weakness, prostration and often death. Petechial and ecchymotic haemorrhages may be observed on the gums or ventral abdomen of some dogs. In chronic cases the fever is not high and there is little jaundice. Anaemia is severe and the affected animals are listless and become very weak and emaciated.

The disease may take on many different clinical forms. Involvement of the circulatory system may produce oedema, purpura and ascites, and there may be stomatitis and gastritis; involvement of the respiratory system may cause catarrh and dyspnoea. CNS involvement causes locomotor disturbances, paresis or epileptiform fits. Cerebral babesiosis may be confused with rabies.

Diagnosis: Examination of blood films, stained with Romanowsky stains such as Giemsa, will reveal the parasites in the red cells. Species identification between large and small *Babesia* is essential with regard to choice of therapeutic drugs.

A range of serological tests have been developed, with IFAT being the most reliable test. Titres exceeding 1/80 are considered to be indicative of infection. Cross-reactivity occurs between species and may also cross-react with *Neospora* and *Toxoplasma*.

Pathology: The spleen is enlarged with dark red soft pulp and prominent splenic corpuscles. The liver is enlarged and jaundiced, with pathological changes ranging from congestion to centrilobular necrosis. The heart, kidneys and muscles are icteric. There may be variable amounts of fluid in the pleural, pericardial and peritoneal cavities. Small haemorrhages are sometimes present on the heart, pleura, bronchi and intestines.

Epidemiology: *B. canis canis* is transmitted by *Dermacentor reticulatus*, *B. canis rossi* by *Haemaphysalis leachi* and *B. canis vogeli* by *Rhipicephalus sanguineus*.

Treatment: In every case, chemotherapy with imidocarb, phenamidine, diminazine aceturate or trypan blue is advisable immediately after clinical diagnosis, since death may occur rapidly (Table 6.13). Diminazine has a low therapeutic index and toxicity appears to be dose-related, although idiosyncratic reactions may occur. In addition to anti-babesial treatment, supportive care should be provided. In dogs with severe anaemia blood transfusion should be considered.

Table 6.13 Babesicides for use in dogs against *B. canis*.

Drug	Recommended dose	Frequency	Comments
Imidocarb diproprionate	5 mg/kg s.c. or i.m.	Two doses at 14-day interval	Pain at injection site
Diminazine (di)aceturate	3.5 mg/kg i.m.	Single	Low therapeutic index
Phenamidine isethionate	15 mg/kg s.c.	Single or repeat 24 hours	Vomiting, CNS signs common side effects
Trypan blue	10 mg/kg i.v.		1% solution, tissue irritant

Control: Prophylaxis depends on regular treatment of dogs with a suitable acaricide, and since *R. sanguineus* may live in kennels, these should also be frequently treated with a suitable acaricide. For dogs visiting tick-endemic regions, tick prevention should be practised, e.g. fipronil application. In addition, a degree of surveillance of dogs exposed to infection is advisable so that treatment can be administered as early as possible. A vaccine has recently been launched in Europe for use against *B. canis*. The vaccine contains surface proteins expressed by cultures of *B. canis* and *B. canis rossi* and provides up to 6 months' protection.

Babesia gibsoni

Common name: Canine piroplasmosis

Predilection site: Blood

Parasite class: Sporozoasida

Family: Babesiidae

Description: Small piroplasm, annular or oval in shape, and no more than one eighth the diameter of the host erythrocyte.

Hosts: Dog

Life cycle: As for *B. canis*

Geographical distribution: Asia, north Africa and occasionally North America

Pathogenesis: Highly pathogenic in dogs causing marked anaemia, remittent fever, haemoglobinuria, constipation, marked splenomegaly and hepatomegaly. The disease is usually chronic with remissions and relapses of fever. Death may not occur for many months.

Clinical signs: Similar to *B. canis*. In acute cases, the first sign is fever, followed by marked anaemia, jaundice, inappetance, marked thirst, weakness, prostration and often death.

Diagnosis: As for *B. canis*

Pathology: As for *B. canis*

Epidemiology: Tick vectors are *Haemaphysalis bispinosa* and *Rhipicephalus sanguineus*.

For both species of *Babesia*, an increasing number of cases are reported in parts of the world such as northern Europe where the disease did not previously exist and may be linked to establishment of ticks in previously non-enzootic regions, and with increasing international pet travel and trade.

Treatment: Diminazine is the drug of choice for the treatment of *B. gibsoni* since imidocarb is less effective against small babesial species (Table 6.14).

Table 6.14 Babesicides for use in dogs against *B. gibsoni*.

Drug	Recommended dose	Frequency	Comments
Diminazine (di)aceturate	3.5 mg/kg i.m.	Single	Low therapeutic index
Phenamidine isethionate	15 mg/kg s.c.	Single or repeat 24 hours	Vomiting, CNS signs common side effects
Parvaquone	20 mg/kg s.c.	Single	

Control: As for *B. canis*. No vaccine is available for this species.

Notes: Phylogenetic analysis of DNA sequences has identified two strains of *Babesia gibsoni*: 'Asia' and 'California'. More recently, *Babesia annae* has been identified and appears to be endemic in Galacia, Spain and transmitted by the tick *Ixodes hexagonus*.

Babesia felis

Synonym: *Nuttallia felis*

Predilection site: Blood

Parasite Class: Sporozoasida

Family: Babesiidae

Description: Small piroplasms, with the majority of merozoites present in erythrocytes, round, irregularly round and 1.5–2 μm in diameter; some are elongate, 2–3 μm long and may form cruciform meronts.

Hosts: Cat

Life cycle: As for *B. canis*

Geographical distribution: Africa

Pathogenesis: Infection usually manifests as an afebrile, chronic low-grade disease.

Clinical signs: Affected animals show anorexia, depression, anaemia, emaciation, constipation and jaundice.

Diagnosis: Examination of blood films, stained with Romanowsky stains such as Giemsa, will reveal the parasites in the red cells. Species identification between large and small *Babesia* is essential with regard to choice of therapeutic drugs. Concurrent infection with other haemoparasites such as *Mycoplasma* (*Haemobartonella*) can be common in endemic areas and complicates the diagnosis.

Pathology: There is splenomegaly and jaundice, and complications are wide ranging and include hepatopathy, renal failure, pulmonary oedema and immune-mediated haemolytic anaemia often associated with feline immunodeficiency disease, feline leukaemia virus or feline infectious anaemia (*Mycoplasma*).

Epidemiology: Natural hosts are wild cats such as the lion and leopard. The highest prevalence is in young adult cats (<3 years old) during the spring and summer in endemic regions. The vectors are unknown, although *Haemaphysalis leachi* has been incriminated in South Africa.

Treatment: The antimalarial drug, primaquine phosphate given at 0.5 mg/kg orally, is the drug of choice for treating *B. felis* infections. Although it reduces the parasitaemia it does not sterilise the infection. Accurate dosing is required in cats to avoid toxicity, although vomiting is a common side effect at this dose rate.

Control: Reducing tick exposure is the best way to prevent infection although this is rarely achievable in endemic areas. Care must be taken in cats with the use of acaricides due to their increased susceptibility to many compounds.

Babesia cati

Predilection site: Blood

Parasite class: Sporozoasida

Family: Babesiidae

Description: Large piroplasms, pyriform in shape

Hosts: Cat

Life cycle: As for other *Babesia* species

Geographical distribution: South Africa, India

Pathogenesis and clinical signs: Not reported

Diagnosis: Examination of blood films, stained with Romanowsky stains such as Giemsa, will reveal the parasites in the red cells. Species identification between large and small *Babesia* is essential with regard to choice of therapeutic drugs. Concurrent infection with other haemoparasites such as *Mycoplasma* (*Haemobartonella*) can be common in endemic areas and complicates the diagnosis.

Treatment and control: Not reported

Cytauxzoon cati

Synonym: *Theileria felis*

Predilection site: Blood

Parasite class: Sporozoasida

Family: Theileriidae

Description: The single signet-ring shaped forms present within erythrocytes are 1–1.2 μm in diameter. Bipolar oval forms, tetrads and dark-staining 'dots' may also be seen.

Hosts: Cat, bobcat (*Lynx rufus*)

Life cycle: The life cycle is poorly understood. Infective sporozoites are injected into the cat from the salivary glands of an infective tick. Meronts develop primarily within tissue histiocytes in many organs and develop to release merozoites, which invade monocytes and erythrocytes.

Geographical distribution: USA

Pathogenesis: Infection of domestic cats with the merogenous stage typically results in a rapidly progressive systemic disease with a high mortality rate. In natural infections with *C. felis* there is an apparent variation in pathogenicity that may be associated with geographical location. During the merogenous phase there is mechanical obstruction to blood flow through various organs, notably the lungs, resulting in a shock-like state. Intravascular and extravascular haemolysis occurs because of erythrocyte invasion by merozoites.

Clinical signs: Soon after infection, affected cats develop non-specific signs, such as anorexia, lymphadenopathy, fever and lethargy, but the course of the disease is usually rapid, with the onset of a severe clinical syndrome characterised by dehydration, pallor, dyspnoea, icterus, recumbency and death. Usually, by the time the cat is presented, it is severely ill. Most cats die within 9–15 days following infection by virulent strains, regardless of treatment.

Diagnosis: Diagnosis is made by the identification of erythrocytic piroplasms in blood smears stained with Wright's stain or Giemsa. Parasitaemias are typically low (1–4%) although in some acute infections as many as 25% of the red cells may be infected. *C. felis* is a small piroplasm that must be differentiated from *Babesia felis*, which is very similar in size and appearance by light microscopy, but differs in geographical location. Dark-staining 'dot' forms may be mistaken for a more common and widespread parasite of cats, *Mycoplasma* (*Haemobartonella*) spp, the cause of feline infectious anaemia. Tissue meronts can be demonstrated in impression smears from bone marrow, spleen or lymph nodes, where they are typically numerous. There is currently no serological assay commercially available.

Pathology: Affected animals are markedly dehydrated, with generalised pallor, jaundice and numerous petechiae and ecchymoses of the epicardium and serosal membranes of the abdominal organs, as well as the visceral pleura of the lungs and mucosa of the urinary bladder. Pulmonary vessels are enlarged and tortuous as a result of vascular occlusion by the tissue stages. The lymph nodes are enlarged, congested, or haemorrhagic and oedematous and the spleen is markedly enlarged. Extra-erythrocytic forms are found within phagocytes in the spleen, lymph nodes, lungs, liver, kidneys and sometimes veins of the heart, urinary bladder and bone marrow and contain hundreds of merozoites or indistinct Koch bodies.

Epidemiology: This species has been found in the erythrocytes and tissues of domestic cats in the USA. It is suspected that *Dermacentor variabilis* is the principal vector. The natural hosts are the North American wild cat species, such as the bobcat, and it is thought that transmission to domestic cats represents inadvertent infection of a dead-end host. The highest incidence of infection occurs during early summer through to autumn when ticks are most active.

Treatment: Once diagnosed, the prognosis is poor and treatment often unsuccessful. Treatment with diminazene aceturate, or imidocarb diproprionate, both at 2 mg/kg i.m., may be used but may result in transient worsening of the condition. Supportive fluid therapy or blood transfusion may also be beneficial.

Control: Reducing tick exposure is the best way to prevent infection although this is rarely achievable in endemic areas. Care must be taken in cats with the use of acaricides due to their increased susceptibility to many compounds.

Hepatozoon spp

Predilection site: Blood

Parasite class: Sporozoasida

Family: Hepatozoidae

Description: Gamonts are found in the cytoplasm of neutrophils and have an ellipsoidal shape, and round or pleomorphic nucleus.

Hosts: Cat

Life cycle: Not known

Geographical distribution: France, Israel, India, South Africa

Pathogenesis: Feline hepatozonosis is characterised by skeletal and myocardial muscle involvement and is commonly associated with immunosuppressive viral disease caused by feline immunodeficiency virus (FIV) and feline leukaemia virus (FeLV). Gamonts are found in peripheral blood neutrophils, although the level of parasitaemia is usually low with less than 1% of neutrophils containing gamonts.

Clinical signs: Infected cats have fever, and may show gait abnormalities, muscular weakness and paresis.

Diagnosis: Diagnosis is based on the detection of the parasite in blood smears.

Epidemiology: The epidemiology of the disease and the vector(s) are unknown.

Treatment and control: Oral administration of doxycycline at 5 mg/kg for 10 days has been used to eliminate gamonts from the blood of domestic cats.

Notes: Hepatozoonosis is a rare infection in cats and the species involved have not been identified.

Anaplasma phagocytophilum

Synonym: *Anoplasma phagocytophilia, Ehrlichia phagocytophilia, Cytoecetes phagocytophilia, Anaplasma platys, Ehrlichia platys*

Common name: Tick-borne fever, pasture fever, canine granulocytic ehrlichiosis, human granulocytic ehrlichiosis, equine granulocyitc erlichiosis, canine infectious thrombocytopenia

Predilection site: Blood

Order: Rickettsiales

Family: Anaplasmataceae

Description: Blood smears stained with Giemsa or Wright's stains reveal one or more loose aggregates (morulae or inclusion bodies, 1.5–5 μm in diameter) of blue–grey to dark blue coccoid, coccobacillary or pleomorphic organisms within the cytoplasm of neutrophils.

Hosts: Sheep, cattle, dog, horse, deer, rodents, man

Life cycle: Obligate intracellular organisms infecting ganulocytes, predominantly neutrophils, appearing within the cytoplasm as membrane-bound vacuoles. Multiplication is by binary fission forming large inclusion bodies (morulae). In untreated animals, the cytoplasmic inclusions can be detected in circulating neutrophils for 1–2 weeks.

Geographical distribution: Probably worldwide, Europe (UK, Norway, Finland, Netherlands and Austria), USA, South America, Australia

Pathogenesis: Organisms enter the dermis via a tick bite and are then spread via the blood and/or the lymph and localise in mature granulocytes, mainly in neutrophils but also in eosinophils, of the peripheral blood. In dogs, severe pulmonary inflammation, alveolar damage and vasculitis of the extremities in the absence of bacterial organisms suggest an immunopathological course of events, such as cytokine-mediated stimulation of host macrophages and non-specific mononuclear phagocyte activity. The infection may also induce an over-active inflammatory response, such as a septic shock-like syndrome, or diffuse alveolar damage leading to respiratory distress syndrome. Phagocytic dysfunction of infected neutrophils may result in a defective host defence and subsequent secondary infections have been reported.

Both animals and humans can be co-infected with various *Anaplasma*, *Ehrlichia*, *Borrelia*, *Bartonella*, *Rickettsia*, *Babesia* and arboviral species. Infection with any of these organisms causes a wide range of clinical and pathological abnormalities, ranging in severity from asymptomatic infection to death. The risk of acquiring one or more tick-borne infections may be dependent on the prevalence of multi-infected vectors. *A. phagocytophilum* and *Borrelia burgdorferi*, for example, share both reservoir hosts and vectors, and in geographical areas where tick-borne fever is endemic, borreliosis is also prevalent.

Clinical signs: In dogs, the spectrum of clinical manifestations caused by *A. phagocytophilum* is wide but most commonly presents as an acute febrile syndrome. The incubation period may vary from 4–14 days, depending on the immune status of the infected individual and the bacterial strain involved. Infected dogs usually present with a history of lethargy and anorexia. Clinical examination commonly reveals fever, reluctance to move and, occasionally, splenomegaly. Less commonly, animals may show lameness, diarrhoea, or nervous signs such as seizures. Systemic manifestations may include haemorrhage, shock and multi-organ failure.

Diagnosis: *A. phagocytophilum* should be considered when an animal presents with an acute febrile illness in an endemic geographic area. Stained blood smears should be examined and with Wright's stain morulae typically appear as dark blue, irregularly stained densities in the cytoplasm of neutrophils. The colour of the morulae is usually darker than that of the cell nucleus. Morulae are often sparse and difficult to detect and a negative blood smear cannot rule out *A. phagocytophilum* infection. Specific diagnostic tests include IFAT, immunoblot analyses, ELISA and PCR analyses. The most widely accepted diagnostic criterion is a four-fold change in titre by IFAT. However, cross-reactivity may occur with other members of the genera *Anaplasma* and *Ehrlichia*. Thrombocytopenia can be a haematological finding although leucopenia has also been reported in rare cases.

Pathology: The disease is characterised by haematological changes typified by thrombocytopenia and leucopenia. The leucopenia is a result of early lymphopenia later accompanied by neutropenia. Thrombocytopenia is one of the most consistent haematological abnormalities in infected dogs. It may be moderate to severe and persists for a few days before returning to normal. Biochemical abnormalities may include mildly elevated serum alkaline phosphatase and alanine aminotransferase activities.

Epidemiology: Rodents as well as domestic and wild ruminants (sheep and deer) have been reported as reservoir hosts of *A. phagocytophilum* in Europe. The predominant reservoir host varies depending on the local natural and agricultural landscape. The vector of *A. phagocytophilum* in Europe is the common sheep tick, *Ixodes ricinus*. The organisms spend part of their normal life cycle within the tick and are transmitted trans-stadially. As the tick vector feeds on a wide range of vertebrate animals, transmission of the infectious agent may take place to multiple host species

Treatment: Doxycycline at 5–10 mg/kg for 3 weeks appears to be the most effective regime for treating infections in dogs and cats. Severe disease may require treatment for longer periods. The most common side effects of doxycycline treatment are nausea and vomiting which are avoided by administering the drug with food.

Control: In dogs and cats, infections can be prevented to some extent by avoiding tick-infested areas. Careful daily inspection for and removal of ticks is recommended in combination with the application of residual acaricidal products. Spray, spot-on liquid or collar formulations are available with residual efficacy of 1 month or more depending on the product.

Notes: The newly reclassified *Anaplasma phagocytophilum* combo nov. (formerly known as three separate ehrlichiae *E. phagocytophila*, *E. equi* and *Anaplasma platys* (formerly known as *E. platys*)) causes canine, equine and human granulocytic ehrlichiosis.

Ehrlichia canis

Common name: Canine monocytic ehrlichiosis, tropical canine pancytopenia

Predilection site: Blood

Order: Rickettsiales

Family: Rickettsiaceae

Description: *Ehrlichia canis* is a small pleomorphic Gram-negative, coccoid, obligatory intracellular bacterium, which parasitises circulating monocytes, intracytoplasmically in clusters (morulae). The earliest stages are small elementary bodies 0.2–0.4 μm in diameter, followed by slightly larger initial bodies 0.5–4 μm diameter, and finally even larger inclusion bodies 4–6 μm diameter. The organisms stain blue with

Romanovsky stain, light red with Machiavello and brown–black by silver stain.

Hosts: Dog

Life cycle: Infection is transmitted to the dog through the bite of an infected *Rhipicephalus sanguineus* tick. Transmission in the tick occurs trans-stadially, but not trans-ovarially. Larvae and nymphs become infected while feeding on rickettsaemic dogs and transmit the infection to the host after moulting to nymphs and adults, respectively.

Geographical distribution: Asia, Europe, Africa, Australia and America

Pathogenesis: Following infection, ehrlichiae organisms enter the bloodstream and lymphatics and localise in macrophages, mainly in the spleen and liver, where they replicate by binary fission. From there, infected macrophages disseminate the infection to other organ systems. The incubation period is 8–20 days and is followed consecutively by an acute, a subclinical and a chronic phase. The acute phase may last 2–4 weeks, and if not treated may enter the subclinical phase of the disease. Dogs in this phase may remain persistent carriers of *E. canis* for months or years. The spleen plays a major role in the pathogenesis of the disease and persistence of infection appears to be within splenic macrophages. Some persistently infected dogs may recover spontaneously, however others subsequently develop the chronic severe form of the disease. Not all dogs develop the chronic phase, and factors leading to the development of this phase remain unclear. The prognosis at this stage is grave, and death may occur as a consequence of haemorrhage and/or secondary infection. Immunological mechanisms appear to be involved in the pathogenesis of the disease through the production of antibodies that bind to the membrane of erythrocytes, and platelet-bound antibodies, which appear to play a role in the pathogenesis of thrombocytopenia. Other mechanisms involved in the development of the thrombocytopenia include increased platelet destruction, shortened platelet half-life during the acute phase and decreased production in the chronic phase. Meningitis and meningioencephalitis are associated with extensive lymphoplasmacytic and monocytic infiltration, perivascular cuffing and gliosis. On rare occasions morulae may be detected in the cerebrospinal fluid of dogs with neurological signs. The finding of circulating immune complexes in sera of naturally infected dogs, suggests that some of the pathological and clinical manifestations are mediated by immune complexes.

Clinical signs: *E. canis* infects all breeds of dogs; however, the German shepherd dog appears to be more susceptible to clinical disease and more severely affected than other breeds, with a higher mortality rate. There is no age predilection, and both sexes are equally affected. The disease is manifested by a wide variety of clinical signs. During the acute phase, clinical signs range from mild and non-specific, to severe and life-threatening. Common non-specific signs in this phase include depression, lethargy, anorexia, pyrexia, tachypnoea and weight loss. Specific clinical signs include lymphadenomegaly, splenomegaly, petechiation and ecchymoses of the skin and mucous membranes, and occasional epistaxis. Less commonly there is vomiting, and serous or purulent oculonasal discharge and dyspnoea. In the chronic severe form of the disease, clinical signs may be similar to those seen in the acute disease but more severe. There may be pallor of the mucous membranes and emaciation, and peripheral oedema, especially of the hind limbs and scrotum, may also be seen. Entire bitches may show prolonged bleeding during oestrus, infertility, abortion and neonatal death. Secondary bacterial and protozoal infections may cause interstitial pneumonia and renal failure.

Ocular signs have been reported to occur during the acute and chronic phases and may manifest as conjunctivitis, petechiae and ecchymoses of the conjunctiva and iris, corneal oedema and panuveitis. Subretinal haemorrhage and retinal detachment resulting in blindness may occur due to a monoclonal gammopathy and hyperviscosity. Neurological signs include ataxia, seizures, paresis, hyperaesthesia and cranial nerve dysfunction, and may be attributed to meningitis or meningoencephalitis, which are more commonly seen during the acute phase.

Systemic manifestations may include haemorrhage, shock and multi-organ failure.

Diagnosis: Diagnosis of *E. canis* infection is based on history, clinical presentation and clinical pathological findings supported by serology. Residence in or travel to known endemic areas, and a history of tick infestation should increase the suspicion of infection.

In general, the *Ehrlichia* can be distinguished by the type of cell they invade. As the name of the disease it causes implies, *E. canis* invades mononuclear cells. Intracytoplasmic *E. canis* morulae may be visualised in monocytes during the acute phase of the disease in some cases. Examination of the buffy coat enhances the chance of visualising morulae in smears. During the acute phase there is an increase in the mean platelet volume, mild leucopenia and anaemia, and megaplatelets appear in the blood smear reflecting active thrombopoiesis. Monocytosis, and reactive monocytes and large granular lymphocytes are also seen. During the subclinical phase a mild thrombocytopenia is a commonly found disease with severe pancytopenia as a result of a suppressed hypocellular bone marrow.

On blood biochemistry there is hypoalbuminaemia and hyperglobulinaemia, the latter due mainly due to hypergammaglobulinaemia, which is usually polyclonal, as determined by serum protein electrophoresis. On rare occasions, monoclonal gammopathy may be noticed and may result in a hyperviscosity syndrome. Pancytopenic dogs reveal significantly lower concentrations of total protein, total globulin and gammaglobulin concentrations as compared to non-pancytopenic dogs. Mild transient increase in serum alanine aminotransferase (AAT) and alkaline phosphatase (AP) may also be present. Anti-platelet antibody test as well as Coombs' test may be positive in infected dogs.

The indirect immunofluorescence antibody test (IFAT) test is the most widely used serological assay for the diagnosis of canine ehrlichiosis, and titres at a dilution equal to or greater than 1:40 are considered evidence of exposure. Two consecutive tests are recommended, 1–2 weeks apart, with a four-fold increase in antibody titre indicative of active infection. In areas endemic for other *Ehrlichia* species, serological cross-reactivity may complicate the diagnosis. Enzyme-linked immunosorbant assays (ELISA) for *E. canis* antibodies have been developed and several commercial dot-ELISA antibody tests have been developed for rapid in-clinic use. Polymerase chain reactions (PCRs) using specific primers for *E. canis* have also been developed. Concurrent infections with other tick-borne pathogens, such as *Babesia* spp and *Hepatozoon canis*, are common in endemic areas and it is therefore important to examine blood smears of infected dogs microscopically and to consider multiple serological or PCR screening for co-infecting organisms.

Pathology: Once present in tissues, *E. canis* organisms continue to invade, persist and replicate in cells. Circulating infected cells may induce vasculitis and subsequent intravascular coagulation, which, in combination with an altered cell-mediated immunity, result in the destruction of platelets. Similar destruction of leucocytes and erythrocytes in combination with decreased erythrocyte production may cause clinical leucopenia and anaemia, respectively. During the subclinical phase, thrombocytopenia, leucopenia and anaemia may continue. Hyperglobinaemia may be observed in the chronic stages, which is unrelated to serum antibody levels. Bone marrow may be impaired during the chronic phase, although the mechanisms for suppression are not completely understood.

Epidemiology: *E. canis* is transmitted by the brown dog-tick, *Rhipicephalus sanguineus*. Transmission has also been shown to occur experimentally with the American dog-tick, *Dermacentor variabilis*. Transmission in the tick occurs trans-stadially, but not transovarially. Larvae and nymphs become infected while feeding on rickettsaemic dogs and transmit the infection to the host after moulting to nymphs and adults, respectively. Adult ticks have been shown to transmit infection 155 days after becoming infected. This phenomenon allows ticks to over-winter and infect hosts in the following spring. The occurrence and geographical distribution of *E. canis* is related to the distribution and biology of its tick vector. *R. sanguineus* ticks are abundant during the warm season, and disease in dogs is seen most commonly during the summer months. Dogs living in endemic regions and those travelling to endemic areas should be considered at risk of infection.

Treatment: Doxycycline at a dose of 10 mg/kg once daily (or 5 mg/kg twice daily) per os, for a minimum period of 3 weeks, is the treatment of choice for acute infections, and most acute cases respond and show clinical improvement within 24–72 hours. Dogs in the subclinical phase may need prolonged treatment, whilst dogs suffering from the chronic severe form of the disease are usually unresponsive to treatment. Other drugs with known efficacy against *E. canis* include tetracycline hydrochloride (22 mg/kg), oxytetracycline (25 mg/kg) and chloramphenicol (50 mg/kg) all given at 8-hourly intervals. Despite treatment, antibody titres may persist for months and even for years. Their persistence may represent an aberrant immune response, or treatment failure, but progressive decrease in the gammaglobulin concentrations is associated with elimination of the rickettsia. *E. canis* antibodies do not provide protection against re-challenge, and seropositive dogs remain susceptible.

Control: No effective anti-*E. canis* vaccine has been developed and tick control remains the most effective preventive measure against infection. Breaking the life cycle of the tick vector at the level of the canine host will eliminate the source of numerous pathogenic agents, in addition to ehrlichiae, that infect dogs, and may decrease the risk of transmission to humans for those tick vectors with broad host ranges. Common acaracides, such as amitraz, fipronil, and pyrethrins, when used according to the manufacturer's instructions, are effective. By targeting the vector, the life cycle and consequently transmission of ehrlichiae will be interrupted. In endemic areas, low-dose oxytetracycline treatment (6.6 mg/kg) once daily has been suggested as an additional prophylactic measure.

Ehrlichia chaffensis

Common name: Canine monocytic ehrlichiosis

Predilection site: Blood

Order: Rickettsiales

Family: Rickettsiaceae

Description: *Ehrlichia chaffensis* is a small pleomorphic Gram-negative, coccoid, obligatory intracellular bacterium, which parasitises circulating monocytes and macrophages, intracytoplasmically in clusters (morulae).

Hosts: Dog, man, deer

Life cycle: As for *E. canis*

Geographical distribution: States of southern USA

Pathogenesis and clinical signs: Experimental infections in dogs have shown fever only. The clinical significance of natural canine infection has yet to be determined.

Diagnosis: The IFA test detects exposure to the rickettsia, however it cannot differentiate between antibodies to other canine ehrlichias. Species identification is by western immunoblot analysis, and PCR using species-specific primers.

Epidemiology: *E. chqffensis* is transmitted by *Amblyomma americanum* (the Lone Star tick) and to a lesser extent by *Dermacentor variabilis*. Persistently infected white-tailed deer (*Odocoileus virginianus*) and possibly canids, serve as reservoirs.

Treatment and control: As for *E. canis*, although treatment is not usually required.

Ehrlichia ewingii

Common name: Canine granulocytic ehrlichiosis

Predilection site: Blood

Order: Rickettsiales

Family: Rickettsiaceae

Description: *Ehrlichia ewingii* is a small pleomorphic Gram-negative, coccoid, obligatory intracellular bacterium, which parasitises circulating neutrophils and eosinophils, intracytoplasmically in clusters (morulae).

Hosts: Dog

Life cycle: Infection is transmitted to the dog through the bite of an infected *Ambylomma americanum* tick. Transmission in the tick occurs trans-stadially, but not trans-ovarially. Larvae and nymphs become infected while feeding on rickettsaemic dogs and transmit the infection to the host after moulting to nymphs and adults, respectively.

Geographical distribution: Southeast and south-central USA

Pathogenesis: Following infection, ehrlichial organisms enter the bloodstream and lymphatics and localise in neutrophils. The pathogenesis of polyarthritis, observed more often with infection by granulocytic ehrlichiae, arises from haemarthrosis and immune complex deposition into the joints.

Clinical signs: The disease is usually an acute mild disease that may lead to polyarthritis in chronically infected dogs. Lameness, joint swelling, stiff gait and fever are common clinical signs. Haematological changes are mild and include thrombocytopenia and anaemia.

Diagnosis: Diagnosis of *E. ewingii* infection is based on history, clinical presentation and clinical pathological findings supported by serology. Residing or travel to known endemic areas, and a history of tick infestation should increase the suspicion of infection. Visualisation of morulae in the respective cell types provides a definitive diagnosis and allows for differentiating between the monocytic and granulocytic ehrlichia. Intracytoplasmic *E. ewingii* morulae may be seen within neutrophils.

The indirect immunofluorescence antibody test (IFAT) is the most widely used serological assay for the diagnosis of canine ehrlichiosis. However, as *E. ewingii* has not yet been cultured *in vitro*, antigen is not readily available for IFAT. In areas endemic for other *Ehrlichia* species, serological cross-reactivity with the monocytic *Ehrlichia* spp may complicate the diagnosis. Anti-*E. ewingii* antibodies strongly cross-react with *E. canis* and *E. chaffensis*, and do not (or weakly) react with *A. phagocytophilum*. The use of western immunoblot and species-specific PCR assays should be used to confirm the ehrlichial species. Species determination is important, as *A. phagocytophilum* is also associated with intra-neutrophilic morula formation and similar clinical signs in dogs.

Pathology: After entering the canine host through the bite of the tick vector, ehrlichial organisms travel through the circulation, invade cells and disseminate to various tissues. Once in tissues, they continue to invade, persist, and replicate in cells. Polyarthritis may arise from haemarthrosis and immune complex deposition into the joints and is often accompanied by neutrophilic inflammation.

Epidemiology: Ehrlichiosis caused by *E. ewingii* has been diagnosed in the USA only. It occurs mainly in the spring and early summer. The main tick vector is *A. americanum* but the organism has been identified in a number of other ticks including *R. sanguineus*, *D. variabilis*, *Ixodes scapularis* and *I. pacificus*.

Treatment: Tetracyclines, especially doxycycline, elicit rapid clinical improvement.

Control: Tick control is the most effective preventive measure against infection. By targeting the vector, the life cycle and consequently transmission of ehrlichiae will be interrupted. Common acaracides, such as amitraz, fipronil, and pyrethrins, when used according to the manufacturer's instructions, are effective in controlling ticks.

Notes: *E. ewingii* and the newly reclassified *Anaplasma phagocytophilum* combo nov. cause canine and human granulocytic ehrlichiosis. *E. ewingii* has been implicated as the cause of human infections in the United States, particularly in immunocompromised people. The role of the dog as a zoonotic reservoir for *E. ewingii* infection is unknown.

Rickettsia rickettsii

Common name: Rocky Mountain spotted fever

Predilection site: Blood vessels

Order: Rickettsiales

Family: Rickettsiaceae

Description: Small pleomorphic Gram-negative, coccoid, obligatory intracellular organisms infecting endothelial cells of smaller blood vessels.

Hosts: Dog, man

Life cycle: Ticks become infected with *R. rickettsii* by feeding on infected small rodents that are the main reservoir of disease. Immature ticks become infected and infection is transmitted trans-stadially and trans-ovarially to later tick stages, which feed on larger mammals.

Geographical distribution: USA, Canada, Central America

Pathogenesis: Following infection the organisms enter the bloodstream and infect endothelial cells causing widespread vasculitis leading to activation of the coagulation and fibrinolytic pathways. Thrombocytopenia occurs through coagulatory and immune-mediated mechanisms. In chronic untreated cases, organs such as the skin, brain, heart and kidneys may develop multiple foci of necrosis and vascular injury leads to leakage of intravascular fluids and oedema. Fluid accumulation in tissues such as the CNS can cause significant brain oedema resulting in a progressive mental and cardiorespiratory depression.

Clinical signs: Infected dogs usually develop fever within several days after tick exposure. This is usually accompanied by signs of lethargy, mental dullness, inappetence, arthralgia and myalgia, manifest as difficulty in rising and eventual reluctance to walk. Lymphadenomegaly of all peripheral lymph nodes is apparent, and subcutaneous oedema and dermal necrosis may develop in severely affected animals. Petechial haemorrhages may occur rarely on the mucous membranes, and more commonly in the ocular fundus. Neurological signs may appear due to meningitis and can include hyperaesthesia, seizures, vestibular dysfunction and a variety of manifestations depending on the lesion localisation. Recovery is rapid and complete in those animals receiving treatment early, before the onset of organ damage or neurological complications. Once the neurological signs have developed, recovery is delayed, or signs may be permanent.

Diagnosis: Clinical laboratory findings are non-specific for a generalised acute phase inflammatory reaction. There is usually a leucopenia in the acute stages followed by a moderate leucocytosis. A left shift and toxic granulation of neutrophils may be observed in animals with the most severe tissue necrosis. Thrombocytopenia is one of the most consistent laboratory findings. Serum biochemical abnormalities include hypoalbuminaemia, elevated serum alkaline phosphatase activity, and variable hyponatraemia and hyperbilirubinaemia. Conduction disturbances related to myocarditis may be seen on electrocardiograph and a diffuse increase in pulmonary interstitial density on radiographs. A micro-immunofluorescence (Micro-IF) test is used to determine specific antibodies. Titres >1/1024 generally indicate recent exposure. PCR specific primers have been used to identify organisms in blood or tissue specimens. Rickettsial isolation involves risk and can only be done in high bio-containment facilities.

Pathology: On postmortem, there are usually widespread petechial and ecchymotic haemorrhages, lymphadenomegaly and splenomegaly. Microscopically, there is a widespread necrotising vasculitis in many organs.

Epidemiology: Two tick species, *Dermacentor andersoni* (wood tick) and *D. variabilis* (dog tick), both three-host ticks, appear to be mainly involved in the transmission of *R. rickettsii*. Only a small proportion of ticks may be infected in the overall population of a given area. In addition to the low prevalence of infection, infected ticks are not immediately infectious but become so following tick attachment and blood feeding for periods of 5–20 hours. Dogs usually develop illness during the warmer months of the year when questing ticks are active. This seasonality is less noticeable at lower latitudes.

Treatment: Left untreated, the disease is highly fatal and treatment should be instituted whenever the disease is suspected. Tetracyclines are the antibiotics of choice and should be administered for at least 7 days, but are only effective if they are given prior to the onset of tissue necrosis or organ failure. Recovery is usually associated with protective immunity.

Control: Prevention can be achieved by tick control and periodic treatment with systemic or topically applied acaricides.

Notes: Rocky Mountain spotted fever is an important zoonotic disease because of its high prevalence and potentially fatal outcome if diagnosis is delayed or missed. Early signs in humans may be vague and misdiagnosis can occur until a rash develops later in the course of disease.

Rickettsia conorii

Common name: Boutonneuse fever, Mediterranean spotted fever, Indian tick typhus, east African tick typhus

Predilection site: Blood

Order: Rickettsiales

Family: Rickettsiaceae

Description: Small pleomorphic Gram-negative, coccoid, obligatory intracellular organisms infecting endothelial cells of smaller blood vessels.

Hosts: Rodents, dog, cattle, sheep, goat, man

Life cycle: Ticks become infected with *R. conorii* by feeding on infected small rodents that are the main reservoir of disease. Immature ticks become infected and infection is transmitted trans-stadially and trans-ovarially to later tick stages, which feed on larger mammals.

Geographical distribution: Southern Europe, Africa, India and the Oriental region

Pathogenesis: Infections appear to be non-pathogenic

Diagnosis: The rickettsiae can be demonstrated by staining blood or organ smears with Giemsa or may be detected serologically.

Epidemiology: The vector of Mediterranean 'boutonneuse' fever is *Rhipicephalus sanguineus*. Apart from dogs, sheep and cattle, other small free-living mammals, such as rats, mice and shrews, are believed to play an important role in the cycle of infection within tick vectors.

Treatment and control: Not usually required although if suspected, tetracyclines are usually effective

Rickettsia felis

Predilection site: Blood vessels

Order: Rickettsiales

Family: Rickettsiaceae

Description: Small pleomorphic Gram-negative, coccoid, obligatory intracellular organisms infecting endothelial cells of smaller blood vessels.

Hosts: Cat, dog, man

Life cycle: Fleas become infected with *R. felis* by feeding on infected animals. Infection in the flea is transmitted trans-stadially and trans-ovarially to later stages, and transmission occurs when the adult flea feeds.

Geographical distribution: North and South America, Europe

Pathogenesis and clinical signs: The pathogenesis of natural infections in dogs and cats is unknown. Cats infected with *R. felis* through exposure to infected fleas develop a subclinical infection.

Epidemiology: In endemic areas of the USA, opposums are major reservoirs for *R. felis*. Infection to dogs and cats is transmitted by the cat flea, *Ctenocephalides felis*.

Table 6.15 Tick-borne *Rickettsia* of dogs.

Disease agents	Disease	Primary tick vectors	Distribution
Ehrlichia canis	Canine monocytic ehrlichiosis	*Rhipicephalus sanguineus*	Worldwide; tropical/temperate
Ehrlichia chaffensis		*Amblyomma americanum*	Worldwide
Ehrlichia ewingii		*Amblyomma americanum*	Southeastern and south-central USA
Anaplasma phagocytophilum (incl *A. platys*)	Canine granulocytic ehrlichiosis	*Ixodes* spp *Rhipicephalus sanguineus*	Worldwide
Rickettsia rickettsii	Rocky Mountain spotted fever	*Dermacentor varabilis* *Dermacentor andersoni*	North and South America
Rickettsia conorii	Boutonneuse fever Mediterranean fever Indian tick typhus East African tick typhus	*Rhipicephalus* sp *Amblyomma* sp *Hyalomma* sp	Europe Asia, Africa

Treatment and control: Treatment with tetracyclines is likely to be effective but seldom indicated. Prevention can be achieved by flea control and periodic treatment with systemic or topically applied insecticides.

Notes: *R. felis* causes flea-transmitted human typhus along with *R. typhus*; the latter is transmitted by rodent fleas.

Haemobartonella felis

Synonym: *Mycoplasma haemofelis*, *Candidatus Mycoplasma turicensis*, *Mycoplasma haemominutum*

Predilection site: Blood

Order: Rickettsiales

Family: Anaplasmataceae

Description: Small pleomorphic Gram-negative, coccoid, obligatory intracellular organisms infecting erythrocytes.

Hosts: Cat

Life cycle: The life cycle is not known but may involve transmission by fleas or lice. Vertical transmission has been implicated.

Geographical distribution: North and South Europe

Pathogenesis: Haemoplasmas induce anaemia by haemolysis and sequestration. The disease may be acute or chronic with periodic recrudescence of clinical signs. Recovered cats may remain carriers. Infection with *Candidatus M. haemominutum* does not often result in clinical signs but a fall in PCV does occur.

Clinical signs: In the acute form, there is intermittent fever with a progressive anaemia.

Diagnosis: The organisms can be detected in blood smears stained with Romanowsky stain.

Pathology: There are no specific or pathognomonic pathological findings, although cats with concurrent FeLV infection develop more pronounced lesions. Tissues are usually pale and on occasions jaundiced. The liver is often pale and jaundiced. Splenomegaly and lymph node enlargement have been reported. Histology of the liver includes centrilobular congestion and degeneration, and in cats with concurrent FeLV there may be haemosiderosis. In the spleen there is congestion, extramedullary haemopoiesis, follicular hyperplasia, erythrophagocytosis and haemosideroisis.

Epidemiology: Transmission of the disease probably depends on arthropods including lice, fleas, ticks and biting flies and, at least in the case of *H. felis*, by ingestion of blood during fighting. Infection is most common in young cats.

Treatment and control: Treatment with tetracyclines is effective. Control of blood sucking arthropods with insecticides and prompt treatment following cat fights.

Notes: The taxonomy of this species is subject to much debate and there is a proposal to re-classify it into the bacterial genus *Mycoplasma* (class Mollicutes) based on 16s rRNA gene sequences and phylogenetic analysis. DNA studies have additionally demonstrated the exitence of two distinct species of *H. felis*; *Mycoplasma haemofelis* (large species) and *Candidatus Mycoplasma haemominutum* (small species). A third species *Candidatus Mycoplasma turicensis* has also been reported.

PARASITES OF THE NERVOUS SYSTEM

Thelazia callipaeda

Common name: Eye worm

Predilection site: Eye, conjunctival sac and lachrymal duct.

Parasite class: Nematoda

Superfamily: Spiruroidea

Description, gross: Small thin white worms 1.0–1.7 cm long; males are 7–11.5 mm and females 7–17 mm.

Description, microscopic: In the male the left spicule is much longer than the right. In the female the vulva is in the oesophageal region.

Final hosts: Dog, cat, occasionally sheep and deer

Intermediate hosts: Muscid flies, particularly *Fannia* spp

Life cycle: The worms are viviparous. The L_1 passed by the female worm into the lachrymal secretion is ingested by the fly intermediate host as it feeds. Development from L_1 to L_3 occurs in the ovarian follicles of the fly during the summer months. L_3 migrate to the mouthparts of the fly and are transferred to the final host when the fly feeds.

Geographical distribution: Far East

Pathogenesis: Lesions are caused by the serrated cuticle of the worm and most damage results from movement by the active young adults causing lachrymation, followed by conjunctivitis. Infection may predispose the host to secondary bacterial infection.

Clinical signs: Conjunctivitis, excessive lachrymation

Diagnosis: This is based on observation of the parasites in the conjunctival sac or on the conjunctiva following local anaesthesia, or finding larvae in the lachrymal secretion (Fig. 6.21).

Pathology: Invasion of the lachrymal gland and ducts may cause inflammation leading to occlusion and

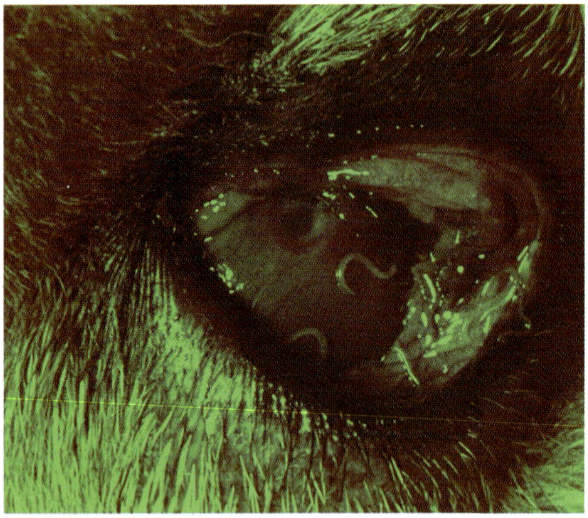

Fig. 6.21 *Thelazia* in the eye of an infected dog.

reduced tear production. Mechanical irritation of the conjunctiva produces inflammation, whilst damage to the cornea leads to opacity, keratitis and corneal ulceration.

Epidemiology: *Thelazia* infections occur seasonally and are linked to periods of maximum fly activity.

Treatment: Surgical removal with forceps following the application of an ocular local anaesthetic. In cases of secondary bacterial infection the use of antibiotic eye preparations may be indicated. Ivermectin at 0.2 mg/kg has been reported to be effective.

Control: Prevention is difficult because of the ubiquitous nature of the fly vectors.

Thelazia californiensis

Common name: Eye worm

Predilection site: Eye, conjunctival sac and lachrymal duct

Parasite class: Nematoda

Superfamily: Spiruroidea

Description, gross: Small thin white worms 1.0–1.5 cm long.

Description, microscopic: A mouth capsule is present and the cuticle has prominent striations at the anterior end.

Final hosts: Dog, cat

Intermediate hosts: Muscid flies

Geographical distribution: North America

All other details as for *T. callipaeda*.

Taenia solium

Synonym: *Cysticercus cellulosae*

Common name: Human pork tapeworm

Predilection site: Small intestine (final host); muscle (intermediate host)

Parasite class: Cestoda

Family: Taeniidae

Description, gross: The adult tapeworm is 3–5 m long with a scolex, typically taeniid, having a rostellum with four suckers and armed with two concentric rows of 22–32 hooks. The uterus of the gravid segment has 7–13 lateral branches. Adults can survive in humans for many years.

Description, microscopic: Cysts are milky white and have a scolex bearing a rostellum and hooks similar to the adult.

Final host: Man

Intermediate hosts: Pig, wild boar, rarely dog and man

Pathogenesis: Dogs that become infected with the metacestode stage can also show signs of cerebral cysticercosis with convulsions.

Encephalitozoon cuniculi

Synonym: *Nosema cuniculi*

Predilection site: Blood

Class: Microsporasida

Family: Nosematidae

Description: Microsporidia are obligate, intracellular, spore-forming protozoa. Trophozoites are 2–2.5 × 0.8–1.2 μm in tissue sections or 4 × 2.5 μm in smears. Spores are about 2 μm long and contain a spirally coiled polar filament with four to five coils.

Hosts: Rabbit, dog, fox (red – *Vulpes vulpes*, blue – *Alopex lagopus*, silver), cat, mouse, rat, man

Life cycle: The infective spore stages are highly resistant and can survive for many years. When spores are ingested, the polar tube is everted and when fully extended the sporoplasm passes through the tube and is innoculated into the cytoplasm of the host cell. There then follows a phase of multiplication by binary or multiple fission (merogony). This is followed by sporogony to form sporoblasts, which then mature into spores.

Geographical distribution: Worldwide

Pathogenesis: The parasite develops within parasitophorous vacuoles in macrophages and other cells, especially vascular endothelial cells.

Clinical signs: Infection in dogs is usually asymptomatic, but there may be loss of condition, posterior weakness, incoordination, apathy and epileptiform seizures.

Diagnosis: Diagnosis in the live animal is difficult and is usually based on identifying the lesions on histopathology and observation of the organisms in Giemsa, Gram or Goodpasture-carbol fuchsin stains. A serum ELISA test is available.

Pathology: In the dog, there has been reported non-suppurative nephritis, encephalitis and vasculitis.

Epidemiology: Not reported in dogs, although in other hosts transmission via urine from infected animals has been described.

Treatment and control: Not reported in dogs

Toxoplasma gondii

See details and description under Parasites of the locomotory system.

Neospora caninum

Synonym: *Histoplasma gondii*

Predilection site: Blood

Order: Sporozoasida

Family: Sarcocystiidae

Description: Tachyzoites measure 6 × 2 μm and are usually located in the cytoplasm of cells. Tissue cysts are oval, 107 μm long, and have a thick wall (up to 4 μm) and are found only in neural tissue.

Intermediate hosts: Cattle, sheep, goat

Final host: Dog

Life cycle: The complete life cycle of *Neospora caninum* has only recently been elucidated. It was previously confused with *Toxoplasma gondii* because of the structural similarity of the asexual stages of the two parasites. Similarities between the two organisms suggested that *N. caninum* was a coccidian parasite whose infective stage was an oocyst. The definitive host has recently been shown to be dogs, which pass small numbers of oocysts in faeces from 8–23 days after infection. Tissue cysts are tachyzoites that can infect a range of animals including cattle, sheep, goats and horses. The dog can also act as an intermediate host.

Geographical distribution: Worldwide

Pathogenesis: Neosporosis occurs most severely in transplacentally infected puppies and is characterised by a progressive ascending paralysis, particularly of the hindlimbs. Polymyositis and hepatitis may also occur. Clinical signs are first noticed at 1–6 months of age but can be seen in adults and older dogs. Sudden death due to myocarditis has been reported.

Clinical signs: Fatal, ascending hindleg paralysis

Diagnosis: History of neurological signs, muscle weakness with a progressive ascending paralysis. An indirect antibody fluorescent test (IFAT) is available.

Pathology: Lesions are most commonly seen in the brain, spinal cord, nerve roots and skeletal muscles, but any organ may be involved including the skin. In the brain, the grey matter is most severely affected, whilst the submeningeal white matter tends to be most severely affected in the spinal cord. Tachyzoite proliferation is associated with focal malacia, suppuration and granulatomous reaction. Chronic lesions are characterised by lymphoplasmacytic, perivascular infiltrations and gliosis. A marked fibrosis may develop, particularly in submeningeal areas of the cerebral and cerebellar cortex. Parasitised muscle fibres undergo rapid necrosis, and there are massive infiltrations of macrophages, lymphocytes and plasma cells. Tissue cysts are scarce and usually found only in the CNS.

Epidemiology: The dog is the intermediate host, and is also a final host in prenatal infections. In cattle, infection can be both vertically transmitted from dam to calf *in utero* and lactogenically, naturally by ingestion of food and water contaminated with dog faeces containing *Neospora caninum* oocysts, or from cow to cow. The mechanisms of repeat congenital transmission are unknown at present.

Treatment: If canine neosporosis is diagnosed early, treatment with trimethoprim, sulphadiazine, pyrimethamine and clindamycin might be useful. Decoquinate has been shown to kill *N. caninum* tachyzoites in cultures.

Control: Dogs should not be allowed to eat aborted fetuses or fetal membranes, and their faeces should be prevented from contaminating bovine feedstuffs.

PARASITES OF THE REPRODUCTIVE/ UROGENITAL SYSTEM

Capillaria plica

Synonym: *Pearsonema plica*

Common name: Bladder hairworm

Predilection site: Urinary bladder, and occasionally the pelvis of the kidney

Parasite class: Nematoda

Superfamily: Trichuroidea

Description, gross: Fine whitish, filamentous worms 1–6 cm long, males measure 13–30 mm and females 30–60 mm.

Description, microscopic: The males have a long thin single spicule and often possess a primitive bursa-like structure. The eggs are barrel-shaped and colourless, 63–68 × 24–27 μm and have thick shells that are slightly striated with bipolar plugs.

Final hosts: Fox, dog and more rarely cat

Intermediate hosts: Earthworms

Life cycle: This parasite requires an earthworm intermediate host, ingested eggs developing to the infective L_3 within 30 days. The prepatent period is around 8 weeks.

Geographical distribution: Many parts of the world

Pathogenesis: It is rarely of pathogenic significance. It can however occasionally induce cystitis where secondary bacterial infection occurs.

Clinical signs: Infections are usually asymptomatic. Cystitis and difficulty in urinating have been observed.

Diagnosis: Diagnosis is based on finding the typical *Capillaria* eggs in urine.

Pathology: Most infections are harmless; the anterior end of the worm embedded in the surface epithelium provokes a light cellular reaction in the lamina propria.

Epidemiology: The route of transmission is via the ingestion of infective larvae present in earthworms.

Treatment: Successful treatment with fenbendazole at 50 mg/kg orally daily for 3 days has been reported.

Control: Care should be taken to ensure that runs are clean, dry and free-draining.

Notes: The taxonomic situation regarding many species of *Capillaria* is complex and recently it has been split into several genera; the old species names are listed with the new proposed generic names.

Dioctophyma renale

Synonym: *Dictophyme renale, Eustrongylus gigas*

Common name: Giant kidney worm

Predilection site: Kidney parenchyma, abdominal cavity

Parasite class: Nematoda

Superfamily: Dioctophymatoidea

Description, gross: *Dioctophyma* is the largest parasitic nematode of domestic animals, the female measuring more than 60 cm in length, with a diameter of around 1.0 cm. The male is about 35 cm long. The worms are deep red–purple in colour. Their size and predilection site are sufficient for identification.

Description, microscopic: The eggs are lemon shaped, yellowish brown, 71–84 × 46–52 μm, with a thick, pitted shell and bipolar plugs, and are unsegmented when passed.

Final hosts: Dog, fox, mink, ferret, otter, pine marten, polecat, mink; sporadically reported in the cat, pig, horse, cattle and man.

Intermediate hosts: Aquatic oligochaetes (annelids), e.g. *Lumbriculus variegatus*

Life cycle: The worms are oviparous. The eggs, in the single-cell stage, are passed in the urine in clumps or chains, and are ingested by the annelid intermediate host in which the two preparasitic moults occur. The development phase in the annelid is about 2–4 months. The final host is infected by swallowing the annelid with the drinking water, or by the ingestion of a paratenic host, such as a frog or fish, which has itself eaten the infected annelid. In the final host, the infective larvae penetrate the intestinal wall, enter the peritoneal cavity and eventually penetrate the kidney. The prepatent period is about 6 months but has been observed to be as long as 2 years.

Geographical distribution: Temperate and subarctic areas; North and South America, Asia. It occurs sporadically in Europe, but has not been recorded in Britain. Its main endemic area is the northern part of North America, chiefly Canada.

Pathogenesis: The final effect of infection is destruction of the kidney. Usually only one kidney is affected, the right being more often involved than the left. The parenchyma is destroyed leaving only the capsule as a distended sac containing the worms; though there may be three or four worms in a kidney, occasionally there is only one. Rarely, the worms may occur in the abdominal cavity, either free or encapsulated, and in the subcutaneous connective tissue.

Clinical signs: The main signs are dysuria with some haematuria, especially at the end of micturition; in a few cases there is lumbar pain. Most cases, however, are completely asymptomatic, even when one kidney has been completely destroyed. Worms in the abdominal cavity can cause a chronic peritonitis.

Diagnosis: The eggs either are quite characteristic, being ovoid and yellowy brown, with pitted shells, and their occurrence in the urine, singly or in clumps or chains, is diagnostic.

Pathology: Adult worms in the renal pelvis are very destructive, causing initially haemorrhagic pyelitis, which becomes suppurative and the parenchyma is eventually destroyed until only the tunic contains the worm and exudate. In the abdominal cavity, the worm often entwines a lobe of the liver and may cause erosion of the hepatic capsule, leading to haemorrhage or infarction and rupture.

Epidemiology: As in many of the parasitic infections of domestic carnivores there is a large reservoir in wild animals from which the intermediate and paratenic hosts are infected. Ranch mink probably acquire infection from their fish diet, and domestic dogs by casual ingestion of infected annelids, frogs or fish.

Treatment: This is rarely called for, although surgery may be attempted in confirmed cases.

Control: Elimination of raw fish from the diet.

Notes: *Dioctophyma* (red scourge) infection in man: this has been mainly recorded in N. America, but other cases have occurred throughout the world. Annelid intermediate hosts in the drinking water are infective and uncooked frogs and fish act as paratenic hosts. The adult worms are found in a thick-walled cyst in the kidney (usually the right) and may cause loin pain and haematuria.

PARASITES OF THE LOCOMOTORY SYSTEM

Trichinella spiralis

See Chapter 5 (Pigs), Parasites of the locomotory system.

Toxoplasma gondii

Predilection site: Muscle, lung, liver, reproductive system, central nervous system

Order: Sporozoasida

Family: Sarcocystiidae

Description: Oocysts in the faeces of cats are unsporulated when passed, spherical and measure 13 × 12 μm (Fig. 6.22). When sporulated, which takes 1–5 days, the oocysts are subspherical and measure 11–14 × 9–11 μm (mean 12.5 × 10 μm), and contain two ellipsoid sporocysts (8.5 × 6 μm), each with four sporozoites, without a Stieda body and with a residuum.

Intermediate hosts: Any mammal, including man, or birds. Note that the final host, the cat, may also be an intermediate host and harbour extra-intestinal stages.

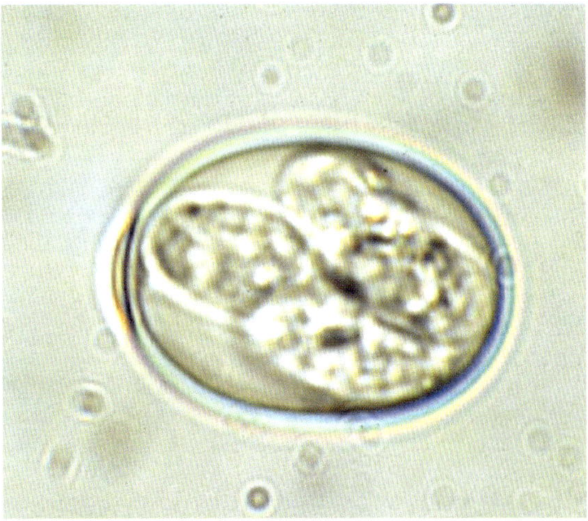

Fig. 6.22 Oocyst of *Toxoplasma gondii.*

Final host: Cat, other felids

Life cycle: The final host is the cat, in which gametogony takes place. Dogs can act as an intermediate host in which the cycle is extra-intestinal and results in the formation of cysts containing thousands of bradyzoites.

Geographical distribution: Worldwide

Pathogenesis: Most *Toxoplasma* infections in animals are light and consequently asymptomatic.

Clinical signs:

- Cats. Despite the fact that cats are frequently infected, clinical disease is rare, although enteritis, enlarged mesenteric lymph nodes, pneumonia, degenerative changes in the central nervous system and encephalitis have been recorded in experimental infections. Congenital transmission, although uncommon, has occurred following activation of bradyzoite cysts during pregnancy.
- Dogs. The onset of illness is marked by fever with lassitude, anorexia and diarrhoea. Pneumonia and neurological manifestations are common. Infection may occur in conjunction with distemper and has also been incriminated in distemper vaccination breakdowns. At necropsy, bradyzoite cysts can be demonstrated in cells in the brain and the respiratory tract; the associated lymph nodes are enlarged.

Diagnosis: Diagnosis is usually based on serological testing by latex agglutination test (LAT) or enzyme-linked immunosorbent assay (ELISA).

Pathology: At necropsy, bradyzoite cysts can be demonstrated in cells in the brain and the respiratory tract; the associated lymph nodes are enlarged.

Epidemiology: Most cats become infected by ingesting *Toxoplasma*-infected animals, usually rodents, whose tissues contain tachyzoites or bradyzoites. Direct transmission of oocysts between cats can also occur. The ingestion of mature bradyzoites is the most important route and results in the shedding of higher numbers of oocysts than when infection is acquired from other stages. Following infection, the cyst wall is digested in the cat's stomach, and in the intestinal epithelium the liberated bradyzoites initiate a cycle of merogonous and gametogonous development culminating in the production of oocysts in 3–10 days. Oocysts are shed for only 1–2 weeks. During this cycle in the intestinal mucosa, the organisms may invade the extra-intestinal organs where the development of tachyzoites and bradyzoites proceeds as in intermediate hosts.

Dogs are infected by the ingestion of undercooked meat containing *Toxoplasma* cysts.

The cat plays a central role in the epidemiology of toxoplasmosis and the disease is virtually absent from areas where cats do not occur. Epidemiological investigations in the USA and elsewhere indicate that 60% of cats are serologically positive to *Toxoplasma* antigen, the majority acquiring infection by predation. As might be expected infections are more prevalent in stray cats. Congenital infection is rare. Following infection, cats shed oocysts for only 1–2 weeks, after which they are resistant to reinfection. However, a proportion remain as carriers, perhaps due to the persistence of some meronts, and reactivation of infection with shedding of oocysts may occur in association with intercurrent disease, during the periparturient period in queens or following corticosteroid therapy. However, the oocysts appear to be very resistant and this compensates for the comparatively short period of oocyst excretion.

Treatment and control: Not indicated

Hepatozoon americanum

Common name: Canine hepatozoonosis

Predilection site: Blood, muscle

Parasite class: Sporozoasida

Family: Hepatozoidae

Description: Gamonts present within neutrophils are ellipsoidal in shape, 8.8×3.9 μm, with a central compact nucleus and enveloped in a thick membrane. The cytoplasm stains pale blue and the nucleus dark reddish with Giemsa stain. Muscle cysts are round to oval, 250–500 μm in diameter with the outer portion made up of concentric layers of fine, pale staining laminar membranes giving the cyst an 'onion skin' structure.

Host: Dog

Life cycle: The life cycle involves two hosts. The tick is a final host in which syngamy occurs, and the dog is an intermediate host in which asexual reproduction occurs. Both larval and nymphal ticks engorge with gamont-infected leucocytes in an infected dog. Following ingestion the gamonts are freed from the leucocytes, associate in pairs in syzygy and transform into male and female gametes leading to the formation of zygotes and oocysts. Each mature oocyst contains numerous sporocysts each containing 10–26 sporozoites. After the tick moults, oocysts are found in the haemocoele and each tick may carry thousands of infective sporozoites. Since the sporozoites remain in the body cavity, the dog is apparently infected by ingesting the tick. Once ingested the sporozoites are released from the oocysts, penetrate the intestinal wall and are transported to target tissues and organs, in the blood and lymph. The parasite infects skeletal and cardiac muscle where it develops between myocytes within host cells of undetermined origin. Mucopolysaccharide layers encyst the infected cells in the muscle where the parasite undergoes merogony. At maturation, the cyst ruptures releasing merozoites into adjacent tissue. Neutrophils and macrophages are recruited to the area and many become infected, leading to pyogranuloma formation with increased vasculation, allowing infected leucocytes containing gamonts to enter the circulation and repeat the asexual reproductive phase at other sites. The cycle is completed when the tick ingests infected blood. The period of development in the dog from infection to the appearance of gamonts is about 32 days.

Geographical distribution: Southeast USA

Pathogenesis: The earliest lesions occur in skeletal muscle with the formation of characteristic 'onion-skin' cysts comprising meronts and mucopolysaccharide lamellar membranes laid down by the host cells. Clinical signs in infected dogs result from the pyogranulomatous inflammatory response that occurs after the encysted mature meront ruptures, releasing merozoites into the surrounding tissue. Some cysts undergo merogony very rapidly while others appear to enter dormancy. Prolonged infection may occur from a single infecting episode perpetuated by repeated merogonic cycles. Infected dogs commonly develop osteoproliferative lesions, most frequently on the diaphysis of long bones. Pain results from both the pyogranulomatous inflammation in skeletal muscle and osteoproliferative lesions. Prolonged infection may persist, perpetuated by prolonged merogony cycles. Muscle atrophy becomes apparent with chronic disease and can result in secondary weakness.

Clinical signs: Dogs infected with *H. americanum* are often presented with fever, generalised pain or hyperaesthesia, muscle atrophy, weakness, depression, reluctance to rise and mucopurulent ocular discharge. Muscle atrophy becomes apparent with chronic disease and can result in secondary weakness. Most dogs maintain a relatively normal appetite, but weight loss is common due to muscle atrophy and chronic cachexia. Mucopurulent ocular discharge is common and is sometimes associated with decreased tear production. Less frequently, clinical signs include polyuria and polydipsia, abnormal lung sounds or cough, pale mucous membranes and lymphadenomegaly.

Diagnosis: Diagnosis based on the identification of gamonts in blood smears is unreliable because of the low numbers present in circulating blood. Blood samples should be examined rapidly using buffy coat smears. Muscle biopsy of the biceps or epaxial muscles is the most consistent method of identification of the characteristic cysts with pyogranuloma formation and the presence of parasites. An ELISA for *H. americanum* has been reported. Infected dogs have a marked neutrophilia, a mild to moderate normocytic, normochromic non-regenerative anaemia and thrombocytosis.

Pathology: On postmortem, chronically infected dogs show cachexia and muscle atrophy, and osteoproliferative lesions may be apparent on bone surfaces. Grossly, pyogranulomas may appear as multiple foci, 1–2 mm in diameter, diffusely scattered predominantly in skeletal and cardiac muscle; they may also be found sporadically in other tissues including adipose tissue, lymph node, intestinal smooth muscle, spleen, skin, kidney, salivary gland, liver, pancreas and lung. Vascular changes in various organs include fibrinoid degeneration of vessel walls, mineralisation and proliferation of vascular intima, and pyogranulomatous vasculitis. Renal lesions are frequently present and include focal pyogranulomatous inflammation with mild glomerulonephritis, lymphoplasmacytic interstitial nephritis, mesangioproliferative glomerulonephritis and occasionally amyloidosis. Amyloid deposits may also be found in spleen, lymph nodes, small intestine and liver. Occasional findings include pulmonary congestion, splenic coagulative necrosis, lymphadenopathy and congestion of the gastric mucosa.

Epidemiology: The main vector of *H. americanum* is the Gulf coast tick, *Amblyomma maculatum*, which is found in southern North America, Central America and the northern parts of South America. Infection is transmitted trans-stadially from nymph to adult stages of the tick vectors. Larval *A. maculatum* can also become infected and transmit *H. americanum* as newly moulted nymphs or adults. Infection appears to be mainly from ingestion of infected ticks. Vertical transmission has been reported.

Treatment: There is no effective treatment capable of eliminating all stages. Clinical remission can be obtained rapidly using a combination of trimethoprim–sulphadiazine (15 mg/kg twice daily), clindamycin (10 mg/kg three times daily) and pyrimethrine (0.25 mg/kg daily) over a period of 14 days. Palliative therapy with non-steroidal anti-inflammatory drugs (NSAIDs) may also be required to reduce fever and pain.

Control: *As for H. canis*

PARASITES OF THE INTEGUMENT

Rhabditis strongyloides

Synonym: *Pelodera strongyloides*

Predilection site: Subcutaneous tissue

Parasite class: Nematoda

Superfamily: Rhabditoidea

Description, gross: Very small worms 1.0–2.8 mm in length with a rhabditiform oesophagus

Description, microscopic: Larvae are approximately 600 μm in length.

Hosts: Dog, cattle, horse

Life cycle: Mainly free living with development through a series of moults at invervals through L_1, L_2, L_3, L_4 to adult.

Geographical distribution: Presumed worldwide

Pathogenesis: Worms invade the hair follicles causing an intense pruritus. Lesions, usually confined to areas of the body in contact with the ground, show hair loss, erythema and pustule formation if infected with bacteria. The intense itching is probably induced by an allergic reaction to the parasite.

Clinical signs: Pruritis, erythema and pustule formation.

Diagnosis: The very small worms, 1.0–2.8 mm in length with a rhabditiform oesophagus, may be recovered from skin scrapings.

Pathology: The worms invade the follicles attracting large numbers of eosinophils. An acute dermatitis develops, commonly with suppurative folliculitis due to secondary bacterial infection.

Epidemiology: These worms are saprophytic, living in warm, moist soil rich in organic matter and significant infections probably require the host's skin to be continually moist and dirty. Cases have been most frequently reported in dogs housed in kennels with damp hay or straw bedding.

Treatment: Treatment is symptomatic.

Control: The condition can be prevented by housing animals on clean, dry bedding.

Dipetalonema reconditum

Predilection site: Subcutaneous tissues, kidney and body cavity

Parasite class: Nematoda

Superfamily: Filarioidea

Description, gross: Male worms measure on average 1.5 cm and females about 2.5 cm.

Description, microscopic: The male spicules are unequal. Microfilariae are 246–292 × 4.7–5.8 μm and have button-hook tails. *D. reconditum* microfilariae are less than 300 μm in length and have a blunt head and a hooked posterior end.

Final hosts: Dogs and various canids

Intermediate hosts: Fleas (*Ctenocephalides canis*, *Ct. felis*, *Pulex irritans*), ticks (*Rhipicephalus sanguineus*), lice (*Heterodoxus spiniger*, *Linognathus setosus*)

Life cycle: Following ingestion of a blood meal the microfilariae develop to the infective stage in about 7–14 days and then migrate to the head. Larvae pass to the host when the intermediate host next feeds. The prepatent period in the dog is 8–10 weeks.

Geographical distribution: Africa, USA, Europe (Italy, UK)

Pathogenesis: The worms are not usually considered pathogenic.

Clinical signs: No associated clinical signs

Diagnosis: *Dipetalonema reconditum* often occurs in the same endemic area as *D. immitis* and the presence of its microfilariae may lead to misdiagnosis on blood examination. The identification of the microfilariae in the blood (samples ideally taken in the early evening) is aided by concentrating the parasites following lysis, filtration and then staining with methylene blue or May–Grunwald Giemsa. Commercial kits are available for this technique. Alternatively one part of blood and nine parts of formalin are centrifuged and the sediment mixed with a blue stain and examined as a microscopic smear. The microfilariae have to be differentiated from those of *D. immitis*, which are more than 300 μm in length and have a tapered head and a straight tail; those of *D. reconditum* are less than 300 μm in length and have a blunt head and a hooked posterior end. More precise differentiation may be achieved by using histochemical stains for acid phosphatase activity. *D. immitis* show distinct red acid-phosphate positive spots at the excretory pore and anus, while *D. reconditum* stains pink overall. Differential diagnosis may be achieved through the application of PCR-based recombinant DNA technology.

Pathology: No associated pathology. The presence of adult worms may occasionally cause subcutaneous abcessation and ulceration.

Epidemiology: Infection is presumably common in areas where the parasite and intermediate hosts co-exist.

Treatment: Drug therapy is not usually indicated.

Control: Preventative measures include control of the intermediate hosts.

Dipetalonema grassi

Synonym: *Acanthocheilonema grassi*

Common name: Subcutaneous filaroidosis

Predilection site: Subcutaneous tissue

Parasite class: Nematoda

Superfamily: Filarioidea

Description, gross: The adult worms are small, the females measuring about 2.5 cm in length.

Description, microscopic: Microfilariae are large, 570 μm in length, with a hook-shaped tail.

Final host: Dog

Intermediate hosts: Ticks and fleas

Life cycle: The life cycle has not been described in detail. Following ingestion of a blood meal, the microfilariae develop to infective larvae in the intermediate host. Larvae pass to the host when the intermediate host next feeds.

Geographical distribution: Southern Europe, Africa

Pathogenesis: *D. grassi* inhabits the thoracic cavity and subcutaneous tissues. It is considered to be of low pathogenicity.

Clinical signs: Infection with this parasite is usually asymptomatic.

Diagnosis: The identification of the microfilariae in the blood (samples ideally taken in the early evening) is aided by concentrating the parasites following lysis, filtration and then staining with methylene blue or May–Grunwald Giemsa. Alternatively, one part of blood and nine parts of formalin are centrifuged and the sediment mixed with a blue stain and examined as a microscopic smear. The microfilariae are large with a hook-shaped tail.

Pathology: No pathology is associated with the infection.

Epidemiology: Infection is presumably common in areas where the parasite and intermediate hosts co-exist.

Treatment and control: Not required

Dipetalonema dracunculoides

Synonym: *Acanthocheilonema dracunculoides*

Predilection site: Peritoneum

Parasite class: Nematoda

Superfamily: Filarioidea

Description, gross: The adult worms are small; male worms are 2.4–3 cm; females are 3.2–6 cm in length.

Description, microscopic: Males have broad, unequal spicules. Microfilariae are not sheathed, 300 µm in length, with a short, blunt tail.

Final host: Dog, hyena

Intermediate hosts: Ticks and fleas

Geographical distribution: Africa (Kenya)

Pathogenesis and clinical signs: Not considered pathogenic

All other details are essentially as for *D. reconditum*.

Dirofilaria repens

Synonym: *Nochtiella repens*

Common name: Cutaneous dirofilariosis

Predilection site: Subcutaneous, intermuscular tissues

Parasite class: Nematoda

Superfamily: Filarioidea

Description, gross: The adults are long slender worms measuring from around 5 cm up to 15 cm in length. Males are 5–7 cm and females 13–17 cm.

Description, microscopic: Microfilariae are 360 × 12 µm.

Final hosts: Dog, cat, fox, bear, occasionally man

Intermediate hosts: Mosquitoes of the genera *Aedes*, *Mansonia*, *Anopheles*, *Culex*

Life cycle: The adults live in subcutaneous nodules and the females release microfilariae, which migrate to the blood and are ingested by female mosquitoes during feeding. Development to L_3 takes place in the mosquito and the final host is infected when the mosquito takes a further blood meal. In the dog the L_3 migrate to the subcutaneous or subserosal tissues and undergo two moults over the next few months. The prepatent period is 27–34 weeks.

Geographical distribution: Mediterranean basin (Italy, Spain, Greece, France, Yugoslavia), Middle East, sub-Saharan Africa, Asia, USA and Canada

Pathogenesis: The adults are found in nodules in subcutaneous and intermuscular tissues and the microfilariae in the blood and lymph. *D. repens* is responsible for cutaneous dirofilariosis, causing mild skin lesions and localised itching. It is of little pathogenic significance in dogs.

In humans, infection is usually asymptomatic. Subcutaneous nodules are found in the breasts, arms, legs, scrotum, eyelid, conjunctivae, penis and testes.

Clinical signs: Itching, mild skin lesions, subcutaneous nodules

Diagnosis: As the microfilariae of *D. repens* and *D. immitis* are morphologically similar, techniques such as isoenzyme characterisation and recombinant DNA application are required to distinguish these species.

Pathology: The presence of the adult parasites causes a local inflammatory reaction with accumulations of eosinophils and mononuclear cells.

Epidemiology: Infection is by biting mosquitoes and transmission is generally confined to warmer months when mosquitoes are active.

Treatment: Treatment is achieved by the surgical removal of the parasites from skin lesions.

Control: Mosquito control is difficult and therefore prophylaxis is based almost entirely on preventative medication with avermectins or milbemycins as used for *D. immitis*.

Cutaneous leishmaniosis

Several species of *Leishmania* are responsible for cutaneous leishmaniosis characterised by a moist ulcerative lesion at the site of insect bites that may become large and granulomatous.

Leishmania infantum

See details and description under Parasites of the liver.

Leishmania tropica

Synonym: *Leishmania tropica* complex

Common name: Cutaneous leishmaniosis, 'dry' oriental sore, Jericho boil

Predilection site: Skin

Parasite class: Zoomastigophorasida

Family: Trypanosomatidae

Description: *Leishmania* amastigotes are small, round or oval bodies, 1.5–3.0 × 2.5–6.5 µm, located within macrophages and possessing a large nucleus and rod-shaped kinetoplast associated with a rudimentary flagellum, which does not extend beyond the cell margin.

Hosts: Man, dog, rock hyrax (*Procavia capensis*)

Life cycle: See *Leishmania infantum*

Geographical distribution: In the dog, *L. tropica* occurs in central and southwest Asia and equatorial and southern Africa, Kenya and Namibia

Pathogenesis: *Leishmania tropica* causes cutaneous leishmaniosis or 'oriental sore', the lesions developing at the site of the insect bite. Gradually the lesion enlarges, remaining red but without heat or pain. Resolution involves immigration of leucocytes, which isolate the infected area leading to necrosis and granuloma formation. Macrophages infected with *Leishmania* organisms are eventually destroyed, and the animal recovers and is immune to reinfection.

Clinical signs: It may take many months or even years for infected dogs to develop clinical signs, so that the disease may only become apparent long after dogs have left endemic areas. Lesions are confined to shallow skin ulcers often on the lip or eyelid, from which recovery is often spontaneous.

Diagnosis: See *Leishmania infantum*

Pathology: The basic lesions are foci of activated proliferating macrophages infected with *Leishmania* organisms. In some cases, these are ultimately surrounded by plasma cells and lymphocytes leading to necrosis and granuloma formation.

Epidemiology: The disease is urban in distribution and dogs are commonly infected. Transmission is by sandflies of the genus *Phlebotomus* (*P. sergenti*, *P. guggisbergi*), particularly in cities and rocky areas in semi-arid areas.

Treatment and control: See *Leishmania infantum*

Other species reported in dogs include:

- *Leishmania aethiopica* found in the Highlands of Ethopia and Kenya
- *Leishmania major* in North Africa, southwest Asia (Algeria to Saudi Arabia) and central Asia (Iran to Uzbekistan), west Africa
- *Leishmania peruviana* found on the mountain slopes of the western Andes in Peru and Bolivia

ECTOPARASITES

LICE

Heavy louse infestation is known as pediculosis. Blood-sucking lice have been implicated in the transmission of disease such as anaplasmosis. However, lice are predominantly of importance because of the direct damage they cause, either by blood-feeding or chewing the skin or hair. Clinical importance is therefore usually a function of their density. Transmission of lice is usually by direct physical contact.

Description: Lice have a segmented body divided into a head, thorax and abdomen. They have three pairs of jointed legs and a pair of short antennae. All lice are dorsoventrally flattened and wingless. The sensory organs are poorly developed; the eyes are vestigial or absent.

Clinical signs: The most notable sign of louse infestation is a scruffy, dry hair or coat. Restlessness, rubbing and damage to the coat suggest that lice are present, and when the hair is parted the parasites will be found.

Diagnosis: The lice and their eggs may be seen within the hair and on the skin when the coat is parted. The lice may be removed and identified under a light microscope.

Pathology: Heavy infestations cause intense pruritus, associated with papulocrustous dermatitis or with patchy alopecia.

Treatment: Lice are killed by most organophosphates (such as chlorpyriphos, malathion or diazinon), amitraz, pyrethroids (for example permethrin) and carbamates (for example carbaryl). Organophosphates and permethrin should not be used in cats; amitraz should be used only with care at half the dose applied to dogs. The more recent products, imidacloprid, fipronil and the macrocyclic lactone, selamectin, may also be particularly effective with high safety margins. However, since the eggs are relatively resistant to most insecticides, repeat treatments 14 days apart may be recommended for some products, to kill newly hatched lice.

Control: Since lice spend their entire life on the host animal, control is readily achieved through the use of topical insecticides on all in-contact animals. Lice can be spread on dirty, shared grooming equipment so appropriate hygiene is essential.

Felicola subrostratus

Synonym: *Felicola subrostrata*

Common name: Cat biting louse

Predilection site: Skin, face, pinnae, back

Parasite class: Insecta

Order: Phthiraptera

Sub-order: Ischnocera

Family: Trichodectidae

Description: This louse is beige or yellow in colour, with transverse brown bands. Adults are an average of 1–1.5 mm in length. The shape of the head is very characteristic, being triangular and pointed anteriorly (Fig. 6.23). Ventrally there is a median longitudinal

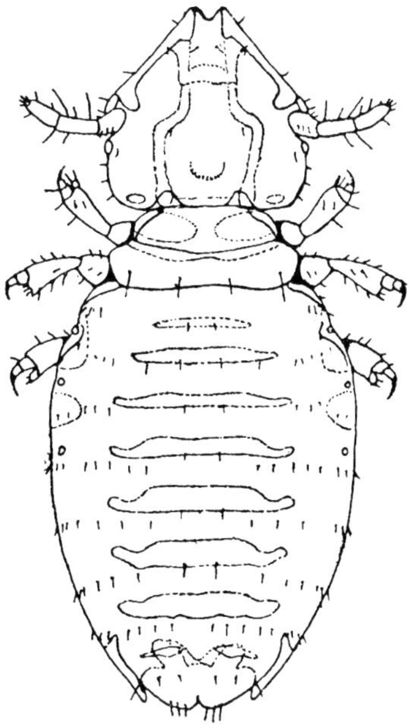

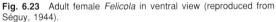

Fig. 6.23 Adult female *Felicola* in ventral view (reproduced from Séguy, 1944).

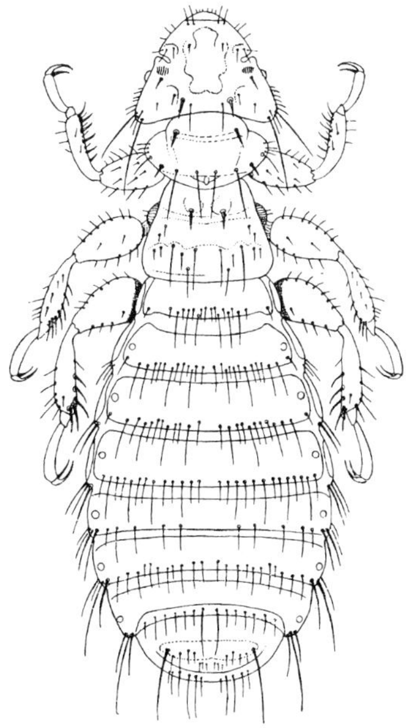

Fig. 6.24 Adult female *Heterodoxus* in ventral view (reproduced from Séguy, 1944).

groove on the head, which fits around the individual hairs of the host. The antennae have three segments, are fully exposed and are similar in both sexes. The legs are small, slender and end in single claws. The abdomen has only three pairs of spiracles and is smooth with few setae.

Hosts: Cat

Life cycle: Eggs are laid on the cat fur and hatch in 10–20 days. The adult stage is reached within 2–3 weeks and the egg-to-adult life cycle requires about 30–40 days.

Geographical distribution: Worldwide

Pathogenesis: This is a chewing louse and is the only species of louse that commonly occurs on cats. Pediculosis is now rare and generally is seen only in elderly or chronically ill animals. It is more problematic in longhaired breeds and pathogenic populations may develop under thickly matted or neglected fur. Infestations most commonly occur on the face, back and pinnae, causing a dull, ruffled coat, scaling, crusts and alopecia.

Epidemiology: Generally, infestation occurs via close bodily contact. This species of louse is highly host specific. Infestations may be common in catteries, where asymptomatic carriers may act as reservoirs. Kittens may be particularly susceptible to infestation.

Heterodoxus spiniger

Predilection site: Skin

Parasite class: Insecta

Order: Phthiraptera

Sub-order: Amblycera

Family: Boopidae

Description: *Heterodoxus spiniger* is a large, slender, yellowish coloured louse. Adults are about 5 mm in length, with a dense covering of thick, medium and long setae (Fig. 6.24). It can easily be distinguished from other lice infesting domestic mammals since the tarsi end in two claws, as opposed to one in the Anoplura and Trichodectidae. It is thought that *H. spiniger* evolved in Australasia as a louse of marsupials that subsequently switched to dingo hosts. It now parasitises a number of canids and other carnivores. *H. spiniger* can be found anywhere on the body of the host.

Hosts: Dog and other carnivores

Life cycle: The life cycle is typical, with eggs giving rise to three nymphal stages followed by the reproductive adult. However, little detail is known.

Geographical distribution: Confined to tropical and subtropical regions between latitudes 40°N and 40°S

Pathogenesis: Lice infestations often accompany manifestations of poor health such as internal parasitism, infectious disease, malnutrition and poor sanitation.

Epidemiology: Infection occurs after direct contact with an infested host animal. Cross-contamination between different host species is possible if the animals have physical contact.

Linognathus setosus

Common name: Dog sucking louse

Predilection site: Skin of head and neck areas

Parasite class: Insecta

Order: Phthiraptera

Sub-order: Anoplura

Family: Linognathidae

Description: This species of louse is up to 2 mm long when fully fed, with a long pointed head. It does not have eyes or ocular points. The second and third pairs of legs are larger than the first pair and end in stout claws. The thoracic sternal plate is absent or if present is weakly developed. Paratergal plates are absent from the abdomen.

Hosts: Dogs and other canids

Life cycle: Adult females lay a single egg per day. Eggs hatch in 10–15 days, giving rise to nymphs that require about 2 weeks to pass through three nymphal stages. The egg-to-adult life cycle requires about 20–40 days.

Geographical distribution: Worldwide

Pathogenesis: *Linognathus setosus* is a common and widespread parasite of dogs, particularly the long ears of breeds such as the spaniel, basset and Afghan hounds. It may cause anaemia and is usually of greater pathogenic significance in younger animals. *Linognathus setosus* is primarily found in the head and neck areas and is especially common under the collar.

Linognathus setosus has been shown to harbour immature stages of the filarial nematode *Dipetalonema reconditum*, which parasitises dogs. However, it is unknown whether the lice act as efficient vectors of these parasites.

Epidemiology: Generally, for the transfer of louse infestation, close bodily contact is necessary. Lice dropped or pulled from the host die in a few days, but eggs that have fallen from the host may continue to hatch over 2–3 weeks in warm weather. Therefore, bedding used by infested hosts should be disinfected.

Trichodectes canis

Common name: Dog biting louse

Predilection site: Skin, head, neck and tail regions

Parasite class: Insecta

Order: Phthiraptera

Sub-order: Ischnocera

Family: Trichodectidae

Description: *Trichodectes canis* is a small, broad, yellowish coloured louse. It is 1–2 mm in length, with dark markings. The head is broader than long and the antennae are three-segmented, short and exposed (Fig. 6.25). The legs are stout and their tarsi bear single claws, with which they tightly grasp the hair of their host. The abdomen has six pairs of spiracles on segments 2–6 and many rows of large, thick setae.

Hosts: Dog, wild canids

Life cycle: *Trichodectes canis* commonly infests the head, neck and tail regions, where it attaches to the base of a hair using its claws or mandibles. The female lays several eggs per day for approximately 30 days. Eggs hatch in 1–2 weeks and give rise to three nymphal stages. The nymphs mature into reproductive adults within about 2 weeks. The egg-to-adult life cycle requires about 30–40 days.

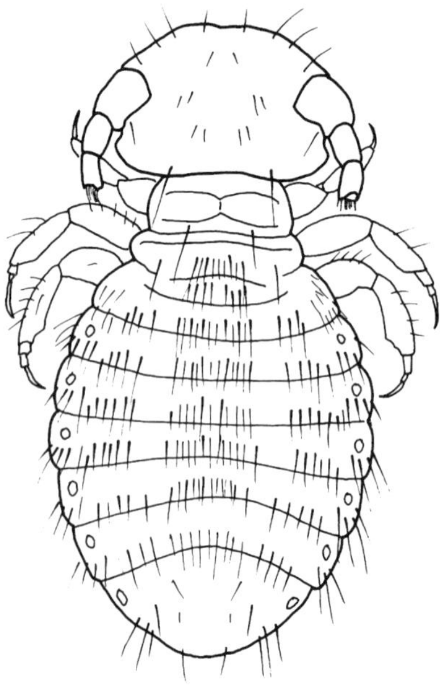

Fig. 6.25 Adult female *Trichodectes* in ventral view (from Séguy, 1944).

Geographical distribution: Worldwide

Pathogenesis: *Trichodectes canis* can be a harmful ectoparasite of dogs, particularly in puppies and old or debilitated dogs. It is most commonly found on the head, neck and tail attached to the base of hairs. It feeds on tissue debris. It is a highly active species and infestation produces intense irritation around predilection sites. Lice often congregate around body orifices or wounds seeking moisture. Intense pruritus, scratching, biting, sleeplessness, nervousness and a matted coat are all typical of *T. canis* infestation. Damage to the skin from scratching results in inflammation, excoriation, alopecia and secondary bacterial involvement.

Trichodectes canis is important as a vector of the tapeworm *Dipylidium caninum*. Lice become infected when they ingest *D. caninum* eggs from dried host faeces. The tapeworm develops into a cysticercoid stage within the louse, where it remains quiescent until the louse is ingested by a dog, during grooming. In the gut of the dog the cystercoid is liberated and develops into an adult tapeworm.

MITES

Infestation by mites is called acariasis and can result in severe dermatitis, known as mange, which may cause significant welfare problems and economic losses.

All mites are small, usually less than 1 mm in length. The body shows no segmentation, although it can have various sutures and grooves. Adult and nymphal mites have four pairs of legs; larvae have only three pairs. The body is usually soft but may carry a number of hardened plates. Eyes are usually absent and, hence, most mites are blind. Hairs, or setae, many of which are sensory in function, cover the body of many species of mite. The mouthparts are highly specialised, consisting of a pair of chelicerae, which may be used for tearing, grasping or piercing.

Cheyletiella blakei

Predilection site: Face, but may occur all over the body

Parasite class: Arachnida

Sub-class: Acari

Order: Acariformes

Sub-order: Trombidiformes (Prostigmata)

Family: Cheyletidae

Description: Adults are about 400 µm in length and ovoid (see Fig. 9.14). They have blade-like chelicerae that are used for piercing their host, and short, strong, opposable palps with curved palpal claws. The palpal femur possesses a long, serrated dorsal seta. The body tends to be slightly elongated with a 'waist'. The legs are short; tarsal claws are lacking and the empodium is a narrow pad with comb-like pulvilli at the ends of the legs. Adults are highly mobile and are able to move about rapidly. The solenidion, on the genu of the first pair of legs, is conical in *C. blakei*. However, this feature can vary in individuals and between life-cycle stages, making identification difficult.

Hosts: Cat

Life cycle: All developmental stages occur on the host animal. Eggs are glued to hairs 2–3 mm above the skin. A prelarva and then a larva develop within the egg, with fully developed octopod nymphs eventually emerging from the egg. The mites then moult through two nymphal stages before the adult stage is reached. The life cycle is completed in approximately 2 weeks. The mites live in the hair and fur, only visiting the skin to feed on lymph and other tissue fluids. They feed on these fluids by piercing the epidermis with their stylet-like chelicerae. Adults can survive for at least 10 days off the host without feeding, or longer in cool environments.

Geographical distribution: Worldwide

Pathogenesis: The mite is not usually highly pathogenic and is more often found in young animals in good physical condition. Long-haired cats tend to be more commonly infested than short-haired cats. This parasite is readily transferred to humans even on short contact, where it causes severe irritation and intense pruritus. A positive diagnosis on a pet may be associated with a history of persistent skin rash in the owner's family. Human cases will resolve spontaneously when the animal source has been treated.

Clinical signs: *Cheyletiella blakei* most commonly infests the facial area of cats, causing mild eczema-like skin conditions and associated pruritus. It is a characteristic of the dermatitis caused by *Cheyletiella* that many skin scales are shed into the fur, giving it a powdery or mealy appearance, and the presence of moving mites among this debris has given it the common name of 'walking dandruff'.

Diagnosis: In any case of excessive scurf or dandruff in the cat *Cheyletiella* should be considered in the differential diagnosis. On parting the coat along the back, and especially over the sacrum, scurf will be seen, and if this is combed out on to dark paper the movement of mites will be detected among the debris. Scraping is not necessary as the mites are always on the skin surface or in the coat.

Pathology: The pathology of *Cheyletiella* infestation is poorly understood. In many cases there is very little skin reaction or pruritus. In the rare severe case, heavy infestations can result in the formation of small, crusty, erythematous papules involving much of the body surface; crusts are formed, but often there is only slight hair loss.

Epidemiology: This highly contagious, although mild, mange can spread rapidly through catteries and kennels. Transmission is usually by direct contact with infested animals, but the adult parasite can survive for over 10 days off the host and therefore bedding and furniture can act as a source of infestation. *Cheyletiella* mites may be phoretic on cat and dog fleas (*Ctenocephalides* spp) and may be transmitted by these ectoparasites.

Treatment: Cats can be treated with a number of topical acaricidal shampoos, such as carbamates (e.g. carbaryl) and fipronil. Selenium sulphide shampoos have also been recommended for cats. With some products, with low residual activity, three successive weekly treatments may be needed.

Control: The cats, all in-contact animals and their surroundings should be treated to control infestation rates. This is particularly important in catteries, which often serve as a source of mite infestation.

Cheyletiella yasguri

Predilection site: Back and head, but may be found all over the body

Parasite class: Arachnida

Sub-class: Acari

Order: Acariformes

Sub-order: Trombidiformes (Prostigmata)

Family: Cheyletidae

Description: Similar in appearance to *C. blakei*, however the solenidion, on the genu of the first pair of legs, is heart-shaped in *C. yasguri* (see Fig. 9.14). Nevertheless, this feature can vary in individuals and between life cycle stages, making identification difficult.

Hosts: Dog

Pathogenesis: The mite is not highly pathogenic and is often found in young animals in good physical condition. *Cheyletiella* may be more common on short-haired breeds of dog and many individuals act as asymptomatic carriers. It is a characteristic of the dermatitis caused by *Cheyletiella* that many skin scales are shed into the hair or fur, giving it a powdery or mealy appearance (Fig. 6.26). There is very little skin reaction or pruritus. In the rare severe case, involving much of the body surface, crusts are formed, but there is only slight hair loss. This parasite is readily transferred to humans even on short contact, where it causes severe irritation and intense pruritus. A positive diagnosis on a pet may be associated with a history of persistent skin rash in the owner's family. Cases will resolve spontaneously when the animal source has been treated.

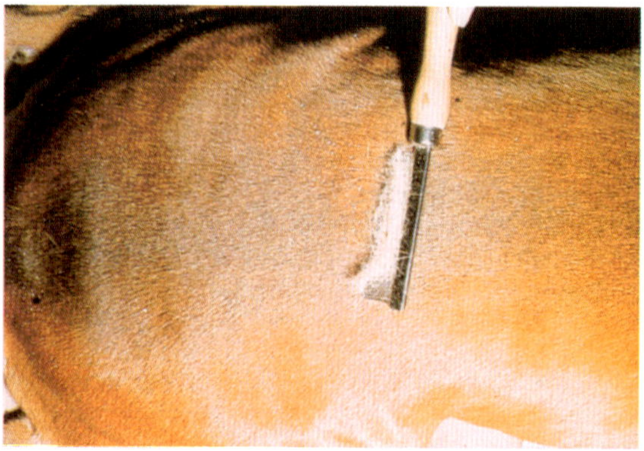

Fig. 6.26 Marked 'dandruff' associated with *Cheyletiella* infection.

Treatment: Dogs can be treated with a number of topical acaricidal shampoos, such as carbamates (e.g. carbaryl), organophosphates (e.g. phosmet, chlorpyriphos, malathion or diazinon), permethrin, amitraz and fipronil. Oral milbemycin may be effective. With some of the older products, with low residual activity, three successive weekly treatments may be needed.

All other details are as for *C. blakei*.

Otodectes cynotis

Common name: Ear mite

Predilection site: External ear canal. May secondarily infest other parts of the body including the head, back, tip of tail and feet.

Parasite class: Arachnida

Sub-class: Acari

Order: Acariformes

Sub-order: Sarcoptiformes (Astigmata)

Family: Psoroptidae

Description: *Otodectes* resembles *Psoroptes* and *Chorioptes* in general conformation, having an ovoid body and projecting legs (Fig. 6.27). Like *Chorioptes* however, it is smaller than *Psoroptes* and does not have jointed pretarsi. The sucker-like pulvillus is cup-shaped, as opposed to trumpet-shaped in *Psoroptes*. In the adult female, the first two pairs of legs carry short, stalked pretarsi, while the third and fourth pairs of legs have a pair of terminal whip-like setae.

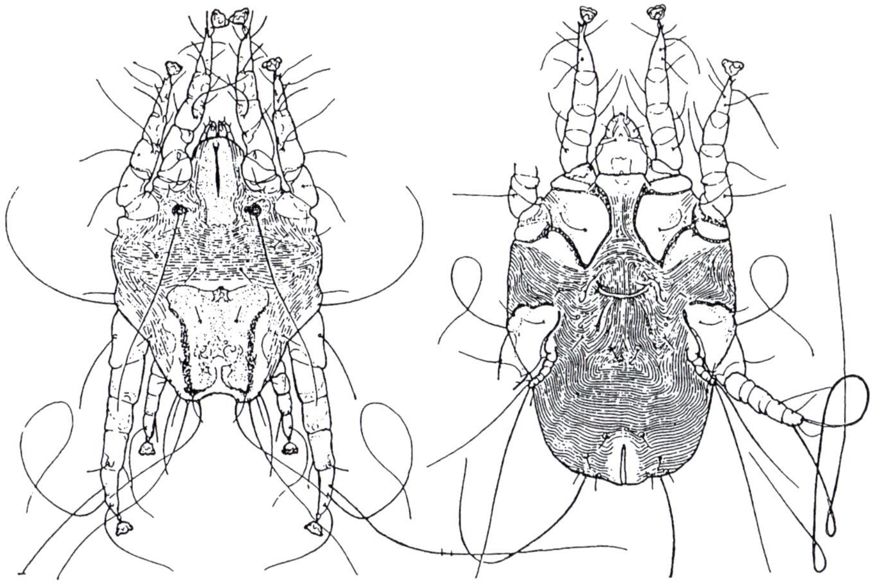

Fig. 6.27 Adult *Otodectes cynotis*. (a) Male, dorsal view. (b) Female ventral view (reproduced from Baker *et al.*, 1956).

The fourth pair is much reduced. The genital opening is transverse. In males all four pairs of legs carry short, stalked pretarsi and pulvilli, but the posterior processes are small.

Hosts: Cat, dog and a number of other small mammals including the ferret and red fox

Life cycle: The life cycle is typical: egg, hexapod larva, followed by octopod protonymph, tritonymph and adult. All developmental stages occur on the host. The complete egg to adult life cycle takes about 3 weeks. Eggs are deposited at a rate of one per day and are attached to the host skin. Adult females produce 15–20 eggs and live for 2–3 weeks. Like *Chorioptes*, this mite feeds superficially on skin debris.

Geographical distribution: Worldwide

Pathogenesis: Most animals harbour this mite, and in adult animals it has almost a commensal association with the host, signs of irritation appearing only sporadically with the transient activity of the mites. The development of clinical signs reflects the development of allergic hypersensitivity by the host to antigenic substances produced by the mites while they are feeding. This can result in responses ranging from asymptomatic to severe otitis and convulsive seizures in different individual hosts. Young animals probably acquire the mites from their mothers during suckling.

Early in infections, there is a brownish waxy exudate in the ear canal, which becomes crusty (Fig. 6.28). The mites live deep in the crust, next to the skin. Secondary bacterial infection may result. Scratching may cause excoriation of the posterior surface of the ear pinna. The resultant violent head shaking and ear scratching are a common cause of aural haematomata. In long-standing cases a severe purulent otitis may result.

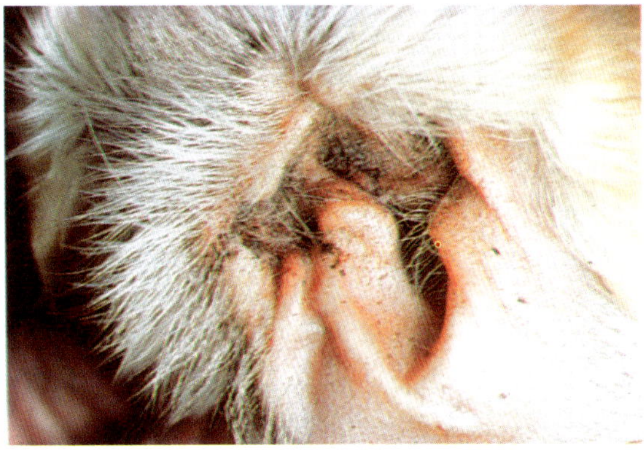

Fig. 6.28 Dark waxy exudate caused by *Otodectes* infection in the dog.

Clinical signs: In general, the ear canals become inflamed and excessively moistened with accumulations of brown–black exudates in cats and grey deposits. This is accompanied by pruritus, intense itching which causes the host to scratch their ears, shake their head or hold it to one side and turn in circles. Signs of severe, untreated cases include emaciation, spasms, self-induced trauma and convulsions, including epileptiform fits. Perforation of the tympanic membrane can result. The clinical signs may be seen in dogs at an earlier stage than in cats and foxes, which do not appear to be affected until the infestation has reached high numbers and the disease is advanced.

Diagnosis: Tentative diagnosis is based on the behaviour of the animal and the presence of dark, waxy deposits and exudate in the ear canal. Confirmation depends on observing the mites either within the ear or by removing some of the deposit and exudate and placing it on a dark surface where the mites will be seen by a hand lens as whitish moving specks.

Pathology: The canal becomes full of cerumen, blood and mite faeces, giving rise to a characteristic otitis externa. Mechanical irritation may account for some of the pruritus, but, in addition, the presence of IgE-like antibodies suggests that hypersensitivity also contributes to the pruritus.

Epidemiology: Transfer may occur through direct contact or from infested female hosts to their pups or kittens.

Treatment: Topical application of systemic selamectin and imidocloprid has been found to give good control in both dogs and cats. There are also many effective preparations available commercially as eardrops, including, in dogs, permethrin, thiabendazole and monosulphiram. With these preparations treatment should be repeated to kill any newly hatched mites. In cats, treatments with milbemycin and ivermectin may be used, and in both cats and dogs fipronil eardrops may be effective. When eardrops are used the ear canal should first be thoroughly cleaned, and after the eardrops have been instilled, the base of the ear massaged to disperse the oily preparation.

Control: Any bedding should be replaced or thoroughly disinfected. In view of the ubiquity and high infectivity of the mite, all dogs or cats in the same household, or those in close contact in kennels and catteries, should be treated at the same time as clinically affected animals. In heavy infestations concurrent whole-body treatment may also be required, to kill any mites that have moved out of the ear canal.

Sarcoptes scabiei

Common name: Scabies

Predilection site: Skin

Parasite class: Arachnida

Sub-class: Acari

Order: Acariformes

Sub-order: Sarcoptiformes (Astigmata)

Family: Sarcoptidae

Description, adults: The adult of this species has a round, ventrally flattened, dorsally convex body (see Fig. 5.12). Adult females are 0.3–0.6 mm long and 0.25–0.4 mm wide, while males are smaller, typically up to 0.3 mm long and 0.1–0.2 mm wide. The posterior two pairs of limbs do not extend beyond the body margin. In both sexes, the pretarsi of the first two pairs of legs bear empodial claws and a sucker-like pulvillus, borne on a long, stalk-like pretarsus. The sucker-like pulvilli help the mite grip the substrate as it moves. The third and fourth pairs of legs in the female and the third pair of legs in the male end in long setae and lack stalked pulvilli. The mouthparts have a rounded appearance. These mites have no eyes or stigmata. The dorsal surface of the body of *S. scabiei* is covered with transverse ridges, but also bears a central patch of triangular scales. The dorsal setae are strong and spine-like. The anus is terminal and only slightly dorsal.

Hosts: All domestic mammals and humans

Geographical distribution: Worldwide

Pathogenesis:

- Dogs. The predilection sites for the mites are thinly haired areas such as the ears (Fig. 6.29), muzzle, face, and elbows but, as in other manges, severe infestations may extend over the whole body. Visually, the condition begins as erythema, with papule formation, and this is followed by scale and crust formation and alopecia (Fig. 6.30). It is a characteristic of this form of mange that there is intense pruritus, which often leads to self-inflicted trauma. After a primary infection dogs begin to

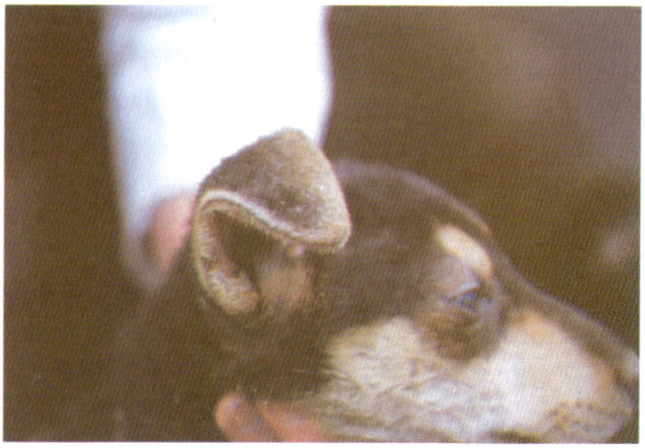

Fig. 6.29 Thickened ear edge characteristic of sarcoptic mange.

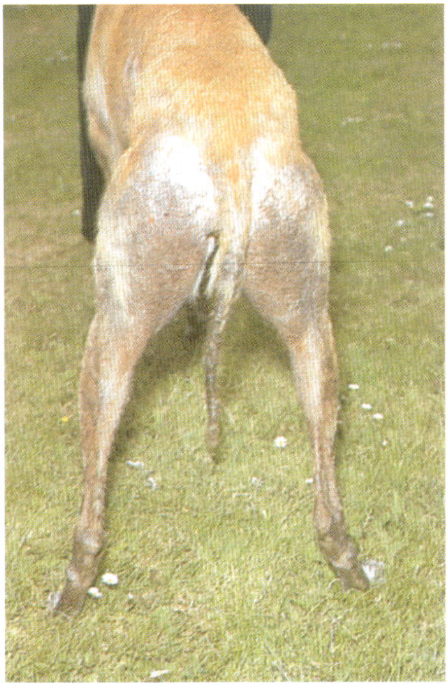

Fig. 6.30 Severe sarcoptic mange in a dog.

scratch within a week, often before lesions are visible. In cases that are neglected for a number of months the whole skin surface may be involved, dogs becoming progressively weak and emaciated. A strong sour odour is a notable feature of this form of mange.

- Cats. Sarcoptic mange is rare in cats. In the few recorded cases, the changes have been similar to those in *Notoedres* infection, with progressive hair loss from the ears, face and neck, extending to the abdomen.

Pathology: Dogs with chronic, generalised disease develop seborrhoea, severe thickening of the skin, crust build-up, peripheral lymphadenopathy and emaciation. However, the lesions associated with canine sarcoptic mange are very non-specific. Usually there is dramatic epidermal hyperplasia and a subtle, diffuse and uniform eosinophilic perivascular dermatitis. However, cases may present with no eosinophilic infiltrate and sacrcoptic mange should be a differential diagnosis for any hyperplastic pruritic dermatitis.

Treatment: Treatment can be either topical or systemic. For topical treatment in dogs effective acaricides include the organochlorines, gamma HCH and bromocyclen, and the organophosphates such as phosmet and amitraz, but the availabilities of some of these compounds is limited or non-existent in some countries. Lime–sulphur is highly effective and safe for use in young animals; several dips 5 days apart are recommended. Many preparations are combined with a surfactant, which aids contact with the mites by removing skin scales and softening crusts and other debris. Selamectin spot-on is effective. Other macrocyclic lactones, such as moxidectin and ivermectin, are not registered for the treatment of sarcoptic mange in dogs, but have been reported to be effective depending on the dosage and route of administration. Hair can be clipped, the crusts and dirt removed by soaking with a good anti-seborrhoeic shampoo, and an acaricidal dip applied.

In cats lime–sulphur dips at 10–day intervals may be used. Selamectin spot-on may give good contol, although this is not an approved application.

Control: Based on the protected location of the parasites, the duration of the life cycle and the necessity of killing all mites, dogs should be bathed weekly with an acaricidal preparation for 4 weeks, or longer if necessary, until lesions have disappeared. Because this is a highly contagious mange, affected dogs should be isolated and it should be explained to owners that rapid cure cannot be expected. To ensure that an outbreak is contained, all dogs on the premises should be treated if possible. In severely distressed dogs, oral or parenteral corticosteroids are valuable in reducing the pruritus and so preventing further excoriation.

For more detailed descriptions see Chapter 5 (Pigs), Parasites of the integument.

Notoedres cati

Common name: Noteodric cat mite

Predilection site: Ears

Parasite class: Arachnida

Sub-class: Acari

Order: Acariformes

Sub-order: Sarcoptiformes (Astigmata)

Family: Sarcoptidae

Description: *Notoedres* closely resembles *Sarcoptes* with a circular outline and short legs with long unjointed pedicels, but it is distinguished by its concentric 'thumb print' striations and absence of spines (Fig. 6.31). The dorsal scales are rounded and arranged transversely. This species is also smaller than *S. scabiei*; females are about 225 μm in length and males about 150 μm, with a short, square rostrum. The anal opening is distinctly dorsal and not posterior. Females have suckers on legs 1 and 2.

Hosts: Largely cat, but may occasionally infest dogs or rabbits, also wild cats, foxes, canids and civets.

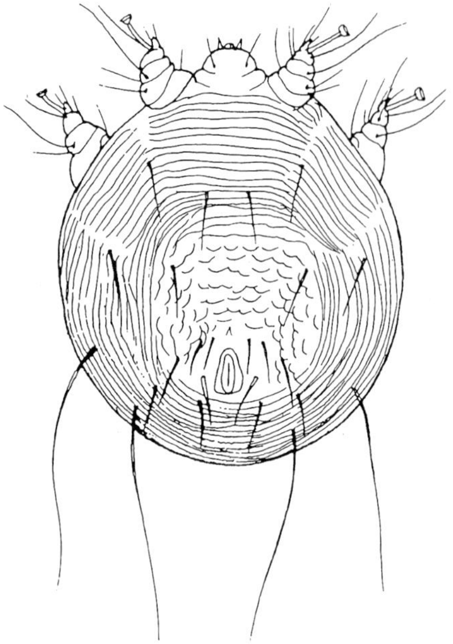

Fig. 6.31 Adult female *Notoedres cati* in dorsal view.

Life cycle: Similar to that of *Sarcoptes*, except that the females in the dermis are usually found in aggregations. The fertilised female creates a winding burrow or tunnel in the upper layers of the epidermis, feeding on liquid oozing from the damaged tissues. The eggs are laid in these tunnels, hatch in 3–5 days, and the six-legged larvae crawl on to the skin surface. These larvae, in turn, burrow into the superficial layers of the skin to create small 'moulting pockets', in which the moults to nymph and adult are completed. Development from egg to adult takes 6–10 days. The adult male then emerges and seeks a female either on the skin surface or in a moulting pocket. After fertilisation the females either produce new tunnels or extend the moulting pocket. New hosts are infected by contact, presumably from transferral of larvae, which are present more superficially than the other stages.

Geographical distribution: Worldwide

Pathogenesis: *Notoedres cati* typically burrows in the stratum corneum and the stratum germinativum, occasionally invading hair follicles and sebaceous glands, causing hyperkeratosis and thickening of the epidermis. The infection appears as dry, encrusted, scaly lesions on the edges of the ears and on the face, the skin thickened and somewhat leathery. Advanced lesions can give cats a wrinkled, thickened skin with hyperkeratinisation and hyperpigmentation casuing an 'old age' appearance. The associated pruritus is often intense, and there may be severe excoriation of the head and neck from scratching. In typical cases the lesions appear first on the medial edge of the ear pinna, and then spread rapidly over the ears, face, eyelids and neck. It may be spread to the feet and tail by contact when the cat grooms and sleeps.

Clinical signs: Intense pruritus, erythema, skin scaling, greyish yellow crusts and loss of hair. Scratching to alleviate itching leads to excoriation of the skin, inflammation and secondary bacterial infections. If untreated, the affected animal can become severely debilitated and notoedric mange may be fatal in 4–6 months.

Diagnosis: *Notoedres cati* occur in clumps in the skin, and are usually initially found around the head and ears causing an ear canker. Transient dermatitis can occur in humans. Diagnosis may initially be based on the intense pruritus, the location of lesions and the rapid spread to involve all kittens in a litter. Confirmation is achieved by finding the mites in skin scrapings.

Pathology: Infestation is associated with erythematous dermatosis, marked epidermal hyperplasia, dermal inflammation consisting principally of mononuclear cells and regional lymphadenopathy.

Epidemiology: Notoedric mange is highly contagious and transmission from host to host is by the spread of larvae or nymphs, but although it occurs in local, limited outbreaks, it is not a frequent cause of skin disease in cats. In Britain, for example, the disease is now rarely encountered.

Treatment: Skin crusts should first be softened with liquid paraffin or soap solution before applying an acaricide. Lime–sulphur dips at 10-day intervals may be used. A 1% solution of selenium sulphide is also recommended for use in cats; treatment should be given at weekly intervals for 4–6 weeks, the prognosis being good. Although not licensed for the treatment of cats, selemectin and ivermectin may prove effective against *Notoedres*, although sudden death in kittens has been reported with the use of ivermectin.

Control: All in-contact animals should be treated and bedding replaced.

Notes: This genus has somewhat similar behaviour and pathogenesis to *Sarcoptes*, but has a more restricted host range.

Demodex canis

Predilection site: Hair follicles and sebaceous glands

Parasite class: Arachnida

Sub-class: Acari

Order: Acariformes

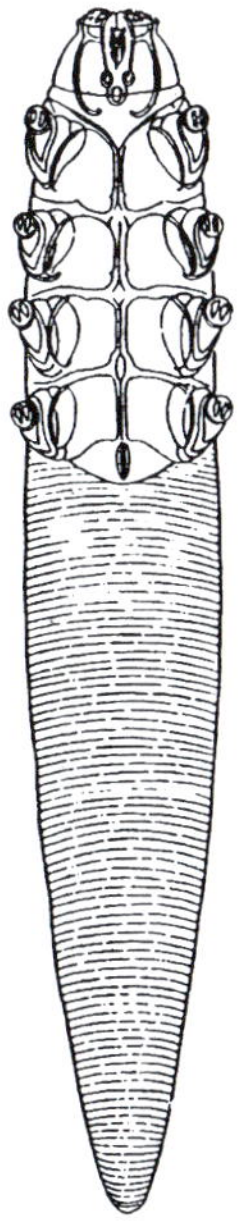

Fig. 6.32 Adult *Demodex* spp ventral view (reproduced from Baker *et al.*, 1956).

Sub-order: Trombidiformes (Prostigmata)

Family: Demodicidae

Description: Species of *Demodex* have an elongate tapering body, up to 0.1–0.4 mm in length, with four pairs of stumpy legs ending in small blunt claws in the adult (Fig. 6.32). Setae are absent from the legs and body. The legs are located at the front of the body, and as such the striated opisthosoma forms at least half the body length.

Hosts: Dog

Life cycle: *Demodex* spp usually live as commensals in the skin, and are highly site-specific, occupying the hair follicles and sebaceous glands. Females lay 20–24 spindle-shaped eggs in the hair follicle that give rise to hexapod larvae, in which each short leg ends in a single, three-pronged claw. Unusually, a second hexapod larval stage follows, in which each leg ends in a pair of three-pronged claws. Octopod protonymph, tritonymph and adult stages then follow. Immature stages and these migrate more deeply into the dermis. One follicle may harbour all life cycle stages concurrently. The life cycle is completed in 18–24 days. In each follicle or gland the mites may occur in large numbers in a characteristic head-downward posture. In the newborn and very young these sites are simple in structure, but later they become compounded by outgrowths. The presence of *Demodex* mites much deeper in the dermis than sarcoptids means that they are much less accessible to surface-acting acaricides. Species of *Demodex* are unable to survive off their host.

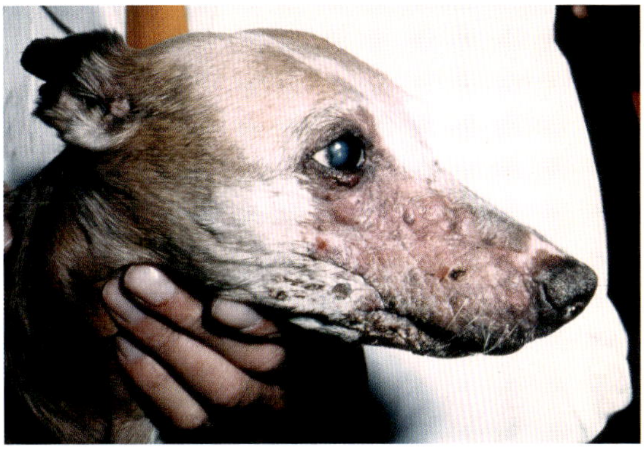

Fig. 6.33 Demodectic mange on the muzzle of a dog.

Geographical distribution: Worldwide

Pathogenesis: For the most part, *Demodex* mites are non-pathogenic and form a normal part of the skin fauna. Occasionally they can cause significant clinical disease, particularly in dogs, where they cause demodectic mange or demodicosis.

Early in infection there is a slight loss of hair on the face and forelimbs, followed by thickening of the skin (Fig. 6.33). The mange may progress no further than the in-contact areas; many of these localised mild infections resolve spontaneously without treatment. On the other hand, lesions may spread over the entire body, and this generalised demodicosis may take one of two forms:

- Squamous demodicosis is the less serious. It is a dry reaction, with little erythema, but widespread alopecia, desquamation and thickening of the skin. In some cases of this type only the face and paws are involved.
- Pustular or follicular demodicosis is the severe form, and follows bacterial invasion of the lesions, often by staphylococci. The skin becomes wrinkled and thickened, with many small pustules from which serum, pus and blood ooze, giving this form its common name of 'red mange' (Fig. 6.34). Affected dogs have an offensive odour. Prolonged treatment is necessary, and survivors may be severely disfigured, so early euthanasia is sometimes requested by owners, and by pedigree breeders.

The pathogenesis of *Demodex* is more complex than that of other mange mites because immune factors appear to play a large part in its occurrence and severity. It is thought that certain bitches carry a genetically controlled factor, which results in immunodeficiency

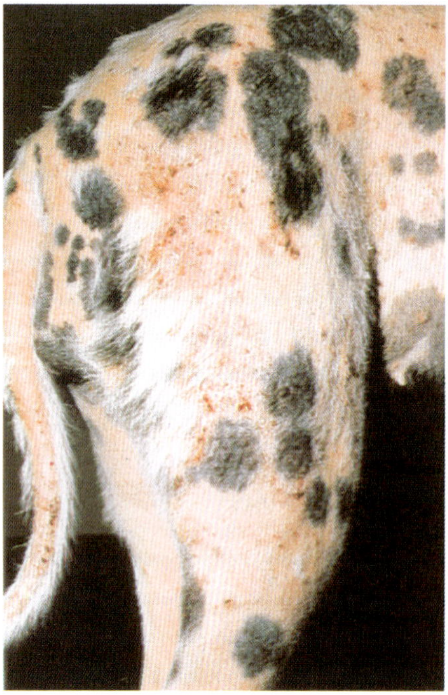

Fig. 6.34 Pustular demodectic mange.

in their offspring, making them more susceptible to mite invasion. It has been observed that litter mates from such a bitch often develop the generalised form of demodectic mange simultaneously, even though they have been reared separately. In addition, *Demodex* itself is thought to cause a cell-mediated immunodeficiency, which suppresses the normal T-lymphocyte response. This defect disappears when the mites have been eradicated from the animal. Demodectic mange may erupt when dogs are given immunosuppressants for other conditions.

Clinical signs: In early infection there is a slight loss of hair on the face and forelimbs, followed by thickening of the skin. Infection may resolve spontaneously or spread over the entire body. A common notable feature of all types of demodectic mange is the absence of pruritus, but this is not universal.

Diagnosis: For confirmatory diagnosis, deep scrapings are necessary to reach the mites deep in the follicles and glands. This is best achieved by taking a fold of skin, applying a drop of liquid paraffin, and scraping until capillary blood appears. Even in normal dogs a few commensal mites may be found in the material, but the presence of a high proportion of larvae and nymphs will indicate a rapidly increasing population, and hence an active infection. Skin biopsy, to detect mites in the follicles, has been used in severely affected dogs, but is rarely necessary.

Pathology: In squamous demodicosis there is little erythema, but widespread alopecia, desquamation and thickening of the skin. In severe pustular or follicular demodicosis the lesions observed are variable and may include comedones, follicular papules and casts. More severely affected patients have deep folliculitis and furunculosis with severe haemorrhagic exudation and thick crusting. Demarcation between affected areas and normal skin is abrupt. Lymphadenopathy is common. There is bacterial invasion of the lesions, often by staphylococci. Dogs with chronic generalised demodicosis have depressed cell-mediated immune responsiveness, associated with the secondary bacterial infections. In some dogs only pododemodicosis is present. Pain and pedal oedema is especially prominent in large dogs.

Epidemiology: Probably because of its location deep in the dermis, it is very difficult to transmit *Demodex* between animals unless there is prolonged contact. It is thought that most infections are acquired in the early weeks of life during suckling. This view is supported by the fact that lesions first appear on the muzzle, face, periorbital region and forelimbs.

Treatment: Of the available acaricides, the most widely used is amitraz although the organophosphate, cythioate, may also be applied. With their deep location in the dermis the mites are not readily accessible to most topically applied acaricides, so repeated treatment is necessary and rapid results should not be expected. In localised squamous mange recovery may be expected in 1–2 months, but in the generalised pustular form the prognosis should indicate that recovery will take at least 3 months, and should, even so, be guarded.

Treatment with oral or injectable ivermectin at 250–300 μg/kg, milbemycin at 2 mg/kg and moxidectin at 400 μg/kg, have all been used successfully for the treatment of generalised canine demodicosis. Ivermectin and moxidectin should be initiated at lower doses and patients monitored for possible adverse effects during therapy. Where pyoderma is severe, antibiotic therapy may be necessary.

Control: In controlling the endemicity of demodicosis, it should be noted that since certain bitches are more prone than others to have susceptible offspring, it may be advisable to discard these from breeding establishments.

Notes: Species of the genus *Demodex* are believed to form a group of closely related sibling species, which are highly specific to particular hosts: *Demodex phylloides* (pig), *Demodex canis* (dog), *Demodex bovis* (cattle), *Demodex equi* (horse), *Demodex musculi* (mouse), *Demodex ratti* (rat), *Demodex caviae* (guinea-pig), *Demodex cati* (cat) and *Demodex folliculorum* and *Demodex brevis* on humans. Various morphological variations may be seen on a host, these are sometimes, probably incorrectly, ascribed separate species status.

Demodex cati

Predilection site: Hair follicles and sebaceous glands

Parasite class: Arachnida

Sub-class: Acari

Order: Acariformes

Sub-order: Trombidiformes (Prostigmata)

Family: Demodicidae

Description: Species of *Demodex* have an elongate tapering body, up to 0.1–0.4 mm in length, with four pairs of stumpy legs ending in small blunt claws in the adult. Setae are absent from the legs and body. The legs are located at the front of the body, and as such the striated opisthosoma forms at least half the body length. Short forms may be found on the cat, sometimes referred to as *Demodex gatoi*; whether these are genuinely a distinct species remains to be determined.

Hosts: Cat

Life cycle: see *D. canis*

Geographical distribution: Worldwide

Pathogenesis: Demodicosis is rare in cats. It takes a localised, self-limiting form, confined to the eyelids and periocular region, and is of the mild squamous type, with some alopecia. Feline demodicosis is usually associated with underlying debilitating disease such as diabetes mellitus, feline leukaemia virus infection and systemic lupus erythematosus.

Clinical signs: Erythema, papules and thickened skin crusts, alopecia. Generalised demodicosis is very rare, but has been reported with variable pruritus, alopecia, scaling, crusting and hyperpigmentation on the head, neck, legs and trunk.

Diagnosis: For confirmatory diagnosis, deep scrapings are necessary to reach the mites deep in the follicles and glands. This is best achieved by taking a fold of skin, applying a drop of liquid paraffin, and scraping until capillary blood appears.

Treatment: In cats, 2% lime–sulphur dips may be effective when given every 5–7 days for six dips; amitraz rinses at 0.0125–0.025% have also been used successfully. In many cases demodicosis in cats spontaneously resolves and treatment is unnecessary.

Control: Control is rarely applied.

A number of non-specific ectoparasites, particularly fleas and ticks, are also found on dogs and cats and are listed in the host–parasite checklist at the end of this chapter. More detailed descriptions of these parasites are found in Chapter 11 (Facultative ectoparasites and arthropod vectors).

In the following checklists, the codes listed below apply:

Helminth classes:
N = Nematoda; T = Trematoda; C = Cestoda; A = Acanthocephala.

Arthropod classes:
I = Insecta; A = Arachnida; P = Pentastomida.

Protozoal classes:
M = Mastigophora; S = Sarcodina; A = Apicomplexa; R = Rickettsia.

Dog parasite checklist.

Section/host system	Helminths		Arthropods		Protozoa	
	Parasite	(Super)family	Parasite	Family	Parasite	Family
Digestive						
Mouth					*Tetratrichomonas canistomae*	Trichomonadidae(M)
Oesophagus	*Spirocerca lupi*	Spiruroidea (N)				
Stomach	*Ollulanus tricuspis*	Trichostrongyloidea (N)				
	Capillaria putorii	Trichuroidea (N)				
	Gnathostoma spinigerum	Spiruroidea (N)				
	Physaloptera praeputialis	Spiruroidea (N)				
	Physaloptera rara	Spiruroidea (N)				
	Spirura ritypleurites	Spiruroidea (N)				
	Spirocerca lupi	Spiruroidea (N)				
Small intestine	*Toxocara canis*	Ascaridoidea (N)			*Isospora canis*	Eimeriidae (A)
	Toxascaris leonina	Ascaridoidea (N)			*Isospora ohioensis*	Eimeriidae (A)
	Trichinella spiralis	Trichuroidea (N)			*Hammondia heydorni*	Sarcocystiidae (A)
	Ancylostoma caninum	Ancylostomatoidea (N)			*Sarcocystis bovicanis*	Sarcocystiidae (A)
	Ancylostoma braziliense	Ancylostomatoidea (N)			*Sarcocystis ovicanis*	Sarcocystiidae (A)
	Ancylostoma ceylanicum	Ancylostomatoidea (N)			*Sarcocystis suicanis*	Sarcocystiidae (A)
	Uncinaria stenocephala	Ancylostomatoidea (N)			*Sarcocystis capracanis*	Sarcocystiidae (A)
	Strongyloides stercoralis	Rhabditoidea (N)				
	Diphyllobothrium latum	Diphyllobothriidae (C)			*Sarcocystis hircicanis*	Sarcocystiidae (A)
	Dipylidium caninum	Dilepididae (C)			*Sarcocystis equicanis*	Sarcocystiidae (A)
	Echinococcus granulosus	Taeniidae (C)			*Sarcocystis fayeri*	Sarcocystiidae (A)
	Echinococcus multilocularis	Taeniidae (C)			*Sarcocystis hovarthi*	Sarcocystiidae (A)
	Echinococcus vogeli	Taeniidae (C)			*Sarcocystis cameli*	Sarcocystiidae (A)
	Spirometra mansoni	Diphyllobothriidae (C)			*Cryptosporidium parvum*	Cryptosporidiidae (A)
	Spirometra mansonoides	Diphyllobothriidae (C)				
	Taenia hydatigena	Taeniidae (C)			*Cryptosporidium canis*	Cryptosporidiidae (A)
	Taenia krabbei	Taeniidae (C)			*Giardia intestinalis*	Diplomonadidae (M)
	Taenia multiceps	Taeniidae (C)				
	Taenia ovis	Taeniidae (C)				
	Taenia pisiformis	Taeniidae (C)				
	Taenia serialis	Taeniidae (C)				
	Taenia skrjabini	Taeniidae (C)				
	Mesocestoides lineatus	Mesocestoididae (C)				
	Alaria alata	Diplostomatidae (T)				
	Alaria americana	Diplostomatidae (T)				
	Alaria canis	Diplostomatidae (T)				
	Alaria michiganensis	Diplostomatidae (T)				

	Heterophyes heterophyes	Heterophyidae (T)				
	Heterophyes nocens	Heterophyidae (T)				
	Metagonimus yokogawai	Heterophyidae (T)				
	Apophallus donicum	Heterophyidae (T)				
	Apophallus muhlingi	Heterophyidae (T)				
	Cryptocotyle lingua	Heterophyidae (T)				
	Echinochasmus perfoliatus	Echinostomatidae (T)				
	Euparyphium ilocanum	Echinostomatidae (T)				
	Nanophyetus salmincola	Troglotrematidae (T)				
	Macracanthorhynchus hirudinaceus	Oligacanthorynchidae (A)				
	Macracanthorhynchus catalinum	Oligacanthorynchidae (A)				
	Onicola canis	Oligacanthorynchidae (A)				
Caecum	*Trichuris vulpis*	Trichuroidea (N)			*Entamoeba histolytica*	Endamoebidae (S)
					Trichomonas intestinalis	Trichomonadidae (M)
Colon					*Pentatrichomonas hominis*	Trichomonadidae (M)
Respiratory						
Nose			*Pneumonyssus caninum*	Halarachnidae (A)		
			Linguatula serrata	Linguatulidae (P)		
Trachea Bronchi						
Lung	*Capillaria aerophila*	Trichuroidea (N)			*Pneumocystis carinii*	Pneumocystidaceae A*
	Crenosoma vulpis	Metastrongyloidea (N)				
	Filaroides hirthi	Metastrongyloidea (N)				
	Filaroides milksi	Metastrongyloidea (N)				
	Oslerus (Filaroides) osleri	Metastrongyloidea (N)				
	Paragonimus westermani	Troglotrematidae (T)				
	Paragonimus kellicotti	Troglotrematidae (T)				
Liver						
	Fasciola hepatica	Fasciolidae (T)			*Leishmania donovani complex*	Trypanosomatidae (M)
	Capillaria hepatica	Trichuroidea (N)			*Hepatozoon canis*	Hepatozoidae (A)
	Opisthorchis sinensis	Opisthorchiidae (T)				
	Opisthorchis felineus	Opisthorchiidae (T)				
	Metorchis albidus	Opisthorchiidae (T)				
	Metorchis conjunctus	Opisthorchiidae (T)				
	Parametorchis complexus	Opisthorchiidae (T)				

(*continued*)

Dog parasite checklist (*continued*).

Section/host system	Helminths: Parasite	Helminths: (Super)family	Arthropods: Parasite	Arthropods: Family	Protozoa: Parasite	Protozoa: Family
Pancreas						
	Pseudamphistomum truncatum	Opisthorchiidae (T)				
Circulatory						
Blood					*Trypanosoma brucei brucei*	Trypanosomatidae (M)
					Trypanosoma congolense	Trypanosomatidae (M)
					Trypanosoma evansi	Trypanosomatidae (M)
					Babesia canis canis	Babesiidae (A)
					Babesia canis rossi	Babesiidae (A)
	Angiostrongylus vasorum	Metastrongyloidea (N)			*Babesia canis vogeli*	Babesiidae (A)
	Dirofilaria immitis	Filarioidea (N)			*Babesia gibsoni*	Babesiidae (A)
Blood vessels	*Schistosoma japonicum*	Schistosomatidae (T)			*Anaplasma phagocytophilum (A. platys)*	Anaplasmataceae (R)
	Schistosoma incognitum	Schistosomatidae (T)				
	Schistosoma rodhaini	Schistosomatidae (T)				
	Schistosoma spindale	Schistosomatidae (T)			*Ehrlichia canis*	Rickettsiaceae (R)
					Ehrlichia chaffensis	Rickettsiaceae (R)
					Ehrlichia ewingii	Rickettsiaceae (R)
Lymphatics	*Brugia pahangi*	Filarioidea (N)			*Rickettsia rickettsii*	Rickettsiaceae (R)
	Brugia malayi	Filarioidea (N)			*Rickettsia conorii*	Rickettsiaceae (R)
					Rickettsia felis	Rickettsiaceae (R)
Nervous						
CNS	*Taenia solium*	Taeniidae (C)			*Encephalitozoon cuniculi*	Nosematidae (M)
					Toxoplasma gondii	Sarcocystiidae (A)
					Neospora caninum	Sarcocystiidae (A)
Eye	*Thelazia callipaeda*	Spiruroidea (N)				
	Thelazia californiensis	Spiruroidea (N)				
Reproductive/ urogenital						
Kidneys						
	Capillaria plica	Trichuroidea (N)				
	Dioctophyma renale	Dioctophymatoidea (N)				

Locomotory						
Muscle	*Toxocara canis*	Ascaridoidea (N)			*Toxoplasma gondii*	Sarcocystiidae (A)
	Trichinella spiralis	Trichuroidea (N)			*Hepatozoon americanum*	Hepatozoidae (A)
Connective tissue						
Integument						
Skin			*Heterodoxus spiniger*	Boopidae (A)	*Leishmania donovani* complex (*L. infantum*)	Trypanosomatidae (M)
			Linognathus setosus	Linognathidae (I)		
			Trichodectes canis	Trichodectidae (I)		
			Cheyletiella yasguri	Cheyletidae (A)	*Leishmania tropica*	Trypanosomatidae (M)
			Otodectes cynotis	Psoroptidae (A)	*Leishmania aethiopica*	Trypanosomatidae (M)
			Sarcoptes scabiei	Sarcoptidae (A)		Trypanosomatidae (M)
			Demodex canis	Demodicidae (A)	*Leishmania major*	Trypanosomatidae (M)
			Dermanyssus gallinae	Dermanyssidae (A)	*Leishmania peruviana*	
			Neotrombicula autumnalis	Trombiculidae (A)		
			Ceratophyllus gallinae	Ceratophyllidae (I)		
			Ctenocephalides canis	Pulicidae (I)		
			Ctenocephalides felis	Pulicidae (I)		
			Pulex irritans	Pulicidae (I)		
			Archaeopsylla erinacei	Pulicidae (I)		
			Spilopsyllus cuniculi	Pulicidae (I)		
			Echidnophaga gallinacea	Pulicidae (I)		
Subcutaneous	*Dipetalonema reconditum*	Filarioidea (N)	*Cordylobia anthropophaga*	Calliphoridae (I)		
	Dipetalonema grassi	Filarioidea (N)	*Cochliomyia hominivorax*	Calliphoridae (I)		
	Dipetalonema dracunculoides	Filarioidea (N)	*Cochliomyia macellaria*	Calliphoridae (I)		
	Dirofilaria repens	Filarioidea (N)	*Chrysomya bezziana*	Calliphoridae (I)		
	Dracunculus medinensis	Dracunculoidea (N)	*Chrysomya megacephala*	Calliphoridae (I)		
	Dracunculus insignis	Dracunculoidea (N)	*Wohlfahrtia magnifica*	Sarcophagidae (I)		
	Rhabditis strongyloides (*Pelodera*)	Rhabditoidea (N)	*Wohlfahrtia meigeni*	Sarcophagidae (I)		
			Wohlfahrtia vigil	Sarcophagidae (I)		
			Dermatobia hominis	Oestridae (I)		

A* = Archiascomycetes.

The following species of flies and ticks are found on dogs. More detailed descriptions are found in Chapter 11: Facultative ectoparasites and arthropod vectors.

Flies of veterinary importance on dogs.

Group	Genus	Species	Family
Blackflies Buffalo gnats	*Simulium*	spp	Simuliidae (I)
Bot flies	*Dermatobia*	*hominis*	Oestridae
Midges	*Culicoides*	spp	Ceratopogonidae (I)
Mosquitoes	*Aedes* *Anopheles* *Culex*	spp spp spp	Culicidae (I)
Muscids	*Musca* *Stomoxys*	*domestica* *calcitrans*	Muscidae (I)
Sandflies	*Phlebotomus*	spp	Psychodidae (I)
Screwworms and blowflies	*Chrysomya* *Cochliomyia* *Cordylobia*	*albiceps* *bezziana* *megacephala* *hominivorax* *macellaria* *anthropophaga*	Calliphoridae (I)
Tabanids	*Chrysops* *Haematopota* *Tabanus*	spp spp spp	Tabanidae (I)

Tick species found on dogs.

Genus	Species	Common name	Family
Otobius	*megnini*	Spinose ear tick	Argasidae (A)
Ornithodoros	*moubata*	Eyed tampan	Argasidae (A)
	porcinus		
Amblyomma	*americanum*	Lone star tick	Ixodidae (A)
	cajennense	Cayenne tick	
	hebraeum	South African bont tick	
	maculatum	Gulf coast tick	
	variegatum	Tropical bont tick	
Boophilus	*annulatus*	Texas cattle fever tick	
	mircoplus	Pantropical cattle tick	
Dermacentor	*andersoni*	Rocky Mountain wood tick	Ixodidae (A)
	pictus		
	reticulatus	Marsh tick	
	variabilis	American dog tick	
	venustus		
Haemaphysalis	*bispinosa*	New Zealand cattle or bush tick	Ixodidae (A)
	concinna		
	leachi	Yellow dog tick	
	punctata		
Hyalomma	*marginatum*	Bont leg ticks	Ixodidae (A)
	dromedarii	Camel *Hyalomma*	
	aegypticum	Tortoise *Hyalomma*	
Ixodes	*canisuga*	British dog tick	Ixodidae (A)
	hexagonus	Hedgehog tick	
	ricinus	Castor bean or European sheep tick	
	holocyclus	Australian paralysis tick	
	pacificus	Western black-legged tick	
	persulcatus	Taiga tick	
	rubicundus	South African paralysis tick	
	scapularis	Shoulder or black-legged tick	
Rhipicephalus	*appendiculatus*	Brown ear tick	Ixodidae (A)
	bursa		
	capensis	Cape brown tick	
	evertsi	Red-legged tick	
	sanguineus	Brown dog or kennel tick	
	simus		

Cat parasite checklist.

Section/host system	Helminths		Arthropods		Protozoa	
	Parasite	(Super)family	Parasite	Family	Parasite	Family
Digestive						
Mouth					*Tetratrichomonas felistomae*	Trichomonadidae (M)
Oesophagus	*Spirocerca lupi*	Spiruroidea (N)				
Stomach	*Ollulanus tricuspis*	Trichostrongyliodea (N)				
	Gnathostoma spinigerum	Spiruroidea (N)				
	Physaloptera praeputialis	Spiruroidea (N)				
	Physaloptera rara	Spiruroidea (N)				
	Spirura ritypleurites	Spiruroidea (N)				
	Capillaria putorii	Trichuroidea (N)				
Small intestine	*Toxascaris leonina*	Ascaridoidea (N)			*Isospora felis*	Eimeriidae (A)
	Toxocara mystax	Ascaridoidea (N)			*Isospora rivolta*	Eimeriidae (A)
	Toxocara malayiensis	Ascaridoidea (N)			*Hammondia hammondi*	Sarcocystiidae (A)
	Ancylostoma braziliense	Ancylostomatoidea (N)				
	Ancylostoma ceylanicum	Ancylostomatoidea (N)			*Sarcocystis bovifelis*	Sarcocystiidae (A)
	Ancylostoma tubaeforme	Ancylostomatoidea (N)			*Sarcocystis ovifelis*	Sarcocystiidae (A)
	Uncinaria stenocephala	Ancylostomatoidea (N)			*Sarcocystis porcifelis*	Sarcocystiidae (A)
	Strongyloides stercoralis	Rhabditoidea (N)			*Sarcocystis hircifelis*	Sarcocystiidae (A)
	Diphyllobothrium latum	Diphyllobothriidae (C)			*Sarcocystis cuniculi*	Sarcocystiidae (A)
	Dipylidium caninum	Dilepididae (C)			*Sarcocystis muris*	Sarcocystiidae (A)
	Echinococcus multilocularis	Taeniidae (C)			*Besnoitia besnoiti*	Sarcocystiidae (A)
	Echinococcus oligarthrus	Taeniidae (C)			*Cryptosporidium felis*	Cryptosporidiidae (A)
	Spirometra mansoni	Diphyllobothriidae (C)			*Giardia intestinalis*	Diplomonadidae (M)
	Spirometra mansonoides	Diphyllobothriidae (C)				
	Spirometra erinacei	Diphyllobothriidae (C)				
	Taenia taeniaeformis	Taeniidae (C)				
	Mesocestoides lineatus	Mesocesoididae (C)				
	Alaria alata	Diplostomatidae (T)				
	Alaria minesotae	Diplostomatidae (T)				
	Alaria marcianae	Diplostomatidae (T)				
	Heterophyes heterophyes	Heterophyidae (T)				
	Metagonimus yokogawai	Heterophyidae (T)				
	Heterophyes nocens	Heterophyidae (T)				
	Apophallus donicum	Heterophyidae (T)				
	Apophallus muhlingi	Heterophyidae (T)				
	Cryptocotyle lingua	Heterophyidae (T)				

	Echinochasmus perfoliatus	Echinostomatidae (T)				
	Euparyphium melis	Echinostomatidae (T)				
	Euparyphium ilocaecum	Echinostomatidae (T)				
	Nanophyetus salmincola	Troglotrematidae (T)				
	Macracanthorhynchus hirodinaceus	Oligacanthorynchidae (A)				
	Macracanthorhynchus catalinum	Oligacanthorynchidae (A)				
	Onicola campanulatus	Oligacanthorynchidae (A)				
Caecum	*Trichuris vulpis*	Trichuroidea (N)			*Entamoeba histolytica*	Endamoebidae (S)
Colon					*Pentatrichomonas hominis*	Trichomonadidae (M)
Respiratory						
Nose			*Linguatula serrata*	Linguatulidae (P)		
Trachea Bronchi						
Lung	*Capillaria aerophila*	Trichuroidea (N)				
	Aelurostrongylus abstrusus	Metastrongyloidea (N)				
	Anafilaroides rostratus	Metastrongyloidea (N)				
	Metathalazia californica	Metastrongyloidea (N)				
	Mammomonogamus ierei	Strongyloidea (N)				
	Mammomonogamus mcgaughei	Strongyloidea (N)				
	Paragonimus westermani	Troglotrematidae (T)				
	Paragonimus kellicotti	Troglotrematidae (T)				
Liver						
	Capillaria hepatica	Trichuroidea (N)	*Linguatula serrata*	Linguatulidae (P)	*Leishmania donovani complex*	Trypanosomatidae (M)
	Fasciola hepatica	Fasciolidae (T)				
	Opisthorcis sinensis	Opisthorchiidae (T)				
	Opisthorcis felineus	Opisthorchiidae (T)				
	Opisthorchis viverrini	Opisthorchiidae (T)				
	Metorchis albidus	Opisthorchiidae (T)				
	Metorchis conjunctus	Opisthorchiidae (T)				
	Parametorchis complexus	Opisthorchiidae (T)				
	Pseudamphistomum truncatum	Opisthorchiidae (T)				
	Eurytrema procyonis	Dicrocoeliidae (T)				
	Platynostomum fastosum	Dicrocoeliidae (T)				

(*continued*)

Cat parasite checklist (*continued*).

Section/host system	Helminths		Arthropods		Protozoa	
	Parasite	(Super)family	Parasite	Family	Parasite	Family
Pancreas						
	Eurytrema procyonis	Dicrocoeliidae (T)				
	Platynosomum fastosum	Dicrocoeliidae (T)				
Circulatory						
Blood					*Trypanosoma brucei brucei*	Trypanosomatidae (M)
					Babesia felis	Babesiidae (A)
					Babesia cati	Babesiidae (A)
					Cytauxzoon cati	Theileriidae (A)
Blood vessels	*Dirofilaria immitis*	Filarioidea (N)			*Hepatozoon* spp	Hepatozoidae (A)
	Schistosoma rodhaini	Schistosomatidae (T)			*Rickettsia felis*	Rickettsiaceae (R)
	Brugia pahangi	Filarioidea (N)			*Haemobartonella felis (syn Mycoplasma haemofelis)*	Anaplasmataceae (R)
	Brugia malayi	Filarioidea (N)				
Lymphatics						
Nervous						
CNS					*Encephalitozoon cuniculi*	Nosematidae (Mi)
					Toxoplasma gondii	Sarcocystiidae (A)
Eye	*Thelazia californiensis*	Spiruroidea (N)				
	Thelazia callipaeda	Spiruroidea (N)				
Reproductive/urogenital						
Kidneys						
	Capillaria plica	Trichuroidea (N)				
	Dioctyphyma renale	Dioctophymatoidea (N)				
Locomotory						
Muscle	*Toxocara mystax*	Ascaridoidea (N)				
	Trichinella spiralis	Trichuroidea (N)			*Toxoplasma gondii*	Sarcocystiidae (A)

Connective tissue						
Integument						
Skin			*Felicola subrostratus*	Trichodectidae (I)	*Leishmania donovani complex*	Trypanosomatidae (M)
			Demodex cati	Demodicidae (A)		
			Otodectes cynotis	Psoroptidae (A)		
			Notoedres cati	Sarcoptidae (A)		
			Sarcoptes scabiei	Sarcoptidae (A)		
			Cheyletiella blakei	Cheyletidae (A)		
			Cheyletiella parasitovorax	Cheyletidae (A)		
			Neotrombicula autumnalis	Trombiculidae (A)		
			Dermanyssus gallinae	Dermanyssidae (A)		
			Ceratphyllus gallinae	Ceratophyllidae (I)		
			Ctenocephalides canis	Pulicidae (I)		
			Ctenocephalides felis	Pulicidae (I)		
			Pulex irritans	Pulicidae (I)		
			Spilopsyllus cuniculi	Pulicidae (I)		
			Archaeopsylla erinacei	Pulicidae (I)		
			Echidnophaga gallinacea	Pulicidae (I)		
Subcutaneous	*Dirofilaria repens*	Filarioidea (N)	*Cordylobia anthropophaga*	Calliphoridae (I)		
			Cochliomyia hominivorax	Calliphoridae (I)		
			Cochliomyia macellaria	Calliphoridae (I)		
			Chrysomya bezziana	Calliphoridae (I)		
			Chrysomya megacephala	Calliphoridae (I)		
			Wohlfahrtia magnifica	Sarcophagidae (I)		
			Wohlfahrtia meigeni	Sarcophagidae (I)		
			Wohlfahrtia vigil	Sarcophagidae (I)		
			Dermatobia hominis	Oestridae (I)		

The following species of flies and ticks are found on cats. More detailed descriptions are found in Chapter 11: Facultative ectoparasites and arthropod vectors.

Flies of veterinary importance on cats.

Group	Genus	Species	Family
Blackflies Buffalo gnats	*Simulium*	spp	Simuliidae (I)
Bot flies	*Dermatobia*	*hominis*	Oestridae
Midges	*Culicoides*	spp	Ceratopogonidae (I)
Mosquitoes	*Aedes* *Anopheles* *Culex*	spp spp spp	Culicidae (I)
Muscids	*Musca* *Stomoxys*	*domestica* *calcitrans*	Muscidae (I)
Sandflies	*Phlebotomus*	spp	Psychodidae (I)
Screwworms and blowflies	*Chrysomya* *Cochliomyia* *Cordylobia*	*albiceps* *bezziana* *megacephala* *hominivorax* *macellaria* *anthropophaga*	Calliphoridae (I)
Tabanids	*Chrysops* *Haematopota* *Tabanus*	spp spp spp	Tabanidae (I)

Tick species found on cats.

Genus	Species	Common name	Family
Otobius	*megnini*	Spinose ear tick	Argasidae (A)
Ornithodoros	*moubata* *porcinus*	Eyed tampan	Argasidae (A)
Amblyomma	*americanum* *cajennense* *hebraeum* *maculatum* *variegatum*	Lone star tick Cayenne tick South African bont tick Gulf Coast tick Tropical bont tick	Ixodidae (A)
Dermacentor	*andersoni* *pictus* *reticulatus* *variabilis* *venustus*	Rocky Mountain wood tick Marsh tick American dog tick 	Ixodidae (A)
Haemaphysalis	*bispinosa* *concinna* *leachi* *punctata*	 Yellow dog tick 	Ixodidae (A)
Ixodes	*dammini* *hexagonus* *ricinus* *holocyclus* *pacificus* *persulcatus* *pilosus* *scapularis*	 Hedgehog tick Castor bean or European sheep tick Australina paralysis tick Western black-legged tick Taiga tick Russet, sourved or bush tick Shoulder or black-legged tick	Ixodidae (A)
Rhipicephalus	*evertsi* *sanguineus* *simus*	Red or red-legged tick Brown dog or kennel tick 	Ixodidae (A)

7
Parasites of poultry and gamebirds

ENDOPARASITES

PARASITES OF THE DIGESTIVE SYSTEM

OESOPHAGUS

Capillaria annulata

Synonym: *Eucoleus annulata*

Common name: Hairworms or threadworms

Predilection site: Oesophagus, crop

Parasite class: Nematoda

Superfamily: Trichuroidea

Description, gross: These are very fine filamentous worms, the narrow stichosome oesophagus occupying about one third to half the body length. Males measure around 15–25 mm and females 37–80 mm.

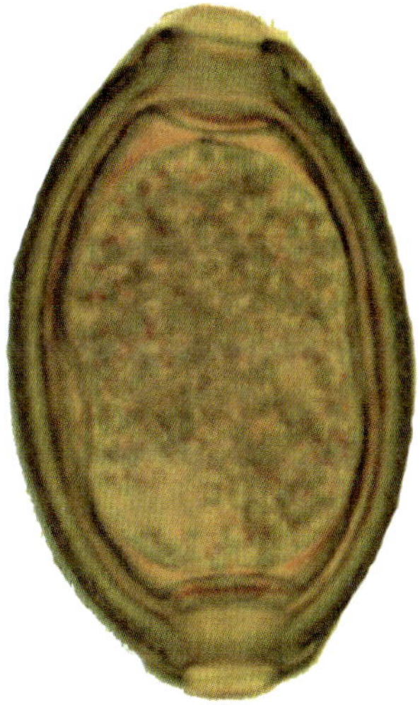

Fig. 7.1 *Capillaria* eggs.

Description, microscopic: The males have a long thin single spicule, with a spiny spicule sheath, and often possess a primitive bursa-like structure. This species has a cuticular swelling at the back of the head. The females contain eggs that resemble those of *Trichuris* in possessing bipolar plugs (Fig. 7.1). The eggs are barrel-shaped and colourless, 60–65 × 25–28 μm, have thick shells that are slightly striated with bipolar plugs.

Final hosts: Chicken, turkey, ducks and wild birds

Intermediate hosts: Earthworms

Life cycle: The life cycle is indirect. Eggs passed in faeces are ingested by earthworms and develop to the infective stage in 2–3 weeks. The prepatent period is about 3–4 weeks in the final host.

Geographical distribution: Worldwide

Pathogenesis: Like *Trichuris* the anterior ends of the parasite are buried in the mucosa and even light infections can produce a catarrhal inflammation and thickening of the oesophagus and crop wall. Heavy infections may cause diphtheritic inflammation and marked thickening of the wall; in such cases mortality may be high.

Clinical signs: Light infections of less than 100 worms may cause poor weight gains and lowered egg production. Heavy infections often induce inappetence and emaciation.

Diagnosis: Because of the non-specific nature of the clinical signs and the fact that, in heavy infections, these may appear before *Capillaria* eggs are present in the faeces, diagnosis depends on necropsy and careful examination of the oesophagus and crop for the presence of the worms. This may be carried out by microscopic examination of mucosal scrapings squeezed between two glass slides; alternatively the contents should be gently washed through a fine sieve and the retained material resuspended in water and examined against a black background.

Pathology: Presence of the adult worms causes catarrhal inflammation and thickening of the oesophagus and crop wall. Heavy infections may cause diphtheritic inflammation and marked thickening of the wall.

Epidemiology: Young birds are most susceptible to *Capillaria* infections while adults may serve as carriers. The epidemiology is largely based on the ubiquity of the earthworm intermediate host.

Treatment: Levamisole in the drinking water is highly effective as are a number of benzimidazoles given in the feed. Elevated oral doses of these anthelmintics, administered over several days, also give high efficacy.

Control: Control depends on regular anthelmintic treatment accompanied, if possible, by moving the birds to fresh ground. Scrubbing and heat treatment of affected surfaces is essential as is the provision of fresh litter in chicken houses.

Notes: The taxonomic situation regarding many species of *Capillaria* is complex and recently it has been split into several genera; the old species names are listed with the new proposed generic names.

Capillaria contorta

See under Crop.

Several spiruroid worms are found in the oesophagus, crop and proventriculus of poultry. The life cycles of these parasites are indirect, involving a range of invertebrate hosts. Infections with these parasites are more common in free-ranging birds. Attempts to control the poultry spiruroids are unlikely to be successful because of the ready availability of the intermediate hosts.

Gongylonema ingluvicola

See under Crop.

Dispharynx nasuta

See under Proventriculus.

Tetrameres americana

See under Proventriculus.

Trichomonas gallinae

Synonym: *Cercomonas gallinae*, *Trichomonas columbae*

Common name: Canker, frounce, roup

Predilection site: Oesophagus, crop, proventriculus

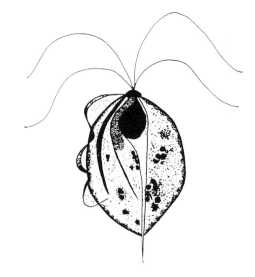

Fig. 7.2 *Trichomonas gallinae.*

Parasite class: Zoomastigophorasida

Family: Trichomonadidae

Description: The body is elongate, ellipsoidal or pyriform, 5–19 × 2–9 μm, with four anterior flagella that arise from the blepharoplast (Fig. 7.2). The undulating membrane does not reach the posterior end of the body and a free posterior flagellum is absent. An accessory filament is present. The axostyle is narrow, protrudes 2–8 μm from the body and its anterior portion is flattened into a spatulate capitulum. There is a crescent-shaped pelta anterior to the axostyle and there is no chromatic ring at its point of emergence. The parabasal body is hook-shaped and has a parabasal filament and the costa is a very fine rod running three quarters the length of the body.

Hosts: Pigeon, turkey, chicken, raptors (hawks, falcons, eagles)

Life cycle: The trichomonads reproduce by longitudinal binary fission. No sexual stages are known and there are no cysts.

Geographical distribution: Worldwide

Pathogenesis: In the turkey and chicken lesions most commonly occur in the crop, oesophagus, pharynx and are uncommon in the mouth.

Clinical signs: Severely affected birds lose weight, stand huddled with ruffled feathers, and may fall over when forced to move. Yellow, necrotic lesions are present in the oesophagus and crop and a greenish fluid containing large numbers of trichomonads may be found in the mouth.

Diagnosis: The clinical signs are pathognomonic and can be confirmed by identifying the characteristic motile trichomonads from samples taken from lesions in the mouth or from fluid.

Pathology: The early lesions in the pharynx, oesophagus and crop are small, whitish to yellowish caseous nodules. These grow in size and may remain circumscribed and separate, or may coalesce to form thick, caseous, necrotic masses that may occlude the lumen. The circumscribed disk-shaped lesions are often described as 'yellow buttons'. The lesions in the liver, lungs and other organs are solid, yellowish, caseous nodules up to 1 cm or more in diameter.

Epidemiology: Turkeys and chickens are infected through drinking contaminated water, the source of contamination being feral pigeons and other wild birds, which also use the water source. Trichomonads enter the water from the mouths, not the faeces, of the wild birds. *T. gallinae* has no cysts and is very sensitive to drying, so direct contamination is necessary.

Treatment: Nitroimidazole compounds, such as dimetridazole and metronidazole, are effective, but their availability has declined in many countries through legislative changes and toxicity concerns.

Control: Control in chickens and turkeys, depends on preventing access of wild pigeons to drinking water.

CROP

Gongylonema ingluvicola

Common name: Gullet worm

Predilection site: Crop, oesophagus and occasionally proventriculus

Parasite class: Nematoda

Superfamily: Spiruroidea

Description, gross: Long, slender worm. The female worm is 32–55 mm long and the males measure around 18 mm.

Description, microscopic: Easily distinguished microscopically by the presence of longitudinal rows of round or oval, cuticular bosses in the anterior region of the body. The eggs measure approximately 58×35 µm.

Final hosts: Chicken, turkey, partridge, pheasant, quail

Intermediate hosts: Cockroaches (*Blatella germanica*) and beetles of the species *Copris minutus*

Life cycle: The life cycle is typically spiruroid. Eggs are passed in faeces and, when eaten by an intermediate host, they hatch and develop to the infective stage within about 30 days. Infection of the definitive host is through the ingestion of infected cockroaches. The adult worms live spirally (in a zipper fashion) embedded in the mucosa or submucosa of the crop with their anterior and/or posterior ends protruding into the lumen. The prepatent period is about 8 weeks.

Geographical distribution: North America, Asia, Africa, Australia and Europe

Pathogenesis: The adult parasites are moderately pathogenic, depending on the number of worms embedded in the epithelium.

Clinical signs: Light infections are often asymptomatic. Heavier infections may produce regurgitation.

Diagnosis: Usually an incidental finding on postmortem.

Pathology: Heavy infections in fowl can induce hypertrophy and cornification of the epithelium of the crop.

Gongylonema crami

Predilection site: Crop

Parasite class: Nematode

Superfamily: Spiruroidea

Final host: Chicken

Details are essentially similar to *Gongylonema ingluvicola*

Trichomonas gallinae

See under Oesophagus.

Capillaria contorta

Synonym: *Eucoleus contorta*

Predilection site: Oesophagus, crop

Parasite class: Nematoda

Superfamily: Trichuroidea

Description: General description as for other *Capillaria* species. Males measure around 12–17 mm and females 27–38 mm. Eggs are $48–56 \times 21–24$ µm.

Final hosts: Chicken, turkey, pheasant, partridge, duck and wild birds

Intermediate hosts: Earthworms.

Life cycle: *C. contorta* appears to be able to develop both directly and indirectly. In the direct life cycle, the infective L_1 develops within the egg in about 3–4 weeks. Infection of the final host is through ingestion of this embryonated infective stage, development to adult worms occurs without a migration phase. In the indirect life cycle, the egg requires to be ingested by an earthworm in which it hatches, the final host being infected by ingestion of the earthworm. The prepatent period is about 3–4 weeks in the final host.

Geographical distribution: Worldwide

Clinical signs: Low infections are frequently asymptomatic, possibly causing some reduction in growth and lower egg production. Severely infected birds often become anaemic, weak and emaciated.

Pathology: Large numbers of worms produce an inflammation varying from catarrhal to diphtheritic.

Epidemiology: Young birds are most susceptible to *Capillaria* infections while adults may serve as carriers. *C. contorta* is important since, having a direct life cycle, it occurs indoors in birds kept on deep litter and outdoors in free-range systems, allowing large numbers of infective eggs to accumulate.

Control: Control depends on regular anthelmintic treatment accompanied if possible by moving the birds to fresh ground. Scrubbing and heat treatment of affected surfaces is essential as is the provision of fresh litter in chicken houses.

Details of the pathogenesis, diagnosis and treatment are as for *C. annulata*.

Capillaria annulata

See under Oesophagus.

PROVENTRICULUS

Tetrameres americana

Synonym: *Tropisurus americana*

Common name: Globular roundworm

Predilection site: Proventriculus

Parasite class: Nematoda

Superfamily: Spiruroidea

Description, gross: The adults show sexual dimorphism. The males are pale white, slender, and only about 5–6 mm long. The females are bright red and almost spherical, with a diameter of about 3.5–5.0 mm (Fig. 7.3).

Description, microscopic: Males have spiny cuticles and no cordons; females have four longitudinal deep furrows on the surface. Eggs are thick-shelled, 42–50 × 24 µm and embryonated when passed.

Final hosts: Chicken, turkey, duck, geese, grouse, quail, pigeon

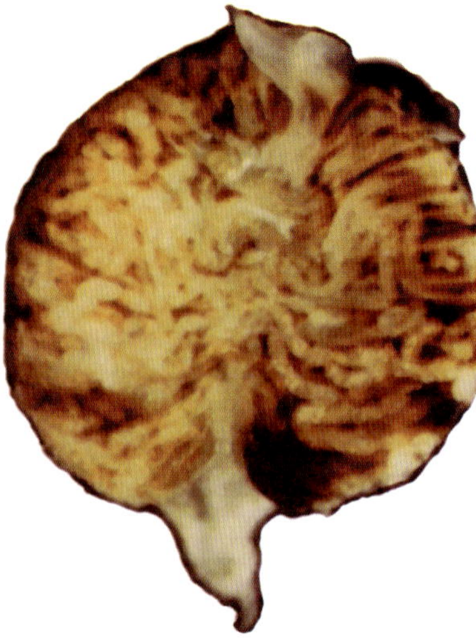

Fig. 7.3 Adult female *Tetrameres americana*.

Intermediate hosts: Cockroaches, grasshoppers and beetles

Life cycle: Eggs are shed with the faeces and hatch when eaten by an intermediate host. The final host becomes infected following ingestion of the intermediate host and the males and females locate in the glands of the proventriculus. Males inhabit the mucosal surface and upper regions of the glands but after mating the males leave the glands and die. The females are embedded deep in the mucosal glands.

Geographical distribution: Commonly occurs in Africa and North America

Pathogenesis: The females in the glands of the proventriculus are bloodsuckers, and can cause anaemia as well as local erosion. Heavy infections may be fatal in chicks, but this genus is usually present only in moderate numbers and is well tolerated. The migration of juvenile stages into the wall of the proventriculus can cause inflammation and thickening.

Clinical signs: Infected fowl may become anaemic and lose condition. Heavy infections, particularly in young chickens, can induce thickening of the proventriculus with oedema and in some instances this can lead to partial blockage of the lumen. Heavy infections can be fatal.

Diagnosis: At necropsy, the female *Tetrameres* appear as dark red spots when viewed from the serosal surface of the proventriculus.

Pathology: The wall of the proventriculus may be thickened to an extent that the lumen is almost obliterated.

Table 7.1 Species of *Tetrameres* found in poultry.

Species	Hosts	Intermediate hosts	Geographical distribution
Tetrameres americana	Chicken, turkey, ducks, geese, grouse, quail, pigeons	Cockroaches, grasshoppers and beetles	Africa and North America
Tetrameres fissipina	Ducks, geese, chicken, turkey, pigeons and wild aquatic birds	Aquatic crustaceans, grasshoppers, earthworms	Most parts of the world
Tetrameres crami	Domestic and wild duck	Amphipods	North America
Tetrameres confusa	Chicken	?	Brazil
Tetrameres mohtedai	Chicken	?	India
Tetrameres pattersoni	Quail	?	?

Epidemiology: Infection is more common in free-ranging birds.

Tetrameres fissispina

Synonym: *Tropisurus fissispina*

Predilection site: Proventriculus

Parasite class: Nematoda

Superfamily: Spiruroidea

Description, gross: See *T. americana*. Males are pale white, slender and 3–6 mm long. The females are bright red, ovoid/spherical, with a diameter varying from around 1.5–6 mm.

Description, microscopic: Males have four longitudinal rows of spines along the median and lateral lines and no cordons; females have four longitudinal deep furrows on the surface. Eggs are thick-shelled, $48–56 \times 26–30$ µm and embryonated when passed.

Final hosts: Duck, goose, chicken, turkey, pigeon and wild aquatic birds

Intermediate hosts: Aquatic crustaceans, such as *Daphnia* and *Gammarus*, grasshoppers, earthworms

Geographical distribution: Most parts of the world

Details of the life cycle, pathogenesis, clinical signs, diagnosis and pathology are as for *T. americana*.

Tetrameres crami

Predilection site: Proventriculus

Parasite class: Nematoda

Superfamily: Spiruroidea

Description, gross: See *T. americana*. Males are white, slender and about 4 mm long. The red ovoid/spherical females measure around 2×1.5 mm.

Final hosts: Domestic and wild duck

Intermediate hosts: Amphipods such as *Gammarus fasciatus* and *Hyalella knickerbockeri*

Geographical distribution: North America

All other details are similar to *T. americana*.

Several other species of *Tetrameres* found in poultry are listed in Table 7.1. Details on pathogenicity in the host species are essentially similar to *T. americana*.

Dispharynx nasuta

Common name: Spiral stomach worm

Synonym: *Dispharynx spiralis*, *Acuaria spiralis*

Predilection site: Oesophagus, proventriculus

Parasite class: Nematoda

Superfamily: Spiruroidea

Description, gross: The body is slender and coiled, particularly the posterior of the male. Males measure up to around 8 mm long and the females 10 mm.

Description, microscopic: The cuticle is ornamented with four wavy cordons that recurve anteriorly and do not fuse. The left spicule is slender and the right spicule shorter and oval-shaped. The eggs are thick-shelled, $33–40 \times 18–25$ µm and embryonated when passed.

Final hosts: Chicken, turkey, pigeon, guinea fowl, grouse, pheasant and other birds

Intermediate hosts: Various isopods such as sowbugs (*Porcellio scaber*) and pillbugs (*Armadillidium vulgare*)

Life cycle: Typically spiruroid. The intermediate host ingests embryonated eggs and development to the L_3 takes place in the body cavity. When the isopod is consumed by the final host, the worms develop to the final stage in the proventriculus or oesophagus.

Geographical distribution: Asia, Africa and the Americas

Pathogenesis: Mild infections usually provoke only a slight nodular inflammatory reaction in the mucosa with excessive mucus production.

Clinical signs: Most mild infections with *Dispharynx* are inapparent. Heavily infected young birds can rapidly lose weight, become emaciated and anaemic. Deaths can be high.

Diagnosis: A tentative diagnosis is based on the presence of spiruroid eggs, which are difficult to differentiate. Species identification is usually based on morphological identification of adult worms on postmortem.

Pathology: In severe infections, deep ulcers and hypertrophy can occur in the mucosa of the proventriculus in which the anterior ends of the worms are embedded.

Echinuria uncinata

Synonym: *Acuaria uncinata*

Predilection site: Oesophagus, proventriculus, gizzard

Parasite class: Nematoda

Superfamily: Spiruroidea

Description, gross: The body is slender and males measure 8–10 mm long and the females 12–18.5 mm.

Description, microscopic: The cuticle is ornamented with four wavy cordons that are non-recurrent and they anastomose in pairs. There are four pairs of pre-cloacal papillae in two groups of two either side, and four pairs of post-cloacal papillae. The left spicule is longer than the right spicule. The eggs are thick-shelled, $37 \times 20\ \mu m$ and embryonated when passed.

Final hosts: Duck, goose, swan and various aquatic birds

Intermediate hosts: *Daphnia* and *Gammarus*

Life cycle: Typically spiruroid. Eggs are passed in the faeces and ingested by water fleas in which they hatch and develop to infective larvae. The parasites continue development when the intermediate host is ingested by an aquatic bird.

Geographical distribution: Worldwide

Pathogenesis: The worms can cause an inflammation of the alimentary tract and the formation of caseous nodules. These nodules can be very large in the gizzard and proventriculus and interfere with the passage of food.

Clinical signs: Infected birds may become weak and emaciated and deaths have been reported.

Hystrichis tricolour

Predilection site: Proventriculus, oesophagus

Parasite class: Nematoda

Superfamily: Dioctophymatoidea

Description, gross: Adult female worms measure up to about 4 cm and males 2.5 cm in length.

Description, microscopic: The cephalic area is expanded, and possesses many regularly positioned spines. The eggs are thick-shelled, coated with tubercles and have truncated poles.

Final hosts: Domestic and wild ducks and anatid birds

Intermediate hosts: Oligochaetes (annelids)

Life cycle: This is indirect. Fowl and other birds become parasitised through ingestion of infected oligochaetes. The adult worms are deeply embedded in the mucosa with their caudal and cephalic regions lying within the lumen of the tract. The prepatent period is around 2 weeks.

Geographical distribution: The extent of the distribution is not known but it occurs occasionally in Europe

Pathogenesis: The parasite induces nodule formation (pea-sized tumours) on the wall of the proventriculus and oesophagus. Sometimes these can perforate to the pleural cavity.

Clinical signs: Low infections are usually asymptomatic but heavy burdens can induce emaciation.

Eustrongyloides papillosus

Predilection site: Oesophagus, proventriculus

Parasite class: Nematoda

Superfamily: Dioctophymatoidea

Description, gross: Females measure about 3 cm in length.

Description, microscopic: The male has a bursal cup with a fringed margin. Eggs are $68 \times 38\ \mu m$.

Final hosts: Duck, goose

Intermediate hosts: Not known, possible oligochaetes

Life cycle: This is not fully known but oligochaetes are likely to be involved as intermediate hosts and various fish as paratenic hosts.

Geographical distribution: Many parts of the world

Pathogenesis: Generally considered to be of low pathogenicity and of little veterinary significance, although the parasites can induce the formation of nodules in the wall of the anterior digestive tract.

Trichomonas gallinae

See under Oesophagus.

For treatment and control, see under Gizzard.

GIZZARD

Several species of gizzard worms are found in ducks and geese. The following applies to all species.

Life cycle: Direct and similar to other strongyles. Infection is via ingestion of L_3, or through skin penetration. Eggs passed in the faeces are already embryonated and develop to the L_3 in the egg. Ingested larvae penetrate the submucosa of the gizzard. Patency is around 2–3 weeks in geese.

Pathogenesis: Adult birds may not show clinical symptoms but act as carriers. These parasites found in the upper alimentary tract, particularly the gizzard, may cause heavy mortality in goslings, ducklings and other young aquatic fowls. Young goslings and ducklings are particularly susceptible. The worms burrow into the mucosa of the gizzard, cause irritation and ingest blood.

Clinical signs: Young fowl may become inappetent, and show diarrhoea and anaemia. Over time the birds become emaciated, weak and, where heavily infected, fatalities can occur. Often older fowl show few clinical signs but act as reservoirs of infection.

Diagnosis: At necropsy, worms may be recovered from the mucosa of the gizzard following incubation in warm saline for 1–2 hours. *Amidostomum* spp are the main trichostrongyloids of the gizzard, which possess a buccal capsule.

Pathology: Severe infections induce haemorrhages on the gizzard mucosa, which may be accompanied by catarrhal inflammation. Heavy infections can cause necrosis of the horny lining of the gizzard, forming reddish brown loose folds containing many embedded worms.

Epidemiology: The infective L_3 requires adequate moisture, such as pond margins, to survive, as they are very susceptible to desiccation.

Treatment: Treatment with one of the modern benzimidazoles or levamisole, often administered in feed or drinking water, is effective.

Control: Gizzard worm infection may be prevented by ensuring that birds do not run on the same ground each year. It is important to restrict access of wild aquatic fowl to areas where geese are raised.

Amidostomum anseris

Synonym: *Amidostomum nodulosum*

Common name: Gizzard worm

Predilection site: Gizzard, occasionally proventriculus, oesophagus

Parasite class: Nematoda

Superfamily: Trichostrongyloidea

Description, gross: The slender adult worms, bright red in colour when fresh, and up to 2.5 cm in length, are easily recognised at necropsy where they predominate in the horny lining of the gizzard. Males measure about 10–17 mm and females 15–25 mm.

Description, microscopic: Characterised by a shallow buccal capsule with three pointed teeth, the middle one being the largest. The male spicules are of equal length and are divided into two branches at the posterior. Eggs are thin-shelled, ellipsoidal and measure around 100×60 µm.

Hosts: Domestic and wild goose, duck and other aquatic fowl

Geographical distribution: Worldwide

Amidostomum skrjabini

Common name: Gizzard worm

Predilection site: Gizzard, occasionally proventriculus, oesophagus

Parasite class: Nematoda

Superfamily: Trichostrongyloidea

Description: Similar to *A. anseris* in possessing a shallow buccal capsule with small teeth. The hatched L_3 require about 5 days in the environment before they are fully infective.

Hosts: Domestic and wild duck

Geographical distribution: Worldwide

Epomidiostomum anatinum

Synonym: *Epomidiostomum uncinatum*, *Strongylus uncinatus*, *Amidostomum anatinum*

Common name: Gizzard worm

Predilection site: Gizzard

Parasite class: Nematoda

Superfamily: Trichostrongyloidea

Description, gross: The body is filiform with a very fine tapering anterior region and yellowish white in colour. Males measure around 6 mm, and females are approximately 10 mm in length.

Description, microscopic: The mouth is surrounded by four protruding papillae. The cuticle bears two lateral epaulets, the posterior edge of which forms a three-toothed fringe. The dark brown spicules are of equal length and the tip comprises three branches. A gubernaculum is absent. The tail of the female has a conical appendage with a small rounded tip. Eggs measure about 80×50 μm.

Hosts: Domestic and wild goose, duck and other aquatic fowl

Geographical distribution: Many parts of the world, especially North America, Africa, Asia and Europe

Notes: A similar species, *Epomidiostomum crami*, is found in Canada geese (*Branta canadensis*) and blue-winged geese (*Chen coeruleus*) in North America.

Epomidiostomum orispinum

Synonym: *Strongylus anseris*, *Strongylus orispinum.*

Common name: Gizzard worm

Predilection site: Gizzard and oesophagus

Parasite class: Nematoda

Superfamily: Trichostrongyloidea

Description, gross: Males measure around 11 mm and females 16 mm in length.

Description, microscopic: The anterior of the worm possesses four posteriorly pointing offshoots and lateral festoons bearing a pair of papillae. Spicules are equal with three shafts pointing distally. The body of the female tapers abruptly, towards the digitate tail.

Hosts: Duck, goose and swan

Geographical distribution: Africa, Europe

Epomidiostomum skrjabini

Common name: Gizzard worm

Predilection site: Gizzard

Parasite class: Nematoda

Superfamily: Trichostrongyloidea

Description, gross: The size of the males and females is similar to that of *E. orispinum*.

Description, microscopic: The head of the worm possesses a cuticular prominence which is armed with four symmetrical, lateral-pointing spines. There are also two epaulet formations.

The mouth is surrounded by four small spines. The bursa has three lobes, the central lobe being poorly developed. Spicules are equal and the posterior ends are split into three sharp-tipped branches. The anterior ends are blunt. The female tail terminates in a finger-like appendage, which is bent venterally.

Hosts: Domestic and wild goose

Geographical distribution: Russia

Cheilospirura hamulosa

Synonym: *Acuaria hamulosa*

Predilection site: Gizzard

Parasite class: Nematoda

Superfamily: Spiruroidea

Description, gross: Males measure up to 15 mm and females 30 mm.

Description, microscopic: The worms have four wavy irregular cuticular cordons that extend to more than half the length of the body. The males have four pairs of pre-cloacal and six pairs of post-cloacal papillae, a short flattened spicule on the right and a longer slender spicule on the left side. Eggs are embryonated when passed.

Final hosts: Chicken, turkey

Intermediate hosts: Grasshoppers (*Melanoplus*), weevils and beetles

Life cycle: Eggs shed in the faeces are ingested by the intermediate host where they develop to the infective stage in about 3 weeks. The final host becomes infected after consuming this intermediate host and the prepatent period is about 3 weeks.

Geographical distribution: Worldwide, in particular Europe, Africa, Asia and the Americas

Pathogenesis: Generally, mild to moderate infections are considered to be of low pathogenicity. In heavy infections, many adult worms penetrate under the keratinised layer of the gizzard where they are found embedded in soft orangy-coloured nodules. The keratinised layer of the gizzard may become necrotic and rupture of the gizzard can occur.

Clinical signs: Mild infections are usually asymptomatic. Severe infections can lead to emaciation, weakness and anaemia.

Diagnosis: This is best achieved through autopsy of an affected chicken, as the eggs of several species of *Cheilospirura* appear very similar.

Pathology: In mild infections, the worms are noticed only if the horny lining of the gizzard is removed, and are found in soft, yellowish red nodules. In severe cases, the horny lining may be partly destroyed, with the worms found below the necrotic material within the altered musculature of the gizzard.

Other species of spiruroid worms found in the gizzard are considered to be of minor significance.

Histiocephalus laticaudatus

Parasite class: Nematoda

Superfamily: Spiruroidea

Hosts: Chicken

Life cycle: Little is known of the life cycle

Geographical distribution: Europe

Streptocara spp

Parasite class: Nematoda

Superfamily: Spiruroidea

Final hosts: Chicken, turkey, duck, goose

Intermediate hosts: Crustaceans (*Daphnia*, *Gammarus*)

SMALL INTESTINE

Ascaridia galli

Predilection site: Small intestine

Parasite class: Nematoda

Superfamily: Ascaridoidea

Description, gross: The worms are stout and densely white, the females measuring up to 12.0 cm in length (Fig. 7.4). *Ascaridia* is by far the largest nematode of poultry.

Description, microscopic: The egg is distinctly oval, with a smooth shell, and cannot easily be distinguished from that of the other common poultry ascaridoid, *Heterakis*.

Hosts: Chicken, turkey, goose, duck, guinea fowl and a number of wild gallifrom birds

Life cycle: The egg becomes infective at optimal temperatures in a minimum of 3 weeks and the parasitic phase is non-migratory, consisting of a transient histotrophic phase in the intestinal mucosa after which the adult parasites inhabit the lumen of the intestine. The egg is sometimes ingested by earthworms, which may act as transport hosts. Eggs can remain viable for

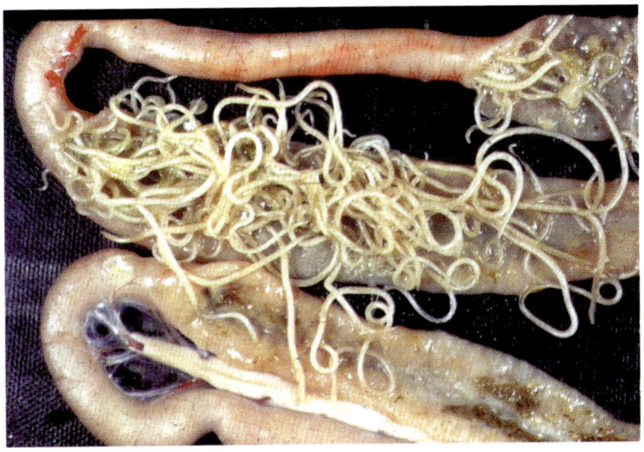

Fig. 7.4 Adult worms of *Ascaridia galli*.

several months under moist cool conditions but are killed by a dry hot environment. The prepatent period ranges from 4–6 weeks in chicks to 8 weeks or more in adult birds. The worms live for about 1 year.

Geographical distribution: Worldwide

Pathogenesis: *Ascaridia* is not a highly pathogenic worm, and any effects are usually seen in young birds of around 1–2 months of age, adults appearing relatively unaffected. The main effect is seen during the prepatent phase, when the larvae are in the duodenal/intestinal mucosa. There they cause enteritis, which is usually catarrhal, but in very heavy infections may be haemorrhagic. In moderate infections the adult worms are tolerated without clinical signs, but when considerable numbers are present the large size of these worms may cause intestinal occlusion and death. Nutritional deficiency may predispose birds to the establishment of infection.

Clinical signs: Heavily infected birds may become anaemic and show intermittent diarrhoea, anorexia, later becoming unthrifty and emaciated. This can lead to a decrease in egg production.

Diagnosis: In infections with adult worms, the eggs will be found in faeces, but since it is often difficult to distinguish these from the slightly smaller eggs of *Heterakis*, confirmation must be made by postmortem examination of a casualty when the large white worms will be found. In the prepatent period, larvae will be found in the intestinal contents and in scrapings of the mucosa.

Pathology: Enteritis or haemorrhagic enteritis may be seen when large numbers of young parasites penetrate the duodenal or jejunal mucosa. The embedded larvae cause haemorrhage and extensive destruction of the glandular epithelium, and proliferation of mucous-secretory cells may result in adhesion of the mucosal villi. Damage to the epithelia may not only be caused by the larvae, but also by the adult worms in the form of pressure atrophy of the villi with occasional necrosis of the mucosal layer. In chronic infections a loss of muscle tonus may be seen, and the intestinal wall may assume a flabby appearance. During the histotropic phase, there is loss of blood, reduced blood sugar and the ureters frequently become distended with urates.

Epidemiology: Adult birds are symptomless carriers, and the reservoir of infection is on the ground, either as free eggs or in earthworm transport hosts. Infection is heaviest in young chicks.

Treatment: Treatment with piperazine salts, levamisole or a benzimidazole, such as flubendazole, mebendazole or fenbendazole, can be administered in the feed (30 ppm over 7 days; 60 ppm over 7 days; 60 ppm over 3 days, respectively). Levamisole is effective at 30 mg/kg given orally, or 300 ppm in the feed.

Control: When birds are reared on a free-range system, and ascaridiosis is a problem, the young birds should, if possible, be segregated and reared on ground previously unused by poultry. Rotation of poultry runs is advisable. Since the nematode may also be a problem in deep litter houses, feeding and watering systems which will limit the contamination of food and water by faeces, should be used.

Ascaridia dissimilis

Predilection site: Small intestine

Parasite class: Nematoda

Superfamily: Ascaridoidea

Description, gross: The worms are stout and densely white, and 3–7 cm in length

Description, microscopic: The egg is distinctly oval, with a smooth shell, and 80–95 μm in size.

Hosts: Turkey

Life cycle: The parasitic phase is non-migratory, consisting of a transient histotrophic phase in the intestinal mucosa after which the adult parasites inhabit the lumen of the intestine. The egg is sometimes ingested by earthworms, which may act as transport hosts. The prepatent period is 6 weeks.

Geographical distribution: Presumed worldwide

Pathogenesis: Considered non-pathogenic

Clinical signs: Moderate infections are frequently inapparent

Diagnosis: Adult worms may be found in the intestine on postmortem or the characteristic ascarid eggs may be seen in faeces.

Pathology: No associated pathology

Epidemiology: Adult birds are symptomless carriers, and the reservoir of infection is on the ground, either as free eggs or in earthworm transport hosts.

Treatment: Not usually required, although treatment with piperazine salts, levamisole or a benzimidazole, such as fenbendazole, is effective.

Control: Strict hygiene and feeding and watering systems, which will limit the contamination of food and water by faeces, should be used

Porrocaecum crassum

Predilection site: Small intestine

Parasite class: Nematoda

Superfamily: Ascaridoidea

Description, gross: The worms are reddish white in colour with males 12–30 mm and female worms 40–55 mm.

Description, microscopic: The tail of the male is conical and there are no caudal alae. The egg is ellipsoidal, and 110 × 85 μm in size.

Hosts: Domestic and wild duck

Life cycle: Similar to other ascarid species

Geographical distribution: Presumed worldwide

Pathogenesis: Considered non-pathogenic

Contracaecum spiculigerum

Predilection site: Small intestine

Parasite class: Nematoda

Superfamily: Ascaridoidea

Description, gross: Males worms are 32–45 mm and female worms 24–64 mm.

Description, microscopic: An oesophageal appendix is present. The egg is spherical, and 50–52 μm in size.

Hosts: Duck, goose, swan and other waterfowl

Life cycle: Similar to other ascarid species

Geographical distribution: Presumed worldwide

Pathogenesis: Considered non-pathogenic

Capillaria caudinflata

Synonym: *Aonchotheca caudinflata*

Predilection site: Small intestine

Parasite class: Nematoda

Superfamily: Trichuroidea

Description: See *C. annulata*. Males measure around 6–12 mm and females up to 25 mm. Females have a characteristic vulval appendage.

Final hosts: Chicken, turkey, goose, pigeon and wild birds

Intermediate hosts: Earthworms

Life cycle: The life cycle of this species is indirect.

Geographical distribution: Worldwide.

Pathogenesis: The anterior ends of the worms are embedded in the mucosa. Light infections can produce a catarrhal inflammation; heavy infections may cause a haemorrhagic enteritis with bloody diarrhoea.

Clinical signs: Heavy infections often induce anaemia and the birds become weak and emaciated.

Capillaria bursata

Predilection site: Small intestine

Parasite class: Nematoda

Superfamily: Trichuroidea

Description, gross: See *C. annulata*. Males measure around 6–12 mm and females up to 25 mm.

Final hosts: Chicken, turkey, pheasant and wild birds

Intermediate hosts: Earthworms

Life cycle: The life cycle of this species is indirect.

Geographical distribution: Worldwide

Capillaria obsignata

Synonym: *Baruscapillaria obsignata*, *Capillaria columbae*

Predilection site: Small intestine

Parasite class: Nematoda

Superfamily: Trichuroidea

Description, gross: See *C. annulata*. Males measure around 10–12 mm and females up to 15 mm.

Description, microscopic: Eggs are barrel-shaped and colourless, 48–53 × 24 μm in size and have thick shells that are slightly striated with bipolar plugs.

Hosts: Pigeon, chicken, turkey, pheasant and wild birds

Life cycle: This species has a direct life cycle. The infective L_1 develops within the egg in about 7–10 days. Infection of the final host is through ingestion of this embryonated infective stage, development to adult worms occurs without a migration phase. The prepatent period is around 3 weeks.

Geographical distribution: Worldwide

Pathogenesis: *C. obsignata* can be highly pathogenic in chickens and pigeons, leading to mortalities. Birds become listless, emaciated and diarrhoeic.

Epidemiology: Young birds are most susceptible to *Capillaria* infections while adults may serve as carriers. *C. obsignata* is important since, having a direct life cycle, it occurs indoors in birds kept on deep litter and outdoors in free-range systems, allowing large numbers of infective eggs to accumulate.

Details of the diagnosis, epidemiology, treatment and control for these species are as for *C. annulata*.

Hartertia gallinarum

Predilection site: Small intestine, gizzard

Parasite class: Nematoda

Superfamily: Spiruroidea

Description, gross: Slender worms that are exceptionally long for a spiruroid. The males measure up to around 40 mm and the females 110 mm.

Description, microscopic: The gross appearance of the worms closely resembles that of *Ascaridia galli*; they have two lateral lips, each divided medially into three lobes. The male has lateral alae, ventral cuticular bosses, four pairs of pre-cloacal and two pairs of post-cloacal papillae. The left spicule is barbed and is larger than the blunt-ended right spicule. Eggs are thick-shelled, 45–53 × 27–33 μm and are embryonated when passed.

Final hosts: Chicken, bustards

Intermediate hosts: Termites

Life cycle: Typically spiruroid. Eggs are passed in faeces and, when ingested by a termite, develop to the infective stage in the body cavity. Following ingestion of an infected intermediate host the larvae develop to maturity in the final host in about 3 weeks.

Geographical distribution: Widespread in Europe, Africa and Asia. It is not found in the New World.

Pathogenesis: Infections are rarely fatal, but when large numbers of worms are present there may be inflammation of the intestine.

Clinical signs: Diarrhoea and emaciation may occur, often accompanied by a decrease in egg production.

Diagnosis: Differentiation of eggs in faeces is difficult as they are morphologically similar to those of other poultry spiruroids. Diagnosis is usually confirmed at necropsy.

Treatment: Not reported

Control: Where feasible, removal of termite nests from areas adjacent to runs used for poultry will be beneficial.

Tapeworms

Tapeworms are a feature of poultry which are reared on pasture, infection being acquired through ingestion of infected intermediate hosts, such as beetles, earthworms, ants, grasshoppers or flies. Infection is uncommon in intensive indoor systems as suitable intermediate hosts are usually absent. The most important and pathogenic species is *Davainea proglottina* which penetrates the duodenal mucosa and in young birds can induce a necrotic haemorrhagic enteritis which can be fatal. *Raillientina echinobothrida* is also pathogenic, inducing a hyperplastic enteritis and multiple caseous nodules where the scolex attaches to the wall of the intestine. Many other tapeworm species produce only mild symptoms, unless infections are heavy, when loss of productivity may be seen. Effective treatment of avian tapeworms is achieved with praziquantel, flubendazole, mebendazole, febantel or niclosamide. The dose rate and duration of administration varies between species of poultry. Control depends on the treatment of infected birds with a suitable anthelmintic and the destruction or removal of intermediate hosts where possible.

Davainea proglottina

Predilection site: Small intestine, particularly the duodenum

Parasite class: Cestoda

Family: Davaineidae

Description, gross: *D. proglottina* is a very small cestode up to 3–4 mm long, and unlike *Amoebotaenia*, usually possesses only four to nine segments (Fig. 7.5). Both the rostellum and suckers bear hooks.

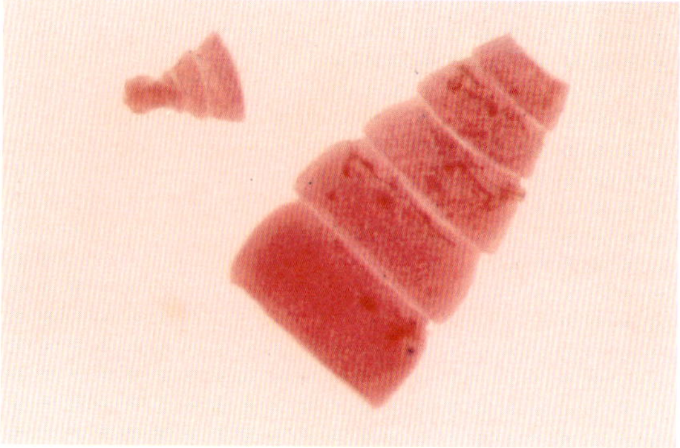

Fig. 7.5 *Davainea proglottina* adult.

Description, microscopic: The genital pores alternate regularly. Eggs measure about 30–40 µm and are found singly within the parenchymatous capsules in the gravid segment.

Final hosts: Chicken, turkey, pigeon and other gallinaceous birds

Intermediate hosts: Gastropod molluscs such as *Agriolimax*, *Arion*, *Cepaea* and *Limax*

Life cycle: Gravid proglottids are shed in faeces and eggs are ingested by various gastropod molluscs, in which they develop to the cysticercoid stage after about 3 weeks. Following ingestion of the mollusc by the final host, the cysticercoids develop into adult tapeworms in about 2 weeks.

Geographical distribution: Most parts of the world

Pathogenesis: This is the most pathogenic of the poultry cestodes, the doubly armed scolex penetrating deeply between the duodenal villi. Heavy infections may cause haemorrhagic enteritis, and light infections retarded growth and weakness.

Clinical signs: Moderate infections can lead to reduced weight gain, innapetance and lowered egg production. Large numbers of parasites may induce emaciation, dyspnoea and even be fatal.

Diagnosis: This is best achieved at necropsy through microscopic examination of mucosal scrapings from the duodenum and anterior small intestine. The tapeworm can easily be overlooked due to its minute size.

Pathology: The mucosal membranes are thickened and haemorrhagic with localised patches of necrosis. Fetid mucus may be present.

Epidemiology: Infection can be common in free-range fowl as suitable intermediate hosts are often available. Young birds tend to be more severely affected than older fowl.

Raillientina cesticillus

Synonym: *Skrjabinia cesticillus*

Predilection site: Small intestine

Parasite class: Cestoda

Family: Davaineidae

Description, gross: A medium-size tapeworm reaching around 10–14 cm in length, but often shorter.

Description, microscopic: The broad scolex is large and the rostellum wide. The unarmed suckers are not prominent and the rostellum is armed with several hundred small hammer-shaped hooks arranged in a double row. The gravid proglottids contain several, thin-walled egg capsules, each housing a single egg. Eggs measure approximately 75 × 90 μm.

Final hosts: Chicken, turkey, guinea fowl

Intermediate hosts: Various genera of beetles, including the families Carabidae, Scarabaeidae, Tenebrionidae, and the meal beetles, *Tribolium* spp.

Life cycle: Gravid proglottids are passed in faeces and eggs are ingested by various intermediate hosts. The embryo hatches from the egg in the intestine and then changes into a cysticercoid in the body cavity. Following ingestion by the final host the activated cysticercoid attaches to the mucosa of the anterior or mid small intestine. The prepatent period is around 2–3 weeks.

Geographical distribution: Worldwide

Pathogenesis: Heavy infections can induce a catarrhal enteritis.

Clinical signs: Reduction in growth rate. Heavy infection can lead to emaciation and weakness.

Diagnosis: This is best achieved at necropsy through microscopic examination of mucosal scrapings from the small intestine.

Pathology: In heavy infections, the embedded scolices of this parasite can produce caseous nodules in the wall of the small intestine.

Epidemiology: Young birds are usually more susceptible to infection than adults. Infection rates depend on the availability of the intermediate hosts. Beetles are numerous for free-range fowl but some beetles may also breed in litter bedding. Eggs are reasonably resistant to environmental conditions and will survive for several months.

Raillietina echinobothrida

Common name: Nodular tapeworm disease

Predilection site: Small intestine

Parasite class: Cestoda

Family: Davaineidae

Description, gross: *Raillietina echinobothrida*, which may be up to 25 cm in length, is similar in shape to *R. tetragona*. The suckers are circular and the rostellum is well endowed with two rows of hooks.

Description, microscopic: The gravid proglottids contain multiple fibrous-walled egg capsules, each housing several eggs. Eggs measure approximately 75 × 95 μm.

Final hosts: Chicken, turkey and other fowl.

Intermediate hosts: Ants of the genera *Pheidole* and *Tetramorium*

Life cycle: See *R. cesticillus*. The prepatent period is around 3 weeks.

Geographical distribution: Worldwide

Pathogenesis: A hyperplastic enteritis may occur at the site of attachment.

Pathology: *R. echinobothrida* is more pathogenic than either *R. cesticillus* or *R. tetragona*. In heavy infections, the embedded scolices of this parasite produce large caseous nodules in the subserous and muscular layers of the wall of the posterior small intestine.

Notes: The lesions in the intestine are similar to those associated with avian tuberculosis.

Raillietina tetragona

Predilection site: Posterior half of small intestine

Parasite class: Cestoda

Family: Davaincidae

Description, gross: A large tapeworm reaching around 20–25 cm in length. The scolex is smaller than that of *R. echinobothridia.*

Description, microscopic: The oval suckers are armed and the rostellum bears one or two rows of hooks (Fig. 7.6). The gravid proglottids contain multiple fibrous-walled egg capsules, each housing many eggs. Eggs measure approximately 65 × 90 μm. *R. tetragona* has a larger number of egg capsules in the gravid proglottid than either *R. cesticillus* or *R. echinobothrida*.

Final hosts: Chicken, guinea fowl and pigeon

Intermediate hosts: Ants of the genera *Pheidole* and *Tetramorium*

Life cycle: See *R. cesticillus*. The prepatent period is around 2–3 weeks.

Geographical distribution: Worldwide

Pathogenesis: In heavy infections, the embedded scolices of this parasite produce large caseous nodules in the wall of the small intestine

Pathology: *R. tetragona* is usually less pathogenic than either *R. echinobothrida* or *R. cesticillus*.

Cotugnia digonopora

Predilection site: Small intestine

Parasite class: Cestoda

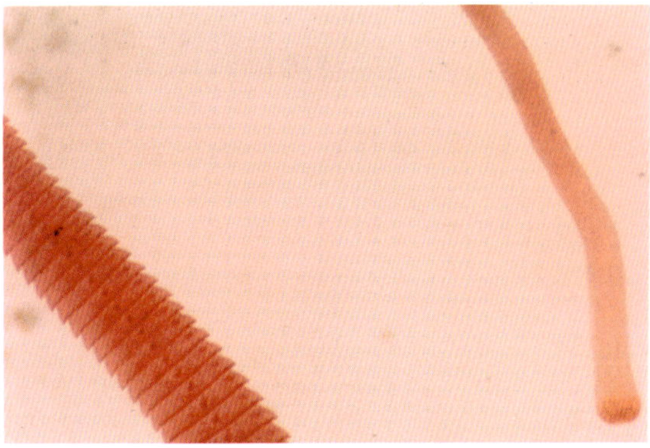

Fig. 7.6 *Raillientina tetragona*: scolex and proglottids.

Family: Davaineidae

Description, gross: The tapeworm is up to 110 mm long. The suckers are large, unarmed and the proglottids are wider than long.

Description, microscopic: The head is large with a small rudimentary retractile rostellum, which is armed with two rows of small hooklets. Segments possess a double set of genital organs.

Final host: Chicken

Life cycle: The life cycle is unknown.

Geographical distribution: Europe, Asia, Africa

Amoebotaenia sphenoides

Synonym: *Amoebotaenia cuneata*

Predilection site: Small intestine

Parasite class: Cestoda

Family: Dilepididae

Description, gross: A small tapeworm, up to 4.0 mm long, with up to 20 proglottids. It is roughly triangular in shape, although the last few segments decrease in size.

Description, microscopic: The rostellum bears a single row of 14 hooks.

Final hosts: Chicken

Intermediate hosts: Earthworms, particularly *Allolobrophora*, *Helodrilus*, *Ocnerodrilus* and *Pheretina* species

Geographical distribution: Most parts of the world

Pathogenesis: Generally considered to be of low pathogenic significance.

Choanotaenia infundibulum

Predilection site: Upper small intestine

Parasite class: Cestoda

Family: Dilepididae

Description, gross: A relatively large tapeworm up to around 20 cm in length and 1.5–3 mm in width. Each segment is wider posteriorly, giving the margin of the tapeworm a 'saw-edge' appearance.

Description, microscopic: The rostellum is ringed with about 18 slender hooks. The genital pores alternate regularly. Eggs measure about 45 × 55 µm and possess a long distinctive filament.

Final hosts: Chicken, turkey and several wild game birds

Intermediate hosts: The housefly, *Musca domestica*, beetles of the genera *Aphodius*, *Calathus*, *Geotrupes* and *Tribolium*, and grasshoppers

Geographical distribution: Most parts of the world

Metroliasthes lucida

Predilection site: Small intestine

Parasite class: Cestoda

Family: Dilepididae

Description, gross: The tapeworm is about 20 cm long and 1.5 mm wide.

Description, microscopic: The scolex has no rostellum or hooks and the suckers are devoid of spines.

Final hosts: Chicken, turkey

Intermediate hosts: Grasshoppers (*Chorthippus*, *Paroxya*, *Melanopus*)

Geographical distribution: North America, India, Africa

Hymenolepis carioca

Predilection site: Small intestine.

Parasite class: Cestoda

Family: Hymenolepididae

Description, gross: This is a slender thread-like tapeworm, reaching a length of up to 8 cm.

Description, microscopic: The scolex is unarmed.

Final hosts: Chicken, turkey and other fowl

Intermediate hosts: Dung and flour beetles and sometimes *Stomoxys* spp

Life cycle: The prepatent period is 3–4 weeks.

Geographical distribution: Most parts of the world, common in the USA

Pathogenesis: Usually considered to be of low pathogenicity.

Clinical signs: Large numbers of tapeworms may cause diarrhoea.

Hymenolepis cantaniana

Common name: Branching tapeworm

Predilection site: Small intestine

Parasite class: Cestoda

Family: Hymenolepididae

Description, gross: A slender tapeworm, reaching a length of up to 2 cm.

Final hosts: Chicken, turkey, pheasant, quail and other fowl

Intermediate hosts: Beetles (Scarabeidae)

Life cycle: The prepatent period is 3–4 weeks.

Geographical distribution: Most parts of the world, particularly Europe, Africa and the USA

Hymenolepis lanceolata

Synonym: *Drepanidotaenia lanceolatum*

Predilection site: Small intestine

Parasite class: Cestoda

Family: Hymenolepididae

Description, gross: This is a slender tapeworm, reaching up to 15–20 cm in length.

Description, microscopic: The proglottids are usually wider than they are long.

Final hosts: Duck and goose

Intermediate hosts: Aquatic copepod crustaceans

Life cycle: The prepatent period is 3–4 weeks.

Geographical distribution: Cosmopolitan

Pathogenesis: Heavy infections can be fatal.

Clinical signs: Large numbers of tapeworms may cause diarrhoea.

Pathology: Moderate to heavy infections can induce a catarrhal enteritis and necrosis of the mucosa.

Fimbriaria fasciolaris

Predilection site: Small intestine

Parasite class: Cestoda

Family: Hymenolepididae

Description, gross: The adult tapeworms measure up to about 4 cm in length by 1.5 mm in width.

Description, microscopic: The scolex possesses a 'pseudoscolex' (a folded expansion) for attachment to the host.

Final hosts: Chicken, duck, goose and wild anseriform birds

Intermediate hosts: Copepods (*Cyclops* and *Diaptomus* spp)

Intestinal flukes

Intestinal flukes are found in both the small and large intestines. The majority of avian intestinal trematodes parasitise aquatic fowl and birds and are of importance where birds forage in habitats that support the snail intermediate hosts.

Eggs passed in the faeces of infected birds hatch to produce a miracidium, which infects the first intermediate snail host. Subsequently cercariae encyst within the snail or are shed and migrate to infect other snails. Cercariae can also encyst in the kidneys of tadpoles and adult frogs. The final host is parasitised by ingesting the infected second intermediate host. The prepatent period is 1–2 weeks.

Large numbers of flukes can irritate the intestinal mucosa inducing a catarrhal, haemorrhagic enteritis and diarrhoea. Young birds are particularly susceptible to infection, showing progressive emaciation, and mortalities can be high. Various anthelmintics are available for treatment. Praziquantel or flubendazole, administered over several days, are effective in aquatic fowl. Niclosamide (not for geese) and fenbendazole are effective against Echinostomatidae.

Echinoparyphium recurvatum

Predilection site: Small intestine, particularly the duodenum

Parasite class: Trematoda

Family: Echinostomatidae

Description, gross: The fluke is about 4×0.7 mm and curved ventrally.

Description, microscopic: Spines are present anterior to the ventral sucker and the head-crown is armed with spines. Eggs measure about 110×82 μm.

Final hosts: Duck, goose, chicken and pigeon

Intermediate hosts: 1. Snails, such as *Lymnaea* spp and *Planorbis* spp. 2. Frogs, tadpoles, snails, such as *Valvata piscinalis* and *Planorbis albus*, freshwater clams and mussels

Geographical distribution: Worldwide, particularly Asia and North Africa

Pathogenesis: Heavy infections may induce weakness, anaemia and emaciation.

Pathology: A catarrhal enteritis is often present and the intestinal mucosa is oedematous.

Hypoderaeum conoideum

Predilection site: Posterior small intestine

Parasite class: Trematoda

Family: Echinostomatidae

Description, gross: The fluke measures around 7–12 mm in length and is up to 2 mm wide. The elongate body possesses spines in the anterior region and tapers towards the posterior.

Description, microscopic: The head-collar is small and armed with about 50 very small spines. Eggs measure about 102 × 65 μm.

Final hosts: Chicken, turkey, duck, goose, swan, pigeon and other aquatic birds

Intermediate hosts: As for *E. recurvatum*

Geographical distribution: Worldwide

Pathogenesis: Enteritis may occur where large numbers of flukes infect the intestine.

Other worms of the small intestine

Polymorphus boschadis

Synonym: *P. minutus*, *Echinorhynchus polymorphus*, *Profilicollis*

Common name: Thorny-headed worm

Predilection site: Small intestine

Parasite phylum: Acanthocephala

Family: Polymorphidae

Description, gross: Males measure around 3 mm and females up to 10 mm in length and are orange coloured when fresh. The anterior region possesses small spines and the cylindrical body has a constriction along its length, about one third from the head.

Description, microscopic: The proboscis has 16 rows of small hooks, their size increasing anteriorly. The spindle-shaped eggs have a thick middle shell and a thin outer shell, the embryo being slightly orange in colour. Eggs measure around 110 × 20 μm.

Final hosts: Duck, goose, chicken, swan and various wild aquatic birds

Intermediate hosts: Crustacean, *Gammarus pulex*, fresh water shrimp and sometimes the crayfish *Potamobius astacus*

Life cycle: The definitive host is infected following ingestion of an intermediate host that contains an infective cystacanth. The adult worm establishes in the posterior small intestine. The prepatent period is 3–4 weeks.

Geographical distribution: Worldwide

Pathogenesis: The worm produces inflammation of the intestinal mucosa and localised haemorrhages, which in heavy infection can induce anaemia.

Diagnosis: Identification of the characteristic eggs in faeces or the adult worms at necropsy.

Pathology: Worms use their armed proboscis to penetrate deep into the mucosa of the intestine and nodules frequently form at the point of attachment. Heavy infections can be fatal.

Filicollis anatis

Common name: Thorny-headed worm

Predilection site: Small intestine

Table 7.2 Intestinal flukes of the family Strigidae.

Parasite	Size (mm)	Predilection site	Definitive host	Intermediate host	Geographical location
Apatemon gracilis	2 × 0.5	Intestine	Duck, pigeon and wild birds	1. Snails 2. Various leeches	Europe, the Americas and Far East
Cotylurus spp	<1.5	Small intestine and rectum	Duck, pigeon and wild birds	1. Snails 2. Snails of the same or other species	Europe, Asia, Africa, North and South America
Parastrigea robusta	2–2.5	Intestine	Duck	?	Europe

Parasite phylum: Acanthocephala

Family: Polymorphidae

Description, gross: The whitish male is about 7 mm in length and the anterior region possesses many small spines. The ovoid proboscis is armed with 18 longitudinal rows of small hooks. The neck of the female worm is elongate, slender and bears a globular-shaped proboscis, the crown of which is armed with 18 rows of minute hooks in a star-shaped pattern.

Description, microscopic: The oval eggs measure approximately 65×20 μm.

Final hosts: Duck, goose, swan and wild aquatic birds

Intermediate hosts: Crustacean, isopod, such as *Asellus aquaticus*

Life cycle: The definitive host is infected following ingestion of an intermediate host that contains an infective cystacanth. The adult worm establishes in the mid to posterior small intestine. The prepatent period is about 4 weeks.

Geographical distribution: Worldwide

Pathogenesis: The worm produces inflammation of the intestinal mucosa and localised haemorrhages.

Clinical signs: Loss of weight, emaciation and, in heavy infections, death

Diagnosis: Identification of the characteristic eggs in faeces or the adult worms at necropsy

Pathology: Male worms penetrate into the mucosa of the intestine and nodules may occur at the point of attachment. The female penetrates deep into the wall of the intestine and often its proboscis is situated directly under the peritoneum, leading to rupture in severe cases.

Treatment and control: Details of the treatment and control are as for *P. boschadis*.

Coccidiosis in chickens

Seven species of *Eimeria* have been identified in chickens; identification is based on location in the intestine and associated pathology. Specific identification is based on the nature and location of the lesions in the intestine together with careful examination of fresh smears for the recognition of the development stages of the parasite.

Diagnosis

Diagnosis is best based on postmortem examination of a few affected birds. This can be made at microscopic level, either by examining the faeces for the presence of oocysts or by examination of scrapings or histological sections of affected tissues. Although oocysts may be detected on faecal examination, it would be wrong to diagnose solely on such evidence for two reasons. First, the major pathogenic effect usually occurs prior to oocyst production, and secondly, depending on the species involved, the presence of large numbers of oocysts is not necessarily correlated with severe pathological changes in the gut. At necropsy, the location and type of lesions present provide a good guide to the species that can be confirmed by examination of the oocysts in the faeces and the meronts and oocysts present in scrapings of the gut. A reliable species diagnosis based on oocyst morphology is not possible as the dimensions and other features overlap between species (see Table 15.11).

Species diagnosis is based on a combination of characteristics, including site of development in the intestinal tract, the type of macroscopic lesions and size of meronts in mucosal smears. The mature meronts may be identified histologically by their location, size and the number of merozoites they contain.

Table 7.3 Predilection sites and prepatent periods of *Eimeria* species in chickens.

Species	Predilection site	Prepatent periods (hours)
E. acervulina	Duodenum	89
E. brunetti	Lower small intestine, caeca, rectum	120
E. maxima	Mid small intestine	120
E. mitis	Small intestine, caeca, rectum	91
E. necatrix	Small intestine	138
E. praecox	Small intestine	84
E. tenella	Caeca	132

Epidemiology

The appearance and development of coccidiosis infections in poultry houses is dependent on a complex interplay of many factors. In fresh litter, few coccidia are present and there may be only a few oocysts scattered around. From the moment a few chicks are infected, rapid multiplication commences and a week later, new oocysts are excreted in large quantities. The infection usually begins to spread at full rate around the third or fourth week after housing. As exposure and immunity increases, the chicks will then gradually recover and withstand the infection. Rearing of thousands of birds on litter-covered floors in enormous houses may result in a tremendous and dangerous build-up of the oocyst population. Whether or not infection leads to the occurrence of disease outbreaks is to a great extent determined by the numbers of oocysts to which birds are exposed. Serious outbreaks of clinical coccidiosis with acute mortality are, however, highly exceptional in modern broiler farms because of the stringent monitoring and control measures employed. Where outbreaks do occur, clinical signs can be ascribed to one, or a combination of two or rarely three coccidial species. Management-related factors, such as stocking density, size of the farm, period of vacancy, quality of the litter, inadequate cleaning, ventilation system, presence of animals of different ages and what anticoccidials are used, will play an important part in influencing the numbers of oocysts that birds will be exposed to, and whether and to what extent the coccidiosis will develop. The occurrence and incidence of disease is also, to a great extent, affected by the type of chicks reared, breed sensitivities to infection, their initial health, acquired immunity and the interference of other diseases. The damaging nature and the location of the coccidia in the intestine will differ to such an extent that ultimately a complex and unique picture will develop on individual poultry farms. A change from litter-covered floors to wire-floored pens greatly reduces the exposure to coccidia. Outbreaks of coccidiosis in laying hens maintained in cages rarely occur. In general, the prophylactic use of anticoccidial drugs is not required if the cages are kept clean and the faeces do not contaminate watering and feeding systems.

Oocysts are disseminated via the faeces and the litter, with dust within the poultry buildings, inside and outside the house by invertebrates and vermin, whilst mechanical ventilation systems serve to scatter the oocysts outside the house. Faecal contamination of vehicles and personnel can spread the infection to other farms. Measures, such as thorough cleaning and disinfecting with oocidal agents, batch depopulation between grow-outs and admitting as few visitors as possible, are essential in order to maintain proper hygiene standards. Today most poultry enterprises rely on floor-rearing methods for broiler production or breeder flocks and use continuous medication programmes. Poultry producers also attempt to control coccidiosis by employing good sanitary programmes. Litters should be kept dry so that oocysts cannot sporulate. Wet litter must be cleaned out and replaced with dry litter. When broiler houses are emptied for a new batch of chickens the litter should be piled up for about 24 hours so that the heat generated can destroy the majority of oocysts. Disinfection is usually impractical since oocysts are resistant to disinfectants used against bacteria, viruses or fungi.

Treatment

This should be introduced as early as possible after a diagnosis has been made. Sulphonamide drugs have been the most widely used and it is recommended that these be given for two periods of 3 days in the drinking water, with an interval of 2 days between treatments. Where resistance has occurred to sulphonamides, mixtures of amprolium and ethopabate have given good results. Toltrazuril has been introduced for the treatment of outbreaks of coccidiosis and its use is restricted to where other treatments have been ineffective.

In the successful treatment of an outbreak of coccidiosis the aim is to treat birds already affected and at the same time allow sufficient merogonous development in the clinically unaffected birds to stimulate their resistance.

Control

Prevention of avian coccidiosis is based on a combination of good management and the use of anticoccidial compounds in the feed or water. Thus, litter should always be kept dry and special attention given to litter near water fonts or feeding troughs. Fonts that prevent water reaching the litter should always be used and they should be placed on drip trays or over the droppings pit. Feeding and watering utensils should be of such a type and height that droppings cannot contaminate them. Good ventilation will also reduce the humidity in the house and help to keep litter dry. Preferably, clean litter should always be provided between batches of birds. If this is not possible, the litter should be heaped and left for 24 hours after it has reached a temperature of 50°C; it should then be forked over again and the process repeated to ensure that all the oocysts in the litter have been destroyed.

The use of anti-coccidial agents depends on the type of management concerned. Broiler chicks are on lifetime-medicated feed and the anticoccidials used are maintained at a level sufficient to prevent merogony. The drugs available for use singly or in various combinations are amprolium, clopidol, diclazuril, ethopabate, halofuginone, lasalocid, maduramicin, monensin, narasin, nicarbazin, robenidine, salinomycin and sulphaquinoxaline. It is recommended that drugs are switched between batches of broilers, the so-called 'rotation programme', or within the lifespan of each batch, the 'shuttle programme'. Most drugs have a minimum period for which they must be withdrawn before the birds can be slaughtered for human consumption. This is usually 5–7 days.

Where replacement laying birds spend their whole life on wire floors, no medication is necessary; if they are reared on litter, for eventual production on wire, then a full level of coccidiostat is given as for broilers. If they are reared on litter, for production on litter, then a programme of anti-coccidials designed to stimulate immunity is used. Preparations frequently used either singly, or in combination, are amprolium, ethopabate, lasalocid, monensin and sulphaquinoxaline. The procedure is to administer these drugs in a decreasing level over the first 16 or 18 weeks of life. This may be done as a two-stage reduction, i.e. between 0 and

8 weeks and 8 and 16 weeks, or, alternatively, as a three-stage reduction, from 0–6 weeks, 6–12 weeks and 12–18 weeks. Using this technique, complete protection against coccidial challenge is maintained in the very young birds and the reduced drug rate in older birds allows limited exposure to developing coccidia so that acquired immunity can develop.

When in-feed coccidiostats are used, there are two further factors to consider. First, outbreaks of coccidiosis may occur in birds on medicated feed either because the level of coccidiostat used is too low or because conditions in the house have changed to allow a massive sporulation of oocysts, which, on ingestion, the level of drug can no longer control. Secondly, the influence of intercurrent infections in affecting appetite, and therefore uptake of coccidiostat, should also be considered.

In the USA, a live 'vaccine' consisting of oocysts of eight species of coccidia is commercially available. Young chicks are given the vaccine in the drinking water, and 10 days later a coccidiostat is introduced into the feed for a period of 3–4 weeks. Successful immunisation has also been achieved with oocysts attenuated by irradiation.

A live, attenuated, oral vaccine is available, as an alternative to coccidiostats, for the control of coccidiosis in chickens. This consists of selected 'precocious' strains of each of the pathogenic species of coccidia that affect poultry; these strains show rapid development *in vivo* with minimal damage to the intestine but stimulate an effective immunity. For success, both techniques depend on subsequent exposure to oocysts to boost immunity and this may not occur unless litter is sufficiently moist to allow sporulation. There is considerable interest in developing more efficient vaccines, in view of the increasing problem of drug resistance in coccidiosis. Various other vaccines have also become available in several countries using either live or attenuated strains of coccidia.

Intestinal coccidiosis

This form of the disease tends to be chronic and may be associated with several species of *Eimeria*. Mortality may not be heavy but morbidity may retard growth significantly. Usually more than one species is present. Specific identification is based on the nature and location of the lesions in the intestine together with careful examination of fresh smears for the recognition of the development stages of the parasite.

Eimeria acervulina

Predilection site: Duodenum (Fig. 7.7)

Parasite class: Sporozoasida

Family: Eimeriidae

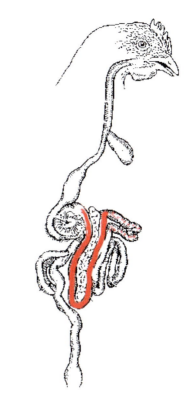

Fig. 7.7 Predilection site of *Eimeria acervulina.*

Description: Oocysts are ovoid, smooth 12–23 × 9–17 μm (mean 18 × 14 μm), without a micropyle or residuum but with a polar granule. The sporocysts are ovoid, with a Stieda body and without a residuum. First-generation meronts are 9–11 μm long and mature in 36–48 hours to produce 8–16 merozoites with a small residuum. Second-generation meronts mature in 41–56 hours to produce 16 merozoites with no residuum; third-generation meronts mature 56–72 hours after inoculation to produce eight merozoites with a residuum and fourth-generation meronts mature 80–96 hours after inoculation and produce 32 merozoites with a large residuum. The macrogamonts are 14.5–19 μm in diameter, and the microgamonts 7–8 μm. The latter produce many tri-flagellate microgametes 2–3 μm long.

Hosts: Chicken

Life cycle: The sporocysts emerge from the oocysts in the gizzard and the sporozoites are activated and emerge in the small intestine. Most enter the duodenum. The meronts are found in the epithelial cells of the villi of the anterior small intestine where they lie above the host nucleus. There are four merogony generations. The first-generation meronts lie at the base of the glands of the crypts of the duodenum.

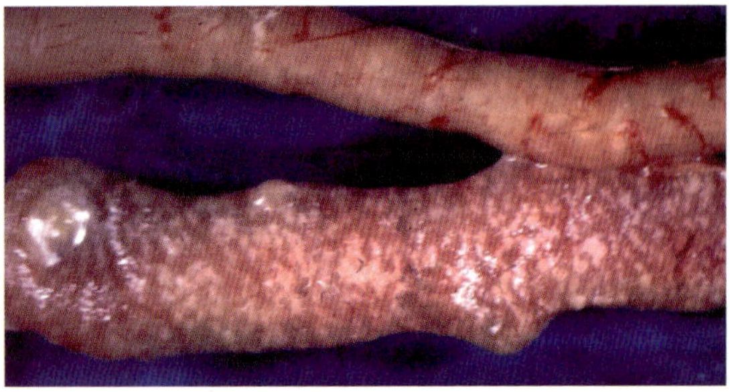

Fig. 7.8 Duodenal lesions of *Eimeria acervulina*.

Second-generation meronts are found at the neck of the glands, third-generation meronts lie at the base of the villi and fourth-generation meronts lie on the sides and the tips of the villi. The sexual stages are found above the host cell nuclei, in the epithelial cells of the villi and to a lesser extent in the gland cells, and are seen 4 days after infection and take 40 hours to mature. The prepatent period is 89 hours. The sporulation time is 24 hours.

Geographical distribution: Worldwide

Pathogenesis: The disease is usually chronic with birds showing poor weight gains but little mortality. Clinical disease occurs about 3 days following the ingestion of large numbers of oocysts.

Clinical signs: *E. acervulina* is generally considered to be moderately pathogenic, and heavy infections can cause severe signs and death. Symptoms include diarrhoea, dejection, ruffled feathers and drooping wings, inappetence, weight loss and depressed weight gain.

Pathology: The lesions in light infections consist of white transverse streaks in the duodenum and upper small intestine (Fig. 7.8). In heavier infections the lesions coalesce and the intestinal wall becomes thickened and congested with marked whitish mucoid exudate. Very large numbers of the characteristic small ovoid oocysts can be seen in smears from the duodenum and on histopathology (Fig. 7.9).

Lesions are scored +1 to +4 as follows:

1. Scattered, white plaque-like lesions containing developing oocysts confined to the duodenum. These lesions are elongated with the longer axis transversely orientated on the thickened intestinal walls like the rungs of a ladder. They may be seen from either the serosal or mucosal intestinal surfaces. The birds would not be affected clinically and weight gains would not be affected.
2. Lesions are much closer together but not coalescent and may extend below the duodenum in young birds. The intestinal walls are not thickened and the gut contents are normal. The birds would show a depression in weight gain.

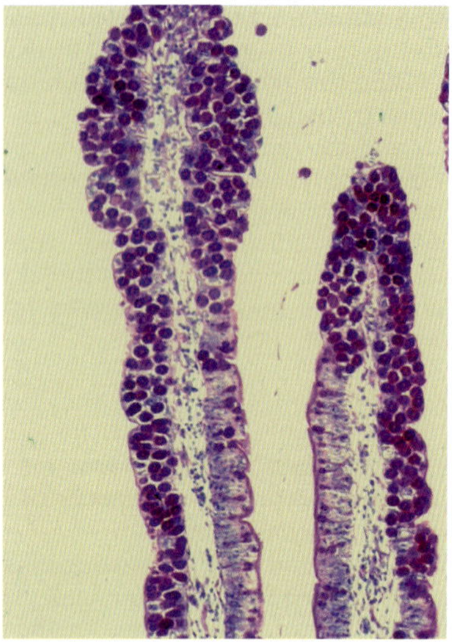

Fig. 7.9 Stages of *Eimeria acervulina* within enterocytes of small intestinal villi.

3. The lesions are clearly recognisable from the mucosal and serosal surfaces, are more numerous and beginning to coalesce. The intestinal wall is thickened and the intestinal contents are watery due to excessive mucus secretion. The birds have diarrhoea, and their weight gains are decreased.
4. The mucosal wall is greyish with colonies completely coalesced. In extremely heavy infections the entire mucosa may be bright red in colour. Individual lesions may be indistinguishable in the upper intestine. Typical ladder-like lesions appear in the middle part of the intestine. The intestinal wall is very much thickened, and the intestine is filled with a creamy exudate, which may contain numbers of oocysts. The birds show diarrhoea, severe weight loss, poor feed conversion and skin de-pigmentation.

Eimeria acervulina

Lesions: Whitish ladder-like streaks to coalescent plaques affecting mainly duodenum (Fig. 7.8).

Mean oocyst size (μm)	Shape and length:width index
18 × 14	Ovoid 1.25
Prepatent period (hours)	**Sporulation time (hours)**
89	24

Eimeria brunetti

Predilection site: Small and large intestine (Fig. 7.10)

Parasite class: Sporozoasida

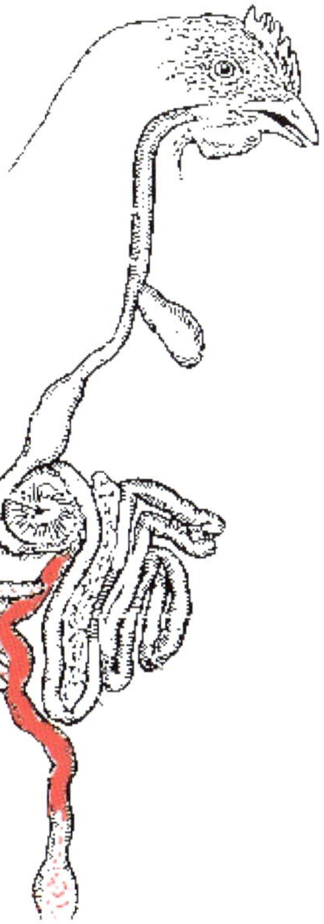

Fig. 7.10 Predilection site of *Eimeria brunetti*.

Family: Eimeriidae

Description: Oocysts are ovoid, smooth 14–34 × 12–26 μm (mean 26 × 22 μm), without a micropyle or residuum but with a polar granule. The sporocysts are ovoid (13 × 7.5 μm), with a Stieda body and a sporocyst residuum. First-generation meronts are 28 × 21 μm long and contain 318 merozoites. Second-generation meronts are smaller than first-generation meronts and contain 15–120 merozoites. The microgamonts contain several centres of microgamete development and are larger than the macrogamonts, which are 25 × 22 μm.

Host: Chicken

Life cycle: The first-generation meronts are found in the epithelial cells in the base of the villi in the mid intestine. There are at least three merogony generations. Second-generation meronts are found subepithelially at the tips of the villi in the lower small intestine 3 days post infection. Third-generation meronts are first seen at 84 hours, and mature by 4 days after infection and are located in the lower small intestine and large intestine. Gamonts are seen from day 5 at the tips and sides of the villi in the lower small intestine and large intestine, either above the host cell nuclei or on the basement membrane. The prepatent period is 120 hours.The sporulation time is 24–48 hours.

Geographical distribution: Worldwide

Pathogenesis: The pathogenicity of this species is high but mortality is variable. Lesions are most pronounced in the posterior small intestine.

Clinical signs: *E. brunetti* is markedly pathogenic, but its effects depend on the degree of infection. Light infections may be asymptomatic. Heavier infections reduce weight gain or cause weight loss. The birds develop fluid droppings containing blood-tinged mucus and mucous casts. The birds become depressed and deaths may occur. The symptoms continue for 5 days before recovery.

Pathology: The gut wall becomes thickened and a pink or blood-tinged catarrhal exudate appears 4–5 days after experimental inoculation. In early or light infections, haemorrhagic, ladder-like streaks are present on the mucosa of the lower small intestine and rectum. In heavy infections, a characteristic necrotic enteritis appears that may involve the entire intestinal tract, but which is more usually found in the lower small intestine, colon and tubular part of the caeca (Fig. 7.11). A patchy or continuous dry, caseous, necrotic membrane may line the intestine, and the intestine may be filled with sloughed, necrotic material. Circumscribed white patches may be visible through the serosa and there may be intestinal perforation with resultant peritonitis.

Lesions are scored +1 to +4 as follows:

1. Gross lesions are very distinct with some greying and reddening of the mucosal surfaces with a few petechiae visible from the serosal surface, appearing as pits on the mucosal surface.
2. Intestinal wall may appear grey in colour and the lower portion may be thickened with flecks of pinkish material sloughed from the intestine. More

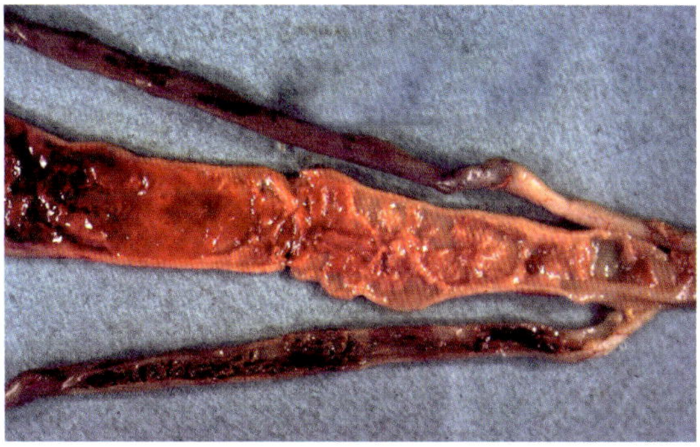

Fig. 7.11 Lesions of *Eimeria brunetti* in lower small intestine.

petechiae are present, with the greatest number appearing on day 5 after infection. They may appear as early as day 3.5 and occur from the yolk stalk posteriorly. Mild mucosal roughening can be detected by feel.

3. Intestinal wall thickened, and a blood-tinged exudate is present. Transverse streaks may be present in the lower rectum with lesions in the caecal tonsils. Weight gains and feed conversion are reduced.
4. Severe coagulative necrosis of the lower intestine can result in erosion of the entire mucosa. This is apparent as a thickening of the intestine wall and in some birds a dry necrotic membrane may line the intestine (pseudomembranous necrosis) and caseous cores may plug the caeca. Lesions may extend into the middle or upper intestine and the necrosis may be severe enough to cause intestinal obstruction and death of the bird.

Eimeria brunetti

Lesions: Coagulation necrosis and bloody enteritis in lower intestine (Fig. 7.11)

Mean oocyst size (μm)	Shape and length:width index
26 × 22	Ovoid 1.31
Prepatent period (hours)	Sporulation time (hours)
120	24–48

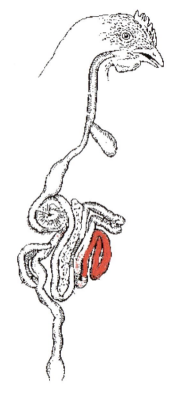

Fig. 7.12 Predilection site of *Eimeria maxima*.

Eimeria maxima

Predilection site: Small intestine (Fig. 7.12)

Parasite class: Sporozoasida

Family: Eimeriidae

Description: Oocysts are ovoid, yellowish and smooth 21–42 × 16–30 μm (mean 30 × 20 μm), without a micropyle or residuum but with a polar granule. Sporocysts are ovoid, 15–19 × 8–9 μm with a Stieda body and without a residuum. The sporozoites are 19 × 4 μm and each has a conspicuous clear globule.

Host: Chicken

Life cycle: The meronts are located above the host cell nuclei (or occasionally beside them) in the epithelial cells of the tips of the villi of the duodenum and upper ileum. There are three asexual generations. The first-generation meronts lie deep in the epithelial cells of the deep glands of the duodenum. They appear 48 hours after inoculation and contain 25–50 loosely packed merozoites. The second-generation meronts are in the epithelial cells of the small intestine villi near the openings of the crypts appearing on the third day after infection and produce about 12 merozoites. Third-generation meronts are in the epithelial cells along the sides of the superficial villi and sometimes near the tips, appearing during the fourth day after infection and produce about 12 merozoites. Gamonts are located below the host cell nuclei and as they enlarge, the host cells are displaced towards the centre of the villi and come to lie in their interior. After fertilisation, an oocyst wall is laid down and the oocysts break out of the villi and are passed in the faeces. The prepatent period is 120 hours. Sporulation time is 30–48 hours.

Geographical distribution: Worldwide

Pathogenesis: Strains of *E. maxima* differ in their pathogenicity, which can be very variable, but some strains can be responsible for high morbidity, and mortality may approach 25%. Lesions occur most frequently in the mid small intestine although the whole of the small intestine may be involved. Clinical disease occurs about 3 days following the ingestion of large numbers of oocysts. Asexual stages cause relatively little damage, with the most serious effects being due to the sexual stages.

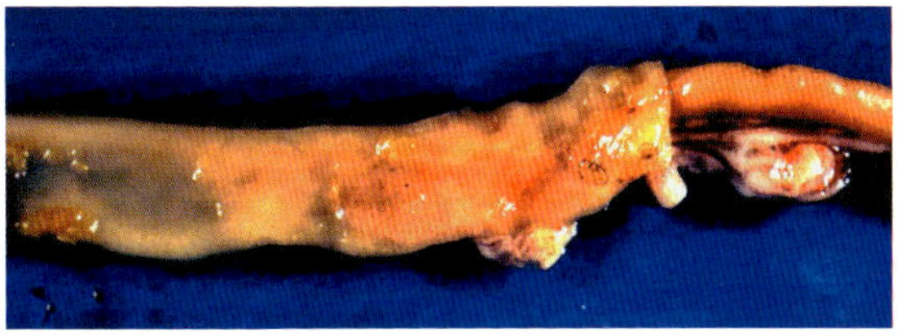

Fig. 7.13 Lesions of *Eimeria maxima*: mid small intestine.

Clinical signs: Symptoms include diarrhoea, depression, ruffled feathers, decreased growth rate or weight loss and, in some cases, death. Birds that recover soon return to normal.

Pathology: The principal lesions are haemorrhages in the mid small intestine. The intestinal muscles lose their tone and the intestine becomes flaccid and dilated with a somewhat thickened wall. There is catarrhal enteritis; the intestinal contents are viscid and mucoid, and are grey–brown or pink–orange in colour (Fig. 7.13). Occasionally there are blood flecks in the intestinal contents, but in heavy infections, haemorrhage may be pronounced and blood may pass into the caeca. Gametocytes or characteristic large yellowish oocysts may be seen in smears from the intestinal mucosa.

Lesions are scored +1 to +4 as follows:

1. Small red petechiae may appear on the serosal side of the mid-intestine surface on the 6th and 7th day of infection. There is no thickening of the intestine, although small amounts of orange mucus may be present. Birds show some weight loss and skin depigmentation.
2. Serosal surface may be speckled with numerous red petechiae. Intestine may be filled with orange mucus, little or no thickening of the intestine.
3. Intestinal wall is ballooned and thickened. The mucosal surface is roughened, intestinal contents filled with pinpoint blood clots and mucus.
4. The intestinal wall may be ballooned for most of its length and, greatly thickened, and contains numerous blood clots and digested red blood cells giving a characteristic colour and putrid odour.

Eimeria maxima

Lesions: thickened mid intestine with petechial haemorrhage and blood-tinged exudate (Fig. 7.13)

Mean oocyst size (μm)	Shape and length:width index
30 × 20	Ovoid 1.47
Prepatent period (hours)	**Sporulation time (hours)**
120	30–48

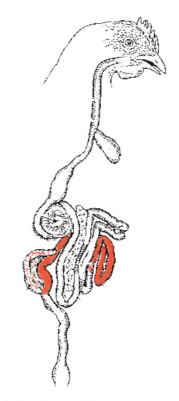

Fig. 7.14 Predilection site of *Eimeria mitis*.

Eimeria mitis

Predilection site: Small and large intestine (Fig. 7.14)

Parasite class: Sporozoasida

Family: Eimeriidae

Description: Oocysts are subspherical, smooth 10–21 × 9–18 μm (mean 16 × 15 μm), without a micropyle or residuum but with a polar granule. The sporocysts are ovoid, 10–16 μm, with a Stieda body and without a residuum. Merogony stages have not been described. The microgamonts are 9–14 μm in diameter, and the microgamonts somewhat larger.

Host: Chicken

Life cycle: The endogenous stages are in the epithelial cells of the villi and occasionally in the crypts of the small intestine; also caeca and rectum. The number of meront generations is unknown. Asexual and sexual stages occur together. The prepatent period is 91 hours. The sporulation time is 18–24 hours.

Geographical distribution: Worldwide

Pathogenesis: No discrete lesions are produced with this species, but infection can cause loss in body weight gain.

Clinical signs: Generally, older chickens are affected by the species found in the small intestine, and clinical signs are similar to those of caecal coccidiosis. Subclinical infections are more common than overt disease and may be suspected when pullets have poor rates of growth and feed conversion, and the onset of egg laying is delayed.

At postmortem examination, the site and severity of the lesions vary according to species and these are summarised in Table 15.10 together with the relevant oocyst morphology and sporulation times.

Pathology: Infection produces little pathology although there may be small petechiae in the lower small intestine and mucoid exudates in the lumen.

Eimeria mitis

Lesions: no discrete lesions, mucoid exudate

Mean oocyst size (μm) 16 × 15	Shape and length:width index Sub-spherical 1.09
Prepatent period (hours) 91	Sporulation time (hours) 18–24

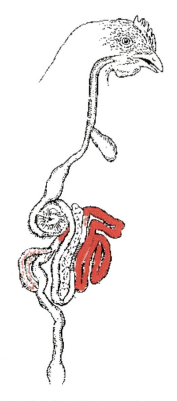

Fig. 7.15 Predilection site of *Eimeria necatrix*.

Eimeria necatrix

Predilection site: Small intestine (Fig. 7.15)

Parasite class: Sporozoasida

Family: Eimeriidae

Description: Oocysts are ovoid, smooth, colourless 12–29 × 11–24 μm (mean 20 × 17 μm), without a micropyle or residuum but with a polar granule. The sporocysts are ovoid, with a Stieda body and without a residuum.

Host: Chicken

Life cycle: Following ingestion of sporulated oocysts, and excystation, sporozoites enter the epithelial cells of the small intestine, pass through the epithelium into the lamina propria at the centre of the villi, and migrate towards the muscularis mucosae. Many sporozoites are engulfed by macrophages during this passage, and are transported to the epithelial cells of the fundus. The macrophages invade these cells and appear to disintegrate leaving the sporozoites unharmed. The sporozoites round up to form first-generation meronts found above the host cell nuclei in the epithelial cells of the crypts of the small intestine. Second-generation meronts develop deep in the mucosa. The prepatent period is 138 hours and the patent period is about 12 days. Sporulation time is 18–24 hours.

Geographical distribution: Worldwide

Pathogenesis: *E. necatrix* is one of the most pathogenic species of coccidia affecting chickens.

Clinical signs: Symptoms seen include diarrhoea (mucoid and sometimes bloody), dejection, ruffled feathers and drooping wings, inappetence, weight loss and depressed weight gain. Death usually occurs 5–7 days after infection, often before oocysts are passed in the faeces. Birds that recover often remain unthrifty and emaciated.

Pathology: The principal lesions are in the small intestine, especially the middle third. Small, white opaque foci are seen by the fourth day after infection. These are the second-generation meronts, and they are often so deep in the mucosa that they are most visible from the serosal surface. Severe haemorrhage may occur by day 5 or 6 and the small intestine may be markedly swollen and filled with clotted or unclotted blood. The wall is thickened, dull red and petechiae are present in the white foci as a result of release of the second-generation merozoites (Fig. 7.16). The gut

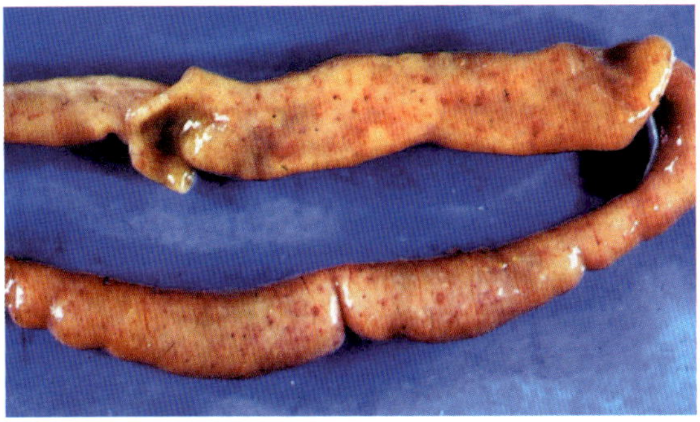

Fig. 7.16 Lesions of *Eimeria necatrix*: mid small intestine.

wall may lose its contractility, become friable, and the epithelium may slough and be replaced by a network of fibrin-containing mononuclear cells. This network is replaced by connective tissue resulting in permanent scarring, which interferes with intestinal absorption.

Lesions are scored +1 to +4 as follows:

1. The presence of small, scattered petechiae and white spots visible from the serosal surface.
2. Numerous petechiae on the serosal surface and some slight ballooning of the intestine.
3. Extensive haemorrhage into the lumen and the presence of red or brown mucus, extensive petechiae on the serosal surface, marked ballooning of the intestine and absence of normal intestinal contents.
4. Ballooning may be extensive and haemorrhage may give an intensive dark colour to the intestinal contents.

Eimeria necatrix

Lesions: ballooning intestine with white spots (meronts), petechiation and blood-filled exudate (Fig. 7.16)

Mean oocyst size (μm)	Shape and length:width index
20 × 17	Sub-spherical 1.19
Prepatent period (hours)	**Sporulation time (hours)**
138	18–24

Eimeria praecox

Predilection site: Small intestine (Fig. 7.17)

Parasite class: Sporozoasida

Family: Eimeriidae

Description: Oocysts are ovoid, smooth, colourless 20–25 × 16–20 μm (mean 21 × 17 μm), without a micropyle or residuum but with a polar granule. The sporocysts are ovoid, with a Stieda body and without a residuum.

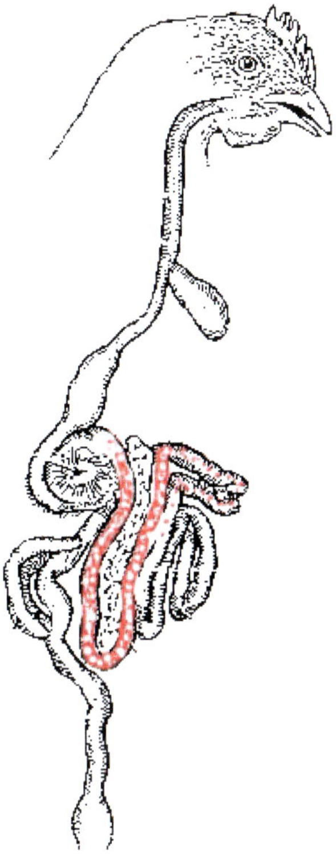

Fig. 7.17 Predilection site of *Eimeria praecox*.

Host: Chicken

Life cycle: The endogenous stages occur in the epithelial cells of the villi, usually along the sides of the villi, and lie below the host cell nucleus. There are at least three, and possibly four, generations of merogony. The second meront generation is seen as early as 36 hours after infection. Later development is irregular, and both asexual and sexual generations are seen together. The prepatent period is 84 hours and the patent period is approximately 4 days. The sporulation time is 48 hours.

Geographical distribution: Worldwide

Pathogenesis: *E. praecox* is considered to be non-pathogenic.

Clinical signs: No associated clinical signs

Pathology: A mucoid exudate is the only lesion seen. Endogenous stages can be detected in the wall of the small intestine by histopathology.

Eimeria praecox	
Lesions: no lesions, mucoid exudate	
Mean oocyst size (μm) 21 × 17	Shape and length:width index Ovoid 1.24
Prepatent period (hours) 84	Sporulation time (hours) 48

Coccidiosis in turkeys

Seven species of *Eimeria* have been identified in turkeys; identification is based on location in the intestine and associated pathology (Table 7.4). Specific identification is based on the nature and location of the lesions in the intestine together with careful examination of fresh smears for the recognition of the development stages of the parasite.

Diagnosis

Diagnosis is best based on postmortem examination of a few affected birds. The oocysts may be identified according to shape and size. At necropsy, the location and type of lesions present provide a good guide to the species, which can be confirmed by examination of the oocysts in the faeces and the meronts and oocysts present in scrapings of the gut.

Epidemiology

The appearance and development of coccidiosis is similar to that described for chickens. Acute infections with pathogenic species occur in young turkey poults 2–10 weeks of age, causing enteritis with variable mortality. Deep-litter houses offer optimal conditions of temperature and humidity for oocyst sporulation, and with overcrowding the risk of heavy infection is further increased.

Table 7.4 Predilection sites and prepatent periods of *Eimeria* species in turkeys.

Species	Predilection site	Prepatent period (hours)
E. adenoides	Lower small intestine, caeca	104–132
E. dispersa	Duodenum, upper small intestine	120–144
E. meleagridis	Caeca	144
E. meleagrimitis	Duodenum	144
E. gallapovonis	Ileum, rectum, caeca	144
E. innocua	Small intestine	120
E. subrotunda	Small intestine	96

Treatment

Anticoccidial drugs, such as lasolocid, monensin, robenidine, amprolium, ethopabate and clopidol/methylbenzoquate, can be used for prophylaxis by incorporating in the feed for the first 12–16 weeks of life. Low doses of anticoccidial drugs can be used to allow immunity to develop, particularly in breeding birds. Monensin should be used under veterinary guidance because of its greater toxicity for turkeys than for chickens.

Control

Prevention of turkey coccidiosis is based on a combination of good management and the use of anticoccidial compounds in the feed or water. Thus, litter should always be kept dry and special attention given to litter near water fonts or feeding troughs. Drinkers that prevent water reaching the litter should always be used and they should be placed on drip trays or over the droppings pit. Feeding and watering utensils should be of such a type and height that droppings cannot contaminate them. Good ventilation will also reduce the humidity in the house and help to keep litter dry. Preferably, clean litter should always be provided between batches of birds. If this is not possible, the litter should be heaped and left for 24 hours after it has reached a temperature of 50°C; it should then be forked over again and the process repeated to ensure that all the oocysts in the litter have been destroyed.

When in-feed coccidiostats are used, there are two further factors to consider. First, outbreaks of coccidiosis may occur in birds on medicated feed either because the level of coccidiostat used is too low or because conditions in the house have changed to allow a massive sporulation of oocysts, which, on ingestion, the level of drug can no longer control. Secondly, the influence of intercurrent infections in affecting appetite, and therefore uptake of coccidiostat, should also be considered.

Intestinal coccidiosis

As with coccidiosis in chickens more than one species is usually present in outbreaks of disease. Specific identification is based on the nature and location of the lesions in the intestine together with careful examination of fresh smears for the recognition of the development stages of the parasite.

Eimeria adenoides

Predilection site: Lower small intestine and caeca

Parasite class: Sporozoasida

Family: Eimeriidae

Description: Oocysts are ellipsoidal or ovoid, smooth, colourless 19–31 × 13–21 μm (mean 26 × 17 μm), with a micropyle, one to three polar granules but with no oocyst residuum. The sporocysts are elongate, with a Stieda body and a residuum and contain a clear globule at the large end. First-generation meronts are 30 × 18 μm when mature (after 30 hours) and contain approximately 700 merozoites, 4–7 × 1.5 μm, with a central nucleus. Second-generation meronts are 10 × 10 μm and produce 12–24 merozoites, 10 × 3 μm, with the nucleus slightly nearer the rounded end. The mature macrogamonts and microgamonts are 20 × 18 μm.

Host: Turkey

Life cycle: *E. adenoides* is found in the lower small intestine, caecae and rectum and has two generations of meronts. First-generation meronts can be seen in the epithelial cells as early as 6 hours after inoculation. Second-generation meronts mature 96–108 hours after inoculation. Sexual stages can be detected as early as 120 hours post infection. The prepatent period is 104–132 hours and the patent period 7–20 days. Sporulation time is 24 hours.

Geographical distribution: Worldwide

Pathogenesis: *E. adenoides* is one of the most pathogenic species of coccidia in turkeys. Clinical signs first appear 4 days after infection, coincident with the rupture of the second-stage meronts. Initially the intestines appear grossly normal until this point; thereafter, the walls of the lower third of the small intestine, caecae and rectum become swollen and oedematous, with petechial haemorrhages visible from the mucosal surface only. The lower intestine becomes filled with mucus. The infected epithelial cells break away, leaving the villi denuded. The blood vessels become engorged and cellular infiltration of the submucosa and epithelium increases progressively. In birds that recover from the disease, and in those that received a low infection, resolution is rapid. Vascularity is greatly reduced and the deep glands are almost free of parasites by the 7th day. The intestine is almost normal by the 9th or 10th day post infection.

Clinical signs: The affected poults are dull, listless, anorexic, stand with ruffled feathers and have their heads tucked under their wings. Their droppings are white and mucoid and may contain blood. Heavy infections can result in mortality.

Pathology: Most of the terminal intestine is congested and contains large numbers of merozoites and long streaks of blood. Caseous material, composed of cellular debris, gametes and a few immature oocysts, accumulates. With time, the caseous exudate is composed largely of oocysts. The faeces in severe cases are relatively fluid and may be blood-tinged and contain mucous casts 2.5–5 cm long. Caseous plugs may be present in the caecae. The terminal intestine may contain creamy white mucus, and petechiae may be present in the mucosa. As recovery proceeds, the intestinal contents appear normal but still contain large numbers of oocysts.

Eimeria dispersa

Predilection site: Duodenum and upper small intestine

Parasite class: Sporozoasida

Family: Eimeriidae

Description: Oocysts are ovoid, smooth, 22–31 × 18–24 μm (mean 26 × 21 μm), with no micropyle, polar granule or oocyst residuum. Sporocysts are ovoid and have a Stieda body.

First-generation meronts are 14 × 13 μm and contain an average of 19 merozoites; second-generation meronts are 8 × 7 μm and contain an average of 13.5 merozoites; third-generation are 9 × 9 μm and contain an average of 15 merozoites; whilst fourth-generation meronts are 12 × 10.5 μm and contain an average of seven merozoites. Mature macrogametes are 18–20 μm in diameter, with microgamonts slightly smaller.

Host: Turkey

Life cycle: First-, second-, third- and fourth-generation meronts are present 30, 48, 72 and 96 hours after infection respectively. Sporozoites and first-generation meronts lie close above the epithelial cell nuclei; second-, third- and fourth-generation meronts are also above the host cell nucleus, but lie near the brush border of the host cell. The mature macro- and microgamonts can be found in the small intestine villar epithelial cells 96 hours after infection. The prepatent period is 120–144 hours. Oocyst sporulation time is 48 hours.

Geographical distribution: Worldwide

Pathogenesis: A mildly pathogenic species that produces creamy, mucoid exudates in the small intestine of young turkeys and depressed weight gains.

Clinical signs: Diarrhoea, weight loss, ruffled feathers, droopiness and growth retardation

Pathology: With pathogenic strains, the most severe lesions occur 5–6 days after infection. The entire small intestine is markedly dilated, and the duodenum and anterior jejunum are creamy white when seen through the serosal surface. The anterior half of the small intestine is filled with creamy, yellowish, sticky, mucoid material. The wall of the anterior intestine is oedematous, but there is little epithelial sloughing. Recovery is rapid and the intestine appears virtually normal 8 days post infection.

Eimeria gallopavonis

Predilection site: Small and large intestine

Parasite class: Sporozoasida

Family: Eimeriidae

Description: Oocysts are ovoid, smooth, 22–31 × 18–24 µm (mean 26 × 21 µm), with no micropyle, polar granule or oocyst residuum. Sporocysts are ovoid and have a Stieda body.

First-generation meronts are 14 × 13 µm and contain an average of 19 merozoites; second-generation meronts are 8 × 7 µm and contain an average of 13.5 merozoites; third-generation are 9 × 9 µm and contain an average of 15 merozoites; whilst fourth-generation meronts are 12 × 10.5 µm and contain an average of seven merozoites. Mature macrogametes are 18–20 µm in diameter with microgamonts slightly smaller.

Host: Turkey

Life cycle: Endogenous stages occur in the epithelial cells at the tips of the villi lying above the host cell nucleus. The first-generation meronts occur in the ileum and rectum. There appear to be two sizes of second-generation meronts, with smaller ones occurring in the rectum and ileum, more rarely the caeca, and larger ones only in the rectum. A few third-generation meronts are found in the rectum producing 10–12 merozoites. These and second-generation meronts develop into gamonts found primarily in the rectum and occasionally, the ileum and caeca. The prepatent period is 144 hours. Oocyst sporulation time is 24 hours.

Geographical distribution: Worldwide

Pathogenesis: Reported to be moderately pathogenic

Clinical signs: Watery or mucoid diarrhoea, depression, ruffled feathers, anorexia

Pathology: This species is found in the ileum, rectum and less commonly the caeca. The intestine is inflamed and oedematous with soft white caseous material in the lumen.

Eimeria meleagrimitis

Predilection site: Duodenum

Parasite class: Sporozoasida

Family: Eimeriidae

Description: Oocysts are subspherical, smooth, colourless 16–27 × 13–22 µm (mean 19 × 16 µm), with no micropyle or oocyst residuum, but with one to three polar granules. The sporocysts are ovoid, with a Stieda body and a residuum and contain a clear globule at the large end. First-generation meronts are 17 × 13 µm when mature (after 48 hours) and contain approximately 80–100 merozoites, 4.5 × 1.5 µm, with a nucleus at the larger end. Second-generation meronts are 8 × 7 µm and produce 8–16 merozoites, 7 × 1.5 µm, with the nucleus slightly near the centre. Third-generation meronts are the same size as the second-generation meronts but differ in possessing a residuum and have a nucleus nearer the large end. The mature macrogamonts and microgamonts are 15 × 11 µm and the macrogamonts contain a residuum.

Host: Turkey

Life cycle: The sporocysts emerge from the oocysts in the gizzard and the sporozoites are activated and emerge from the sporocysts in the small intestine. The sporozoites invade the tips of the villi and migrate down the villi in the lamina propria until they reach the glands. First-generation meronts can be found in the gland epithelial cells as early as 12 hours after infection and are mature by 48 hours. The first-generation merozoites invade the adjacent epithelial cells forming colonies of second-generation meronts that mature at about 66 hours after infection. Third-generation meronts may appear as early as 72 hours after inoculation and are mature by 96 hours. Macrogametes and microgamonts appear 114 hours after infection. The prepatent period is 144 hours. Oocyst sporulation time is 24–72 hours.

Geographical distribution: Worldwide

Pathogenesis: *E. meleagrimitis* is moderately to markedly pathogenic and has three generations of merogony with disease occurring following the rupture of the third-stage meronts, at about 4 days after infection. It is usually located in the small intestine anterior to the yolk stalk, but may extend throughout the intestine.

Clinical signs: Disease is seen in turkey poults 2–10 weeks of age and rarely in older birds because of acquired immunity. The affected poults are dull, listless, stand with ruffled feathers and have their heads tucked under their wings. Feed consumption drops following infection and affected birds are huddled together with closed eyes, drooping wings and ruffled feathers. Their droppings are white and mucoid and, at the peak of the disease, intestinal cores may be passed and the faeces may contain a few flecks of blood. Death occurs 5–7 days after infection, particularly in young poults under 6 weeks old.

Pathology: Lesions are seen from the end of the 4th day after infection. The jejunum is slightly thickened, dilated and contains an excessive amount of clear, colourless fluid, or mucus containing merozoites, small amounts of blood and other cells. By days 5–6 after infection, the duodenum is enlarged and its blood vessels are engorged. It contains a reddish brown, necrotic core that is firmly adherent to the mucosa and extends a little way into the upper small intestine. The remainder of the intestine is congested and petechial haemorrhages may be present in the mucosa of most of the small intestine. The mucosa begins to regenerate on the 6th or 7th day after infection. A few petechiae are present in the duodenum and jejunum. There are small streaks of haemorrhage and spotty congestion in the ileum. The posterior part of the jejunum and ileum may contain greenish, mucoid casts, 5–10 cm long and 3–6 mm in diameter. Necrotic material may be found in the ileum or faeces.

The following two non-pathogenic species of coccidia in turkeys are uncommon.

Eimeria innocua

Predilection site: Small intestine

Parasite class: Sporozoasida

Family: Eimeriidae

Description: Oocysts are subspherical, smooth, 16–26 × 17–25 μm (mean 22 × 21 μm), without a micropyle or polar granules.

Hosts: Turkey

Life cycle: Endogenous stages occur in the epithelial cells at the tips of the villi, which are heavily parasitised. The prepatent period is 120 hours and patency is 9 days. The sporulation time is 48 hours.

Geographical distribution: North America, Bulgaria

Eimeria subrotunda

Predilection site: Small intestine

Parasite class: Sporozoasida

Family: Eimeriidae

Description: Oocysts are subspherical, smooth, 16–26 × 14–24 μm (mean 22 × 20 μm), without a micropyle or polar granules.

Host: Turkey

Life cycle: Endogenous stages occur in the epithelial cells at the tips of the villi, extending along the side of the villi to some extent. The prepatent period is 96 hours and patency is 12–13 days. The sporulation time is 48 hours.

Geographical distribution: North America

Coccidiosis in ducks and geese

Eimeria anseris

Predilection site: Small and large intestine

Parasite class: Sporozoasida

Family: Eimeriidae

Description: Oocysts are small and pear-shaped, with a truncated cone, smooth, colourless, 16–24 × 13–19 μm (mean 21 × 17 μm), with a micropyle, and without a polar granule but with a residuum just beneath the micropyle. Sporocysts are ovoid and almost completely fill the oocysts, 8–12 × 7–9 μm, with a slightly thickened wall at the small end and with a residuum. Mature meronts are 12 × 20 μm and contain approximately 15–25 merozoites. The macrogametes are usually spherical and 12–26 × 10–15 μm. The microgamonts are 12–66 × 8–18 μm.

Hosts: Domestic goose, blue goose (*Anser caerulescens*), Richardson's Canada goose (*Branta canadensis hutchinsi*)

Life cycle: The life cycle is typically coccidian although precise details of the life cycle are lacking. There appears to be only one merogony generation. Endogenous stages occur in compact clumps under the intestinal epithelium near the muscularis mucosa and also in the epithelial cells of the villi of the small intestine, and in heavy infections also in the caeca and rectum. The gamonts are mostly in the subepithelial tissues but invade the epithelium in heavy infections. The prepatent period is 6–7 days and patent period 2–8 days.

Geographical distribution: Europe

Pathogenesis: There is comparatively little information on coccidiosis of ducks and geese. *E. anseris* has been reported as causing acute intestinal coccidiosis with haemorrhage in goslings.

Clinical signs: Diarrhoea with mucus and haemorrhage

Diagnosis: Diagnosis is best based on postmortem examination of a few affected birds. At necropsy the location and type of lesions present provide a good guide to the species, which can be confirmed by examination of the oocysts in the faeces and the meronts and oocysts present in scrapings of the gut.

Pathology: There may be intestinal hyperaemia, mucus production with flecks of coagulated blood within the gut lumen. Oocysts are found in small discrete papilliform lesions.

Epidemiology: *E. anseris* occurs in young birds and is associated with birds that are kept under intensive conditions.

Treatment: Little is known about treatment, but by analogy with other hosts, one of the sulphonamide drugs should be tried.

Control: Prevention is based on good management, avoidance of overcrowding and stress, and attention to hygiene. Contact with wild geese should be avoided wherever possible.

Eimeria nocens

Predilection site: Small intestine

Parasite class: Sporozoasida

Family: Eimeriidae

Description: Oocysts are ellipsoidal or ovoid, thick-walled, brown, 25–33 × 17–24 μm (mean 29 × 20 μm), with a distinct micropyle, which is covered by the outer layer of the oocyst wall. Mature meronts are 15 × 30 μm and contain approximately 15–35 merozoites. The macrogametes are usually ellipsoidal or irregularly spherical and 20–25 × 16–21 μm. The microgamonts are spherical or ellipsoidal and 28–36 × 23–31 μm.

Hosts: Domestic goose, blue goose (*Anser caerulescens*)

Life cycle: Precise details of the life cycle are lacking. Developmental stages occur in the epithelial cells of the tips of villi at the posterior part of the small intestine but may also occur beneath the epithelium. The younger developmental stages lie near the host cell nuclei, and as they grow they displace the nuclei and eventually destroy the cell and come to lie free and partly beneath the epithelium. The prepatent period is 4–9 days.

Geographical distribution: Europe, North America

Pathogenesis: *E. nocens* has been reported as causing acute intestinal coccidiosis in goslings.

Clinical signs: Diarrhoea with mucus and flecks of blood

Diagnosis: As for *E. anseris*

Pathology: There may be intestinal hyperaemia and mucus production with small flecks of coagulated blood within the gut lumen.

Epidemiology: *E. nocens* occurs in young birds and is associated with birds that are kept intensively under conditions which offer optimal conditions of temperature and humidity for oocyst sporulation. Overcrowding further exacerbates infection levels and risks from disease.

Treatment and control: As for *E. anseris*

Tyzzeria perniciosa

Predilection site: Small intestine

Parasite class: Sporozoasida

Family: Eimeriidae

Description: Oocysts are ellipsoidal, colourless, 10–13 × 9–11 μm (mean 12 × 10 μm), without a micropyle and with a residuum. First-generation meronts are 12 × 8 μm and contain only a few merozoites. Further meront generations are 15–16 × 14–15 μm and contain more and larger merozoites.

Hosts: Domestic duck, pintail duck, diving duck (*Aythya erythropus*)

Life cycle: The life cycle is typically coccidian and there appear to be at least three merogony generations. The endogenous stages are in the mucosal and submucosal cells of the small intestine. The prepatent period is 5 days. Oocyst sporulation time is 1 day.

Geographical distribution: Presumed worldwide

Pathogenesis: *T. perniciosa* is highly pathogenic for ducklings. Infected birds stop eating, lose weight and become weak; there can be a high mortality.

Clinical signs: Anorexia, diarrhoea with mucus and haemorrhage

Diagnosis: Diagnosis is best based on postmortem examination and by examination of the oocysts in the faeces. Masses of very small rounded oocysts are present in smears and scrapings of the gut.

Pathology: On postmortem, inflammation and haemorrhagic areas are seen throughout the small intestine and especially in the upper part of the intestine. The intestinal wall is thickened and round white spots are visible through the serosal surface. In severe cases, the lumen is filled with blood and often cheesy exudates. The intestinal epithelium sloughs off in long pieces often forming a lifting 'tube'.

Treatment and control: As for *E. anseris*

Eimeria anatis

Predilection site: Small intestine

Parasite class: Sporozoasida

Family: Eimeriidae

Description: Oocysts are ovoid, smooth, colourless, 14–19 × 11–16 μm (mean 17 × 14 μm), with thickened ring-forming shoulders around the micropyle, and without a polar granule or residuum. Sporocysts are ovoid or ellipsoidal, with a slight thickening at the small end and with a few residual granules.

Hosts: Duck and wild mallard (*Anas platyrhynchos*)

Life cycle: The life cycle has not been described.

Geographical distribution: Europe (Germany, Russia and CIS states)

Pathogenicity: Unknown

Tyzzeria anseris

Synonym: *Tyzzera parvula*

Predilection site: Small intestine

Parasite class: Sporozoasida

Family: Eimeriidae

Description: Oocysts are ellipsoidal, colourless, 10–16 × 9–14 μm without a micropyle or residuum.

Hosts: Domestic goose, Canada goose and other wild geese

Geographical distribution: Worldwide

Coccidiosis in gamebirds

Pheasants

The development of intensive management systems by pheasant-rearing farms has led to an increase in coccidiosis. The significance of coccidiosis in wild pheasants is difficult to assess because natural predators and scavengers deal promptly with weak or dead birds. Treatment with clopidol, lasalocid, amprolium or potentiated sulphonamides (sulphaquinolaxaline or sulphadimidine) is generally effective, although specific efficacy data are lacking.

Apart from the usual measures of isolation and rigorous hygiene, the use of preventive medication in intensively reared pheasants provides a means of controlling the disease where outbreaks occur.

Eimeria colchici

Predilection site: Caeca

Parasite class: Sporozoasida

Family: Eimeriidae

Description: Oocysts are elongate, ellipsoidal with one side less rounded than the other, colourless, 19–33 × 11–21 (mean 27 × 17 μm) with an inconspicuous micropyle, a polar granule but no oocyst residuum (Fig. 7.18). Sporocysts are elongate, 11.5–15.5 × 6–7.5 (mean 14.6 × 6.6 μm). Sporozoites are arranged head to tail in the sporocysts and possess a single large refractive globule. First-generation meronts are 18 × 13 μm and contain 50–100 elongate merozoites; second-generation meronts are 28 × 21 μm and contain large numbers of merozoites and third-generation meronts measure 8.5 × 7 μm and contain on average 19 merozoites.

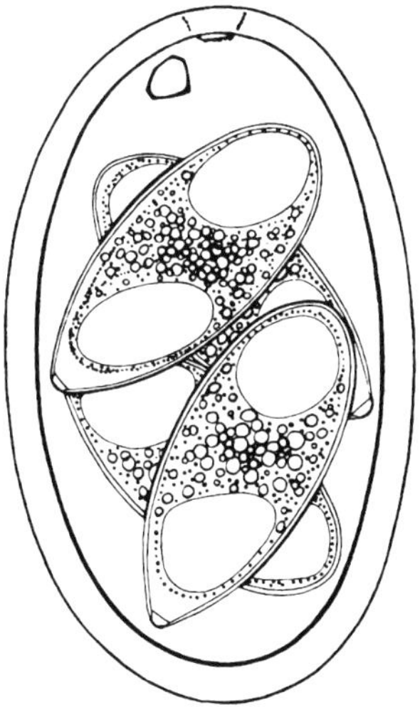

Fig. 7.18 Oocyst of *Eimeria colchici*.

Life cycle: The life cycle is typically coccidian. First-generation meronts are found deep in the glands of the mucosal lining of the mid small intestine; second-generation meronts appear in colonies in the lamina propria at the base of the villi; small third-generation meronts develop in the glands of the caeca. The gametocytes develop in the epithelial cells lining the caecal mucosa. The prepatent period is 6 days. Sporulation time is 2 days.

Geographical distribution: USA, Europe (UK, Bulgaria, Czech Republic, Slovakia)

Pathogenesis: *E. colchici* is the most pathogenic species of coccidia in pheasants, producing weight loss and mortality in infected birds.

Clinical signs: Diarrhoea and white soiling around the vent

Diagnosis: Postmortem examination of affected birds reveals the characteristic white cores and examination of scrapings or histological sections of affected tissues shows large numbers of gametocytes in the caeca. On faecal examination there are large numbers of oocysts in a white caseous exudate (Fig. 7.19).

Pathology: There is hyperaemia and mucoid enteritis in the small intestine caused by the second-generation meronts. Dead birds have soft white cores in the caeca and lower small intestine. In the caeca there is extensive invasion of the mucosa by gametocytes with the entire epithelium and subepithelial cells of the lamina propria infected. The cores are composed of oocysts, necrotic debris and food material.

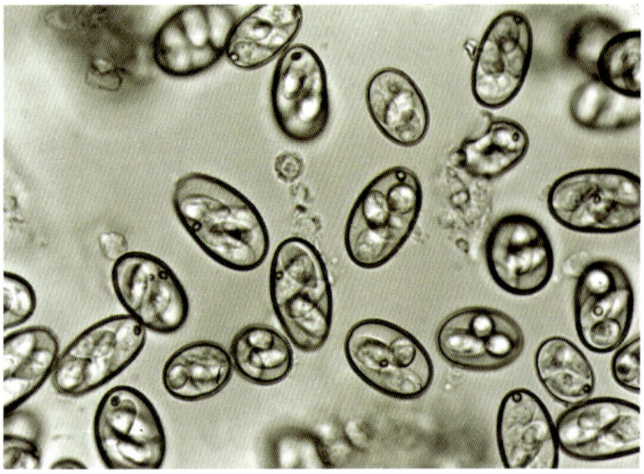

Fig. 7.19 Oocysts of *Eimeria colchici* found on faecal examination.

Eimeria duodenalis

Predilection site: Small intestine

Parasite class: Sporozoasida

Family: Eimeriidae

Description: Oocysts are subspherical to broadly ellipsoidal, smooth, colourless to pale yellowish brown, 18–24 × 15.4–21.4 μm (mean 21.2 × 18.6 μm), with no micropyle and no oocyst residuum (Fig. 7.20). The ellipsoidal sporocysts measure 11.6–13.6 × 6.1–6.8 μm (mean 12.6 × 6.7 μm). There is a small Stieda body and a larger sub-Stieda body. The sporocyst residuum largely obscures the sporozoites, which possess a large refractile body and occasionally a second smaller one.

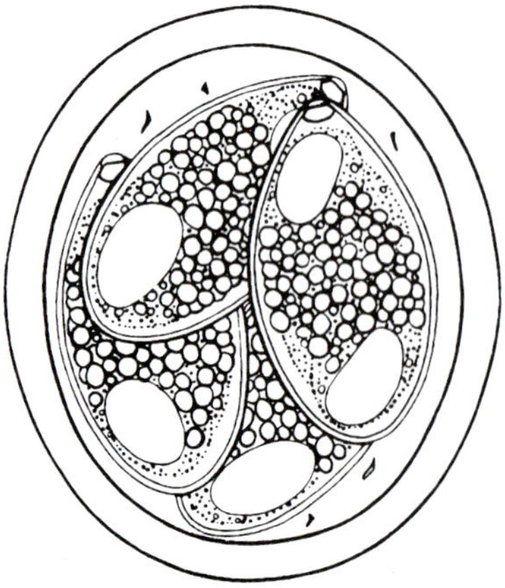

Fig. 7.20 Oocyst of *Eimeria duodenalis*.

Life cycle: First-generation meronts appear in the epithelial cells towards the tips of the duodenal villi. Second- and third-generation meronts follow on quickly in the same site but extending further along the intestinal tract. Gametocytes and third-generation meronts are both present together, and the infection may extend throughout the entire small intestine with the villi heavily parasitised, and multiple infection of individual epithelial cells occurring frequently. The prepatent period is 5 days. Sporulation time is 1–2 days.

Geographical distribution: Europe (UK, France, Lithuania, Kazakhstan), USA

Pathogenesis: As the specific name implies, this parasite develops in the duodenum and upper small intestine where it can cause a mucoid enteritis.

Clinical signs: Light infections are generally asymptomatic but heavier infections may cause a mucoid enteritis.

Diagnosis: Postmortem examination of affected birds reveals a mucoid enteritis in the duodenum and upper small intestine and examination of scrapings or histological sections of affected tissues shows large numbers of small subspherical oocysts in the small intestine.

Pathology: The intestines of the birds that die are congested and contain a pinkish mucoid exudate, whilst the caeca may be distended with a foamy yellow fluid. Scrapings from the small intestine show masses of small subspherical oocysts.

Epidemiology: Coccidiosis in pheasants occurs most frequently in young birds reared under intensive conditions. Disease surveys carried out in the UK showed that *E. duodenalis* accounted for 10–15% of the coccidiosis cases where species identification was possible.

Eimeria megalostoma

Predilection site: Unknown

Parasite class: Sporozoasida

Family: Eimeriidae

Description: Oocysts are ovoid, yellowish brown, 24 × 19 μm with a thick oocyst wall and prominent micropyle.

Life cycle: Not described

Geographical distribution: North America, UK, Kazakhstan

Pathogenesis: No information available. Occurs only rarely in small numbers and has not been associated with outbreaks of disease.

Clinical signs: Not reported

Diagnosis: Diagnosis is based on oocyst morphology from faecal samples. Where possible, postmortem examination of affected birds and examination of scrapings or histological sections of affected tissues should be undertaken.

Pathology: Not described.

Epidemiology: The significance of coccidiosis in wild pheasants is difficult to assess because natural predators and scavengers deal promptly with weak or dead birds.

Eimeria pacifica

Predilection site: Small intestine, caeca

Parasite class: Sporozoasida

Family: Eimeriidae

Description: Oocysts are ovoid, 17–26 × 14–20 μm with a mammilated oocyst wall.

Life cycle: The life cycle is typically coccidian. Endogenous stages have been reported to occur in the epithelial cells of the duodenum but have also been reported in the caeca.

Geographical distribution: North America, Kazakhstan, Lithuania

Pathogenesis: Infection produces mucoid enteritis with low mortality but high morbidity

Clinical signs: Mucoid diarrhoea

Diagnosis: Postmortem examination of affected birds reveals a mucoid enteritis and examination of scrapings or histological sections of affected tissues shows large numbers of small sub-spherical oocysts in the small intestine and caeca.

Pathology: Not described

Epidemiology: As for other species of coccidia

Eimeria phasiani

Predilection site: Small and large intestine

Parasite class: Sporozoasida

Family: Eimeriidae

Description: Oocysts are ellipsoidal, smooth, yellowish, 20.1–30.9 × 13.4–20.5 μm (mean 25 × 17 μm), with no micropyle and no oocyst residuum, but with one to three polar granules. Sporocysts are elongate, pyriform, each with a prominent Stieda body, 12.9–15.9 × 5.6–7.4 μm (mean 14.3 × 6.7 μm). Sporozoites contain a single refractile body.

Life cycle: Development of the endogenous stages occurs in the small intestine and there is a gradual spread down the gut as the infection proceeds. First-generation meronts develop in the epithelial cells lining the glands of the ascending duodenum and the upper small intestine. Second-generation meronts are most numerous towards the tips of the villi in the upper small intestine. Third-generation meronts and gametocytes are found throughout the small intestine and also in the proximal part of the caeca, being most numerous towards the tips of the villi.

The prepatent period is 5 days. Sporulation time is 2 days.

Geographical distribution: Europe (UK, France, Germany, Czech Republic, Slovakia, Lithuania, Kazakhstan), USA

Pathogenesis: Mortality can reach 50% in 2- or 3-week-old pheasants.

Clinical signs: Infection can result in anorexia, depression and a reduction in weight gain and in heavy infections causes liquid faeces with mucus and a little blood.

Diagnosis: Postmortem examination of affected birds reveals a mucoid enteritis and examination of scrapings or histological sections of affected tissues shows large numbers of gametocytes in the small intestine and proximal part of the caeca.

Pathology: The main lesions consist of mucoid enteritis in the small intestine. The intestines of heavily infected birds are hyperaemic and show petechial haemorrhages, whilst the lumen may be filled with blood-streaked mucus (Fig. 7.21). The developmental stages of *E. phasiani* occur below the nucleus of the host cell, causing 'ballooning' of the infected cell with enlargement of the nucleus. Oocysts occur throughout the small intestine and in the proximal part of the caeca.

Epidemiology: Coccidiosis in pheasants occurs most frequently in young birds reared under intensive conditions.

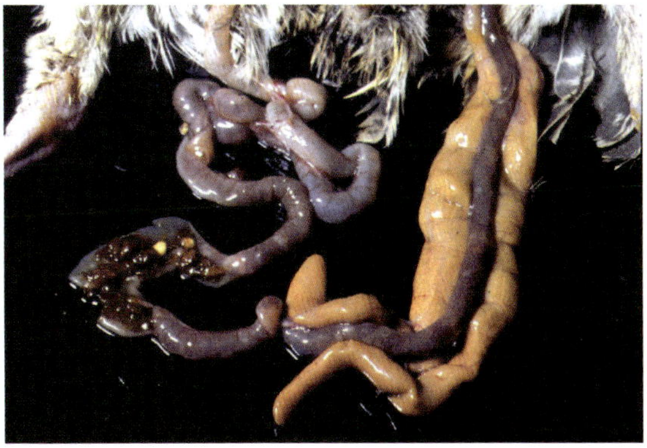

Fig. 7.21 Caecal lesions of *Eimeria phasiani*.

Disease surveys carried out in the UK showed that *E. phasiani* accounted for approximately 15% of the coccidiosis cases where species identification was possible. In studies conducted in the Czech Republic/ Slovakia, *E. phasiani* occurred less frequently than *E. colchici* in wild pheasants but was most prevalent during the winter and spring when it was identified in 18–41% of the samples examined.

Partridge

Several species of coccidia have been described in partridge, based mainly on oocyst morphology. Details on life cycle, pathogenesis, treatment and control are lacking. Prevention, as with other hosts, should be based on good management, avoidance of overcrowding and stress, and attention to hygiene.

Eimeria caucasica

Predilection site: Unknown

Parasite class: Sporozoasida

Family: Eimeriidae

Description: Oocysts elongate, rarely ovoid, 25–36 × 14–21 μm (mean 33 × 19 μm).

Hosts: Rock partridge (*Alectoris graeca*)

Geographical distribution: Eastern Europe, Kazakhstan

Notes: Thought to be a *nomen nudum* (fails to qualify as a valid scientific name because of an inadequate description).

Eimeria procera

Predilection site: Unknown

Parasite class: Sporozoasida

Family: Eimeriidae

Description: Oocysts elongate–ellipse, 28–31 × 16–17 μm (mean 29.5 × 16.5 μm).

Hosts: Grey partridge (*Perdix perdix*)

Geographical distribution: Unknown

Eimeria koifoidi

Predilection site: Small intestine

Parasite class: Sporozoasida

Family: Eimeriidae

Description: Oocysts ovoid, 16–25 × 14–20 μm (mean 20 × 18 μm)

Hosts: Grey partridge (*Perdix perdix*), Chukar partridge (*Alectoris chukar*), Rock partridge (*Alectoris graeca*)

Geographical distribution: Unknown. Reported in UK and Bulgaria.

Eimeria legionensis

Predilection site: Small intestine

Parasite class: Sporozoasida

Family: Eimeriidae

Description: Oocysts elliptic, almost symmetrical, sometimes slightly flattened, 18–24 × 12–16 μm (mean 21.3 × 14.6 μm).

Hosts: Red-legged partridge (*Alectoris rufa*), Rock partridge (*Alectoris graeca*)

Geographical distribution: Unknown. Reported in UK and Bulgaria

Diagnosis: Postmortem examination of affected birds reveals the characteristic white cores and examination of scrapings or histological sections of affected tissues shows large numbers of gametocytes in the caeca. On faecal examination there are large numbers of oocysts in a white caseous exudate.

Pathology: Dead birds have soft white cores in the caeca and lower small intestine. In the caeca there is extensive invasion of the mucosa by gametocytes with the entire epithelium and subepithelial cells of the lamina propria infected. The cores are composed of oocysts, necrotic debris and food material.

Quail

Several species of coccidia have been described in these species, based mainly on oocyst morphology. Details on life cycle, pathogenesis, treatment and control are lacking.

Eimeria bateri

Predilection site: Unknown

Parasite class: Sporozoasida

Family: Eimeriidae

Description: Oocysts are ellipsoid, ovoid or infrequently round, 15–28 × 14–23 μm (mean 23 × 18 μm).

Hosts: Japanese quail (*Corturnix japonica*), Corturnix quail (*Corturnix corturix*)

Geographical distribution: Unknown

Eimeria coturnicus

Predilection site: Unknown

Parasite class: Sporozoasida

Family: Eimeriidae

Description: Oocysts are oval, 26–39 × 20–26 μm (mean 32.5 × 23 μm).

Hosts: Coturnix quail (*Coturnix coturnix*)

Geographical distribution: Unknown

Eimeria taldykurganica

Predilection site: Unknown

Parasite class: Sporozoasida

Family: Eimeriidae

Description: Oocysts ovoid, 21.9–25.4 × 11.9–13.1 μm (mean 23.65 × 12.5 μm).

Hosts: Japanese quail (*Corturnix japonica*), Corturnix quail (*Corturnix corturix*)

Geographical distribution: Japan, USA

Eimeria tsunodai

Predilection site: Caeca

Parasite class: Sporozoasida

Family: Eimeriidae

Description: Oocysts are ovoid, 15.5–22.5 × 16.5–18.5 μm (mean 19 × 17.5 μm).

Hosts: Japanese quail (*Corturnix japonica*)

Geographical distribution: Japan, USA

Pathogenesis and clinical signs: Produces a distinctive haemorrhagic caecal coccidiosis with bloody diarrhoea.

Eimeria uzura

Predilection site: unknown

Parasite class: Sporozoasida

Family: Eimeriidae

Description: Oocysts are broad elliptic or ovoid, 19–30 × 15–23 μm (mean 24.4 × 18.7 μm).

Hosts: Japanese quail (*Corturnix japonica*)

Geographical distribution: Japan, USA

Pathogenesis and clinical signs: Reported to cause outbreak of coccidiosis in commercially reared Japanese quail in USA

Guinea fowl

Eimeria grenieri

Predilection site: Small intestine

Parasite class: Sporozoasida

Family: Eimeriidae

Description: Oocysts are ellipsoidal, smooth, 15–27 × 12–18 μm (mean 21 × 15 μm), with a micropyle and polar granules but without a residuum. Sporocysts are ovoid, with a Stieda body and a residuum.

Hosts: Guinea fowl

Life cycle: The life cycle is typically coccidian and there appear to be three merogony generations. First-generation meronts are in the epithelial cells of the crypts below the host cell nucleus near the muscularis mucosae of the duodenum. Second-generation meronts are in the crypts of the lower part of the villi of the upper and middle small intestine. Third-generation meronts are in the middle to tips of the villi of the middle to lower small intestine. The gamonts are in the caecal epithelium. The prepatent period is 4–5 days and patent period 3 days.

Geographical distribution: Europe, Africa

Pathogenesis and clinical signs: *E. grenieri* has been reported to cause disease in guinea fowl, causing diarrhoea and weight loss.

Eimeria numidae

Predilection site: Small and large intestine

Parasite class: Sporozoasida

Family: Eimeriidae

Description: Oocysts are ellipsoidal, smooth, 15–21 × 12–17 μm, with a button-shaped micropyle, a polar granule but without a residuum. Sporocysts are elongate, pointed at one end without a Stieda body.

Hosts: Guinea fowl

Life cycle: First-generation meronts are in the epithelial cells of the duodenum. Second-generation meronts are in the epithelial cells of the jejunum and ileum and also in the large intestine as far as the rectum. Some of the second-generation meronts form third-generation meronts. The prepatent period is 5 days. Sporulation time is 1–2 days.

Geographical distribution: Europe (Hungary)

Pathogenesis and clinical signs: Not considered markedly pathogenic, although may cause mortality in heavy infections. Symptoms include mucous diarrhoea and depression.

Other protozoa

Cryptosporidium baileyi

See under Large intestine.

Cryptosporidium meleagridis

Predilection site: Small intestine

Parasite class: Sporozoasida

Family: Cryptosporidiidae

Description: Oocysts are ellipsoid, 5.6–6.3 × 4.5–4.8 μm (mean 6.2 × 4.6 μm).

Hosts: Turkey, chicken, duck, parrot

Life cycle: Oocysts, each with four sporozoites, are liberated in the faeces. Following ingestion, the sporozoites invade the microvillous brush border of the proventriculus, intestines and lungs and the trophozoites rapidly differentiate to form meronts with four to eight merozoites. Only a single merogony generation has been reported.

Geographical distribution: Presumed worldwide

Pathogenesis: Infection with this parasite has been associated with diarrhoea and a low death rate in 10- to 14-day-old turkey poults. *C. meleagridis* also infects other avian hosts (for example, parrots) and is also the third most common *Cryptosporidium* parasite in humans.

Clinical signs: Diarrhoea

Diagnosis: Oocysts may be demonstrated using Ziehl–Nielsen-stained faecal smears in which the sporozoites appear as bright red granules. Speciation of *Cryptosporidium* is difficult, if not impossible, using conventional techniques. A range of molecular and immunological techniques has been developed, that include the use of immunofluorescence (IF) or enzyme-linked immunosorbent assays (ELISA). More recently, DNA-based techniques have been used for the molecular characterisations of *Cryptosporidium* species.

Pathology: There is villous atrophy and crypt hyperplasia in the ileum of affected turkeys and humans.

Epidemiology: Transmission appears to be mainly by the faecal–oral route.

Treatment and control: There is no reported effective treatment. Good hygiene and management are important in preventing disease from cryptosporidiosis. Thus, litter should always be kept dry and special attention given to litter near water fonts or feeding troughs. Fonts that prevent water reaching the litter should always be used and they should be placed on drip trays or over the droppings pit. Feeding and watering utensils should be of such a type and height that droppings cannot contaminate them. Batch rearing of birds, depopulation and adequate disinfection procedures should help limit levels of infection. Antibiotics to control secondary bacterial infections of the respiratory form may be required. Good ventilation in poultry houses is also essential.

Spironucleus meleagridis

Synonym: *Hexamita meleagridis*

Common name: Infectious catarrhal enteritis, hexamitosis, spironucleosis

Predilection site: Small intestine, caeca

Parasite class: Zoomastigophorasida

Family: Diplomonadidiiae

Description: This protozoan is bilaterally symmetrical in that it possesses two nuclei, two sets of three anterior flagella and two flagella, which pass through the body to emerge posteriorly (Fig. 7.22).

Hosts: Turkey, game birds (pheasant, quail, partridge)

Life cycle: Trophozoites are formed by binary fission. Cyst stages are thought to occur.

Geographical distribution: Worldwide

Pathogenesis: Spironucelosis is a disease of young birds with adult birds symptomless carriers. The mortality in a flock varies and can be as high as 80%, reaching a peak in the flock at 7–10 days after the first bird dies, but heavy losses seldom occur in birds over 10 weeks old. The incubation period is 4–7 days.

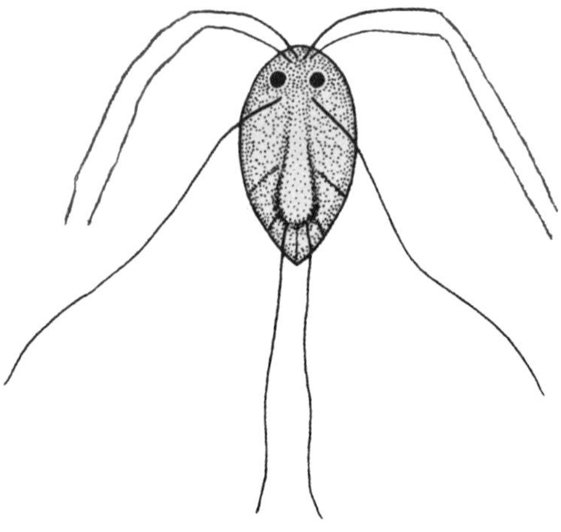

Fig. 7.22 *Spironucleus meleagridis.*

Clinical signs: Affected birds are ruffled, have a foamy, watery diarrhoea, lose weight rapidly and may become weak and die.

Diagnosis: Infection can be diagnosed by finding the characteristic motile protozoa in fresh scrapings from the small intestine. The organism can be differentiated from other flagellates in the gut by its small size, absence of an undulating membrane and characteristic motion. The organism can also be demonstrated in Giemsa-stained smears from the small intestine.

Epidemiology: Infection is transmitted through contaminated feed and water. Carrier adult birds are the most important sources of infection for young poults. Wild gamebirds may be a source of infection to birds reared outdoors in natural pens. Hot weather and overcrowding predispose to infection and the severity of a disease outbreak.

Treatment: Dimetridazole at 27 g/100 litres of drinking water for 12 days or 54 g/100 litres for 3–5 days then 27 g/100 litres for 12 days are effective treatments. However, in many countries products containing dimetridazole are becoming unavailable for legislative reasons.

Control: Control depends on good management and hygiene. Young birds should be raised in batches away from others birds of different age groups. Separate utensils should be used for different groups of birds and kept raised or on wire mesh floors. Outdoor natural pens should be moved periodically and contact with pheasants, quail or partridge prevented. Dimetridazole at 125–200 g/tonne in feed or 12 g/l in drinking water for up to 15 days can be used in prevention. However, see the note above regarding availability.

LARGE INTESTINE

Several species of *Heterakis* are found in poultry. Gross examination readily indicates the genus, but for specific identification microscopic examination is necessary to demonstrate the spicules.

Heterakis gallinarum

Synonym: *Heterakis papillosa*, *Heterakis gallinae*, *Heterakis vesicularis*

Common name: Poultry caecal worm

Predilection site: Caeca; rarely large and small intestine

Parasite class: Nematoda

Superfamily: Ascaridoidea

Description, gross: Whitish worms up to 1.5 cm long, with elongated pointed tails. The male is 7–13 mm long and the female is 10–15 mm. Gross examination readily indicates the genus, but for specific identification microscopic examination is necessary to determinate the shape of the oesophagus and the size and shape of spicules.

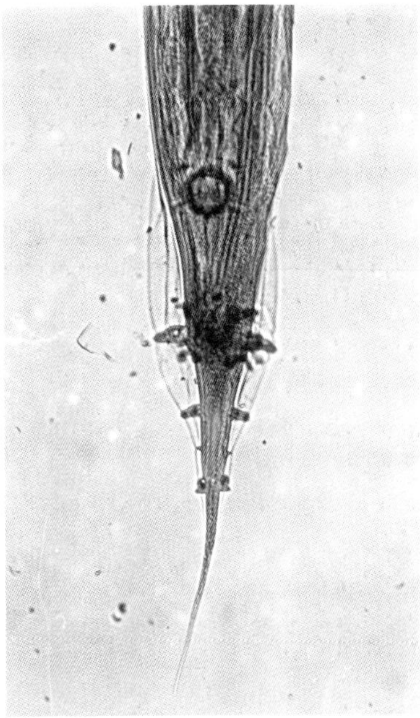

Fig. 7.23 Posterior of a male *Heterakis gallinarum* showing the pre-cloacal sucker and caudal alae supported by caudal papillae.

Description, microscopic: The oesophagus has a large posterior bulb. Generic identity may be confirmed by the presence of a large circular pre-cloacal sucker in the male and prominent caudal alae supported by 12 pairs of caudal papillae (Fig. 7.23). The spicules are unequal in length, the left (about 0.7 mm) has broad alae and the right is slender (about 2 mm). The egg is ovoid, 65–80 × 35–46 μm, thick and smooth-shelled, and is difficult to distinguish from that of *Ascaridia*.

Hosts: Chicken, turkey, pigeon, pheasant, partridge, grouse, quail, guinea fowl, duck, goose and a number of wild galliform birds

Life cycle: The direct life cycle is similar to that of *Ascaridia* spp. The egg is infective on the ground in about 2 weeks at optimal temperatures. Eggs may remain viable in the soil for several months. Earthworms may be transport hosts, the eggs simply passing through the gut, or paratenic hosts in which the egg hatches and the L_3 travels to the tissues to await ingestion by the fowl. In *H. gallinarum* all parasitic moults appear to occur in the caecal lumen. The prepatent period of the genus is about 4 weeks. Longevity is about 12 months.

Geographical distribution: Worldwide

Pathogenesis: *H. gallinarum* is the commonest nematode parasite of poultry, and is usually regarded as being non-pathogenic, although heavy infections can induce thickening of the caecal mucosa. Its chief pathogenic importance is as a vector of the protozoan, *Histomonas meleagridis*, the causal agent of 'blackhead' (enterohepatitis) in turkeys. The organism can be transmitted from fowl to fowl in the egg of *Heterakis* and in earthworms containing hatched larvae of the worm.

Clinical signs: Frequently, *H. gallinarum* alone produces an asymptomatic infection.

Diagnosis: *H. gallinarum* infection is usually only diagnosed accidentally, by the finding of eggs in faeces or the presence of worms at necropsy. Differentiation between the three species of *Heterakis* is based on the shape of the oesophagus and the length and shape of the spicules.

Pathology: The caeca may show marked inflammation and thickening of the mucosa with petechial haemorrhages.

Epidemiology: *H. gallinarum* is widespread in most poultry flocks and is of little pathogenic significance in itself, but is of great importance in the epidemiology of *Histomonas*. Larvated eggs can remain viable in soil for about 1 year and can be a source of infection in free-range birds. Additionally, paratenic hosts such as earthworms can transmit infection.

Treatment: Treatment with piperazine salts, levamisole or a benzimidazole, such as flubendazole, mebendazole or fenbendazole, can be administered in the feed (30 ppm over 7 days; 60 ppm over 7 days; 60 ppm over 3 days; respectively). Levamisole is effective at 30 mg/kg orally or 300 ppm in the feed.

Control: Control of *H. gallinarum* is only necessary when histomonosis is a problem in turkeys. It is largely based on hygiene, and in backyard flocks two main points are: the segregation of turkeys from other domestic poultry, and the removal and disposal of litter from poultry houses. Where the problem is serious and continuous, it may be advisable to administer either piperazine or levamisole intermittently in the feed or water in addition to continuous *Histomonas* chemoprophylaxis.

Heterakis isolonche

Common name: Caecal worm

Predilection site: Caeca; rarely large and small intestine

Parasite class: Nematoda

Superfamily: Ascaridoidea

Description, gross: Whitish worms up to 1.5 cm long, with elongated pointed tails. The male is 7–13 mm long and the female is 10–15 mm. Gross examination readily indicates the genus, but for specific identification microscopic examination is necessary to demonstrate the spicules.

Description, microscopic: The spicules are asymetrical and generic identity may be confirmed by the presence of a large circular pre-cloacal sucker in the male and prominent caudal alae supported by large caudal papillae. The egg is ovoid, thick and smooth-shelled, about $65–75 \times 38–45$ μm and is difficult to distinguish from that of *Ascaridia*.

Hosts: Pheasant, grouse, quail, duck, chicken

Life cycle: As for *H. gallinarum*. In *H. isolonche* infection, the hatched larvae enter the caecal mucosa, and develop to maturity in nodules. Each nodule has an opening into the gut through which the eggs reach the lumen.

Geographical distribution: Worldwide

Pathogenesis: *H. isolonche* of game birds is in itself pathogenic, causing a severe inflammation of the caeca with nodules projecting from both peritoneal and mucosal surfaces. These can cause ulceration of the mucosa and diarrhoea with progressive emaciation and there may be high mortality in heavily infected flocks.

Clinical signs: Infections with *H. isolonche* may produce nodular typhlitis, diarrhoea, emaciation and death.

Diagnosis: *H. isolonche* infection is diagnosed at necropsy by the finding of caecal nodules containing adult worms, and if necessary, confirmed microscopically by examination of the spicules.

Pathology: The caeca may show marked inflammation and thickening of the mucosa with nodule formation and petechial haemorrhages.

Epidemiology: Infection is common in birds raised in permanent grass pens. Larvated eggs can remain viable in soil for about 1 year. Additionally, paratenic hosts such as earthworms can transmit infection.

Treatment: As for *H. gallinarum*

Control: Where *H. isolonche* infection is endemic in pheasantries, the runs should be abandoned and pheasant chicks reared on fresh ground.

Heterakis dispar

Predilection site: Caeca; rarely large and small intestine

Parasite class: Nematoda

Superfamily: Ascaridoidea

Description, gross: Refer to *H. gallinarum*, though *H. dispar* is larger than either *H. gallinarum* or *H. isolonche*; males measure 11–18 mm and females 16–23 mm in length.

Description, microscopic: The male spicules are of sub-equal length (40–50 μm).

Hosts: Duck, goose, chicken

Life cycle: The direct life cycle is similar to that of *Ascaridia* spp. The egg is infective on the ground in about 2 weeks at optimal temperatures. Eggs may remain viable in the soil for several months. Earthworms may be transport hosts, the eggs simply passing through the gut, or paratenic hosts in which the egg hatches and the L_3 travels to the tissues to await ingestion by the host. The prepatent period is about 4 weeks. Longevity is about 12 months.

Geographical distribution: Many parts of the world

Heterakis brevispeculum

Predilection site: Caeca; rarely large and small intestine

Parasite class: Nematoda

Superfamily: Ascaridoidea

Description: See *H. gallinarum* for general information. The spicules are of equal length (about 0.5 mm) and possess a barb near the tip.

Hosts: Duck, goose, guinea fowl, chicken

Geographical distribution: Worldwide

Trichostrongylus tenuis

Predilection site: Small intestine, caeca

Parasite class: Nematoda

Superfamily: Trichostrongyloidea

Description, gross: The adults are small and hair-like. Males measure around 5.0–6.5 mm and females 7–9 mm in length. The spicules are curved.

Description, microscopic: The worms have no buccal capsule. A useful generic character is the distinct excretory notch in the oesophageal region.

Hosts: Game birds (grouse, partridge and pheasant), chicken, duck, goose, turkey, emu

Life cycle: This is direct and the pre-parasitic phase is typically trichostrongyloid. Infection is through ingestion of infective L_3 from the environment. The parasitic phase is non-migratory and the prepatent period is short, only 7–10 days.

Geographical distribution: North America, Asia and Europe

Pathogenesis: *T. tenuis* has been implicated in outbreaks of severe enteritis in game birds. Moderate to severe infections cause diarrhoea, which is often fatal. Lighter infections result in a chronic syndrome characterised by anaemia and emaciation.

Clinical signs: These are reduced appetite, anaemia and general emaciation.

Diagnosis: Identification of the adult worms on postmortem

Pathology: Light infections cause little pathological effects but heavy infections can induce an acute haemorrhagic typhlitis

Epidemiology: High stocking densities can lead to build-up of large numbers of infective larvae with associated high morbidity and mortality, particularly in grouse.

Treatment: On game farms, therapy with levamisole in the drinking water has proved useful. Formulations of fenbendazole and flubendazole are available for incorporation into feed.

Control: Where game are farmed, the pens should be moved regularly to prevent the accumulation of larvae and, if possible, the runs should not be placed in the same areas in successive years.

Capillaria anatis

Synonym: *Capillaria brevicollis*, *C. collaris*, *C. anseris*, *C. mergi*

Predilection site: Caeca

Parasite class: Nematoda

Superfamily: Trichuroidea

Description, gross: See *C. annulata*. Males measure around 16–24 mm and females 28–38 mm.

Description, microscopic: The males have a long thin single spicule and often possess a primitive bursa-like structure. The eggs are barrel-shaped, colourless and have thick shells that are slightly striated with bipolar plugs.

Hosts: Chicken, turkey, gallinaceous birds (pheasant, partridge), pigeon, duck, goose

Life cycle: The life cycle is direct. The infective L_1 develops within the egg in about 3–4 weeks. Infection of the final host is through ingestion of this embryonated infective stage, development to adult worms occurs without a migration phase. The prepatent period is 3–4 weeks.

Table 7.5 Species of *Capillaria* found in gamebirds.

Species	Hosts	Location
Capillaria (*Eucoleus*) *contorta*	Chicken, turkey, duck and wild birds	Oesophagus, crop
Capillaria (*Eucoleus*) *annulata*	Chicken, turkey, duck and wild birds	Oesophagus, crop
Capillaria (*Eucoleus*) *perforans*	Pheasant, guinea fowl	Oesophagus, crop
Capillaria uropapillata	Pheasant	Oesophagus, crop
Capillaria phasianina	Pheasant, grey partridge	Small intestine, caeca
Capillaria anatis	Chicken, turkey, gallinaceous birds (pheasant, partridge), pigeon, duck, goose	Caeca

Geographical distribution: Worldwide

Pathogenesis: The anterior ends of the worms are embedded in the mucosa. Heavy infection can induce haemorrhagic enteritis with bloody diarrhoea. The caecal wall is often thickened.

Clinical signs: Infected birds may become weak and emaciated and be anaemic.

Pathology: Chronically infected birds have thickened intestinal walls covered with a catarrhal exudate.

Treatment and control is as for other *Capillaria* species.

The following two species of *Subulura* found in the large intestine are considered to be of minor significance. Intermediate hosts are cockroaches and beetles. Treatment and control is not usually required. Note that current taxonomic revision suggests this genus falls within its own superfamily: the Subuluroidea.

Subulura suctoria

Synonym: *Allodapa suctoria*, *Subulura brumpti*

Predilection site: Caeca

Parasite class: Nematoda

Superfamily: Oxyuroidea

Description, gross: The males measure around 8–10 mm and the females up to 18 mm.

Description, microscopic: The small buccal capsule has three teeth at its base. The oesophagus is dilated posteriorly, followed by a bulb. The tail of the male has large lateral alae and is curved ventrad. A slit-like pre-cloacal sucker is present, surrounded by radiating muscle fibres. In the female, the vulva is situated just anterior to the middle of the body. Eggs are thin-shelled and spherical, 52–64 × 41–49 mm, and embryonated when laid.

Final hosts: Chicken, turkey, guinea fowl, quail, grouse, pheasant and various galliform birds such as ducks

Intermediate hosts: Include various cockroaches, beetles and earwigs

Life cycle: Eggs passed in faeces are ingested by the intermediate host where they develop to the infective L_3 stage after about 2 weeks. Following ingestion by the final host the larvae migrate to the lumen of the caeca. The prepatent period is 6–8 weeks.

Geographical distribution: Asia, Africa and the Americas, Hawaii, parts of Europe (Spain)

Subulura differens

Predilection site: Caeca

Parasite class: Nematoda

Superfamily: Oxyuroidea

Final hosts: Chicken, guinea fowl

Geographical distribution: Europe, Africa, Brazil

Strongyloides avium

Common name: Threadworm

Predilection site: Caeca, small intestine

Parasite class: Nematoda

Superfamily: Rhabditoidea

Description, gross: Slender, hair-like worms 2.2 mm long. Only females are parasitic.

Description, microscopic: The long oesophagus may occupy up to one third of the body length and the uterus is intertwined with the intestine, giving the appearance of twisted thread. Unlike other intestinal parasites of similar size the tail has a blunt point. *Strongyloides* eggs are oval, thin-shelled and small, 52–56 × 36–40 µm, being half the size of typical strongyle eggs. The larvated egg is usually passed in the faeces.

Hosts: Chicken, turkey, goose, quail, wild birds

Life cycle: *Strongyloides* is unique among the nematodes of veterinary importance, being capable of both parasitic and free-living reproductive cycles. The parasitic phase is composed entirely of female worms in the caeca and these produce larvated eggs by parthenogenesis. After hatching, larvae may develop through four larval stages into free-living adult male and female worms and this can be followed by a succession of free-living generations. Infection is generally direct, but percutaneous infection can occur. The prepatent period is from 8–14 days.

Geographical distribution: Worldwide

Pathogenesis: *Strongyloides* can be a serious pathogen in young floor-reared birds.

Clinical signs: Acute, heavy infections cause weakness, emaciation and bloody, slimy diarrhoea.

Diagnosis: Small embryonated eggs may be found in the faeces. Adult parasites can be demonstrated in mucosal scrapings from the caecal mucosa on postmortem.

Pathology: Mature parasites in the caeca, if present in large numbers, may cause inflammation with oedema and erosion of the epithelium.

Epidemiology: *Strongyloides* infective larvae are not ensheathed and are susceptible to extreme climatic conditions. However warmth and moisture favour development and allow the accumulation of large numbers of infective stages.

Treatment and control: No information is available.

Caecal flukes

See general comments under Intestinal flukes.

Notocotylus attenuatus

Predilection site: Caecum, rectum

Parasite class: Trematoda

Family: Notocotylidae

Description, gross: The adult fluke is 2–5 mm long by 0.7–1.5 mm wide and is narrow anteriorly.

Description, microscopic: Eggs are small and measure 20 × 10 µm and possess two long filaments, which are up to 200 µm in length.

Final hosts: Chicken, duck, goose, and other aquatic birds

Intermediate hosts: Snails, such as *Planorbis* spp, *Lymnaea* spp and *Bulinus*

Geographical distribution: Worldwide

Catatropis verrucosa

Predilection site: Caecum

Parasite class: Trematoda

Family: Notocotylidae

Description, gross: The fluke is 2–6 mm long by 0.8–2 mm wide.

Description, microscopic: Eggs measure around 20–25 µm in length and possess two filaments, 160–200 µm long.

Final hosts: Chicken, duck, goose and other aquatic birds

Intermediate hosts: Snails, such as *Planorbis* spp

Geographical distribution: Worldwide

Brachylaemus commutatus

Synonym: *Harmostomum commutatus*

Predilection site: Caeca

Parasite class: Trematoda

Family: Brachylaemidae

Description, gross: The elongate fluke measures around 4–7 mm in length by 1–2 mm in width.

Description, microscopic: Eggs are approximately 30 × 15 µm

Final hosts: Chicken, turkey, other fowl, pigeon and pheasant

Intermediate hosts: Land snails

Geographical distribution: Southern Europe, Africa, parts of Asia

Echinostoma revolutum

Predilection site: Caeca and rectum

Parasite class: Trematoda

Family: Echinostomatidae

Description, gross: *E. revolutum* can measure up to around 2 cm in length but is often 1.0–1.5 cm by about 2 mm in width.

Table 7.6 Caecal flukes found in poultry.

Parasite	Family	Size (mm)	Predilection site	Definitive host	Intermediate hosts	Geographical location
Notocotylus attenuatus	Notocotylidae	2–5 × 1	Caeca and rectum	Chicken, duck, goose and wild aquatic birds	Various snails	Many parts of the world
Catatropis verrucosa	Notocotylidae	2–6 × 1–2	Caeca	Chicken, duck, goose and wild aquatic birds	Various snails	Worldwide
Brachylaemus commutatus	Brachylaemidae	4–7 × 1–2	Caeca	Chicken, turkey, other fowl, pigeon and pheasant	Land snails	Southern Europe, Africa, parts of Asia
Postharmostomum commutatum syn. *P. gallinarum*	Brachylaemidae syn. Harmostomidae		Caeca	Chicken, turkey, guinea fowl, pheasant and pigeon	Various snails	North Africa, North America, southern Europe and parts of southeast Asia
Echinostoma revolutum	Echinostomatidae	1–1.5 × 2	Caeca and rectum	Duck, goose, pigeon, various fowl and aquatic birds	1. Aquatic snails 2. Various aquatic snails and tadpoles	Worldwide

Description, microscopic: The adult fluke possesses a head-collar, which is armed with spines and the anterior tegument is spiny. Eggs measure about 110 × 65 μm.

Final hosts: Duck, goose, pigeon, various fowl and aquatic birds

Geographical distribution: Worldwide

Notes: *E. revolutum* can also infect man. *E. paraulum* occurs in the small intestine of duck and pigeon and can cause weakness, inappetence and diarrhoea in the latter.

Chicken caecal coccidiosis

Two species of coccidia are found in the chicken, of which *Eimeria tenella* is the most important throughout the world.

Eimeria tenella

Predilection site: Caeca (Fig. 7.24)

Parasite class: Sporozoasida

Family: Eimeriidae

Description: Oocysts are ovoid, smooth, colourless 14–31 × 9–25 μm (mean 25 × 19 μm), without a micropyle or residuum but with a polar granule. The sporocysts are ovoid, with a Stieda body and without a residuum.

Host: Chicken

Life cycle: Following ingestion, the oocyst wall breaks in the gizzard releasing the sporocysts. The sporozoites are activated by bile or trypsin when the sporocysts reach the small intestine, and they escape from the sporocysts. The sporozoites enter the epithelial cells either directly or following ingestion by a macrophage. Each schizont rounds up to form a first-generation meront each containing about 900 merozoites, approximately 2–4 μm long. These emerge into the caeca about 2.5–3 days after infection and invade new host cells. Second-generation meronts are formed, and these lie above the host cell nucleus producing 200–350 merozoites, which are approximately 16 μm long, and which are found 5 days after inoculation. They invade new host cells to either form the third-generation meronts (which lie beneath the host cell nucleus and produce 4–30 third-generation merozoites which are about 7 μm long and which invade new cells to form gamonts) or to form the gamonts directly. The macrogametes and microgamonts lie below the host cell nuclei. The microgamonts form many biflagellate microgametes, which fertilise the macrogametes. The resulting oocysts lay down a

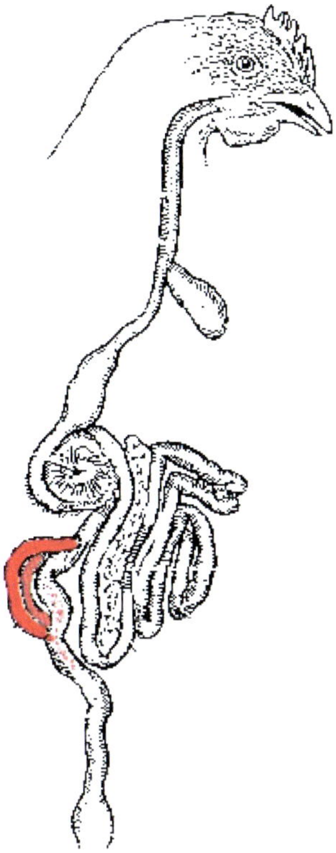

Fig. 7.24 Predilection site of *Eimeria tenella*.

resistant wall, break out of the cells into the gut lumen and are then passed in the faeces. The prepatent period is 132 hours. Sporulation time is 18–48 hours.

Geographical distribution: Worldwide

Pathogenesis: The first-stage meronts of this species develop deep in the glands. The second-stage meronts are also unusual in that the epithelial cells in which they develop leave the mucosa and migrate into the lamina propria and submucosa. When these meronts mature and rupture, about 72 hours after ingestion of oocysts, haemorrhage occurs, the mucosal surface is largely detached and clinical signs become apparent.

Clinical signs: Clinical disease occurs when large numbers of oocysts are ingested over a short period and is characterised by the presence of soft faeces often containing blood. The chicks are dull and listless, with drooping feathers. In subclinical infections, there are poor weight gains and food conversion rates.

Pathology: At postmortem, the caeca are often found to be dilated and contain a mixture of clotted, and unclotted blood (Fig. 7.25). In longer-standing infections, the caecal contents become caseous and adherent to the mucosa. As regeneration of the mucosa

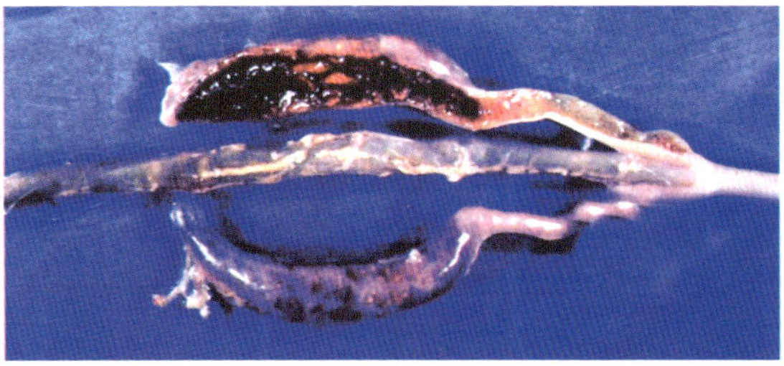

Fig. 7.25 Lesions of *Eimeria tenella* in caeca.

occurs these caecal plugs are detached and caseous material is shed in the faeces.

Lesions are scored +1 to +4 as follows:

1. Very few small scattered petechiae on the caecal wall with no thickening of the caecal walls and normal caecal contents.
2. Lesions more numerous with noticeable blood in the caecal contents. The caecal wall is somewhat thickened with normal caecal contents.
3. Large amounts of blood and caecal cores present. The caecal walls are greatly thickened with little, if any, faecal contents in the caeca.
4. Caecal walls are greatly distended with blood or large caseous cores.

Epidemiology: *E. tenella* is the species primarily responsible for caecal coccidiosis. Coccidiosis due to *E. tenella* occurs principally in chickens of 3–7 weeks of age. The prevalence of disease due to this species, and caecal coccidiosis, has declined since many of the anticoccidial drugs in general use were developed specifically to control this pathogenic species.

Eimeria tenella

Lesions: Haemorrhage in caecal lumen followed by thickening of mucosa and formation of caecal cores with clotted blood (Fig. 7.25)

Mean oocyst size (μm)	Shape and length:width index
25 × 19	Ovoid 1.16
Prepatent period (hours)	**Sporulation time (hours)**
132	18–48

Wenyonella gallinae

Predilection site: Caeca, rectum

Parasite class: Sporozoasida

Family: Eimeriidae

Description: Oocysts are ovoid, rough, punctate 29–34 × 20–23 μm (mean 31 × 21 μm). There are four sporocysts, which are flask-shaped, 19 × 8 μm, and each contain four sporozoites

Hosts: Chicken

Life cycle: Details of the life cycle have not been described. The prepatent period is 7–8 days and patent period 3 days. The sporulation time is 4–6 days.

Geographical distribution: India

Pathogenesis and clinical signs: May cause diarrhoea with blackish green, semi-solid excreta.

Diagnosis: Diagnosis is based on postmortem examination and by examining the faeces for the presence of oocysts or by examination of scrapings or histological sections of affected tissues. At necropsy, the location and type of lesions present provide a good guide to the species that can be confirmed by examination of the sporulated oocysts, which contain four sporocysts each with four sporozoites.

Pathology: The terminal part of the intestine is thickened and congested with pinpoint haemorrhages in the mucosa.

Epidemiology: Not described

Treatment and control: Prevention of infection is based on good management. Chicken rearing areas should always be kept dry and special attention given to litter near water drinkers and feeders. Anticoccidial compounds used for control of *Eimeria* species in chickens should be equally effective.

Turkey caecal coccidiosis

Eimeria adenoides

See Small intestine.

Eimeria gallopavonis

See Small intestine.

Eimeria meleagrimitis

Predilection site: Caeca

Parasite class: Sporozoasida

Family: Eimeriidae

Description: Oocysts are ellipsoidal, smooth, 19–31 × 14–23 μm (mean 23 × 16 μm) with no micropyle and no oocyst residuum but with one to two polar granules. Sporocysts are ovoid with a Stieda body and a residuum. First-generation meronts are 20 × 15 μm and contain 50–100 merozoites; second-generation meronts are approximately 9 μm in diameter and contain 8–16 merozoites. Mature gamonts are 18 × 13 μm.

Hosts: Turkey

Life cycle: There are two to three merogony stages. The first-generation meronts appear in the middle small intestine 2–5 days after infection; second-generation meronts appear 60 hours after infection in the caeca, and are mature by 70 hours. There may be a third asexual generation, but most of the second-generation merozoites develop into sexual stages. Gamonts appear in the caeca, rectum, and to a small extent, the ileum and the prepatent period is 144 hours. The sporulation time is 15–72 hours.

Geographical distribution: Worldwide

Pathogenesis: A relatively non-pathogenic species, producing masses of ovoid oocysts in a white discharge from the caeca and lower small intestine.

Clinical signs: Infection is not associated with clinical signs.

Pathology: Non-pathogenic. The endogenous stages can be seen on histopathology in the caeca.

Cryptosporidium baileyi

Predilection site: Small and large intestine, cloaca, bursa of Fabricius, nasopharyx, sinuses, trachea, conjunctiva

Parasite class: Sporozoasida

Family: Cryptosporidiidae

Description: Oocysts are ellipsoid, 5.6–6.3 × 4.5–4.8 μm (mean 6.2 × 4.6 μm).

Hosts: Chicken, turkey, duck, cockatiel, quail, ostrich

Life cycle: Oocysts, each with four sporozoites, are liberated in the faeces. Following ingestion, the sporozoites invade the microvillous brush border of the proventriculus, intestines and lungs and the trophozoites rapidly differentiate to form meronts with four to eight merozoites. There appear to be three merogony generations and both thin- and thick-walled oocysts have been observed. The prepatent period is 3 days and patent period 10–20 days.

Geographical distribution: Presumed worldwide

Pathogenesis: *Cryptosporidium baileyi* cryptosporidiosis is a disease of the epithelial lining of the bursa of Fabricius and cloaca of chicken, although the trachea and conjunctiva are lesser sites of infection. The presence of developmental stages in the microvillus region of enterocytes of the ileum and large intestines are not

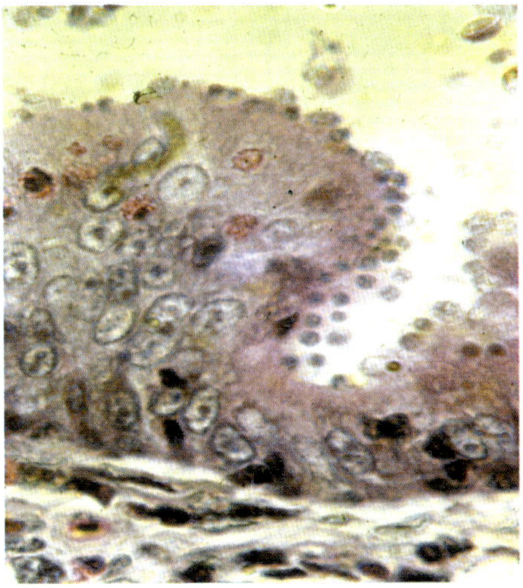

Fig. 7.26 *Cryptosporidium baileyi*: cloacal bursa.

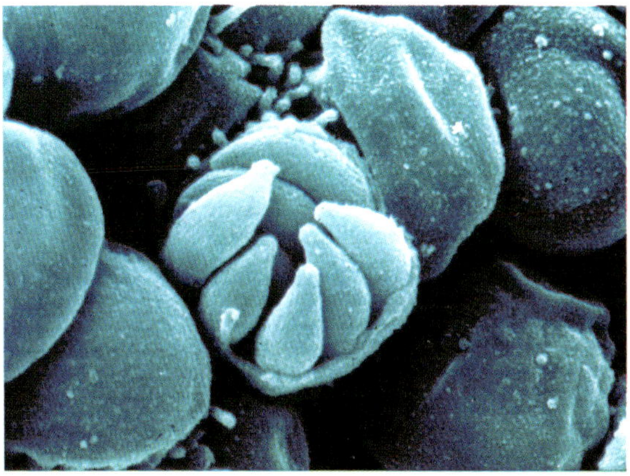

Fig. 7.28 Scanning electron micrograph of meront of *Cryptosporidium baileyi*.

usually associated with clinical signs. Similarly, heavy infection of the bursa of Fabricius and cloaca does not appear to result in clinical illness (Figs 7.26, 7.27, 7.28). In the respiratory form of infection, up to 50% of a broiler flock may show clinical signs, and mortalities may reach 10%. Conjunctivitis in several species of birds has been reported.

Clinical signs: Enteric infections are not associated with clinical signs. In the respiratory form, initially disease is accompanied by sneezing and coughing, followed by head extension to facilitate breathing. Severe signs of respiratory disease last up to 4 weeks post-infection.

Diagnosis: As for *C. meleagridis*

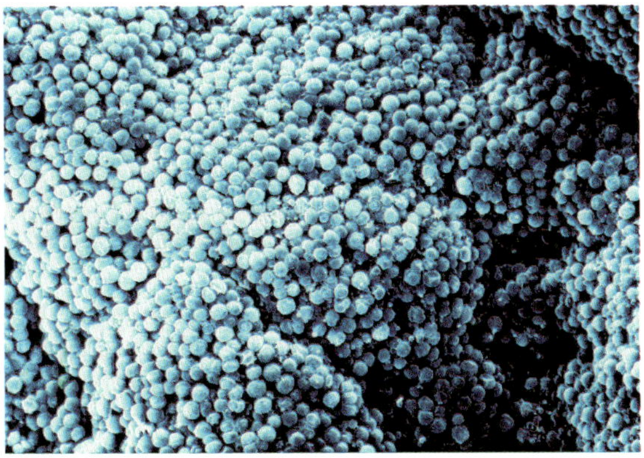

Fig. 7.27 Scanning electron micrograph of cloacal bursa, showing numerous stages of *Cryptosporidium baileyi*.

Pathology: Villous atrophy, shortening of microvilli and enterocyte detachment are the major pathological changes associated with intestinal cryptosporidiosis. In respiratory cryptosporidiosis, gross lesions consist of excess mucus in the trachea, nasal mucosal congestion and atrophic bursa of Fabricius. Cryptosporidia are found in the nasopharynges, trachea, bronchi and bursa, but are not seen in the small intestine. With the respiratory form of cryptosporidiosis, there is epithelial cell deciliation and hyperplasia, mucosal thickening and discharge of mucocellular exudate into the airways in young broilers. Bronchopneumonia may be present in severely infected birds.

Epidemiology: Transmission appears to be mainly by the faecal–oral route although in the respiratory form, infection may be spread by coughing and sneezing.

Treatment and control: As for *C. mealeagridis*

Histomonas meleagridis

See Parasites of the liver.

The following flagellate infections are not associated with disease, with the possible exception of *T. gallinarum*. Numbers of these protozoa can increase considerably in association with other gut enteropathies, and disruption of the normal bacterial flora.

Trichomonads reproduce by longitudinal binary fission. No sexual stages are known and there are no cysts, with the exception of *Chilomastix*.

Diagnosis: Trichomonads are differentiated by morphological identification of the organisms from fresh and stained faecal preparations. The organisms can also be cultured in a range of media used for trichomonads.

Epidemiology: Birds become infected by ingestion of trichomonads, and cysts in the case of *Chilomastix gallinarum*, in contaminated water or feed.

Treatment and control: Not required

Tetratrichomonas gallinarum

Synonym: *Trichomonas gallinarum, Trichomonas pullorum*

Predilection site: Caeca

Parasite class: Zoomastigophorasida

Family: Trichomonadidae

Description: The body is piriform and is 7–15 × 3–9 µm. There are four anterior flagella, and a posterior flagellum, which runs along the undulation membrane and extends beyond it. An accessory filament is present. The axostyle is long, pointed and slender, and lacks a chromatic ring at its point of emergence. Supracostal granules are present, but there are no subcostal or endoaxostylar granules. The pelta is elaborate and terminates in a short ventral extension which is more or less free from the ventral edge of the axostyle. The parabasal body usually consists of a ring of variously spaced granules plus one or two fibrils or rami.

Hosts: Chicken, turkey, guinea fowl, quail, pheasant, partridge

Geographical distribution: Worldwide

Tritrichomonas eberthi

Synonym: *Trichomonas eberthi*

Predilection site: Caeca

Parasite class: Zoomastigophorasida

Family: Trichomonadidae

Description: The body is elongate, 8–14 × 4–7 µm, with vaculolated cytoplasm and 3 anterior flagella (Fig. 7.29). The undulating membrane is prominent and extends the full length of the body. The posterior flagellum extends about half the length of the body beyond the undulating membrane. An accessory filament is present. The blepharoplast is composed of four granules; the axostyle is massive and hyaline, and its anterior end is broadened to form a capitulum and a ring of chromatin granules is present at the point that the axostyle emerges from the body. The parabasal body is shaped like a flattened rod and is of variable length.

Hosts: Chicken, turkey

Geographical distribution: Worldwide

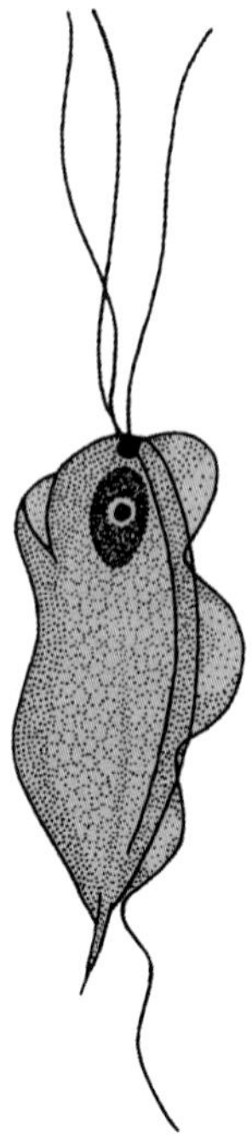

Fig. 7.29 *Tritrichomonas eberthi.*

Tetratrichomonas anatis

Synonym: *Trichomonas anatis*

Predilection site: Small and large intestine

Parasite class: Zoomastigophorasida

Family: Trichomonadidae

Description: The body is broadly beet-shaped, 13–27 × 8–18 µm, with four anterior flagella, and an undulating membrane that extends most of the length of the body and terminates in a free posterior flagellum. There is a costa and a slender, fibrillar axostyle.

Hosts: Duck

Geographical distribution: Worldwide

Tetratrichomonas anseris

Synonym: *Trichomonas anseris*

Predilection site: Caeca

Parasite class: Zoomastigophorasida

Family: Trichomonadidae

Description: The body is elongate, 8–14 × 4–7 µm, with vaculolated cytoplasm and three anterior flagella. The undulating membrane is prominent and extends the full length of the body. The posterior flagellum extends about half the length of the body beyond the undulating membrane. An accessory filament is present. The blepharoplast is composed of four granules; the axostyle is massive and hyaline, and its anterior end is broadened to form a capitulum and a ring of chromatin granules is present at the point that the axostyle emerges from the body. The parabasal body is shaped like a flattened rod and is of variable length.

Hosts: Goose

Geographical distribution: Worldwide

Chilomastix gallinarum

Predilection site: Caeca

Parasite class: Zoomastigophorasida

Family: Trichomonadidae

Description: The body is pear-shaped, 11–20 × 5–12 μm with a nucleus at the anterior end of the body (Fig. 7.30). There are three anterior flagella and a short fourth flagellum that undulates within a cytosomal cleft that is shaped like a figure 8, which is located on the ventral body spiralling to the left and extending half to two thirds of the body length. Cysts are lemon-shaped, 7–9 × 4–6 μm, with a single nucleus.

Hosts: Chicken, turkey

Life cycle: Trophozoites are formed by binary fission. Cyst stages are formed.

Geographical distribution: Worldwide

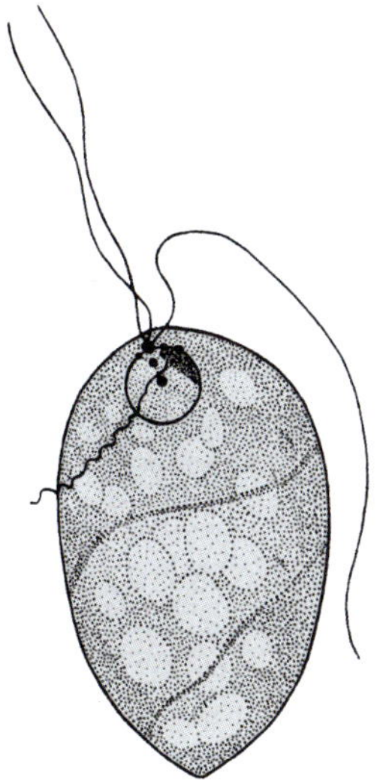

Fig. 7.30 *Chilomastix gallinarum.*

Cochlosoma anatis

Synonym: *Cochlosoma rostratum*

Predilection site: Large intestine, cloaca, caeca

Parasite class: Zoomastigophorasida

Family: Cochlosomatidae

Description: The body is beet-shaped, 6–12 × 4–7 μm, with a nucleus in the middle of the body. There are six flagella of unequal length arising from a blepharoplast at the anterior end, and two trailing flagella lying in a longitudinal groove. A sucker covers one third to one half of the body length.

Hosts: Duck, muscovy duck, mallard and other wild ducks

Geographical distribution: Presumed worldwide

Pathogenicity: Unknown

PARASITES OF THE RESPIRATORY SYSTEM

Syngamus trachea

Synonym: *Syngamus parvis*, *Syngamus gracilis*

Common name: Gapeworm

Predilection site: Trachea or lungs

Parasite class: Nematoda

Superfamily: Strongyloidea

Description, gross: The reddish large female, around 1–3 cm, and the small whitish male (up to 0.5 cm) worms, are permanently in copula forming a Y shape: they are the only parasites found in the trachea of domestic birds (Fig. 7.31). Males possess two spicules.

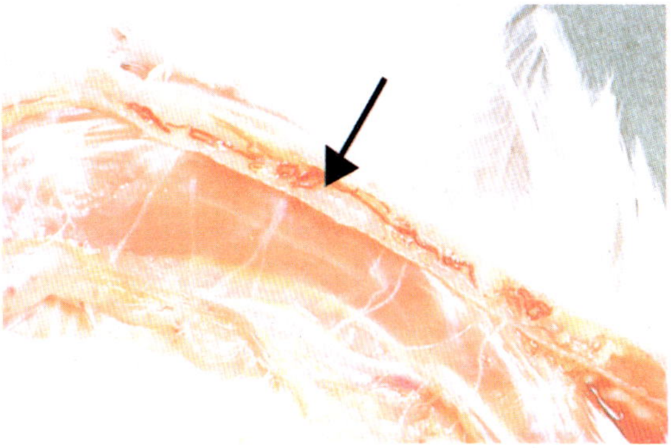

Fig. 7.31 Adult *Syngamus trachea* in situ (arrow).

Description, microscopic: The worms have large shallow cup-shaped buccal capsules, which have up to ten teeth at their base. There are no leaf-crowns. The ellipsoidal thin-shelled eggs are 70–100 × 43–46 μm with a thick operculum at both ends.

Hosts: Chicken, turkey, game birds (pheasant, partridge, guinea fowl), pigeon and various wild birds

Life cycle: Eggs escape under the bursa of the male and are carried up the trachea in the excess mucus produced in response to infection: they are then swallowed and passed in the faeces. Unlike other strongyloids the L_3 develops within the egg. Infection may occur by one of three ways, firstly by ingestion of the L_3 in the egg, secondly by ingestion of the hatched L_3 or thirdly by ingestion of a transport (paratenic) host containing the L_3. The most common paratenic host is the common earthworm, but a variety of other invertebrates including slugs, snails, beetles and some flies may act as transport hosts. After penetrating the intestine of the final host the L_3 travel, via the liver, to the lungs, probably in the blood since they are found in the alveoli 4–6 hours after experimental infection. The two parasitic moults take place in the lungs within 5 days by which time the parasites are 1.0–2.0 mm long. Copulation occurs around day 7 in the trachea or bronchi after which the female grows rapidly. The prepatent period is 16–20 days. Longevity is around 9 months.

Geographical distribution: Worldwide

Pathogenesis: The effects of *S. trachea* are most severe in young birds, especially game chicks and turkey poults. In these, migration through the lungs in heavy infections may cause emphysema, oedema and result in pneumonia and death. In less severe infections the adult worms cause a haemorrhagic tracheitis with excess mucus production, which may lead to partial occlusion of the airways and difficulty in breathing. In turkeys, the male worms can be substantially embedded in the mucosa of the trachea, inducing the formation of nodules.

Clinical signs: These are most commonly seen in young chicks and poults. Pneumonia during the prepatent phase may cause signs of dyspnoea and depression, whereas the presence of adult worms and excess mucus in the trachea lead to signs of respiratory distress, asphyxia or suffocation with the bird gasping for air; often there is a great deal of head shaking and coughing as it tries to rid itself of the obstruction. The clinical picture of 'gapes' may thus range from gasping, dyspnoea and death to, in less severely affected animals, weakness, anaemia and emaciation.

Diagnosis: This is based on clinical signs and the finding of eggs in the faeces. Disease is probably best confirmed by postmortem examination of selected cases when reddish worms will be found attached to the tracheal mucosa. The infected trachea often contains an increased amount of mucus.

Pathology: The carcases of infected birds are emaciated and anaemic and worms are found in the posterior part of the trachea, attached to the mucosa and surrounded by mucus, which may be streaked with blood. In turkeys, male worms become deeply embedded in the wall of the trachea, causing the development of nodules.

Epidemiology: Gapeworm infection primarily affects young domestic chickens of less than 2–3 months of age, but turkeys of all ages are susceptible, the adults often acting as carriers. All ages of other passeriform and galliform species are susceptible to infection. Infrequently *S. trachea* can infect anseriform birds. Eggs may survive for up to 9 months in soil and L_3 for years within the earthworm or other transport hosts. Disease is seen most frequently in breeding and rearing establishments where outdoor pens, such as are used for breeding pheasants, are in use. Eggs, passed by wild birds such as rooks and blackbirds, may initiate infection; these may also infect earthworms. Infection is usually highest during the summer when earthworms are active. Infected chicks normally develop an age resistance by 2–3 months of age and markedly reduce their worm burdens. Partial immunity to reinfection is established.

Treatment: In-feed, modern benzimidazoles are effective, administered usually over a period of several days. Birds need to be monitored, as severely affected ones may not ingest adequate anthelmintic. Nitroxynil and levamisole are also very efficacious when given in the water.

Control: Young birds should not be reared with adults, especially turkeys, and to prevent infection becoming established runs or yards should be kept dry and contact with wild birds prevented. Avoid the continuous rearing of birds on the same ground. Drug prophylaxis may be practised over the period when outbreaks are normally expected. It is not usually feasible to eliminate the paratenic hosts.

Syngamus bronchialis

Synonym: *Cyathostoma bronchialis*

Common name: Gapeworm

Predilection site: Trachea, bronchi

Parasite class: Nematoda

Superfamily: Strongyloidea

Description, gross: Adult worms are 0.4–3 cm long; males are 4–5.8 mm and females 16–31 mm.

Description, microscopic: The buccal capsule is cup-shaped with six to seven teeth at its base. The male bursa is well developed but worms in this species are not permanently in copula, which contrasts to the situation with *Syngamus trachea*. Eggs are 74–83 × 49–62 μm.

Hosts: Goose, duck, swan

Geographical distribution: Worldwide

Pathogenesis: Young birds are most susceptible to disease and heavy infections can be pathogenic, leading to emaciation and death.

Clinical signs: In heavy infections these may include depression of food intake, asphyxia and dyspnoea.

Epidemiology: Severe infections are often associated with the ingestion of transport hosts such as earthworms, slugs, snails and invertebrates. Larvae may encyst and survive for years within invertebrate hosts. Infections often occur seasonally, when, for instance, large numbers of earthworms occur on the surface after heavy rain.

Typhlocoelum cymbium

Synonym: *Tracheophilus sisowi*

Predilection site: Trachea, bronchi

Parasite class: Trematoda

Family: Cyclocoelidae

Description, gross: Adult fluke are 6–11.5 mm by 3 mm. The body has rounded ends and is wide in the middle.

Description, microscopic: Eggs are 122 × 63 μm.

Hosts: Duck

Intermediate hosts: Snails of the genera *Helisoma* and *Planorbis*

Life cycle: Eggs are coughed up and swallowed in the faeces. A miracidium, containing a single redia, hatches from the egg. The redia, not the miracidium, enters a snail and after 11 days produces small numbers of cercariae. There is no sporocyst stage. The cercariae are retained within the snail and encyst. Birds are infected by eating infected snails. The larval fluke reach the bronchi via the bloodstream.

Geographical distribution: Europe, Asia, Central America

Pathogenesis and clinical signs: The parasites cause obstruction of the trachea and affected birds may die of asphyxia.

Treatment and control: There is no reported treatment. Control is impractical.

Typhlocoelum cucumerinum

Synonym: *Distoma cumumerinum*, *Typhloceolum obovlae*

Predilection site: Trachea, air sacs, oesophagus

Parasite class: Trematoda

Family: Cyclocoelidae

Description, gross: Adult fluke are 6–12 × 2–5 mm. The body is oval and blunter anteriorly than posteriorly.

Description, microscopic: Eggs are 156 × 85 μm.

Hosts: Duck

Intermediate hosts: Snails

Geographical distribution: Europe, North and South America

Pathogenesis and clinical signs: Affected birds suffer from dyspnoea and asphyxia.

Hyptiasmus tumidus

Synonym: *Hyptiasmus arcuatus*, *Cyclocoelum arcuatum*

Predilection site: Nasal and orbital sinuses

Parasite class: Trematoda

Family: Cyclocoelidae

Hosts: Duck, goose

Description, gross: Adult fluke are 7–20 × 2–5 mm. The body is pyriform and more rounded posteriorly.

Description, microscopic: Eggs are 95 × 55 μm.

Geographical distribution: Europe, Japan

Pathogenesis and clinical signs: Infection causes nasal catarrh.

Cytodites nudus

Common name: Air sac mite

Predilection site: Lung, air sac

Parasite class: Arachnida

Sub-class: Acari

Order: Acariformes

Sub-order: Sarcoptiformes (Astigmata)

Family: Cytoditidae

Description: The air-sac mite, *Cytodites nudus*, is found in the air passages and lungs of wild birds, poultry and canaries. The mite is oval and about

500 μm long, with a smooth cuticle. The chelicerae are absent and the palps are fused to form a soft, sucking organ through which fluids are imbibed. Legs are stout and unmodified, ending in a pair of stalked suckers and a pair of small claws.

Hosts: Birds, particularly poultry and canaries

Life cycle: Larval, nymphal and adult stages take place on the surface of the respiratory tract of the host, with the complete life cycle of the mite requiring 14–21 days.

Geographical distribution: Worldwide

Pathogenesis: Small infestations may have no obvious effect on the animal; large infestations may cause accumulation of mucus in the trachea and bronchi, leading to coughing and respiratory difficulties, air saculitis and weight loss. Balance may be affected in infested birds. Weakness, emaciation and death have been described with heavy infections.

Clinical signs: Coughing, respiratory difficulties, pulmonary oedema, weight loss, loss of balance or coordination.

Diagnosis: Positive diagnosis is only possible at post-mortem, when necropsy reveals white spots on the surface of air sacs.

Pathology: Death is usually associated with peritonitis, enteritis, emaciation and respiratory complications.

Epidemiology: Infestation may be spread by the host through coughing.

Treatment: Treatment with topical moxidectin every 3 weeks as necessary may be effective.

Control: It is important to treat all the birds in an aviary when commencing a preventative programme.

PARASITES OF THE LIVER

Histomonas meleagridis

Common name: 'Blackhead', infectious enterohepatitis

Predilection site: Caeca, liver

Parasite class: Zoomastigophorasida

Family: Monocercomonadidae

Description: A pleomorphic organism the morphology depending on the organ location and the stage of disease. In the caecum, the organism is round or oval, amoeboid, with clear ectoplasm and granular endoplasm, 6.0–20 μm in diameter, and bears a single flagellum (Fig. 7.32) although this appears to be lost when in the mucosal tissue or the liver. The nucleus is vesicular and a flagellum arises from a small blepharoplast near the nucleus. In the caecal mucosa and liver, the organism is found singly or in clusters and is amoeboid, 8–15 μm in diameter, with no flagellum. Both luminal and tissue stages exhibit pseudopodial movement.

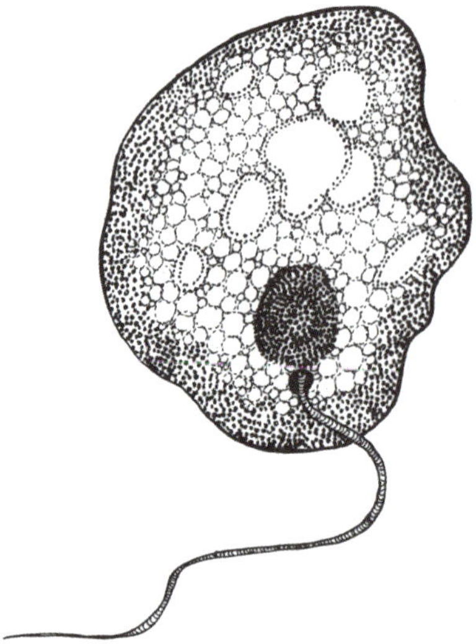

Fig. 7.32 *Histomonas meleagridis.*

Hosts: Turkey, game birds (pheasant, partridge), occasionally chickens

Life cycle: Birds become infected by ingestion of the embryonated egg of the caecal worm, *Heterakis gallinarum*, the flagellate being carried in the unhatched larva. When the egg hatches, the histomonads are released from the larva and enter the caecal mucosa where they cause ulceration and necrosis. They reach the liver in the portal stream and colonise the liver parenchyma, producing circular necrotic foci, which increase in size as the parasites multiply in the periphery of the lesion. The next phase of the life cycle is not clear, but it is presumed that the *Heterakis* worms become infected with the caecal histomonads, possibly by ingestion, and that these subsequently reach the ovary of the worm. It is certainly established that the histomonads become incorporated in a proportion of the *Heterakis* eggs, and thus reach the exterior. Infection of birds may also result from the ingestion of earthworms, which are transport hosts for *Heterakis* eggs and larvae.

Geographical distribution: Worldwide

Pathogenesis: The disease is essentially one of young turkeys up to 14 weeks old and is characterised by necrotic lesions in the caecae and liver. The earliest lesions are small ulcers in the caeca, but these quickly enlarge and coalesce so that the entire mucosa becomes necrotic and detaches, forming, with the caecal contents, a caseous plug. The liver lesions are circular and up to 1.0 cm in diameter with yellow depressed centres; they are found both on the surface and in the substance of the liver.

Mortality in poults may reach 100% and in birds which recover the caecum and liver may be permanently scarred.

Clinical signs: Infection is often mild and asymptomatic in chickens. Turkey poults become dull, the feathers are ruffled and the faeces become sulphur-yellow in colour 8 or more days after infection. Unless treated, the birds usually die within 1 or 2 weeks.

In older turkeys, the disease is more usually a chronic, wasting syndrome followed by recovery and subsequent immunity. The name 'blackhead' was first coined to describe the disease when cyanosis of the head and wattles was thought to be a characteristic feature. However, this sign is not necessarily present, and anyway is not confined to histomonosis.

Diagnosis: This is based on history, clinical signs and necropsy findings. Although rarely necessary, histological sections of liver or caecum may be prepared for specialist examination.

Pathology: The principal lesions of histomonosis appear in the caecum and liver. One or both caeca may be affected with small, raised pin-point ulcers, which subsequently enlarge and may affect the whole mucosa, occasionally ulcerating and perforating the caecal wall causing peritonitis. The mucosa becomes thickened and necrotic and may be covered with a characteristic, foul-smelling yellowish exudate that can eventually form hard dry caecal cores adhering to the caecal wall. The caeca are markedly inflamed and often enlarged. Liver lesions are pathognomonic and consist of circular, depressed, yellowish areas of necrosis and tissue degeneration, varying in size up to 1cm or more and extending deeply into the liver (Fig. 7.33). In older birds the lesions may be confluent and other organs such as the kidney and lung may occasionally be involved. The parasites can be readily found on histopathological examination. Affected lesions are hyperaemic, haemorrhagic and necrotic with lymphocytic and macrophage infiltration and the presence of giant cells.

Epidemiology: Although showing no signs of *Histomonas* infection, the domestic chicken is commonly infected with *H. gallinarum*, whose eggs, if fed to turkeys, will regularly produce histomonosis. Typically, histomonosis occurs when turkey poults are reared on ground shared, or recently vacated, by domestic chickens. However, since the organism may survive in embryonated *Heterakis* eggs in soil, or as larvae in earthworms, for over 2 years, outbreaks may arise on apparently clean ground. Young turkeys may also become infected when reared by broody hens, which are carriers.

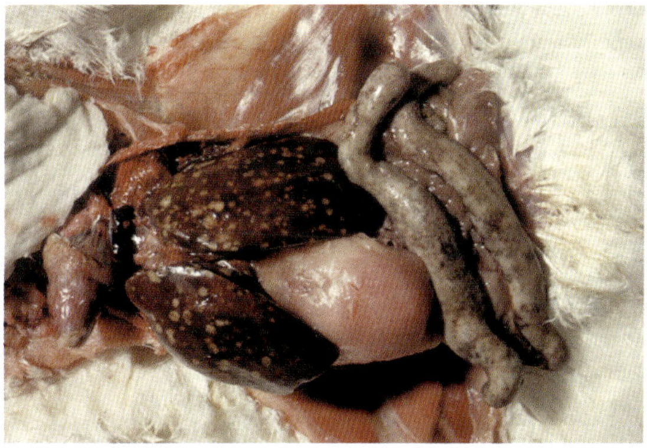

Fig. 7.33 Liver lesions due to *Histomonas meleagridis*.

Treatment: A number of drugs are effective, particularly the nitro-imidazole compounds, such as dimetridazole. These have been withdrawn in many countries because of concerns over human toxicity and carcinogenicity, and as such, few, if any, effective treatments are available.

Control: Histomoniosis can be prevented through good management. Turkeys should be reared on ground not used by domestic chickens for at least 2 years, or on fresh litter or wire floors raised above the ground. In game bird rearing facilities (pheasant, partridge), young birds should be raised in raised pens and their droppings removed regularly. When poults are old enough to be moved to rearing pens they should be placed on clean ground where birds have not been previously kept for at least 2 years, as *Heterakis* eggs may remain viable in soil or earthworms for some time, depending on the climate and soil type. The use of anthelmintics for the control of *Heterakis* worms can be an effective control measure in limiting infection and spread.

PARASITES OF THE CIRCULATORY SYSTEM

Bilharziella polonica

Predilection site: Mesenteric and pelvic veins

Parasite class: Trematoda

Family: Schistosomatidae

Description, gross: The body is lancet-shaped posteriorly and the sexes are separate. Males about are 4 mm and females 2 mm.

Description, microscopic: The female genital pore is just behind the ventral sucker and the short uterus contains one egg at a time. The eggs have a long, narrow and elongate anterior end and a swollen posterior end with a terminal spine, and measure 400 × 100 μm.

Hosts: Duck

Intermediate hosts: Snails of the genera *Planorbis*

Life cycle: Eggs are laid in the small vessels of the intestinal wall through which they penetrate and are passed out in the faeces. Development takes place in the snail intermediate host leading to the release of cercariae, which infect the intermediate host either percutaneously, or following ingestion.

Geographical distribution: Europe, North America

Pathogenesis and clinical signs: Generally considered to be non-pathogenic. Eggs in the wall of the intestine may produce inflammation. Parasites have been found in the pancreas, spleen and kidneys, but in these organs they eventually die.

Treatment and control: Not required

Leucocytozoon caulleryi

Predilection site: Blood

Parasite class: Sporozoasida

Family: Plasmodiidae

Description: Gamonts present in erythrocytes when mature are round, 15.5 × 15 μm, and distort the host cell causing the host cell nucleus to form a narrow, dark band extending about one third of the way around the parasite. Meglomeronts present within tissues are 26–300 μm in diameter.

Hosts: Chicken, guinea fowl

Life cycle: Sporozoites are introduced into a new host by the feeding insects. Parasites undergo merogony in the endothelial cells of the liver, heart, kidney, spleen, thymus, pancreas and other organs of the avian host. The meronts are spherical or lobed and divide at first into cytomeres, which eventually fuse forming meglomeronts, which produce a great number of merozoites. Gamonts appear in the blood about 14 days post infection and are found in erythrocytes or sometimes erythroblasts, and the infected host cells become distorted and assume a spindle-shape. When mature the parasites break out of the host cell and lie free in the plasma. When ingested during blood feeding by the vector insect, *Culicoides* spp, a zygote is formed which elongates into an ookinete about 21 μm long, which passes through the midgut wall to form subspherical oocysts on the midgut outer wall. Sporozoites are formed and pass to the salivary glands and are introduced to the new host when the midges bite them.

Geographical distribution: Asia

Pathogenesis: Some strains of *L. caulleryi* are non-pathogenic and others are highly pathogenic, killing a high percentage of chickens in a flock.

Clinical signs: Affected chickens are listless, diarrhoeic and anaemic with pallid combs and wattles.

Diagnosis: Gamonts can be seen in Giemsa-stained bloodsmears, the gamont being rounded in *L. caulleryi*. There are no pigment granules. On postmortem there are haemorrhages, splenomegaly and hepatomegaly and many organs have grossly visible white dots due to the presence of the meronts.

Pathology: There is marked haemorrhage in the lungs, livers and kidneys and there may be gross haemorrhage from the kidney lesions into the peritoneal cavity due to the presence of megalomeronts, which cause haemorrhage on rupture.

Epidemiology: The incidence of disease is linked to the presence and relative abundance of the midge vectors, *Culicoides* spp. In Japan, outbreaks occur frequently in June when the rice paddy fields are ready for planting and offer ideal conditions for midges to breed.

Treatment: Treatment is not usually effective although pyrimethamine (1 ppm) and sulphadimethoxine (10 ppm) or clopidol at 125 ppm in feed may prevent but not cure infections of *L. caulleryi.*

Control: Control requires eliminating the arthropod vector from the environment of the host. Insecticidal sprays and repellents sprayed within houses may be used to reduce the insect populations.

Leucocytozoon sabrazesi

Synonym: *Leucocytozoon schueffneri*, *Leucocytozoon macleani*

Predilection site: Blood

Parasite class: Sporozoasida

Family: Plasmodiidae

Description: Gamonts present in erythrocytes when mature are elongate, 22–24 × 4–7 μm, and distort the host cell, which becomes spindle-shaped, 67 × 6 μm, with long cytoplasmic horns extending beyond the parasites. The host cell nucleus forms a narrow, darkly staining band along one side of the parasite.

Hosts: Chicken, guinea fowl

Life cycle: As for *Leucocytozoon caulleryi*

Geographical distribution: Southeast Asia, Indonesia

Pathogenesis: Occurs uncommonly but can cause significant losses in flocks.

Clinical signs: Clinical signs include pyrexia, diarrhoea, leg paralysis, discharge from the mouth and anaemia.

Diagnosis: Gamonts can be seen in Giemsa-stained blood smears, the gamont being elongate in *L. sabrazesi*. On postmortem there are haemorrhages, splenomegaly and hepatomegaly and many organs have grossly visible white dots due to the presence of the meronts.

Pathology: As for *L. caulleryi*

Epidemiology: The incidence of disease is linked to the presence and relative abundance of the midge vectors, *Culicoides* spp.

Treatment: Treatment is not usually effective.

Leucocytozoon smithi

Synonym: *Leucocytozoon schueffneri*, *Leucocytozoon macleani*

Predilection site: Blood

Parasite class: Sporozoasida

Family: Plasmodiidae

Description: The mature gamonts are rounded at first but later become elongate, averaging 20–22 μm in length. Their host cells are elongate, averaging 45 × 14 μm, with pale cytoplasmic horns extending out beyond the enclosed parasite. The host cell nucleus is elongate, forming a long, thin, dark band along one side of the parasite, often splitting to form a band on each side of the parasite. Hepatic meronts in the hepatocytes are 10–20 × 7–14 μm (mean 13.5 × 10.5 μm).

Hosts: Turkey

Life cycle: Birds become infected when bitten by a blackfly vector. The sporozoites enter the bloodstream, invade various tissue cells, round up, and become meronts. Hepatic meronts occur in the liver cells, the earliest stage containing round and crescent-shaped, basophilic cytomeres, which develop into masses of deeply staining merozoites that completely fill the host cell cytoplasm. Megalomeronts have not been seen but eventually merozoites enter blood cells and form gamonts. In the blackfly's midgut, microgametes are formed and develop into oocysts to produce sporozoites, which break out of the oocysts and pass to the salivary glands, where they accumulate. The prepatent period is 9 days.

Geographical distribution: Europe, North America

Pathogenesis: *L. smithi is* markedly pathogenic for turkeys, and extremely heavy losses have been reported. Adult birds are less seriously affected than poults, and the disease runs a slower course, but even they may die. Recovered birds continue to carry parasites in their blood. Some birds recover completely, but in other birds persistent infection may lead to lethargy, lack of libido in male birds and persistent coughing. Sudden stress in these birds may lead to death.

Clinical signs: Affected poults are anorexic, lethargic and have difficulty in moving; in the later stages there may be incoordination, and the birds may suddenly collapse, become comatose and die. Birds surviving for 2–3 days after signs of disease appeared, tend to recover.

Diagnosis: Diagnosis is based on finding and identifying the gamonts in Giemsa-stained blood smears, or the meronts in tissue sections.

Pathology: Affected birds are anaemic and emaciated. The spleen and liver are enlarged, and there is enteritis involving the duodenum, sometimes extending throughout the small intestine.

Epidemiology: The vectors of *L. smithi* are blackflies of the genus *Simulium* and disease occurs in domestic and wild turkeys in North America and Europe in mountainous or hilly areas where suitable blackfly breeding habitats occur.

Treatment: No effective treatment has been reported.

Control: Prevention depends on blackfly control. Ideally, turkeys should not be raised in areas where blackflies occur in significant numbers, or they should be raised under conditions that prevent them from being bitten by blackflies by rearing in screened quarters using 32–36 mesh screening.

Leucocytozoon simondi

Predilection site: Blood

Parasite class: Sporozoasida

Family: Plasmodiidae

Description: Mature macrogametes and microgamonts are elongate, sometimes rounded, 14–22 μm long, and present within erythrocytes or leucocytes, which become elongate, up to 45–55 μm long, with their nucleus forming a long, thin, dark band along one side. Infected host cells have pale cytoplasmic horns extending out beyond the parasite and the nucleus. Hepatic meronts are 11–18 μm in diameter; megalomeronts found in various tissues of the body are 6–164 μm in diameter when mature.

Hosts: Duck, goose

Life cycle: Birds become infected when bitten by a blackfly vector. The sporozoites enter the bloodstream, invade various tissue cells, round up, and become meronts. Two types of meront occur in the duck. Hepatic meronts occur in the liver cells, forming a number of cytomeres, which in turn form small merozoites

Table 7.7 Avian sub-genera of *Plasmodium*.

Sub-genus	Description
Parasites lacking pigment	
Plasmodioides	Gametocytes and meronts large; mature parasites displace host cell nucleus; present only in circulating leucocytes
Parasites with pigment	
Haemamoeba	Gametocytes round or ovoid; mature parasites typically displace host cell nucleus towards pole
Huffia	Gametocytes elongate; mature forms do not displace host cell nucleus towards pole; meronts present in circulating erythrocyte precursors, not in mature erythrocytes
Giovannolaia	Gametocytes elongate; mature forms do not displace host cell nucleus towards pole; meronts present in mature erythrocytes, not in circulating erythrocyte precursors; erythrocytic meronts generally larger than erythrocyte nucleus and contain noticeable amount of cytoplasm
Novyella	Gametocytes elongate; mature forms do not displace host cell nucleus towards pole; meronts present in mature erythrocytes, not in circulating erythrocyte precursors; erythrocytic meronts smaller than host cell nucleus; without noticeable cytoplasm

by multiple fission. Megalomeronts are found in the brain, lungs, liver, heart, kidney, gizzard, intestine, and lymphoid tissues 4–6 days after exposure. They are more common than the hepatic meronts. Each megalomeront produces many thousands of bipolar merozoites. The merozoites enter blood cells and form gamonts. Merogony continues in the internal organs for an indefinite, long time, although at a much reduced rate. During this relapse phase adult birds are not seriously affected but they are the source of infection for the new crop of ducklings. In the blackfly's midgut four to eight microgametes are formed by exflagellation from the microgamonts. These fertilise the macrogametes to form a motile zygote or ookinete about 33 × 5 μm. Ookinetes are present in the blackfly midgut 2–6 hours after ingestion of infected blood. They develop into oocysts both in the midgut wall and in the midgut itself and produce several slender sporozoites 5–10 μm long, with one end rounded and the other pointed. They break out of the oocysts and pass to the salivary glands, where they accumulate. Viable sporozoites can be found for at least 18 days after an infective feeding.

Geographical distribution: Northern USA, Canada, Europe, Vietnam

Pathogenesis: *L. simondi is* markedly pathogenic for ducks and geese. The heaviest losses occur among young birds with very rapid onset. Adult birds are more chronically affected, and the disease develops more slowly in them. Mortality is low but if it does occur is seldom less than 4 days after the appearance of signs. Death usually occurs as the peripheral parasitism approaches its peak, 10–12 days after infection. Ducklings that recover often fail to grow normally, and recovered birds remain carriers.

Clinical signs: Acutely affected ducklings are listless and inappetent, with rapid, laboured breathing due to obstruction of the lung capillaries with meronts. They may go through a short period of nervous excitement just before death. Adult birds are thin and listless.

Diagnosis: Diagnosis is based on finding and identifying the gamonts in Giemsa-stained blood smears, or the meronts in tissue sections.

Pathology: The principal lesions are splenomegaly with liver hypertrophy and degeneration. Anaemia and leucocytosis are present, and the blood clots poorly.

Epidemiology: The vectors of *L. simondi* are various species of blackflies (*Simulium* and other simuliids) and disease occurs commonly in domestic ducks and geese in mountainous or hilly areas where cold, rapid streams act as suitable blackfly breeding habitats.

Treatment: No effective treatment has been reported.

Control: Prevention depends on blackfly control. Ideally, ducks and geese should not be raised in areas where blackflies occur in significant numbers, or, raising them under conditions that prevent them from being bitten by blackflies by rearing in screened quarters using 32–36 mesh screening. Since wild ducks and geese are reservoirs of infection for domestic birds, the latter should not be raised close to places where wild birds congregate.

Plasmodium gallinaceum

Subgenus: *Haemamoeba*

Synonym: *Plasmodium metataticum*

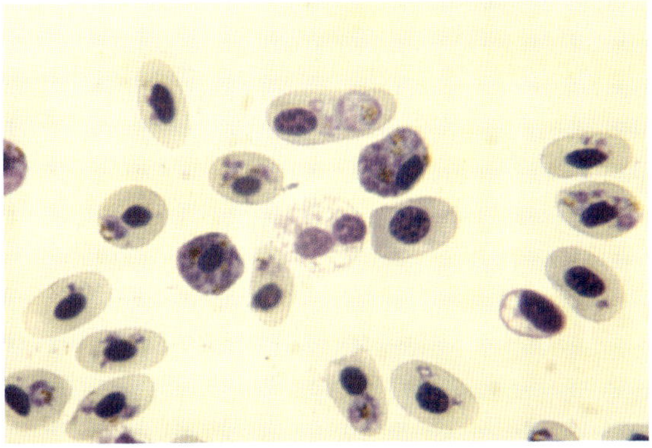

Fig. 7.34 Intraerythrocytic stages of *Plasmodium gallinaceum*.

Common name: Avian malaria

Predilection site: Blood

Parasite class: Sporozoasida

Family: Plasmodiidae

Description: The trophozoite is a small rounded form containing a large vacuole, which displaces the cytoplasm of the parasite to the periphery of the red blood cell. The nucleus is situated at one of the poles, giving the young form a 'signet ring' appearance when stained by Giemsa. Both gametocytes and meronts of *P. gallinaceum* can be round, oval or irregular in shape. The nucleus of host cells is rarely expelled during infection, but may be displaced by the parasite (Fig. 7.34). Each meront produces from eight to thirty-six merozoites and on average there are 16–20 merozoites in erythrocytic meronts.

Hosts: Chicken, guinea fowl

Life cycle: Following the introduction of the sporozoites from infected mosquitoes, numerous pre-erythrocytic meronts (cryptozoites) are found in the macrophages and fibroblasts of the skin near the point of entry. Merozoites from this first generation of pre-erythrocytic meronts form a second generation of pre-erythrocytic meronts, the metacryptozoites, which reach maturity at about 72 hours. Merozoites from the metacryptozoites enter erythrocytes and cells of the lymphoid–macrophage system in the skin, spleen, lungs and capillary endothelial cells of the major organs. In this species, the exoerythrocytic developmental stages may be added to by forms which are derived from the erythrocytic cycle. These are known as phanerozoites, being derived from the merozoites of the meronts in the erythrocytic cycle.

The erythrocytic cycle is initiated 7–10 days after infection by merozoites from metacryptozoites and at other times by merozoites from exoerythrocytic meronts located, according to species, in the endothelial or haemopoietic cells. On entering the erythrocyte, the merozoite rounds up to form a trophozoite. The early trophozoites undergo merogony to produce merozoites, which are released from the meronts synchronously. After a number of asexual generations have occurred, some merozoites undergo sexual development with the formation of microgametocytes and macrogametocytes, the latter being generally more numerous, and stain more intensely blue with Giemsa than do the microgametocytes. Further development of the gametocyte stages can take place only when a suitable mosquito host ingests the blood. Development in the mosquito is rapid. Following ingestion, the nucleus of the microgametocyte divides, and through a process of exflagellation, 6–8 μm long, thin, flagella-like microgametes are extruded from the parent cell, become detached and swim away to find, and fertilise, the macrogamete. The resulting zygote (ookinete) is motile and penetrates the midgut mucosa and comes to lie on the outer surface of the stomach, forming an early oocyst about 50–60 μm in diameter. The nucleus of the oocyst divides repeatedly to produce a very large number of sporozoites. Maturation of the oocyst takes a variable period of time depending on the species of parasite, temperature and the species of mosquito; but in general, it is 10–20 days. When mature, the oocyst ruptures, liberating the sporozoites into the body cavity of the mosquito, which then migrate all over the body of the mosquito but eventually reach the salivary glands and are now infective to a new host, infection occurring when the mosquito takes a blood meal. A mosquito remains infected for its lifespan, transmitting malarial parasites every time it takes a blood meal.

Geographical distribution: Southeast Asia, Indonesia, Malaysia, Borneo, India, Sri Lanka. The distribution in domestic chickens coincides with the natural host, the jungle fowl.

Pathogenesis: *Plasmodium gallinaceum* can be highly pathogenic in domestic chickens, particularly when European breeds are introduced into endemic areas where the cycle is maintained in wild red jungle fowl. Anaemia is caused by destruction of circulating erythrocytes by developing meronts. Neurological complications are caused by obstruction of capillaries in the brain by extra-erythrocytic meronts.

Clinical signs: Birds with acute infection may be lethargic, anaemic with pale combs, diarrhoeic and show partial or total paralysis.

Diagnosis: Parasites can be seen in Giemsa-stained blood smears. The presence of meronts with numerous merozoites and round gametocytes that displace the host cell nucleus are distinctive for *P. gallinaceum*.

Pathology: There may be pallor of the carcase due to anaemia, brown-tinged skin and mucous membranes due to pigment deposition, splenomegaly, and darkening of the viscera, especially liver, spleen, lungs and brain due to accumulation of pigment. Microscopic lesions are most evident in the blood. In the kidneys there may be accumulation of pigment in macrophages, fatty degeneration of the parenchyma and possibly immune complex glomerulonephritis. In the lungs there may be accumulation of pigment in macrophages in the capillaries, obstruction of the blood vessels and lymphatics and pulmonary oedema.

Epidemiology: In Sri Lanka the mosquito vector is *Mansonia crassipes*. In other areas of its geographical range, the vectors are unknown and detailed epidemiological studies have not been conducted. A range of anopholine species of the genera *Anopheles*, *Armigeres*, *Culex*, *Culiseta* and *Mansonia* have been shown experimentally to be capable of transmitting infection.

Treatment: Sulphonamide drugs (sulphachloropyrazine, sulphamonomethozine) and halofuginone have been shown to be effective in the laboratory.

Control: Mosquito control can potentially reduce transmission of this parasite but detailed control methods have not been studied. More potentially effective measures include keeping poultry in mosquito-proof buildings or keeping domestic chickens in areas away from the wild reservoir hosts.

Plasmodium juxtanucleare

Subgenus: *Novyella*

Synonym: *Plasmodium japonicum*

Common name: Avian malaria

Predilection site: Blood

Parasite class: Sporozoasida

Family: Plasmodiidae

Description: Meronts are small, round, ovoid or irregular and usually in contact with the erythrocyte host cell nucleus and produce two to seven (mean four) merozoites. Gamonts are round, ovoid, irregular or elongate pyriform leading to the host erythrocyte often being distorted.

Hosts: Chicken, red jungle fowl (*Gallus gallus*) in Sri Lanka, greywing francolin (*Francolinus africanus*) in South Africa, bamboo partridge (*Bambusicola thoracica*) in Taiwan

Life cycle: Details on the pre-erythrocytic development following inoculation by a mosquito vector are not known. Extraerythrocytic meronts have been reported in lymphoid–macrophage cells of the spleen, liver, kidney, heart, lung, bone marrow, testes, pancreas and brain, being most common in the spleen. Erythrocytic cycles peak at 6–8 days with merozoites undergoing sexual development with the formation of microgametocytes and macrogametocytes; the latter are generally more numerous, and stain more intensely blue with Giemsa than do the microgametocytes. Further development of the gametocyte stages can take place only when a suitable mosquito host ingests the blood. Development in the mosquito is similar to other species.

Geographical distribution: South and Central America (Mexico, Brazil, Uruguay), Asia (Sri Lanka, Philipines, Taiwan, Japan, Malaysia), east Africa (Tanzania) and South Africa

Pathogenesis: This species is highly pathogenic, causing severe anaemia through erythrocyte destruction and organ damage due to massive numbers of exo-erythrocytic forms. Central nervous system signs are associated with exo-erythrocytic forms causing damage to endothelial cells of the brain capillaries.

Clinical signs: Affected birds are lethargic, depressed, progressively emaciated and anaemic. Severely affected birds have a protruding abdomen caused by splenic and hepatic enlargement and ocular haemorrhage may occur. Affected birds may show paralysis or central nervous system signs. Coma and death occur in heavy infections after a short period of time.

Diagnosis: Giemsa-stained blood smears usually reveal numerous meronts and gamonts in the erythrocytes and infected cells also have dark pigment granules (digested haemoglobin). As blood samples cool, motile microgametes may be seen in the plasma in wet smears. This species can be distinguished from *P. gallinaceum* by its more elongate gametocytes and by tendency of the meront stages to cling closely to the host cell nucleus.

Pathology: The liver and spleen are enlarged and dark brown–black in colour. Exo-erythrocytic stages can be seen in the endothelial cells and reticuloendothelial cells of the liver, spleen and brain.

Epidemiology: *P. juxtanucleare* is a parasite of wild birds that infects domestic chickens when wild reservoir birds and mosquito vectors are present. Infection is spread by culicine mosquitoes of the genus *Culex* (*C. sitiens*, *C. annulus*, *C. gelidus* and *C. tritaeniorynchus* in Malaysia; *C. saltanensis* in Brazil). Natural vectors in other parts of its range are unknown and detailed epidemiological studies have not been undertaken.

Treatment: Affected birds or flocks may be treated with primaquine at 100 mg/kg orally or sulphonamide–trimethoprim combinations may be tried. Sulphonamide drugs (sulphachloropyrazine, sulphamonomethozine) and halofuginone, which are effective against other *Plasmodium* species in birds, may also be effective.

Control: Since mosquitoes spread malaria, prevention depends on mosquito control. Residual spraying of poultry houses with insecticides may be effective. Birds can also be raised in screened quarters in areas where mosquitoes are particularly prevalent.

Notes: Closely related species that occur in cage birds, pigeon, waterfowl, Guinea fowl, pheasant, quail and turkey include *P. vaughani*, *P. rouxi*, *P. nucleophilum*, *P. kempi*, *P. leanucleus* and *P. dissanaikei*.

Plasmodium durae

Subgenus: *Giovannolaia*

Synonym: *Plasmodium japonicum*

Common name: Avian malaria

Predilection site: Blood

Parasite class: Sporozoasida

Family: Plasmodiidae

Description: Trophozoites are amoeboid in appearance. Mature meronts rarely displace the host cell nucleus and contain 6–14 (mean eight) merozoites. Gamonts are elongate, at the end or side of the host cell, and often displace the host cell nucleus, although the host cell is not usually enlarged. Pigment granules are usually large, round and black.

Hosts: Turkey, francolins (*Francolinus leucoscepus*, *F. levaillantii levaillantii*)

Life cycle: The detailed life cycle has not been described. Exo-erythrocytic meronts have been found in capillary endothelial cells of lung, liver, spleen and brain tissue, but are especially numerous in the brain. In turkeys, parasitaemias peak between 15 and 25 days post infection. On entering the erythrocytes, the merozoites round up to form trophozoites. The early trophozoites undergo merogony to produce merozoites, which are released from the meronts synchronously. After a number of asexual generations, some merozoites undergo sexual development with the formation of microgametocytes and macrogametocytes. Further development of the gametocyte stages can take place only when a suitable mosquito host ingests the blood. Development in the mosquito is similar to other species.

Geographical distribution: Sub-Saharan Africa (Kenya, Nigeria, Zimbabwe, South Africa)

Pathogenesis: *Plasmodium durae* is highly pathogenic in domestic turkeys, and depending on strain and geographic location, cause death in up to 90% of young turkey poults. Adult birds often develop right pulmonary hypertension as a consequence of hypoxic pulmonary arterial hypertension. Developing exo-erythrocytic meronts may block cerebral capillaries such that infected birds can exhibit neurological signs and paralysis before death.

Clinical signs: Young poults show few clinical signs until immediately prior to death, when severe convulsions may occur. Adult birds are lethargic, anorexic and may develop oedematous legs and gangrene of the wattles.

Diagnosis: The parasites can be identified in Giemsa-stained thin blood smears. Meronts are small and rounded and the gametocytes are elongate and do not curve around the host erythrocyte nucleus.

Pathology: As for *P. juxtanucleare*

Epidemiology: The vectors involved in transmission are not fully known.

Treatment: Sulphonamide drugs (sulphachloropyrazine, sulphamonomethozine) and halofuginone may be effective in treatment. Sulphamonomethozine does not provide full protection from mortality when given after the appearance of circulating parasites and sulphachloropyrazine, whilst reducing mortality, has no effect on the parasitaemia, suggesting activity against exo-erythrocytic meronts.

Control: As for other avian malaria species.

Notes: Closely related species of the subgenus *Giovannolaia* reported in duck, goose, turkey, francolin, Guinea fowl, quail, partridge and pigeon include *P. fallax*, *P. circumflexum*, *P. polare*, *P. lophurae*, *P. gabaldoni*, *P. pinotti*, *P. pediocetti*, *P. formosanum*, *P. anasum* and *P. hegneri*.

Haemoproteus meleagridis

Predilection site: Blood

Parasite class: Sporozoasida

Family: Plasmodiidae

Description: Macrogametes and microgametes present in erythrocytes are elongate and curve around the host cell nucleus, occupying about half to three quarters of the host cell. The nucleus of macrogametocytes is generally more compact, the cytoplasm denser, and melanin granules more evenly distributed compared with the polar clustering in microgametocytes.

Hosts: Turkey

Life cycle: Details of the life cycle are incomplete. Sporozoites in the salivary gland of the insect vector enter the circulation of the host when the insect bites. Meronts occur in the vascular epithelium of the lung, liver, kidney and spleen. Merozoites develop within the meront in clusters and when mature are released into the circulation as tiny round bodies which transform into macrogametes and microgamonts within erythrocytes.

Geographical distribution: North America

Pathogenesis and clinical signs: Generally considered non-pathogenic, or only slightly pathogenic.

Epidemiology: Vectors are thought to be midges (*Culicoides*) or hippoboscids.

Treatment and control: Not usually required although general insect control or preventative measures may limit infection.

Haemoproteus nettionis

Synonym: *Haemoproteus anatis*, *Haemoproteus anseris*, *Haemoproteus hermani*

Predilection site: Blood

Parasite class: Sporozoasida

Family: Plasmodiidae

Description: Macrogametes and microgametes present in erythrocytes are elongate and curve around the host cell nucleus, partially encircling the host cell nucleus and often displacing it. They contain a few to 30 or more pigment granules, which are usually coarse and round and often grouped at the ends of the cell. The host cell is not enlarged.

Hosts: Duck, goose, wild duck and swans

Life cycle: As for *Haemoproteus meleagridis*

Geographical distribution: Worldwide

Pathogenesis and clinical signs: As for *Haemoproteus meleagridis*

Diagnosis: As for *Haemoproteus meleagridis*

Epidemiology: Vectors are midges (*Culicoides*). The parasite is essentially a parasite of wild waterfowl and may infect domestic birds in endemic areas.

Treatment and control: As for *Haemoproteus meleagridis*

Trypanosoma gallinarum

Predilection site: Blood

Parasite class: Zoomastigophorasida

Family: Trypanosomatidae

Description: Pleomorphic organisms, 26–29 μm long, or even longer, with a free flagellum

Hosts: Chicken

Life cycle: Multiplication occurs in the avian host by longitudinal binary fission of the epimastigote form in various tissues. Following ingestion by the invertebrate host, they multiply in the midgut before migrating forward to the salivary glands, forming tryptomastigotes. Metacyclic trypanosomes are inoculated into the new host when the arthropod feeds.

Geographical distribution: Africa

Trypanosoma avium

Predilection site: Blood

Parasite class: Zoomastigophorasida

Family: Trypanosomatidae

Description: As for *T. gallinarum*.

Pathogenesis: Avian trypanosomes are considered non-pathogenic.

Diagnosis: Detection is by examination of Giemsa-stained thin blood smears or examination of buffy coat from a microhaematocrit tube following centrifugation (Fig. 7.35).

Epidemiology: Species are transmitted by a variety of blood-sucking arthropods including mosquitoes, simuliids, hippoboscids and red mites. Trypanosomes persist during periods of adverse conditions in the bone marrow and reappear in the spring.

Treatment and control: Not required

Aegyptianella pullorum

Predilection site: Blood

Parasite order: Rickettsiales

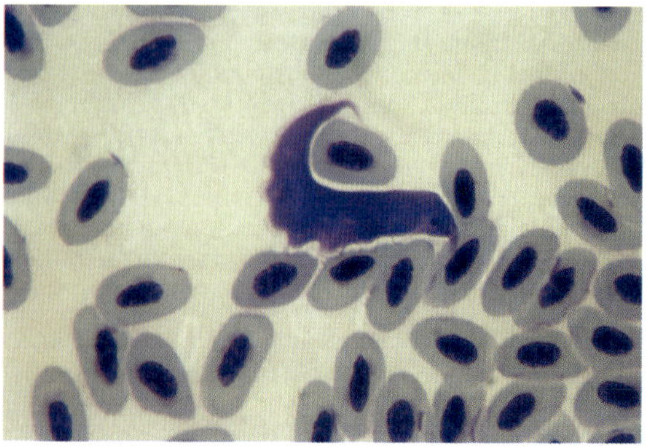

Fig. 7.35 Tryptomastigote of *Trypanosoma avium*.

Family: Anaplasmataceae

Description: *Anaplasma*-like bodies of various sizes found in the cytoplasm of erythrocytes. The organisms occur as initial bodies followed by development forms and marginal bodies ('signet-ring') in the cytoplasm of erythrocytes. The early trophozoites or initial bodies occur in erythrocytes, are small (0.5–1.0 μm) and round to oval. Spherical bodies up to 4 μm containing up to 25 small granules may occur.

Hosts: Chicken, turkey, goose, duck

Life cycle: The life cycle is simple with multiplication of the organisms within erythrocytes. Transmission is by the soft tick, *Argas persicus*.

Geographical distribution: Africa, Asia, southern Europe

Aegyptianella moshkovskii

Predilection site: Blood

Parasite order: Rickettsiales

Family: Anaplasmataceae

Description: The organism usually produces four to six trophozoites. The early trophozoites within the erythrocytes are small (0.2–0.6 μm). Larger mature forms are 2.1 × 1.4 μm with large oval or irregular forms (0.9–5.3 μm).

Hosts: Chicken, turkey, pheasant, wild birds

Life cycle: As for *A. pullorum*

Geographical distribution: Africa, India, southeast Asia, Egypt, Russia and parts of eastern CIS states

Pathogenesis: Both species of *Aegyptianella* are pathogenic. The following descriptions apply to both species.

The intra-erythrocytic parasites cause severe anaemia, jaundice and frequent death. The incubation period is 12–15 days.

Clinical signs: Affected animals show ruffled feathers, anorexia, droopiness and diarrhoea and hyperthermia may be found. The clinical condition is often complicated by fowl spirochaetosis, which is also transmitted by *Argas persicus*.

Diagnosis: Diagnosis is based on the demonstration of organisms in Giemsa-stained bloodsmears. Intraerythrocytic forms (marginal bodies) and extra-erythrocytic forms may be seen in leucocytes, lymphocytes, monocytes and also in the plasma.

Pathology: Anaemia, jaundice, enlargement of the liver and the spleen, yellow–green kidneys and petechial haemorrhage of the serosa may be seen at necropsy.

Epidemiology: Infection is tick transmitted by the soft tick, *Argas persicus*. Indigenous poultry rarely suffer the acute disease, but freshly introduced stock are especially susceptible and may die within a few days. Recovered birds are frequently carriers.

Treatment: Tetracycline compounds (oxytetracycline, chlortetracycline, 15–30 mg/kg per os) are effective and usually recommended for treatment.

Control: Tick control and treatment of premises, where adults and nymphal ticks may hide in cracks and crevices. After cleaning, premises should be treated with an acaracide, such as carbaryl, coumaphos or malathion.

PARASITES OF THE NERVOUS SYSTEM

Oxyspirura mansoni

Synonym: *Oxyspirura parvorum*

Common name: Eye worm

Predilection site: Eye

Parasite class: Nematoda

Superfamily: Spiruroidea

Description, gross: These are slender worms with a smooth cuticle and a globular-shaped pharynx. The males measure around 10–15 mm and the females 14–20 mm.

Description, microscopic: The tail of the male is curved ventrally and alae are absent. Spicules are uneven; the right being short and stubby, the left long and slender.

Final hosts: Chicken, turkey, guineafowl, peafowl

Intermediate hosts: Cockroaches (*Pycnoscelus surinamensis*)

Life cycle: The life cycle is indirect. Eggs pass through the lachrymal duct, are swallowed and shed in the faeces. These are ingested by an intermediate host and development to the infective stage occurs. Following consumption of the intermediate host by the definitive host the larvae migrate from the oesophagus and pharynx to the eye via the lachrymal duct.

Geographical distribution: Many areas of the world, particularly the tropical and subtropical regions. It is not present in Europe.

Pathogenesis: It occurs on the conjunctiva, under the nictitating membrane, or in the nasal–lachrymal ducts or the conjunctival sacs. Although not a highly pathogenic genus, moderate infections can induce an inflammation of the eye with the nictitating membrane becoming oedematous. Heavy infections may cause blindness or occlusion of the nasal passages.

Clinical signs: Birds may be observed scratching the eyes if they become irritated. Affected birds develop opthalmitis, which becomes inflamed with watery eyes.

Diagnosis: A definitive diagnosis is made by finding the parasite in the conjunctival sac. It may be necessary to instill local anaesthetic into the eye to allow removal. Examination of lacrimal secretions may reveal eggs or first-stage larvae.

Pathology: Untreated heavy infections can cause ophthalmia with erosion of the eyeball.

Treatment: Oral or topical levamisole or tetramisole and ivermectin have been used successfully to treat infections. Removal with fine forceps after instillation of local anaesthetic has been reported.

Control: Attempts to control the poultry spiruroids are unlikely to be fully successful because of the ready availability of the intermediate hosts. Reduction and restriction of cockroaches will be beneficial.

Notes: The genus *Oxyspirura* in birds is the equivalent of *Thelazia* in mammals.

PARASITES OF THE REPRODUCTIVE/ UROGENITAL SYSTEM

Prosthogonimus pellucidus

Synonym: *Prosthogonimus intercalandus*, *Prosthogonimus cuneatus*

Common name: Oviduct fluke

Predilection site: Cloaca, oviduct and bursa of Fabricius

Parasite class: Trematoda

Family: Prosthogonimidae

Description, gross: Adults are pear-shaped, semi-transparent, pale orange when fresh and measure around 9–12 mm in length, being broader towards the posterior. Two suckers are present.

Description, microscopic: Eggs are around 29 × 13 µm in size, dark brown and have a small spine at the opposite pole to the operculum.

Final hosts: Chicken, turkey, other fowl, goose and duck

Intermediate hosts: 1. Aquatic snails such as *Bithynia teutaculata*. 2. Nymphal stage of various dragonflies

Life cycle: Eggs are passed in faeces and hatch to produce a miracidium, which penetrates a snail to form a mother sporocyst, which produces daughter sporocysts. These directly produce cercariae, there being no redial development, and the cercariae are shed from the snail and will enter dragonfly larvae via the rectal respiratory chamber where they eventually encyst as the metacercaria stage in the haemocoele. Infection of the final host occurs through ingestion of the infected nymphal stage or the adult dragonfly. The immature trematodes then migrate to the cloaca and bursa of Fabricius or enter the oviduct. The fluke is mature after about a week.

Geographical distribution: Worldwide

Pathogenesis: *Prosthogonimus* is considered to be the most pathogenic of the trematodes that infect poultry and ducks in America and Europe. Usually chickens are mainly affected. Even moderate infections can inflame the oviduct resulting in the formation of eggs with a soft shell or lacking a shell. Large numbers of flukes can be fatal.

Clinical signs: Infected birds may have an enlarged flaccid abdomen, become listless, show discharge of a limey secretion from the cloaca and may lay abnormally formed eggs. The feathers around the cloaca become soiled. Sometimes there is complete cessation of egg laying.

Diagnosis: Fluke eggs can be identified in secretions from the cloaca or found in the abdominal cavity at necropsy.

Pathology: The oviduct is often severely inflamed with a thick yellow–white secretion in the lumen. Irritation in the oviduct can cause a reversal of peristalsis, resulting in egg, bacteria and parasite material entering the abdominal cavity and causing peritonitis. The comb and wattles can become cyanotic in chronically infected birds. Sometimes there is a whitish milky discharge from the cloaca.

Epidemiology: The occurrence is seasonal with the main peak of infection in the spring and summer in temperate regions.

Treatment: Albendazole, fenbendazole, flubendazole at 5 mg/kg or praziquantel at 5–10 mg/kg.

Control: Reduction of snails and their habitats will limit infection in the final hosts and where possible flocks should be denied access to the margins of ponds and lakes.

Prosthogonimus macrorchis

Common name: Oviduct fluke

Predilection site: Cloaca, oviduct, and bursa of Fabricius

Parasite class: Trematoda

Family: Prosthogonimidae

Description, gross: Adults are pear-shaped, semi-transparent, reddish coloured and measure around 7–8 mm in length, being broader towards the posterior.

Description, microscopic: The testes are larger than in *P. pellucidus*. Eggs are around 25 μm and have a small spine at the opposite pole to the operculum.

Final hosts: Chicken, turkey, other fowl and duck

Intermediate hosts: As for *P. pellucidus*

Geographical distribution: North America

Prosthogonimus ovatus

Common name: Oviduct fluke

Predilection site: Cloaca, oviduct and bursa of Fabricius

Parasite class: Trematoda

Family: Prosthogonimidae

Description, gross: Adults are pear-shaped, semi-transparent and smaller than *P. pellucidus* and *P. macrorchis* measuring about 4–6 mm in length. The cuticle is covered with spines.

Description, microscopic: Eggs are around 23 × 13 μm in size and have a small spine at the opposite pole to the operculum.

Final hosts: Chicken, turkey, other fowl and goose

Intermediate hosts: As for *P. pellucidus*

Geographical distribution: Europe, Asia, Africa and North and South America

Plagiorchis arcuatus

Synonym: *Leptoderma arcuatus*

Predilection site: Oviduct and bursa of Fabricius

Parasite class: Trematoda

Family: Plagiorchidae

Description, gross: The fluke is oval, about 4–5 mm in length by 1.5 mm in breadth, and tapers to a point at both ends.

Description, microscopic: The cuticle possesses small spines, which are more numerous in the anterior region.

Final hosts: Chicken and other poultry

Intermediate hosts: 1. Snails, particularly *Lymnaea* and *Physa* spp. 2. Various crustacea, molluscs and insects

Geographical distribution: Parts of Europe and Russia

Details of the life cycle, pathogenesis, clinical signs, diagnosis, pathology, epidemiology, treatment and control for these species are as for *P. pellucidus*.

Eimeria truncata

Predilection site: Kidney

Parasite class: Sporozoasida

Family: Eimeriidae

Description: Oocysts are ovoid, smooth, with a narrow truncate small end, 14–27 × 12–22 μm with a micropyle and micropylar cap, sometimes with a residuum. Mature meronts in the renal epithelial cells are 13 μm in diameter and contain 20–30 merozoites. Macrogametes are 12–18 × 11–15 μm and microgamonts are 15–22 × 13–18 μm.

Hosts: Domestic goose, greylag goose (*Anser anser*), Canada goose (*Branta canadensis*), Ross' goose (*Anser rossi*)

Life cycle: Complete details on the life cycle are lacking. Meronts and gamonts occur in the epithelial cells of the kidney tubules. The prepatent period is 5–14 days. Sporulation time is 1–5 days.

Geographical distribution: Worldwide

Pathogenesis: *E. truncata*, found in the kidneys of geese, can cause an acute nephritis especially where domestic geese are reared intensively. It is highly pathogenic for young goslings and can cause up to 100% mortality within a few days of onset of clinical symptoms. Outbreaks have also been recorded in geese in wildfowl sanctuaries.

Clinical signs: Marked weakness, emaciation, polydipsia, muscular incoordination and death

Diagnosis: Infection is diagnosed by identification of oocysts in urates or by the characterised kidney lesions on postmortem or histopathology.

Pathology: The kidneys are markedly enlarged, light in colour, and show numerous small, white nodules, streaks and lines on the surface and throughout the cortex and medulla of the kidney. Infected cells are eventually destroyed and the adjacent cells show pressure atrophy and destruction. Affected tubules are packed with urates, oocysts and gamonts in various stages of development and may be enlarged up to 5–10 times the diameter of normal tubules.

Epidemiology: *E. truncata* occurs as a sporadic parasite in domestic geese and is most likely to occur when geese are kept in crowded, unsanitary conditions. Contact with wild geese may introduce the infection.

Treatment: Little is known about treatment, but by analogy with other hosts, one of the sulphonamide drugs should be tried.

Control: Prevention is based on good management, avoidance of overcrowding and stress, and attention to hygiene. Contact with wild geese should be avoided wherever possible.

PARASITES OF THE LOCOMOTORY SYSTEM

Sarcocystis horvarthi

Synonym: *Sarcocystis gallinarum*

Order: Sporozoasida

Family: Sarcocystiidae

Description: In the chicken, the tissue cysts are 1–10 mm long with striated walls and are found in skeletal muscles of the breast, thigh, neck and oesophagus.

Final host: Dog

Intermediate hosts: Chicken

Life cycle: Infection in the chicken is by ingestion of sporocysts in dog faeces. Complete details of the merogony phase of development are not known. Ultimately, merozoites penetrate muscle cells where they encyst giving rise to broad banana-shaped bradyzoites contained within a sarcocyst, which is the infective stage for the carnivorous final host.

Geographical distribution: Unknown, presumed worldwide

Pathogenesis: Infections in chickens are generally inapparent, but have been reported to cause severe myositis or muscular dystrophy.

Clinical signs: Muscle weakness and inability to stand have been reported.

Diagnosis: Antemortem diagnosis is difficult and most cases of *Sarcocystis* infection are only revealed at postmortem when grossly visible sarcocysts in the muscle are discovered or detected by microscopic examination.

Epidemiology: Little is known of the epidemiology, but it is clear that where dogs are kept in close association with chickens or their feed, then transmission is likely.

Treatment and control: Treatment is not indicated. The only control measures possible are those of simple hygiene. Farm dogs should not be housed in, or allowed access to, fodder stores nor should they be allowed to defecate in pens where chickens are housed. It is also important that dogs are not fed raw or uncooked chicken.

Toxoplasma gondii

Predilection site: Muscle, lung, liver, reproductive system, central nervous system

Order: Sporozoasida

Family: Sarcocystiidae

Description: Tachyzoites are found developing in vacuoles in many cell types, for example fibroblasts, hepatocytes, reticular cells and myocardial cells. In any one cell there may be 8–16 organisms, each measuring 6.0–8.0 μm. Tissue cysts, measuring up to 100 μm in diameter, are found mainly in the muscle, liver, lung and brain may contain several thousand lancet-shaped bradyzoites.

Final hosts: Cat, other felids

Intermediate hosts: All warm-blooded mammals and birds

Life cycle: The definitive host is the cat in which gametogony takes place (see Chapter 6). Birds act as an intermediate host in which the cycle is extra-intestinal and results in the formation of tachyzoites and bradyzoites, which are the only forms found in non-feline hosts.

Geographical distribution: Worldwide

Pathogenesis and clinical signs: Most *Toxoplasma* infections in animals are light and consequently asymptomatic. Toxoplasmosis has been occasionally reported in poultry and is usually mild and unnoticed.

Diagnosis: Tachyzoites of *Toxoplasma gondii* are often difficult to find in tissue sections, but are more likely to be present in sections of brain and placenta. Identification can be confirmed by immunohistochemistry, while the polymerase chain reaction may be used to identify parasite DNA in tissues.

Epidemiology: The cat plays a central role in the epidemiology of toxoplasmosis and infection in poultry may occur through ingestion of feed contaminated with cat faeces or through ingestion of bradyzoites and tachyzoites in the flesh of another intermediate host, such as rats.

Treatment and control: As for *Sarcocystis hovarthi*

PARASITES OF THE INTEGUMENT

Avioserpens taiwana

Synonym: *Filaria taiwana*, *Oshimaia taiwana*, *Avioserpens denticulophasma*, *Petroviprocta vigissi*

Predilection site: Subcutaneous tissue

Parasite class: Nematoda

Superfamily: Dracunculoidea

Description, gross: The male is unknown. The female is up to 25 cm long by 0.8 mm in width.

Description, microscopic: The anterior end is rounded, the mouth being surrounded by a chitinous rim bearing two prominent lateral papillae. There are four smaller papillae further back on the head. The uterus is large and filled with larvae. The vagina, vulva and anus are atrophied and the tail ends in a conical papilla.

Final host: Duck

Intermediate hosts: Copepods (*Cyclops*)

Life cycle: Larvae are released into water and infective stages have been shown to occur in *Cyclops* in Taiwan. Infection of the final host occurs through the ingestion of the intermediate host.

Geographical distribution: China, Taiwan

Pathogenesis: The worms cause the formation of swellings under the mandible, which are at first soft and movable and, after about 1 month, hard and painful and may reach the size of a large nut. They interfere with swallowing and respiration and may cause death from inanition or asphyxia. Occasionally the swellings occur on the shoulders and legs and interfere with the bird's movements. Numerous microfilariae are found in the blood. The adult worms eventually rupture and disintegrate and healing occurs, although if the worms die in the swellings, abscesses may form. The disease lasts about 11 months.

Clinical signs: Hard, painful swellings located under the mandible, and occasionally on the shoulders and legs. Surviving birds have poor growth rates.

Diagnosis: Identification of the adult worms within subcutaneous swellings

Pathology: Not described

Epidemiology: Found in domesticated ducks in China, mainly in the dry season (January to April), and in Taiwan, where disease may also occur in September to October. It affects ducks 3 weeks to 2 months old.

Treatment: Removal of the worms through an incision into the most prominent part of the swelling and antiseptic treatment of the swelling is effective.

Control: Ducklings should be provided with water free from *Cyclops* and should not be allowed access to marshland.

Collyriclum faba

Common name: Skin or cystic fluke

Predilection site: Skin, subcutaneous tissues, particularly around the cloacal opening

Parasite class: Trematoda

Family: Troglotrematidae

Description, gross: This fluke has a spiny tegument, is dorsally convex and ventrally flattened and measures about 4 × 5 mm. There is no ventral sucker.

Description, microscopic: Eggs are very small, measuring about 20 × 10 μm.

Final hosts: Chicken, turkey and wild birds

Intermediate hosts: 1. Snails. 2. Dragonfly nymphs

Life cycle: Eggs are passed through an opening in the wall of the cyst and hatch in the environment to produce a miracidium, which penetrates a snail. These directly produce cercariae, there being no redial development, and the cercariae are shed from the snail and will enter dragonfly larvae, where they encyst to the metacercaria stage. Infection of the final host occurs through ingestion of the infected dragonfly. The immature trematodes then migrate to the subcutaneous tissues.

Geographical distribution: Europe, Asia, North and South America

Pathogenesis: Commonly found in tissue around the cloaca but in heavy infections flukes may also be present along the thorax, abdomen, beak and neck. Such infections produce anaemia and loss of body condition and can be fatal.

Clinical signs: Young birds may show difficulty in moving, inappetance, anaemia, emaciation and even death. The presence of cysts can lead to disfigurement of the skin.

Diagnosis: Typical cysts are found around the cloacal opening and along the thorax and abdomen. Each cyst has a central opening and a pair of flukes.

Pathology: The flukes are located in hard whitish grey subcutaneous cysts, which can measure around 3–10 mm in diameter. These cysts have a central pore and contain a pair of flukes and are usually filled with dark fluid and eggs.

Epidemiology: Only birds with access to marshy areas where the intermediate hosts occur are likely to become infected.

Treatment: Surgical removal is the only effective treatment.

Control: Birds should be restricted from entering marshy areas.

ECTOPARASITES

LICE

Heavy louse infestation is known as pediculosis and is particularly common in poultry. All species on birds are chewing lice and therefore are of importance because of the direct damage they cause by chewing the skin or feathers, although some blood-feeding may occur when the base of feathers are damaged. Clinical importance is therefore usually a function of the density of the lice present. Transmission is usually by direct physical contact.

Description: Lice have a segmented body divided into a head, thorax and abdomen. They have three pairs of jointed legs and a pair of short antennae. All lice are dorsoventrally flattened and wingless. The sensory organs are poorly developed; the eyes are vestigial or absent.

Life cycle: The general life cycle of poultry lice is relatively uniform across the various species. During a lifespan of approximately a month the female lays 200–300 operculate eggs ('nits'). These are usually whitish, and are glued singly to the feathers where they may be seen with the naked eye. Eggs hatch within 5–7 days. The nymph that hatches from the egg is similar to, although much smaller than, the adult. The nymph moults three times over 2–3 weeks before giving rise to the adult. The lice normally feed on bits of skin or feather products. Adult lice may live for several weeks on the host but can remain alive only for about 1 week off the host. The bird lice can digest keratin; biting off pieces of feather, breaking these up with comb-like structures in their crops, and digesting them with secretions aided by bacterial action. They will ingest not only the sheaths of growing feathers, but also down and skin scabs.

Clinical signs: Restlessness, feather damage, emaciation and markedly reduced performance are all symptoms of severe pediculosis. Infected birds are unable to rest, cease feeding and may injure themselves by scratching and feather plucking, with results often more serious than any immediate damage by the lice.

Pathogenesis: Although there are differences in pathogenicity between the species of louse found on poultry, the effects of avian pediculosis are broadly similar, varying only in degree. Heavy infestations decrease reproductive potential in males, egg production in females and weight gain in growing chickens. The skin lesions are also sites for secondary bacterial infections. While most lice are not highly pathogenic to mature birds in low numbers, they may be fatal to chicks. As in the other pediculoses, the condition in domestic birds is often itself a symptom of ill-health from other causes, such as other infection, malnutrition or inadequate, overcrowded and unhygienic housing. Chewing lice may occasionally cause severe anaemia by puncturing small feathers and feeding on the blood that oozes out.

Diagnosis: Adult lice and eggs can be seen on the skin and feathers and removed for microscopic examination and indentification.

Pathology: The pathology of louse infestation is highly variable. In heavy infestations the skin becomes inflamed, erythematous and eventually covered by scabs and blood clots, involving much of the body surface.

Epidemiology: Infection occurs after direct contact with an infested host animal. Cross-contamination between different host species is possible if the animals have physical contact.

Treatment: Topical insecticidal compounds, such as permethrin, carbaryl, malathion, cypermethrin or rotenone, can be used to kill lice. However, as the insecticides are unable to kill the eggs, two applications are necessary with a 10–14-day interval. Deep-litter or free-range birds may be more easily treated by scattering carbaryl, coumaphos, malathion or stirophos dust on the litter.

Control: Regular checking and spraying of birds will enable infestation rates to be controlled. In addition, cross-contamination should be avoided. This is achieved by treating any birds in the environment of the chickens and restricting contact between wild birds and poultry. The housing and nesting should be thoroughly cleaned to eliminate sources of reinfestation such as egg-laden feathers. As would be expected, the practice of de-beaking allows an increase in infestations by preventing birds from preening and grooming.

Cuclotogaster heterographus

Common name: Head louse

Predilection site: Skin and feathers of the head and neck

Parasite class: Insecta

Order: Phthiraptera

Sub-order: Ischnocera

Family: Philopteridae

Description, gross: A grey, slow-moving louse found close to the skin. *Cuclotogaster heterographus* has a rounded body with a large, slender head, which is rounded at the front (Fig. 7.36). Adult males measure approximately 2.5 mm and females 2.6 mm in length.

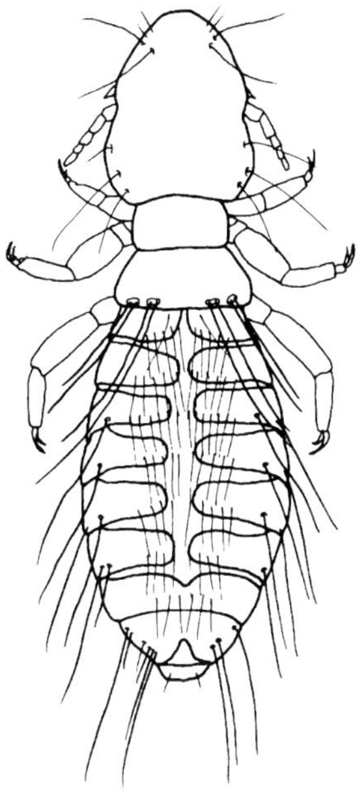

Fig. 7.36 Adult female *Cuclotogaster heterographus* (dorsal view).

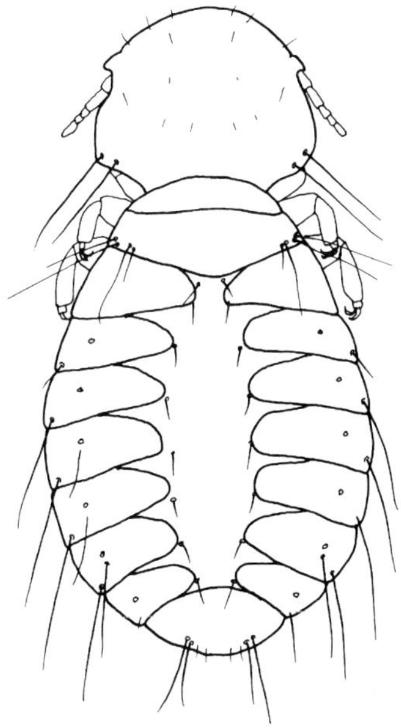

Fig. 7.37 Adult female *Goniocotes gallinae* (dorsal view).

Description, microscopic: The first segment of the antennae of males is long and thick and bears a posterior process. The abdomen is elongate in the male and barrel-shaped in the female, with dark brown lateral tergal plates. Three long bristles project from each side of the dorsal surface of the head and the five-segmented antennae are fully exposed. Each leg has two tarsal claws.

Hosts: Chicken, other poultry

Geographical distribution: Worldwide

Pathogenesis: As the common name, chicken head louse, suggests, *Cuclotogaster heterographus* occurs mainly on the skin and feathers of the head, although it occurs occasionally on the neck and elsewhere. *C. heterographus* feeds on tissue debris; skin scales and scabs and can digest keratin from feathers and down. Infestation with *C. heterographus* is particularly important in young birds. Infestations of young birds and chicks may be pathogenic and sometimes fatal; the birds become weak and droopy and may die within a month. When birds become fairly well feathered, head lice infestation decreases, but can increase again when the birds reach maturity.

Goniocotes gallinae

Common name: Fluff louse

Predilection site: Feathers

Parasite class: Insecta

Order: Phthiraptera

Sub-order: Ischnocera

Family: Philopteridae

Description, gross: The fluff louse, *Goniocotes gallinae*, is one of the smallest lice found on poultry, at about 0.7–1.3 mm in length. It has a pale yellow, almost circular body (Fig. 7.37).

Description, microscopic: The head is rounded and carries two large bristles projecting from each side of its dorsal surface. The antennae are five-segmented, fully exposed and the same in both sexes. There are two tarsal claws on each leg and few hairs on the dorsal abdomen.

Hosts: Chicken

Geographical distribution: Worldwide

Pathogenesis: *Goniocotes gallinae* may occur on the down feathers anywhere on the body, but are often found in the fluff at the bases of feathers, the preferred sites being the back and the rump. These lice generally occur in low densities and so have little effect on the host. However, cases of severe *Goniocotes* infestation can cause restlessness, damaged plumage, anaemia and markedly reduced performance.

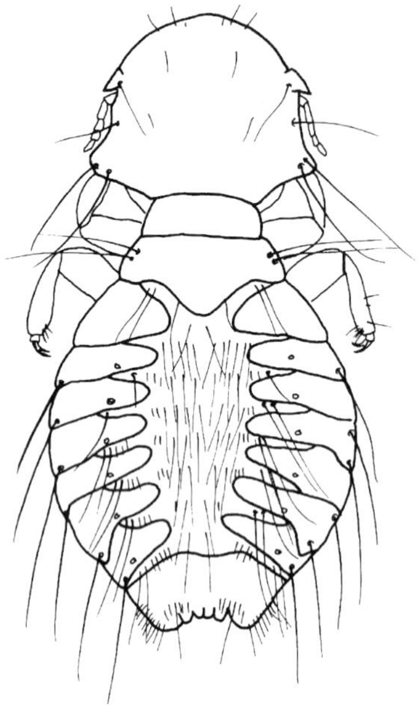

Fig. 7.38 Adult female *Goniodes dissimilis* (dorsal view).

Goniodes dissimilis

Common name: Brown chicken louse

Predilection site: Skin and body feathers

Parasite class: Insecta

Order: Phthiraptera

Sub-order: Ischnocera

Family: Philopteridae

Description, gross: *Goniodes dissimilis* are large lice, about 3 mm in length and brown in colour (Fig. 7.38).

Description, microscopic: The broad head is posteriorly concave, producing marked angular corners at the posterior margins. The head carries two large bristles projecting from each side of its dorsal surface. The antennae have five segments and are fully exposed. Each leg has two tarsal claws.

Hosts: Chicken

Geographical distribution: Worldwide

Pathogenesis: *Goniodes dissimilis* is more abundant in temperate habitats. Birds are unable to rest, cease feeding and may injure themselves by scratching and feather plucking. In general young birds suffer more severely, with loss of body weight, debility and perhaps death.

Goniodes gigas

Common name: Large chicken louse

Predilection site: Skin and body feathers

Parasite class: Insecta

Order: Phthiraptera

Sub-order: Ischnocera

Family: Philopteridae

Description, gross: Very large, brown lice occurring on the body and feathers of the fowl. Males measure 3–4 mm and females 5 mm in length.

Description, microscopic: They have a broad head, which is concave posteriorly, producing marked angular corners at the posterior margins. The head bears two large bristles, which project from each side of its dorsal surface. The antennae have five segments and are fully exposed. Each leg has two tarsal claws.

Hosts: Chicken

Geographical distribution: Worldwide, but *Goniodes gigas* is more abundant in tropical areas.

Goniodes meleagridis

Predilection site: Skin and body feathers

Parasite class: Insecta

Order: Phthiraptera

Sub-order: Ischnocera

Family: Philopteridae

Description: These lice are characterised by broad mandibles located ventrally on the head, short antennae (three to five segments) and a dorsoventrally flattened body. They are large lice, the adults reaching up to 5 mm in length.

Hosts: Turkey

Life cycle: During a lifespan of about a month the female lays 200–300 operculate eggs ('nits'). These are usually whitish, and are glued to the hair or feathers, where they may be seen with the naked eye. The eggs hatch within 4–7 days and the lice spend their entire life cycle on the host, feeding on feather debris. The nymph that hatches from the egg is similar to, although much smaller than, the adult. The nymph moults three times over 2–3 weeks before giving rise to the reproductive adult.

Geographical distribution: Worldwide

Pathogenesis: Birds are unable to rest, cease feeding and may injure themselves by scratching and feather plucking, with results often more serious than any immediate damage by the lice. This species of louse is commonest in adult birds, but young birds that do become infested suffer more severely, with loss of body weight, debility and perhaps death. The bird lice can digest keratin, biting off pieces of feather, breaking these up with comb-like structures in their crops, and digesting them with secretions aided by bacterial action. They will ingest not only the sheaths of growing feathers, but also down and skin scabs.

Clinical signs: In general, young birds suffer more severely, with loss of body weight, debility, and perhaps death. In adult laying birds the effect on body weight is slight, and the main loss is in depression of egg production.

Epidemiology: Infection occurs after direct contact with an infested host animal. Cross-contamination between different host species is possible if the animals have physical contact.

Lipeurus caponis

Common name: Wing louse

Predilection site: Skin, wing and tail feathers

Parasite class: Insecta

Order: Phthiraptera

Sub-order: Ischnocera

Family: Philopteridae

Description: Grey, slow-moving lice found close to the skin on the under-side of the large wing feathers. These lice are slender and elongate in shape. *Lipeurus caponis* is an elongated, narrow species, about 2.2 mm in length and 0.3 mm in width (Fig. 7.39). The head is long and rounded at the front, and the antennae are five-segmented and fully exposed. The legs are narrow and bear two tarsal claws. Characteristically the hind legs are about twice as long as the first two pairs of legs. There are characteristic small angular projections on the head in front of the antennae. There are relatively few dorsal hairs on the abdomen.

Hosts: Chicken

Geographical distribution: Worldwide

Pathogenesis: *L. caponis* is common on the underside of the wing and tail feathers of chicken and other fowl throughout the world. Pathogenic effects are usually slight in healthy animals and include restlessness, irritation and general unthriftiness. Young birds may be susceptible to heavy infestation, especially where underlying disease or malnutrition is debilitating.

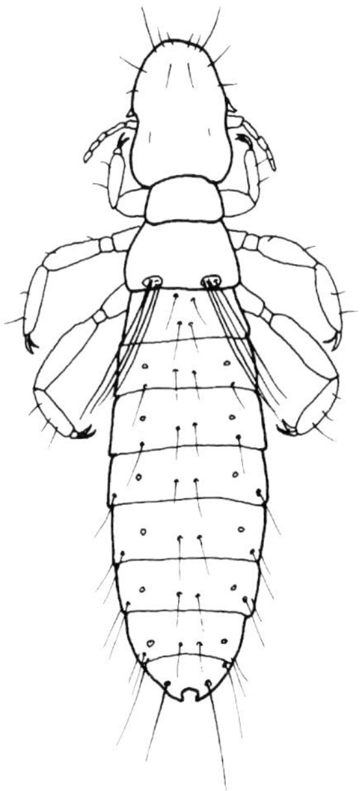

Fig. 7.39 Adult *Lipeurus caponis* (dorsal view).

Menacanthus stramineus

Common name: Yellow body or chicken body louse

Predilection site: Skin

Parasite class: Insecta

Order: Phthiraptera

Sub-order: Amblycera

Family: Menoponidae

Description, gross: The chicken body louse or yellow body louse, *Menacanthus stramineus*, is relatively large; the male measures approximately 2.8 mm in length and the female 3.3 mm (Fig. 7.40).

Description, microscopic: The head is almost triangular in shape and the ventral portion of the front of the head is armed with a pair of spine-like processes. The palps and four-segmented antennae are distinct. The antennae are club-shaped and mostly concealed beneath the head. The flattened abdomen is elongated and broadly rounded posteriorly with two dorsal rows of setae on each abdominal segment. There are three pairs of short, two-clawed legs. The eggs have characteristic filaments on the anterior half of the shell and on the operculum.

Hosts: Chicken, turkey, guinea fowl, peafowl, pheasant, quail, cage birds (canary)

Geographical distribution: Worldwide

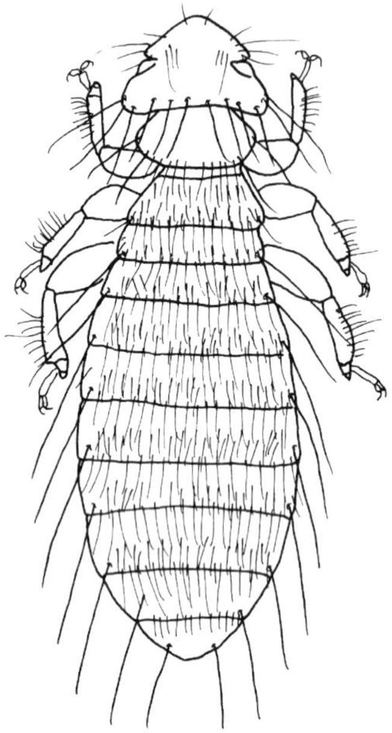

Fig. 7.40 Adult *Menacanthus stramineus* (dorsal view).

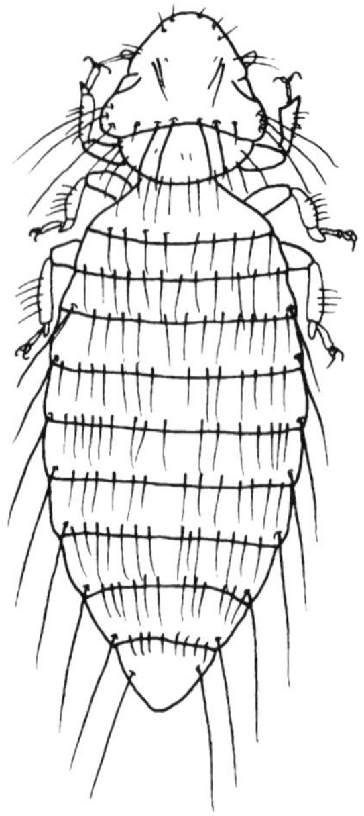

Fig. 7.41 Adult *Menopon gallinae* (dorsal view).

Pathogenesis: *Menacanthus stramineus* is the most pathogenic louse of adult birds, and may lead to fatalities in chicks. It is an extremely active species which lays its eggs in clusters mainly in the anal region. Infestation can result in severe irritation, causing skin inflammation and localised scabs and blood clots, especially in the region of the vent, and in young birds, on the head and throat. Birds become restless and do not digest their food properly. Ultimately infestation may result in decreased hen weight, decreased clutch size and death in young birds and chicks. Populations may reach as many as 35 000 lice per bird. Lice infestations often accompany manifestations of poor health such as internal parasitism, infectious disease, malnutrition and poor sanitation. Although found naturally infected with the virus of eastern encephalomyelitis, it is not considered an important vector.

Epidemiology: This species is the most common and destructive louse of domestic chickens. It is widespread and often reaches pest proportions. It is most common on the breast, thighs and around the vent. In heavy infestations, the lice may also be found under the wings and on other parts of the body, including the head. After introduction into a flock *Menacanthus stramineus* spreads from bird to bird by contact. Cross-contamination between different host species is possible if the animals have physical contact. Large populations are particularly common on caged layers.

Menopon gallinae

Common name: Shaft louse

Predilection site: Skin and feathers

Parasite class: Insecta

Order: Phthiraptera

Sub-order: Amblycera

Family: Menoponidae

Description: Pale yellow, rapidly moving louse. It is a small louse; adults measure approximately 2 mm in length. *Menopon gallinae* has small palps and a pair of four-segmented antennae, folded into grooves in the head (Fig. 7.41). The abdomen is tapered posteriorly in the female but rounded in the male and has a sparse covering of small to medium-length setae on its dorsal surface.

Hosts: Chicken, turkey, duck

Geographical distribution: Worldwide

Pathogenesis: This louse feeds only on feathers, and, although common, is rarely a serious parasite in adult birds. The shaft louse does not usually infest young birds until they are well feathered, but heavy infestations in young birds may prove fatal. *Menopon gallinae* rests on the body feather shafts of chickens and feeds on parts of the feathers. The louse occurs largely on the thigh and breast. It may also infest turkeys and ducks, particularly if kept in close association with chickens.

Menopon leucoxanthum

Common name: Shaft louse

Predilection site: Skin and feathers

Parasite class: Insecta

Order: Phthiraptera

Sub-order: Amblycera

Family: Menoponidae

Description: A small, rapidly moving louse which especially favours the preen gland, inhibiting production of the oily secretion and causing 'wet feather'.

Hosts: Ducks

Life cycle: The nymph moults three times over 2–3 weeks before giving rise to the reproductive adult. Individuals are highly mobile and move rapidly.

Geographical distribution: worldwide

Pathogenesis: Partly due to irritation birds preen continuously, but without the oily secretion the feathers cannot be waterproofed. Unable to repel water and injured by constant preening, the plumage becomes tattered and dirty, with the feathers broken. Water can penetrate to the skin, and when much of the body is affected the birds are soaked, and may die of pneumonia following chilling. Though the damaged plumage may be replaced at the annual moult it soon degenerates, as a result of the excessive preening, into its former sodden condition.

Clinical signs: Wet damaged plumage

Diagnosis: Lice and their eggs are visible on the skin and feathers of the host animal.

Pathology: The pathology of louse infestation is highly variable. In heavy infestations the skin becomes inflamed, erythematous and eventually covered by scabs and blood clots.

Epidemiology: Infection occurs after direct contact with an infested host animal. Cross-contamination between different host species is possible if the animals have physical contact.

Treatment: Topical insecticidal compounds such as permethrin, carbaryl, malathion, cypermethrin or rotenone can be used to kill lice. However as the insecticides are unable to kill the eggs, two applications are necessary with a 10-day interval.

Control: Although methods such as dusting the nesting material or providing insecticide-treated laying boxes can be used to avoid undue handling of birds, the results obtained from treating individual birds are undoubtedly better.

There is a large number of closely related species of lice that may be found on ducks, geese and other waterfowl. Of epidemiological significance is that these species are amongst the least specific of all lice. The lice can be found on the skin and feathers in all areas of the body. In ducks, infection with lice can damage feathers affecting water resistance and insulation so that the birds may die from cold. Treatment and control are as for *Menopon leucoxanthum*

MITES

Infestation by mites is called acariasis and can result in severe dermatitis, known as mange, which may cause significant welfare problems and economic losses.

Table 7.8 Lice of ducks, geese and other wildfowl.

Family	Genus	Key representative species
Philopteridae	*Anaticola*	*Anaticola anseris, Anaticola crassicornis, Anaticola tadornae, Anaticola thoracicus*
Philopteridae	*Acidoproctus*	*Acidoproctus rostratus*
Philopteridae	*Anatoecus*	*Anatoecus dentatus, Anatoecus brunneiceps, Anatoecus cygni, Anatoecus icterodes*
Philopteridae	*Ornithobius*	*Ornithobius cygni, Ornithobius mathisi, Ornithobius waterstoni*
Menoponidae	*Holomenopon*	*Holomenopon leucoxanthum*
Menoponidae	*Ciconiphilus*	*Ciconiphilus decimfasciatus, Ciconiphilus parvus, Ciconiphilus pectiniventris, Ciconiphilus cygni, Ciconiphilus quadripustulatus*
Menoponidae	*Trinoton*	*Trinoton anserium, Trinoton squalidurn, Trinoton querquedula*

Table 7.9 Lice of gamebirds.

Family	Genus	Key representative species
Philopteridae	*Goniocotes*	*Goniocotes chryocephalus, Goniocotes obscurus, Goniocotes microthorax*
Philopteridae	*Goniodes*	*Goniodes colchici, Goniodes dispar*
Philopteridae	*Lipeurus*	*Liperus maculosus*
Philopteridae	*Cuclotogaster*	*Cuclotogaster heterogrammicus, Cuclotogaster obsuricor*
Menoponidae	*Amyrsidea*	*Amyrsidea perdicis*
Menoponidae	*Menacanthus*	*Menacanthus stramineus, Menacanthus layali*
Menoponidae	*Menopon*	*Menopon pallens*
Degeeriellidae	*Lagopoecus*	*Lagopoecus colchicus*

Clinical signs: This mite causes feeding lesions most commonly seen on the breast or legs of the bird. The feeding nymphs and adults cause irritation, restlessness and debility, and in heavy infections there may be severe, and occasionally fatal, anaemia. Newly hatched chicks may die rapidly as a result of mite activity. Egg production may decrease significantly.

Diagnosis: The mites may be found in poultry housing during the day, particularly in cracks or where roost poles touch supports, or on birds at night. The mites can be observed in these locations with the naked eye, particularly after feeding when they appear red. Masses of mites may be found in the nasopharyngeal system of dead birds.

Pathology: The effects of mites are highly variable, but may include hyperkeratosis, acanthosis, epidermitis, dermatitis, poor feather growth and loss of feathers.

Dermanyssus gallinae

Common name: Poultry red mite, roost mite

Predilection site: Skin

Class: Arachnida

Sub-class: Acari

Order: Parasitiformes

Sub-order: Mesostigmata

Family: Dermanyssidae

Description: The red mite or chicken mite, *Dermanyssus gallinae*, is one of the most common mites of poultry. It is a mesostigmatid mite that feeds off the blood of fowl, pigeons, caged birds and many other wild birds. It occasionally bites mammals, including humans, if the usual hosts are unavailable. The adults are relatively large at 0.75–1 mm in length, with long legs (Fig. 7.42). The body is usually grey–white, becoming red to black when engorged. A single dorsal shield is present, which tapers posteriorly but is truncated at its posterior margin. The anal shield is relatively large and is at least as wide as the genitoventral plate. Three anal setae are present. The chelicerae are elongate and stylet-like.

Hosts: Domestic poultry and wild birds; occasionally parasitic on mammals, including humans.

Life cycle: This mite spends much of its life cycle away from its host; the adult and nymph only visiting birds to feed, mainly at night. The favoured habitats are poultry houses, usually of timber construction, in the crevices of which the eggs are laid. The life cycle can be completed in a minimum of a week, allowing large populations to develop rapidly, although during cold weather the cycle is slower. Approximately 1 day after feeding, batches of eggs are laid in hiding places, detritus or near nests and roosts. Within 2–3 days the eggs hatch into six-legged larvae. The larvae do not feed before moulting, and become an octopod protonymph 1–2 days later. Within another couple of days they moult again, and soon afterwards they complete their final moult to become an adult. Both nymphal stages feed, as do the adult mites. The adult can survive for several months without feeding, so a reservoir population can persist in unoccupied poultry houses and aviaries.

Geographical distribution: Worldwide

Pathogenesis: The mite is a particular threat to fowl housed in old buildings. It causes feeding lesions, which are most likely to be seen on the breast or legs of the bird. The mites can directly cause irritation and anaemia, and can lower egg production and weight gain. Newly hatched chicks may rapidly die as a result of mite activity. Infestation of pigeons is common. Cats and dogs may become infested as a result of contact with poultry, and human carriers are also important. In Australia, *Dermanyssus gallinae*

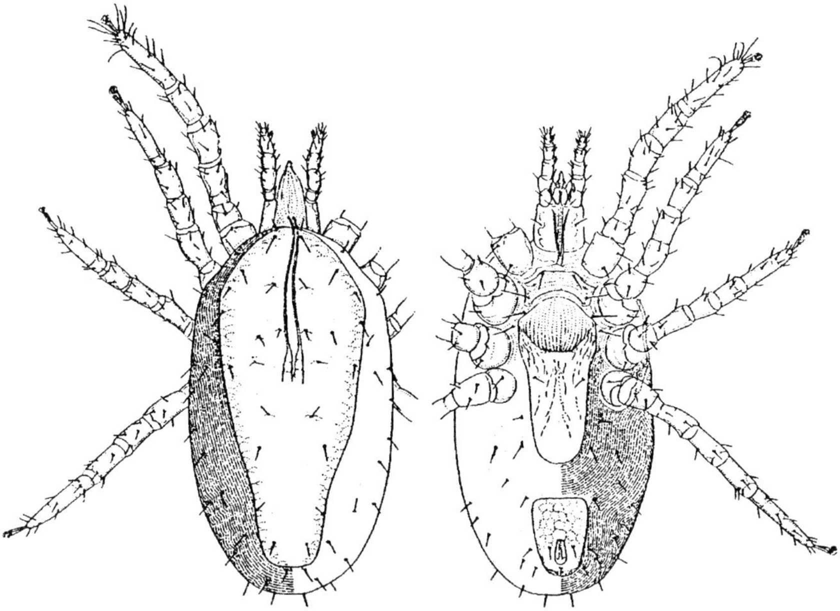

Fig. 7.42 Adult female of the red mite, *Dermanyssus gallinae*. (a) Dorsal view. (b) Ventral view (reproduced from Baker *et al.*, 1956).

is a vector of *Borrelia anserina*, the cause of avian spirochaetosis.

Epidemiology: Populations generally increase during the winter months and decrease in the summer months, and infestation intensity increases during the host breeding period. The presence of nestlings may stimulate rapid reproduction and an exponential increase in mite numbers, so that at the time of fledging there are a significantly higher proportion of nymphs in the nest than adults. Mites are transmitted by mite dispersion between farms (through the transport of crates, egg flats or even on humans themselves), or by direct contact between birds. *Dermanyssus gallinae* may be an important pest of poultry flocks maintained on the floor in barn or deep-litter systems, but is less important in caged production facilities. Since *Dermanyssus* can survive for long periods in the absence of a host, a poultry house may remain infested several months after birds are removed.

Treatment: Treatment of birds is only palliative, and attention should be paid to the mite habitats in buildings. Individual birds may be treated by spraying or dusting the birds with an acaricide such as a pyrethroid or carbaryl, coumaphos, malathion or stirofos. Systemic control with repeated treatment with ivermectin (1.8–5.4 mg/kg) or moxidectin (8 mg/kg) is effective for short periods.

Control: Buildings and equipment should be cleaned, scalded with boiling water and treated with an acaricide such as carbaryl or synergised pyrethroids. Dimethoate and fenthion may be used as residual house sprays when poultry are not present. Where the mites have invaded dwelling houses their ability to survive in nests, without feeding for several months, makes these important as reservoir sites, and all nests should be removed from eaves once the fledglings have departed. Buying-in mite-free birds and using good sanitation practices are important to prevent a build-up of mite populations.

Notes: *Dermanyssus* readily infects other animals, and can cause erythema and intense pruritus in cats that occupy old wooden poultry houses. Humans may develop skin lesions when mites enter rooms from wild birds' nests in the eaves of houses.

Ornithonyssus sylviarum

Synonym: *Liponyssus*

Common name: Northern fowl mite

Predilection site: Base of the feathers, particularly the vent area

Parasite class: Arachnida

Sub-class: Acari

Order: Parasitiformes

Sub-order: Mesostigmata

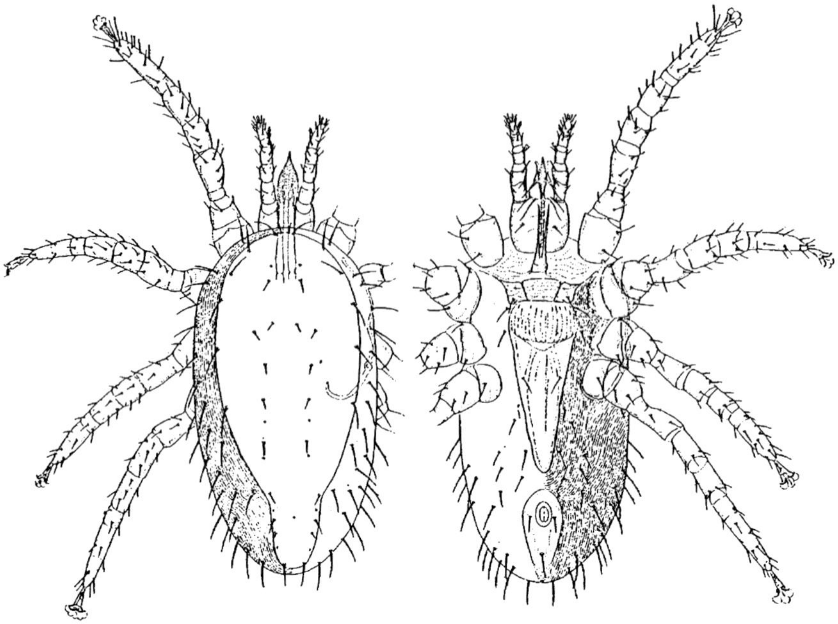

Fig. 7.43 Adult females *Ornithonyssus sylviarum* (northern fowl mite). (a) Dorsal view. (b) Ventral view (reproduced from Baker *et al.*, 1956).

Family: Macronyssidae

Description: The adults are relatively large, oval-shaped, 0.75–1 mm in length with long legs that allow it to move rapidly (Fig. 7.43). The body is usually greyish-white, becoming red to black when engorged. A single dorsal shield is wide for two-thirds of its length, then tapers posteriorly to become about half as wide, and is truncated at its posterior margin. The female typically has only two pairs of setae on the sternal shield. The anal shield is relatively large and at least as wide as the genitoventral plate. Three anal setae are present. The chelicerae are elongate and stylet-like. The body carries many long setae and is much more hairy than *Dermanyssus.*

Hosts: Poultry and wild birds

Life cycle: Unlike *Dermanyssus*, *Ornithonyssus* spends its entire life on the bird and can only survive for about 10 days away from a host. The female lays one to five sticky, whitish eggs on the host at the base of the feathers, primarily in the vent area, after a blood-meal. The eggs hatch within approximately a day to produce hexapod larvae. The larvae do not feed, and moult to become protonymphs. The protonymphs feed on blood from the host, before moulting over to become tritonymphs. The tritonymphs do not feed, and moult to the adult stage. The entire life cycle can be completed in 5–12 days under optimal conditions, but usually takes longer. Due to the short generation times large populations can develop rapidly on the birds.

Geographical distribution: Present in temperate areas throughout the world

Pathogenesis: *Ornithonyssus sylviarum* is a blood-sucking ectoparasite. It occasionally bites mammals, including humans, if the usual hosts are unavailable. This mite is capable of transmitting fowlpox, St Louis encephalitis, Newcastle disease, chlamydiosis and western equine encephalomyelitis. The viruses that cause western equine encephalitis and St. Louis encephalitis have both been detected in *O. sylviarum* from nests of wild birds in North America, and it is likely that this mite acts a vector for their transmission among avian hosts. They may bite humans, causing pruritus.

Clinical signs: White or off-white eggs can be seen in the vent area on feather shafts. Feathers may become matted and severe scabbing may develop, particularly around the vent. Infested chickens show a grey–black discoloration of the feathers due to the large number of mites present. In heavy infections, birds are restless and lose weight from irritation, egg production may be reduced, and there may be severe anaemia. Common signs, apart from debility, are thickened, crusty skin and soiled feathers around the vent.

Diagnosis: The mites are found on the birds or in their nesting and housing. Although similar in superficial morphology to the common chicken mite, *Dermanyssus gallinae*, *Ornithonyssus sylviarum* can be distinguished behaviourally by the fact that it is present on birds in large numbers during the day.

Pathology: Feeding causes pruritus, feather damage, weakness, anaemia and death. Scratching of the bites may result in secondary bacterial infection.

Epidemiology: As *Ornithonyssus sylviarum* is almost a permanent parasite, infection occurs via contact or by placing birds in accommodation recently vacated by infected stock.

Treatment and control: See *D. gallinae*

Ornithonyssus bursa

Synonym: *Liponyssus bursa*

Common name: Tropical fowl mite

Predilection site: Skin

Parasite class: Arachnida

Sub-class: Acari

Order: Parasitiformes

Sub-order: Mesostigmata

Family: Macronyssidae

Description: Similar to *O. sylviarum*. However, the ventral plate bears three pairs of setae, while in *O. sylvarium* and *D. gallinae* only two pairs of setae are on the ventral plate.

Hosts: Poultry and wild birds

Geographical distribution: Tropical: Southern Africa, India, China, Australia, Columbia, Panama and USA

Epidemiology: In warmer climates *O. bursa* is thought to replace the northern fowl mite, *O. sylviarum*.
For details see *O. sylviarum*

Knemidokoptes gallinae

Synonym: *Knemidokoptes laevis gallinae*, *Cnemidocoptes*, *Neocnemidocoptes*

Common name: Depluming itch mite

Predilection site: Feathered areas

Parasite class: Arachnida

Sub-class: Acari

Order: Acariformes

Sub-order: Sarcoptiformes (Astigmata)

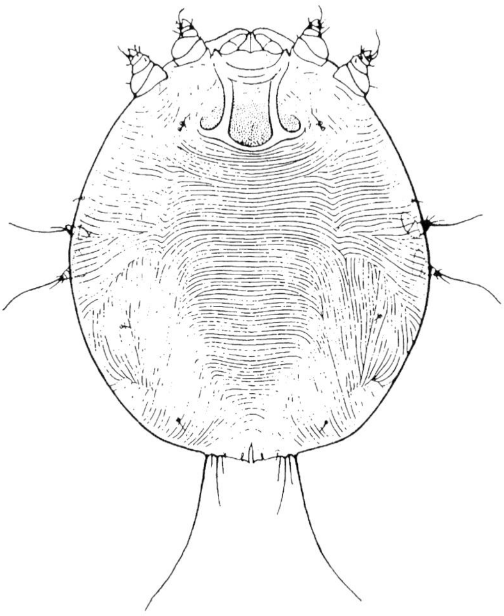

Fig. 7.44 Adult female of *Knemidokoptes gallinae*, dorsal view (reproduced from Hirst, 1922).

Family: Knemidokoptidae

Description: This is the only burrowing genus of mites on domestic birds, and resembles *Sarcoptes* in many respects. The circular body and short, stubby legs and the avian host are usually sufficient for generic diagnosis (Fig. 7.44). Although similar in appearance to *Knemidokoptes mutans*, individuals are typically smaller, and the pattern of dorsal striations is unbroken.

Hosts: Chicken, turkey, pheasants and geese

Life cycle: The fertilised female creates a winding burrow or tunnel in the upper layers of the epidermis, feeding on liquid oozing from the damaged tissues. Females are ovo-viviparous, giving birth to live hexapod larvae, which crawl onto the skin surface. These larvae, in turn, burrow into the superficial layers of the skin to create small 'moulting pockets', in which the moults to protonymph, tritonymph and adult are completed. The adult male then emerges and seeks a female either on the skin surface or in a moulting pocket. After fertilisation the females either produce new tunnels or extend the moulting pocket. The entire life cycle is spent on the host and is completed in 17–21 days.

Geographical distribution: Worldwide

Pathogenesis: The parts of the body most commonly infected are the head, neck, back, abdomen and upper legs. Severe cases can result in emaciation and death.

Clinical signs: *Knemidokoptes gallinae* burrows into the feather shafts, and the intense pain and irritation cause the bird to pull out body feathers. This is known as 'depluming itch'. The condition is characterised by intense scratching and feather loss over extended areas of the body. Feathers fall out, break off or are pulled out by the bird. Mites may be found embedded in the tissue at the base of feather quills, causing scaling, papules and thickening of the skin.

Diagnosis: The progressive feather loss and scratching indicate the presence of the parasite. Identification of the mite species can be achieved through examination of mites found on feather shafts or skin scrapings taken from the edge of lesions.

Pathology: The burrowing activity of the mites causes hyperkeratosis, thickening and wrinkling of the skin, and sloughing of the keratinous layers. Proliferative skin lesions may be observed on the legs, with digit necrosis observed in some birds.

Epidemiology: Infestation is especially prevalent in spring and summer and may disappear in autumn. New hosts are infected by contact. Infection may remain latent for a long time with a small static mite population until stress, such as chill or movement to a strange cage, occurs and the population increases.

Treatment: Malathion and sevin dusts may be applied. Birds may also be treated with ivermectin; two to three treatments at 10-day intervals may be required to completely eliminate the mites. The ivermectin may be applied on the skin behind the neck, orally or injected. For individual birds repeated topical application of paraffin may also be effective, if time consuming.

Control: Repeated treatments of acaricides will prevent reinfestations. All housing should be thoroughly disinfected.

Knemidokoptes mutans

Synonym: *Cnemidocoptes*

Common name: Scaly leg mite

Predilection site: Beneath the scales of the feet and legs

Parasite class: Arachnida

Sub-class: Acari

Order: Acariformes

Sub-order: Sarcoptiformes (Astigmata)

Family: Knemidokoptidae

Description and life cycle: Details are as for *K. gallinae*

Hosts: Chicken, turkey

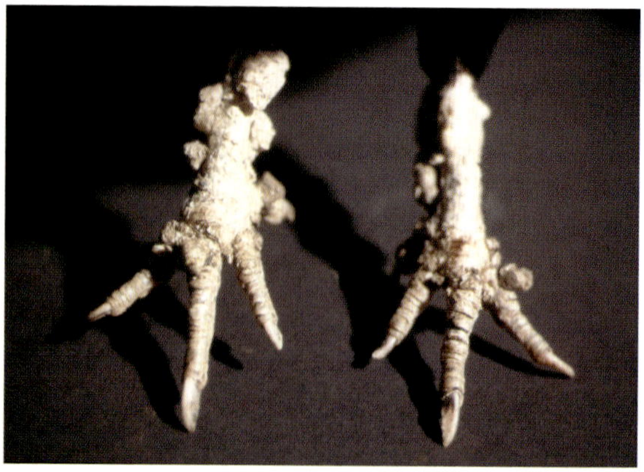

Fig. 7.45 Damage to the scales of the legs and feet caused by burrowing of the mite *Knemidokoptes mutans*.

Pathogenesis: In poultry, *Knemidokoptes mutans* affects the skin beneath the leg scales, causing the scales to loosen and rise, and giving a ragged appearance to the usually smooth limbs and toes (Fig. 7.45). Lameness and distortion of the feet and claws may be evident. The mites get onto the feet of the birds from the ground, and the lesions develop from the toes upwards.

Clinical signs: Raised scales on the feet and legs. The infestation may result in lameness and malformation of the feet. Occasionally the neck and comb may be affected. As the disease progresses over the course of several months, birds stop feeding and eventually die.

Diagnosis: The raised scales on the legs and feet indicate the presence of the parasite. Confirmation is achieved by finding the mites in skin scrapings taken from lesions. Mature adult mites are often found beneath the crusts.

Pathology: The parasites pierce the skin underneath the scale, causing an inflammation with exudate that hardens on the surface and displaces the scales.

Epidemiology: Infection may remain latent for a long time with a small static mite population until stress, such as chill or movement to a new environment, occurs, and the population increases. The condition is more common in birds allowed access to the ground and, therefore, tends to be more prevalent in barnyard and deep-litter systems rather than in caged production facilities. The mites are highly contagious.

Treatment: For 'scaly leg', the legs should be dipped into an acaricide solution. The treatment should be repeated several times at 10-day intervals. Birds can be treated by dipping the legs in a bath containing HCH (0.1%), sulphur solution (10%) or sodium fluoride (0.5%). Oral or topical ivermectin may also be effective.

Table 7.10 Mites of domestic and wild birds: there are a large number of closely related species of feather, follicle and quill mites that may be found on a wide range of birds. Quill mites may be found within the shaft of living feathers whereas feather mites are located externally, usually at the base of the feather. Feather follicle mites are found in the feather follicles of the skin. The mites cause restlessness and feather plucking. Treatment and control may be achieved through the application of acaricides such as pyrethrum, trichlorfon, dichlorvos; oral or topical ivermectin or selamectin may also be effective.

Family	Genus	Key representative species
Dermoglyphidae	*Dermoglyphus*	*Dermoglyphus elongatus, D. passerinus*
Freyanidae	*Freyana*	*Freyana largifolia, F. anatina*
Epidermoptidae	*Epidermoptes* *Microlichus* *Promyialges*	*Epidermoptes bilobatus* *Microlichus avus* *Promyialges macdonaldi, P. pari, P. uncus*
Pterolichidae	*Pterolichus* *Sideroferus*	*Pterolichus bolus* *Sideroferus lunula*
Hypoderidae	*Hypodectes*	*Hypodectes propus*
Trombiculidae	*Neoschongastia*	*Neoschongastia americana, N. kallipygos*
Syringophilidae	*Syringophilus*	*Syringophilus bipectinatus*

Control: The poultry house should be thoroughly cleaned and the perches and nesting boxes sprayed with acaricide.

Megninia ginglymura

Common name: Feather mites

Parasite class: Arachnida

Sub-class: Acari

Order: Acariformes

Sub-order: Sarcoptiformes (Astigmata)

Family: Analgidae

Predilection site: At the base of the feathers of the body and wings. Some species in this genus may also occur beneath the skin.

Description and life cycle: In *Megninia ginglymura* the male has greatly enlarged third legs and large posterior lobes with copulatory suckers. The female has all legs of similar size.

Hosts: A wide range of birds including chickens, pigeons and passeriformes

Clinical signs: *Megninia ginglymura* may cause feather-pulling activity in pullets. Birds may become weak and irritated with damaged feathers.

Pathology: Dermatitis with secretion. Records of economic damage by these mites are rare, but up to 20% decrease in egg production has been reported with heavy infestation.

Epidemiology: More than 25 species of the superfamily Analgoidea are found on domestic poultry throughout the world, including *Megninia cubitalis. Megninia columbae* may be found on pigeons.

Treatment: The application of acaricides such as pyrethrum, trichlorfon, dichlorvos or oral or topical ivermectin or selamectin may be effective.

Laminosioptes cysticola

Common name: Subcutaneous mite, fowl cyst mite

Predilection site: Subcutaneous tissues, lung, peritoneum

Parasite class: Arachnida

Sub-class: Acari

Order: Acariformes

Sub-order: Sarcoptiformes (Astigmata)

Family: Laminosioptidae

Description, gross: *Laminosioptes cysticola* is a small, oval mite, approximately 250 μm in length.

Description, microscopic: The posterior two pairs of legs end in claws and suckerless pedicels, while the anterior two pairs of legs end in claws (Fig. 7.46). This mite has a smooth, elongated body and few setae. The gnathosoma is small and not visible when viewed from above.

Hosts: Chicken, turkey and pigeons, occasionally in wild birds

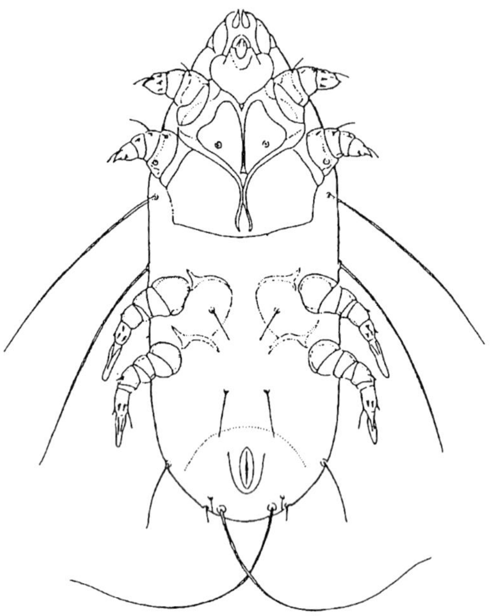

Fig. 7.46 Adult female *Laminosioptes cysticola*, ventral view (reproduced from Baker *et al.*, 1956).

Life cycle: The life cycle is typical: egg, hexapod larva, followed by octopod protonymph, tritonymph and adult. All developmental stages occur on the host. However, life cycle details are lacking. The mites are found in the subcutaneous muscle fascia and in deeper tissues in the lungs, peritoneum, muscle and abdominal viscera.

Geographical distribution: Worldwide. It is abundant in Europe and is also found in the USA, South America and Australia

Pathogenesis: *Laminosioptes* is not usually associated with clinical signs and is only discovered at meat inspection, when infected carcases are condemned partly on aesthetic grounds and partly because the infection appears somewhat similar to avian tuberculosis.

Clinical signs: The parasites are not usually regarded as pathogenic although occasionally neurological signs including circling, loss of balance, wing droop, and death have been reported.

Diagnosis: The nodules may be seen in living birds by parting the breast feathers and sliding the skin back and forth with the fingertips. Examination of the nodules under a dissection microscope usually allows the identification of the mite species.

Pathology: Aggregations of these small, oval mites are found in yellow nodules, several millimetres in diameter, in the subcutaneous muscle fascia and in deeper tissues in the lungs, peritoneum, muscle and abdominal viscera. The subcutaneous nodules are often calcified, but these only contain dead mites as the calcareous deposits are produced around the mites after they have died. Active mites occur in the deep tissues. The nodules created by the mites reduce the value of meat intended for human consumption.

Epidemiology: It is estimated that around 1% of free-living urban pigeons harbour *Laminosioptes cysticola*. The mode of transmission of this mite is unknown.

Treatment: Ivermectin may be effective, but euthanasia may be required for rapid elimination of infected birds.

Control: Destroying or quarantining infected birds reduces infestations within the flock.

Notes: It has been reported that the fowl cyst mite may cause a granulomatous pneumonia in dogs.

Several generalist ectoparasites are found on poultry and are listed in the host–parasite checklist at the end of this chapter. More detailed descriptions of these parasites are found in Chapter 11 (Facultative ectoparasites and arthropod vectors).

In the following checklists, the codes listed below apply:

Helminth classes:
N = Nematoda; T = Trematoda; C = Cestoda; A = Acanthocephala.

Arthropod classes:
I = Insecta; A = Arachnida.

Protozoal classes:
M = Mastigophora; S = Sarcodina; A = Apicomplexa; R = Rickettsia.

Chicken parasite checklist.

Section/host system	Helminths		Arthropods		Protozoa	
	Parasite	(Super)family	Parasite	Family	Parasite	Family
Digestive						
Pharynx					*Trichomonas gallinae*	Trichomonadidae (M)
Oesophagus	*Gongylonema ingluvicola*	Spiruroidea (N)			*Trichomonas gallinae*	Trichomonadidae (M)
	Dispharynx nasuta	Spiruroidea (N)				
	Capillaria (Eucoleus) annulata	Trichuroidea (N)				
	Capillaria (Eucoleus) contorta	Trichuroidea (N)				
Crop	*Gongylonema ingluvicola*	Spiruroidea (N)			*Trichomonas gallinae*	Trichomonadidae (M)
	Gongylonema crami	Spiruroidea (N)				
	Capillaria (Eucoleus) annulata	Trichuroidea (N)				
	Capillaria (Eucoleus) contorta	Trichuroidea (N)				
Proventriculus	*Gongylonema ingluvicola*	Spiruroidea (N)			*Trichomonas gallinae*	Trichomonadidae (M)
	Dispharynx nasuta	Spiruroidea (N)				
	Tetrameres americana	Spiruroidea (N)				
	Tetrameres fissispina	Spiruroidea (N)				
	Tetrameres confusa	Spiruroidea (N)				
	Tetrameres mohtedai	Spiruroidea (N)				
Gizzard	*Cheilospirura hamulosa*	Spiruroidea (N)				
	Histiocephalus laticaudatus	Spiruroidea (N)				
	Streptocara spp	Spiruroidea (N)				
Small intestine	*Capillaria caudinflata*	Trichuroidea (N)			*Eimeria acervulina*	Eimeriidae (A)
	Capillaria bursata	Trichuroidea (N)			*Eimeria brunetti*	Eimeriidae (A)
	Capillaria obsignata	Trichuroidea (N)			*Eimeria maxima*	Eimeriidae (A)
	Ascaridia galli	Ascaridoidea (N)			*Eimeria mitis*	Eimeriidae (A)
	Hartertia gallinarum	Spiruroidea (N)			*Eimeria necatrix*	Eimeriidae (A)
	Raillietina echinobothrida	Davaineidae (C)			*Eimeria praecox*	Eimeriidae (A)
	Raillietina tetragona	Davaineidae (C)			*Cryptosporidium meleagridis*	Cryptosporidiidae (A)
	Raillietina cesticillus	Davaineidae (C)				
	Davainea proglottina	Davaineidae (C)				
	Cotugnia digonopora	Davaineidae (C)				
	Amoebotaenia cuneata	Dilepididae (C)				
	Amoebotaenia sphenoides	Dilepididae (C)				

(*continued*)

Chicken parasite checklist (*continued*).

Section/host system	Helminths		Arthropods		Protozoa	
	Parasite	(Super)family	Parasite	Family	Parasite	Family
	Choanotaenia infundibulum	Dilepididae (C)				
	Metroliasthes lucida	Dilepididae (C)				
	Fimbriaria fasciolaris	Hymenolepididae (C)				
	Hymenolepis carioca	Hymenolepididae (C)				
	Hymenolepis cantaniana	Hymenolepididae (C)				
	Echinoparyphium recurvatum	Echinostomatidae (T)				
	Hypoderaeum conoideum	Echinostomatidae (T)				
	Polymorphus boschadis	Polymorphidae (A)				
	Catatropis verrucosa	Notocotylidae (T)				
	Brachylaemus commutatus	Brachylaemidae (T)				
	Posthermostomum commutatum	Brachylaemidae (T)				
Caeca	*Capillaria anatis*	Trichuroidea (N)			*Eimeria tenella*	Eimeriidae (A)
	Heterakis gallinarum	Ascaridoidea (N)			*Wenyonella gallinae*	Eimeriidae (A)
	Heterakis isolonche	Ascaridoidea (N)			*Cryptosporidium baileyi*	Cryptosporidiidae (A)
	Heterakis dispar	Ascaridoidea (N)				
	Heterakis brevispeculum	Ascaridoidea (N)			*Histomonas meleagridis*	Monocercomonadidae (M)
	Trichostrongylus tenuis	Trichostrongyloidea (N)			*Tetratrichomonas gallinarum*	Trichomonadidae (M)
	Subulura brumpti	Oxyuroidea (N)				
	Subulura suctoria	Oxyuroidea (N)			*Tritrichomonas eberthi*	Trichomonadidae (M)
	Subulura differens	Oxyuroidea (N)			*Chilomastix gallinarum*	Trichomonadidae (M)
	Strongyloides avium	Rhabditoidea (N)				
	Echinostoma revolutum	Echinostomatidae (T)				
	Notocotylus attenuatus	Notocotylidae (T)				
	Catatropis verrucosa	Notocotylidae (T)				
	Brachylaemus commutatus	Brachylaemidae (T)				
Large intestine	*Prosthogonimus pellucidus*	Prosthogonimidae (T)			*Cryptosporidium baileyi*	Cryptosporidiidae (A)
Cloacal bursa	*Prosthogonimus macrorchis*	Prosthogonimidae (T)				
Rectum	*Prosthogonimus ovatus*	Prosthogonimidae (T)				
	Plagiorchis arcuatus	Plagiorchidae (T)				
	Notocotylus attenuatus	Notocotylidae (T)				
Respiratory						
Nares						

Trachea Bronchi	*Syngamus trachea*	Strongyloidea (N)	*Cytodites nudus*	Cytoditidae (A)		
Lung						
Air sacs						
Liver					*Histomonas meleagridis*	Monocercomonadidae (M)
Pancreas						
Circulatory						
Blood					*Leucocytozoon caulleryi*	Plasmodiidae (A)
					Leucocytozoon sabrazesi	Plasmodiidae (A)
					Plasmodium gallinaceum	Plasmodiidae (A)
					Plasmodium juxtanucleare	Plasmodiidae (A)
					Trypanosoma avium	Trypanosomatidae (M)
					Trypanosoma gallinarum	Trypanosomatidae (M)
					Aegyptianella pullorum	Anaplasmataceae (R)
					Aegyptianella moshkovskii	Anaplasmataceae (R)
Blood vessels						
Nervous						
CNS						
Eye	*Oxyspirura mansoni*	Spiruroidea (N)				
Reproductive/ urogenital						
Oviduct	*Plagiorchis arcuatus*	Plagiorchidae (T)				
	Prosthogonimus pellucidus	Prosthogonimidae (T)				
	Prosthogonimus macrorchis	Prosthogonimidae (T)				
	Prosthogonimus ovatus	Prosthogonimidae (T)				
Locomotory						
Muscle					*Sarcocystis hovarthi*	Sarcocystiidae (A)
					Toxoplasma gondii	Sarcocystiidae (A)
Connective tissue						

(continued)

Chicken parasite checklist (*continued*).

Section/host system	Helminths		Arthropods		Protozoa	
	Parasite	(Super)family	Parasite	Family	Parasite	Family
Kidneys						
Integument						
Skin	*Collyriclum faba*	Troglotrematidae (T)	*Dermanyssus gallinae*	Dermanyssidae (A)		
	Dithrydium variable	Mesocestoididae (C)	*Ornithonyssus bursa*	Macronyssidae (A)		
			Ornithonyssus sylvarium	Macronyssidae (A)		
			Knemidokoptes mutans	Knemidokoptidae (A)		
			Knemidokoptes gallinae	Knemidokoptidae (A)		
			Epidermoptes bilobatus	Epidermoptidae (A)		
			Rivoltasia bifurcata	Epidermoptidae (A)		
			Megninia cubitalis	Analgidae (A)		
			Megninia ginglymura	Analgidae (A)		
			Megninia ortari	Analgidae (A)		
			Pterolichus obtusus	Pterolichidae (A)		
			Neotrombicula autumnalis	Trombiculidae (A)		
			Neoschongastia americana	Trombiculidae (A)		
			Androlaelaps casalis	Laelapidae (A)		
			Syringophilus bipectinatus	Syringophilidae (A)		
			Dermoglyphus elongatus	Dermoglyphidae (A)		
			Cuclotogaster heterographus	Philopteridae (I)		
			Goniocotes gallinae	Philopteridae (I)		
			Goniodes gigas	Philopteridae (I)		
			Goniodes dissimilis	Philopteridae (I)		
			Lipeurus caponis	Philopteridae (I)		
			Numidilipeurus tropicalis	Philopteridae (I)		
			Menacanthus stramineus	Menoponidae (I)		
			Menopon gallinae	Menoponidae (I)		
			Echidnophaga gallinacea	Pulicidae (I)		
			Ctenocephalides felis	Pulicidae (I)		
			Ceratophyllus gallinae	Ceratophyllidae (I)		
			Ceratophyllus columbae	Ceratophyllidae (I)		
			Cimex lectularis	Cimicidae (I)		
			Wohlfahrtia magnifica	Sarcophagidae (I)		
			Cochliomyia hominivorax	Calliphoridae (I)		
Subcutaneous	*Collyriclum faba*	Troglotrematidae (T)	*Laminosioptes cysticola*	Laminosioptidae (A)		

The following species of flies and ticks are found on poultry. More detailed descriptions are found in Chapter 11: Facultative ectoparasites and arthropod vectors.

Flies of veterinary importance on poultry.

Group	Genus	Species	Family
Blackflies Buffalo gnats	*Simulium*	spp	Simuliidae (I)
Midges	*Culicoides*	spp	Ceratopogonidae (I)
Mosquitoes	*Aedes* *Anopheles* *Culex*	spp spp spp	Culicidae (I)
Muscids	*Musca* *Stomoxys*	*domestica* *calcitrans*	Muscidae (I)
Sandflies	*Phlebotomus*	spp	Psychodidae (I)
Screwworms and blowflies	*Chrysomya*	*albiceps* *bezziana* *megacephala*	Calliphoridae (I)
	Cochliomyia	*hominivorax* *macellaria*	
	Cordylobia	*anthropophaga*	
	Wohlfahrtia	*magnifica*	Sarcophagidae (I)

Tick species found on poultry.

Genus	Species	Common name	Family
Argas	*persicus*	Fowl tick	Argasidae
	walkerae		Argasidae
	reflexus		Argasidae
Ornithodoros	*moubata*	Eyeless tampan	Argasidae
	savignyi	Eyed tampan	Argasidae
Haemaphysalis	*cinnabarina*		Ixodidae
	leporispalustris		Ixodidae
Amblyomma	*hebraeum*		Ixodidae
	americanum		Ixodidae
Ixodes	*ricinus*	European sheep, castor bean tick	Ixodidae
	holocyclus		Ixodidae

Turkey parasite checklist.

Section/host system	Helminths		Arthropods		Protozoa	
	Parasite	(Super)family	Parasite	Family	Parasite	Family
Digestive						
Pharynx					*Trichomonas gallinae*	Trichomonadidae (M)
Oesophagus	*Capillaria (Eucoleus) annulata*	Trichuroidea (N)			*Trichomonas gallinae*	Trichomonadidae (M)
	Capillaria contorta	Trichuroidea (N)				
	Gongylonema ingluvicola	Spiruroidea (N)				
	Dispharynx nasuta	Spiruroidea (N)				
Crop	*Capillaria annulata*	Trichuroidea (N)			*Trichomonas gallinae*	Trichomonadidae (M)
	Capillaria contorta	Trichuroidea (N)				
	Gongylonema ingluvicola	Spiruroidea (N)				
Proventriculus	*Gongylonema ingluvicola*	Spiruroidea (N)			*Trichomonas gallinae*	Trichomonadidae (M)
	Dispharynx nasuta	Spiruroidea (N)				
	Tetrameres americana	Spiruroidea (N)				
	Tetrameres fissispina	Spiruroidea (N)				
Gizzard	*Cheilospirura hamulosa*	Spiruroidea (N)				
	Streptocara spp	Spiruroidea (N)				
Small intestine	*Capillaria obsignata*	Trichuroidea (N)			*Eimeria adenoides*	Eimeriidae (A)
	Capillaria caudinflata	Trichuroidea (N)			*Eimeria dispersa*	Eimeriidae (A)
	Capillaria bursata	Trichuroidea (N)			*Eimeria gallopavonis*	Eimeriidae (A)
	Ascaridia galli	Ascaridoidea (N)			*Eimeria innocua*	Eimeriidae (A)
	Ascaridia dissimilis	Ascaridoidea (N)			*Eimeria meleagrimitis*	Eimeriidae (A)
	Raillietina cesticillus	Davaineidae (C)			*Eimieria subrotunda*	Eimeriidae (A)
	Raillietina echinobothrida	Davaineidae (C)			*Cryptosporidium meleagridis*	Cryptosporidiidae (A)
	Davainea proglottina	Davaineidae (C)			*Spironucleus (Hexamita) meleagridis*	Diplomonadidae (M)
	Choanotaenia infundibulum	Dilepididae (C)				
	Metroliasthes lucida	Dilepididae (C)				
	Hymenolepis carioca	Hymenolepidae (C)				
	Hymenolepis cantaniana	Hymenolepidae (C)				
	Hypoderaeum conoideum	Echinostomatidae (C)				
Caeca	*Capillaria anatis*	Trichuroidea (N)			*Eimeria adenoides*	Eimeriidae (A)
	Heterakis gallinarum	Ascaridoidea (N)			*Eimeria gallopavonis*	Eimeriidae (A)
	Trichostrongylus tenuis	Trichostrongyloidea (N)			*Eimeria meleagrimitis*	Eimeriidae (A)
	Subulura brumpti	Oxyuroidea (N)			*Histomonas meleagridis*	Monocercomonadidae (M)
	Subulura suctoria	Oxyuroidea (N)			*Tetratrichomonas gallinarum*	Trichomonadidae (M)
	Strongyloides avium	Rhabditoidea (N)			*Tritrichomonas eberthi*	Trichomonadidae (M)
	Brachylaemus commutatus	Brachylaemidae (T)			*Chilomastix gallinarum*	Trichomonadidae (M)
	Postharmostomum commutatum	Brachylaemidae (T)			*Cryptosporidium baileyi*	Cryptosporidiidae (A)

Large intestine	*Prosthogonimus pellucidus*	Prosthogonimidae (T)			*Cryptosporidium baileyi*	Cryptosporidiidae (A)
Cloacal bursa	*Prosthogonimus macrorchis*	Prosthogonimidae (T)				
Rectum	*Prosthogonimus ovatus*	Prosthogonimidae (T)				
	Plagiorchis arcuatus	Plagiorchidae (T)				
Respiratory						
Nares						
Trachea	*Syngamus trachea*	Strongyloidea (N)	*Cytodites nudus*	Cytoditidae (A)		
Bronchi						
Lung						
Air sacs						
Liver					*Histomonas meleagridis*	Monocercomonadidae (M)
Pancreas						
Circulatory						
Blood					*Haemoproteus meleagridis*	Plasmodiidae (A)
					Leucocytozoon smithi	Plasmodiidae (A)
					Plasmodium durae	Plasmodiidae (A)
Blood vessels					*Aegyptianella pullorum*	Anaplasmataceae (R)
					Aegyptianella moshkovskii	Anaplasmataceae (R)
Nervous						
CNS						
Eye	*Oxyspirura mansoni*	Spiruroidea (N)				
Reproductive/ urogenital						

(*continued*)

Turkey parasite checklist (*continued*).

Section/host system	Helminths		Arthropods		Protozoa	
	Parasite	(Super)family	Parasite	Family	Parasite	Family
Oviduct						
	Prosthogonimus pellucidus	Prosthogonimidae (T)				
	Prosthogonimus macrorchis	Prosthogonimidae (T)				
	Prosthogonimus ovatus	Prosthogonimidae (T)				
	Plagiorchis arcuatus	Plagiorchidae (T)				
	Notocotylus attenuatus	Notocotylidae (T)				
Kidneys						
Locomotory						
Connective tissue					*Toxoplasma gondii*	Sarcocystiidae (A)
Integument						
Skin	*Collyriclum faba*	Troglotrematidae (T)	*Dermanyssus gallinae*	Dermanyssidae (A)		
	Dithyridium variable	Mesocestoididae (C)	*Ornithonyssus bursa*	Macronyssidae (A)		
			Ornithonyssus sylvarium	Macronyssidae (A)		
			Knemidokoptes gallinae	Knemidokoptidae (A)		
			Knemidokoptes mutans	Knemidokoptidae (A)		
			Megninia ginglymura	Analgidae (A)		
			Androlaelaps casalis	Laelapidae (A)		
			Freyana chanayi	Dermoglyphidae (A)		
			Pterolichus obtusus	Pterolichidae (A)		
			Neotrombicula autumnalis	Trombiculidae (A)		
			Neoschongastia americana	Trombiculidae (A)		
			Syringophilus bipectinatus	Syringophilidae (A)		
			Goniodes meleagridis	Philopteridae (I)		
			Menacanthus stramineus	Menoponidae (I)		
			Menopon gallinae	Menoponidae (I)		
			Cuclotogaster heterographus	Philopteridae (I)		
			Lipeurus caponis	Philopteridae (I)		
			Echidnophaga gallinacea	Pulicidae (I)		
			Ceratophyllus gallinae	Ceratophyllidae (I)		
			Wohlfahrtia magnifica	Sarcophagidae (I)		
Subcutaneous	*Collyriclum faba*	Troglotrematidae (T)	*Laminosioptes cysticola*	Laminosioptidae (A)		
			Cochliomyia hominivorax	Calliphoridae (I)		

Flies of veterinary importance on turkeys.

Group	Genus	Species	Family
Blackflies Buffalo gnats	*Simulium*	spp	Simuliidae (I)
Midges	*Culicoides*	spp	Ceratopogonidae (I)
Mosquitoes	*Aedes* *Anopheles* *Culex*	spp spp spp	Culicidae (I)
Muscids	*Musca* *Stomoxys*	*domestica* *calcitrans*	Muscidae (I)
Sandflies	*Phlebotomus*	spp	Psychodidae (I)
Screwworms and blowflies	*Chrysomya*	*albiceps* *bezziana* *megacephala*	Calliphoridae (I)
	Cochliomyia	*hominivorax* *macellaria*	
	Cordylobia	*anthropophaga*	
	Wohlfahrtia	*magnifica*	Sarcophagidae (I)

Tick species found on turkeys.

Genus	Species	Common name	Family
Argas	*persicus*	Fowl tick	Argasidae
	walkerae		Argasidae
	reflexus		Argasidae
Ornithodoros	*moubata*	Eyeless tampan	Argasidae
	savignyi	Eyed tampan	Argasidae
Haemaphysalis	*cinnabarina*		Ixodidae
	leporispalustris		Ixodidae
Amblyomma	*hebraeum*		Ixodidae
	americanum		Ixodidae
Ixodes	*ricinus*	European sheep, castor bean tick	Ixodidae
	holocyclus		Ixodidae

Duck parasite checklist.

Section/host system	Helminths		Arthropods		Protozoa	
	Parasite	(Super)family	Parasite	Family	Parasite	Family
Digestive						
Pharynx						
Oesophagus	*Capillaria (Eucoleus) annulata*	Trichuroidea (N)				
	Capillaria contorta	Trichuroidea (N)				
	Echinuria (Acuaria) uncinata	Spiruroidea (N)				
	Typhlocoelum cucumerinum	Cyclocoelidae (T)				
Crop	*Capillaria contorta*	Trichuroidea (N)				
Proventriculus	*Echinuria (Acuaria) uncinata*	Spiruroidea (N)				
	Tetrameres americana	Spiruroidea (N)				
	Tetrameres crami	Spiruroidea (N)				
	Tetrameres fissispina	Spiruroidea (N)				
	Hystrichis tricolor	Dioctophymatoidea (N)				
	Eustrongyloides papillosus	Dioctophymatoidea (N)				
Gizzard	*Amidostomum anseris*	Trichostrongyloidea (N)				
	Amidostomum skrjabini	Trichostrongyloidea (N)				
	Epomidiostomum anatinum	Trichostrongyloidea (N)				
	Epomidiostomum orispinum	Trichostrongyloidea (N)				
	Epomidostomum skrjabini	Trichostrongyloidea (N)				
	Echinuria (Acuaria) uncinata	Spiruroidea (N)				
	Steptocera spp	Spiruroidea (N)				
Small intestine	*Ascaridia galli*	Ascaridoidea (N)			*Eimeria anatis*	Eimeriidae (A)
	Porrocaecum crassum	Ascaridoidea (N)			*Tyzzeria perniciosa*	Eimeriidae (A)
	Contracaecum spiculigerum	Ascaridoidea (N)			*Spironucleus (Hexamita) meleagridis*	Diplomonadidae (M)
	Polymorphus boschadis	Polymorphidae (A)				
	Filicollis anatis	Polymorphidae (A)				
	Echinoparyphium recurvatum	Echinostomatidae (T)			*Cryptosporidium meleagridis*	Cryptosporidiidae (A)
	Hypoderaeum conoideum	Echinostomatidae (T)				
	Apatemon gracilis	Strigeidae (T)				
	Parastrigea robusta	Strigeidae (T)				
	Cotylurus cornutus	Strigeidae (T)				
	Cotylurus flabelliformis	Strigeidae (T)				
	Hymenolepis lanceolata	Hymenolepididae (C)				
	Fimbriaria fasciolaris	Hymenolepididae (C)				

Caeca	*Heterakis dispar*	Ascaridoidea (N)	*Tetratrichomonas anatis*	Trichomonadidae (M)
	Heterakis isolonche	Ascaridoidea (N)	*Cochlosoma anatis*	Cochlosomatidae (M)
	Heterakis gallinarum	Ascaridoidea (N)		
	Heterakis brevispeculum	Ascaridoidea (N)		
	Trichostrongylus tenuis	Trichostrongyloidea (N)		
	Capillaria anatis	Trichuroidea (N)		
	Subulura suctoria	Oxyuroidea (N)		
	Echinostoma revolutum	Echinostomatidae (T)		
	Notocotylus attenuatus	Notocotylidae (T)		
	Catatropis verrucosa	Notocotylidae (T)		
Large intestine	*Prosthogonimus pellucidus*	Prosthogonimidae (T)	*Cryptosporidium baileyi*	Cryptosporidiidae
	Prosthogonimus macrorchis	Prosthogonimidae (T)		
Cloacal bursa	*Prosthogonimus ovatus*	Prosthogonimidae (T)	*Cryptosporidium baileyi*	Cryptosporidiidae
Rectum	*Notocotylus attenuatus*	Notocotylidae (T)		
Respiratory				
Nares	*Hyptiasmus tumidus*	Cyclocoelidae (T)		
Trachea	*Syngamus bronchialis*	Strongyloidea (N)		
Bronchi	*Typhlocoelum cymbium*	Cyclocoelidae (T)		
	Typhlocoelum cucumerinum	Cyclocoelidae (T)		
Lung				
Air sacs	*Typhlocoelum cucumerinum*	Cyclocoelidae (T)		
Liver				
Pancreas				
Circulatory				
Blood			*Leucocytozoon simondi*	Plasmodiidae (A)
			Haemoproteus nettionis	Plasmodiidae (A)
			Aegyptianella pullorum	Anaplasmataceae (R)
Blood vessels	*Bilharziella polonica*	Schistosomatidae (T)		
Nervous				
CNS				
Eye				
Reproductive/urogenital				
Oviduct	*Prosthogonimus pellucidus*	Prosthogonimidae (T)		
	Prosthogonimus macrorchis	Prosthogonimidae (T)		
	Prosthogonimus ovatus	Prosthogonimidae (T)		
Kidneys			*Eimeria truncata*	Eimeriidae (A)

(continued)

Duck parasite checklist (*continued*).

Section/host system	Helminths		Arthropods		Protozoa	
	Parasite	(Super)family	Parasite	Family	Parasite	Family
Locomotory						
Connective tissue					*Toxoplasma gondii*	Sarcocystiidae (A)
Integument						
Skin	*Avioserpens taiwana*	Dracunculoidea (N)	*Trinotron anserium*	Philopteridae (I)		
	Collyriclum faba	Troglotrematidae (T)	*Anaticola anseris*	Philopteridae (I)		
			Anaticola crassicornis	Philopteridae (I)		
			Anaticola tadornae	Philopteridae (I)		
			Anaticola thoracicus	Philopteridae (I)		
			Acidoproctus rostratus	Philopteridae (I)		
			Anatoecus dentatus	Philopteridae (I)		
			Anatoecus brunneiceps	Philopteridae (I)		
			Anatoecus cygni	Philopteridae (I)		
			Anatoecus icterodes	Philopteridae (I)		
			Ornithobius cygni	Philopteridae (I)		
			Ornithobius mathisi	Philopteridae (I)		
			Ornithobius waterstoni	Philopteridae (I)		
			Menopon gallinae	Menoponidae (I)		
			Menopon leucoxanthum	Menoponidae (I)		
			Holomenopon leucoxanthum	Menoponidae (I)		
			Ciconiphilus decimfasciatus	Menoponidae (I)		
			Ciconiphilus parvus	Menoponidae (I)		
			Ciconiphilus pectinventris	Menoponidae (I)		
			Ciconiphilus cygni	Menoponidae (I)		
			Ciconiphilus quadripustulatus	Menoponidae (I)		
			Trinoton ansertium	Menoponidae (I)		
			Trinoton squalidum	Menoponidae (I)		
			Trinoton querquedula	Menoponidae (I)		
Subcutaneous	*Avioserpens taiwana*	Dracunculoidea (N)				
	Collyriclum faba	Troglotrematidae (T)				
	Ornithofilaria fallisensis	Filarioidea (N)				

Goose parasite checklist.

Section/host system	Helminths		Arthropods		Protozoa	
	Parasite	(Super)family	Parasite	Family	Parasite	Family
Digestive						
Pharynx						
Oesophagus	*Echinuria (Acuaria) uncinata*	Spiruroidea (N)				
Crop						
Proventriculus	*Echinuria (Acuaria) uncinata*	Spiruroidea (N)				
	Tetrameres americana	Spiruroidea (N)				
	Tetrameres fissispina	Spiruroidea (N)				
	Eustrongyloides papillosus	Dioctophymatoidea (N)				
Gizzard	*Amidostomum anseris*	Trichostrongyloidea (N)				
	Epomidiostomum anatinum	Trichostrongyloidea (N)				
	Epomidiostomum orispinum	Trichostrongyloidea (N)				
	Epomidiostomum skrjabini	Trichostrongyloidea (N)				
	Echinuria (Acuaria) uncinata	Spiruroidea (N)				
	Steptocara spp	Spiruroidea (N)				
Small intestine	*Ascaridia galli*	Ascaridoidea (N)			*Eimeria anseris*	Eimeriidae (A)
	Contracaecum spiculigerum	Ascaridoidea (N)			*Eimeria nocens*	Eimeriidae (A)
	Capillaria caudinflata	Trichuroidea (N)			*Tyzzeria anseris*	Eimeriidae (A)
	Polymorphus boschadis	Polymorphidae (A)				
	Filicollis anatis	Polymorphidae (A)				
	Hypoderaeum conoideum	Echinostomatidae (T)				
	Echinoparyphium recurvatum	Echinostomatidae (T)				
	Hymenolepis lanceolata	Hymenolepididae (C)				
	Fimbriaria fasciolaris	Hymenolepididae (C)				
Caeca	*Heterakis gallinarum*	Ascaridoidea (N)			*Tetratrichomonas anseris*	Trichomonadidae (M)
	Heterakis dispar	Ascaridoidea (N)				
	Heterakis brevispeculum	Ascaridoidea (N)				
	Capillaria anatis	Trichuroidea (N)				
	Trichostrongylus tenuis	Trichostrongyloidea (N)				
	Strongyloides avium	Rhabditoidea (N)				
	Echinostoma revolutum	Echinostomatidae (T)				
	Notocotylus attenuatus	Notocotylidae (T)				
	Catatropis verrucosa	Notocotylidae (T)				

(*continued*)

Goose parasite checklist (*continued*).

Section/host system	Helminths		Arthropods		Protozoa	
	Parasite	(Super)family	Parasite	Family	Parasite	Family
Large intestine Cloacal bursa Rectum	*Prosthogonimus ovatus*	Prosthogonimidae (T)				
	Notocotylus attenuatus	Notocotylidae (T)				
Respiratory						
Nares	*Hyptiasmus tumidus*	Cyclocoelidae (T)				
Trachea Bronchi	*Syngamus bronchialis*	Strongyloidea (N)				
	Syngamus skrjabinomorpha	Strongyloidea (N)				
Lung						
Air sacs						
Liver						
Pancreas						
Circulatory						
Blood					*Leucocytozoon simondi*	Plasmodiidae (A)
					Haemoproteus nettionis	Plasmodiidae (A)
					Aegyptianella pullorum	Anaplasmataceae (R)
Blood vessels						
Nervous						
CNS						
Eye						
Reproductive/urogenital						
Oviduct	*Prosthogonimus pellucidus*	Prosthogonimidae (T)				
	Prosthogonimus ovatus	Prosthogonimidae (T)				
Kidneys					*Eimeria truncata*	Eimeriidae (A)

Locomotory						
Connective tissue					*Toxoplasma gondii*	Sarcocystiidae (A)
Integument						
Skin	*Collyriclum faba*	Troglotrematidae (T)	*Anaticola anseris*	Philopteridae (I)		
	Dithyridium variable	Mesocestoididae (C)	*Anaticola anseris*	Philopteridae (I)		
			Anaticola crassicornis	Philopteridae (I)		
			Anaticola tadornae	Philopteridae (I)		
			Anaticola thoracicus	Philopteridae (I)		
			Acidoproctus rostratus	Philopteridae (I)		
			Anatoecus dentatus	Philopteridae (I)		
			Anatoecus brunneiceps	Philopteridae (I)		
			Anatoecus cygni	Philopteridae (I)		
			Anatoecus icterodes	Philopteridae (I)		
			Ornithobius cygni	Philopteridae (I)		
			Ornithobius mathisi	Philopteridae (I)		
			Ornithobius waterstoni	Philopteridae (I)		
			Holomenopon leucoxanthum	Menoponidae (I)		
			Ciconiphilus decimfasciatus	Menoponidae (I)		
			Ciconiphilus parvus	Menoponidae (I)		
			Ciconiphilus pectinventris	Menoponidae (I)		
			Ciconiphilus cygni	Menoponidae (I)		
			Ciconiphilus quadripustulatus	Menoponidae (I)		
			Trinoton ansertium	Menoponidae (I)		
			Trinoton squalidum	Menoponidae (I)		
			Trinoton querquedula	Menoponidae (I)		
			Knemidokoptes gallinae	Knemidokoptidae (A)		
Subcutaneous	*Collyriclum faba*	Troglotrematidae (T)				
	Ornithofilaria fallisensis	Filarioidea (N)				

Pheasant parasite checklist.

Section/host system	Helminths		Arthropods		Protozoa	
	Parasite	(Super)family	Parasite	Family	Parasite	Family
Digestive						
Pharynx						
Oesophagus	*Capillaria* (*Eucoleus*) *perforans*	Trichuroidea (N)				
	Capillaria (*Eucoleus*) *annulata*	Trichuroidea (N)				
	Capillaria (*Eucoleus*) *contorta*	Trichuroidea (N)				
	Capillaria uropapillata	Trichuroidea (N)				
	Dispharynx nasuta	Spiruroidea (N)				
	Gongylonema ingluvicola	Spiruroidea (N)				
Crop	*Capillaria* (*Eucoleus*) *perforans*	Trichuroidea (N)				
	Capillaria (*Eucoleus*) *annulata*	Trichuroidea (N)				
	Capillaria (*Eucoleus*) *contorta*	Trichuroidea (N)				
	Capillaria uropapillata	Trichuroidea (N)				
	Gongylonema ingluvicola	Spiruroidea (N)				
Proventriculus	*Dispharynx nasuta*	Spiruroidea (N)				
	Gongylonema ingluvicola	Spiruroidea (N)				
Gizzard						
Small intestine	*Ascaridia galli*	Ascaridoidea (N)			*Eimeria colchici*	Eimeriidae (A)
	Capillaria caudinflata	Trichuroidea (N)			*Eimeria duodenalis*	Eimeriidae (A)
	Capillaria obsignata	Trichuroidea (N)			*Eimeria megalostoma*	Eimeriidae (A)
	Capillaria phasianina	Trichuroidea (N)			*Eimeria pacifica*	Eimeriidae (A)
	Capillaria bursata	Trichuroidea (N)			*Eimeria phasiani*	Eimeriidae (A)
	Hymenolepis cantaniana	Hymenolepididae (C)				
Caeca	*Heterakis gallinarum*	Ascaridoidea (N)			*Tetratrichomonas gallinarum*	Trichomonadidae (M)
	Heterakis isolonche	Ascaridoidea (N)				
	Capillaria phasianina	Trichuroidea (N)			*Spironucleus meleagridis*	Diplomonadidae (M)
	Capillaria anatis	Trichuroidea (N)				
	Trichostrongylus tenuis	Trichostrongyloidea (N)				
	Postharmostomum commutatum	Brachylaemidae (T)				
	Brachylaemus commutatus	Brachylaemidae (T)				
	Subulura suctoria	Oxyuroidea (N)				
Large intestine						
Cloacal bursa						
Rectum						
Respiratory						
Nares						

Trachea	*Syngamus trachea*	Strongyloidea (N)				
Bronchi						
Lung						
Air sacs						
Liver					*Histomonas meleagridis*	Monocercomonadidae (M)
Pancreas						
Circulatory						
Blood					*Leucocytozoon simondi*	Plasmodiidae (A)
					Haemoproteus nettionis	Plasmodiidae (A)
					Aegyptianella pullorum	Anaplasmataceae (R)
					Aegyptianella moshkovskii	Anaplasmataceae (R)
Blood vessels						
Nervous						
CNS						
Eye						
Reproductive/ urogenital						
Oviduct						
Kidneys						
Locomotory						
Muscle					*Toxoplasma gondii*	Sarcocystiidae (A)
Connective tissue						
Integument						
Skin	*Dithyridium variable*	Mesocestoididae (C)	*Dermanyssus gallinae*	Dermanyssidae (A)		
			Amyrsidea perdicis	Menoponidae (I)		
			Goniocotes chryocephalus	Philopteridae (I)		
			Gonoides colchici	Philopteridae (I)		
			Liperus maculosus	Philopteridae (I)		
			Lagopoecus colchicus	Degeeriellidae (I)		
			Knemidokoptes gallinae	Knemidokoptidae (A)		
Subcutaneous						

Red-legged and grey partridge parasite checklist (R: red-legged partridge; G: grey partridge).

Section/host system	Helminths		Arthropods		Protozoa	
	Parasite	(Super)family	Parasite	Family	Parasite	Family
Digestive						
Pharynx						
Oesophagus	*Capillaria* (*Eucoleus*) *perforans*	Trichuroidea (N)				
	Capillaria (*Eucoleus*) *annulata*	Trichuroidea (N)				
	Capillaria (*Eucoleus*) *contorta*	Trichuroidea (N)				
	Capillaria uropapillata	Trichuroidea (N)				
	Dispharynx nasuta	Spiruroidea (N)				
	Gongylonema ingluvicola	Spiruroidea (N)				
Crop	*Capillaria* (*Eucoleus*) *perforans*	Trichuroidea (N)				
	Capillaria (*Eucoleus*) *annulata*	Trichuroidea (N)				
	Capillaria (*Eucoleus*) *contorta*	Trichuroidea (N)				
	Capillaria uropapillata	Trichuroidea (N)				
	Gongylonema ingluvicola	Spiruroidea (N)				
Proventriculus	*Dispharynx nasuta*	Spiruroidea (N)				
	Gongylonema ingluvicola	Spiruroidea (N)				
Gizzard						
Small intestine	*Ascaridia galli*	Ascaridoidea (N)			*Eimeria caucasica*	Eimeriidae (A)
	Capillaria caudinflata	Trichuroidea (N)			*Eimeria procera* (G)	Eimeriidae (A)
	Capillaria obsignata	Trichuroidea (N)			*Eimeria koifoidi* (G)	Eimeriidae (A)
	Capillaria phasianina	Trichuroidea (N)			*Eimeria legionensis* (R)	Eimeriidae (A)
					Spironucleus meleagridis	Diplomonadidae (M)
Caeca	*Heterakis gallinarum*	Ascaridoidea (N)			*Tetratrichomonas gallinarum*	Trichomonadidae (M)
	Capillaria anatis	Trichuroidea (N)				
	Capillaria phasianina	Trichuroidea (N)				
	Trichostrongylus tenuis	Trichostrongyloidea (N)				
Large intestine						
Cloacal bursa						
Rectum						
Respiratory						
Nares						
Trachea	*Syngamus trachea*	Strongyloidea (N)				
Bronchi						
Lung						
Air sacs						

Liver					*Histomonas meleagridis*	Monocercomonadidae (M)
Pancreas						
Circulatory						
Blood						
Blood vessels						
Nervous						
CNS						
Eye						
Reproductive/ urogenital						
Oviduct						
Kidneys						
Locomotory						
Muscle					*Toxoplasma gondii*	Sarcocystiidae (A)
Connective tissue						
Integument						
Skin	*Dithyridium variable*	Mesocestoididae (C)	*Dermanyssus gallinae*	Dermanyssidae (A)		
			Goniocotes microthorax (G)	Philopteridae (I)		
			Goniocotes obscurus (R)	Philopteridae (I)		
			Goniodes dispar	Philopteridae (I)		
			Amyrsidea perdicis	Menoponidae (I)		
			Menacanthus layali (R)	Menoponidae (I)		
			Menacanthus stramineus	Menoponidae (I)		
			Menopon pallens	Menoponidae (I)		
			Lipeurus maculosus (G)	Philopteridae (I)		
			Cuclotogaster heterogrammicus (G)	Philopteridae (I)		
			Cuclotogaster obsuricor (R)	Philopteridae (I)		
			Lagopoecus colchicus	Degeeriellidae (I)		
Subcutaneous						

Quail parasite checklist.

Section/host system	Helminths		Arthropods		Protozoa	
	Parasite	(Super)family	Parasite	Family	Parasite	Family
Digestive						
Pharynx						
Oesophagus	*Capillaria (Eucoleus) annulata*	Trichuroidea (N)				
	Capillaria (Eucoleus) contorta	Trichuroidea (N)				
	Gongylonema ingluvicola	Spiruroidea (N)				
Crop	*Capillaria (Eucoleus) annulata*	Trichuroidea (N)				
	Capillaria (Eucoleus) contorta	Trichuroidea (N)				
	Gongylonema ingluvicola	Spiruroidea (N)				
Proventriculus	*Dispharynx nasuta*	Spiruroidea (N)				
	Tetrameres pattersoni	Spiruroidea (N)				
	Gongylonema ingluvicola	Spiruroidea (N)				
Gizzard						
Small intestine	*Ascaridia galli*	Ascaridoidea (N)			*Eimeria bateri*	Eimeriidae (A)
	Hymenolepis cantaniana	Hymenolepididae (C)			*Eimeria coturnicus*	Eimeriidae (A)
	Strongyloides avium	Rhabditoidea (N)			*Eimeria taldykurganica*	Eimeriidae (A)
					Eimeria tsunodai	Eimeriidae (A)
					Eimeria uzura	Eimeriidae (A)
					Spironucleus meleagridis	Diplomonadidae (M)
Caeca	*Heterakis gallinarum*	Ascaridoidea (N)			*Tetratrichomonas gallinarum*	Trichomonadidae (M)
	Heterakis isolonche	Ascaridoidea (N)				
	Capillaria anatis	Trichuroidea (N)				
	Subulura suctoria	Oxyuroidea (N)				
	Strongyloides avium	Rhabditoidea (N)				
Large intestine					*Cryptosporidium baileyi*	Cryptosporidiidae (A)
Cloacal bursa						
Rectum						
Respiratory						
Nares						
Trachea						
Bronchi						
Lung						
Air sacs						

Liver		
Pancreas		
Circulatory		
Blood		
Blood vessels		
Nervous		
CNS		
Eye		
Reproductive/ urogenital		
Oviduct		
Kidneys		
Locomotory		
Connective tissue		
	Toxoplasma gondii	Sarcocystiidae (A)
Integument		
Skin		
Subcutaneous		

Guinea fowl parasite checklist.

Section/host system	Helminths		Arthropods		Protozoa	
	Parasite	(Super)family	Parasite	Family	Parasite	Family
Digestive						
Pharynx						
Oesophagus	*Capillaria* (*Eucoleus*) *perforans* *Capillaria* (*Eucoleus*) *annulata* *Capillaria* (*Eucoleus*) *contorta*	Trichuroidea (N) Trichuroidea (N) Trichuroidea (N)				
Crop	*Capillaria* (*Eucoleus*) *perforans* *Capillaria* (*Eucoleus*) *annulata* *Capillaria* (*Eucoleus*) *contorta*	Trichuroidea (N) Trichuroidea (N) Trichuroidea (N)				
Proventriculus	*Dispharynx nasuta*	Spiruroidea (N)				
Gizzard						
Small intestine	*Ascaridia galli* *Raillientina tetragona* *Raillientina cesticillus*	Ascaridoidea (N) Davaineidae (C) Davaineidae (C)			*Eimeria grenieri* *Eimeria numidae*	Eimeriidae (A) Eimeriidae (A)
Caeca	*Heterakis gallinarum* *Heterakis brevispeculum* *Trichostrongylus tenuis* *Subulura suctoria*	Ascaridoidea (N) Ascaridoidea (N) Trichostrongyloidea (N) Oxyuroidea (N)			*Tetratrichomonas gallinarum*	Trichomonadidae (M)
Large intestine Cloacal bursa Rectum						
Respiratory						
Nares						
Trachea Bronchi	*Syngamus trachea*	Strongyloidea (N)				
Lung						
Air sacs						

Liver						
Pancreas						
Circulatory						
Blood					*Leucocytozoon caulleryi*	Plasmodiidae (A)
					Leucocytozoon sabrazesi	Plasmodiidae (A)
					Plasmodium gallinaceum	Plasmodiidae (A)
Blood vessels						
Nervous						
CNS						
Eye	*Oxyspirura mansoni*	Spiruroidea (N)				
Reproductive/ urogenital						
Oviduct						
Kidneys						
Locomotory						
Muscle					*Toxoplasma gondii*	Sarcocystiidae (A)
Connective tissue						
Integument						
Skin			*Menopon gallinae*	Menoponidae (I)		
			Goniocotes gallinae	Philopteridae (I)		
			Lipeurus maculosus	Philopteridae (I)		
Subcutaneous						

8
Parasites of ungulates

DEER

PARASITES OF THE DIGESTIVE SYSTEM

Gongylonema pulchrum

Synonym: *G. scutatum*

Common name: Gullet worm

Predilection site: Oesophagus, rumen

Parasite class: Nematoda

Superfamily: Spiruroidea

Final host: Sheep, goat, cattle, pig, buffalo, horse, donkey, deer, camel, man

Intermediate host: Coprophagous beetles, cockroaches

Geographical distribution: Probably worldwide

For more details see Chapter 3 (Sheep and goats).

Paramphistomum cervi

Synonym: *Paramphistomum explanatum*

Common name: Rumen fluke

Predilection site: Rumen

Parasite class: Trematoda

Family: Paramphistomatidae

Definitive hosts: Cattle, sheep, goat, deer, buffalo, antelope

Intermediate hosts: Water snails, principally *Planorbis* and *Bulinus*

Geographical distribution: Worldwide

Gongylonema verrucosum

Common name: Rumen gullet worm

Predilection site: Rumen, reticulum, omasum

Parasite class: Nematoda

Superfamily: Spiruroidea

Ceylonocotyle streptocoelium

Common name: Rumen fluke

Synonym: *Paramphistomum streptocoelium*

Predilection site: Rumen

Parasite class: Trematoda

Superfamily: Paramphistomatidae

Definitive hosts: Cattle, sheep, goat and wild ruminants

Geographical distribution: Africa

For more details see Chapter 2 (Cattle).

ABOMASUM

A number of ostertagian parasites are found in the abomasa of various deer hosts. The identification of individual species is beyond the scope of this book and interested readers will need to consult a relevant taxonomic specialist. There are several species of cattle or sheep nematodes, which are described in more detail under the chapters for these hosts (Table 8.1). There have been no specific studies on the pathogenesis of abomasal parasites in deer. Worm burdens in deer are generally light with lesions in the abomasum resembling those of ostertagiosis in cattle. Clinical disease is uncommon in free-ranging deer and occurs uncommonly in captive animals. For most anthelmintics, the dose rate in deer is that recommended for cattle or higher. Both benzimidazoles and macrocyclic lactones have been shown to be effective against gastrointestinal nematodes in deer.

Spiculopteragia asymmetrica

Predilection site: Abomasum

Parasite class: Nematoda

Table 8.1 Cattle and sheep nematodes found in the abomasum of deer.

Species	(Super)family	Hosts	Geographical distribution
Ostertagia ostertagi	Trichostrongyloidea	Cattle, roe deer (*Capreolus capreolus*)	Worldwide
Teladorsagia circumcincta	Trichostrongyloidea	Cattle, sheep, goat, deer, camel, llama	Worldwide
Haemonchus contortus	Trichostrongyloidea	Sheep, goat, cattle, deer, camel, llama	Worldwide
Trichostrongylus axei	Trichostrongyloidea	Cattle, sheep, goat, deer, horse, donkey, pig and occasionally man	Worldwide
Parabronema skrjabini	Spiruroidea	Sheep, goat, cattle, camel	Central and east Africa, Asia, and some Mediterranean countries, notably Cyprus

Superfamily: Trichostrongyloidea

Hosts: Fallow deer (*Dama dama*), roe deer (*Capreolus capreolus*)

Spiculopteragia spiculoptera

Synonym: *Ostertagia spiculoptera*, *Spiculopteragia bohmi*

Predilection site: Abomasum

Parasite class: Nematoda

Superfamily: Trichostrongyloidea

Hosts: Red deer (*Cervus elaphus*)

Apteragia quadrispiculata

Predilection site: Abomasum

Parasite class: Nematoda

Superfamily: Trichostrongyloidea

Hosts: Roe deer (*Capreolus capreolus*), red deer (*Cervus elaphus*), sika deer (*Cervus nippon*), fallow deer (*Dama dama*), moose (*Alces alces*), reindeer (*Rangifer tarandus*)

Rinadia mathevossiani

Predilection site: Abomasum

Parasite class: Nematoda

Superfamily: Trichostrongyloidea

Hosts: Red deer (*Cervus elaphus*), roe deer (*Capreolus capreolus*), sika deer (*Cervus nippon*), fallow deer (*Dama dama*), moose (*Alces alces*), reindeer (*Rangifer tarandus*)

Ostertagia leptospicularis

Synonym: *Skrjabinagia kolchida*, *Grosspiculagia podjapolskyi*, *Ostertagia crimensis*

Predilection site: Abomasum

Parasite class: Nematoda

Superfamily: Trichostrongyloidea

Hosts: Fallow deer (*Dama dama*), roe deer (*Capreolus capreolus*), red deer (*Cervus elaphus*), sika deer (*Cervus nippon*), moose (*Alces alces*), reindeer (*Rangifer tarandus*), cattle, sheep, goat, camel

Notes: Considered to be a polymorphic species with two male morphs, *Ostertagia leptospicularis* and *Skrjabinagia kolchida* (*Grosspiculagia podjapolskyi*).

This species is described in more detail in Chapter 2 (Cattle).

SMALL INTESTINE

A number of intestinal species have been reported in deer (Table 8.2) but are generally of little clinical significance. The majority of these are parasites of cattle or sheep and are described in more detail under the chapters for these hosts.

A range of protozoa similar to those present in other ruminants is found in the intestine of deer. A number of *Eimeria* species have been reported in several species of deer but their significance is not known (Table 8.3).

Table 8.2 Intestinal helminths in deer.

Species	(Super)family	Hosts	Geographical distribution
Small intestine			
Trichostrongylus vitrinus	Trichostrongyloidea	Sheep, goat, deer and occasionally pig and man	Mainly temperate regions of the world
Trichostrongylus longispicularis	Trichostrongyloidea	Cattle, sheep, goat, deer, camel, llama	Ruminants in Australia; and cattle in America and parts of Europe
Nematodirus spathiger	Trichostrongyloidea	Sheep, goat, occasionally cattle and other ruminants	Cosmopolitan, but more prevalent in temperate zones
Nematodirus filicollis	Trichostrongyloidea	Sheep, goat, occasionally cattle and deer	Cosmopolitan, but more prevalent in temperate zones
Cooperia curticei	Trichostrongyloidea	Sheep, goat, deer	Worldwide
Cooperia onchophora	Trichostrongyloidea	Cattle, sheep, goat, deer	Worldwide
Cooperia punctata	Trichostrongyloidea	Cattle, deer	Worldwide
Cooperia pectinata	Trichostrongyloidea	Cattle, deer	Worldwide
Bunostomum trigonocephalum	Ancylostomatoidea	Sheep, goat, camel, deer	Worldwide
Capillaria bovis Syn: *C. brevipes*	Trichuroidea	Cattle, Sheep, goat, deer	Worldwide
Moniezia benedeni	Anoplocephalidae	Cattle, red deer, roe deer, camel. Intermediate hosts: forage mites	Worldwide
Large intestine			
Oesophagostomum venulosum	Strongyloidea	Sheep, goat, deer, camel	Worldwide
Oesophagostomum columbianum	Strongyloidea	Sheep, goat, deer, camel	Worldwide; more important in tropical and subtropical areas
Chabertia ovina	Strongyloidea	Sheep, goat occasionally deer, cattle and other ruminants	Worldwide but more prevalent in temperate regions
Trichuris ovis	Trichuroidea	Sheep, goats, occasionally cattle and other ruminants	Worldwide
Trichuris globulosa	Trichuroidea	Cattle, occasionally sheep, goats, camels and other ruminants	Worldwide
Trichuris capreoli	Trichuroidea	Deer	?

PARASITES OF THE RESPIRATORY SYSTEM

Cephenemyia trompe

Common name: Reindeer throat bot

Predilection site: Nasopharynx

Parasite class: Insecta

Family: Oestridae

Description, gross: The adult is bee-like in appearance, 14–16 mm in length and covered in long, yellowish and black hairs overlying a shining black body. Developing larvae are white, while fully developed larvae are about 25–40 mm long and yellow–brown. The entire larval body is covered by bands of short spines on both sides and narrows posteriorly.

Hosts: Reindeer, deer, moose and caribou

Table 8.3 *Eimeria* spp of deer.

Roe deer (*Capreolus capreolus*)	Red deer/wapiti (*Cervus elaphus*)	Reindeer (*Rangifer tarandus*)
Eimeria capreoli	*Eimeria asymmetrica*	*Eimeria arctica*
Eimeria catubrina	*Eimeria austriaca*	*Eimeria mayeri*
Eimeria panda	*Eimeria cervi*	*Eimeria tarandi*
Eimeria patavina	*Eimeria elaphi*	
Eimeria ponderosa	*Eimeria robusta*	
Eimeria rotunda	*Eimeria sordida*	
Eimeria superba	*Eimeria wapiti*	

Life cycle: The adult flies are active from June to September and, like *Oestrus*, the females are viviparous. The fly hovers close to the animal, then darts in and ejects larvae in fluid into the nostrils of the host animal. The larvae migrate to the retropharyngeal pouches. There they become attached in clusters and develop. Further development occurs in the nasopharynx, as the larvae migrate to and crowd in the retropharangeal pouches that lie on either side of the throat at the base of the tongue. Fully developed, third-stage larvae, which may be 40 mm in length, crawl to the anterior nasal passages and are sneezed out. Pupation occurs on the ground under surface debris. The pupation period is about 4 weeks. The adult flies have no mouthparts for feeding so they are short-lived and mate shortly after emerging.

Geographical distribution: Throughout the northern holarctic region including Europe and North America

Pathogenesis: Although the larvae occasionally cause death from suffocation, their general effect is loss of condition. The adult flies cause disturbance and avoidance responses, which reduce feeding and result in loss of condition. In summer, keratitis and blindness may occur in reindeer if larvae are deposited in the eye.

Clinical signs: There are few external signs of the presence of deer nose bots, although there may be some nasal discharge. Occasionally, heavy infections may cause death by suffocation. Behaviour such as snorting and lowering or shaking of the head may indicate the migration of mature larvae within the nasal passages or oviposition activity of the adult fly.

Diagnosis: Occasionally a larva may be found on the ground after a severe sneezing attack, but often a positive diagnosis can only be made at necropsy.

Pathology: The retropharyngeal pouch may be enlarged and the epithelium of the pouch may be pitted or eroded and become partly detached, necrotic and oedematous in infected deer.

Epidemiology: *C. trompe* is considered to be a serious problem in domestic reindeer management in Scandinavia. It is estimated that in Sweden the losses due to *C. trompe* and the warble fly *Oedemagena tarandi* equate to approximately 15% of the income from reindeer production.

Treatment: Nose bots are generally well tolerated in wild hosts and treatment is not usually required.

Dictyocaulus viviparus

Predilection site: Bronchi, trachea

Parasite class: Nematoda

Superfamily: Trichostrongyloidea

Description, gross: The adults are slender thread-like worms; males measure around 4.0–5.5 cm and females 6–8 cm in length.

Description, microscopic: The buccal ring is triangular in shape. First-stage larvae are 300–360 μm with the intestinal cells containing numerous chromatin granules.

Hosts: Cattle, buffalo, deer (red deer) and camel

Geographical distribution: Worldwide, but especially important in temperate climates with a high rainfall

Table 8.4 Other species of bot flies (family: Oestridae).

Genus	Species	Host(s)	Region
Pharyngomyia	*picta*	Red deer (*Cervus elaphus*); sika deer (*Cervus nippon*); fallow deer (*Dama dama*); roe deer (*Capreolus capreolus*)	Europe, central Asia
Cephenemyia	*auribarbis*	Red deer (*Cervus elaphus*); fallow deer (*Dama dama*); mule deer, white-tailed deer (*Odocoileus* spp)	Europe, North America
	jellisoni	Moose (Alces alces); elk (*Cervus elaphus*);	North America
	stimulator	Roe deer (*Capreolus capreolus*)	Eurasia

Life cycle: The life cycle is as described under cattle. The prepatent period in red deer is 20–24 days and larvae are excreted for approximately 25 days.

Geographical distribution: Worldwide

Pathogenesis: Larval migration produces only a mild inflammatory response in the lungs. Thus, larger numbers of immature worms reach the pulmonary bronchi and heavy burdens of mature worms are well tolerated.

Clinical signs: In contrast with *D. viviparus* infection in cattle, coughing is not a common sign of affected red deer. Clinical signs commonly associated with lungworm infection are loss of condition, dull coat as well as inappetence, reduced weight gains, fever, increased tachycardia and tachypnoea, dyspnoea and death in severe cases.

Diagnosis: Presumptive diagnosis of infection can be made on clinical signs if young susceptible deer develop respiratory problems or inappetence. On postmortem examination, the diagnosis is confirmed by finding large numbers of lungworms and mucus in pulmonary airways and pneumonic changes in the lungs. Mature *D. viviparus* infection can be detected by recovery of first-stage larvae from faecal samples by the Baermann technique (see Chapter 15).

Pathology: Gross pathological changes in lungs are consolidation of the dorsal portion of the diaphragmatic lobes, excess mucus and lungworms in the trachea, bronchi and bronchioles, and enlarged bronchial lymph nodes. Death results from asphyxiation due to obstruction of the trachea and bronchi with adult lungworms and mucus.

Epidemiology: Clinical disease is more prevalent in autumn in deer calves kept under intensive conditions.

Treatment: Benzimidazole anthelmintics and macrocylic lactones are generally effective at increased dose rates.

Control: The importance and widespread occurrence of *D. viviparus* infection in farmed red deer has prompted a number of recommendations for its control. Clinical disease is exacerbated by stressors such as malnutrition and transport and often associated with high stocking densities. These conditions should be avoided as should grazing on pasture where cattle have grazed. Any introduced deer should be treated on arrival and then 3 and 6 weeks later. Live lungworm vaccine has been used as a preventative.

Dictyocaulus eckerti

Synonym: *Dictyocaulus noerneri*

Predilection site: Bronchi, trachea

Parasite class: Nematoda

Superfamily: Trichostrongyloidea

Hosts: Roe deer (*Capreolus capreolus*), fallow deer (*Dama dama*) and various other deer

Description, gross: Similar to *D. viviparus*

Description, microscopic: The buccal ring is kidney-shaped.

Geographical distribution: Worldwide, but especially important in temperate climates with high rainfall.

The following metastrongylid parasites have been reported in the lungs of various deer hosts. Control is impractical and rarely, if ever, indicated. For more details of these species see Chapter 3 (Sheep and goats).

Protostrongylus rufescens

Common name: Small lungworm

Predilection site: Small bronchioles

Parasite class: Nematoda

Superfamily: Metastrongyloidea

Definitive hosts: Sheep, goat, deer and wild small ruminants

Intermediate hosts: Snails (*Helicella*, *Theba*, *Abida*, *Zebrina*, *Arianta*)

Muellerius capillaris

Common name: Nodular lungworms

Predilection site: Lung

Parasite class: Nematoda

Superfamily: Metastrongyloidea

Definitive hosts: Sheep, goat, deer and wild small ruminants

Intermediate hosts: Snails (*Helix*, *Succinea*) and slugs (*Limax*, *Agriolimax*, *Arion*)

Cystocaulus ocreatus

Common name: Small lungworm

Predilection site: Lung

Parasite class: Nematoda

Superfamily: Metastrongyloidea

Definitive hosts: Sheep, goat, deer and wild small ruminants

Intermediate hosts: Snails (*Helicella*, *Helix*, *Theba*, *Cepaea*, *Monacha*)

Geographical distribution: Worldwide

Varestrongylus sagittatus

Synonym: *Bicaulus sagittatus*

Common name: Small lungworm

Predilection site: Lung

Parasite class: Nematoda

Superfamily: Metastrongyloidea

Description: Adult worms are slender, small worms, 1.4–3.4 cm long.

Final hosts: Red deer (*Cervus elaphus*), fallow deer (*Dama dama*)

Intermediate hosts: Slugs and snails

Life cycle: Ingested third-stage larvae present within the intermediate host, migrate through the intestinal wall to the lymph nodes, migrating via the lymph and blood to the lungs. They then form 'breeding clusters' in which they grow to sexual maturity. Female worms are ovoviviparous with first-stage larvae coughed up and swallowed. When ingested by a molluscan intermediate host the larvae develop to infective L_3 in 3–4 weeks

Geographical distribution: Europe

Pathogenesis and clinical signs: Infection can cause pulmonary oedema, emphysema and inflammation of the lungs. Secondary bacterial infection can lead to pneumonia, emaciation and death.

Diagnosis: *Varestrongylus* first-stage larvae have a dorsal, posteriorly directed spine.

Treatment: Treatment with fenbendazole or mebendazole given over 3–5 days has been reported to be effective.

Varestrongylus capreoli

Synonym: *Capreocaulus capreoli*

Predilection site: Lung

Parasite class: Nematoda

Superfamily: Metastrongyloidea

Final hosts: Roe deer (*Capreolus capreolus*)

All other details similar to *V. sagittatus*.

Echinococcus granulosus

See Parasites of the liver.

PARASITES OF THE LIVER

Fascioloides magna

Common name: Large American liver fluke

Predilection site: Liver and bile ducts

Parasite class: Trematoda

Family: Fasciolidae

Description, gross: Flukes are large and thick and measure up to 10 × 2.5 cm. The flukes are oval, with a rounded posterior end. They possess no anterior cone and when fresh are flesh-coloured (Fig. 8.1).

Description, microscopic: Eggs are large, operculate, measure 109–168 × 75–96 μm and have a protoplasmic appendage at the pole opposite the operculum.

Final hosts: Deer, cattle, sheep, goat, pig, horse

Intermediate hosts: A variety of freshwater snails, *Fossaria* spp, *Lymnaea* spp, *Stagnicola* spp

Life cycle: The life cycle is similar to that of *F. hepatica*. The eggs hatch to miracidia after 4 weeks or longer. Development in the snail takes 7–8 weeks. The prepatent period in deer is around 30 weeks.

Geographical distribution: Mainly occurs in North America, central, eastern and southwestern Europe, South Africa and Mexico

Pathogenesis: In deer (and cattle), the flukes are frequently encapsulated in thin-walled fibrous cysts in the liver parenchyma and this restricted migration results in low pathogenicity.

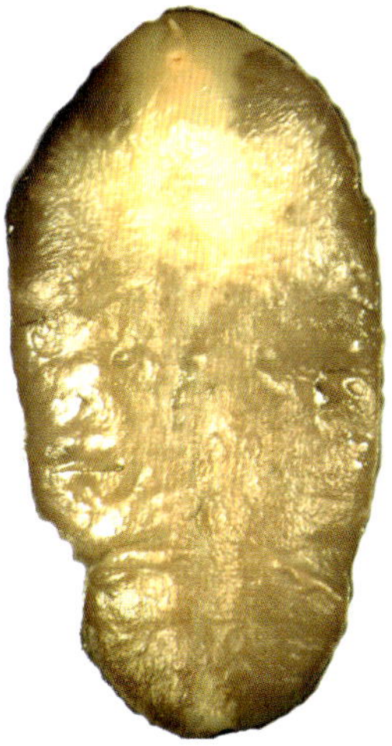

Fig. 8.1 *Fascioloides magna.*

Clinical signs: In deer and cattle the parasites can cause hepatic damage on reaching the liver but the flukes rapidly become encapsulated by the host reaction and clinical signs are minimal.

Diagnosis: This is based primarily on clinical signs. The presence of cysts and the large flukes are usually seen on postmortem examination. Faecal examination for the presence of fluke eggs is a useful aid to diagnosis.

Pathology: In deer, encapsulated thin-walled fibrous cysts are found in the liver parenchyma.

Epidemiology: The various snail intermediate hosts tend to occur in stagnant semi-permanent water that contains large amounts of dead or dying vegetation, swamp areas, or pools and streams. *F. magna* is indigenous to North America and is common in Canada and the Great Lake areas where the white-tailed deer and the elk are commonly infected.

Treatment: For cattle and sheep the commonly used flukicides such as triclabendazole, closantel, clorsulon and albendazole are effective. Mature *F. magna* are susceptible to oxyclosanide.

Control: Elimination of the snail intermediate hosts is difficult due to their varied habitats.

Notes: *F. magna* is primarily a parasite of deer (Cervidae) and is commonly found in white-tailed deer, elk and moose.

Fasciola hepatica

Common name: Liver fluke

Predilection site: Liver

Parasite class: Trematoda

Family: Fasciolidae

Definitive hosts: Sheep, cattle, goat, horse, deer, man and other mammals

Dicrocoelium dendriticum

Synonym: *Dicrocoelium lanceolatum*

Common name: Small lanceolate fluke

Predilection site: Liver

Parasite class: Trematoda

Family: Dicrocoeliidae

Final hosts: Sheep, goats, cattle, deer and rabbits, occasionally in the horse and pig

Intermediate hosts: Two are required. 1. Land snails of many genera, principally *Cionella lubrica* in N. America and *Zebrina detrita* in Europe. Some 29 other species have been reported to serve as first intermediate hosts of the genera *Abida*, *Theba*, *Helicella* and *Xerophila*. 2. Brown ants of the genus *Formica*, frequently *F. fusca*

Geographical distribution: Worldwide except for South Africa and Australia. In Europe the prevalence is high but in the British Isles prevalence is low, being confined to small foci throughout the country.

Dicrocoelium hospes

Predilection site: Liver

Parasite class: Trematoda

Family: Dicrocoeliidae

Hosts: Cattle and deer

Geographical distribution: Parts of Africa

Notes: Details are essentially similar to *D. dendriticum*

Stilesia hepatica

Predilection site: Bile ducts

Parasite class: Cestoda

Family: Thysanosomidae

Final hosts: Sheep, deer and other ruminants

Intermediate hosts: The intermediate host is probably an oribatid mite

Geographical distribution: Africa and Asia

Taenia hydatigena

Synonym: *Taenia marginata*, *Cysticercus tenuicollis*

Predilection site: Abdominal cavity, liver (intermediate hosts); small intestine (definitive hosts)

Parasite class: Cestoda

Family: Taeniidae

Final hosts: Dog, fox, weasel, stoat, polecat, wolf, hyena

Intermediate hosts: Sheep, cattle, deer, pig, horse

Echinococcus granulosus

Common name: Dwarf dog tapeworm, hydatidosis

Predilection site: Mainly liver and lungs (intermediate hosts); small intestine (definitive host)

Parasite class: Cestoda

Family: Taeniidae

Description: Hydatid cysts are large fluid-filled vesicles, 5–10 cm in diameter, with a thick concentrically laminated cuticle and an internal germinal layer.

Final hosts: Dog and many wild canids

Intermediate hosts: Domestic and wild ruminants, deer, man and primates, pig and lagomorphs; horses and donkeys are resistant

Geographical distribution: Worldwide

For more details of these species see Chapter 3 (Sheep and goats).

PARASITES OF THE CIRCULATORY SYSTEM

Babesia bovis

Synonym: *Babesia argentina*

Predilection site: Blood

Parasite class: Sporozoasida

Family: Babesiidae

Hosts: Cattle, buffalo, deer

Geographical distribution: Australia, Africa, Central and South America, Asia and southern Europe

For more details see Chapter 2 (Cattle).

Theileria cervi

Synonym: *Theileria tarandi*

Predilection site: Blood, lymph nodes

Parasite class: Sporozoasida

Family: Theileriidae

Hosts: Fallow deer, red deer, sika deer, white-tailed deer, reindeer

Notes: Little information is available on this species

Anaplasma marginale

Predilection site: Blood

Order: Rickettsiales

Family: Anaplasmataceae

Hosts: Cattle, sheep, goat, deer, camel, wild ruminants

Geographical distribution: Africa, southern Europe, Australia, South America, Asia, former Soviet States and USA

Anaplasma centrale

Predilection site: Blood

Order: Rickettsiales

Family: Anaplasmataceae

Hosts: Cattle, deer, wild ruminants, and perhaps sheep, may act as reservoirs of infection

Geographical distribution: Africa, southern Europe, Australia, South America, Asia, former Soviet States and USA

For more details of these species see Chapter 2 (Cattle).

PARASITES OF THE NERVOUS SYSTEM

Elaphostrongylus cervi

Synonym: *Elaphostrongylus rangiferi*

Predilection site: Connective tissue, CNS

Parasite class: Nematoda

Superfamily: Metastrongyloidea

Description, gross: The mature worms are long and slender. Males are up to 40 mm long; and females up to 60 mm long.

Description, microscopic: First-stage larvae have a dorsal spine on the tail.

Final hosts: Red deer (*Cervus elaphus*), roe deer (*Capreolus capreolus*), sika deer (*Cervus nippon*)

Intermediate hosts: Various land and freshwater snails and slugs

Life cycle: Female worms lay eggs that either hatch *in situ* or are carried to the lungs via the boodstream and then hatch. Larvae migrate through the lungs to the airways and are then swallowed and pass out in the faeces. The larvae may survive in the environment for up to 2 years before infecting a molluscan intermediate host. The parasites develop through the second-stage larvae to the infective, third-stage larvae in the mollusc within 27–50 days and can retain their infectivity for up to another 2 years. Deer become infected when they ingest snails containing infective larvae. After ingestion, the larvae burrow through the gut wall and migrate to the final tissue site, at the same time developing into adult worms. The prepatent period is about 112 days.

Geographical distribution: *E. cervi* is present in most countries of northern and central Europe and the CIS States. It is also present in New Zealand.

Pathogenesis: The severity of clinical disease is very much influenced by the level of infection and location in the body. Light infections are usually subclinical. Three clinical syndromes are described:

- Acute disease characterised by hindlimb paralysis and perhaps blindness resulting from damage to the central nervous system.
- Chronic ill-thrift, resulting from connective tissue damage.
- Verminous pneumonia, resulting from larval migration.

Additionally, there may be economic losses through trimming, downgrading or condemnation of carcases.

Clinical signs: Most infections are inapparent. Clinical signs include exercise intolerance, hindlimb incoordination and nervous disorders.

Diagnosis: Diagnosis is based on finding the infective larvae in faeces using the Baermann method. The first-stage larvae have a characteristic dorsal spine on their tails and look very like the protostrongylid larvae of *Muellerius* spp that infest sheep.

Pathology: Connective tissue lesions are most likely to be found in the muscles of the neck, shoulders, flanks and loins. These consist of green discoloration of fascial sheets, and chronic granulomata with encapsulated, degenerated worms. Similar lesions may he seen in regional lymph nodes. Worms associated with central nervous system lesions are most likely to be seen in the subdural and subarachnoid spaces. Pulmonary lesions consist of a diffuse interstitial pneumonia with focal emphysema and consolidation.

Epidemiology: This parasite affects a number of deer species and the prevalence of infection is generally high in both wild and farmed deer.

Treatment and control: Fenbendazole given on 3 consecutive days has been reported to be effective. Control is difficult given the ubiquitous nature of the intermediate hosts.

Notes: The nomenclature of this parasite remains controversial.

Parelaphostrongylus tenuis

Synonym: *Odocoileostrongylus tenuis*, *Elaphostrongylus tenuis*

Common names: Cerebrospinal nematodiosis, meningeal worm, moose sickness, moose disease

Predilection site: Veins and venous sinuses of cranial meninges, CNS

Parasite class: Nematoda

Superfamily: Metastrongyloidea

Description, gross: The mature worms are long and thread-like; males are up to 40 mm and females up to about 90 mm.

Description, microscopic: First-stage larvae have a dorsal spine on the tail.

Final hosts: White-tailed deer (*Odocoileus virginianus*), moose (*Alces alces*), wapiti (*Cervus canadensis*), other deer species, llama, guanaco, alpaca

Intermediate hosts: Snails and slugs

Life cycle: Unembryonated eggs are released into the bloodstream and travel to the lungs where they lodge in the capillaries and complete their development to L_1 before moving to the alveoli from where they are coughed up and swallowed and passed in the faeces. To develop further they must penetrate or be eaten by a slug or snail. In the foot of the snail the larvae develop through the second-stage larvae to the infective, third-stage larvae. Deer become infected when they accidentally ingest slugs or snails containing infective larvae. After ingestion, the larvae burrow through the gut wall and migrate to the CNS via the spinal nerves and spinal cord, at the same time developing into adult worms. The prepatent period is about 82–137 days.

Pathogenesis: In the white-tailed deer the parasite causes little clinical effect but in other cervids and camelids can cause debilitating neurological signs and in North America is the causative agent of 'moose sickness'. Llamas and their relatives are susceptible to *P. tenuis*.

Clinical signs: Signs of infection are rare in white-tailed deer. Infected moose may show swaying, paraparesis, torticollis, circling, blindness, ataxia, paresis, difficulty in standing, weight loss and death. In red deer (wapiti), there is progressive neurological disease and death.

Diagnosis: Diagnosis is based on finding adult worms in the CNS.

Epidemiology: *P. tenuis* is a common parasite of white-tailed deer in North America. Infection occurs in moose that share the same range as white-tailed deer.

Treatment and control: Not practical. Strict management of national and international deer translocations should be practised wherever possible.

PARASITES OF THE REPRODUCTIVE/ UROGENITAL SYSTEM

No parasites of veterinary significance reported.

PARASITES OF THE LOCOMOTORY SYSTEM

Taenia cervi

Synonym: *Cysticercus cervi*, *Taenia krabbei*, *Cysticercus tarandi*

Predilection site: Small intestine (definitive host); muscle (intermediate host)

Parasite class: Cestoda

Family: Taeniidae

Final hosts: Wolf, red fox, artic fox

Intermediate hosts: Red deer (*Cervus elaphus*), roe deer (*Capreolus capreolus*), reindeer (*Rangifer tarandus*)

Life cycle: Wild canids are infested by consuming the cysticercus in the intermediate host. The intermediate host is infected through the ingestion of tapeworm eggs that hatch in the intestine.

Geographical distribution: Worldwide

Pathogenesis: Cysticerci may cause economic loss through condemnation at meat inspection.

Clinical signs: Adult tapeworms are considered to be of little pathogenic importance. Infected intermediate hosts do not usually show clinical signs of disease.

Diagnosis: Diagnosis is through the identification of cysts at postmortem.

Pathology: The mature, ovoid white cysticerci are grossly visible in the muscle, heart, lung, liver and brain.

Epidemiology: Deer are infected by grazing pasture and forages contaminated with carnivore faeces harbouring taenid eggs.

Treatment and control: Control is not practical.

Notes: The correct nomenclature for the intermediate host stage is the 'metacestode stage of *Taenia cervi*' rather than '*Cysticercus cervi*'. It is unclear whether *Taenia krabbei* found mainly in reindeer is synonymous with *T. cervi*, which is found mainly in red deer and roe deer, and that they are one and the same species present in different hosts.

Several species of *Sarcocystis* have been reported in deer (Table 8.5). Specific details are beyond the scope of this book.

PARASITES OF THE CONNECTIVE TISSUE

Elaeophora schneideri

Common name: Filarial dermatosis, 'sore head'

Predilection site: Blood vessels

Parasite class: Nematoda

Superfamily: Filarioidea

Definitive hosts: Sheep, goat, deer (elk, moose, mule deer)
For more details see Chapter 3 (Sheep and goats).

Hypoderma diana

Common name: Warble fly

Predilection site: Subcutaneous skin

Parasite class: Insecta

Family: Oestridae

Description, adults: Adult female *Hypoderma diana* are about 15 mm in length and bee-like in appearance; the abdomen is covered with yellow–orange hairs with a broad band of black hairs around the middle. The adults have no functioning mouthparts.

Description, larvae: The mature larvae are thick and somewhat barrel-shaped, tapering anteriorly. When mature they are 25–30 mm in length and most segments bear short spines. Larvae are dirty white in colour when newly emerged from the host, but rapidly turn dark brown. The pupa is almost black. The larvae are relatively host specific and live as subcutaneous parasites of deer.

Hosts: Deer

Life cycle: Females emerge with all their eggs fully developed. They have a relatively short lifespan in which they do not feed, and are able to mate and oviposit soon after emergence. Mating takes place off the host at aggregation points where females are intercepted in flight. The female lays between 300–600 eggs on the lower regions of the legs and lower body of the host animal, where they are glued to the hairs.

The first-stage larvae are less than 1 mm in length, hatch within a week and crawl down the hairs, either burrowing directly into the skin or into the hair follicles. The larvae then continue to burrow beneath the skin. *Hypoderma diana* migrates below the skin along nerves to the spinal cord. After about 4 months, usually by autumn, larvae reach the epidural fat of the spine in the region of the thoracic and lumbar vertebrae, where they overwinter. Next spring, migration is resumed until, about 9 months after oviposition, the larvae reach the skin of the back. A characteristic small swelling (the 'warble') is formed and a small hole is cut to the surface. A cystic nodule then begins to form around each larva. The larva reverses its position and rests with its two posterior spiracles close to the opening in the warble, allowing the larva to breathe. In this location the larva moults twice, during which time it grows rapidly, more than doubling in length.

Table 8.5 *Sarcocystis* species found in deer.

Species	Deer host(s)	Final hosts	Distribution
Sarcocystis cervicanis	Red deer (*Cervus elaphus*)	Dog	Europe
Sarcocystis grueneri	Red deer (*Cervus elaphus*), reindeer (*Rangifer tarandus*)	Dog, fox (*Vulpes vulpes*), coyote (*Canis latrans*)	Eurasia
Sarcocystis wapiti	Red deer (*Cervus elaphus*), roe deer (*Capreolus capreolus*)	Dog, coyote (*Canis latrans*)	North America
Sarcocystis sybillensis	Red deer (*Cervus elaphus*), roe deer (*Capreolus capreolus*)	Dog	North America
Sarcocystis hofmani	Red deer (*Cervus elaphus*), roe deer (*Capreolus capreolus*), fallow deer (*Dama dama*), sika deer (*Cervus nippon*)	Dog, raccoon dog (*Nyctereutes procyanoides*)	Eurasia
Sarcocystis capreolicanis	Roe deer (*Capreolus capreolus*)	Dog, fox (*Vulpes vulpes*)	Europe
Sarcocystis gracilis	Roe deer (*Capreolus capreolus*)	Dog, fox (*Vulpes vulpes*)	Eurasia
Sarcocystis rangi	Reindeer (*Rangifer tarandus*)	Dog	Europe
Sarcocystis tarandivulpis	Reindeer (*Rangifer tarandus*)	Dog, fox (*Vulpes vulpes*), raccoon dog (*Nyctereutes procyanoides*)	Europe
Sarcocystis tarandi	Reindeer (*Rangifer tarandus*)	Unknown	Europe
Sarcocystis rangiferi	Reindeer (*Rangifer tarandus*)	Unknown	Europe
Sarcocystis alceslatranis	Moose (*Alces alces*)	Dog, coyote (*Canis latrans*)	North America Europe
Sarcocystis jorrini	Fallow deer (*Dama dama*)		Europe

Larval migration and growth take place in the host until April. The larvae then drop off the host animal and pupate in soil. The fly emerges after approximately 36 days. The duration of pupation depends on ambient temperature and ground cover; higher pupal survival occurs when there is at least some grass cover and where the ground does not freeze.

Geographical distribution: Northern hemisphere

Pathogenesis: The fly is most active in May and June, but it is not recognised as a cause of 'gadding' in deer. The mature larvae occur subcutaneously along the back, and hide damage occurs with linear perforations.

Clinical signs: Except for poor growth in severe cases, the hosts show no symptoms until the larvae appear along the back, when the swellings can be seen and felt. The larval migration is not usually noticed clinically, but heavy infestations may reduce growth. Occasionally the pressure of larvae on the spinal cord can cause paralysis. When the larvae reach the skin on the animal's back, large, soft, painful swellings of up to 3 mm diameter develop. The larvae lie in cysts containing yellow purulent fluid.

Diagnosis: The presence of the larvae under the skin of the back of deer allows diagnosis of warble flies. The eggs may also be found on the hairs of the animals in the summer.

Pathology: Warble larvae induce a pronounced tissue inflammation. The cellular reacton is predominantly eosinophilic and lymphocytic. The presence of the larvae also induces the production of a thickened connective-tissue lined cavity, surrounding the larva, filled with with inflammatory cells, particularly eosinophils.

Epidemiology: *Hypoderma diana* is present in a great variety of habitats, overlapping the territory of its hosts. It is spread throughout Europe and Asia, from 30° to 60° north, living in several different ecological zones, such as mixed, deciduous and coniferous forests, wooded steppes and wetlands. The adult fly is most active in May and June, particularly on warm, sunny days. The main factors influencing the flight and oviposition of female flies are ambient air temperature and light, as a result of which they are most active at midday. As in other species, the extent of parasitism and prevalence are higher in younger animals, possibly due to a measure of resistance in adults built up through repeated contact with the parasite. The degree of parasitism in male deer is usually higher than in females and castrated animals.

Treatment: Like other species, *Hypoderma diana* is highly susceptible to systemically active organophosphorus insecticides and to the macrocyclic lactones ivermectin, doramectin, eprinomectin and moxidectin.

Control: For farm-raised deer a control programme may be implemented, with regular treatment timed in relation to the local population dynamics of *Hypoderma*. Animals may be given some protection by being herded into corrals, shelters or shaded areas to reduce the risk of infestation when adult flies are active.

It is more difficult to develop effective control measures for diseases in wild and semi-wild deer. Here it is important that any attempted parasite controls do not have an effect on the environment in which the animals live. For free-range deer that cannot be captured, food may be supplemented with oral forms of antiparasitic preparations. However, care must be taken in selecting a suitable food medium for the antiparasitic agent, since it cannot be freely distributed around the environment because it may be eaten by other animals; neither can the volume ingested be controlled.

Notes: With the success of control measures against warbles in cattle it is important to realise that *H. diana*, although capable of infecting many species of deer, will not infect cattle. As a consequence of this, even in areas where (as is commonly the case) almost all the deer carry the parasitic larvae, cattle are not at risk.

Hypoderma tarandi

Synonym: *Oedemagena tarandi*

Common name: Reindeer warble

Predilection site: Subcutaneous connective tissue

Parasite class: Insecta

Family: Oestridae

Description: Large, hairy flies with reddish yellow hairy abdomens. Mature, third-stage larvae are approximately 25 mm in length.

Hosts: Reindeer, musk ox and caribou

Life cycle: The life cycle of *Hypoderma tarandi* resembles that of other species in the genus *Hypoderma*. They are active in July and August, each female laying between 500 and 700 eggs, which are attached to the downy undercoat rather than the outer hair. The flanks, legs, and rump are preferential laying sites. After approximately 6 days the egg hatches on the skin, and the larva then burrows into and under the skin. Unlike other *Hypoderma*, however, the L_1 migrates directly to the back in the subcutaneous connective tissue via the spine. When the larva comes to rest in about September to October, a swelling (warble) is created around it where it feeds on the animal's blood and body fluids. The L_3 makes a cutaneous perforation and the larvae breathe by applying their spiracles to the aperture. When growth is completed in the spring, the larva leaves the reindeer through its air hole and drops to the ground to pupate. It then emerges as an adult fly, completing the cycle.

Geographical distribution: Circum-arctic and subarctic regions of Europe, Asiatic Russia and America

Pathogenesis: The adult flies cause gadding, and the newly hatched larvae may cause dermatitis with local oedema when they penetrate the skin. The main importance of this genus, however, is economic, from damage to hides by the L_3. In Sweden this loss can amount to a fifth of the total income from reindeer herds. Up to two hundred holes may be found in typically infested reindeer skins in Russia.

Clinical signs: Except for poor growth in severe cases, the hosts show no symptoms until the larvae appear along the back, when the swellings can be seen and felt. The larval migration is not usually noticed clinically, but heavy infestations may reduce growth. Occasionally the pressure of larvae on the spinal cord can cause paralysis. When the larvae reach the skin on the animal's back, large, soft, painful swellings may be observed. The larvae lie in cysts containing yellow purulent fluid. Attacks by warble flies laying eggs can cause irritation to reindeer. Host animals may injure themselves as a result.

Diagnosis: The presence of the larvae under the skin of the back allows diagnosis of warble flies. The eggs may also be found on the hairs of the animals in the summer.

Pathology: Warble larvae induce a pronounced tissue inflammation. The cellular reacton is predominantly eosinophilic and lymphocytic. The presence of the larvae also induces the production of a thickened connective tissue lined cavity surrounding the larva, filled with with inflammatory cells, particularly eosinophils.

Epidemiology: Fawns and yearlings are most affected by this parasite, which produces large oedematous swellings. These swellings may suppurate and attract blowflies, which then oviposit in the wound.

Treatment: Injectable ivermectin, doramectin, eprinomectin or moxidectin administered between November and January is extremely effective in eliminating these parasites.

Control: In control schemes a single annual treatment in autumn is usually recommended before the larvae have reached the back and perforated the hide.

Notes: Limited geographical distribution but of local veterinary importance

PARASITES OF THE INTEGUMENT

Besnoitia tarandi

Predilection site: Skin, conjunctiva

Order: Sporozoasida

Family: Sarcocystiidae

Intermediate hosts: Reindeer, caribou

Final host: Unknown

ECTOPARASITES

LICE

Lice infestations are frequently encountered in deer. It is beyond the scope of this book to provide detailed descriptions of all the species of lice that may be encountered on deer throughout the world. Some of the more common species that may be encountered are provided in Table 8.6.

Treatments with insecticides, such as carbaryl, cypermethrin, deltamethrin, diazinon, lindane, and malathion, are usually effective in controlling lice on deer. Insecticidal dust bags or 'back rubbers' can be used as self-dosing rubbing stations for deer, and other ungulates. Because louse populations on most temperate ungulates increase during the cooler months, insecticides should ideally be administered to them in the autumn/winter months. Avermectins are generally less effective against chewing lice but may be effective against sucking lice. Animals destined to be introduced into established herds should be quarantined and where necessary treated.

MITES

Sarcoptes scabiei

Predilection site: Skin

Parasite class: Arachnida

Sub-class: Acari

Order: Acariformes

Sub-order: Sarcoptiformes (Astigmata)

Family: Sarcoptidae

Hosts: Red deer, roe deer, moose, reindeer

For more details see Chapter 5 (Pigs).

Table 8.6 Lice on deer.

Lice	Family	Host(s)	Region
Bovicola longicornis	Trichodectidae	Red deer (*Cervus elaphus*)	Europe
Solenopotes burmeisteri	Linognathidae	Red deer (*Cervus elaphus*)	Eurasia
Solenopotes ferrisi	Linognathidae	Elk (*Cervus elaphus*)	North America
Bovicola tibialis	Trichodectidae	Fallow deer (*Dama dama*)	Europe
Bovicola meyeri	Trichodectidae	Roe deer (*Capreolus capreolus*)	Eurasia
Solenopotes capreoli	Linognathidae	Roe deer (*Capreolus capreolus*)	Eurasia
Bovicola maai	Trichodectidae	Sika deer (*Cervus nippon*)	Eurasia
Solenopotes burmeisteri	Linognathidae	Sika deer (*Cervus nippon*)	Eurasia
Bovicola forficula	Trichodectidae	Muntjac (*Muntiacus muntjak*)	Asia
Tricholipeurus indicus	Trichodectidae	Muntjac (*Muntiacus muntjak*)	Asia
Solenopotes muntiacus	Linognathidae	Muntjac (*Muntiacus muntjak*)	South Asia
Solenopotes tarandi	Linognathidae	Reindeer, caribou (*Rangifer tarandus*)	Eurasia, North America
Solenopotes binipilosus	Linognathidae	White-tailed deer, black-tailed deer, mule deer (*Odocoileus* spp)	North, Central and South America

A number of non-obligate ectoparasites are found on deer and these are listed in the host–parasite checklist at the end of this chapter. More detailed descriptions of these parasites are found in Chapter 11 (Facultative ectoparasites and arthropod vectors).

CAMELS

PARASITES OF THE DIGESTIVE SYSTEM

Gongylonema pulchrum

Common name: Gullet worm

Predilection site: Oesophagus, rumen

Parasite class: Nematoda

Superfamily: Spiruroidea

Final host: Sheep, goat, cattle, pig, buffalo, horse, donkey, deer, camel, man

Intermediate host: Coprophagous beetles, cockroaches

Geographical distribution: Probably worldwide

For more details see Chapter 3 (Sheep and goats).

Gongylonema verrucosum

Common name: Rumen gullet worm

Predilection site: Rumen, reticulum, omasum

Parasite class: Nematoda

Superfamily: Spiruroidea

Final host: Cattle, sheep, goat, deer, camel

Intermediate hosts: Coprophagous beetles and cockroaches

For more details see Chapter 3 (Sheep and goats).

Studies on the helminth parasites of camels are few, and published information consists mainly of case reports and lists of reported helminths. Many of the species reported are accidental infections with parasite species of domestic ruminants and their significance and pathogenicity are generally not known. The most important species, against which treatment is targeted, is the camel stomach worm *Haemonchus longistipes*. This nematode, either alone or in mixed infections with *Trichostrongylus* spp, may cause a debilitating and sometimes fatal condition. Limited information is available on the efficacy of anthelmintics against gastrointestinal nematodes in camels. Benzimidazoles and ivermectin given at cattle dose rates have reported efficacy against a number of gastrointestinal nematode species found in camels. Ivermectin has been reported as less effective against *Nematodirus* and *Trichuris* spp.

Monthly treatments of young animals during the rainy season can help reduce parasitic burdens. Removal of faeces around watering points and keeping these areas dry can also reduce numbers of infective larvae.

ABOMASUM

Haemonchus longistipes

Common name: Camel stomach worm

Predilection site: Abomasum

Parasite class: Nematoda

Superfamily: Trichostrongyloidea

Description, gross: Relatively small worms; males are 10–20 mm and females 18–30 mm.

Description, microscopic: Females have a reduced knob-like vulval flap (c.f. *H. contortus* which has a well developed linguiform vulvar flap).

Hosts: Camel

Life cycle: As for *H. contortus* in cattle and sheep

Geographical distribution: Africa, Middle East

Pathogenesis and clinical signs: *H. longistipes* worms are voracious blood-suckers producing symptoms similar to *H. contortus* in domestic ruminants. Infection has been reported to cause anaemia, oedema, emaciation and death.

Epidemiology: The epidemiology is similar to that reported with haemonchosis in domestic ruminants. The prevalence of this parasite varies from region to region and from season to season in the same region. Higher prevalence rates have been reported during the rainy season with a drop in prevalence during the dry season.

Camelostrongylus mentulatus

Predilection site: Abomasum, small intestine

Parasite class: Nematoda

Superfamily: Trichostrongyloidea

Description, gross: *C. mentulatus* is similar in size to *Ostertagia ostertagi*. Males are 6.5–7.5 mm long and females are 8–10 mm long.

Description, microscopic: The bursa possesses two large lateral lobes and the spicules are narrow, long, denticulated and of equal length. Eggs measure about 80 × 45 μm.

Hosts: Camel, llama, sheep, goat

Geographical distribution: Common in the Middle East and Australia; South America

Pathogenesis: Generally of low pathogenicity and considered of little importance.

Pathology: Heavy infections can produce a gastric hyperplasia and increase in abomasal pH, similar to that seen in *Ostertagia* infection.

Impalaia tuberculata

Predilection site: Abomasum

Parasite class: Nematoda

Superfamily: Trichostrongyloidea

Description, gross: Males are 7–9 mm and females 14–18 mm long.

Description, microscopic: The cervical cuticle is studded with papillae. Eggs measure about 60 × 32 μm.

Hosts: Wild ruminants, camel

Geographical distribution: India

Impalaia nudicollis

Predilection site: Abomasum

Parasite class: Nematoda

Superfamily: Trichostrongyloidea

Description, gross: Males are 7.5–8.2 mm and females 14.8–16.7 mm long.

Description, microscopic: Males have long spicules and a long gubernaculum. Eggs measure about 60 × 32 μm.

Hosts: Wild ruminants, camel

Geographical distribution: Africa, India

Other parasites of cattle or sheep and wild ruminants have been reported in the abomasum of camels (Table 8.7). More details of these species are found in Chapters 2 and 3.

Species of nematodes and cestodes reported in the small intestines of camels are generally of little clinical significance and only brief details are listed below. Cattle or sheep parasites found in the small intestine are listed in Table 8.8, and those of the large intestine are given in Table 8.9. Further details of these parasites can be found in Chapters 2 and 3. A more detailed list of helminth species found in camels is provided in the parasite checklist at the end of the chapter.

SMALL INTESTINE

Nematodirus mauritanicus

Predilection site: Small intestine

Parasite class: Nematoda

Superfamily: Trichostrongyloidea

Table 8.7 Cattle and sheep parasites found in the abomasum of camels.

Species	(Super)family	Hosts	Geographical distribution
Teladorsagia circumcincta	Trichostrongyloidea	Cattle, sheep, goat, deer, camel, llama	Worldwide
Ostertagia leptospicularis	Trichostrongyloidea	Deer (roe deer), cattle, sheep, goat, camel	Many parts of the world, particularly Europe and New Zealand
Haemonchus contortus	Trichostrongyloidea	Sheep, goat, cattle, deer, camel, llama	Worldwide
Marshallagia marshalli	Trichostrongyloidea	Sheep, goats, camel and wild small ruminants	Tropics and subtropics including southern Europe, USA, South America, India and Russia
Trichostrongylus axei	Trichostrongyloidea	Cattle, sheep, goat, deer, horse, donkey, pig, camel and occasionally man	Worldwide
Parabronema skrjabini	Spiruroidea	Sheep, goat, cattle, camel	Central and east Africa, Asia, and some Mediterranean countries, notably Cyprus

Table 8.8 Cattle and sheep parasites found in the small intestine of camels.

Species	(Super)family	Hosts	Geographical distribution
Nematodes			
Trichostrongylus longispicularis	Trichostrongyloidea	Cattle, sheep, goat, deer, camel, llama	Ruminants in Australia; and cattle in America and parts of Europe
Trichostrongylus vitrinus	Trichostrongyloidea	Sheep, goat, deer, camel, occasionally pig and man	Mainly temperate regions of the world
Trichostrongylus colubriformis	Trichostrongyloidea	Sheep, goat, cattle, camel and occasionally pig and man	Worldwide
Trichostrongylus probolorus	Trichostrongyloidea	Sheep, camel, man	?
Nematodirus spathiger	Trichostrongyloidea	Sheep, goat, occasionally cattle and other ruminants	Cosmopolitan, but more prevalent in temperate zones
Nematodirus helvetianus	Trichostrongyloidea	Cattle, occasionally sheep, goat and other ruminants, camel	
Nematodirus abnormalis	Trichostrongyloidea	Sheep, goat, camel	Europe, Asia, North America, Australia and Russia
Cooperia oncophora	Trichostrongyloidea	Cattle, sheep, goat, deer, camel	Worldwide
Cooperia surnabada (syn *C. mcmasteri*)	Trichostrongyloidea	Cattle, sheep, camel	Parts of Europe, North America and Australia
Bunostomum trigonocephalum	Ancylostomatoidea	Sheep, goat, camel	Worldwide
Strongyloides papillosus	Rhabditoidea	Sheep, cattle, other ruminants, camel and rabbits	Worldwide
Cestodes			
Moniezia benedeni	Anoplocephalidae	Cattle, red deer, roe deer, camel Intermediate hosts: forage mites	Worldwide
Moniezia expansa	Anoplocephalidae	Sheep, goats, camel, occasionally cattle Intermediate hosts: forage mites	Worldwide
Thysaniezia ovilla (syn *T. giardia*)	Thysanosomidae	Cattle, sheep, goat, camel and wild ruminants Intermediate hosts: Oribatid mites and psocids	Southern Africa
Avitellina centripunctata	Thysanosomidae	Sheep and other ruminants, camel Intermediate hosts: oribatid mites or psocid lice	Europe, Africa and Asia. Widespread in camels in Asia and Africa
Stilesia globipunctata	Thysanosomidae	Sheep, cattle and other ruminants, camel Intermediate hosts: oribatid mites or psocid lice	Southern Europe, Africa and Asia

Description, gross: Females are 21–24 mm and males 13–15 mm long.

Description, microscopic: Male spicules are joined for part of their length with the tips enclosed in a thin lanceolate membrane.

Hosts: Camel

Nematodirella dromedarii

Predilection site: Small intestine

Parasite class: Nematoda

Superfamily: Trichostrongyloidea

Table 8.9 Cattle and sheep parasites found in the large intestine of camels.

Species	(Super)family	Hosts	Geographical distribution
Oesophagostomum virginimembrum syn *Oe. venulosum*	Strongyloidea	Sheep, goat, deer, camel	Worldwide
Oesophagostomum columbianum	Strongyloidea	Sheep, goat, deer, camel	Worldwide; more important in tropical and subtropical areas
Chabertia ovina	Strongyloidea	Sheep, goat, camel, occasionally deer, cattle and other ruminants	Worldwide but more prevalent in temperate regions
Trichuris ovis	Trichuroidea	Sheep, goat, camel, occasionally cattle and other ruminants	Worldwide
Trichuris globulosa	Trichuroidea	Cattle, occasionally sheep, goat, camel and other ruminants	Worldwide

Description, gross: The anterior of the worm is narrow and is similar to *Nematodirus*. Males are 10–15 mm, and females 10–29 mm long.

Description, microscopic: The very long spicules can measure up to half the body length and are equal in size (Fig. 8.2). Eggs are large, measuring about 250 × 125 μm.

Hosts: Dromedary camel

Life cycle: This is thought to be similar to that of *Nematodirus* spp (not *N. battus*).

Geographical distribution: Presumed throughout the host range of Asia and north Africa

Nematodirella cameli

Predilection site: Small intestine

Parasite class: Nematoda

Superfamily: Trichostrongyloidea

Hosts: Camel, reindeer

Geographical distribution: Russia and CIS countries

Avitellina woodlandi

Predilection site: Small intestine

Parasite class: Cestoda

Family: Thysanosomidae

Hosts: Camel

Intermediate hosts: Thought to be oribatid mites

Notes: This parasite has only been described from dromedaries in Africa

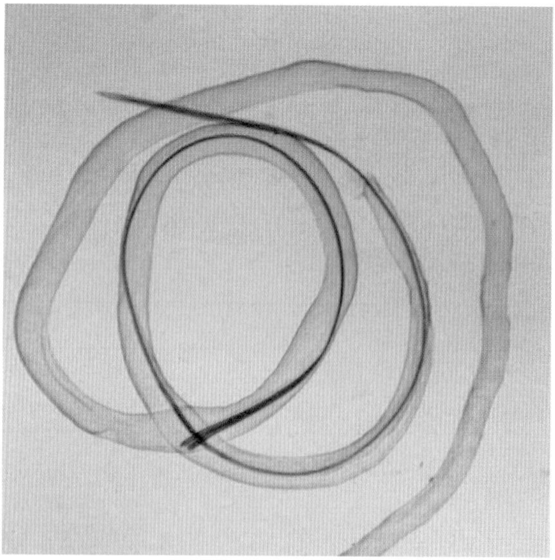

Fig. 8.2 *Nematodirella dromedarii* showing the very long male spicules.

Stilesia vittata

Predilection site: Small intestine

Parasite class: Cestoda

Family: Thysanosomidae

Description, gross: 18–23 cm long

Description, microscopic: The scolex is 0.5–0.6 mm in size; mature proglottids contain 10–14 testicles.

Hosts: Camel

Eimeria bactriani

Synonym: *Eimeria nolleri*

Predilection site: Small intestine

Parasite class: Sporozoasida

Family: Eimeriidae

Host: Camel (Bactrian, dromedary)

Description: The oocysts are spherical to ellipsoidal, pale yellow–brown, smooth, 21–34 × 20–28 μm with a micropyle but without micropylar cap and oocyst residuum. Sporocysts are spherical or elongate, 8–9 × 6–9 μm with a residuum. Meronts in the small intestine are 16 × 10 μm and contain 20–24 merozoites; mature microgamonts are 25 × 20 μm.

Life cycle: The life cycle is typically coccidian with endogenous stages found in the small intestine, although the number of merogony stages is unknown. Sporulation time is 9–15 days.

Geographical distribution: Germany, CIS (Russia and former Soviet States)

Pathogenesis and clinical signs: Not reported

Diagnosis: Diagnosis is based on clinical signs and the demonstration of oocysts in diarrhoeic faeces.

Epidemiology: Unknown

Treatment and control: Little is known about treatment, but by analogy with other hosts, one of the sulphonamide drugs should be tried if disease is suspected. Prevention is based on good management, avoidance of overcrowding and stress, and attention to hygiene, particularly watering areas, which should be protected from faecal contamination.

Notes: There is controversy regarding the specific name of this coccidium. In some texts it is referred to as *E. nolleri*.

Eimeria cameli

Predilection site: Small and large intestine

Parasite class: Sporozoasida

Family: Eimeriidae

Host: Camel (Bactrian, dromedary)

Description: The oocysts are large, pyriform, 80–100 × 55–94 μm with a rough brown wall, with a micropyle, with or without a micropylar cap, and without an oocyst residuum. Sporocysts are elongate or ellipsoidal, pointed at both ends, 30–50 × 14–20 μm without a Stieda body, but with a residuum. Sporozoites are comma-shaped, lie lengthwise head to tail in the sporocyst, and have a clear globule at the large end. Giant meronts in the small intestine are up to 350 μm and contain many merozoites.

Life cycle: Giant meronts are found in the small intestine and gamonts are found in the ileum and occasionally the caecum. Sporulation time is 9–15 days.

Geographical distribution: Worldwide

Pathogenesis and clinical signs: Infections can produce severe enteritis leading to progressive weight loss and emaciation. Watery diarrhoea, sometimes containing blood, has been found in heavy infections. Diarrhoea and secondary bacterial infections may aggravate the condition leading to death in young camels.

Pathology: Presence of the parasite may cause inflammatory lesions in the small intestine and giant meronts may be visible with the naked eye. Cystic structures containing oocysts may be seen in the mucosa on histopathology.

Epidemiology: Young camels are much more susceptible to infection.

Treatment and control: As for *E. bactriani*

Notes: This is the most frequently encountered *Eimeria* species in camels in north Africa.

Eimeria dromedarii

Predilection site: Small intestine

Parasite class: Sporozoasida

Family: Eimeriidae

Host: Camel (Bactrian, dromedary)

Description: The oocysts are ovoid, 23–33 × 20–25 μm with a brown wall, with a micropylar cap, but without a polar granule or oocyst residuum (Fig. 8.3). Sporocysts are ovoid or spherical, 8–11 × 6–9 μm without a Stieda body, or residuum. Sporozoites are comma-shaped, with one to two clear globules.

Life cycle: Giant meronts are found in the small intestine and gamonts are found in the ileum and occasionally the caecum. Sporulation time is 15–17 days.

Geographical distribution: Worldwide

Pathogenesis and clinical signs: As for *E. cameli*

Notes: This species is found frequently, often together with *E. cameli*.

Eimeria pellerdyi

Predilection site: Unknown

Parasite class: Sporozoasida

Family: Eimeriidae

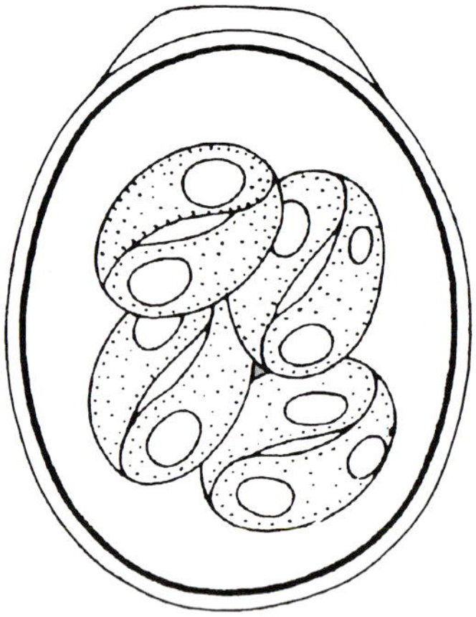

Fig. 8.3 Oocyst of *Eimeria dromedarii*.

Host: Camel (Bactrian)

Description: The oocysts are ovoid or ellipsoidal, smooth, colourless, 22–24 × 12–14 μm without a micropyle, polar granule or oocyst residuum. Sporocysts are ovoid, 9–11 × 4–6 μm with a small Stieda body and a residuum. Sporozoites are club-shaped, 8–10 × 1–3 μm with a clear globule at the large end.

Life cycle: Unknown

Geographical distribution: Unknown

Pathogenesis and clinical signs: Unknown

Eimeria rajasthani

Predilection site: Unknown

Parasite class: Sporozoasida

Family: Eimeriidae

Host: Camel (dromedary)

Description: The oocysts are ellipsoidal, light yellowish green, 34–39 × 25–27 μm with a micropylar cap, but without a polar granule, or oocyst residuum. Sporocysts are ovoid, 14–15 × 8–11 μm with a Stieda body and a residuum. Sporozoites are elongate, 10–14 × 3–4 μm with two or more clear globules.

Life cycle: Unknown

Geographical distribution: Unknown

Pathogenesis and clinical signs: Unknown

Isospora orlovi

Predilection site: Unknown

Parasite class: Sporozoasida

Family: Eimeriidae

Host: Camel

Description: Oocysts contain two sporocysts each with four sporozoites. The oocysts are ellipsoidal, oval, cylindrical or figure-of-eight-shaped, smooth, 27–35 × 15–20 μm without a polar granule, micropyle or residuum. Sporocysts are ellipsoidal, ovoid (15–20 × 13–17 μm) or spherical (13–15 μm diameter) without a Stieda body, but with a residuum.

Life cycle: Unknown

Geographical distribution: Russia, former Soviet States

Pathogenesis and clinical signs: Unknown

Notes: Another species, *Isospora cameli*, has been reported in India. It is not clear if these species are valid.

Cryptosporidium parvum

Predilection site: Small intestine

Parasite class: Sporozoasida

Family: Cryptosporidiidae

For more details see Chapter 2 (Cattle).

LARGE INTESTINE

Buxtonella sulcata

Predilection site: Large intestine

Parasite class: Ciliophora

Family: Pycnotrichidae

Description: The body is ovoid, 100 × 72 μm, and uniformly ciliated with a prominent curved groove bordered by two ridges running from end to end with a cyathostome at the anterior end, and an oval or bean-shaped macronucleus, 28 × 14 μm in size.

Geographical distribution: Worldwide

PARASITES OF THE RESPIRATORY SYSTEM

Cephalopina titillator

Synonym: *Cephalopsis titillator*

Common name: Camel nasal bot fly

Predilection site: Nasal cavity

Parasite class: Insecta

Family: Oestridae

Description, adult: The adult fly measures 8–10 mm in length. It is relatively robust and has a powdery grey appearance. The head is large, orange above and yellow below. The eyes are broadly separated, especially in the female. The thorax is reddish brown, with a black pattern. The abdomen has irregular black blotches and white hairs. The legs are yellow.

Description, larvae: The first-stage larvae are about 0.7 mm in length and have long spines on the lateral edges of the segments. L_2 are about 15 mm in length and the L_3 25–35 mm in length, the latter being characterised by smooth fleshy lobes on each segment and large mouth-hooks.

Hosts: Camels

Life cycle: Eggs are laid around the nasal area. Larvae hatch and migrate into the nasal cavity, frontal sinus and pharynx of their host, where they spend several months feeding and moulting. When mature, the larvae make their way back to the nose, considerably irritating the camel in the process. As a result they are sneezed out on to the ground, and from here the larvae burrow into the ground and pupate. Pupation takes about 25 days.

Geographical distribution: Occurs over entire range of both species of camels: sub-Saharan Africa, Middle East, Australia and Asia.

Pathogenesis: The larvae irritate and damage the mucosa. Camels snort, sneeze and are restless, and may even stop feeding, especially during the emergence of mature larvae from the nostrils. When large numbers of larvae are present the animals' breathing and working capacity may be severely impaired. Unlike many oestrids, adult *Cephalopina* do not panic the animals, and large numbers are often seen resting on the head and around the nostrils.

Clinical signs: Snorting, sneezing, increased grooming, nasal discharge, bleeding from the nostrils, coughing and reduced milk production and body weight.

Diagnosis: The adult flies may be visible and recognisable on the host. The eggs are also easily identifiable on the host. Larvae present in the pharynx may be seen on direct inspection.

Pathology: The larval phase usually occupies about 11 months, and is associated with inflammation, sometimes purulent, of the nasopharyngeal mucosa.

Epidemiology: Infestation of up to 90% of camel herds has been recorded.

Treatment: Macrocyclic lactones, rafoxanide, trichlorphon and nitroxynil have all been reported to be effective against the larvae of *Cephalopina titillator*.

Control: The most effective means of control of this parasite is to remove the eggs from the host's coat. This requires, where possible, daily examination of the animal, paying particular attention to the area around the nostrils.

Oestrus ovis

Common name: Sheep nasal bot

Predilection site: Nasal passages

Parasite class: Insecta

Family: Oestridae

Hosts: Primarily sheep and goat, but also ibex, camel and humans

For more details see Chapter 3 (Sheep and goats).

Dictyocaulus filaria

Predilection site: Lungs

Parasite class: Nematoda

Superfamily: Trichostrongyloidea

Hosts: Sheep, goat, camel and a few wild ruminants

Geographical distribution: Worldwide

Pathogenesis and clinical signs: Severe infections cause depression, coughing, dyspnoea and loss of condition.

Epidemiology: *D. filaria* is found in the respiratory tract of camels in Africa.

Treatment and control: Benzimidazoles, levamisole and avermectins are all reported to be effective against this species in camels.

For more details see Chapter 3 (Sheep and goats).

Dictyocaulus viviparus

Synonym: *Dictyocaulus cameli*

Predilection site: Lungs

Parasite class: Nematoda

Superfamily: Trichostrongyloidea

Hosts: Cattle, deer, camel

Geographical distribution: Worldwide

Pathogenesis and clinical signs: As for *D. filaria*

For more details see Chapter 2 (Cattle).

Echinococcus granulosus

See Parasites of the liver.

PARASITES OF THE LIVER

Fasciola hepatica

Common name: Liver fluke

Predilection site: Liver

Parasite class: Trematoda

Family: Fasciolidae

Definitive hosts: Sheep, cattle, goat, horse, deer, man and other mammals

For more details see Chapter 3 (Sheep and goats).

Echinococcus granulosus

Predilection site: Mainly liver and lungs (intermediate hosts)

Parasite class: Cestoda

Family: Taeniidae

Definitive hosts: Dog and many wild canids

Intermediate hosts: Domestic and wild ruminants, man and primates, pig and lagomorphs

For more details see Chapter 3 (Sheep and goats).

Fasciola gigantica

Common name: Tropical large liver fluke

Predilection site: Liver

Parasite class: Trematoda

Family: Fasciolidae

Final hosts: Cattle, buffalo, sheep, goat, pig, camel, deer, man

For more details see Chapter 2 (Cattle).

PARASITES OF THE PANCREAS

Eurytrema pancreaticum

Common name: Pancreatic fluke

Predilection site: Pancreatic ducts

Parasite class: Trematoda

Family: Dicrocoeliidae

For more details see Chapter 3 (Sheep and goats).

PARASITES OF THE CIRCULATORY SYSTEM

Dipetalonema evansi

Synonym: *Deraiophoronema evansi*

Common name: Subcutaneous filaroidosis

Predilection site: Heart, arteries and veins, pulmonary arteries, spermatic arteries, lymph nodes

Parasite class: Nematoda

Superfamily: Filarioidea

Description, gross: Fairly large filarial worms; adult male worms are 8–11 cm; adult females are 14.5–18.5 cm.

Description, microscopic: Microfilariae are ensheathed, 200–315 μm in length and found in the peripheral blood.

Final host: Camel

Intermediate hosts: Mosquitoes of the genus *Aedes*

Life cycle: The life cycle has not been described in detail but *Aedes* mosquitoes are thought to act as intermediate hosts. Following ingestion of a blood meal the microfilariae develop to infective larvae in the intermediate host. Larvae pass to the host when the intermediate host next feeds.

Geographical distribution: North Africa, Asia, eastern Russia, Australia

Pathogenesis: Light infections are inapparent. Heavy infections can cause emaciation, arteriosclerosis and heart insufficiency and parasitic orchitis in the spermatic vessels.

Clinical signs: Emaciation, lethargy, orchitis

Diagnosis: Filarial nematodes within arteries cannot be detected clinically. The identification of the microfilariae in the blood (samples ideally taken in the early evening) is aided by concentrating the parasites following lysis, filtration and then staining with methylene blue or May–Grunwald Giemsa. Alternatively, one part of blood and nine parts of formalin are centrifuged and the sediment mixed with a blue stain and examined as a microscopic smear.

Pathology: The presence of the parasites in an artery or vein leads to inflammation of the vessel wall and thrombosis may occur. Fibrosis leads to a granulomatous arteritis or phlebitis, and possible occlusion of the vessel lumen. Aneurysms may occur in the spermatic vessels.

Epidemiology: Infection is presumably common in areas where the parasite and intermediate hosts co-exist.

In the eastern former Soviet States infection may occur in up to 80% of camels.

Treatment: Stibophen, at 0.5 mg/kg i.v., is effective both therapeutically and prophylactically as a prevention during the periods of mosquito activity.

Control: Mosquito control methods, such as the use of insect repellents, may limit exposure. Stibophen used prophylactically as described above may help limit infection. Ivermectin at 200 µg/kg can be used to eliminate microfilariae.

Schistosoma bovis

Common name: Blood fluke, bilharziosis

Predilection site: Portal and mesenteric veins, urogenital veins

Parasite class: Trematoda

Family: Schistosomatidae

Final hosts: Cattle, sheep, goat, camel (dromedary)

Intermediate hosts: Snails (*Bulinus contortus*, *B. truncates*, *Physopsis africana*, *P. nasuta*)

Geographical distribution: Africa, Middle East, southern Asia, southern Europe

Schistosoma mattheei

Predilection site: Portal, mesenteric and bladder veins

Parasite class: Trematoda

Family: Schistosomatidae

Final hosts: Cattle, sheep, goat, camel, man

Intermediate hosts: Snails (*Bulinus*)

Geographical distribution: South and central Africa, Middle East

Notes: Thought to be synonymous with *S. bovis* but differs on morphological and pathological grounds and is restricted to the alimentary canal.

Trypanosoma brucei brucei

Subgenus: *Trypanozoon*

Common name: Nagana

Predilection site: Blood. *T. brucei bucei* is also found extravascularly in, for example, the myocardium, CNS and reproductive tract.

Parasite class: Zoomastigophorasida

Family: Trypanosomatidae

Hosts: Cattle, horse, donkey, zebu, sheep, goat, camel, pig, dog, cat, wild game species, particularly antelope

Geographical distribution: Approximately 10 million square kilometres of sub-Saharan Africa between latitudes 14°N and 29°S

Treatment: The two drugs in common use in camels are diaminazine aceturate and suramin. Treatment should be followed by surveillance since reinfection, followed by clinical signs and parasitaemia, may occur within a week or two.

Notes: Antelope are the natural host species and are reservoirs of infection for domestic animals. Horses, mules and donkeys are very susceptible, and the disease is very severe in sheep, goats, camels and dogs (see respective hosts).

For more details see Chapter 2 (Cattle).

Trypanosoma brucei evansi

Subgenus: *Trypanozoon*

Synonym: *Trypanosoma evansi*, *T. equinum*

Common name: Surra, el debab, mbori, murrina, mal de caderas, doukane, dioufar, thaga

Predilection site: Blood

Parasite class: Zoomastigophorasida

Family: Trypanosomatidae

Hosts: Horse, donkey, camel, cattle, zebu, goat, pig, dog, water buffalo, elephant, capybara, tapir, mongoose, ocelot, deer and other wild animals. Many laboratory and wild animals can be infected experimentally.

Geographical distribution: North Africa, Central and South America, central and southern Russia, parts of Asia (India, Burma, Malaysia, southern China, Indonesia, Phillipines)

Treatment and control: Suramin or quinapyramine (Trypacide) are the drugs of choice for treatment and also confer a short period of prophylaxis. For more prolonged protection a modified quinapyramine known as 'Trypacide Pro-Salt' is also available. Unfortunately, drug resistance, at least to suramin, is not uncommon. Currently in camels, isometamidium is administered intravenously because of local tissue reactions.

Notes: The original distribution of this parasite coincided with that of the camel, and is often associated with arid desserts and semiarid steppes.

For more details see Chapter 4 (Horses).

Trypanosoma congolense

Subspecies: *congolense*

Subgenus: *Nannomonas*

Common name: Nagana, paranagana, Gambia fever, ghindi, gobial

Predilection site: Blood

Parasite class: Zoomastigophorasida

Family: Trypanosomatidae

Hosts: Cattle, sheep, goat, horse, camel, dog, pig. Reservoir hosts include antelope, giraffe, zebra, elephant and warthog.

Geographical distribution: Widely distributed in tropical Africa between latitudes 15°N and 25°S.

Pathogenesis: With *T. congolense*, there are many strains, which differ markedly in virulence. The signs caused by this species are similar to those caused by other trypanosomes, but the central nervous system is not affected.

Treatment and control: Isometidium is the drug of choice but is administered intravenously because of local tissue reactions. Diaminazine is contraindicated in the camel.

For more details see Chapter 2 (Cattle).

Trypanosoma vivax

Subspecies: *vivax*

Subgenus: *Duttonella*

Common name: Nagana, souma

Predilection site: Blood

Parasite class: Zoomastigophorasida

Family: Trypanosomatidae

Hosts: Cattle, sheep, goat, camel, horse, antelope and giraffe are reservoirs

Geographical distribution: Central Africa, West Indies, Central and South America (Brazil, Venezuela, Bolivia, Columbia, Guyana, French Guyana), Mauritius.

For more details see Chapter 2 (Cattle).

Theileria camelensis

Predilection site: Blood, lymph nodes

Parasite class: Sporozoasida

Family: Theileriidae

Description: Trophozoite forms in the erythrocyte are predominantly round.

Hosts: Camel

Life cycle: Not described although probably similar to *Theileria* spp in cattle and sheep.

Geographical distribution: North Africa

Pathogenesis and clinical signs: Non-pathogenic

Diagnosis: Presence of erythrocytic forms in blood smears.

Pathology: No associated pathology

Epidemiology: Transmitted by *Hyalomma dromedarii.*

Treatment and control: Not required

Notes: The validity of this species is questionable

Theileria dromederi

Predilection site: Blood, lymph nodes

Parasite class: Sporozoasida

Family: Theileriidae

Description: Trophozoite forms in the erythrocyte are predominantly round.

Hosts: Camel

Anaplasma marginale

Predilection site: Blood

Order: Rickettsiales

Family: Anaplasmataceae

Hosts: Cattle, sheep, goat, camel, wild ruminants

Geographical distribution: Africa, southern Europe, Australia, South America, Asia, former Soviet states and USA

For more details see Chapter 2 (Cattle).

Anaplasma centrale

Predilection site: Blood

Order: Rickettsiales

Family: Anaplasmataceae

Hosts: Cattle, wild ruminants, and perhaps sheep, may act as reservoirs of infection.

Geographical distribution: Africa, southern Europe, Australia, South America, Asia, former Soviet states and USA

For more details see Chapter 2 (Cattle).

PARASITES OF THE NERVOUS SYSTEM

Thelazia leesi

Common name: Eyeworm

Predilection site: Conjunctival sac

Parasite class: Nematoda

Superfamily: Spiruroidea

Final host: Camel

Intermediate host: Muscid flies

Geographical distribution: Africa, Asia, Russia

Pathogenesis and clinical signs: Heavy infections may cause irritation and keratitis with epiphora

Thelazia rhodesi

Common name: Cattle eyeworm

Predilection site: Eye, conjunctival sac, lachrymal duct

Parasite class: Nematoda

Superfamily: Spiruroidea

Final host: Cattle, buffalo, occasionally sheep, goat, camel

Intermediate host: Muscid flies, particularly *Fannia* spp

For more details see Chapter 2 (Cattle).

PARASITES OF THE LOCOMOTORY SYSTEM

Taenia hyaenae

Synonym: *Cysticercus dromedarii*, *Cysticercus cameli*

Common name: Cysticercosis

Predilection site: Muscle, liver and other organs

Parasite class: Cestoda

Family: Taeniidae

Description, gross: Cysts are 12–18 mm in length.

Description, microscopic: The cysticercus of *T. hyaenae* has an armed protoscolex with a double row of hooks.

Definitive host: Hyena

Intermediate hosts: Camel, cattle, goat, rarely sheep and various antelopes

Life cycle: Eggs passed by hyenas are ingested by the intermediate hosts in which the oncospheres migrate to the muscles via the blood before developing to infective cycticerci.

Geographical distribution: Tropical Africa

Pathogenesis and clinical signs: Infection is usually asymptomatic.

Sarcocystis cameli

Predilection site: Muscle

Order: Sporozoasida

Family: Sarcocystiidae

Description: In the camel, the tissue cysts are compartmented up to 12 mm long with striated walls and are found in oesophageal, skeletal and cardiac muscle.

Intermediate hosts: Camel (Bactrian and dromedary)

Final host: Dog

Life cycle: Infection in the camel is by ingestion of sporocysts in dog faeces. Complete details of the merogony phase of development are not known.

Geographical distribution: North Africa (Egypt, Morocco, Sudan), Asia

Pathogenesis and clinical signs: The pathogenic significance is unknown. The parasite is widespread within its endemic range with a high percentage of camels found to be infected at slaughter. Myocardial lesions and emaciation have both been attributed to infection.

Diagnosis: Antemortem diagnosis is difficult and most cases of *Sarcocystis* infection are only revealed at postmortem when the grossly visible sarcocysts in the muscle are discovered.

Pathology: The tissue cysts may be visible to the naked eye but are more likely to be detected on histopathology.

Epidemiology: Little is known of the epidemiology, but, from the high prevalence of symptomless infections observed in abattoirs, it is clear that where dogs are kept in close association with camels or their feed, then transmission is likely.

Treatment and control: Treatment is not usually indicated. The only control measures possible are those of simple hygiene. Dogs should not be fed raw or uncooked camel meat.

Sarcocystis ippeni

Predilection site: Muscle

Order: Sporozoasida

Family: Sarcocystiidae

Intermediate hosts: Camel (dromedary)

Final host: Unknown

Toxoplasma gondii

Predilection site: Muscle, lung, liver, reproductive system, central nervous system

Order: Sporozoasida

Family: Sarcocystiidae

For more details see Chapter 5 (Pig).

PARASITES OF THE CONNECTIVE TISSUE

Three species of filarial worms have been reported in camel causing skin nodules, 0.5–4 cm in diameter, on various parts of the body. The intermediate hosts are various species of biting flies.

Elaeophora schneideri

Common name: Filarial dermatosis, 'sore head'

Predilection site: Blood vessels

Parasite class: Nematoda

Superfamily: Filarioidea

Definitive hosts: Sheep, goat, deer, camel (elk, moose, mule deer)

For more details see Chapter 3 (Sheep and goats).

Onchocerca fasciata

Predilection site: Connective tissue, ligamentum nuchae

Parasite class: Nematoda

Superfamily: Filarioidea

Final host: Camel

Geographical distribution: Africa

Onchocerca gutturosa

Predilection site: Connective tissue, ligamentum nuchae

Parasite class: Nematoda

Superfamily: Filarioidea

Final host: Cattle, camel

ECTOPARASITES

Microthoracius cameli

Common name: Camel sucking louse

Predilection site: Skin

Parasite class: Insecta

Family: Microthoraciidae

Description: *Microthoracius cameli* have a very characteristic elongated, spindle-shaped head, which is almost as long as its swollen, rounded abdomen (Fig. 8.5). The entire body is 1–2 mm in length.

Hosts: Camel

Life cycle: The life cycle is typical, with eggs giving rise to three nymphal stages followed by the reproductive adult. However, little precise detail is known.

Geographical distribution: Worldwide, in association with its host

Pathogenesis: These lice are blood-feeders and heavy infestations can significantly reduce weight gain and milk production.

Clinical signs: The signs of infestation are variable. Light infestation may have no obvious effects, but pruritis, dermatitis and hair loss are usually evident at heavier parasite loads.

Diagnosis: The lice and their eggs can be seen on the skin of the host animal when the hair is parted.

Epidemiology: Infection occurs after direct contact with an infested host animal. Cross-contamination between different host species is possible if the animals have physical contact.

Treatment and control: Macrocyclic lactones, such as moxidectin, in a repeated treatment programme of 7–10 days may be effective.

Notes: Microthoraciidae contains four species in the genus *Microthoracius*. Three species parasitise llamas. The fourth species *Microthoracius cameli* is parasitic on camels. The closely related *Microthoracius mazzai* is an economically important parasite of alpacas (see later).

Hippobosca camelina

Common name: Camel fly

Predilection site: Skin

Parasite class: Insect

Family: Hippoboscidae

Description: Adult flies are approximately 10 mm in length and are generally pale reddish brown with yellow spots on the indistinctly segmented abdomen. They have one pair of wings, the veins of which are crowded together towards the anterior margin. Both sexes of adult are blood feeders. The mature larvae are rarely seen and measure about 5 mm in length.

Hosts: Camels

Life cycle: Gravid female flies mature a single larvae within the oviduct. When fully developed the mature third-stage larva is larviposited on the host. These larvae drop to the ground and pupate almost immediately When pupation is completed, the newly emerged winged adults locate a suitable host animal on which they blood-feed, remaining on the host for long periods. Each female can produce only five or six larvae in its lifetime.

Geographical distribution: Sub-Saharan Africa

Pathogenesis: This species is primarily a nuisance and a cause of disturbance. There is no evidence that it plays any role in the transmission of camel trypanosomiasis.

Clinical signs: The adult flies are clearly visible when feeding on the host animal. Irritation at the feeding sites may be observed.

Diagnosis: Observation of adult flies on the host animal

Epidemiology: The adult flies are most abundant on the host during the summer months.

Treatment and control: This is best achieved by topical application of insecticides, preferably those with some repellent and residual effect, such as the synthetic pyrethroids, permethrin and deltamethrin.

Wohlfahrtia nuba

Common name: Flesh flies

Predilection site: Skin wounds

Parasite class: Insecta

Family: Sarcophagidae

Hosts: Camels

Geographical distribution: Primarily north Africa and the Near East

For more details see Chapter 11 (Facultative ectoparasites and arthropod vectors).

Sarcoptes scabiei

Subspecies: *cameli*

Common name: Camel mange, 'jarab'

Predilection site: Skin

Parasite class: Arachnida

Sub-class: Acari

Order: Acariformes

Sub-order: Sarcoptiformes (Astigmata)

Family: Sarcoptidae

Hosts: Camels

Geographical distribution: Africa, Asia

Pathogenesis and clinical signs: Host reaction starts on the head, neck, mammary glands, prepuce and flanks. The first lesions appear as erythema, papules and intense pruritis with hair loss, which becomes reddened and moist. The lesions may become generalised with hyperkeratosis on the neck and legs, with intense pruritis leading to loss of appetite, weight loss and emaciation.

Epidemiology: New hosts are infected by contact with infected individuals, presumably by the transfer of larvae, which are commonly present more superficially on the skin surface. Transmission occurs between mature animals and also from mother to offspring at birth.

Treatment and control: Spray treatments of lindane or organophosphates repeated after 1–2 weeks and ivermectin given twice at 2-week intervals been reported to be effective. It is important to treat the whole herd and new introductions.

Notes: Sarcoptic mange is one of the most important diseases of camels and can also be transmitted to humans.

Chorioptes bovis

Synonym: *Chorioptes ovis*, *Chorioptes equi*, *Chorioptes caprae*, *Chorioptes cuniculi*

Predilection site: Skin; particularly the legs, feet, base of tail and upper rear surface of the udder.

Parasite class: Arachnida

Sub-class: Acari

Order: Acariformes

Sub-order: Sarcoptiformes (Astigmata)

Family: Psoroptidae

Hosts: Cattle, sheep, horse, goat, camel, llama, rabbit

Notes: Has been reported in dromedary camels in zoos

For more details see Chapter 2 (Cattle).

Hyalomma dromedarii

Common name: Camel tick

Predilection site: All over the body but especially the axilla, inguinal region, face and ears

Parasite class: Arachnida

Sub-class: Acari

Order: Parasitiformes

Sub-order: Ixodida (Metastigmata)

Family: Ixodidae

Hosts: Camels, but may also be of veterinary significance in ruminants and horses

For more details see Chapter 11 (Facultative ectoparasites and arthropod vectors).

A number of non-obligate ectoparasites are found on camels and these are listed in the host–parasite checklist at the end of this chapter. More detailed descriptions of these parasites are found in Chapter 11.

LLAMAS, ALPACAS, GUANACOS, VICUNA

PARASITES OF THE DIGESTIVE SYSTEM

Gongylonema pulchrum

Common name: Gullet worm

Predilection site: Oesophagus, rumen

Parasite class: Nematoda

Superfamily: Spiruroidea

Final host: Sheep, goat, cattle, pig, buffalo, horse, donkey, deer, camel, camelids, man

Intermediate host: Coprophagous beetles, cockroaches

Geographical distribution: Probably worldwide

For more details see Chapter 3 (Sheep and goats).

ABOMASUM

The following nematode species have been reported in the abomasum of camelids in their country of origin, Peru. Their pathogenicities are unknown

Graphinema aucheniae

Predilection site: Abomasum

Parasite class: Nematoda

Superfamily: Trichostrongyloidea

Hosts: Alpaca

Spiculopteragia peruvianus

Predilection site: Abomasum

Parasite class: Nematoda

Superfamily: Trichostrongyloidea

Hosts: Alpaca

Camelostrongylus mentulatus

Predilection site: Abomasum, small intestine

Parasite class: Nematoda

Superfamily: Trichostrongyloidea

Geographical distribution: Common in the Middle East and Australia; South America

Additionally several cattle and sheep nematode species have been reported in farmed camelids (Table 8.10).

SMALL INTESTINE

Intestinal species reported in camelids are generally of little clinical significance. Many of the species listed are parasites of cattle or sheep and are described in more detail under the chapters for these hosts.

Table 8.10 Cattle and sheep parasites found in the abomasum of camelids.

Species	(Super)family	Hosts	Geographical distribution
Teladorsagia circumcincta	Trichostrongyloidea	Cattle, sheep, goat, deer, camel, llama	Worldwide
Ostertagia leptospicularis	Trichostrongyloidea	Deer (roe deer), cattle, sheep, goat, camel	Many parts of the world, particularly Europe and New Zealand
Haemonchus contortus	Trichostrongyloidea	Sheep, goat, cattle, deer, camel, llama	Worldwide
Marshallagia marshalli	Trichostrongyloidea	Sheep, goats and wild small ruminants	Tropics and subtropics including southern Europe, USA, South America, India and Russia
Trichostrongylus axei	Trichostrongyloidea	Cattle, sheep, goat, deer, horse, donkey, pig and occasionally man	Worldwide

Lamanema chavezi

Predilection site: Small intestine

Parasite class: Nematoda

Superfamily: Trichostrongyloidea

Host: Alpaca (*Lama pacos*), vicuna (*Vicugna vicugna*)

Description, gross: Small worms, males 8–9 mm long; females 14–18 mm.

Description, microscopic: Shallow buccal capsule with dorsal tooth and two small lateroventral teeth at the base. In the male, the lateral lobes are large; the dorsal lobe is small. There are short spicules and large gubernaculums.

Nematodirus lamae

Predilection site: Small intestine

Parasite class: Nematoda

Superfamily: Trichostrongyloidea

Hosts: Alpaca (*Lama pacos*), llama, vicuna (*Vicugna vicugna*)

Description, gross: Small worms, males 10–13 mm long; females 14–20 mm.

Description, microscopic: Male worms have a deeply emarginated dorsal lobe with two distinct lobules; there are long spicules with enlarged distal ends terminating in two distinct bifurcated medioventral processes.

Geographical distribution: South America

Pathogenicity: Not reported

Table 8.11 lists parasites of cattle or sheep which have been reported in the small intestine of camelids.

The following species of *Eimeria* have been described from the faeces of alpacas in their native country of Peru. Details of their life cycle, pathogenicity, etc. are not known.

Eimeria lamae

Predilection site: Unknown

Parasite class: Sporozoasida

Family: Eimeriidae

Host: Alpaca

Description: The oocysts are ellipsoidal, to ovoid, smooth, bluish to greenish yellow, 30–40 × 21–30 μm with a micropyle and micropylar cap, with or without a polar granule, but without an oocyst residuum (Fig. 8.4). Sporocysts are elongate ovoid, 13–16 ×

Table 8.11 Cattle and sheep parasites found in the small intestine of camelids.

Species	(Super)family	Hosts	Geographical distribution
Nematodes			
Trichostrongylus vitrinus	Trichostrongyloidea	Sheep, goat, deer, llama and occasionally pig and man	Worldwide
Trichostrongylus colubriformis	Trichostrongyloidea	Sheep, goat, cattle, camel and occasionally pig and man	Worldwide
Trichostrongylus longispicularis	Trichostrongyloidea	Cattle, sheep, goat, deer, camel, llama	Australia; America and parts of Europe
Nematodirus helvetianus	Trichostrongyloidea	Cattle, occasionally sheep, goat and other ruminants	Worldwide
Cooperia surnabada (syn *C. mcmasteri*)	Trichostrongyloidea	Cattle, sheep, camel	Parts of Europe, North America and Australia
Bunostomum trigonocephalum	Ancylostomatoidea	Sheep, goat, camel	Worldwide
Strongyloides papillosus	Rhabditoidea	Sheep, cattle, other ruminants and rabbits	Worldwide
Cestodes			
Moniezia expansa	Anoplocephalidae	Sheep, goats, occasionally cattle Intermediate hosts: forage mites	Worldwide

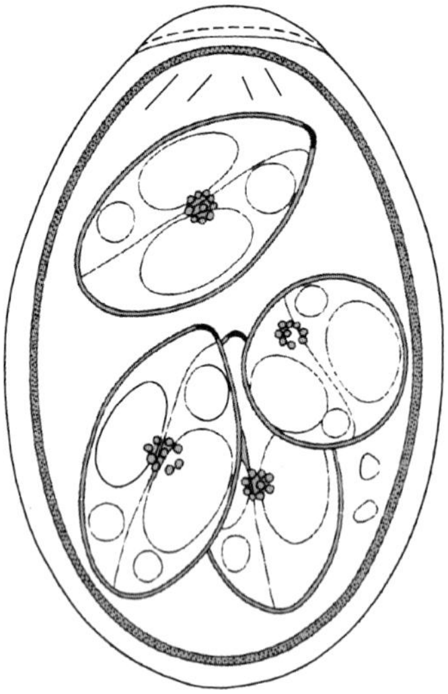

Fig. 8.4 Oocyst of *Eimeria lamae.*

8–10 µm with a Stieda body and a residuum. Sporozoites are elongate, with one to three clear globules.

Eimeria alpacae

Predilection site: Unknown

Parasite class: Sporozoasida

Family: Eimeriidae

Host: Alpaca

Description: The oocysts are ellipsoidal, rarely ovoid, pale green–blue, smooth, 22–26 × 18–21 µm with a micropyle and micropyle cap, with or without polar granules and without an oocyst residuum. Sporocysts are ovoid, 10–13 × 7–8 µm with a faint Stieda body and a residuum. Sporozoites are elongate and lie lengthwise head to tail in the sporocyst with one to three clear granules.

Eimeria punoensis

Predilection site: Unknown

Parasite class: Sporozoasida

Family: Eimeriidae

Host: Alpaca

Description: Oocysts are ellipsoidal, smooth, 17–22 × 14–19 µm (mean 19.9 × 16.4 µm), with a micropyle, micropylar cap and polar granules. Sporocysts are elongate, 9.2 × 6.1 µm with a faint Stieda body and a sporocyst residuum.

Eimeria macusaniensis

Predilection site: Unknown

Parasite class: Sporozoasida

Family: Eimeriidae

Host: Alpaca

Description: The oocysts are ovoid, sometimes pyriform, colourless, 81–107 × 61–80 µm, with a micropyle and micropylar cap, but without a polar granule, or oocyst residuum. Sporocysts are elongate ovoid, 33–40 × 16–20 µm, with a faint Stieda body and a residuum. Sporozoites are elongate, with a clear globule at the large end, and a small one at the small end.

Cryptosporidium parvum

For more details see Chapter 2 (Cattle).

LARGE INTESTINE (see Table 8.12)

Table 8.12 Cattle and sheep parasites found in the large intestine of camelids.

Species	(Super)family	Hosts	Geographical distribution
Oesophagostomum venulosum	Strongyloidea	Sheep, goat, deer, camel	Worldwide
Oesophagostomum columbianum	Strongyloidea	Sheep, goat, deer, camel	Worldwide; more important in tropical and subtropical areas
Chabertia ovina	Strongyloidea	Sheep, goat, occasionally deer, cattle and other ruminants	Worldwide but more prevalent in temperate regions
Trichuris ovis	Trichuroidea	Sheep, goats, occasionally cattle and other ruminants	Worldwide
Skrjabinema ovis	Oxyuroidea	Sheep, goat, guanaco	Worldwide

PARASITES OF THE RESPIRATORY SYSTEM

Dictyocaulus filaria

Predilection site: Lungs

Parasite class: Nematoda

Superfamily: Trichostrongyloidea

Hosts: Sheep, goat, camelids and a few wild ruminants

Geographical distribution: Worldwide

Pathogenesis and clinical signs: Severe infections cause depression, coughing, dyspnoea and loss of condition.

Epidemiology: *D. filaria* is found in the respiratory tract of camelids in many areas of the world.

Treatment and control: Benzimidazoles, levamisole and avermectins are all reported to be effective against this species in camels.

For more details of these species see Chapter 3 (Sheep and goats).

Dictyocaulus viviparus

Synonym: *Dictyocaulus cameli*

Predilection site: Lungs

Parasite class: Nematoda

Superfamily: Trichostrongyloidea

Hosts: Cattle, deer, camel, camelids

Geographical distribution: Worldwide

Pathogenesis and clinical signs: As for *D. filaria*

For more details see Chapter 2 (Cattle).

PARASITES OF THE LIVER

Fasciola hepatica

Common name: Liver fluke

Predilection site: Liver

Parasite class: Trematoda

Family: Fasciolidae

Definitive hosts: Sheep, cattle, goat, horse, deer, llama, man and other mammals

For more details see Chapter 3 (Sheep and goats).

Dicrocoelium dendriticum

Synonym: *Dicrocoelium lanceolatum*

Common name: Small lanceolate fluke

Predilection site: Liver

Parasite class: Trematoda

Family: Dicrocoeliidae

Definitive hosts: Sheep, goats, cattle, deer, llama and rabbits; occasionally in the horse and pig

Geographical distribution: Worldwide except for South Africa and Australia

For more details see Chapter 3 (Sheep and goats).

Echinococcus granulosus

Predilection site: Mainly liver and lungs (intermediate hosts)

Parasite class: Cestoda

Family: Taeniidae

Definitive hosts: Dog and many wild canids

Intermediate hosts: Domestic and wild ruminants, man and primates, pig, camelids and lagomorphs

For more details see Chapter 3 (Sheep and goats).

Fasciola gigantica

Common name: Tropical large liver fluke

Predilection site: Liver

Parasite class: Trematoda

Family: Fasciolidae

Final hosts: Cattle, buffalo, sheep, goat, pig, camel, deer, llama, man

For more details see Chapter 2 (Cattle).

Fascioloides magna

See Deer.

PARASITES OF THE NERVOUS SYSTEM

Parelaphostrongylus tenuis

Synonym: *Odocoileostrongylus tenuis, Elaphostrongylus tenuis*

Common names: Cerebrospinal nematodiosis, meningeal worm, moose sickness, moose disease

Predilection site: Veins and venous sinuses of cranial meninges, CNS

Parasite class: Nematoda

Superfamily: Metastrongyloidea

Table 8.13 *Sarcocystis* species found in camelids.

Species	Camelid host (s)	Final hosts	Distribution
Sarcocystis aucheniae Syn. *S. tiopodi* *S. guanicocanis*	Llama, guanaco, alpaca	Dog	South America
Sarcocystis lamacenis	Llama	Unknown	South America

Final hosts: White-tailed deer (*Odocoileus virginianus*), moose (*Alces alces*), wapiti (*Cervus canadensis*), other deer species, llama, guanaco, alpaca

Intermediate hosts: Snails and slugs

For more details see Deer.

PARASITES OF THE REPRODUCTIVE/UROGENITAL SYSTEM

No parasites of veterinary significance reported.

PARASITES OF THE LOCOMOTORY SYSTEM

Toxoplasma gondii

See Camels.

ECTOPARASITES

Microthoracius mazzai

Common name: Llama louse

Predilection site: Hair, particularly around the face

Parasite class: Insecta

Family: Microthoraciidae

Description: *Microthoracius mazzai* have a very characteristic elongated, spindle-shaped head, which is almost as long as its swollen, rounded abdomen (Fig. 8.5). The entire body is 1–2 mm in length.

Hosts: Alpaca, llamas and relatives

Life cycle: The life cycle is typical, with eggs giving rise to three nymphal stages followed by the reproductive adult. The life cycle may be completed in as little as 2 weeks, and adults may live for up to 6 weeks.

Geographical distribution: Worldwide, in association with its host

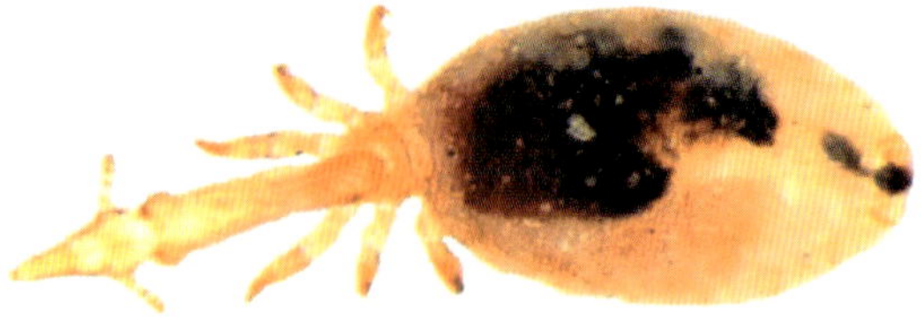

Fig. 8.5 *Microthoracius* spp (photograph courtesy of Kevin Floate and R. Spooner).

Pathogenesis: These lice are blood-feeders and heavy infestations can significantly reduce weight gain and milk production.

Clinical signs: The signs of infestation are variable. Light infestation may have no obvious effects, but pruritis, dermatitis and hair loss are usually evident at heavier parasite loads. Anaemia may be seen in young animals with heavy infestations.

Diagnosis: The lice can be seen in the hair of the host animal when the hair is parted. The eggs (nits) may be seen glued to hair shafts.

Epidemiology: Infection usually occurs after direct contact with an infested host animal. Cross-contamination between different host species is possible if the animals have physical contact. Transfer may occur from a contaminated environment or grooming equipment as the lice can survive for short periods off the host.

Treatment and control: Dips, dusts and sprays containing coumaphos, malathion or permethrin may be effective, particularly if applied after shearing. Macrocyclic lactones, such as ivermectin, doramectin and moxidectin, given in a repeated treatment programme of 7–10 days may also be highly effective.

Notes: Microthoraciidae contains four species in the genus *Microthoracius*. Three species parasitise llamas: *M. mazzai*, *M. minor* and *M. praelongiceps*. The fourth species *Microthoracius cameli* is parasitic on camels (see Camel ectoparasites).

Psoroptes ovis

Synonym: *Psoroptes communis* var *ovis*, *Psoroptes cuniculi*, *Psoroptes cervinus*, *Psoroptes bovis*, *Psoroptes equi*, *Psoroptes aucheniae*

Common name: Scab mite

Predilection site: Skin

Parasite class: Arachnida

Sub-class: Acari

Order: Acariformes

Sub-order: Sarcoptiformes (Astigmata)

Family: Psoroptidae

Hosts: Sheep, cattle, goat, horse, rabbit, camelids

Life cycle: The eggs of *P. ovis* are relatively large, about 250 µm in length, and oval.

Geographical distribution: Worldwide; particularly Europe and South America

For more details see Chapter 3 (Sheep and goats).

Chorioptes bovis

Synonym: *Chorioptes ovis*, *Chorioptes equi*, *Chorioptes caprae*, *Chorioptes cuniculi*

Predilection site: Skin; particularly the legs, feet, base of tail and upper rear surface of the udder

Parasite class: Arachnida

Sub-class: Acari

Order: Acariformes

Sub-order: Sarcoptiformes (Astigmata)

Family: Psoroptidae

Hosts: Cattle, sheep, horse, goat, camel, llama, rabbit

For more details see Chapter 2 (Cattle).

Sarcoptes scabiei

Predilection site: Skin

Parasite class: Arachnida

Sub-class: Acari

Order: Acariformes

Sub-order: Sarcoptiformes (Astigmata)

Family: Sarcoptidae

Hosts: Llama, guanaco, alpaca, vicuna

For more details see Chapter 5 (Pigs).

A number of non-obligate ectoparasites are found on camelids and these are listed in the host–parasite checklist at the end of this chapter. More detailed descriptions of these parasites are found in Chapter 11 (Facultative ectoparasites and arthropod vectors).

In the following checklists, the codes listed below apply:

Helminth classes:
N = Nematoda; T = Trematoda; C = Cestoda.

Arthropod classes:
I = Insecta; A = Arachnida.

Protozoal classes:
M = Mastigophora; S = Sarcodina; A = Apicomplexa; R = Rickettsia.

Deer parasite checklist.

Section/host system	Helminths		Arthropods		Protozoa	
	Parasite	(Super)family	Parasite	Family	Parasite	Family
Digestive						
Oesophagus	*Gongylonema pulchrum*	Spiruroidea (N)				
Rumen/reticulum	*Gongylonema verrucosum*	Spiruroidea (N)				
	Paramphistomum cervi	Paramphistomatidae (T)				
	Paramphistomum ichikawai	Paramphistomatidae (T)				
	Ceylonocotyle streptocoelium	Paramphistomatidae (T)				
Abomasum	*Spiculopteragia asymmetrica*	Trichostrongyloidea (N)				
	Spiculopteragia spiculoptera	Trichostrongyloidea (N)				
	Apteragia quadrispiculata	Trichostrongyloidea (N)				
	Rinadia mathevossiani	Trichostrongyloidea (N)				
	Ostertagia leptospicularis	Trichostrongyloidea (N)				
	Ostertagia ostertagi	Trichostrongyloidea (N)				
	Teladorsagia circumcincta	Trichostrongyloidea (N)				
	Haemonchus contortus	Trichostrongyloidea (N)				
	Trichostrongylus axei	Trichostrongyloidea (N)				
	Parabronema skrjabini	Spiruroidea (N)				
	Physocephalus cristatus	Spiruroidea (N)				
Small intestine	*Trichostrongylus vitrinus*	Trichostrongyloidea (N)			*Eimeria capreoli*	Eimeriidae (A)
	Trichostrongylus longispicularis	Trichostrongyloidea (N)			*Eimeria catubrina*	Eimeriidae (A)
	Nematodirus helvetianus	Trichostrongyloidea (N)			*Eimeria panda*	Eimeriidae (A)
	Nematodirus spathiger	Trichostrongyloidea (N)			*Eimeria patavina*	Eimeriidae (A)
	Nematodirus filicollis	Trichostrongyloidea (N)			*Eimeria ponderosa*	Eimeriidae (A)
	Cooperia oncophora	Trichostrongyloidea (N)			*Eimeria rotunda*	Eimeriidae (A)
	Cooperia curticei	Trichostrongyloidea (N)			*Eimeria superba*	Eimeriidae (A)
	Cooperia pectinata	Trichostrongyloidea (N)			*Eimeria asymmetrica*	Eimeriidae (A)
	Cooperia punctata	Trichostrongyloidea (N)			*Eimeria austriaca*	Eimeriidae (A)
	Bunostomum trigonocephalum	Strongyloidea (N)			*Eimeria cervi*	Eimeriidae (A)
	Capillaria bovis	Trichuroidea (N)			*Eimeria elaphi*	Eimeriidae (A)
	Moniezia benedeni	Anoplocephalidae (C)			*Eimeria robusta*	Eimeriidae (A)
					Eimeria sordida	Eimeriidae (A)
					Eimeria wapiti	Eimeriidae (A)
					Eimeria arctica	Eimeriidae (A)
					Eimeria mayeri	Eimeriidae (A)
					Eimeria tarandi	Eimeriidae (A)
					Cryptosporidium parvum	Cryptosporidiidae (A)

Caecum	*Chabertia ovina*	Strongyloidea (N)					
Colon	*Oesophagostomum columbianum*	Strongyloidea (N)					
	Oesophagostomum venulosum	Strongyloidea (N)					
	Trichuris ovis	Trichuroidea (N)					
	Trichuris globulosa	Trichuroidea (N)					
	Trichuris capreoli	Trichuroidea (N)					
Respiratory							
Nasopharynx				*Cephenemyia trompe*	Oestridae (I)		
				Cephenemyia auribarbis	Oestridae (I)		
				Cephenemyia jellisoni	Oestridae (I)		
				Cephenemyia stimulator	Oestridae (I)		
				Pharyngomyia picta	Oestridae (I)		
Trachea							
Bronchi							
Lung	*Dictyocaulus viviparus*	Trichostrongyloidea (N)					
	Dictyocaulus eckerti	Trichostrongyloidea (N)					
	Protostrongylus rufescens	Metastrongyloidea (N)					
	Muellerius capillaris	Metastrongyloidea (N)					
	Cystocaulus ocreatus	Metastrongyloidea (N)					
	Varestrongylus sagittatus	Metastrongyloidea (N)					
	Varestrongylus capreoli	Metastrongyloidea (N)					
	Echinococcus granulosus	Taeniidae (C)					
Liver							
	Fasciola hepatica	Fasciolidae (T)					
	Fasciola gigantica	Fasciolidae (T)					
	Fascioloides magna	Fasciolidae (T)					
	Dicrocoelium dendriticum	Dicrocoeliidae (T)					
	Dicrocoelium hospes	Dicrocoeliidae (T)					
	Stilesia hepatica	Thysanosomidae (C)					
	Echinococcus granulosus	Taeniidae (C)					
	Cysticercus tenuicollis (metacestode – *Taenia hydatigena*)	Taeniidae (C)					

(*continued*)

Deer parasite checklist (*continued*).

Section/host system	Helminths		Arthropods		Protozoa	
	Parasite	(Super)family	Parasite	Family	Parasite	Family
Pancreas						
Circulatory						
Blood					*Babesia bovis*	Babesiidae (A)
					Theileria cervi	Theileriidae (A)
					Anaplasma marginale	Anaplasmataceae (R)
					Anaplasma centrale	Anaplasmataceae (R)
Blood vessels						
Nervous						
CNS	*Elaphostrongylus cervi*	Metastrongyloidea (N)				
	Parelaphostrongylus tenuis	Metastrongyloidea (N)				
Eye						
Reproductive/ urogenital						
Locomotory						
Muscle	*Cysticercus cervi* (metacestode – *Taenia cervi*)	Taeniidae (C)			*Toxoplasma gondii*	Sarcocystiidae (A)
					Sarcocystis cervicanis	Sarcocystiidae (A)
					Sarcocystis grueneri	Sarcocystiidae (A)
					Sarcocystis wapiti	Sarcocystiidae (A)
					Sarcocystis sybillensis	Sarcocystiidae (A)
					Sarcocystis hofmani	Sarcocystiidae (A)
					Sarcocystis capreolicanis	Sarcocystiidae (A)
					Sarcocystis gracilis	Sarcocystiidae (A)
					Sarcocystis rangi	Sarcocystiidae (A)
					Sarcocystis tarandivulpis	Sarcocystiidae (A)
					Sarcocystis tarandi	Sarcocystiidae (A)
					Sarcocystis rangiferi	Sarcocystiidae (A)
					Sarcocystis alceslatranis	Sarcocystiidae (A)
					Sarcocystis jorrini	Sarcocystiidae (A)

Connective tissue	*Elaeophora schneideri*	Filarioidea (N)	*Hypoderma diana*	Oestridae (I)		
			Hypoderma tarandi	Oestridae (I)		
Integument						
Skin			*Bovicola longicornis*	Trichodectidae (I)		
			Bovicola tibialis	Trichodectidae (I)	*Besnoitia tarandi*	Sarcocystiidae (A)
			Bovicola meyeri	Trichodectidae (I)		
			Bovicola maai	Trichodectidae (I)		
			Bovicola forficula	Trichodectidae (I)		
			Tricholipeurus indicus	Trichodectidae (I)		
			Solenopotes burmeisteri	Linognathidae (I)		
			Solenopotes capreoli	Linognathidae (I)		
			Solenopotes ferrisi	Linognathidae (I)		
			Solenopotes muntiacus	Linognathidae (I)		
			Solenopotes tarandi	Linognathidae (I)		
			Solenopotes binipilosus	Linognathidae (I)		
			Sarcoptes scabiei	Sarcoptidae (A)		
Subcutaneous			*Lucilia* spp	Calliphoridae (I)		
			Cordylobia anthropophaga	Calliphoridae (I)		
			Cochliomyia hominivorax	Calliphoridae (I)		
			Chrysomya bezziana	Calliphoridae (I)		
			Chrysomya megacephala	Calliphoridae (I)		
			Wohlfahrtia magnifica	Sarcophagidae (I)		
			Wohlfahrtia nuba	Sarcophagidae (I)		
			Sarcophaga dux	Sarcophagidae (I)		
			Dermatobia hominis	Oestridae (I)		

The following species of flies and ticks are found on deer. More detailed descriptions are found in Chapter 11: Facultative ectoparasites and arthropod vectors.

Flies of veterinary importance on deer.

Group	Genus	Species	Family
Blackflies Buffalo gnats	*Simulium*	spp	Simuliidae (I)
Bot flies	*Cephenemyia* *Dermatobia*	*trompe* *hominis*	Oestridae (I) Oestridae (I)
Flesh flies	*Sarcophaga* *Wohlfahrtia*	*dux* *magnifica* *nuba*	Sarcophagidae (I)
Hippoboscids	*Lipoptena*	*depressa* *cervi*	
Midges	*Culicoides*	spp	Ceratopogonidae (I)
Mosquitoes	*Aedes* *Anopheles* *Culex*	spp spp spp	Culicidae (I)
Muscids	*Musca* *Stomoxys*	spp *calcitrans*	Muscidae (I)
Sandflies	*Phlebotomus*	spp	Psychodidae (I)
Screwworms and blowflies	*Chrysomya* *Cochliomyia* *Cordylobia* *Calliphora* *Lucilia*	*bezziana* *megacephala* *rufifaces* *albiceps* *hominivorax* *macellaria* *anthropophaga* spp spp	Calliphoridae (I)
Tabanids	*Chrysops* *Haematopota* *Tabanus*	spp spp spp	Tabanidae (I)

Tick species found on deer.

Genus	Species	Common name	Family
Ornithodoros	*hermsi*	Sand tampan	Argasidae (A)
	savignyi		
	turicata		
Otobius	*megnini*	Spinose ear tick	Argasidae (A)
Amblyomma	*americanum*	Lone star tick	Ixodidae (A)
	cajennense	Cayenne tick	
	maculatum	Gulf coast tick	
Boophilus	*annulatus*	Blue cattle tick	Ixodidae (A)
	microplus	Tropical cattle tick	
Dermacentor	*andersoni*	Rocky Mountain wood tick	
	variablilis	American dog tick	
	albipictus	Moose tick	
	marginatus	Sheep tick	
	nitens	Tropical horse tick	
	reticulatus	Marsh tick	
	silvarum		
	occidentalis	Pacific coast tick	
Haemaphysalis	*punctata*		
	longicornis		
	bispinosa	Bush tick	
	concinna	Bush tick	
Hyalomma	*anatolicum*	Bont legged tick	Ixodidae (A)
	excavatum	Brown ear tick	
	marginatum	Mediterranean *Hyalomma*	
	scupense		
Ixodes	*ricinus*	Castor bean or European sheep tick	Ixodidae (A)
	holocyclus		
	persulcatus	Taiga tick	
	pacificus	Western black legged tick	
	rubicundus	Karoo paralysis tick	
	scapularis		
Rhipicephalus	*bursa*		Ixodidae (A)
	capensis	Cape brown tick	
	sanguineus	Brown dog or kennel tick	

Camel parasite checklist.

Section/host system	Helminths		Arthropods		Protozoa	
	Parasite	(Super)family	Parasite	Family	Parasite	Family
Digestive						
Oesophagus	*Gongylonema pulchrum*	Spiruroidea (N)				
Rumen/ reticulum	*Gongylonema pulchrum*	Spiruroidea (N)				
	Gongylonema verrucosum	Spiruroidea (N)				
Abomasum	*Haemonchus longistipes*	Trichostrongyloidea (N)				
	Haemonchus contortus	Trichostrongyloidea (N)				
	Teladorsagia circumcincta	Trichostrongyloidea (N)				
	Ostertagia trifurcata	Trichostrongyloidea (N)				
	Ostertagia leptospicularis	Trichostrongyloidea (N)				
	Camelostrongylus mentulatus	Trichostrongyloidea (N)				
	Marshallagia marshalli	Trichostrongyloidea (N)				
	Marshallagia mongolica	Trichostrongyloidea (N)				
	Trichostrongylus axei	Trichostrongyloidea (N)				
	Impalaia nudicollis	Trichostrongyloidea (N)				
	Impalaia tuberculata	Trichostrongyloidea (N)				
	Parabronema skrjabini	Spiruroidea (N)				
	Physocephalus cristatus	Spiruroidea (N)				
Small intestine	*Nematodirus abnormalis*	Trichostrongyloidea (N)			*Eimeria bactriani*	Eimeriidae (A)
	Nematodirus dromedarii	Trichostrongyloidea (N)			*Eimeria cameli*	Eimeriidae (A)
	Nematodirus helvetianus	Trichostrongyloidea (N)			*Eimeria dromedarii*	Eimeriidae (A)
	Nematodirus mauritanicus	Trichostrongyloidea (N)			*Eimeria pellerdyi*	Eimeriidae (A)
	Nematodirus spathiger	Trichostrongyloidea (N)			*Eimeria rajasthani*	Eimeriidae (A)
	Nematodirella dromedarii	Trichostrongyloidea (N)			*Isospora orlovi*	Eimeriidae (A)
	Nematodirella cameli	Trichostrongyloidea (N)			*Cryptosporidium parvum*	Cryptosporidiidae (A)
	Cooperia oncophora	Trichostrongyloidea (N)				
	Cooperia surnabada	Trichostrongyloidea (N)				
	Trichostrongylus colubriformis	Trichostrongyloidea (N)				
	Trichostrongylus longispicularis	Trichostrongyloidea (N)				
	Trichostrongylus probolorus	Trichostrongyloidea (N)				
	Trichostrongylus vitrinus	Trichostrongyloidea (N)				
	Bunostomum trigonocephalum	Strongyloidea (N)				
	Strongyloides papillosus	Rhabditoidea (N)				
	Moniezia benedeni	Anoplocephalidae (C)				
	Moniezia expansa	Anoplocephalidae (C)				
	Thysaniezia giardi	Anoplocephalidae (C)				
	Avitellina centripunctata	Thysanosomidae (C)				
	Avitellina woodlandi	Thysanosomidae (C)				
	Stilesia globipunctata	Thysanosomidae (C)				
	Stilesia vittata	Thysanosomidae (C)				
	Thysaniezia ovilla	Thysanosomidae (C)				

Caecum	*Chabertia ovina*	Strongyloidea (N)			*Balantidium coli*	Balantiidae (C)
Colon	*Oesophagostomum columbianum*	Strongyloidea (N)			*Buxtonella sulcata*	Pycnotrichidae (C)
	Oesophagostomum venulosum	Strongyloidea (N)				
	Oesophagostomum virginimembrum	Strongyloidea (N)				
	Trichuris ovis	Trichuroidea (N)				
	Trichuris globulosa	Trichuroidea (N)				
	Trichuris cameli	Trichuroidea (N)				
Respiratory						
Nose			*Cephalopina titillator*	Oestridae (I)		
			Oestrus ovis	Oestridae (I)		
Trachea Bronchi						
Lung	*Dictyocaulus filaria*	Trichostrongyloidea (N)				
	Dictyocaulus viviparus	Trichostrongyloidea (N)				
	Echinococcus granulosus	Taeniidae (C)				
Liver						
	Fasciola hepatica	Fasciolidae (T)				
	Fasciola gigantica	Fasciolidae (T)				
	Dicrocoelium dendriticum	Dicrocoeliidae (T)				
	Dicrocoelium hospes	Dicrocoeliidae (T)				
	Stilesia hepatica	Thysanosomidae (C)				
	Echinococcus granulosus	Taeniidae (C)				
	Cysticercus tenuicollis (metacestode – *Taenia hydatigena*)	Taeniidae (C)				
Pancreas						
	Eurytrema pancreaticum	Dicrocoeliidae (T)				
Circulatory						
Blood	*Schistosoma bovis*	Schistosomatidae (T)			*Trypanosoma brucei brucei*	Trypanosomatidae (M)
	Schistosoma mattheei	Schistosomatidae (T)			*Trypanosoma congolense*	Trypanosomatidae (M)
					Trypanosoma vivax	Trypanosomatidae (M)
					Trypanosoma evansi	Trypanosomatidae (M)
					Theileria camelensis	Theileriidae (A)
					Theileria dromedari	Theileriidae (A)
	Dipetalonema evansi	Filarioidea (N)			*Anaplasma centrale*	Anaplasmataceae (R)
	Onchocerca armillatai	Filarioidea (N)			*Anaplasma marginale*	Anaplasmataceae (R)
Blood vessels						

(continued)

Camel parasite checklist (*continued*).

Section/host system	Helminths		Arthropods		Protozoa	
	Parasite	(Super)family	Parasite	Family	Parasite	Family
Nervous						
CNS	*Coenurus cerebralis* (*Taenia multiceps*)	Taeniidae (C)				
Eye	*Thelazia rhodesi*	Spiruroidea (N)				
	Thelazia leesi	Spiruroidea (N)				
Reproductive/urogenital						
Locomotory						
Muscle	*Cysticercus bovis*	Taeniidae (C)			*Sarcocystis cameli*	Sarcocystiidae (A)
	Cysticercus dromedarii (metacestode – *Taenia hyaenae*)	Taeniidae (C)			*Sarcocystis ippeni*	Sarcocystiidae (A)
					Toxoplasma gondii	Sarcocystiidae (A)
Connective tissue	*Onchocerca fasciata*	Filarioidea (N)				
	Onchocerca gutturosa	Filarioidea (N)				
Integument						
Skin	*Stephanofilaria* spp	Filarioidea (N)	*Sacoptes scabiei*	Sarcoptidae (A)		
			Chorioptes bovis	Psoroptidae (A)		
			Microthoracius cameli	Microthoraciidae (I)		
Subcutaneous	*Onchocerca fasciata*	Filarioidea (N)	*Lucilia cuprina*	Calliphoridae (I)		
	Onchocerca gibsoni	Filarioidea (N)	*Cordylobia anthropophaga*	Calliphoridae (I)		
	Onchocerca gutturosa	Filarioidea (N)	*Cochliomyia hominivorax*	Calliphoridae (I)		
			Chrysomya bezziana	Calliphoridae (I)		
			Chrysomya megacephala	Calliphoridae (I)		
			Wohlfahrtia magnifica	Sarcophagidae (I)		
			Wohlfahrtia nuba	Sarcophagidae (I)		
			Sarcophaga dux	Sarcophagidae (I)		
			Dermatobia hominis	Oestridae (I)		

The following species of flies and ticks are found on camels. More detailed descriptions are found in Chapter 11: Facultative ectoparasites and arthropod vectors.

Flies of veterinary importance on camels.

Group	Genus	Species	Family
Blackflies Buffalo gnats	*Simulium*	spp	Simuliidae (I)
Bot flies	*Cephalopina*	*titillator*	Oestridae (I)
Flesh flies	*Sarcophaga* *Wohlfahrtia*	*dux* *magnifica* *nuba*	Sarcophagidae (I)
Hippoboscids	*Hippobosca*	*camelina* *maculata*	Hippoboscidae (I)
Midges	*Culicoides*	spp	Ceratopogonidae (I)
Mosquitoes	*Aedes* *Anopheles* *Culex*	spp spp spp	Culicidae (I)
Muscids	*Haematobia* *Musca* *Stomoxys*	*irritans* *autumnalis* *domestica* *calcitrans*	Muscidae (I)
Sandflies	*Phlebotomus*	spp	Psychodidae (I)
Screwworms and blowflies	*Chrysomya* *Cochliomyia* *Cordylobia* *Calliphora* *Lucilia*	*bezziana* *hominivorax* *anthropophaga* spp spp	Calliphoridae (I) Calliphoridae (I)
Tabanids	*Chrysops* *Haematopota* *Tabanus*	spp spp spp	Tabanidae (I)
Tsetse flies	*Glossina*	*fusca* *morsitans* *palpalis*	Glossinidae (I)

Tick species found on camels.

Genus	Species	Common name	Family
Ornithodoros	*savignyi*	Eyed or sand tampan	Argasidae (A)
Otobius	*megnini*	Spinose ear tick	Argasidae (A)
Amblyomma	*lepidum* *gemma* *variegatum*		Ixodidae (A)
Boophilus	*decoloratus*	Blue tick	Ixodidae (A)
Dermacentor	*marginatus* *reticulatus* *silvarum*	Sheep tick Marsh tick	
Haemaphysalis	*punctata* *sulcata* *persulcatus*	Bush tick	
Hyalomma	*anatolicum* *dromedarii* *detritum* *impressum* *marginatum* *plumbeum* *rufipes*	Camel *Hyalomma* Mediterranean *Hyalomma*	Ixodidae (A)
Ixodes	*ricinus* *holocyclus* *rubicundus* *scapularis*	Castor bean or European sheep tick Karoo paralysis tick	Ixodidae (A)
Rhipicephalus	*bursa* *evertsi* *pulchellus* *sanguineus*	 Red or red-legged tick Brown dog or kennel tick	Ixodidae (A)

Camelid (llama, alpaca, guanaco, vicuna) parasite checklist.

Section/host system	Helminths		Arthropods		Protozoa	
	Parasite	(Super)family	Parasite	Family	Parasite	Family
Digestive						
Oesophagus	*Gongylonema pulchrum*	Spiruroidea (N)				
Rumen/reticulum	*Gongylonema pulchrum*	Spiruroidea (N)				
Stomach	*Graphinema aucheniae*	Trichostrongyloidea (N)				
	Spiculopteragia peruvianus	Trichostrongyloidea (N)				
	Camelostrongylus mentulatus	Trichostrongyloidea (N)				
	Teladorsagia circumcincta	Trichostrongyloidea (N)				
	Marshallagia marshalli	Trichostrongyloidea (N)				
	Haemonchus contortus	Trichostrongyloidea (N)				
	Trichostrongylus axei	Trichostrongyloidea (N)				
	Ostertagia leptospicularis	Trichostrongyloidea (N)				
Small intestine	*Lamanema chavezi*	Trichostrongyloidea (N)			*Eimeria lamae*	Eimeriidae (A)
	Nematodirus lamae	Trichostrongyloidea (N)			*Eimeria alpacae*	Eimeriidae (A)
	Nematodirus helvetianus	Trichostrongyloidea (N)			*Eimeria punoensis*	Eimeriidae (A)
	Nematodirus battus	Trichostrongyloidea (N)			*Eimeria macusaniensis*	Eimeriidae (A)
	Trichostrongylus vitrinus	Trichostrongyloidea (N)				
	Trichostrongylus colubriformis	Trichostrongyloidea (N)			*Cryptosporidium parvum*	Cryptosporidiidae (A)
	Trichostrongylus longispicularis	Trichostrongyloidea (N)			*Giardia intestinalis*	Diplomonadidae (M)
	Cooperia surnabada	Trichostrongyloidea (N)				
	Bunostomum trigonocephalum	Ancylostomatoidea (N)				
	Strongyloides papillosus	Rhabditoidea (N)				
	Moniezia expansa	Anoplocephalidae (C)				
Caecum	*Oesophagostomum* sp	Strongyloidea (N)				
Colon	*Chabertia ovina*	Strongyloidea (N)				
	Trichuris ovis	Trichuroidea (N)				
	Skrjabinema ovis	Oxyuroidea (N)				
Respiratory						
Nose						
Trachea	*Dictyocaulus viviparus*	Trichostrongyloidea (N)				
Bronchi	*Dictyocaulus filaria*	Trichostrongyloidea (N)				
Lung						

(continued)

Camelid (llama, alpaca, guanaco, vicuna) parasite checklist (*continued*).

Section/host system	Helminths		Arthropods		Protozoa	
	Parasite	(Super)family	Parasite	Family	Parasite	Family
Liver						
	Fasciola hepatica	Fasciolidae (T)				
	Fasciola gigantica	Fasciolidae (T)				
	Fascioloides magna	Fasciolidae (T)				
	Dicrocoelium dendriticum	Dicrocoeliidae (T)				
	Echinococcus granulosus	Taeniidae (C)				
Pancreas						
Circulatory						
Blood						
Blood vessels						
Nervous						
CNS	*Parelaphostrongylus tenuis*	Metastrongyloidea (N)				
Eye	*Thelazia rhodesi*	Spiruroidea (N)				
Reproductive/urogenital						
Locomotory						
Muscle					*Toxoplasma gondii*	Sarcocystiidae (A)
					Sarcocystis aucheniae	Sarcocystiidae (A)
					Sarcocystis lamacenis	Sarcocystiidae (A)
Connective tissue						
Integument						
Skin			*Microthoracius mazzai*	Microthoraciidae (I)		
			Sarcoptes scabiei	Sarcoptidae (A)		
			Psoroptes ovis	Psoroptidae (A)		
			Chorioptes bovis	Psoroptidae (A)		
			Bovicola breviceps	Trichodectidae (I)		
Subcutaneous			*Cochliomyia hominivorax*	Calliphoridae (I)		

Flies of veterinary importance on camelids.

Group	Genus	Species	Family
Midges	*Culicoides*	spp	Ceratopogonidae (I)
Mosquitoes	*Aedes* *Anopheles* *Culex*	spp spp spp	Culicidae (I)
Muscids	*Musca* *Stomoxys*	*domestica* *calcitrans*	Muscidae (I)

Tick species found on camelids.

Genus	Species	Common name	Family
Otobius	*megnini*	Spinose ear tick	Argasidae (A)
Amblyomma	*americanum* *cajennense* *hebraeum* *maculatum* *variegatum*	Lone star tick Cayenne tick South African bont tick Gulf Coast tick	Ixodidae (A)
Boophilus	*annulatus* *decoloratus* *microplus*	Texas cattle fever tick Blue tick Tropical cattle tick	Ixodidae (A)
Dermacentor	*andersoni* *marginatus* *reticulatus* *occidentalis* *varabilis*	Rocky Mountain wood tick Sheep tick Marsh tick Pacific coast tick American dog tick	Ixodidae (A)
Haemaphysalis	*punctata* *concinna* *bispinosa* *longicornis*	 Bush tick Bush tick	Ixodidae (A)
Hyalomma	*dromedarii* *marginatum*	Camel *Hyalomma* Mediterranean *Hyalomma*	Ixodidae (A)
Ixodes	*ricinus* *holocyclus* *rubicundus* *scapularis*	Castor bean or European sheep tick Karoo paralysis tick	Ixodidae (A)
Rhipicephalus	*evertsi* *sanguineus* *simus*	Red or red-legged tick Brown dog or kennel tick Glossy tick	Ixodidae (A)

9
Parasites of laboratory animals

RABBITS

PARASITES OF THE DIGESTIVE SYSTEM

Helminth infections are rarely seen in domestic rabbits unless they are kept in conditions that expose them to the infective stages resultant from contact with wild rabbits. The following species, with the exception of *Passalurus*, are therefore generally only found in wild rabbits and treatment of domesticated rabbits for many of these parasites is therefore rarely indicated. When treatment is required, fenbendazole and mebendazole are effective. In-feed medication with flubendazole can also be given over 10 days.

A more detailed list of helminth species found in both domesticated and wild rabbits is provided in the parasite checklist at the end of the chapter.

Graphidium strigosum

Common name: Rabbit strongyle

Predilection site: Stomach

Parasite class: Nematoda

Superfamily: Trichostrongyloidea

Description, gross: The adults are reddish worms when fresh, with 40–60 longitudinal lines and fine, transverse striations. The male is 8–16 mm, and female 11–20 mm long.

Description, microscopic: The male bursa has large lateral lobes and a small dorsal lobe. Spicules are long, slender and each ends distally in several points. Eggs are typically trichostrongyle, ovoid and 98–106 × 50–58 μm.

Hosts: Rabbit, hares

Life cycle: The life cycle is direct. Infection is by ingestion of infective larvae, which develop to the adult stage in the stomach in about 12 days.

Geographical distribution: Europe

Pathogenesis and clinical signs: Light infections cause little effect, but heavy infections cause destruction of the gastric mucosa, diarrhoea, anaemia, emaciation and sometimes death if untreated.

Diagnosis: This is based on identification of the eggs in the faeces or adult worms in the stomach on postmortem.

Obeliscoides cuniculi

Predilection site: Stomach

Parasite class: Nematoda

Superfamily: Trichostrongyloidea

Description, gross: The adults are brownish red worms; the male is 10–16 mm, and female 15–18 mm long.

Description, microscopic: The male spicules are brown, and bifurcated at the distal end. The body of the female is tapered over the posterior 20% of its length. Eggs are typically trichostrongyle, ovoid and 76–86 × 44–45 μm.

Hosts: Rabbit, hare and occasionally white-tailed deer

Life cycle: The life cycle is direct. Infection is by ingestion of infective larvae, which develop to the adult stage in the stomach in about 19 days.

Geographical distribution: USA

Pathogenesis and clinical signs: Similar to *G. strigosum*

Diagnosis: This is based on identification of the eggs in the faeces or adult worms in the stomach on postmortem.

Epidemiology: The parasite can undergo hypobiosis on some occasions.

Trichostrongylus retortaeformis

Predilection site: Small intestine

Parasite class: Nematoda

Superfamily: Trichostrongyloidea

Description, gross: The adults are small, white and hair-like, usually less than 7.0 mm long and difficult to see with the naked eye.

Description, microscopic: In the male, the ventro-ventral ray tends to be disparate from the other rays and spicules are stout, unequal in length and terminate in a barb-like tip (see Table 3.1). The females possess double ovejectors.

Hosts: Rabbits, hares

Life cycle: The life cycle is direct and typically trichostrongyle.

Geographical distribution: Worldwide

Pathogenesis and clinical signs: The parasites penetrate into the mucosa, causing desquamation, and in heavy infections inflammation of the intestine with excess mucous exudate.

Diagnosis: This is based on clinical signs, seasonal occurrence of disease and, if possible, lesions at post-mortem examination. Faecal egg counts are a useful aid to diagnosis, although faecal cultures are necessary for generic identification of larvae.

TAPEWORMS

Gross: Tapeworms of the genus *Cittotaenia* are up to 80 cm long and 1 cm wide.

Microscopic: Proglottids are broader than long and each contains two sets of genital organs. Eggs are about 64 μm in diameter and have a pyriform apparatus.

Intermediate hosts: Forage mites, mainly of the family Oribatidae.

Life cycle: Mature proglottids or eggs are passed in the faeces and on to pasture where the oncospheres are ingested by forage mites. The embryos migrate into the body cavity of the mite where they develop to cysticercoids. Infection of the final host is by ingestion of infected mites during grazing.

Epidemiology: Infection may occur in domesticated rabbits, grazing contaminated grass.

Pathogenesis and clinical signs: Heavy infections may cause digestive disturbances, emaciation and occasionally death in affected rabbits.

Diagnosis: This is based largely on the presence of mature proglottids in the faeces.

Cittotaenia ctenoides

Predilection site: Small intestine

Parasite class: Cestoda

Family: Anoplocephalidae

Description, microscopic: The scolex is about 0.5 mm wide

Final hosts: Rabbit

Geographical distribution: Europe

Cittotaenia pectinata

Predilection site: Small intestine

Parasite class: Cestoda

Family: Anoplocephalidae

Description, microscopic: The scolex is smaller (0.25 mm) than that of *C. ctenoides*.

Final hosts: Rabbit, hare

Geographical distribution: Europe, Asia, America

OXYURID WORMS

Passalurus ambiguus

Common name: Rabbit pinworm

Predilection site: Caecum, colon

Class: Nematoda

Superfamily: Oxyuridoidea

Description, gross: Adult worms are 4–11 mm in size and semitransparent; males are 4–5 mm and females 9–11 mm.

Description, microscopic: The oesophagus has the typical oxyurid oesophageal bulb. Eggs are thin-walled, with slightly flattened walls on one side and measure 95–103 × 43 μm

Hosts: Rabbit, hare

Life cycle: Development is direct and infection occurs through the ingestion of infective eggs. Immature stages are found in the mucosa of the small intestine and caecum.

Geographical distribution: Worldwide

Pathogenesis: Rabbits can harbour large numbers of oxyurid worms with no clinical signs. These worms can be a problem in rabbit colonies.

Treatment and control: Single treatments are not very effective because of the direct life cycle and rapidity of reinfection. Fenbendazole at 50 mg/kg in feed for 5 days is effective.

COCCIDIOSIS

There are 11 species of coccidia affecting rabbits (Table 9.1). The intestinal species, *E. flavescens* and

Table 9.1 *Eimeria* species in rabbits.

Species	Predilection site	Prepatent periods (days)
E. flavescens	Small and large intestine	9
E. intestinalis	Small intestine	9–10
E. exigua	Small intestine	7
E. perforans	Small intestine	5
E. irresidua	Small intestine	9
E. media	Small intestine	5–6
E. vejdovskyi	Small intestine	10
E. coecicola	Small intestine	9–11
E. magna	Small intestine	7
E. piriformis	Colon	9
E. stiedai	Liver, bile ducts	18

E. intestinalis, are the most pathogenic causing the destruction of crypts in the intestine resulting in diarrhoea and emaciation with disease commonest around weaning. Coccidial infections are seen commonly on commercial rabbit farms.

Diagnosis: As in other hosts, diagnosis is best made by a postmortem examination. Species identification is based on pathological lesions and location within the intestine. Identification is possible on oocysts recovered from faeces following sporulation. In practice, the demonstration of many oocysts in the faeces is often used as an indication that rabbits require treatment.

Treatment and control: A number of coccidiostats are available for prophylactic use, including robenidine and clopidol. Sulphonamides (sulphadimidine or sulphaquinoxaline) are used for treatment, usually given as two 7-day courses in drinking water, 1 week apart to allow for the possibility of reinfection. Control of rabbit coccidiosis involves the daily cleaning of cages, hutches or pens and the provision of clean feeding troughs. In many large units, control is achieved by rearing animals on wire floors, or alternatively, coccidiostats such as amprolium, clopidol or robenidine are incorporated in the feed.

Eimeria flavescens

Predilection site: Small and large intestine (Fig. 9.1)

Parasite class: Sporozoasida

Family: Eimeriidae

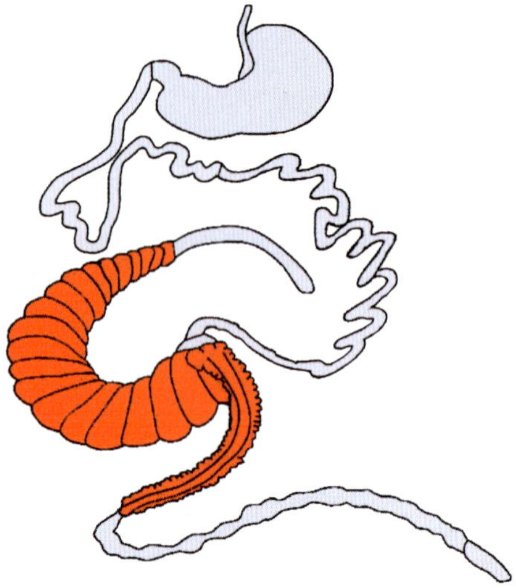

Fig. 9.1 Predilection site of *Eimeria flavescens*.

Life cycle: There are five merogony stages. The first-generation meronts are in the glands of the lower small intestine, the second- to fifth-generation meronts are in the caecum and colon. The second-, third- and fourth-generation meronts are in the superficial epithelium, and the fifth-generation meronts and the gamonts are in the crypts. Gamonts and gametes appear about 7 days, and oocysts appear in the faces about 9 days after infection. Sporulation time is 4 days.

Geographical distribution: Worldwide

Pathogenesis and clinical signs: *E. flavescens* is highly pathogenic for young rabbits, causing high morbidity and mortality and is a major problem on commercial rabbit farms.

Pathology: There is thickening of the intestinal wall of the caecum and colon with petechial haemorrhages and loss of epithelium in the caecum and colon.

Eimeria intestinalis

Predilection site: Small intestine (Fig. 9.2)

Parasite class: Sporozoasida

Family: Eimeriidae

Life cycle: There are three merogony stages. First-generation meronts are at the base of the villi in the lower ileum. There appear to be two types of second-generation meronts in the distal part of the villi, followed by third-generation meronts in the same location on the villi. Gamonts begin developing 8 days post infection, and are located above the host cell nucleus in the epithelial cells of the villi. The prepatent

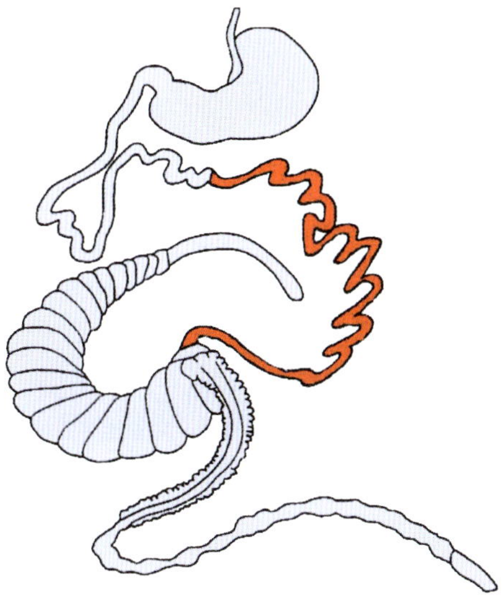

Fig. 9.2 Predilection site of *Eimeria intestinalis*.

period is 9–10 days and the patent period 6–10 days. Sporulation time is 3 days.

Geographical distribution: Worldwide

Pathogenesis and clinical signs: *E. intestinalis* is highly pathogenic, causing diarrhoea and emaciation.

Pathology: There is oedema of the intestinal wall with destruction of the crypts in the ileum and lower jejunum. Greyish white foci may coalesce forming a sticky purulent layer in the small intestine.

Eimeria exigua

Predilection site: Small intestine (Fig. 9.3)

Parasite class: Sporozoasida

Family: Eimeriidae

Life cycle: Development takes place in the ileum and lower jejunum but details of the life cycle are unknown. The prepatent period is 7 days. The sporulation time is 1 day.

Geographical distribution: Unknown, probably worldwide

Pathogenesis and clinical signs: This species is not considered pathogenic or only slightly pathogenic. Infections are usually asymptomatic but heavy infections may cause slight depression of growth.

Eimeria perforans

Predilection site: Small intestine (Fig. 9.4)

Parasite class: Sporozoasida

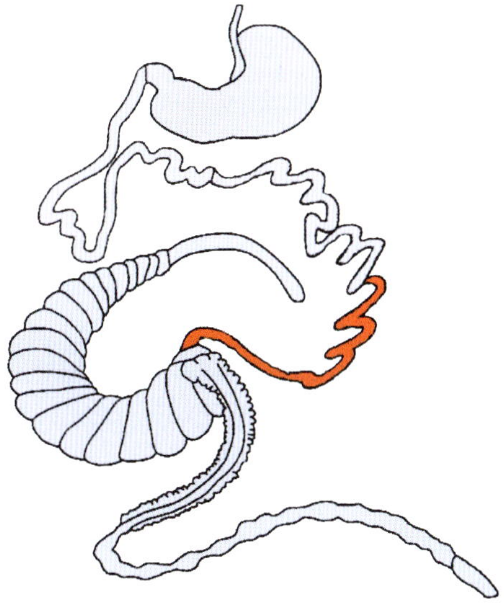

Fig. 9.3 Predilection site of *Eimeria exigua*.

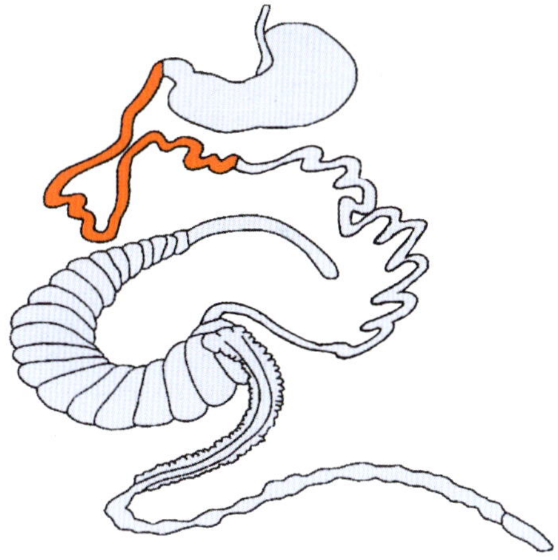

Fig. 9.4 Predilection site of *Eimeria perforans*.

Family: Eimeriidae

Life cycle: The endogenous stages are found in the epithelial cells of the villi and crypts of the small intestine, especially the middle section. There are two asexual generations, followed by gametogony. The prepatent period is 5 days and the patent period is 12–32 days. Sporulation time is 1.5–2 days.

Geographical distribution: Worldwide

Pathogenesis and clinical signs: *E. perforans* is one of the less pathogenic intestinal coccidia of rabbits, but it may cause mild to moderate signs in a heavy infection. Symptoms are usually mild, but in heavy infections there may be anorexia, diarrhoea, weakness, weight loss and growth retardation.

Pathology: The duodenum may be enlarged and oedematous, and may appear a chalky white colour. The jejunum and ileum may contain white spots and streaks and petechiae have been observed in the caecum.

Eimeria irresidua

Predilection site: Small intestine (Fig. 9.5)

Parasite class: Sporozoasida

Family: Eimeriidae

Life cycle: There are four merogony stages. First-generation meronts are in the crypts, second-generation meronts are in the lamina propria, and third- and fourth-generation meronts and gamonts are in the villous epithelium in the jejunum, and to a lesser extent the ileum. The prepatent period is 9 days. Sporulation time is 4 days.

Geographical distribution: Worldwide

Pathogenesis and clinical signs: Mildly pathogenic causing a depression in weight gain and in some cases diarrhoea. During this time, there is a reduction in food and water consumption as well as faecal excretion. Occasionally causes mortality depending on the level of infection.

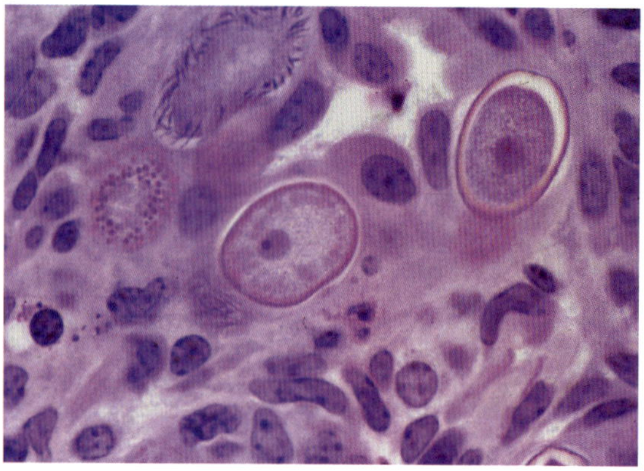

Fig. 9.6 Gamonts of *Eimeria irresidua*.

Pathology: Catarrhal inflammation of the small intestine, particularly the jejunum, may be seen. On postmortem there may be enteritis, with gross thickening of the intestine. Large numbers of meronts and gamonts may be found in mucosal scrapings. Histopathological examination shows a congested and thickened mucosa with villous atrophy, villous fusion and crypt hyperplasia with numerous parasite stages present within the mucosa (Fig. 9.6).

Eimeria media

Predilection site: Small intestine (Fig. 9.7)

Parasite class: Sporozoasida

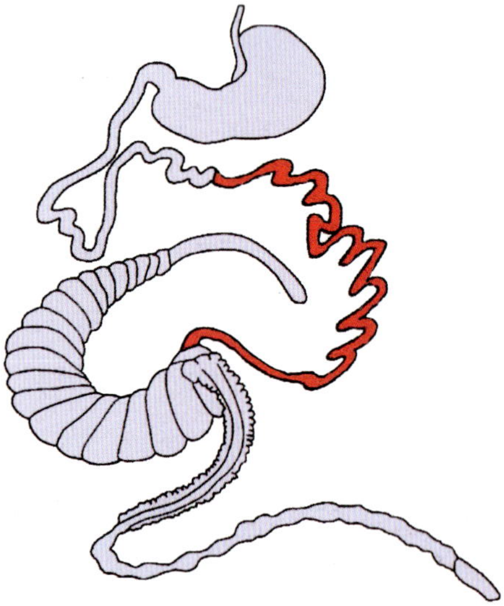

Fig. 9.5 Predilection site of *Eimeria irresidua*.

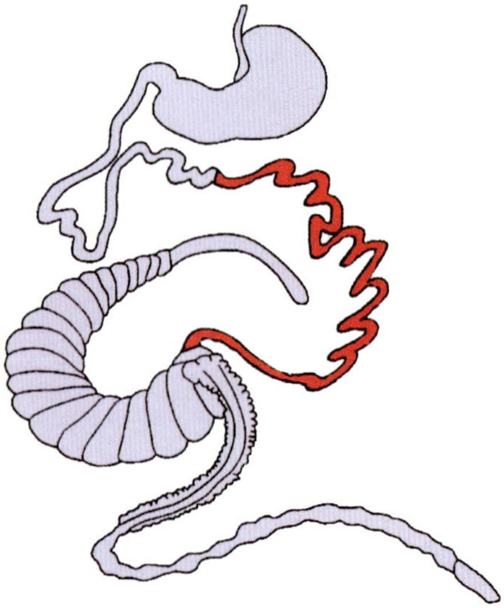

Fig. 9.7 Predilection site of *Eimeria media*.

Family: Eimeriidae

Life cycle: There are two merogony stages. The endogenous stages are found above or below the host cell nuclei of the epithelial cells and submucosa of the villi of the small intestine, mainly jejunum and ileum. The prepatent period is 5–6 days and the patent period is 15–18 days. Sporulation time is 2 days.

Geographical distribution: Worldwide

Pathogenesis and clinical signs: *E. media* is slightly to moderately pathogenic, causing a depression in weight gain and in some cases diarrhoea. During this time, there is a reduction in food and water consumption as well as faecal excretion.

Pathology: The affected parts of the intestine, mainly the duodenum, are oedematous with greyish foci. In heavy infections, the lesions may extend into the large intestine.

Eimeria vejdovskyi

Predilection site: Small intestine (Fig. 9.8)

Parasite class: Sporozoasida

Family: Eimeriidae

Life cycle: Development takes place in the ileum and lower jejunum but details of the life cycle are unknown. The prepatent period is 10 days. The sporulation time is 2 days.

Geographical distribution: Unknown, probably worldwide

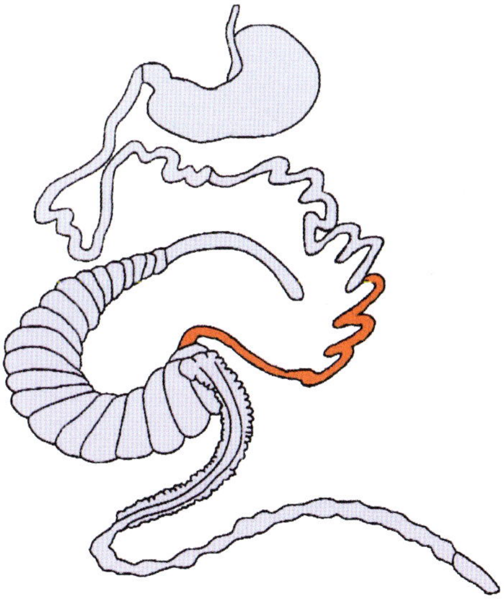

Fig. 9.8 Predilection site of *Eimeria vejdovskyi*.

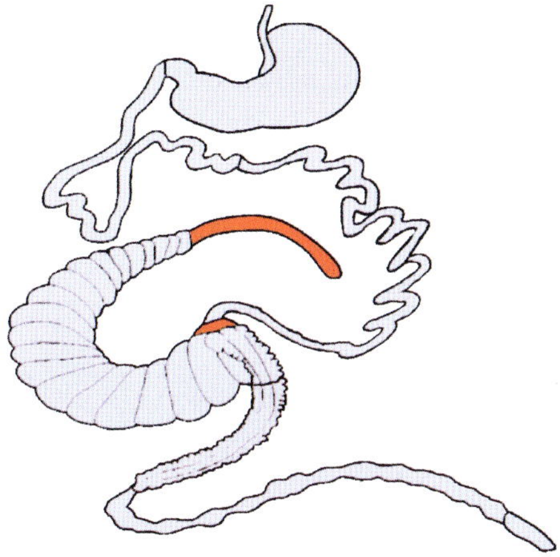

Fig. 9.9 Predilection site of *Eimeria coecicola*.

Pathogenesis and clinical signs: This species is considered only slightly pathogenic. Infections are usually asymptomatic but heavy infections may cause slight depression of growth.

Pathology: Lesions occur only in the ileum and distal jejunum following heavy infection.

Eimeria coecicola

Predilection site: Large intestine (Fig. 9.9)

Parasite class: Sporozoasida

Family: Eimeriidae

Life cycle: The number of generations is unknown. The meronts are in the epithelial cells of the ileum and the gamonts in the epithelial cells of the vermiform process of the caecum. The gamonts are usually sited beneath the host cell nucleus. The prepatent period is 9–11 days, the patent period 7–9 days. Sporulation time is 4 days.

Geographical distribution: Worldwide

Pathogenesis and clinical signs: This species is not considered pathogenic and infection is not associated with clinical signs.

Pathology: In heavy infections, lesions may be seen in the crypts of the vermiform appendix.

Eimeria magna

Predilection site: Small intestine (Fig. 9.10)

Parasite class: Sporozoasida

Family: Eimeriidae

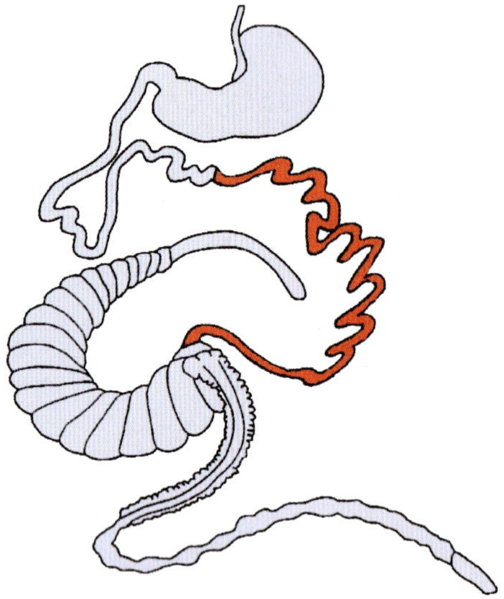

Fig. 9.10 Predilection site of *Eimeria magna*.

Life cycle: There are two or three merogony stages. The meronts develop in the villar epithelial cells from the middle of the jejunum to the posterior end of the ileum. They lie either above or below the host cell nucleus. The prepatent period is 7 days and the patent period 12–21 days. Sporulation time is 2–3 days.

Geographical distribution: Worldwide

Pathogenesis and clinical signs: *E. magna* is mildly to moderately pathogenic, causing a depression in weight gain and in some cases diarrhoea. During this time, there is a reduction in food and water consumption as well as faecal excretion. A large amount of mucus may be passed in the faeces. Mortality may occur depending on the level of infection.

Pathology: The intestinal mucosa is hyperaemic and inflamed. Epithelial sloughing may occur. Large numbers of meronts and gamonts may be found in mucosal scrapings. Histopathological examination shows a congested and thickened mucosa with villous atrophy, villous fusion and crypt hyperplasia.

Eimeria piriformis

Predilection site: Colon (Fig. 9.11)

Parasite class: Sporozoasida

Family: Eimeriidae

Life cycle: There are three generations of meronts found in the proximal and distal colon. The prepatent period is 9 days and the patent period is 5–10 days. Sporulation time is 4 days.

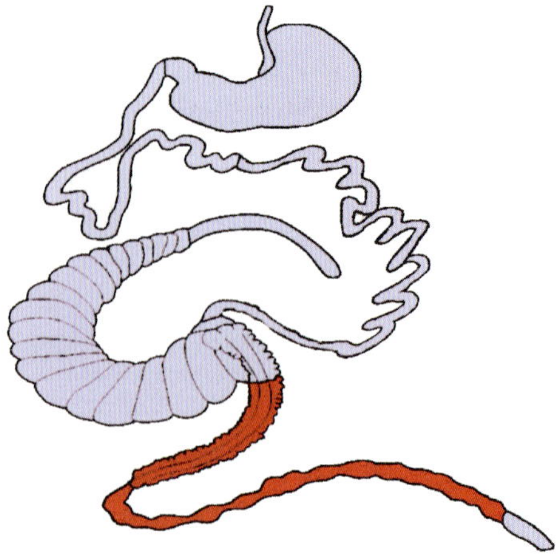

Fig. 9.11 Predilection site of *Eimeria piriformis*.

Geographical distribution: Worldwide

Pathogenesis and clinical signs: *E. piriformis* is mildly to moderately pathogenic. Infection causes anorexia, diarrhoea, weakness, weight loss and growth retardation, and in heavy infections can result in death.

Pathology: Endogenous stages are found in the wall of the large intestine on histopathology.

Entamoeba cuniculi

Predilection site: Caecum

Parasite sub-phylum: Sarcodina

Family: Endamoebidae

Description: Trophozoites are 20–30 μm in diameter. The cysts are 10–33 μm in diameter and contain a single nucleus.

Hosts: Rabbit

Life cycle: Trophozoites divide by binary fission. Before encysting the amoebae round up, become smaller and lay down a cyst wall. Each cyst has one nucleus. Amoebae emerge from the cysts and grow into trophozoites

Geographical distribution: Worldwide

Pathogenesis: Non-pathogenic

Retortamonas cuniculi

Synonym: *Embadomonas cuniculi*

Predilection site: Caecum

Parasite sub-phylum: Mastigophora

Family: Retortamonadorididae

Description: Trophozoites are ovoid, 7–13 × 5–10 µm, with an anterior flagella and a posterior trailing flagella emerging from the cytosomal groove and occasionally have a tail-like process. Cysts are pyriform or ovoid, 5–7 × 3–4 µm.

Hosts: Rabbit

Life cycle: Reproduction is by binary fission. Infection occurs by ingestion of the cyst stage.

Geographical distribution: Worldwide

Pathogenesis: Non-pathogenic

Diagnosis: Diagnosis is based on the identification of the characteristic trophozoites.

PARASITES OF THE RESPIRATORY SYSTEM

Several protostrongylid nematodes are found in the lungs of wild rabbits. These are listed in the parasite checklist at the end of the chapter.

Echinococcus granulosus

See Chapter 3 (Sheep and goats).

PARASITES OF THE LIVER

Capillaria hepatica

Synonym: *Callodium hepatica*, *Hepaticola hepatica*

Predilection site: Liver

Parasite class: Nematoda

Superfamily: Trichuroidea

Hosts: Rat, mouse, squirrel, rabbit and farmed mustelids; occasionally dog, cat and man

Taenia serialis

Synonym: *Coenurus serialis*

Predilection site: Small intestine (definitive host; intramuscular and subcutaneous connective tissue (intermediate host)

Parasite class: Cestoda

Family: Taeniidae

Final hosts: Dog, fox and other canids

Intermediate hosts: Rabbit, hare and rarely rodents and man.

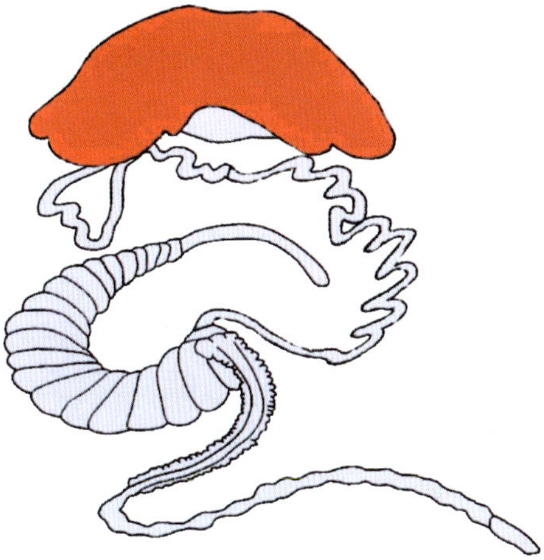

Fig. 9.12 Predilection site of *Eimeria stiedai*.

Geographical distribution: Worldwide

For more information see Chapter 6 (Dogs and cats).

Eimeria stiedai

Predilection site: Liver, bile ducts (Fig. 9.12)

Parasite class: Sporozoasida

Family: Eimeriidae

Life cycle: The sporozoites emerge from the sporocysts in the small intestine and migrate to the liver via the lymph vessels. Merogony occurs above the host cell nucleus in the epithelial cells of the bile ducts. The number of asexual generations is uncertain, but there appear to be at least six. In due course, some merozoites form macrogametes and others form microgamonts. The latter produce large numbers of comma-shaped biflagellate microgametes. These fertilise the macrogametes which lay down an oocyst wall, break out of the host cell and pass into the intestine with the bile, and then out in the faeces. The prepatent period is 18 days and the patent period 21–30 days. The sporulation time is 2–3 days.

Geographical distribution: Worldwide

Pathogenesis and clinical signs: This species, which occurs in the bile ducts, reaches the liver via the portal vein and then locates in the epithelium of the bile ducts where it results in a severe cholangitis. Grossly the liver is enlarged and studded with white nodules. Some of the symptoms seen are due to interference with liver function. Mild cases may be asymptomatic. In more severe infections the animals become inappetant and lose weight. There may be diarrhoea, jaundice, ascites

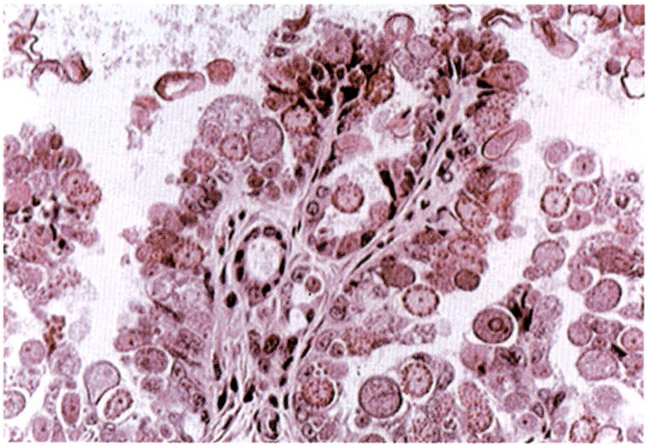

Fig. 9.13 Gamonts of *Eimeria stiedai* within hyperplastic bile duct epithelium.

and polyuria. The symptoms may become chronic, or death may occur in 21–30 days. Clinical signs of *E. stiedai* infection include wasting, diarrhoea, ascites and polyuria.

Pathology: The liver may become markedly enlarged, and white circular nodules or elongated cords may be visible. These nodules are sharply initially circumscribed, but later coalesce. The bile ducts are grossly enlarged and are filled with developing parasites. There is pronounced hyperplasia of the bile duct epithelial cells, and the epithelium is thrown into folds. Each cell contains one or more parasites (Fig. 9.13).

Other helminths found in the liver of wild rabbits are listed in the parasite checklist at the end of the chapter.

PARASITES OF THE CIRCULATORY SYSTEM

Rickettsia conorii

Common name: Boutonneuse fever, Mediterranean spotted fever, Indian tick typhus, east African tick typhus

Predilection site: Blood

Order: Rickettsiales

Family: Rickettsiaceae

For a more detailed description see Chapter 6 (Dogs and cats).

Hepatozoon cuniculi

Predilection site: Spleen

Parasite class: Sporozoasida

Family: Hepatozoidae

Description: Merocysts may reach 4–6 mm in diameter.

Hosts: Rabbit

Life cycle: The life cycle is unknown. Meronts are found in the spleen and gamonts within leucocytes.

Geographical distribution: Reported in Italy

Pathogenesis: Not known

PARASITES OF THE NERVOUS SYSTEM

Encephalitozoon cuniculi

Synonym: *Nosema cuniculi*

Predilection site: Blood

Class: Microsporasida

Family: Nosematidae

Description: Microsporidia are obligate, intracellular, spore-forming protozoa. Trophozoites are 2–2.5 × 0.8–1.2 μm in tissue sections or 4 × 2.5 μm in smears. Spores are about 2 μm long and contain a spirally coiled polar filament with four to five coils.

Hosts: Rabbit, dog, red fox (*Vulpes vulpes*), blue fox (*Alopex lagopus*), silver fox, cat, mouse, rat, man

Life cycle: The infective spore stages are highly resistant and can survive for many years. When spores are ingested, the polar tube is everted and when fully extended the sporoplasm passes through the tube and is innoculated into the cytoplasm of the host cell. There then follows a phase of multiplication by binary or multiple fission (merogony). This is followed by sporogony to form sporoblasts, which then mature into spores.

Geographical distribution: Worldwide

Pathogenesis: In rabbits, infection is very common causing granuloma formation in the kidneys, liver and brain. Infection in the brain causes convulsions, tremors, torticollis, ataxia, urinary incontinence, coma and death.

Clinical signs: Many infected rabbits are asymptomatic, although clinical signs such as head tilt, urinary incontinence, posterior paresis and anterior uveitis have been reported.

Diagnosis: Diagnosis in the live animal is difficult and is usually based on identifying the lesions on histopathology and observation of the organisms in Giemsa, Gram's or Goodpasture-carbol fuchsin stains. A serum ELISA test is available.

Pathology: In the rabbit, microscopic lesions consist of focal granulomas and pseudocysts in the brain and kidneys, with occasional severe, focal interstitial nephritis.

Epidemiology: Transplacental infection occurs in rabbits and rodents, but is probably rare with most infections in these animals acquired by ingestion of spores. Evidence suggests that in many countries, infection in rabbits is common.

Treatment: Treatment with benzimidazoles (fenbendazole, oxfendazole and albendazole) has been reported in rabbits. Fenbendazole is given at 20 mg/kg and albendazole 15 mg/kg for 28 days. Corticosteroids may suppress granulomata formation, and should be used with caution.

Control: Control in rabbits depends on testing individuals, isolation and treatment. The primary source of infection is urinary excretion and ingestion of spores. Strict hygiene should therefore be followed with raised food dishes and use of water bottles rather than bowls. Rabbits should not be housed in tiered hutches where urine contamination of cages below is common.

Notes: There are reports of *E. cuniculi* acting as a zoonosis, particularly in immunocompromised individuals.

PARASITES OF THE REPRODUCTIVE/UROGENITAL SYSTEM

No parasites of veterinary significance reported.

PARASITES OF THE LOCOMOTORY SYSTEM

Toxoplasma gondii

Predilection site: Muscle, lung, liver, reproductive system, central nervous system

Order: Sporozoasida

Family: Sarcocystiidae

Intermediate hosts: Any mammal, including man, or birds.

Final host: Cat, other felids

For more details see Chapter 3 (Sheep and goats).

Sarcocystis cuniculi

Predilection site: Muscle

Order: Sporozoasida

Family: Sarcocystiidae

Description: In the rabbit, the sarcocysts are elongate, compartmented and up to 5 mm × 5 mm. The cyst wall has numerous fine projections up to 11 μm long, packed into a tight pile. Metrocytes are 4–5 μm in diameter.

Final host: Cat

Intermediate host: Rabbit

Life cycle: Infection in the rabbit is by ingestion of sporocysts in cat faeces. Complete details of the merogony phase of development are not known. Ultimately, merozoites penetrate muscle cells where they encyst, giving rise to broad banana-shaped bradyzoites contained within a sarcocyst, which is the infective stage for the carnivorous final host.

Geographical distribution: Worldwide

Pathogenesis and clinical signs: Non-pathogenic.

Diagnosis: Diagnosis is made by microscopic identification of the characteristic cysts. They may be sometimes visible macroscopically.

Epidemiology: Little is known of the epidemiology, but it is clear that where cats are able to hunt or catch rabbits then transmission is likely. The longevity of the sporocysts shed in the faeces is not known.

Treatment and control: Not necessary

ECTOPARASITES

MITES

Psoroptes cuniculi

Synonym: *Psoroptes ovis*, *Psoroptes cervinus*, *Psoroptes bovis*, *Psoroptes equi*

Common name: Ear canker mite

Predilection site: Ears

Parasite class: Arachnida

Sub-class: Acari

Order: Acariformes

Sub-order: Sarcoptiformes (Astigmata)

Family: Psoroptidae

Description: Mites of the genus *Psoroptes* are non-burrowing mites, up to 0.75 mm in length and oval in shape (Fig. 3.43). All the legs project beyond the body margin. Its most important recognition features are the pointed mouthparts and the three-jointed pretarsi (pedicels) bearing funnel-shaped suckers (pulvilli).

Adult females have jointed pretarsi and pulvilli on the first, second and fourth pairs of legs and long, whip-like setae on the third pair. In contrast, the smaller adult males, which are recognisable by their copulatory suckers and paired posterior lobes, have pulvilli on the first three pairs of legs and setae on the fourth pair. The legs of adult females are approximately the same length, whereas in males the fourth pair is extremely short.

The *Psoroptes* mite described as *P. cuniculi* is found primarily in rabbits, where it is usually localised in the ears, causing ear mange (psoroptic otocariasis). *P. cuniculi* may also be found in the ears of sheep and horses, causing irritation and head shaking, and also in sheep associated with haematomas.

In adult *Psoroptes cuniculi,* the outer opisthosomal setae are, on average, slightly shorter than those seen in *P. ovis*. Nevertheless, the usefulness of this character is questionable, since there is considerable variation and overlap in the lengths of the setae between the two groups, and the mean length of the setae of mites is known to decrease with the age of a body lesion. It appears very likely that *P. cuniculi* is simply a host-adapted population of the species *P. ovis*.

Hosts: Rabbit, goat, sheep and horse

Life cycle: The eggs of *Psoroptes cuniculi* are relatively large (about 250 μm in length) and oval. The hexapod larva, which hatches from the egg, is about 330 μm long. The larva moults into a protonymph, the protonymph moults into a tritonymph and the tritonymph moults to become an adult. Egg, larval, protonymph and tritonymph stages and the adult pre-oviposition period each require a minimum of 2 days to be completed, giving a mean egg to adult time of about 10 days.

Geographical distribution: Worldwide

Pathogenesis: *Psoroptes cuniculi* localises in the ears, where the mites may occur at relatively low intensities, but occasionally proliferate causing severe mange in which the auditory canal may be completely blocked with greyish debris. If untreated, the infection may extend over the rest of the body with scabs, loss of hair and excoriation from scratching. The initial preclinical stages may last for several months, during which the infestation is difficult to spot and causes little obvious problems to the infested rabbit. Mites are non-burrowing and therefore are found only in exudate, not in tissue.

Clinical signs: In the initial stages of the infection, small skin scales appear deep in the ear canal. These yellow–grey scales can be relatively thick; they contain large numbers of parasites, mite eggs, skin cells and blood. If untreated the scales begin to crust and may eventually grow to a thickness of 10 mm and fill the ear in severe cases. Scratching behaviour and shaking of the head may occur, and scabs and loss of hair may be observed in the ears. Eventually the mites may spread out of the ear and over the rest of the body.

Diagnosis: A sample of scab should be taken from the infected area. When placed in a glass jar or beaker the highly mobile mites will leave the scab and start to migrate up the sides of the jar. Mites can then be collected and examined under a microscope for key features: oval outline, all legs projecting beyond the body margin, three-jointed pre-tarsus.

Pathology: At low population densities, little pathology may be evident. In a rapidly expanding population, however, there may be chronic erosive and proliferative eosinophilic dermatitis.

Epidemiology: When in its preclinical phase deep in the ear, transmission is uncommon. However once the infestation has spread transmission is more likely, primarily through physical contact but also may occur via the environment.

Treatment: Treatment is as for otodectic mange of cats and dogs. Insecticidal preparations such diazinon applied daily for 4 days, and repeated in 10 days have been found to be effective. Treatment with injected ivermectin is highly successful. The infected bedding should be burnt and the housing thoroughly disinfected. The crust will resolve itself, without the need to clean the ears, falling off approximately 10 days after the first treatment.

Control: All in-contact animals should be treated. The housing must be disinfected to prevent reinfection. Regular inspection of the animal, paying particular attention to the ears, should help to control the parasite and reduce the effects of subsequent infestations.

Cheyletiella parasitivorax

Common name: Rabbit fur mite

Predilection site: Most commonly found on the dorsum, above the tail and on the neck, but may occur all over the body.

Parasite class: Arachnida

Sub-class: Acari

Order: Acariformes

Sub-order: Trombidiformes (Prostigmata)

Family: Cheyletidae

Description: Adults are about 400 μm in length and ovoid (Fig. 9.14). They have blade-like chelicerae that are used for piercing their host, and short, strong, opposable palps with curved palpal claws. The palpal femur possesses a long, serrated dorsal seta. The body tends to be slightly elongated with a 'waist'. The

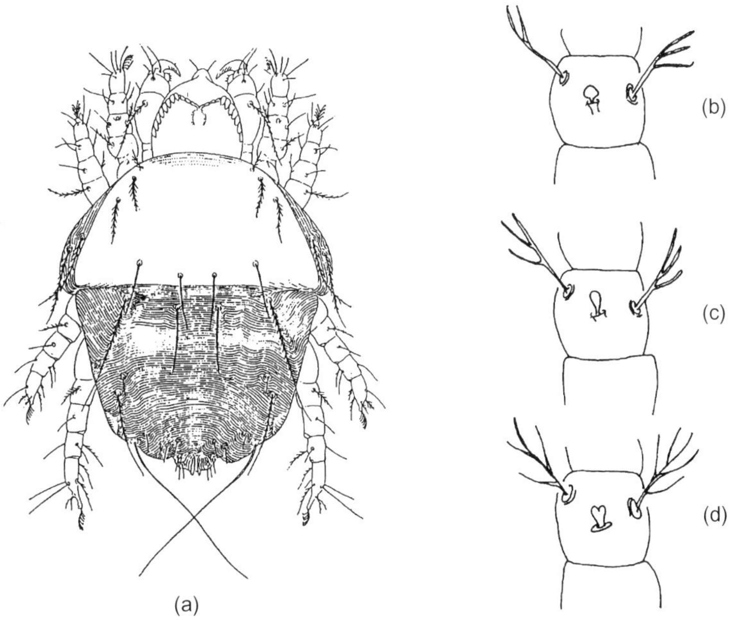

Fig. 9.14 (a) Adult female *Cheyletiella parasitovorax*, dorsal view (reproduced from Baker *et al.*, 1956). Genu of the first pair of legs of adult females of (b) *Cheyletiella parasitovorax*, (c) *Cheyletiella blakei* and (d) *Cheyletiella yasguri*.

legs are short; tarsal claws are lacking and the empodium is a narrow pad with comb-like pulvilli at the ends of the legs. Adults are highly mobile and are able to move about rapidly.

Three very similar species of *Cheyletiella* are of veterinary importance and are common: *Cheyletiella yasguri* on dogs, *C. blakei* on cats and *C. parasitivorax* on rabbits. All three species are morphologically very similar. However, the solenidion, on the genu of the first pair of legs, is described as globose in *C. parasitivorax,* conical in *C. blakei* and heart-shaped in *C. yasguri*. Nevertheless, this feature can vary in individuals and between life cycle stages, making precise identification difficult. Identification to genus and knowledge of the host is usually sufficient for diagnosis, but it is important to be aware of the potential for cross-transmission of the various species of *Cheyletiella* from other in-contact hosts.

Host: Rabbit

Life cycle: All developmental stages occur on the host animal. Eggs are glued to hairs 2–3 mm above the skin. A prelarva and then a larva develop within the egg, with fully developed octopod nymphs eventually emerging from the egg. The mites then moult through two nymphal stages before the adult stage is reached. The life cycle is completed in approximately two weeks. The mites live in the hair and fur, only visiting the skin to feed on lymph and other tissue fluids. They feed on these fluids by piercing the epidermis with their stylet-like chelicerae. Adults can survive for at least 10 days off the host without feeding, or longer in cool environments.

Geographical distribution: Worldwide, particularly North America, Europe, Asia, Australia and New Zealand.

Pathogenesis: *Cheyletiella* is relatively common in rabbits, but the mite is not highly pathogenic at low densities and is often found in young animals in good physical condition. It is a characteristic of the dermatitis caused by *Cheyletiella* that many skin scales are shed into the fur, giving it a powdery or mealy appearance, and the presence of moving mites among this debris has given it the common name of 'walking dandruff'. There is usually very little skin reaction or pruritus. In the rare severe case, involving much of the body surface, crusts are formed. *Cheyletiella parasitivorax* is capable of transmitting the myxomatosis virus among European rabbits.

Clinical signs: Infestation can result in eczema-like skin conditions and associated pruritus and hair loss. Severe cases may show serous exudate and extensive alopecia.

Diagnosis: In any case of excessive scurf or dandruff, *Cheyletiella* should be considered in the differential diagnosis. On parting the coat along the back, and especially over the sacrum, scurf will be seen, and if this is combed out on to dark paper the movement of mites will be detected among the debris. Skin scraping is not necessary as the mites are always on the skin surface or in the coat.

Pathology: The pathology of *Cheyletiella* infestation is poorly understood. In many cases there is very little skin reaction or pruritus. However, in severe cases rabbits may show alopecia with red, scaly skin and dermatitis with hyperkeratosis.

Epidemiology: *Cheyletiella parasitivorax* is a common fur mite of rabbits. It is highly contagious and can spread rapidly through rabbit colonies. Transmission is usually by direct contact with infested animals although the parasite can survive for over 10 days off the host, therefore bedding and housing can act as a source of infestation.

Treatment: Topical acaricides, such as pyrethrin and dichlorvos-containing sprays, are effective against *Cheyletiella*. Systemic treatment with ivermectin on three occasions, 7 days apart, is effective. Selamectin spot-on has also been used effectively. Fipronil should only be used with great caution because it has been associated with deaths in some cases.

Control: All in-contact animals should be treated, bedding replaced and housing disinfected.

Notes: Of all the mite infestations of domestic animals, this is one of the most readily transferable to humans. The mites can penetrate clothing and are easily transferred, even on short periods of contact. It is often found that when a positive diagnosis has been made on a pet, there is a history of persistent skin rash in the owner's family. In contrast to the condition in its natural hosts, the infestation in humans causes severe irritation and intense pruritus. The early sign is an erythema, which may progress to a vesicular and pustular eruption. Cases in humans invariably clear up spontaneously when the animal source has been treated.

Listrophorus gibbus

Common name: Fur mite

Predilection site: Skin

Parasite class: Arachnida

Sub-class: Acari

Order: Acariformes

Sub-order: Sarcoptiformes (Astigmata)

Family: Listrophoridae

Description: *L. gibbus* is a small, brown non-burrowing mite, occasionally present at low to moderate densities on domestic rabbits.

Table 9.2 Occasional mite parasites of rabbits.

Notoedres cati	See Chapter 6: Dogs and cats
Chorioptes bovis	See Chapter 2: Cattle
Sarcoptes scabiei	See Chapter 5: Pigs
Neotrombicula autumnalis	See Chapter 11: Facultative ectoparasites and arthropod vectors
Dermanyssus gallinae	See Chapter 7: Poultry and gamebirds

Host: Rabbit

Geographical distribution: Worldwide

Life cycle: It is an obligate parasite, completing all stages of the life cycle (egg, larva, nymph, adult) on the host.

Pathogenesis and clinical signs: *L. gibbus* may co-occur with *C. parasitivorax*. This mite is generally considered to be non-pathogenic and is found primarily on the back and abdomen.

Diagnosis: Hair plucks can be examined under a dissecting microscope or with hand lens for the characteristic brown mite or its eggs.

Treatment and control: As for *C. parasitivorax*

FLEAS

Spilopsyllus cuniculi

Common name: Rabbit flea, European rabbit flea

Predilection site: Ears

Parasite class: Insecta

Parasite order: Siphonaptera

Family: Pulicidae

Description: The rabbit flea, *S. cuniculi*, has both pronotal and genal ctenidia, the latter being composed of four to six oblique spines. Adults are dark brown, and females are, on average, 1 mm in length; males are slightly smaller. Eyes are present and the frons at the front of the head is rounded with the frontal tubercle conspicuous. There are two stout spines beneath the eye (Fig. 11.27).

Hosts: Rabbit, hare, dog, cat

Life cycle: The rabbit flea, *S. cuniculi*, occurs largely on the ears. It is more sedentary than most other species of flea and remains for long periods with its mouthparts embedded in the host. The life cycle of this species is believed to be mediated by host hormones imbibed with the host blood. The presence of progesterones inhibits or delays flea maturation. Following mating, the adult female rabbit ovulates and, about 10 days before parturition, the levels of oestrogens and corticosteroids in the blood increase. These hormones cause the fleas to attach tightly to their host and stimulate development of the eggs of the female flea. Reproductive hormones of the pregnant female host stimulate maturation of the ovaries and oocytes of feeding female fleas and testicular development in males. These fleas can only reproduce after feeding on a pregnant doe. This serves to synchronise the life cycles of the flea and its host and results in the emergence of adult fleas at the same time as a new litter of host animals are born. The adult fleas become ready to mate when the litter is born: an airborne kairomone emanating from the newborn rabbits and their urine boosts copulation. The hormones of the host also cause adult fleas to increase the rate of feeding and defecation by about five times. This provides an abundance of food in the burrow for the newly hatched larvae. Oviposition occurs soon after adults have transferred on to the newborn young. The larvae feed on organic matter in the nest debris and mature 15–45 days later when they infest the host littermates before they disperse from the burrow. Populations of *S. cuniculi* may increase dramatically during the rabbit breeding season.

Adult female fleas on bucks or non-pregnant does are more mobile and will move to pregnant does if able. The rise in ear temperatures during rabbit mating will also stimulate movement of fleas from one rabbit to another.

Geographical distribution: Worldwide

Pathogenesis: When rabbits are not breeding, the distribution of *S. cuniculi* is related to skin temperature, with fleas usually congregating on the ears. Because they assemble here in large numbers, the intensity of bites may cause considerable irritation and tissue damage.

The rabbit flea may also be found on cats and dogs, which hunt or frequent rabbit habitats. On these hosts they are commonly found on the face and attached to the pinneal margin.

Spilopsyllus cuniculi is the main vector of myxomatosis and it also transmits the non-pathogenic *Trypanosoma nabiasi*.

Clinical signs: These fleas may cause a great deal of irritation and tissue damage at the congregation sites on the ears.

Diagnosis: The fleas may be seen on the skin of the host animal, particularly around the ears. They have a more sedentary habit than most fleas, and will remain on the ear even when it is handled.

Epidemiology: The fleas can survive for up to 9 months at low temperatures without feeding. The main method of transmission is from the mother to her young.

Treatment: Imidacloprid may be used in rabbits to kill adult fleas on contact. Fipronil should only be used with extreme care in rabbits due to its potential toxicity.

Control: Not usually necessary. In case of repeated infestation the source should be identified and contact prevented; all in-contact animals should be treated; bedding should be replaced and housing disinfected.

Table 9.3 lists species of fleas which have also been found on rabbits. For more details see Chapter 11 (Facultative ectoparasites and arthropod vectors).

Table 9.3 Occasional flea parasites of rabbits.

Ctenocephalides felis	See Chapter 6: Dogs and cats
Ctenocephalides canis	See Chapter 6: Dogs and cats
Echidnophaga gallinacea	See Chapter 7: Poultry and gamebirds

FLIES

Lucilia sericata

Synonym: *Phaenicia sericata*

Common name: Greenbottle, sheep blowfly

Predilection site: Skin wounds

Parasite class: Insecta

Family: Calliphoridae

Description, adults: *Lucilia sericata* blowflies measure up to 10 mm in length and are characterised by a metallic greenish to bronze sheen.

Description, larvae: Larvae are smooth, segmented, and measure 10–14 mm in length. They possess a pair of oral hooks at the anterior extremity, and at the posterior peritremes bearing spiracles.

Hosts: Mainly sheep, but a range of other domestic and wild animals may be affected including humans.

Life cycle: Female blowflies lays clusters of 225–250 yellowish cream eggs on wounds or soiled hair, attracted by the its odour. The eggs hatch into larvae in about 12 hours. The larvae then feed, grow rapidly and moult twice to become fully mature maggots in 3 days.

Geographical distribution: Worldwide

Pathogenesis: Blowfly strike of domestic rabbits and occasionally other domestic mammals and birds may be very common, particularly if dirty, debilitated by clinical disease or wounded. Strike is a very serious condition in rabbits and death may result within a few days.

Clinical signs: Infested animals show extensive skin ulceration, shock, weakness, depression, lethargy and anorexia.

Diagnosis: This is based on the clinical signs and recognition of maggots in the lesion.

Pathology: Struck animals have a rapid increase in body temperature and respiratory rate. The animals show extensive tissue damage, become anaemic and suffer severe toxaemia.

Epidemiology: Predominantly a summer problem in temperate areas, but may occur all year round in more tropical regions.

Treatment: Once the problem is diagnosed, affected rabbits should be separated and the area surrounding the lesion clipped. Where possible larvae should be removed. The rabbit may require sedation, intravenous fluid therapy and analgesia. Ivermectin may be used to kill any remaining feeding larvae. Unless caught in its early stages the prognosis must be guarded, since myiasis can be extremely damaging to rabbits relatively quickly.

Control: To prevent fly-strike, formulations of pour-on cyromazine are available specifically for rabbits. They offer prevention for up to 8–10 weeks. Longer term steps should be taken to prevent diarrhoea and faecal contamination of the hair, either through worm control or diet as required.

Note: Several other species of blowfly or fleshfly may also strike rabbits in various parts of the world. The treatment is as described above for *L. sericata*.

Cuterebra

See Rats.

GUINEA PIGS

PARASITES OF THE DIGESTIVE SYSTEM

SMALL INTESTINE

Hymenolepis diminuta

See Rats and mice.

Rodentolepis nana

See Rats and mice.

Eimeria caviae

Predilection site: Large intestine

Parasite class: Sporozoasida

Family: Eimeriidae

Description: Oocysts are ellipsoidal or ovoid, smooth, brown, 13–26 × 12–23 μm, without a micropyle, or polar granule but with a residuum.

Life cycle: Following ingestion of oocysts, sporozoites enter the intestinal epithelium to become first-generation meronts. Following a further three merogony generations gamonts appear in epithelial cells of the large intestine leading the excretion of oocysts in the faeces. The prepatent period is about 7 days and the patent period approximately 4–5 days.

Geographical distribution: Worldwide

Pathogenesis and clinical signs: *E. caviae* is usually non-pathogenic but may occasionally cause diarrhoea and mortality. Clinical signs include unthriftiness, poor weight gain in young animals; droppings are slimy and contain blood.

Diagnosis: Diagnosis is based on identification of oocysts in the faeces in association with clinical and pathological findings.

Pathology: Lesions seen at postmortem occur in the mucosa of the colon and consist of small white, or pale yellow plaques and petechial haemorrhages. In severe infections the whole mucosa may be destroyed. There have also been reports of hepatomegaly with focal necrosis containing oocysts.

Epidemiology: Crowding and lack of good sanitation promote spread of coccidiosis. Breeding establishments and rescue centres are potential sources of infection. Older guinea pigs are generally immune from disease but may seed the environment with oocysts leading to infection in young animals that have no previous exposure.

Treatment: Information on treatment in the guinea pig is scanty, although by analogy with other host species, the use of sulphonamides, such as sulphamezathine, should be tried.

Control: Good sanitation and isolation are effective measures in preventing coccidiosis. If possible, guinea pigs should be housed on wire floor cages to reduce the incidence of infection. Standard disinfectants are ineffective against coccidial oocysts but ammonia-based products are effective.

Cryptosporidium wrairi

Predilection site: Small intestine

Parasite class: Sporozoasida

Family: Cryptosporidiidae

Description: Mature oocysts are ovoid, 4.8–5.6 × 4.0–5.0 µm (mean 5.40 × 4.6 µm), with a length:width ratio of 1.17. First-generation meronts are 3.4–4.4 µm when mature and contain eight merozoites; second-generation meronts contain four merozoites. Developing macrogametes are 4–7.0 µm in size.

Life cycle: Oocysts, each with four sporozoites, are liberated in the faeces. Following ingestion, the sporozoites invade the microvillous brush border of the enterocytes and the trophozoites rapidly differentiate in 3–4 days to form meronts with eight merozoites followed by a second merogony stage containing four merozoites. Gametogony follows after two generations of meronts usually around 13–15 days post infection. The prepatent period has not been reported.

Geographical distribution: Unknown

Pathogenesis and clinical signs: The infection has only been reported in small guinea pigs (weighing 200–300 g) and is not associated with diarrhoea or overt signs of disease. Clinical signs are usually inapparent.

Diagnosis: Oocysts may be demonstrated using Ziehl–Nielsen-stained faecal smears in which the sporozoites appear as bright red granules. Speciation of *Cryptosporidium* is difficult, if not impossible, using conventional techniques. A range of molecular and immunological techniques has been developed, that include the use of immunofluorescence (IF) or enzyme-linked immunosorbent assays (ELISA). More recently, DNA-based techniques have been used for the molecular characterisations of *Cryptosporidium* species.

Pathology: There may be chronic enteritis depending on the severity of infection. Lesions are usually focal when only limited areas of the intestine are affected. The organisms are more numerous in the posterior ileum and are distributed over the entire surface of the intestinal villi but are more numerous towards the tips and absent in the crypts.

Epidemiology: The primary route of infection is mainly direct animal-to-animal transmission by the faecal–oral route.

Treatment and control: Not required

Giardia intestinalis

See Chapter 6 (Dogs and cats).

LARGE INTESTINE

Paraspidodera uncinata

Predilection site: Large intestine

Parasite class: Nematoda

Superfamily: Ascaridoidea

Description, gross: Male worms are 16–17 mm and females 18–21 mm.

Description, microscopic: The egg is ellipsoidal, 43 × 31 µm

Host: Guinea pig

Life cycle: The life cycle is direct. Eggs passed in the faeces are infective after 3–5 days. When ingested they migrate to the caecum and colon and mature in about 45 days.

Geographical distribution: Worldwide

Pathogenesis and clinical signs: Generally considered non-pathogenic, although heavy infections may cause weight loss, debility and diarrhoea.

Diagnosis: Diagnosis is based on identification of eggs in the faeces or adult worms in the large intestine.

Epidemiology: This caecal worm occurs naturally in the caecum and colon of the wild guinea pig in South America and in laboratory guinea pigs around the world. Infection is usually associated with guinea pigs housed in outdoor runs.

Treatment and control: Piperazine at 3 g/l in the drinking water for 7 days is effective. Ivermectin at 200–500 µg given subcutaneously is also likely to be effective. Control is based on good hygiene and management.

A number of protozoa are found in the caecum of the guinea pig. All are considered non-pathogenic. *Entamoeba caviae* and *Tritrichomonas caviae* are common in the caeca of laboratory guinea pigs.

Entamoeba caviae

Predilection site: Caecum

Parasite class: Sarcodina

Family: Endamoebidae

Description: Trophozoites are 10–20 µm in diameter. The nucleus, when stained has a central or eccentric endostome with a ring of relatively coarse peripheral granules. The cysts, which are rare, are 11–17 µm in size and contain eight nuclei when mature.

Tritrichomonas caviae

Predilection site: Caecum

Parasite class: Zoomastigophorasida

Family: Trichomonadidae

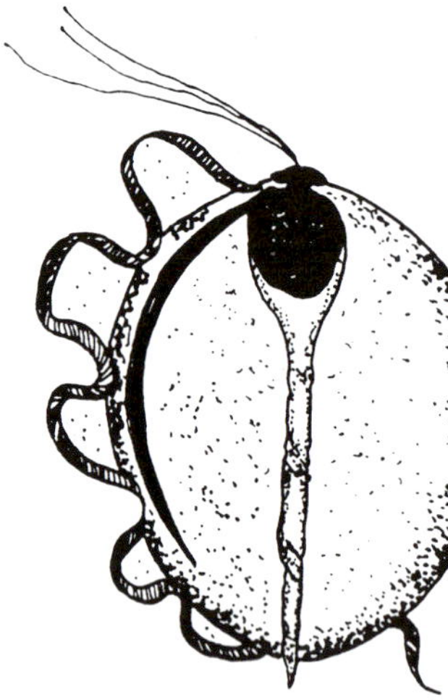

Fig. 9.15 *Tritrichomonas caviae.*

Description: The body is 10–22 μm long with a flat cylindrical nucleus, three anterior flagella and a prominent undulating membrane extending the length of the body (Fig. 9.15). The axostyle is well defined with a prominent costa.

Other species of flagellate protozoa found in the caecum of the guinea pig are shown in the host–parasite checklist at the end of this chapter.

PARASITES OF THE RESPIRATORY SYSTEM

No parasites of veterinary significance reported.

PARASITES OF THE LIVER

No parasites of veterinary significance reported.

PARASITES OF THE CIRCULATORY SYSTEM

No parasites of veterinary significance reported.

PARASITES OF THE NERVOUS SYSTEM

No parasites of veterinary significance reported.

PARASITES OF THE REPRODUCTIVE/ UROGENITAL SYSTEM

Klossiella cobayae

Predilection site: Kidney

Parasite class: Sporozoasida

Family: Klossiellidae

Description: The mature zygote is 30–40 μm in diameter and produces 30 or more sporocysts each containing about 30 sporozoites.

Host: Guinea pig

Life cycle: The life cycle is not clearly understood. Within epithelial cells of kidney tubules, trophozoites form meronts and merozoites. Merozoites enter the epithelial cells of the convoluted tubules of the kidney, where they form gamonts. Fertilised gametes are believed to develop into sporonts, which bud to form sporoblasts. Each of these sporoblasts undergoes successive divisions to form sporocysts that contain sporozoites. Mature sporocysts are surrounded by a thick wall and pass from the body in the urine. When ingested by another host, the sporozoites are released from the sporocyst, move to the kidney, where they enter epithelial cells and initiate the cycle.

Geographical distribution: Worldwide

Pathogenesis and clinical signs: Although usually considered non-pathogenic, a chronic to subacute nephritis with degenerative lesions has been described.

Diagnosis: Sporocysts may be detected in urine sediments or trophozoite stages may be found on postmortem in the kidney. The site and location are pathognomonic.

Pathology: Only heavily parasitised kidneys have gross lesions, which appear as tiny grey foci on the cortical surface. Microscopically these foci are areas of necrosis, with perivascular infiltration of inflammatory cells, especially lymphocytes, with an increase in interstitial fibroblasts.

Epidemiology: Sporocysts are passed in the urine and infection takes place by the ingestion of the sporulated sporocysts.

Treatment and control: Not required

PARASITES OF THE LOCOMOTORY SYSTEM

Toxoplasma gondii

See Parasites of the locomotory system of the rabbit.

PARASITES OF THE INTEGUMENT

No parasites reported.

ECTOPARASITES

LICE

Gyropus ovalis

Common name: Guinea pig louse

Predilection site: Skin, especially the ears and neck

Parasite class: Insecta

Parasite order: Phthiraptera

Parasite sub-order: Amblycera

Family: Gyropidae

Description: *Gyropus ovalis* is a chewing louse with club-shaped antennae positioned within grooves in the head (Fig. 9.16). It has a broad, rounded head with four-segmented maxillary palps and stout mandibles. The body is pale yellow in colour, oval in shape and 1–1.5 mm in length.

Hosts: Guinea pig and rodents

Life cycle: The life cycle is typical, with eggs giving rise to three nymphal stages followed by the reproductive adult. However, little precise detail is known.

Geographical distribution: Worldwide

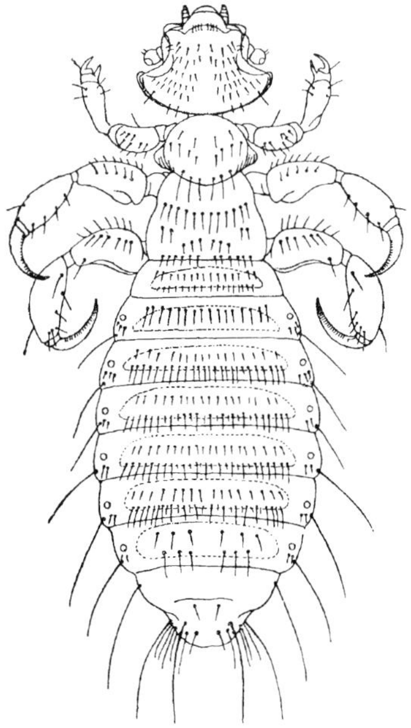

Fig. 9.16 Adult female *Gyropus ovalis* (from Séguy, 1944).

Pathogenesis: This species tears pieces of skin until blood pools and then feeds from these pools. Underlying skin may be dry or oily and thickened or crusty. Severely infected animals may show secondary bacterial infection and stress, including weight loss. Infestation often accompanies manifestations of poor health, such as internal parasitism, infectious disease, malnutrition and poor sanitation.

Clinical signs: The signs of infestation are variable. Light infestation may have no obvious effects, but pruritis, dermatitis, scratching and hair loss are usually evident at heavier parasite loads.

Diagnosis: The lice and their eggs can be seen on the skin of the host animal when the hair is parted.

Epidemiology: Infection occurs after direct contact with an infested host animal. Cross-contamination between different host species is possible if the animals have physical contact.

Treatment: Since lice spend their entire life on the host animal, control is readily achieved through the use of topical insecticides. Treatment of *G. ovalis* involves dusting of the guinea pig and bedding with carbaryl (5%) powder lightly once per week, dipping in 2.5% lime–sulphur solution once per weeks for 4–6 weeks, or treatment with ivermectin. However, since the eggs are quite resistant to most insecticides, repeat treatments 14 days apart are recommended to kill newly hatched nymphs. Imidacloprid is very safe and effective treatment for guinea pig lice and can be used on pregnant females and newly weaned young. One application lasts for 30 days.

Control: Prevention of infestation includes the use of clean bedding, which should be changed regularly. The cage and other areas where guinea pigs roam should be cleaned and rinsed thoroughly with a diluted bleach solution.

Notes: Closely related to the very similar *Gliricola porcelli.*

Gliricola porcelli

Common name: Guinea pig louse

Predilection site: Body fur

Parasite class: Insecta

Parasite order: Phthiraptera

Parasite sub-order: Amblycera

Family: Gyropidae

Description: A very similar species to *Gyropus ovalis.* However, *G. porcelli* is a slender, yellow louse, typically measuring 1–2 mm in length and 0.3–0.4 mm in

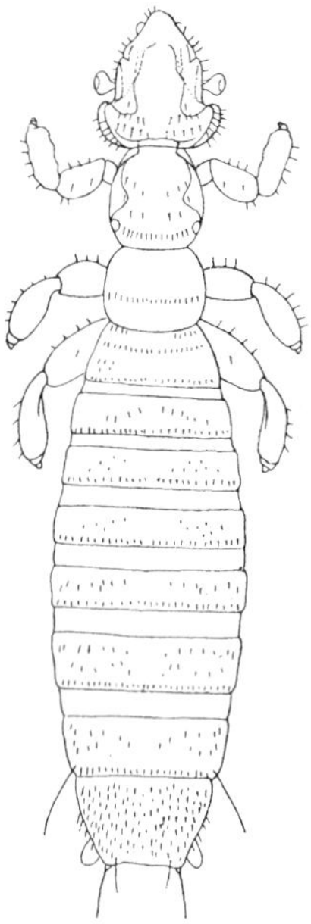

Fig. 9.17 Adult female *Gliricola porcelli* (from Séguy, 1944).

width (Fig. 9.17). The head is longer than it is wide and is rounded posteriorly. The maxillary palps have two segments. Antennae are four-segmented with pedicellate terminal segments and are almost concealed by the antennal fossae. The five pairs of abdominal spiracles are located ventrally within distinct, sclerotised spiraclar plates. The stout legs are modified for grasping hair but have no tarsal claws. A ventral furrow on the abdomen aids attachment to hair.

Hosts: Guinea pigs

Pathogenesis: As for *Gyropus ovalis*

Treatment and control: As for *Gyropus ovalis*

Trimenopon hispidium

Common name: Guinea pig louse

Predilection site: Hair

Parasite class: Phthiraptera

Sub-order: Amblycera

Family: Trimenoponidae

Pathogenesis: Lice of this genus are very rare and light infestations are easily overlooked. Occasional, heavy infestations may cause excessive scratching leading to alopecia and a roughened coat.

Hosts: Guinea pigs

Treatment and control: as for *Gyropus ovalis*

MITES

Chirodiscoides caviae

Synonym: *Campylochirus caviae*

Predilection site: Skin

Parasite class: Arachnida

Sub-class: Acari

Order: Acariformes

Sub-order: Sarcoptiformes (Astigmata)

Family: Listrophoridae

Description: Mites of the family Listrophoridae are soft-bodied, strongly striated with a distinct dorsal shield, and have mouthparts and legs modified for grasping hairs. Females of *Chirodiscoides caviae* are about 500 μm and males about 400 μm in length. The gnathosoma is distinctly triangular. The propodosomal sternal shield is strongly striated and used to clasp hairs (Fig. 9.18). The body is flattened dorsoventrally. All legs are slender and well developed, with legs I and II strongly modified for clasping to hair.

Hosts: Guinea pigs

Life cycle: *Chirodiscoides caviae* spends its entire life on the hair of the host rather than on the skin, feeding at the base of the hair and gluing its eggs to the hairs. The life cycle is typical: egg, hexapod larva, followed by octopod protonymph, tritonymph and adult. All developmental stages occur on the host. The entire life cycle requires approximately 14 days.

Geographical distribution: Worldwide

Pathogenesis: *Chirodiscoides caviae* is commonly found on guinea pigs. Light infestations probably have little effect and are easily overlooked. The mites may cause inflammation, scaling, crusting and pruritic dermatitis, leading to scratching and alopecia.

Clinical signs: Subclinical cases may be asymptomatic; clinical cases show pruritus and alopecia usually along the posterior trunk of the body.

Diagnosis: For confirmatory diagnosis, coat brushings must be examined; *C. caviae* are found only in the fur.

Epidemiology: New hosts are infected by contact with infected individuals.

Treatment: Systemic treatment with ivermectin on three occasions, 7 days apart, may be effective.

Control: All in-contact animals should be treated and the cage or housing should be cleaned.

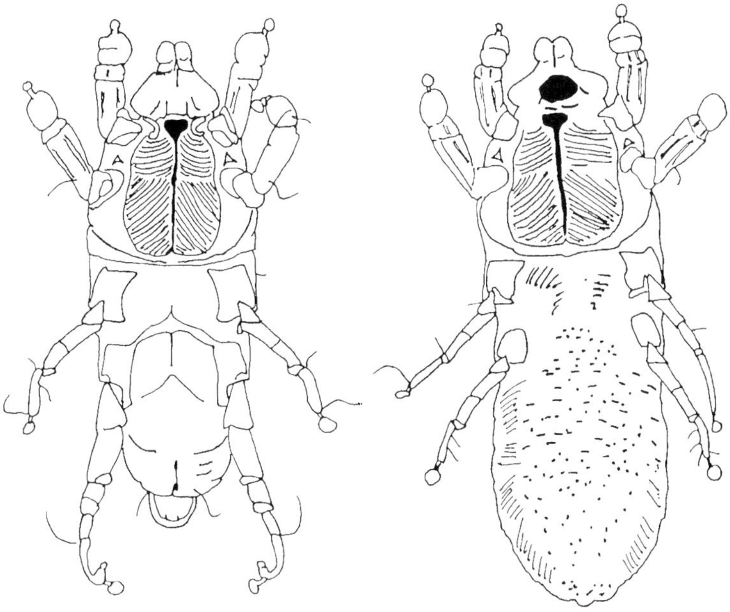

Fig. 9.18 Adults of *Chirodiscoides caviae*. (a) Male ventral view. (b) Female ventral view.

Trixicarus caviae

Common name: Guinea pig mite

Predilection site: Skin, body

Parasite class: Arachnida

Sub-class: Acari

Order: Acariformes

Sub-order: Sarcoptiformes (Astigmata)

Family: Sarcoptidae

Description: *Trixicarus caviae* superficially resembles *S. scabiei* (Fig. 9.19). The dorsal striations of the idiosoma of *T. caviae* are similar to those of *S. scabiei* (Table 9.4). However, the dorsal scales, which break the striations, are more sharply pointed and the dorsal setae are simple and not spine-like. Like *N. cati*, the anus is located on the dorsal surface. *Trixicarus caviae* is also smaller than *S. scabiei* and similar in size to *N. cati*; females are about 240 μm in length and 230 μm in breadth.

Hosts: Guinea pigs

Life cycle: The life cycle is believed to be similar to that of *S. scabiei*.

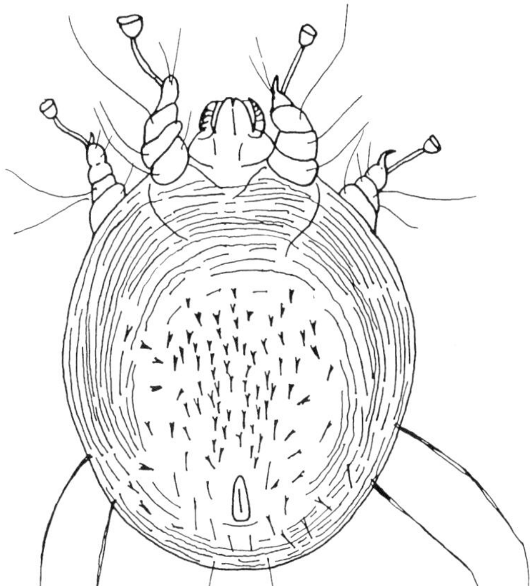

Fig. 9.19 Adult female of *Trixicarus caviae* (dorsal view).

Table 9.4 Differentiation between adult female *Sarcoptes scabiei*, *Notoedres cati* and *Trixicarus caviae*.

Parameter	*Sarcoptes scabiei*	*Notoedres cati*	*Trixicarus caviae*
Length (μm)	400–430	225–250	230–240
Anus position	Terminal	Dorsal	Dorsal
Dorsal setae	Some stout dorsal spines	All dorsal setae simple (not spine-like)	All dorsal setae simple (not spine-like)
Dorsal scales	Many, pointed	Few, rounded	Many, pointed

Geographical distribution: Originated in South America but has now spread worldwide.

Pathogenesis: These are burrowing mites, and the burrowing activity results in irritation, inflammation and pruritus, causing biting, scratching and rubbing of the infested areas and leading to alopecia. The infestation spreads quickly from the initial lesions to cause more generalised mange. Death may occur within 3–4 months of infestation. Transmission is by close physical contact and from mother to offspring.

Clinical signs: Infestation causes irritation, biting, scratching, rubbing and general restlessness.

Diagnosis: Confirmatory diagnosis is by examination of skin scrapings for the presence of mites. However, since these are sometimes difficult to demonstrate, a negative finding should not preclude a tentative diagnosis of mange and initiation of treatment.

Pathology: Affected areas display marked acanthosis and hyperkeratosis and may become secondarily infected with bacteria.

Treatment: Ivermectin may be administered twice at 7- to 10-day intervals.

Control: All bedding must be replaced, and housing and the guinea pig's local environment thoroughly cleaned.

For further details about *Sarcoptes* mites, see Chapter 5 (Pigs).

Psoroptes cuniculi

Synonym: *Psoroptes ovis*, *Psoroptes cervinus*, *Psoroptes bovis*, *Psoroptes equi*

Common name: Ear canker mite

Predilection site: Ears

Parasite class: Arachnida

Sub-class: Acari

Order: Acariformes

Sub-order: Sarcoptiformes (Astigmata)

Family: Psoroptidae

For detail see Rabbits

Guinea pigs may also be affected by the cat flea, *Ctenocephalides felis*. For details see, Chapter 11 (Facultative ectoparasites and arthropod vectors).

RATS AND MICE

PARASITES OF THE DIGESTIVE SYSTEM

SMALL INTESTINE

Nippostrongylus brasiliensis

Synonym: *Nippostrongylus muris*, *Heligmosomum muris*

Predilection site: Small intestine

Parasite class: Nematoda

Superfamily: Trichostrongyloidea

Description, gross: Adults are filiform and reddish in colour; males measure 2.1–4.5 mm and females 2.5–6 mm.

Description, microscopic: Eggs are ellipsoidal, thin-shelled and measure $52–63 \times 28–35$ μm.

Hosts: Rat, mouse, hamster, gerbil, rabbit, chinchilla

Life cycle: The life cycle is direct and typically trichostrongyloid. Infection is usually percutaneous and larvae migrate via the lungs. Worms are adult by around 5 days post infection and are usually short-lived. The prepatent period is 5–6 days.

Geographical distribution: Worldwide

Pathogenesis and clinical signs: Initial light infections cause inflammation of the skin, lungs and intestines. Severe infections cause verminous pneumonia and death.

Diagnosis: Diagnosis depends on the identification of the eggs in faeces or adult worms in the intestine on postmortem.

Epidemiology: This parasite is common in wild rats but can become problematical in animal colonies where management and sanitation are poor.

Treatment: Piperazine in the drinking water (5 g/l) and ivermectin by injection are effective.

Control: In laboratory colonies of rodents, eradication depends on strict hygiene and good management.

Nematospiroides dubius

Synonym: *Heligmosomoides polygyrus*

Predilection site: Small intestine

Parasite class: Nematoda

Superfamily: Trichostrongyloidea

Description, gross: Adults are long red worms 0.6–1.3 cm long, with a coiled tail.

Description, microscopic: Worms possess a cephalic vesicle. Eggs are ovoid and measure 68×43 μm.

Hosts: Rat, mouse

Life cycle: Typically trichostrongyloid with infection via the L_3. The prepatent period is 9 days and patency may last for up to 8 months.

Geographical distribution: North America, Europe

Pathogenesis: Infections are usually asymptomatic but may produce small cysts in the intestinal wall.

Diagnosis: Identification of the eggs in faeces or the adult worms in the small intestine.

Epidemiology: Internal autoinfection occurs in humans; but infection in rodents usually involves an intermediate host.

Treatment and control: As for *N. brasiliensis*

Notes: *N. dubius* is widely used as a laboratory model for nematode infection studies.

Rodentolepis nana

Synonym: *Hymenolepis nana*, *Hymenolepis fratern*, *Vampirolepis nana*

Common name: Dwarf tapeworm

Predilection site: Small intestine

Parasite class: Cestoda

Family: Hymenolepididae

Description, gross: The tapeworm is small, 2.5–4 cm in length and has a characteristically slender strobila with about 200 segments.

Description, microscopic: The scolex has four suckers and is armed with a retractable rostellum bearing a single row of 20–30 hooks. The genitalia are single and the segments are wider than they are long. Eggs are small, round or oval in shape, $44–62 \times 30–55$ μm, and contain a lemon-shaped embryophore with protruding polar plugs and an embryo with three small hooks.

Final hosts: Rat, mouse, birds, man

Intermediate hosts: Flour beetles (*Tenebrio*) or fleas

Life cycle: The life cycle can be direct, the cysticercoids developing in the villi of the small intestine of the final host and then emerging to develop to the adult tapeworm in the intestinal lumen. Otherwise flour beetles or fleas can serve as intermediate hosts.

Geographical distribution: Worldwide. Common in Asia, Africa, South America and in parts of southern Europe.

Pathogenesis and clinical signs: Infections in laboratory rodents are relatively uncommon and usually asymptomatic, although heavy infestations can cause weight loss, vomiting and occasionally obstruction of the intestine. Heavy infections in humans may cause enteritis, anorexia and anal pruritis.

Diagnosis: Identification of the eggs in faeces or the adult worms in the small intestine.

Epidemiology: Internal autoinfection occurs in humans; but infection in rodents usually involves an intermediate host. Under conditions of poor hygiene infected rodents will contaminate food with their faeces, leading to human infection. In addition such an environment will support the intermediate hosts. Human prevalence is highest in children.

Treatment: Not usually indicated. Niclosamide mixed in powdered feed at 10 mg/100 mg bodyweight for two 7-day periods, 1 week apart, has been reported to be effective; or praziquantel (5–10 mg/kg) repeated in 10 days.

Control: In laboratory colonies of rodents, eradication depends on strict hygiene, and elimination of potential intermediate hosts.

Notes: *Rodentolepis nana* is of peripheral veterinary importance in that it is a common tapeworm of man and of laboratory and wild rodents. This is the only species of tapeworm for which an intermediate host is not required.

Hymenolepis diminuta

Common name: Rat tapeworm

Predilection site: Small intestine

Parasite class: Cestoda

Family: Hymenolepididae

Description, gross: A small tapeworm, about 20–60 mm in length

Description, microscopic: The rostellum does not possess hooks. The eggs are larger than *R. nana*, measuring about 60 μm, and the outer membrane is darker and may be striated.

Final hosts: Rat, mouse, man

Intermediate hosts: Larvae, nymphs and adults of various species of moths, cockroaches, fleas, beetles, millipedes and moths

All other details as for *R. nana*.

Coccidia

Eimeria nieschulzi

Synonym: *Eimeria halli*

Predilection site: Small intestine

Parasite class: Sporozoasida

Family: Eimeriidae

Description: Oocysts are ellipsoidal or ovoid, smooth, colourless or yellowish, 16–26 × 13–21 μm, without a micropyle, or oocyst residuum but with a polar granule. Sporocysts are elongate, ovoid and have a small Stieda body and residuum. Sporozoites contain a central nucleus with an eosinophilic globule at each end.

Hosts: Rat (*Rattus norvegicus*, *Rattus rattus*)

Life cycle: Infection is by ingestion of sporulated oocysts. First-generation meronts occur after 36 hours followed by three further merogony generations and gametogony within the epithelial cells of the small intestine. The prepatent period is 7 days and patency 4–5 days. Sporulation time is approximately 72 hours.

Geographical distribution: Worldwide

Pathogenesis and clinical signs: *E. nieschulzi* primarily affects young animals causing weakness, diarrhoea and emaciation. Animals that recover are immune but disease may occur in adults under periods of stress.

Diagnosis: Diagnosis is based on identification of oocysts in the faeces in association with clinical and pathological findings.

Epidemiology: Crowding and lack of good sanitation promote spread of coccidiosis.

Treatment: None of the available anticoccidials have been reported as effective in the rat.

Control: Infection is usually self-limiting in the individual and colony. Good sanitation and isolation are effective measures in preventing coccidiosis. Wherever possible, rats should be housed on wire floor cages to reduce the incidence of infection. Standard disinfectants are ineffective against coccidial oocysts but ammonia-based products are effective.

Eimeria falciformis

Predilection site: Small and large intestine

Parasite class: Sporozoasida

Family: Eimeriidae

Description: Oocysts are broadly ellipsoidal, smooth, colourless, 14–26 × 13–24 μm, without a micropyle or oocyst residuum. Sporocysts are elongate, have a Stieda body and residuum. Sporozoites lie longitudinally within the sporocyst.

Host: Mouse (*Mus muscularis*)

Life cycle: Infection is by ingestion of sporulated oocysts. The number of merogony stages has not been determined. The prepatent period is 4 days.

Geographical distribution: Worldwide

Pathogenesis and clinical signs: Mild infections have little effect, but severe ones cause anorexia, diarrhoea and sometimes death.

Diagnosis: Diagnosis is based on identification of oocysts in the faeces in association with clinical and pathological findings.

Pathology: Catarrhal enteritis, haemorrhage and epithelial sloughing have been reported.

Epidemiology: Crowding and lack of good sanitation promote spread of coccidiosis. Breeding establishments and laboratory mice are potential sources of infection. In one study, 8 out of 10 conventional laboratory mouse colonies were found to be infected.

Treatment: None of the available anticoccidials have been reported as effective in the mouse.

Control: Control depends on good hygiene and isolation as effective measures in preventing coccidiosis. Wherever possible, laboratory mice should be housed on wire floor cages to reduce the incidence of infection. Standard disinfectants are ineffective against coccidial oocysts but ammonia-based products are effective. Deriving a new colony by Caesarean section can eliminate infection.

Several other species of coccidia are found in rats and mice worldwide but are generally considered non-pathogenic and control measures are not usually required.

Eimeria hasei

Predilection site: Unknown

Parasite class: Sporozoasida

Family: Eimeriidae

Description: Oocysts are ellipsoidal or ovoid, ellipsoidal or spherical, 16–20 × 12–17 μm, without a micropyle, or oocyst residuum but with a polar granule. Sporocysts are 9 × 5 μm.

Hosts: Rat (*Rattus rattus*)

Geographical distribution: Russia

Eimeria nochti

Predilection site: Unknown

Parasite class: Sporozoasida

Family: Eimeriidae

Description: Oocysts are ovoid, 15–24 × 12–22 μm, without a micropyle, oocyst residuum or polar granule.

Hosts: Rat (*Rattus rattus*, *Rattus norwegicus*)

Geographical distribution: Russia

Eimeria ratti

Predilection site: Unknown

Parasite class: Sporozoasida

Family: Eimeriidae

Description: Oocysts are cylindrical to ovoid, 16–28 × 15–16 μm, without a micropyle, oocyst residuum but with a polar granule.

Hosts: Rat (*Rattus rattus*)

Geographical distribution: Russia

Eimeria musculi

Predilection site: Unknown

Parasite class: Sporozoasida

Family: Eimeriidae

Description: Oocysts are spherical, smooth, greenish, 21–26 μm in diameter, without a micropyle or oocyst residuum. Sporocysts are broadly ovoid.

Hosts: Mouse (*Mus muscularis*)

Geographical distribution: Russia, Kazakhstan

Eimeria scheuffneri

Predilection site: Unknown

Parasite class: Sporozoasida

Family: Eimeriidae

Description: Oocysts are ellipsoidal, smooth, colourless or yellowish, 18–23 × 13–16 μm, without a micropyle or oocyst residuum. Sporocysts are ovoid.

Hosts: Mouse (*Mus muscularis*)

Geographical distribution: Russia

Eimeria krijgsmanni

Predilection site: Unknown

Parasite class: Sporozoasida

Family: Eimeriidae

Description: Oocysts are cylindrical, smooth, colourless, 18–26 × 15–16 μm, without a micropyle or oocyst residuum. Sporocysts are ovoid.

Hosts: Mouse (*Mus muscularis*)

Geographical distribution: Russia, Kazakhstan

Eimeria keilini

Predilection site: Unknown

Parasite class: Sporozoasida

Family: Eimeriidae

Description: Oocysts are ellipsoidal, smooth, yellowish, 24–32 × 18–121 μm, without a micropyle or oocyst residuum.

Hosts: Mouse (*Mus muscularis*)

Geographical distribution: Russia

Eimeria hindlei

Predilection site: Unknown

Parasite class: Sporozoasida

Family: Eimeriidae

Description: Oocysts are ovoid, smooth, greenish, 22–27 × 18–21 μm, without a micropyle or oocyst residuum.

Hosts: Mouse (*Mus muscularis*)

Geographical distribution: Russia

Cryptosporidium muris

Predilection site: Small intestine

Parasite class: Sporozoasida

Family: Cryptosporidiidae

Description: Oocysts are small, ovoid, 7.4 × 5.6 μm and contain four free sporozoites.

Trophozoites attached to the surface of a gland cell consist of a small amount of cytoplasm with a nucleus, and often appear to be surrounded by a cyst wall (peritrophic membrane). The maturing first-generation meronts reach a maximum size of 7 × 6 μm and contain eight merozoites. Microgametocytes are 5 × 4 μm and contain 16 microgametes; macrogametocytes are 7 × 5 μm.

Hosts: Rat, mouse, hamster, squirrel, Siberian chipmunk, wood mouse (*Apodemus sylvaticus*), bank vole (*Clethrionomys glareolus*), *Dolichotis patagonum*, rock hyrax, Bactrian camel, mountain goat, man and cynomolgus monkey

Life cycle: Oocysts, each with four sporozoites, are liberated in the faeces. Following ingestion, the sporozoites invade the microvillous brush border of the gastric glands and the trophozoites rapidly differentiate to form meronts with four to eight merozoites. Gametogony follows after two generations of meronts and oocysts are produced in 10–18 days post infection.

Geographical distribution: Worldwide

Pathogenesis and clinical signs: Infections in rodents appear to cause few pathogenic effects and infections are usually asymptomatic.

Diagnosis: Oocysts may be demonstrated using Ziehl–Nielsen-stained faecal smears in which the sporozoites appear as bright red granules. Speciation of *Cryptosporidium* is difficult, if not impossible, using conventional techniques. A range of molecular and immunological techniques has been developed, that include the use of ELISA. More recently, DNA-based techniques have been used for the molecular characterisations of *Cryptosporidium* species.

Pathology: In heavy infections there may be large numbers of parasites within the gastric glands of the stomach (pars glandularis) with meronts and gamonts extending from the isthmus down to the base of each gland (Fig. 9.20). Infection results in thickening of the glandular mucosa with some glands becoming dilated and hypertrophied, and parasitised glands lined with undifferentiated cells.

Epidemiology: Transmission appears to be mainly by the faecal–oral route.

Treatment and control: Not required

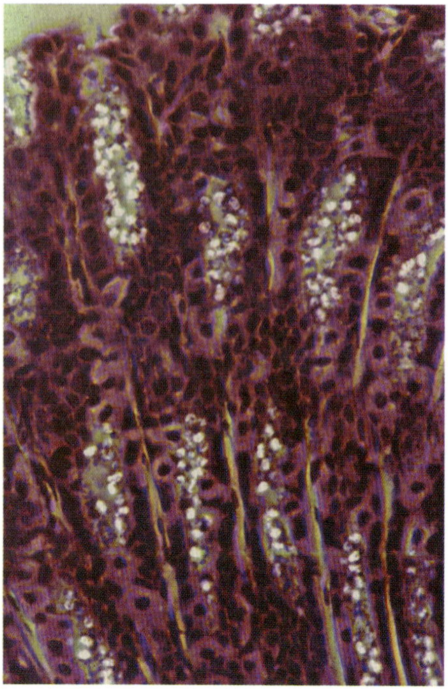

Fig. 9.20 *Cryptosporidium muris* in gastric mucosa of mouse.

Other protozoa

Giardia muris

Predilection site: Small intestine

Parasite class: Zoomastigophorasida

Family: Diplomonadidae

Description: The trophozoite has a pyriform to ellipsoidal, bilaterally symmetrical body; 7–13 μm long by 5–10 μm wide. The dorsal side is convex and there is a large sucking disk on the ventral side. There are two anterior nuclei, two slender axostyles, eight flagellae in four pairs and a pair of small and rounded median bodies.

Hosts: Rodents (mouse, rat, hamster)

Life cycle: The life cycle is simple and direct, the trophozoite stage dividing by binary fission to produce further trophozoites. Intermittently, trophozoites encyst forming resistant cyst stages that pass out in the faeces of the host.

Geographical distribution: Worldwide

Pathogenesis and clinical signs: Infections are generally asymptomatic but have been reported to cause chronic enteritis in young mice.

Diagnosis: *Giardia* cysts can be detected in faeces by a number of methods. Traditional methods of identification involve direct examination of faecal smears, or faecal concentration by formalin-ethyl acetate or zinc sulphate methods and subsequent microscopic examination. It is generally recommended that three consecutive samples be examined as cysts are excreted intermittently.

Pathology: The pathology has not been described. There may be villous atrophy, crypt hypertrophy and an increased number of intraepithelial lymphocytes. Trophozoites may be seen between villi, attached by their concave surface to the brush border of epithelial cells.

Epidemiology: Limited epidemiological studies suggest that direct animal-to-animal contact and faecal contamination are the most likely methods of transmission, although water contamination can also be considered as a possible route.

Treatment and control: Metronidazole at 0.5% in the drinking water for 10 days is reported to be effective. As infection is transmitted by the faecal–oral route, good hygiene and prevention of faecal contamination of feed and water are essential.

Spironucleus muris

Synonym: *Hexamita muris, Octomitus muris, Syndyomita muris*

Predilection site: Small intestine, caecum

Parasite class: Zoomastigophorasida

Family: Diplomonadidae

Description: The body is pyriform, 7–9 × 2–3 μm with two nuclei near the anterior end, and six anterior and two posterior flagella. There is no cytostome.

Hosts: Mouse, rat, hamster

Pathogenesis and clinical signs: Infection causes enteritis and diarrhoea in laboratory rodents. With chronic infections there is weight loss and listlessness and diarrhoea is uncommon.

Diagnosis: Identification of characteristic trophozoites in mucosal smears or on histopathology. Cysts may be seen in fresh faecal smears or in smears stained with Giemsa.

Pathology: Lesions are generally confined to the anterior small intestine with inflammation of the duodenum, and the duodenal crypts are cystic and filled with trophozoites of *S. muris*.

Epidemiology: Infection is common in some rodent colonies. Transmission presumably occurs by ingestion of trophozoites or cysts from faeces or by faecal contamination.

Treatment and control: Control relies mainly on good hygiene and management in rodent colonies and culling of animals with symptoms of diarrhoea unresponsive to treatment, or those showing chronic weight loss.

LARGE INTESTINE

Pinworms

Life cycle: The life cycle is direct. Females deposit embryonated eggs on the perineal skin. Infection occurs in three ways:

1. Directly by ingestion of embryonated eggs from the perineum
2. Indirectly with food
3. By retro-infection when eggs hatch in the perineal region and migrate back via the anus.

Pathogenesis and clinical signs: Pinworms are relatively common but non-pathogenic parasites in the large intestine of laboratory rodents.

Diagnosis: Diagnosis is based on identification of oocysts in the faeces.

Epidemiology: Crowding and lack of good sanitation promote spread of infection.

Treatment: Treatment can be with either piperazine (4–7 g/ml) given as three separate 7-day courses in drinking water; or ivermectin at 0.4 mg/kg by injection or orally twice 5 days apart; or fenbendazole at 0.1% in feed for 3–4 weeks.

Control: Eradication is extremely difficult and repeat anthelmintic treatment may be required.

Notes: Human infections have been reported with *Syphacia* spp in laboratory workers.

Syphacia obvelata

Common name: Mouse pinworm

Predilection site: Caecum, colon

Parasite class: Nematoda

Superfamily: Oxyuroidea

Desription, gross: Small worms, up to 6 mm in size; male are 1–1.5 mm, and females 3.4–6 mm.

Desription, microscopic: The mouth has three distinct lips without a buccal capsule.The oesophagus has a pre-bulbular swelling and a posterior globular bulb. Small cervical alae are present. Egg are asymmetrically flattened, larvated and larger than those of *S. muris*, measuring 118–153 × 33–55 μm (Fig. 9.21).

Hosts: Mouse, rat

Geographical distribution: Worldwide

Aspicularis tetraptera

Common name: Mouse pinworm

Predilection site: Caecum, colon

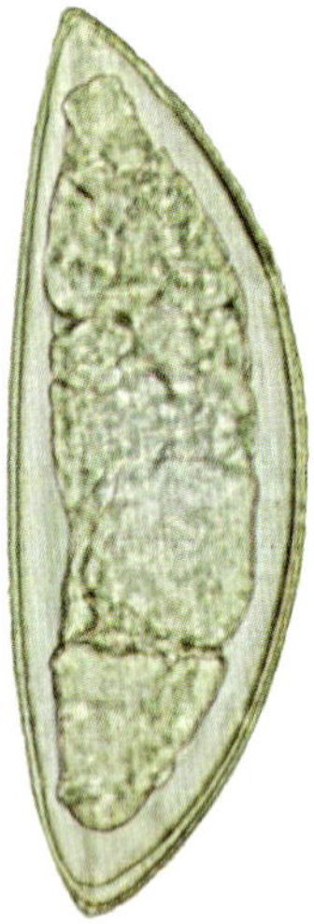

Fig. 9.21 Egg of *Syphacia obvelata*.

Parasite class: Nematoda

Superfamily: Oxyuroidea

Description, gross: Small worms, males are 2–4 mm, and females 3–4 mm.

Description, microscopic: The oesophageal bulb is oval and the oesophagus club-shaped. Broad cervical alae are present. Egg are asymmetrically flattened, larvated and larger than those of *S. muris*, measuring 89–93 × 36–42 μm.

Hosts: Mouse, rat

Geographical distribution: Worldwide

Life cycle: The life cycle differs from *Syphacia* in that the eggs are passed in the faeces and are not found on the perineum. Infection is by ingestion of infected eggs.

Syphacia muris

Common name: Rat pinworm

Predilection site: Caecum, colon

Parasite class: Nematoda

Superfamily: Oxyuroidea

Description, gross: Small worms, up to 4 mm in size; males are 1.2–1.3 mm, and females 2.8–4 mm.

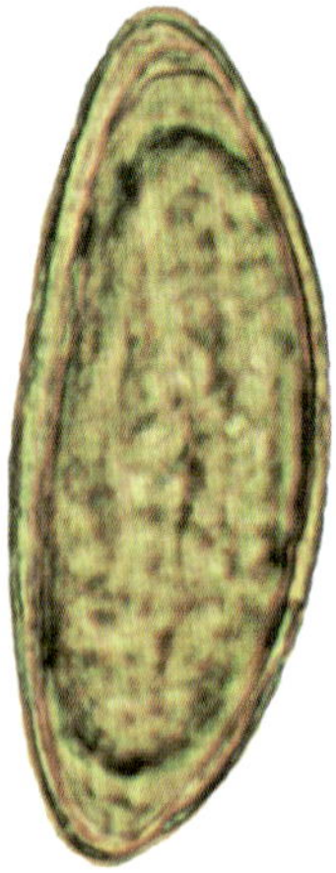

Fig. 9.22 Egg of *Syphacia muris*.

Description, microscopic: Eggs are asymmetrically flattened, larvated and measure 72–82 × 25–36 μm (Fig. 9.22).

Hosts: Rat, mouse

Others

Trichuris muris

Common name: Whipworms

Predilection site: Large intestine

Parasite class: Nematoda

Superfamily: Trichuroidea

Description, microscopic: Eggs are lemon-shaped, 67–70 × 31–34 μm, with two protruding polar plugs.

Hosts: Rat, mouse

Eimeria separata

Predilection site: Large intestine

Parasite class: Sporozoasida

Family: Eimeriidae

Description: Oocysts are ellipsoidal or ovoid, smooth, colourless or yellowish, 10–19 × 10–17 μm, without a micropyle or oocyst residuum, but with one to three polar granules. Sporocysts are ellipsoidal and have a small Stieda body and residuum.

Hosts: Rat (*Rattus norvegicus*)

Geographical distribution: North America, Europe, Asia, Africa

Entamoeba muris

Predilection site: Large intestine

Parasite class: Sarcodina

Family: Endamoebidae

Description: Trophozoites are 8–30 μm long. The nucleus, when stained, has a central or eccentric endostome with a ring of relatively coarse peripheral granules. The cysts are 9–20 μm in size and contain eight nuclei when mature.

Hosts: Rat, house mouse, golden hamster, wild rodents

Tritrichomonas muris

Predilection site: Large intestine

Synonym: *Trichomonas criceti*

Parasite class: Zoomastigophorasida

Family: Trichomonadidae

Description: The body is pyriform 12–20 μm long and there are three anterior flagella, which arise from a conspicuous blepharoplast. The undulating membrane is prominent and extends the length of the body in ribbon-like folds bounded by a thick marginal filament, which extends beyond the body as a free trailing flagellum. The costa is well developed and the axostyle is present as a thick tubular structure and has a short posterior extension.

Hosts: Mouse, rat, vole

Tritrichomonas minuta

Predilection site: Large intestine

Parasite class: Zoomastigophorasida

Family: Trichomonadidae

Description: The body is 4–9 μm long and there are three anterior flagella. The undulating membrane extends almost the length of the body and there is a trailing posterior flagellum.

Hosts: Rat, mouse, hamster

Tritrichomonas wenyoni

Predilection site: Large intestine

Parasite class: Zoomastigophorasida

Family: Trichomonadidae

Description: The body is 4–16 μm long and there are three anterior flagella. The undulating membrane extends the length of the body and has a long trailing posterior flagellum. The axostyle is broad and hyaline.

Hosts: Rat, mouse, hamster, monkey

Tetratrichomonas microti

Predilection site: Large intestine

Synonym: *Trichomonas microti*

Parasite class: Zoomastigophorasida

Family: Trichomonadidae

Description: The body is 4–9 μm long and there are four anterior flagella. The undulating membrane extends almost the length of the body and there is a trailing posterior flagellum (Fig. 9.23). The axostyle is slender.

Hosts: Rat, house mouse, golden hamster, vole (*Microtus pennsylvanicus*), wild rodents

PARASITES OF THE RESPIRATORY SYSTEM

Angiostrongylus cantonensis

Synonym: *Parastrongylus cantonensis*

Common name: Rat lungworm

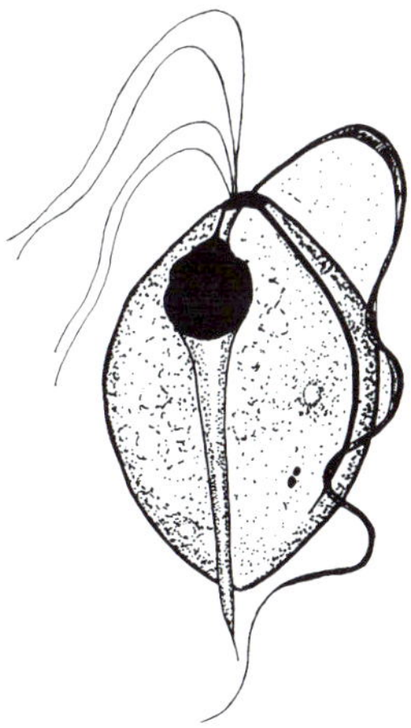

Fig. 9.23 *Tetratrichomonas microti.*

Predilection site: Pulmonary veins

Parasite class: Nematoda

Superfamily: Metastrongyloidea

Description, gross: The body is filariform and tapered at both ends. Males measure about 18 mm and females 23 mm in length. Fresh female worms have a 'barber's pole' appearance as the white uterine tubules spiral round the blood-filled intestine.

Description, microscopic: The slender spicules are of equal length and are striated. A gubernaculum is present. The ovoid eggs laid in the pulmonary arteries are thin-shelled, transparent and unembryonated.

Final hosts: Rat, human

Intermediate hosts: Molluscs; land snails of the genera *Agrolimax*, *Limax*, *Deroceras.* Crustaceans such as prawns and crabs can act as paratenic hosts.

Life cycle: Infection is aquired through the ingestion of a mollusc containing L_3 larvae. The larvae are released in the digestive tract and migrate via the hepatic portal system and lungs to the central nervous system where they undergo two moults. The young worms eventually migrate via the cerebral vein to the pulmonary arteries. The adult worms mate, lay eggs which pass to the capillaries and embryonate, hatch and L_1 larvae enter the alveoli and eventually are coughed up, swallowed and pass out in the faeces. The L_1 are ingested by or penetrate the intermediate host. The prepatent period is around 6 weeks.

Geographical distribution: Asia and Pacific Islands, Australia, India, Africa, Caribbean, parts of USA

Pathogenesis and clinical signs: Light infections are usually asymptomatic. Heavy infestations can lead to uncoordinated movement and weakness. There may be blood-stained fluid from the eyes and a bloody nasal discharge. The presence of parasites in the lung can cause coughing and sneezing. In man, signs may incude a stiff neck, headache, paraesthesia, nausea, vomiting and fever.

Diagnosis: The presence of larvae in faeces

Pathology: The migration of larvae is accompanied by an eosinophilic reaction and in the lung there may be intra-alveolar haemorrhages and in the brain, granulomatous reactions, haemorrhage and abscesses. The lung parenchyma may become consolidated.

Epidemiology: Rate of infection in rats and in the intermediate hosts is usually highest during the rainy seasons.

Treatment and control: Mebendazole and albendazole have been used. Anthelmintic treatment is not usually recommended for treatment of infection in man. Control in man is through education and cooking of the snail hosts and thorough washing of raw vegetables and salad greens.

Notes: Humans can be a paratenic host following the ingestion of infective intermediate hosts. *A. cantonensis* can cause meningitis and meningoencephalitis with mild to moderate symptoms, often of sudden onset, with intense headaches, vomiting, moderate intermittent fever and in about 50% of cases, coughing, anorexia, malaise, constipation and somnolence, and in severe cases coma and death.

PARASITES OF THE LIVER

Capillaria hepatica

Synonym: *Callodium hepatica*, *Hepaticola hepatica*

Predilection site: Liver

Parasite class: Nematoda

Superfamily: Trichuroidea

Hosts: Rat, mouse, squirrel, rabbit and farmed mustelids; occasionally dog, cat and man

For more information see Chapter 6 (Dogs and cats).

Taenia taeniaeformis

Synonym: *Hydatigera taeniaeformis*, *Taenia crassicollis*, *Cysticercus fasciolaris*, *Strobilocercus fasciolaris*

Predilection site: Small intestine (definitive host); liver (intermediate host)

Parasite class: Cestoda

Family: Taeniidae

Description, microscopic: The metacestode stage is a small vesicle in which the scolex is not invaginated but connected to the vesicle by a semented strobila so that the whole larva looks like a small tapeworm (a strobilocercus – *Cysticercus fasciolaris*).

Definitive hosts: Cat, lynx, stoat, fox

Intermediate hosts: Mouse, rat, rabbit, squirrel

Geographical distribution: Cosmopolitan

Pathology: Each strobilocercus is found within a pea-sized nodule partially embedded in the liver parenchyma.

Epidemiology: Rodents are infected by grazing pasture and forages contaminated with cat faeces harbouring eggs of *T. taeniaeformis*. Two cycles can occur. An urban cycle that involves the domestic cat and house and field rodents, and a sylvatic cycle that in North America uses bobcats and wild rodents.

Notes: The correct nomenclature for the intermediate host stage is the 'metacestode stage of *Taenia taeniaeformis*' rather than '*Cysticercus fasciolaris*'.

Hepatozoon muris

Synonym: *Hepatozoon perniciosum*, *Leucocytozoon muris*, *Leucocytozoon ratti*

Parasite class: Sporozoasida

Family: Hepatozoidae

Description: Meronts in the liver are 10–30 µm in diameter. Gamonts in the lymphocytes appear in stained blood smears as elongated, oval bodies, 8–12 × 3–6 µm.

Hosts: Rat

Life cycle: Rats become infected by ingesting the invertebrate host, the spiny rat mite, *Echinolaelaps echidninus*. Sporozoites are released in the intestine, enter the hepatic portal system and are transported to the liver. Merogony takes place in the liver parenchymal cells. Merozoites enter the lymphocytes in the blood and become gamonts. Fertilisation and sporogony occur in the arthropod vector following ingestion.

Geographical distribution: France, Israel, India, South Africa

Pathogenesis and clinical signs: Non-pathogenic

Diagnosis: Diagnosis is based on the detection of the gamonts in blood smears.

Pathology: Anaemia, emaciation, splenomegaly and hepatic degeneration have been reported in rats with severe infections but these changes may have been caused by a concurrent heavy infection with the mite vector.

Epidemiology: The vector is the spiny rat mite, *Echinolaelaps echidninusi.*

Treatment and control: No effective treatment has been reported. Control of the mites will prevent transmission of the parasite.

PARASITES OF THE CIRCULATORY SYSTEM

Angiostrongylus costaricensis

Predilection site: Mesenteric arteries and arterioles

Parasite class: Nematoda

Superfamily: Metastrongyloidea

Description, gross: The worms are tapered at both ends and are filiform in shape. Males measure about 20 mm and females 30–40 mm in length. The spicules are equal in length, slender and striated.

Description, microscopic: The cephalic ends of the spicules are blunt and the caudal tips are pointed. A gubernaculum is present. The ovoid eggs layed in the mesenteric arterioles are thin-shelled, transparent and unembryonated. The embryonated eggs shed in faeces measure around 90 µm.

Definitive hosts: Rodents, common in the cotton rat. Can also infect man.

Intermediate hosts: Terrestrial molluscs such as slugs and snails. The slug *Vaginulus plebius* is the main intermediate host for infection in the cotton rat and man.

Life cycle: Larvae are shed in the faeces of the rodent and are ingested by a mollusc in which development to the L_3 stage takes place. Following ingestion of the mollusc by rats, or ingestion of vegetation that is contaminated with infective mucous trails, the L_3 migrate via the lymphatics. After two moults the worms migrate to the ileocaecal arteries where they mature, reproduce and lay eggs, which are then carried to the intestinal wall. Eggs embryonate, hatch to L_1 larvae and migrate to the lumen of the intestine and pass out in the faeces. The prepatent period is around 3–4 weeks.

Geographical distribution: Mainly the Americas, in particular Costa Rica. Infection has occasionally been reported in other parts of the world.

Pathogenesis and clinical signs: Heavy infections with adult worms in rats can cause obstruction and necrosis of the gut wall and the mesentery and may sometimes be fatal. In man, infection causes anorexia, vomiting, diarrhoea and fever.

Diagnosis: The L_1 larvae may be detected in faeces. At necropsy, adult worms can often be seen in the mesenteric vessels.

Pathology: Large infections can induce local haemorrhages in the arterioles. In cases where large numbers of eggs have been shed into the mesenteric capillaries the serosal surface can have a yellowish coloration. In man, the adult parasites are frequently present in the ileocaecocolic arteries where they induce a thickening of the intestinal wall and a granulomatous eosinophilic inflammatory response. The syndrome is termed abdominal angiostrongylosis.

Epidemiology: The cotton rat (*Sigmodon hispidus*) is the most common definitive host in the Americas. Infection of man in endemic areas is probably through accidental ingestion of infected slugs on vegetables or salads or via infected mucous trails on green vegetation.

Treatment: Anthelmintic treatment is not advised in man.

Control: This is not practical in rodents. Control of slugs and rodents and greater public awareness of the zoonotic disease should reduce infection in man. Thorough washing of vegetables and salad greens is important.

Notes: Other *Angiostrongylus* species are found in wild rodents, such as *A. mackerrasae* (rats in Australia) and *A. schmidti* (rice rat in the USA).

PARASITES OF THE NERVOUS SYSTEM

No parasites of veterinary significance reported.

PARASITES OF THE REPRODUCTIVE/ UROGENITAL SYSTEM

Trichosomoides crasicauda

Common name: Bladder threadworm

Predilection site: Bladder

Parasite class: Nematoda

Superfamily: Trichuroidea

Description: The female is about 10 mm long; males are 1.5–3.5 mm, a permanent hyperparasite living within the reproductive tract of the female.

Hosts: Rat

Life cycle: Infection is by ingestion of embryonated eggs voided in the urine. Eggs hatch in the stomach, penetrate the stomach wall and are carried in the blood to the lungs and other parts of the body. Only those larvae that reach the kidneys or urinary bladder survive. The life cycle takes 8–9 weeks and the prepatent period is 8–12 weeks.

Pathogenesis and clinical signs: The parasite is generally considered non-pathogenic although there have been reports of urinary calculi and bladder tumours associated with infection.

Pathology: The female worms occur either free in the urinary bladder or are embedded in the bladder wall. The presence of the worms can cause granulomatous lesions in the lungs, and white nodules in the bladder wall.

Epidemiology: Transmission in laboratory animals occurs from parents to offspring.

Treatment and control: Not reported

Klossiella muris

Predilection site: Kidney

Parasite class: Sporozoasida

Family: Klossiellidae

Description: Sporocysts measure 16×13 μm and contain 25–34 sporozoites.

Hosts: Mouse

Life cycle: The life cycle is not clearly understood. Within epithelial cells of kidney tubules, trophozoites form meronts and merozoites, of which there are two types. One forms 8–12 merozoites and the other 40–60 merozoites. Merozoites enter the epithelial cells of the convoluted tubules of the kidney, where they form gamonts. Fertilised gametes are believed to develop into sporonts, which bud to form sporoblasts. Each of these sporoblasts undergoes successive divisions to form sporocysts that contain sporozoites. Mature sporocysts are surrounded by a thick wall and pass from the body in the urine. When ingested by another host, the sporozoites are released from the sporocyst, move to the kidney, where they enter epithelial cells and initiate the cycle.

Geographical distribution: Worldwide

Pathogenesis and clinical signs: Infections in mice appear to cause few pathogenic effects and are usually asymptomatic.

Diagnosis: Sporocysts may be detected in urine sediments or trophozoite stages may be found on postmortem in the kidney. The site and location are pathognomonic.

Pathology: Only heavily parasitised kidneys have gross lesions, which appear as tiny grey foci on the cortical surface. Microscopically these foci are areas of necrosis, with perivascular infiltration of inflammatory cells, especially lymphocytes with an increase in interstitial fibroblasts.

Epidemiology: Sporocysts are passed in the urine and infection takes place by the ingestion of the sporulated sporocysts.

Treatment and control: Not required

PARASITES OF THE LOCOMOTORY SYSTEM

Toxoplasma gondii

See Parasites of the locomotory system of the rabbit.

ECTOPARASITES

MITES

Ornithonyssus bacoti

Synonym: *Liponyssus bacoti, Macronyssus bacoti*

Common name: Tropical rat mite

Predilection site: Skin

Parasite class: Arachnida

Sub-class: Acari

Order: Parasitiformes

Suborder: Mesostigmata

Family: Macronyssidae

Description: This rapidly moving, long-legged mite has an oval body, of about 1.0 mm in length. Both sexes blood-feed. The colour varies from white to reddish black depending on the amount of blood it has ingested. It is similar in appearance and life cycle to the fowl mite, *Ornithonyssus sylviarum*. The body carries many long setae and is much more hairy than the red mite of poultry *Dermanyssus gallinae*. The adult female survives for around 70 days, during which it feeds every 2 or 3 days and lays about 100 eggs.

Hosts: Rats, mice, hamsters and a wide variety of mammals and birds

Life cycle: *Ornithonyssus bacoti* spends its entire life on the host and can only survive for about 10 days away from a host.

Geographical distribution: Worldwide

Pathogenesis: Bites are painful and in heavy infections hosts are restless and lose weight from irritation and there may be severe anaemia.

Clinical signs: Skin irritation and dermatitis

Diagnosis: White or off-white eggs can be seen in the hair. Mites should be collected and identified under a dissecting microscope.

Pathology: Feeding results in severely pruritic papular dermatitis, thickened, crusty skin and soiled fur.

Epidemiology: A common parasite worldwide, despite its name. It is particularly common in laboratory rodent colonies. Being an almost permanent parasite, infection is by contact or contamination from accommodation recently vacated by infected stock.

Treatment and control: Treatment includes the application of topical acaricides such as pyrethrin or systemic ivermectin given orally or topically. Repeat treatments will be required to kill newly hatched nymphs.

Myocoptes musculinus

Predilection site: Fur

Parasite class: Arachnida

Sub-class: Acari

Order: Acariformes

Sub-order: Sarcoptiformes (Astigmata)

Family: Listrophoridae

Description: These mites are soft-bodied, strongly striated with a distinct dorsal shield, and have mouthparts and legs modified for grasping hairs (Fig. 9.24). Adult female *Myocoptes musculinus* are elongated ventrally, about 300 μm in length, and the propodosomal body striations have spine-like projections. The genital opening is a transverse slit. The anal opening is posterior and ventral. Legs I and II are normal, possessing short-stalked, flap-like pretarsi. Legs III and IV are highly modified for clasping hair. Males are smaller than females, about 190 μm in length with less pronounced striations and a greatly enlarged fourth pair of legs for grasping the female during copulation. The posterior of the male is bilobed.

Hosts: Mouse, but will also infest guinea pigs.

Life cycle: *Myocoptes musculinus* spends its entire life on the hair of the host rather than on the skin, feeding at the base of the hair and gluing its eggs to the hairs. The life cycle is typical: egg, hexapod larva, followed by octopod protonymph, tritonymph and adult. All developmental stages occur on the host. The entire life cycle requires around 14 days.

Geographical distribution: Worldwide

Pathogenesis: This mite causes myocoptic mange in wild and laboratory mice. It is extremely widespread but is usually of little pathogenic significance. Problems may occur, however, in crowded laboratory colonies or in animals in poor condition. Lesions are often found along the head and neck and between the shoulder blades. With heavy infestation, mice may scratch constantly, leading to self-induced skin trauma and alopecia.

Clinical signs: Infestation may be asymptomatic, or the mite may cause inflammation, scaling, crusting, and pruritic dermatitis, leading to scratching and alopecia.

Diagnosis: For confirmatory diagnosis, skin scrapings or coat brushings must be examined for eggs and mites.

Pathology: Infestations may be asymptomatic, but the mite may cause erythema, inflammation, scaling, crusting, pruritic dermatitis with secondary alopecia. Chronic cases may develop secondary bacterial infection.

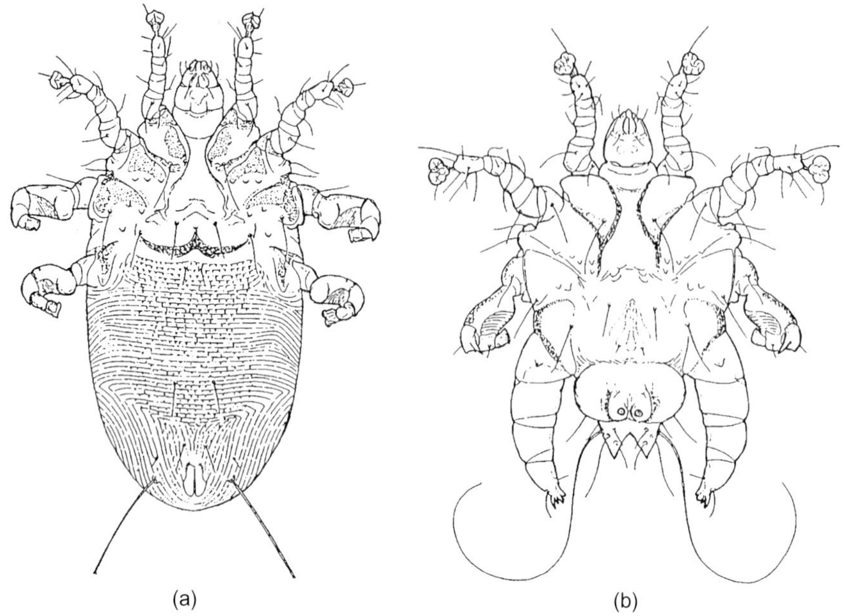

Fig. 9.24 Adults of *Myocoptes musculinus*. (a) Female ventral view. (b) Male ventral view (from Baker *et al*., 1956).

Epidemiology: New hosts are infected by contact with infected individuals.

Treatment: Application of pyrethrin dusts, oral or systemic ivermectin on three occasions, 7 days apart, may be effective. Adverse reactions to ivermectin have been reported in some strains of mice.

Control: All in-contact animals should be treated and the cage or housing should be cleaned.

Leptotrombidium deliense

Common name: Scrub typhus mite, chigger

Predilection site: Fur

Parasite class: Arachnida

Sub-class: Acari

Order: Acariformes

Sub-order: Trombidiformes (Prostigmata)

Family: Trombiculidae

Hosts: Ground dwelling rodents

Geographical distribution: Southeast Asia and Japan

Pathogenesis: Only the larvae blood feed. Infestation causes pruritus, erythema and scratching, though there may be considerable individual variation in response. The larvae of this species are vectors of scrub typhus caused by *Rickettsia tsutsugamushi*.

Notes: There are several closely related species in the genus *Leptotrombidium*. For further details see Chapter 11 (Facultative ectoparasites and arthropod vectors).

Myobia musculi

Predilection site: Fur

Parasite class: Arachnida

Sub-class: Acari

Order: Acariformes

Sub-order: Sarcoptiformes (Astigmata)

Family: Myobidae

Description: The fur mite of mice is a small, translucent mite, typically around 300 μm in length and 190 μm wide (Fig. 9.25). The body is broadly rounded at the rear with transverse striations on the integument. The gnathosoma is small and simple with stylet-like chelicerae. Between the second, third and fourth pairs of legs there are lateral bulges and each tarsus bears an empodial claw. The anus is dorsal and flanked by a long pair of setae.

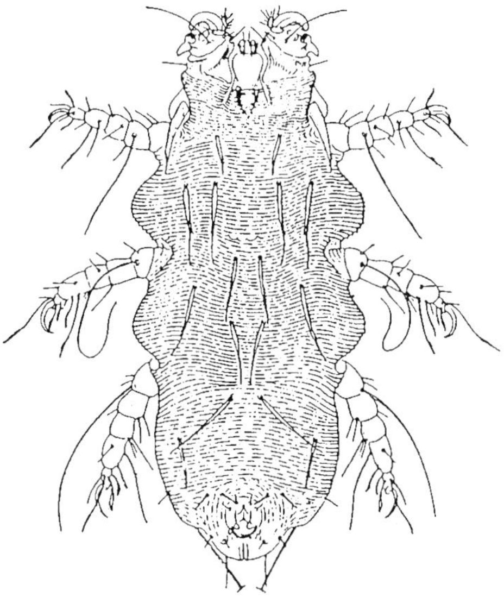

Fig. 9.25 Adult female *Myobia musculi* (dorsal view) (from Baker *et al.*, 1956).

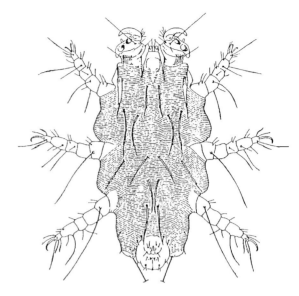

Fig. 9.26 Adult female *Radfordia ensifera* (dorsal view) (from Baker *et al.*, 1956).

Life cycle: The female oviposits amongst the fur, cementing the eggs to the base of the hairs. Eggs hatch within 8 days, and the larvae moult four days later. The egg-to-adult life cycle requires a minimum period of 12 days. All stages feed on extracellular fluids.

Geographical distribution: Worldwide

Pathogenesis and clinical signs: Light infestations are asymptomatic and hence often go unnoticed. Larger mite populations result in alopecia, dermatitis, pruritus and a harsh coat. The preferred site of infestation is the head and the underside of the neck. *Myobia musculi* has a worldwide distribution.

Treatment and control: As for *Myocoptes musculinus*.

Notes: *Radfordia ensifera* and *R. affinis* are closely related species of Myobidae, normally found on rats and mice, respectively. They are morphologically similar to *M. musculi*, but can be distinguished by the presence of two tarsal claws as opposed to just one (Fig. 9.26). *Radfordia ensifera* produces intense itching, leading to scabs most frequently seen on the shoulders, neck, and the face.

A large number of other closely related species of mites may also occasionally be found on rats and mice (Table 9.5); treatment and control are as for *Myocoptes musculinus*. Distinguishing between individual genera and species is beyond the scope of this text.

LICE

Polyplax spinulosa

Predilection site: Fur

Parasite class: Insecta

Parasite order: Phthiraptera

Parasite sub-order: Anoplura

Family: Polyplacidae

Description: These lice are slender, 0.6–1.5 mm in length and yellow–brown in colour. The head bears prominent, five-segmented antennae, no eyes and no ocular points (Fig. 9.27). There is a distinct sternal plate on the ventral surface of the thorax. The forelegs are small and the hindlegs are large with large claws and tibial spurs. The abdomen has 7–13 dorsal plates, and approximately seven lateral plates on each side. The egg is elongated, with a cone-like operculum.

Hosts: Mouse, rat

Life cycle: The lice spend their entire life cycle in the host and transmission occurs by direct contact. The eggs hatch in about 5–6 days to give rise to three nymphal stages, followed by the reproductive adult. The first nymphal stage is found on the entire body, while older stages are found predominantly on the front of

Table 9.5 Species of mites found on rats and mice.

Species	Family	Details
Psorergates simplex	Psorergatidae	A follicular mite that causes small white intradermal nodules. Closely related to the more pathogenically important *Psorergates ovis*; see Chapter 3: Sheep and goats
Demodex musculi *Demodex ratticola*	Demodicidae	Largely non-pathogenic but may occasionally cause follicular dermatitis; see *Demodex*, Chapter 6: Dogs and cats
Notoedres muris	Sarcoptidae	An ear mite of rats. It is relatively rare. It burrows into skin, and may result in yellowish crusty-looking warts on edges of ears and nose; see *Notoedres cati*, Chapter 6: Dogs and cats
Ornithonyssus sylviarum	Macronyssidae	See Chapter 7: Poultry and gamebirds
Dermanyssus gallinae	Dermanyssidae	See Chapter 7: Poultry and gamebirds
Liponyssoides sanguineus	Dermanyssidae	House mouse mite. A blood-feeding mite of mice and rats found worldwide. It readily bites humans and may act as a vector of rickettsial pox caused by infection with *Rickettsia akari*. Distinguished from *D. gallinae* by more pointed posterior of dermal shield
Laelaps nuttalli *Hirstionyssus isabellinus* *Haemogamasus pontiger* *Eulaelaps stabularis*	Laelapidae	Adults have a single dorsal shield and the sternal plates are wider than long. Though capable of biting, they more commonly feed on skin debris and serous exudate, infesting already abraded areas of skin
Laelaps echidninus		The spiny rat mite. A known vector of a number of disease agents such as *Francisella tularensis* and *Hepatozoon muris*
Androlaelaps casalis		Common on a wide variety of rodents; there are several species within this genus (e.g. *A. rotundus*, *A. frontalis* and *A. sinuosa*). *Androlaelaps casalis* may also cause dermatitis of humans

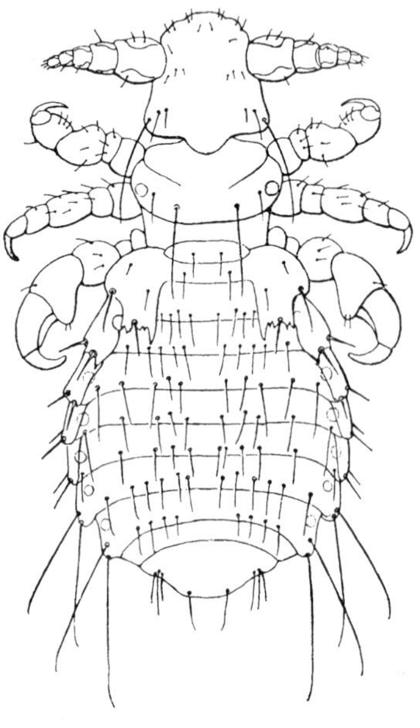

Fig. 9.27 Adult female *Polyplax* in dorsal view.

the body. The entire life cycle is completed in about 2 weeks.

Geographical distribution: Worldwide

Pathogenesis: These blood-sucking lice are commonly encountered in wild rats and mice, but rarely seen in laboratory rodents. They cause irritation, restlessness and constant scratching, particularly behind the ears. Anaemia, unthrifty appearance and debilitation occur in heavy infestations.

Clinical signs: Pruritus, restlessness, debilitation and anaemia.

Diagnosis: Adult lice, nymphs or eggs may be found on the fur.

Treatment and control: Lice may be killed by most organophosphates (such as diazinon, malathion methoxychlor) and pyrethroids (such as permethrin). Topical application of fipronil or imidocloprid or systemic ivermectin may also be highly effective, but care must be taken because adverse effects to ivermectin have been reported in some strains of mice.

Polyplax serrata

Common name: Spined rat louse

Predilection site: Fur

Parasite class: Insecta

Parasite order: Phthiraptera

Parasite sub-order: Anoplura

Family: Polyplacidae

Hosts: Mouse

Pathogenicity: *P. serrata* may be a vector for murine eperythrozoonosis.

Treatment and control: As for *P. spinulosa*

FLEAS

Nosopsyllus fasciatus

Common name: Northern rat flea

Predilection site: Fur and skin

Parasite class: Insecta

Parasite order: Siphonaptera

Family: Ceratophyllidae

Description: The northern rat flea has a pronotal ctenidium with 18–20 spines (Fig. 9.28). A genal ctenidium is absent. Eyes are present, and the head carries a row of three setae below the eye. The frontal tubercle on the head of both sexes is conspicuous. There are three or four bristles on the inner surface of the hind femur. The body is elongated and about 3–4 mm in length.

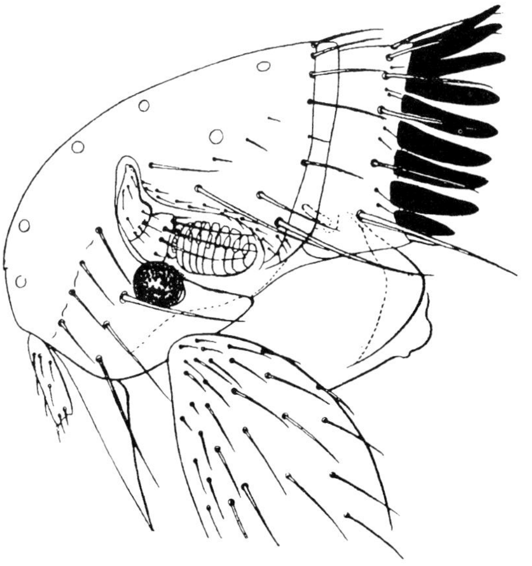

Fig. 9.28 The northern rat flea, *Nosopsyllus fasciatus*, male head (after Smart, 1943).

Hosts: Rat, mouse, humans

Life cycle: The life cycle is typical: egg, three larval stages, pupa and adult. Life cycle development may be completed at temperatures as low as 5°C. Larval stages are found only in the nest or burrow. The larvae of this species may pursue and solicit faecal blood meals from adult fleas. The larvae grasp the adult in the region of the sensilium using their large mandibles. Adults respond by defecating stored semi-liquid blood, which is then imbibed by the larvae directly from the anus.

Geographical distribution: Although originally European in distribution, the northern rat flea, *Nosopsyllus fasciatus*, has now been transported to temperate habitats worldwide.

Pathogenesis: Its main hosts are rodents, particularly the Norway rat, *Rattus norvegicus*. However, it has also been found on house mice, gophers and many other hosts. The northern rat flea will attack and feed on humans, although it is not thought to be an important vector of plague. It is known to be a vector of *Hymenolepis diminuta* in parts of Europe, Australia and South America.

Clinical signs: Symptoms include restlessness and scratching of affected areas. The bites may be visible on the skin. Allergic dermatitis may be seen, but should be differentiated from other similar conditions such as sarcoptic mange.

Diagnosis: Diagnosis is not easy as adults may leave the host and eggs and larvae are difficult to find. The bites of these fleas are similar to those of mosquitoes, lice and mites, with inflammation and itchiness.

Epidemiology: *Nosopsyllus fasciatus* fleas are not host specific and may attack any available mammal or bird for a blood meal. As they are able to survive off the host, transmission can occur from the bedding and housing. This flea is highly mobile on the host and can be especially common in host nesting material.

Treatment: Several organophosphorus, carbamate and pyrethrin-based insecticides are effective. Imidacloprid and fipronil may be highly effective and kill adult fleas on contact.

Control: Should this species become established in pet rats or mice the animal should be treated, all litter and bedding should be removed and burnt and the cage sprayed with an insecticide. If there is invasion of other domestic hosts or humans from wild animals, the source must be eradicated.

Xenopsylla cheopis

Common name: Oriental or black rat flea

Predilection site: Skin

Parasite class: Insecta

Parasite order: Siphonaptera

Family: Pulicidae

Description: *Xenospylla cheopis* resembles *P. irritans* in that both genal and pronotal ctenidia are absent (Fig. 9.29). The head is smoothly rounded anteriorly. The flea has a light amber coloration. The maxillary laciniae reach nearly to the end of the forecoxae. Eyes are present, yet it can only see very bright light. Immediately behind the eyes are two short antennae. The segments of the thorax appear relatively large and the pleural ridge is present in the mesopleuron of the thorax. There is a conspicuous row of bristles along the rear margin of the head and a stout ocular bristle in front of the eye.

Hosts: Rat, humans; this species may also infest mice, cottontail rabbits and ground squirrels.

Life cycle: The life cycle of *X. cheopis* is typical: egg, three larval stages, pupa and adult. Eggs are usually laid in the environment rather than on the animal host. Eggs are laid in batches of about 3–25 a day, with a female laying 300–1000 eggs over a lifespan that may be from 10 days to more than a year. Eggs hatch after about 5 days (range 2–14 days depending upon local conditions). The larva that emerges avoids light and feeds actively on organic debris. The duration of the larval stage depends upon local conditions. The most important environmental variable is humidity and larvae may die if they move outside a narrow range; humidities above 60–70% and temperatures above 12°C and are required for life cycle development in this species.

The larval period may last 12–84 days, and the pupal and pharate adult period in the cocoon, from 7–182 days, depending on the availability of a suitable host. Adults may survive for up to 100 days if a host is available, and up to 38 days without food, if humidity is high. Adult males and females can take several blood meals a day. If the host dies, the flea moves almost immediately to find a new one.

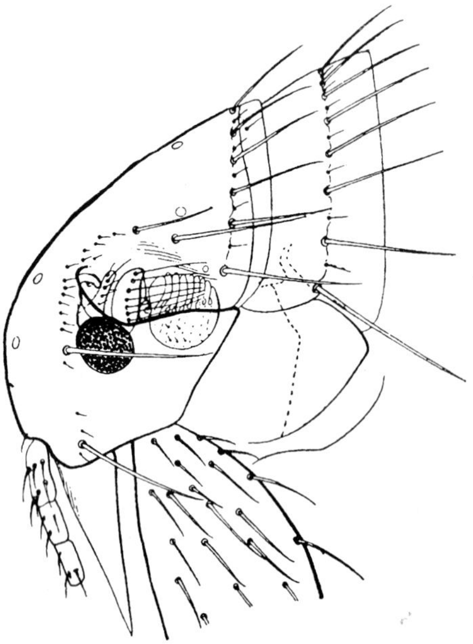

Fig. 9.29 The Oriental rat flea, *Xenopsylla cheopis*, male head (after Smart, 1943).

Geographical distribution: Worldwide. The distribution of the Oriental rat flea, *X. cheopis*, largely follows that of its primary host the black rat, *Rattus rattus*. It has a worldwide distribution and is one of the most abundant fleas in the southern states of the US. It is particularly common in urban areas.

Pathogenesis: The bites of the flea may prove irritating to the host animal causing it to scratch and rub itself. *Xenopsylla cheopis* is also an intermediate host of helminths, such as *Hymenolepis diminuta* and *H. nana*. *Xenopsylla cheopis* is the main vector of *Yersinia pestis*, the cause of bubonic plague in man. *X. cheopis* acquires *Y. pestis* when feeding on its usual hosts. When the bacilli multiply in its gut the proventriculus becomes blocked so that blood cannot be ingested; the hungry flea moves from host to host in attempts to feed, and in its wanderings the infection may be transferred from its endemic base in rodents to the human population. Bacteria secreted in faeces may also enter a host through abrasions. Though now rare in humans, plague still exists in wild rodents ('sylvatic plague') in parts of Africa, Asia, South America and the western states of the USA. *Xenosylla cheopis* is also a vector of murine typhis (*Rickettsia typhi*). In the case of typhus, the disease is only transmitted by rickettsia in faeces. However, the pathogen can invade the ovary, leading to its transovarial transmission, via eggs.

Clinical signs: The adult fleas may be seen on the skin and coat of the host animal. Other signs are the host scratching affected areas.

Diagnosis: Diagnosis can be achieved by identifying the flea species on the host.

Epidemiology: The fleas are able to survive off the host for long periods, making infection possible from the enviroment. They are uncommon in laboratory or pet rats and mice so their presence may indicate that there is contamination by wild rodents.

Pathology: Flea feeding does not appear to produce histopathology at the flea feeding sites nor does the elevated basophilic blood response of infested rats affect subsequent feeding or longevity of the fleas.

Treatment: A wide range of products is available to treat infested hosts. Imidacloprid and fipronil may be used in rats to kill adult fleas on contact. Growth regulators such as methoprene or pyriproxyfen are another effective longer-term alternative.

Control: For optimal control nesting material must be removed and replaced, the housing treated and reinfestation from the environment or introduced animals prevented.

Leptopsylla segnis

Common name: Mouse flea

Predilection site: Fur

Parasite class: Insecta

Parasite order: Siphonaptera

Family: Leptopsyllidae

Description: In the adult there are both genal and pronotol ctenidia, and the genal ctenidium contains only four spines.

Hosts: Mice and rats

Life cycle: The life cycle is typical: egg, three larval stages, pupa and adult. Eggs and larvae are found in the hosts nest and the adults are obligate blood-feeders on the host animal. The adult fleas live for approximately 20 days on the host. The entire life cycle may be completed in 3–4 weeks under ideal conditions or 2 years under adverse conditions.

Geographic distribution: Europe and on the east and west coasts of the United States

Pathogenicity: bites cause irritation causing the host to scratch and rub and may provoke allergic responses. This species of flea has been infected experimentally with plague and murine typhus, but generally it is considered a poor disease vector.

Epidemiology: Found largely in temperate areas and it does not survive hot dry conditions.

Treatment and control: As for *Xenopsylla cheopis*

FLIES

Cuterebra

Common name: New World skin bot flies

Predilection site: Skin

Parasite class: Insecta

Family: Oestridae (sub-family Cuterebrinae)

Description, adults: The adults are large flies (up to 30 mm in length) covered by dense, short hairs, and have a blue–black-coloured abdomen. They have small, non-functional mouthparts and do not feed as adults.

Description, larvae: Larvae have strongly curved mouth-hooks and numerous strong body spines.

Hosts: Rodents and rabbits, but may occasionally infest dogs and cats.

Life cycle: Females lay eggs on the ground near or within the entrance of host nests, or on grass near trails used by hosts. These are picked up by the passing host. The larvae enter the body, directly through the skin or through one of the orifices such as the nose, and then migrate subdermally. At their final, species-specific resting site the larvae eventually form a warble-like swelling. In rodents the warble is often formed near the anus, scrotum or tail. Larval development may require between 3 and 7 weeks. When mature, the larvae leave the host and drop to the ground where they pupate.

Geographical distribution: New World

Pathogenesis: Species of the genus *Cuterebra* are largely dermal parasites of rodents and rabbits, but may occasionally infest dogs and cats. The larvae cause subdermal nodules. They are not commonly seen in laboratory colonies, but may be found in animals maintained out of doors.

Clinical signs: Symptoms include the swellings and lesions made by larvae.

Diagnosis: The presence of one or more superficially situated swellings with central openings indicates myiasis. Specific diagnosis can only be made after extraction and identification of the larvae.

Pathology: In the warble formed around each larva, a thin layer of necrotic tissue develops and the larva feeds off the tissue debris and exudate. In general, the cuterebrid species are of little economic veterinary importance. However, occasional fatal cases of infestation have been recorded in cats and dogs.

Epidemiology: 26 species are known to occur in the USA and Canada. They are also found in Mexico and the neotropical regions; however, the taxonomy of this genus is not yet clearly defined. In most regions there is only a single generation per year, adults are active in spring and summer and they overwinter as pupae in the ground.

Treatment: Surgical removal of larvae can be performed relatively easily if required for infected captive animals. The cyst opening should be enlarged by incision and the parasite excised. The wound should then be rinsed with an antiseptic solution and a topical antibiotic administered.

Control: Area-wide control is impractical and for long-term management areas of known fly activity should be avoided.

In the following checklists, the codes listed below apply:

Helminth classes:
N = Nematoda; T = Trematoda; C = Cestoda.

Arthropod classes:
I = Insecta; A = Arachnida.

Protozoal classes:
M = Mastigophora; S = Sarcodina; A = Apicomplexa; R = Rickettsia.

Rabbit parasite checklist.

Section/host system	Helminths		Arthropods		Protozoa	
	Parasite	(Super)family	Parasite	Family	Parasite	Family
Digestive						
Oesophagus						
Stomach	*Graphidium strigosum*	Trichostrongyloidea (N)				
	Obeliscoides cuniculi	Trichostrongyloidea (N)				
Small intestine	*Trichostrongylus retortaeformis*	Trichostrongyloidea (N)			*Eimeria fluorescens*	Eimeriidae (A)
	Trichostrongylus calcaratus	Trichostrongyloidea (N)			*Eimeria exigua*	Eimeriidae (A)
	Trichostrongylus colubriformis	Trichostrongyloidea (N)			*Eimeria intestinalis*	Eimeriidae (A)
	Trichostrongylus vitrinus	Trichostrongyloidea (N)			*Eimeria irresidua*	Eimeriidae (A)
	Nematodirus leporis	Trichostrongyloidea (N)			*Eimeria magna*	Eimeriidae (A)
	Strongyloides papillosus	Rhabditoidea (N)			*Eimeria media*	Eimeriidae (A)
	Cittotaenia ctenoides	Anoplocephalidae (C)			*Eimeria perforans*	Eimeriidae (A)
	Cittotaenia variables	Anoplocephalidae (C)			*Eimeria vejdovskyi*	Eimeriidae (A)
	Cittotaenia pectinata	Anoplocephalidae (C)				
	Paranoplocephala cunniculi	Anoplocephalidae (C)				
	Mosgovoyia ctenoides	Anoplocephalidae (C)				
Caecum Colon	*Passalurus ambiguus*	Oxyuroidea (N)			*Eimeria piriformis*	Eimeriidae (A)
	Passalurus nonannulatus	Oxyuroidea (N)			*Eimeria coecicola*	Eimeriidae (A)
	Dermatoxys veligera	Oxyuroidea (N)			*Eimeria flavescens*	Eimeriidae (A)
	Trichuris leporis	Trichuroidea (N)			*Entamoeba cuniculi*	Endamoebidae (S)
					Retortamonas cuniculi	Retortamonadoridae (M)
Respiratory						
Nose						
Trachea Bronchi						
Lung	*Protostrongylus tauricus*	Metastrongyloidea (N)				
	Protostrongylus pulmonaris	Metastrongyloidea (N)				
	Protostrongylus oryctolagi	Metastrongyloidea (N)				
	Echinococcus granulosus	Taeniidae (C)				

(*continued*)

Rabbit parasite checklist (*continued*).

Section/host system	Helminths		Arthropods		Protozoa	
	Parasite	(Super)family	Parasite	Family	Parasite	Family
Liver						
	Capillaria hepatica	Trichuroidea (N)			*Eimeria stiedai*	Eimeriidae (A)
	Fasciola hepatica	Fasciolidae (T)				
	Echinococcus granulosus	Taeniidae (C)				
	Cysticercus serialis (metacestode – *Taenia serialis*)	Taeniidae (C)				
Pancreas						
Peritoneum	*Cysticercus serialis* (metacestode – *Taenia serialis*)	Taeniidae (C)				
Circulatory						
Blood						
Blood vessels					*Rickettsia conorii*	Rickettsiaceae (R)
					Hepatozoon cuniculi	Hepatozoidae (A)
Spleen						
Nervous						
CNS					*Encephalitozoon cuniculi*	Nosematidae (Mi)
Eye						
Ear			*Psoroptes cuniculi*	Psoroptidae (A)		

Mi = Microsporidia.

Reproductive/ urogenital						
Kidneys						
Locomotory						
Muscle					*Sarcocystis cuniculi*	Sarcocystiidae (A)
					Toxoplasma gondii	Sarcocystiidae (A)
Connective tissue	*Coenurus serialis* (metacestode – *Taenia serialis*)	Taeniidae (C)				
Integument						
Skin			*Listrophorus gibbus*	Listrophoridae (A)		
			Notoedres cati	Sarcoptidae (A)		
			Sarcoptes scabiei	Sarcoptidae (A)		
			Chorioptes bovis	Psoroptidae (A)		
			Cheyletiella parasitovorax	Cheyletidae (A)		
			Neotrombicula autumnalis	Trombiculidae (A)		
			Dermanyssus gallinae	Dermanyssidae (A)		
			Spilopsyllus cuniculi	Pulicidae (I)		
			Ctenocephalides felis	Pulicidae (I)		
			Ctenocephalides canis	Pulicidae (I)		
			Echidnophaga gallinacea	Pulicidae (I)		
			Lucilia sericata	Calliphoridae (I)		
Subcutaneous			*Cordylobia anthropophaga*	Calliphoridae (I)		
			Cordylobia rhodaini	Calliphoridae (I)		
			Dermatobia hominis	Oestridae (I)		

Guinea pig parasite checklist.

Section/host system	Helminths		Arthropods		Protozoa	
	Parasite	(Super)family	Parasite	Family	Parasite	Family
Digestive						
Oesophagus						
Stomach						
Small intestine	*Hymenolepis diminuta*	Hymenolepididae (C)			*Eimeria caviae*	Eimeriidae (A)
	Rodentolepis nana	Hymenolepididae (C)			*Cryptosporidium wrairi*	Cryptosporidiidae (A)
					Giardia intestinalis	Diplomonadidae (M)
Caecum	*Paraspidodera uncinata*	Ascaridoidea (N)			*Entamoeba caviae*	Endamoebidae (S)
Colon					*Caviomonas mobilis*	Diplomonadidae (M)
					Monocercomonoides caviae	Diplomonadidae (M)
					Monocercomonoides quadrifunilis	Diplomonadidae (M)
					Monocercomonoides wenrichi	Diplomonadidae (M)
					Monocercomonoides exilis	Diplomonadidae (M)
					Protomonas brevifilia	Diplomonadidae (M)
					Hexamastix caviae	Diplomonadidae (M)
					Chilomitus caviae	Diplomonadidae (M)
					Chilomitus conexus	Diplomonadidae (M)
					Retortamonas caviae	Retortamonadoridae (M)
					Tritrichomonas caviae	Trichomonadidae (M)
Respiratory						
Nose						
Trachea Bronchi						
Lung						

Liver				
Pancreas				
Circulatory				
Blood				
Blood vessels				
Nervous				
CNS				
Eye				
Reproductive/ urogenital				
Kidneys			*Klossiella cobayae*	Klossiellidae (A)
Locomotory				
Muscle			*Toxoplasma gondii*	Sarcocystiidae (A)
Connective tissue				
Integument				
Skin	*Trixicarus caviae*	Sarcoptidae (A)		
	Demodex caviae	Demodicidae (A)		
	Chirodiscoides caviae	Listrophoridae (I)		
	Gliricola porcelli	Gyropidae (I)		
	Gyropus ovalis	Gyropidae (I)		
	Trimenopon hispidium	Trimenoponidae (I)		
	Ctenocephalides felis	Pulicidae (I)		
Subcutaneous	*Cuterebra* spp	Oestridae (I)		

Rat parasite checklist.

Section/host system	Helminths		Arthropods		Protozoa	
	Parasite	(Super)family	Parasite	Family	Parasite	Family
Digestive						
Oesophagus						
Stomach						
Small intestine	*Nematospiroides dubius*	Trichostrongyloidea (N)			*Eimeria nieschulzi*	Eimeriidae (A)
	Nippostrongylus brasiliensis	Trichostrongyloidea (N)			*Eimeria hasei*	Eimeriidae (A)
	Hymenolepis diminuta	Hymenolepididae (C)			*Eimeria nochti*	Eimeriidae (A)
	Rodentolepis nana	Hymenolepididae (C)			*Eimeria ratti*	Eimeriidae (A)
					Cryptosporidium muris	Cryptosporidiidae (A)
					Giardia muris	Diplomonadidae (M)
					Spironucleus muris	Diplomonadidae (M)
Caecum Colon	*Aspicularis tetraptera*	Oxyuroidea (N)			*Eimeria separata*	Eimeriidae (A)
	Syphacia muris	Oxyuroidea (N)			*Tetratrichomonas microti*	Trichomonadidae (M)
	Syphacia obvelata	Oxyuroidea (N)			*Tritrichomonas muris*	Trichomonadidae (M)
	Trichuris muris	Trichuroidea (N)			*Tritrichomonas minuta*	Trichomonadidae (M)
					Tritrichomonas wenyoni	Trichomonadidae (M)
					Entamoeba muris	Endamoebidae (S)
Respiratory						
Nose						
Trachea Bronchi						
Lung	*Angiostrongylus cantonensis*	Metastrongyloidea (N)				
Liver	*Capillaria hepatica*	Trichuroidea (N)			*Hepatozoon muris*	Hepatozoidae (A)
	Cysticercus fasciolaris (metacestode – *Taenia taeniaeformis*)	Taeniidae (C)				
Pancreas						
Circulatory						
Blood	*Angiostrongylus costaricensis*	Metastrongyloidea (N)				
Blood vessels						

Nervous						
CNS						
Eye						
Reproductive/ urogenital						
Kidneys						
	Trichosomoides crasicauda	Trichuroidea (N)				
Locomotory						
Muscle					*Toxoplasma gondii*	Sarcocystiidae (A)
Connective tissue						
Integument						
Skin			*Notoedres muris*	Sarcoptidae (A)		
			Demodex ratticola	Demodecidae (A)		
			Radfordia ensifera	Myobidae (A)		
			Leptotrombidium deliense	Trombiculidae (A)		
			Dermanysssus gallinae	Dermanyssidae (A)		
			Liponyssoides sanguineus	Dermanyssidae (A)		
			Haemogamasus pontiger	Laelapidae (A)		
			Androlaelpas casalis	Laelapidae (A)		
			Laelaps echidnina	Laelapidae (A)		
			Ornithonyssus sylviarum	Macronyssidae (A)		
			Ornithonyssus bacoti	Macronyssidae (A)		
			Trimenopon jenningsi	Trimenoponidae (A)		
			Polyplax spinulosa	Polyplacidae (I)		
			Xenopsylla cheopis	Pulicidae (I)		
			Nosopsyllus fasciatus	Ceratopyllidae (I)		
			Leptopsylla segnis	Leptopsyllidae (I)		
Subcutaneous			*Cuterebra* spp	Oestridae (I)		

Mouse parasite checklist.

Section/host system	Helminths		Arthropods		Protozoa	
	Parasite	(Super)family	Parasite	Family	Parasite	Family
Digestive						
Oesophagus						
Stomach						
Small intestine	*Nematospiroides dubius*	Trichostrongyloidea (N)			*Cryptosporidium muris*	Cryptosporidiidae (A)
	Nippostrongylus brasiliensis	Trichostrongyloidea (N)			*Giardia muris*	Diplomonadidae (M)
					Spironucleus muris	Diplomonadidae (M)
	Hymenolepis diminuta	Hymenolepididae (C)			*Eimeria falciformis*	Eimeriidae (A)
	Rodentolepis nana	Hymenolepididae (C)			*Eimeria musculi*	Eimeriidae (A)
					Eimeria scheuffneri	Eimeriidae (A)
					Eimeria krijgsmanni	Eimeriidae (A)
					Eimeria keilini	Eimeriidae (A)
					Eimeria hindlei	Eimeriidae (A)
Caecum Colon	*Aspicularis tetraptera*	Oxyuroidea (N)			*Tetratrichomonas microti*	Trichomonadidae (M)
	Syphacia muris	Oxyuroidea (N)				
	Syphacia obvelata	Oxyuroidea (N)			*Tritrichomonas muris*	Trichomonadidae (M)
	Trichuris muris	Trichuroidea (N)			*Tritrichomonas minuta*	Trichomonadidae (M)
					Tritrichomonas wenyoni	Trichomonadidae (M)
					Entamoeba muris	Endamoebidae (S)
Respiratory						
Nose						
Trachea Bronchi						
Lung						
Liver						
	Capillaria hepatica	Trichuroidea (N)				
	Cysticercus fasciolaris (metacestode – *Taenia taeniaeformis*)	Taeniidae (C)				
	Echinococcus multilocularis	Taeniidae (C)				

Pancreas				
Circulatory				
Blood				
Blood vessels				
Nervous				
CNS				
Eye				
Reproductive/ urogenital				
Kidneys			*Klossiella muris*	Klossiellidae (A)
Locomotory				
Muscle			*Toxoplasma gondii*	Sarcocystiidae (A)
			Sarcocystis muris	Sarcocystiidae (A)
Connective tissue				
Integument				
Skin	*Myobia musculi*	Myobidae (A)		
	Myocoptes musculinus	Listrophoridae (A)		
	Radfordia affinis	Myobidae (A)		
	Demodex musculi	Demodecidae (A)		
	Psorogates simplex	Psorogatidae (A)		
	Ornithonyssus bacoti	Macronyssidae (A)		
	Trichoecius romboutsi	Myocoptidae (A)		
	Lipponyssoides sanguineus	Dermanyssidae (A)		
	Haemogamasus pontiger	Laelapidae (A)		
	Laelaps echidninus	Laelapidae (A)		
	Leptotrombidium deliense	Trombiculidae (A)		
	Polyplax serrata	Polyplacidae (I)		
	Xenopsylla cheopis	Pulicidae (I)		
	Nosopsyllus fasciatus	Ceratopyllidae (I)		
	Leptopsylla segnis	Leptopsyllidae (I)		
Subcutaneous	*Cuterebra* spp	Oestridae (I)		

10
Parasites of exotics

PIGEONS

PARASITES OF THE DIGESTIVE SYSTEM

CROP, PROVENTRICULUS

Trichomonas gallinae

Synonym: *Cercomonas gallinae, Trichomonas columbae*

Common name: Canker, frounce, roup

Predilection site: Phayrnx, oesophagus, crop, proventriculus

Parasite class: Zoomastigophorasida

Family: Trichomonadidae

Description: The body is elongate, ellipsoidal or pyriform, 5–19 × 2–9 μm, with four anterior flagella that arise from the blepharoplast. The undulating membrane does not reach the posterior end of the body and a free posterior flagellum is absent. An accessory filament is present. The axostyle is narrow, protrudes 2–8 μm from the body and its anterior portion is flattened into a spatulate capitulum. There is a crescent-shaped pelta anterior to the axostyle and there is no chromatic ring at its point of emergence. The parabasal body is hook-shaped and has a parabasal filament and the costa is a very fine rod running three quarters the length of the body.

Hosts: Pigeon, turkey, chicken, raptors (hawks, falcons, eagles)

Life cycle: The trichomonads reproduce by longitudinal binary fission. No sexual stages are known and there are no cysts.

Geographical distribution: Worldwide

Pathogenesis: The domestic pigeon is the primary host, but the parasite has been found in birds of prey that feed on pigeons, and it has been experimentally established in a wide range of other birds. *T. gallinae* is extremely common in domestic pigeons and often causes serious losses. Previous infection leads to a varying degree of immunity, and adult pigeons, that have survived infection as squabs, are symptomless carriers. Infection with a relatively harmless strain produces immunity against virulent strains. Injection of plasma from infected pigeons also confers immunity.

In pigeons, trichomoniosis is essentially a disease of young birds; 80–90% of the adults are infected but show no signs of disease. Trichomoniosis varies from a mild condition to a rapidly fatal one with death 4–18 days after infection (there are strain differences in virulence).

Clinical signs: Severely affected birds lose weight, stand huddled with ruffled feathers and may fall over when forced to move. Yellow, necrotic lesions are present in the mouth, oesophagus and crop of pigeon squabs and a greenish fluid containing large numbers of trichomonads may be found in the mouth. The condition is often fatal.

Diagnosis: The clinical signs are pathognomonic and can be confirmed by identifying the characteristic motile trichomonads from samples taken from lesions in the mouth or from fluid.

Pathology: The early lesions in the pharynx, oesophagus and crop are small, whitish to yellowish caseous nodules. These grow in size and may remain circumscribed and separate, or may coalesce to form thick, caseous, necrotic masses that may occlude the lumen. The circumscribed disk-shaped lesions are often described as ‘yellow buttons’. The lesions in the liver, lungs and other organs are solid, yellowish, caseous nodules up to 1 cm or more in diameter.

Epidemiology: In pigeons and doves, trichomoniosis is transmitted from the adults to the squabs in the ‘pigeon milk’ which is produced in the crop. The squabs become infected within minutes of hatching. Hawks and wild raptors become infected by eating infected birds.

Treatment: Carnidazole is used for the treatment and prophylaxis of trichomoniosis in pigeons at a dose rate of 10 mg for adult birds and 5 mg for squabs. Other nitroimidazole compounds, such as dimetridazole and metronidazole, are also effective, but their availability has declined in many countries through legislative changes and toxicity concerns.

Control: Control of trichomoniosis in pigeons depends on the elimination of the infection from the adult birds by drug therapy.

Notes: *Trichomonas gallinae* parasitises the mouth, sinuses, orbital region, pharynx, oesophagus, crop and even proventriculus, but is not found beyond the proventriculus. It often occurs in the liver, and to a lesser extent in other organs including the lungs, air sacs, heart, pancreas, and more rarely spleen, kidneys, trachea and bone marrow.

Spiruroid nematodes

Several species of spiruroid worms belonging to the genera *Tetrameres* and *Dyspharynx* are found in the proventriculus of pigeons. These species have been described in detail in Chapter 7 (Poultry and gamebirds).

Tetrameres americana

Synonym: *Tropisurus americana*

Predilection site: Proventriculus

Parasite class: Nematoda

Superfamily: Spiruroidea

Final hosts: Chicken, turkey, duck, goose, grouse, quail, pigeon

Intermediate hosts: Cockroaches, grasshoppers and beetles

Geographical distribution: Africa and North America

Tetrameres fissispina

Synonym: *Tropisurus fissispina*

Predilection site: Proventriculus

Parasite class: Nematoda

Superfamily: Spiruroidea

Final hosts: Duck, goose, chicken, turkey, pigeon and wild aquatic birds

Intermediate hosts: Aquatic crustaceans such as *Daphnia* and *Gammarus*; grasshoppers, earthworms

Geographical distribution: Most parts of the world

Dispharynx nasuta

Synonym: *Dispharynx spiralis, Acuaria spiralis*

Predilection site: Oesophagus, proventriculus

Parasite class: Nematoda

Superfamily: Spiruroidea

Final hosts: Chicken, turkey, pigeon, guinea fowl, grouse, pheasant and other birds

Intermediate hosts: Various isopods such as sowbugs (*Porcellio scaber*) and pillbugs (*Armadillidium vulgare*).

Geographical distribution: Asia, Africa and the Americas

Others

Ascaridia columbae

Synonym: *Ascaridia maculosa*

Predilection site: Small intestine

Parasite class: Nematoda

Superfamily: Ascaridoidea

Description, gross: The worms are stout and densely white; males are 1.6–7 cm and females measure 2–9.5 cm in length.

Description, microscopic: The egg is distinctly oval, with a smooth shell, and measures $80–90 \times 40–50$ μm.

Hosts: Pigeon

Life cycle: The parasitic phase is non-migratory, consisting of a transient histotrophic phase in the intestinal mucosa after which the adult parasites inhabit the lumen of the intestine. The egg is sometimes ingested by earthworms, which may act as transport hosts. The prepatent period is 6 weeks.

Geographical distribution: Presumed worldwide

Pathogenesis: Non-pathogenic

Clinical signs: Large numbers of worms produce no clinical signs.

Diagnosis: Adult worms may be found in the intestine on postmortem or the characteristic ascarid eggs may be seen in faeces.

Pathology: No associated pathology

Epidemiology: Adult birds are symptomless carriers, and the reservoir of infection is on the ground, either as free eggs or in earthworm transport hosts. Infection is heaviest in young squabs.

Treatment: Not usually required although treatment with piperazine salts, levamisole or a benzimidazole, such as fenbendazole, is effective. Capsules containing fenbendazole or cambendazole are effective and can be given by mouth to pigeons.

Control: Strict hygiene and feeding and watering systems, which will limit the contamination of food and water by faeces, should be used.

Ornithostrongylus quadriradiatus

Predilection site: Crop, proventriculus, small intestine

Parasite class: Nematoda

Superfamily: Trichostrongyloidea

Description, gross: The adult worms, which measure up to 2.5 cm, are bloodsuckers, have a reddish colour and can be seen by the naked eye.

Description, microscopic: In the male bursa, the ventral rays are close together and the dorsal ray is short. Spicules end in three pointed processes. Eggs are ovoid and measure $70–75 \times 38–40\ \mu m$

Hosts: Pigeon

Life cycle: The life cycle is direct and typically trichostrongyle.

Geographical distribution: North America, South Africa, Australia, Europe

Pathogenesis: The worms are voracious blood feeders and burrow into the mucosa and in severe infections cause a catarrhal enteritis.

Clinical signs: Causes an enteritis and anaemia, which in heavy infections may result in severe mortality in domestic pigeons.

Diagnosis: Identification of the worms on postmortem or eggs in the faeces.

Pathology: Haemorrhagic enteritis with ulceration and necrosis may occur in severe infections.

Epidemiology: The parasite may be responsible for heavy losses in breeding establishments.

Treatment: Oral benzimidazoles used for other nematode species should be effective.

Control: Where pigeons or doves are kept should be cleaned regularly to avoid build-up of eggs and infective larvae.

The following helminths have been reported in the intestines of pigeons and have been described in detail under Chapter 7 (Poultry and gamebirds).

Capillaria caudinflata

Synonym: *Aonchotheca caudinflata*

Predilection site: Small intestine

Parasite class: Nematoda

Superfamily: Trichuroidea

Final hosts: Chicken, turkey, goose, pigeon and wild birds

Intermediate hosts: Earthworms

Life cycle: The life cycle of this species is indirect.

Geographical distribution: Worldwide

Treatment and control: Oral capsules containing fenbendazole or cambendazole are effective.

Capillaria obsignata

Synonym: *Baruscapillaria obsignata, Capillaria columbae*

Predilection site: Small intestine

Parasite class: Nematoda

Superfamily: Trichuroidea

Hosts: Pigeon, chicken, turkey, and wild birds

Geographical distribution: Worldwide

Davainea proglottina

Predilection site: Small intestine, particularly the duodenum

Parasite class: Cestoda

Family: Davaineidae

Final hosts: Chicken, turkey, pigeon and other gallinaceous birds

Intermediate hosts: Gastropod molluscs such as *Agriolimax*, *Arion*, *Cepaea* and *Limax*

Geographical distribution: Most parts of the world

Raillietina tetragona

Predilection site: Posterior half of small intestine

Parasite class: Cestoda

Family: Davaineidae

Final hosts: Chicken, Guinea fowl and pigeons

Intermediate hosts: Ants of the genera *Pheidole* and *Tetramorium*

Geographical distribution: Worldwide

Echinoparyphium recurvatum

Predilection site: Small intestine, particularly the duodenum

Parasite class: Trematoda

Family: Echinostomatidae

Final hosts: Duck, goose, chicken and pigeon

Intermediate hosts: 1. Snails, such as *Lymnaea* spp and *Planorbis* spp. 2. Frogs, tadpoles and snails, such as *Valvata piscinalis* and *Planorbis albus*

Geographical distribution: Worldwide, particularly Asia and North Africa

Hypoderaeum conoideum

Predilection site: Posterior small intestine

Parasite class: Trematoda

Family: Echinostomatidae

Final hosts: Chicken, turkey, duck, goose, swan, pigeon and other aquatic birds

Intermediate hosts: As for *E. recurvatum*

Geographical distribution: Worldwide

Heterakis gallinarum

Synonym: *Heterakis papillosa, Heterakis gallinae, Heterakis vesicularis*

Common name: Poultry caecal worm

Predilection site: Caeca; rarely large and small intestine

Parasite class: Nematoda

Superfamily: Ascaridoidea

Hosts: Chicken, turkey, pigeon, pheasant, partridge, grouse, quail, guinea fowl, duck, goose and a number of wild galliform birds

Geographical distribution: Worldwide

Capillaria anatis

Synonym: *Capillaria brevicollis, C. collaris, C. anseris, C. mergi*

Predilection site: Caeca

Parasite class: Nematoda

Superfamily: Trichuroidea

Hosts: Chicken, turkey, gallinaceous birds (pheasant, partridge), pigeon, duck, goose

Geographical distribution: Worldwide

Brachylaemus commutatus

Synonym: *Harmostomum commutatus*

Predilection site: Caeca

Parasite class: Trematoda

Family: Brachylaemidae

Final hosts: Chicken, turkey, other fowl, pigeon and pheasant

Intermediate hosts: Land snails

Geographical distribution: Southern Europe, Africa, parts of Asia

Echinostoma revolutum

Predilection site: Caeca and rectum

Parasite class: Trematoda

Family: Echinostomatidae

Final hosts: Duck, goose, pigeon, various fowl and aquatic birds

Geographical distribution: Worldwide

Notes: *E. revolutum* can also infect man. *E. paraulum* occurs in the small intestine of duck and pigeon and can cause weakness, inappetence and diarrhoea in the latter.

Eimeria labbeana

Synonym: *Eimeria peifferi, Eimeria columbarum*

Predilection site: Small intestine

Parasite class: Sporozoasida

Family: Eimeriidae

Description: Oocysts are sub-spherical to spherical, smooth, colourless or slightly yellowish brown, 13–24 × 12–23 μm, without a micropyle or a residuum but with a polar granule. Sporocysts are elongate ovoid, with a Stieda body and residuum. The sporozoites are slightly crescent-shaped with one end wider than the other, lie lengthwise head to tail in the sporocysts, and have a clear globule at each end.

Hosts: Pigeon (*Columba domestica*), rock dove (*Columba livia*), collared dove (*Streptopelia decaoto*)

Life cycle: After the sporulated oocysts are ingested, the sporozoites are released and invade the epithelial cells of the intestine. First generation meronts are present 20–48 hours after infection in the epithelial cells of the anterior ileum. Mature second-generation meronts are present 96 hours, and mature third-generation meronts are present 144 hours after infection. The macrogametes are in the epithelial cells of the ileum. The prepatent period is about 5 days. The sporulation time is 4 days or less.

Geographical distribution: Worldwide

Pathogenesis: *E. labbeana* is slightly to markedly pathogenic, depending on the strain of parasite and age of the birds. Adults are fairly resistant, although fatal infections have been seen. The birds become weak and emaciated, eat little but drink a great deal, and have a greenish diarrhoea. The heaviest losses occur among squabs in the nest. A high percentage of the squabs may die, and those that recover are often somewhat stunted.

Clinical signs: Light infections are usually asymptomatic. In heavier infections, birds are listless, have a puffed-up appearance, and show weakness, emaciation and diarrhoea.

Diagnosis: Diagnosis is based on identification of oocysts in the faeces in association with any clinical and pathological findings.

Pathology: In severe infections there is inflammation of the intestinal mucosa with the lumen filled with a haemorrhagic exudate.

Epidemiology: Transmission is via the faecal–oral route and is more common in young birds. Sources of infection include dirty contaminated baskets, eating or drinking contaminated food or water or drinking from contaminated water in roosts such as roof guttering.

Treatment: Sulphonamides administered in the drinking water (e.g. sulphamethoxine 120 g per 2000 ml), are effective in treating infection. Clazuril also is effective at 2.5 mg given as an oral tablet per pigeon, regardless of weight. All birds in the same loft are usually treated simultaneously to prevent reinfection of untreated birds.

Control: Prevention is based on good management, avoidance of overcrowding and stress, and attention to hygiene.

Two other species of coccidia have been described in pigeons in India although details of the life cycle and pathogenicity are lacking. In *Eimeria columbae*, the oocysts are subspherical, 16 × 14 μm without a micropyle, but with an oocyst residuum. In *Wenyonella columbae*, oocysts are spherical or slightly ovoid, 21–27 × 21–26 μm without a micropyle, polar granule or oocyst residuum.

Spironucleus columbae

Predilection site: Small intestine

Parasite class: Zoomastigophorasida

Family: Diplomonadidae

Description: Trophozoites are small 5–9 × 2.5–7 μm.

Hosts: Pigeon

Geographical distribution: Worldwide

Pathogenesis and clinical signs: Infection may cause enteritis in pigeons.

Treatment and control: As for *Trichomonas gallinae*

PARASITES OF THE RESPIRATORY SYSTEM

Syngamus trachea

Synonym: *Syngamus parvis, Syngamus gracilis*

Common name: Gapeworm

Predilection site: Trachea or lungs

Parasite class: Nematoda

Superfamily: Strongyloidea

Hosts: Chicken, turkey, game birds (pheasant, partridge, guinea fowl), pigeon and various wild birds

Geographical distribution: Worldwide

For more details see Chapter 7 (Poultry and gamebirds).

Cytodites nudus

Common name: Air sac mite

Predilection site: Lung, air sac

Parasite class: Arachnida

Sub-class: Acari

Order: Acariformes

Sub-order: Sarcoptiformes (Astigmata)

Family: Cytoditidae

Description, gross: The mite is oval and about 500 μm long, with a smooth cuticle (Fig. 10.1).

Description, microscopic: The chelicerae are absent and the palps are fused to form a soft, sucking organ through which fluids are imbibed. Legs are stout and unmodified, ending in a pair of stalked suckers and a pair of small claws.

Hosts: Birds, particularly poultry and canaries

Life cycle: Larval, nymphal and adult stages take place on the surface of the respiratory tract of the host, with the complete life cycle of the mite requiring 14–21 days.

Geographical distribution: Worldwide

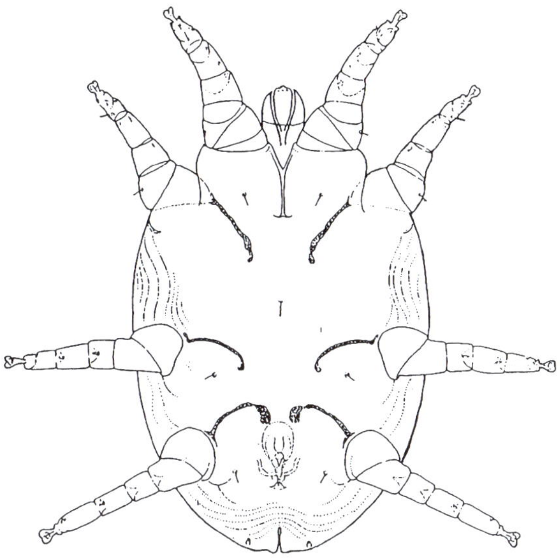

Fig. 10.1 Adult *Cytodites nudus*, ventral view (reproduced from Baker *et al.*, 1956).

Pathogenesis: Small infestations may have no obvious effect on the animal; large infestations may cause accumulation of mucus in the trachea and bronchi, leading to coughing and respiratory difficulties, air saculitis and weight loss. Balance may be affected in infested birds. Weakness, emaciation and death have been described with heavy infections.

Clinical signs: Coughing, respiratory difficulties, pulmonary oedema, weight loss, loss of balance or coordination.

Diagnosis: Positive diagnosis is only possible at post-mortem, when necropsy reveals white spots on the surface of air sacs.

Pathology: Death is usually associated with peritonitis, enteritis, emaciation and respiratory complications.

Epidemiology: Infestation may be spread through coughing.

Treatment: Treatment with topical moxidectin every 3 weeks as necessary may be effective.

PARASITES OF THE CIRCULATORY SYSTEM

Leucocytozoon marchouxi

Synonym: *Leucocytozoon turtur*

Predilection site: Blood

Parasite class: Sporozoasida

Family: Plasmodiidae

Description: Macrogametes are rounded or elliptical, stain dark blue with Giemsa and have a compact, reddish nucleus. This species forms rounded megaloshizonts in nearly all internal organs.

Hosts: Pigeons and doves

Life cycle: Sporozoites are introduced into a new host by the feeding insects. Parasites undergo merogony in the endothelial cells of internal organs forming megaloschizonts. These lead to the production of gametocytes in the blood, which, after ingestion by the vector insect, form zygote and oocysts. These undergo sporogony leading to the formation of sporozoites, which pass to the salivary glands and are introduced to the new host when the insect vectors feed.

Geographical distribution: Worldwide

Pathogenesis and clinical signs: Until recently this species was considered non-pathogenic in pigeons and doves but the species has been shown to be pathogenic to pink pigeons (*Columba mayeri*).

Diagnosis: Demonstration of gametocytes in blood smears

Epidemiology: Vectors are members of the genus *Simulium* (blackflies).

Treatment and control: Not usually required although general insect control or preventative measures may limit infection.

Haemoproteus columbae

Predilection site: Blood

Parasite class: Sporozoasida

Family: Plasmodiidae

Description: Macrogametes and microgametes present in erythrocytes range from tiny ring forms to elongate crescent-shapes that curve around the host cell nucleus in the form of a halter. Macrogametes stain dark blue with Giemsa stains, the nucleus is red to dark purple and compact, and pigment granules are dispersed throughout the cytoplasm.

Hosts: Domestic and wild pigeon, dove and other wild birds

Life cycle: Sporozoites in the salivary gland of the fly enter the circulation of the host when the insect bites and penetrate endothelial cells of blood vessels where they develop into meronts forming 15 or more cytomeres, each producing large numbers of merozoites. When merozoites are mature they are released into the circulation as tiny round bodies which transform into macrogametes and microgamonts within erythrocytes.

Further development takes place in the insect host after blood feeding. After fertilisation, a zygote forms in the insect midgut where sporogony takes place, forming sporozoites. These are liberated in the body cavity and pass to the salivary glands.

Geographical distribution: North America

Pathogenesis and clinical signs: Generally considered to be of low pathogenicity in adult birds, but an acute form of infection has been reported in sqabs. Clinical signs included anorexia and anaemia.

Diagnosis: Demonstration of gametocytes in blood smears

Epidemiology: Vectors are hippoboscid flies, *Pseudolynchia*.

Treatment and control: Not usually required although general insect control or preventative measures may limit infection

Haemoproteus sacharovi

Predilection site: Blood

Parasite class: Sporozoasida

Family: Plasmodiidae

Description: Macrogametes and microgametes are present in erythrocytes and completely fill the host cell when mature, distorting and pushing the nucleus to one side. Pigment granules are sparse compared with other species.

Hosts: Domestic pigeon, dove

Pathogenesis: Low pathogenicity although there have been reports of hepatomegaly in sqabs.

All other details are essentially similar to *H. columbae* although the vector(s) have not been identified.

PARASITES OF THE NERVOUS SYSTEM

No parasites of veterinary significance.

PARASITES OF THE REPRODUCTIVE/ UROGENITAL SYSTEM

No parasites of veterinary significance.

PARASITES OF THE LOCOMOTORY SYSTEM

Toxoplasma gondii

See Chapter 7 (Poultry and gamebirds), for more details.

PARASITES OF THE INTEGUMENT

Laminosioptes cysticola

Common name: Subcutaneous mite, fowl cyst mite

Predilection site: Subcutaneous tissues, lung, perotoneum

Parasite class: Arachnida

Sub-class: Acari

Order: Acariformes

Sub-order: Sarcoptiformes (Astigmata)

Family: Laminosioptidae

Description, gross: *Laminosioptes cysticola* is a small, oval mite, approximately 250 μm in length (Fig. 7.46).

Description, microscopic: The posterior two pairs of legs end in a claw and suckerless pedicels, while the anterior two pairs of legs end in claws. This mite has a smooth, elongated body and few setae. The gnathosoma is small and not visible when viewed from above.

Hosts: Chicken, turkey and pigeon, occasionally in wild birds

Life cycle: The life cycle is typical: egg, hexapod larva, followed by octopod protonymph, tritonymph and adult. All developmental stages occur on the host. However, life cycle details are lacking. The mites are found in the subcutaneous muscle fascia and in deeper tissues in the lungs, peritoneum, muscle and abdominal viscera.

Geographical distribution: Worldwide. It is abundant in Europe and is also found in the United States, South America and Australia.

Pathogenesis: *Laminosioptes* is not usually associated with clinical signs and is only discovered in pigeons at postmortem. Active mites occur in the deep tissues. The nodules created by the mites reduce the value of meat intended for human consumption.

Clinical signs: The parasites are not usually regarded as pathogenic.

Diagnosis: The nodules may be seen in living birds by parting the breast feathers and sliding the skin back and forth with the fingertips. Examination of the nodules under a dissection microscope usually allows the identification of the mite species.

Pathology: Aggregations of these small, oval mites are found in yellow nodules, several millimetres in diameter, in the subcutaneous muscle fascia and in deeper tissues in the lungs, peritoneum, muscle and abdominal viscera. The subcutaneous nodules are often calcified, but these only contain dead mites as the calcareous deposits are produced around the mites after they have died.

Epidemiology: It is estimated that around 1% of free-living urban pigeons harbour *Laminosioptes cysticola*. The mode of transmission of this mite is unknown.

Treatment: Macrocyclic lactones may be effective.

Control: Destroying or quarantining the infected birds may be required to achieve long-term reduction in infestations within a flock.

ECTOPARASITES

Colombicola columbae

Common name: Slender pigeon louse

Predilection site: Wings or anterior part of the body

Parasite class: Insecta

Parasite order: Phthiraptera

Parasite sub-order: Ischnocera

Family: Philopteridae

Description: A pale yellow, slender louse usually 2–3 μm in length.

Hosts: Pigeons and doves

Life cycle: Eggs of this species are usually attached to the feathers close to the skin. There are three nymphal stages similar to, although much smaller than, the adult. Development of the final stage gives rise to the fully mature reproductive adult.

Geographical distribution: Probably worldwide

Pathogenesis: Infection may cause a mild pruritus, and in common with most pediculoses, heavy infestations are usually seen only in diseased and debilitated birds causing feather damage and irritation.

Clinical signs: Feather damage and irritation

Diagnosis: Adult lice may be seen moving around the plumage or eggs may be seen attached to feathers.

Pathology: Lice are rarely linked to significant pathology.

Epidemiology: Infection occurs after direct contact with an infested host animal. Cross-contamination between different host species is possible if the animals have physical contact.

Treatment: Topical insecticidal compounds, such as permethrin, carbaryl, malathion, cypermethrin or rotenone, can be used to kill lice. However, as the insecticides are unable to kill the eggs, two applications are necessary with a 10-day interval.

Control: Although methods such as dusting the litter or providing insecticide-treated laying boxes are used to avoid undue handling of birds, the results obtained from treating individual birds are undoubtedly better. Regular checking and spraying of birds will enable infestation rates to be controlled. In addition, cross-contamination should be avoided. This is achieved by treating any birds in the environment of the pigeons and restricting contact between wild birds and pigeons. The housing and nesting should be thoroughly cleaned to eliminate sources of reinfestation such as egg-laden feathers.

Pseudolynchia canariensis

Common name: Pigeon fly

Predilection site: Skin

Parasite class: Insecta

Family: Hippoboscidae

Description: Adult flies are approximately 10 mm in length and are generally pale reddish brown with yellow spots on the indistinctly segmented abdomen. They have one pair of wings, the veins of which are crowded together towards the anterior margin. Both sexes of adult are blood feeders. The larvae are rarely seen and measure about 5 mm in length.

Hosts: Mainly pigeons but other domestic birds may also be infested.

Life cycle: Gravid female flies mature larvae singly. Each female can produce only five or six larvae in its lifetime. These larvae pupate almost immediately after larviposition. When pupation is completed, the newly emerged winged adults locate a suitable host animal on which they blood-feed, remaining on the host for long periods. In temperate areas, flies are most abundant in the summer months.

Geographical distribution: Worldwide

Pathogenesis: The adult flies bite and blood-feed, resulting in a nuisance and disturbance. Heavily infested birds may be restless, emaciated and become susceptible to secondary infections. They may act as vectors of *Haemoproteus columbae* and *H. sacharovi*.

Clinical signs: The adult flies are clearly visible when feeding on the host animal. Irritation at the feeding sites may be observed.

Diagnosis: The adult flies may be found on the host animal.

Epidemiology: The adult flies are most abundant on the host during the summer months.

Treatment and control: This is best achieved by topical application of insecticides, preferably those with some repellent and residual effect such as the synthetic pyrethroids, permethrin and deltamethrin.

Ceratophyllus columbae

Common name: Pigeon flea

Predilection site: Skin

Parasite class: Insecta

Parasite order: Siphonaptera

Family: Ceratophyllidae

Description: Adults of *Ceratophyllus columbae* are typically 2–2.5 mm long with no antennal fossae. Eyes are present. There is a pronotal comb carrying more than 24 teeth, while the genal comb is absent. There is a lateral row of four to six bristles on the inner surface of the hind femur, and there are no spines on the basal section of the legs. Detailed description of individual species in this genus is beyond the scope of this text.

Hosts: Pigeon

Life cycle: The life cycle is typical: egg, three larval stages, pupa and adult. Before the female can begin ovipositing it needs to feed on the host several times. Unlike most other fleas, which often remain on the host and feed for long periods, pigeon fleas spend most of their time in the nest of the host, and only move on to the birds to feed for short periods.

The larvae feed on detritus amongst the nest material, bird droppings and on undigested blood from the adult faeces. The larval stages are completed in a few weeks, before the pupal cocoon is spun. The flea overwinters in the cocoon and emerges in an old nest in spring as temperatures rise. Large numbers may occur in the nests of passerine birds, and they may complete their life cycle during the period of nest occupation by these birds. Work has shown a negative correlation between flea abundance and mean body mass of the brood being parasitised.

If the nest is reused by birds the following year, the newly emerged adults will locate the new hosts, feed and continue the cycle. If the nest is not reused, the newly emerged adults will make their way to the nest entrance, where they may be able to attach to a bird that is examining the old nest as a potential nest site. Alternatively, they may climb up trees and bushes, where they stop periodically and face the brightest source of light, jumping in response to a shadow passing in front of the light.

Geographical distribution: Found predominantly in the Old World, but has been introduced into the Americas.

Pathogenesis: Feeding activity may cause irritation, restlessness and, with heavy infestations, anaemia. In wild birds, flea reproduction and feeding activity is synchronised with the breeding season. Adult *C. columbae* may also feed on humans and domestic pets.

Clinical signs: Symptoms include restlessness and scratching of affected areas. The bites may be visible on the skin. Allergic dermatitis may be seen.

Diagnosis: Diagnosis is not easy as adults may leave the host and eggs and larvae are difficult to find. The bites of these fleas are similar to those of mosquitoes, lice and mites, with inflammation and itchiness.

Epidemiology: These fleas are not host specific and may attack any available mammal or bird for a blood-meal. As they are able to survive off the host, transmission can occur from the bedding and housing. This flea is highly mobile on the host and can be especially common in host nesting material. *Ceratophyllus columbae* feeds readily on humans and domestic pets, and is often acquired in the handling of pigeons and wild birds. It has also been known to migrate into rooms from nests under adjacent eaves. When such nests are removed they should be incinerated; otherwise the underfed fleas may parasitise domestic pets and humans.

Treatment: Topical treatment of the affected birds with insecticidal products such as permethrin, carbaryl, malathion and rotenone is effective.

Control: Should fleas become established, drastic measures may have to be adopted to get rid of them. All litter and nest material should be removed and burnt, and the housing sprayed with an insecticide.

Argas reflexus

Common name: Pigeon tick

Predilection site: Skin

Parasite class: Arachnida

Sub-class: Acari

Order: Parasitiformes

Sub-order: Ixodida (Metastigmata)

Family: Argasidae

Description: Species of the genus are usually dorsoventrally flattened, with definite margins, which can be seen even when the tick is engorged. The cuticle is wrinkled and leathery. Most species are nocturnal and are parasites of birds, bats, reptiles or, occasionally, small insectivorous mammals. Most species seldom attack humans. Species of this genus are usually found in dry, arid habitats.

The adult *Argas reflexus* is between 6 and 11 mm in length. It may be distinguished from the fowl tick, *Argas persicus*, by its body margin, which is composed of irregular grooves, and by the hypostome, which is not notched apically. It is reddish brown in colour with paler legs.

Hosts: Birds, mainly pigeons

Life cycle: *Argas reflexus* is nocturnal and breeds and shelters in cracks and crevices in the roost structure. Females deposit batches of 50–100 eggs in these cracks and crevices. After hatching, larvae locate and attach to a host, where they remain and feed for several days. After feeding they detach, leave the host and shelter in the pigeon lofts or roosts. Several days later they moult to become first-stage nymphs. They then proceed through two nymphal stages, interspersed with frequent feeds, before moulting to the adult stage. Adult males and females feed about once a month. Females can become completely engorged within 30–45 minutes. All stages of these ticks remain around the roosting area, quiescent in the day and actively feeding at night. *Argas reflexus* can survive in empty roosts for more than a year. Engorged females diapause between July and August. If oviposition has already commenced, egg-laying stops and resumes the following year without the need for another blood meal.

Geographical distribution: Europe, Russia, Asia, north and west Africa.

Pathogenesis: Infestation may cause irritation, sleeplessness, loss of egg productivity and anaemia, which can prove fatal. Heavy infestations can take enough blood to bring about the death of their host. This species transmits *Borrelia anserina*, the cause of fowl spirochaetosis, and *Aegyptianella pullorum*, a rickettsial infection. It may also be a vector of west Nile and chenuda virus and the quaranfil virus group.

Clinical signs: Inflammation and raised areas will be present from tick bites. Larvae may be found living in the feathers. These ticks can cause sleeplessness, loss of productivity and anaemia, which can prove fatal.

Diagnosis: The adult ticks, particularly the engorged larvae, may be seen on the skin. Nymphs and adult ticks may be found in cracks of the woodwork. Red spots may be seen on the skin where the ticks have fed.

Pathology: Small granulomatous reactions may form at the site of tick bites consisting of a mixed inflammatory cell response with fibrosis.

Epidemiology: *Argas reflexus* eggs show limited levels of cold tolerance; winter temperatures of 3°C cause approximately 50% mortality. This limits its northern distribution through Europe.

Treatment: Argasid ticks, which exist in lofts and enclosures, can be controlled by application of an acaricide to their environment coupled with treatment of the population on the host. Environmental treatment of roosts and lofts may be effected using acaricidal sprays or emulsions containing organophosphates or pyrethroids. All niches and crevices in affected buildings should be sprayed, and nesting boxes and perches should also be painted with acaricides. At the same time as premises are treated, birds should be dusted with a suitable acaricide or, in the case of larger animals, sprayed or dipped. Treatment should be repeated at monthly intervals.

Control: All new animals should be treated prior to introduction into an existing flock.

RATITES (OSTRICH, RHEA, EMU)

PARASITES OF THE DIGESTIVE SYSTEM

PROVENTRICULUS, GIZZARD

Libyostrongylus

Life cycle: The life cycle is typically strongyle. Following ingestion, infective larvae burrow into the proventricular glands and under the kaolin layer of both proventriculus and gizzard where they develop into adult worms 4–5 weeks later

Pathogenesis: The young worms penetrate deeply into the mucosa of the glands of the proventriculus. Adults live on the surface of the epithelium (Fig. 10.2) where they feed on blood, causing a severe inflammatory reaction and anaemia.

Clinical signs: Chicks are most susceptible to infection and become anaemic, weak and emaciated with heavy mortality in untreated cases.

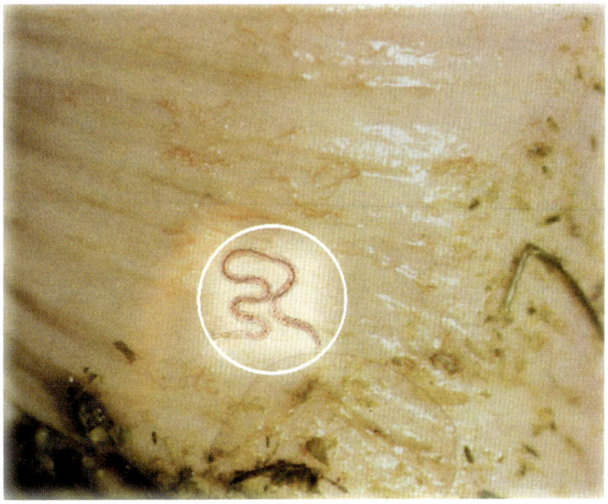

Fig. 10.2 *Libyostrongylus douglassi*: mucosal surface of proventriculus. Insert shows magnified worm.

Diagnosis: Diagnosis is based on finding eggs in the faeces or by identifying the worms in the proventriculus and gizzard on postmortem.

Treatment: Levamisole (30 mg/kg), fenbendazole (15 mg/kg) and ivermectin (200 μg/kg) are effective in the treatment of wireworm infection in young ostrich.

Control: Appropriate hygiene and husbandry measures, including removal of faeces aimed at limiting pasture contamination, help limit exposure to dangerous levels of infective larvae. It is important to isolate and treat all new birds to prevent introduction of infection on ostrich farms.

Libyostrongylus douglassi

Common name: Wireworm

Predilection site: Proventriculus, gizzard

Parasite class: Nematoda

Superfamily: Trichostrongyloidea

Description, gross: Small yellowish red nematodes; males 4–6 mm and females 5–6 mm

Description, microscopic: The male bursa is well developed; the dorsal ray is long and split in its distal half forming three small branches either side. The spicules each end in a large and small spine. Eggs measure 59–74 × 36–44 mm. Third-stage larvae are characterised by a small knob at the tip of the tail.

Hosts: Ostrich

Geographical distribution: Africa, North America, Europe

Libyostrongylus dentatus

Common name: Wireworm

Predilection site: Proventriculus, gizzard

Parasite class: Nematoda

Superfamily: Trichostrongyloidea

Description, gross: Males 6–8 mm and females 10–12 mm

Description, microscopic: There is a prominent dorsal oesophageal tooth. There is a large bursa; the dorsal ray is long and bifurcated extending into a rounded lobe of the bursal membrane. A spicule with dorsal process arises two thirds from the anterior and the main shaft ends in a rounded point capped by a hyaline sheath.

Hosts: Ostrich

Geographical distribution: Africa, North America

Spiruroid nematodes

Several species of spiruroid worms belonging to the genera *Spiura* and *Odontospiura* are found in the proventriculus of rheas. These species are essentially similar to spiruroid worm species found in the proventriculus of poultry (see Chapter 7). The identification of individual species is beyond the scope of this book and interested readers will need to consult a relevant taxonomic specialist. Diagnosis is based on the presence of spiruroid eggs in the faeces or the presence of the worms in the proventriculus on postmortem.

Spiruria uncinipenis

Synonym: *Sicarius uncinipenis*

Predilection site: Proventriculus

Parasite class: Nematoda

Superfamily: Spiruroidea

Description, gross: Males measure 15–20 mm and females 16–26 mm.

Description, microscopic: The spicules are short and unequal in length.

Final hosts: Rhea

Geographical distribution: South America

Spiruria zschokkei

Synonym: *Vaznema zschokkei*

Predilection site: Proventriculus

Parasite class: Nematoda

Superfamily: Spiruroidea

Description, gross: Males measure 16–17 mm; female worms are 17–25 mm in length.

Description, microscopic: The spicules are long and filiform.

Final hosts: Rhea

Geographical distribution: South America

Odontospiruria cetiopenis

Predilection site: Proventriculus, gizzard

Parasite class: Nematoda

Superfamily: Spiruroidea

Description, gross: Males measure 15–17 mm; female worms are 20–23 mm.

Final hosts: Rhea

Geographical distribution: South America

SMALL INTESTINE

Deletrocephalus dimidiatus

Predilection site: Small intestine

Parasite class: Nematoda

Superfamily: Strongyloidea

Description, gross: Adult worms are stout and robust with a well developed buccal capsule. Male worms are 9–11 mm and females 14–16 mm long.

Description, microscopic: Males are bursate with long, thin spicules. The eggs are $160 \times 70\,\mu m$. Third-stage larvae are approximately 720 µm long with a rounded head, 28–31 intestinal cells and a short to medium tail.

Final hosts: Greater rhea (*Rhea Americana*), lesser rhea (*Pterocnemia pennata*)

Life cycle: The life cycle is thought to be direct, with birds ingesting infective larvae whilst foraging.

Geographical distribution: South America, North America, Europe

Pathogenesis and clinical signs: There are limited reports on the distribution and pathogenicity of this parasite in rheas. The parasite has become established in domesticated rheas and has been reported to cause weak, diarrhoeic chicks in heavy infections.

Diagnosis: Diagnosis is based on finding eggs in the faeces or by identifying the worms in the intestine on postmortem.

Treatment and control: There is little information on the treatment of this parasite in rheas. Benzimidazoles and ivermectin have been used in the treatment of nematodes in ostrich, and therefore may be of benefit. Rearing of chicks away from adult birds and regular cleaning of pens may help limit infection.

Paradeletrocephalus minor

Predilection site: Small intestine

Parasite class: Nematoda

Superfamily: Strongyloidea

Description, gross: Adult worms are similar in size to *Deletrocephalus* spp.

Description, microscopic: The buccal capsule has vertical ridges and there are no external or internal coronary rings.

Final hosts: Greater rhea (*Rhea Americana*), lesser rhea (*Pterocnemia pennata*)

Geographical distribution: South America

Hottuynia struthionis

Predilection site: Small intestine

Parasite class: Cestoda

Family: Davaineidae

Description, gross: These are large tapeworms (60–120 cm).

Description, microscopic: The scolex is 1–2 mm wide and bears a double row of about 160 large and small hooks. Genital pores are unilateral.

Final hosts: Ostrich, rhea

Life cycle: The life cycle is unknown.

Geographical distribution: Africa, South America

Pathogenesis: The tapeworm is seen especially in ostrich chicks but has also been reported in rheas, causing unthriftiness, emaciation and diarrhoea.

Clinical signs: Affected chicks lose their appetite and may die.

Diagnosis: Diagnosis is based on finding eggs in the faeces or by identifying the worms in the proventriculus and gizzard on postmortem.

Treatment: Praziquantel at 7.5 mg/kg is effective.

Control: As the intermediate host is not known, specific control measures are not possible. Rearing of chicks away from adult birds, regular cleaning of pens and insect control would seem expedient.

LARGE INTESTINE

Codiostomum struthionis

Predilection site: Large intestine

Parasite class: Nematoda

Superfamily: Strongyloidea

Description, gross: These strongylid worms are 13–17 mm in length.

Description, microscopic: The large buccal capsule is sub-globular with external and internal leaf crowns but no teeth. The male bursa has a large projecting dorsal lobe.

Hosts: Ostrich

Life cycle: The life cycle is unknown.

Geographical distribution: Africa

Pathogenesis and clinical signs: Potentially a pathogenic worm causing anaemia and poor growth rates.

Diagnosis: The eggs are identical to *L. douglassi* and diagnosis is based on identification of the adult worms in the caeca and colon.

Treatment and control: As for *Libyostrongylus*

Trichostrongylus tenuis

Predilection site: Small intestine, caeca.

Parasite class: Nematoda

Superfamily: Trichostrongyloidea

Hosts: Game birds (grouse, partridge and pheasant), chicken, duck, goose, turkey, emu

Geographical distribution: North America, Asia and Europe

Epidemiology: A common parasite of various galliform and anseriform birds

For more details see Chapter 7 (Poultry and gamebirds).

Other parasites reported in the intestines of ratites are listed in the parasite checklist at the end of this chapter.

PARASITES OF THE RESPIRATORY SYSTEM

Paronchocerca struthionis

Predilection site: Pulmonary arteries, lungs

Parasite class: Nematoda

Superfamily: Filarioidea

Description, gross: Long abursate nematodes, 3–5 cm in length with bluntly rounded extremities.

Description, microscopic: Male spicules are dissimilar in length; a gubernaculum is absent. Microfilariae are 100–125 μm long with a rounded posterior extremity.

Hosts: Ostrich

Geographical distribution: Africa

Pathogenicity: Not reported

Syngamus trachea

Common name: Gapeworm

Predilection site: Trachea

Parasite class: Nematoda

Superfamily: Strongyloidea

Hosts: Chicken, turkey, game birds (pheasant, partridge, guinea-fowl), various wild birds

Geographical distribution: Worldwide

For more details see Chapter 7 (Poultry and gamebirds).

Cyathostoma variegatum

Common name: Gapeworm

Predilection site: Trachea, bronchi

Parasite class: Nematoda

Superfamily: Strongyloidea

Description, gross: Adult worms are 0.4–3 cm long; males are 4–5.8 mm and females 16–31 mm.

Description, microscopic: The buccal capsule is cup-shaped with six to seven teeth at its base. The male bursa is well developed but worms in this species are not permanently in copula, which contrasts to the situation with *Syngamus trachea*. Eggs are 74–83 × 49–62 μm.

Hosts: Duck, emu

Life cycle: The life cycle is thought to be similar to that of *Syngamus*

Geographical distribution: Australia

Pathogenicity: Has been reported to cause severe respiratory distress in young emus.

Epidemiology: A number of paratenic hosts may be involved in transmission.

Treatment and control: Ivermectin is likely to be effective.

PARASITES OF THE CIRCULATORY SYSTEM

Leucocytozoon struthionis

Predilection site: Blood

Parasite class: Sporozoasida

Family: Plasmodiidae

Description: Gamonts are round and present within erythrocytes

Final host: Ostrich

Intermediate host: Blackflies (*Simulium*)

Geographical distribution: Africa

Pathogenesis and clinical signs: Thought to be of low pathogenicity although it has been found in association with myocarditis in young ostrich chicks and may cause anaemia during early parasitaemia.

Epidemiology: A common parasite of ostrich chicks in South Africa transmitted by blackflies, *Simulium*

Diagnosis: Identification of either gamonts in blood or megalomeronts in tissue.

Treatment and control: Not reported

Plasmodium struthionis

Predilection site: Blood

Parasite class: Sporozoasida

Family: Plasmodiidae

Pathogenesis: Reported in ostrich as causing an asymptomatic low, chronic parasitaemia.

PARASITES OF THE NERVOUS SYSTEM

No parasites of veterinary significance reported.

ECTOPARASITES

Struthiolipeurus struthionis

Common name: Ostrich louse

Predilection site: Feathers and skin

Parasite class: Ischnocera

Family: Philopteridae

Description: Narrow-bodied louse with a large head (Fig. 10.3)

Hosts: Ostrich

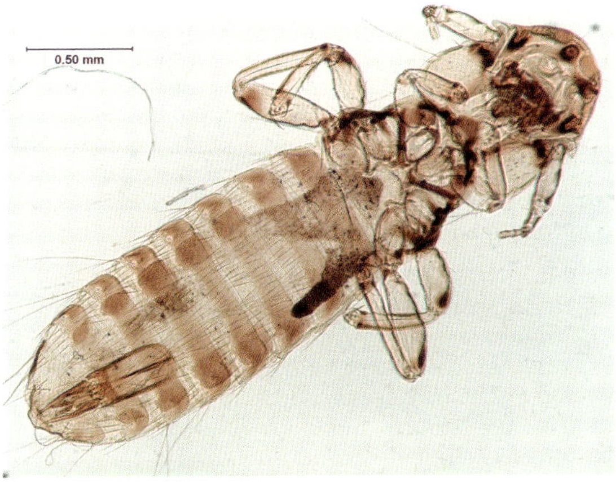

Fig. 10.3 *Struthiolipeurus struthionis* (photograph courtesy of Dr Vince Smith).

Life cycle: The biology of these lice has not been fully studied, but is thought to be typical: egg, several nymphal stages and adult requiring about 1 month for completion.

Pathogenesis and clinical signs: This is a chewing louse, which damages the feathers, reducing the value of especially white plumes. The damage causes the feathers to have a moth-eaten appearance.

Diagnosis: Lice and eggs may be found in the feathers close to the skin.

Treatment and control: Treatment with pyrethroid is recommended; carbaryl dust (5%) may also be effective.

A variety of other lice may also be found on Ostrich including *Struthiolipeurus nandu* and *Struthiolipeurus stresemanni*. *Struthiolipeurus rhea*, *Meinertzhageniella lata* and *Meinertzhageniella schubarti* have been reported in rheas; and *Dahlemhornia asymmetrica* in emus.

Gabucinia spp

Common name: Shaft or quill mites

Predilection site: These mites can be found in the ventral groove of the feather shaft.

Parasite class: Arachnida

Family: Gabuciniidae

Description: These are pale elongated mites, about 0.5 μm in length. The dorsal idiosoma appears patterned or sculpted. The first two pairs of legs protrude anteriorly.

Hosts: Ostrich

Life cycle: Typical: egg, nymphal stages and reproductive adult. Knowledge of the biology of these quill mites is very limited. Under intensive conditions this parasite is able to multiply rapidly on ostriches reaching high densities.

Pathogenesis and clinical signs: Quill mites are very common, but occasionally become a problem in ostriches kept under intensive conditions. Large numbers of mites cause severe feather damage, causing scarring of the skin and a reduction in the economic value of the infested animal.

Diagnosis: Mites may be observed at the base of the feathers.

Treatment and control: Treatment with ivermectin has been reported to be effective.

Notes: There are several species in this genus, which infest a range of wild birds, but *Gabucinia sculpturata* and *Gabucinia (Pterolinchus) bicaudatus* are the most common and well described in ostrich.

Numerous species of tick have also been reported to infest ostriches in their native ranges. These are summarised in the parasite checklist at the end of this chapter.

REPTILES

Reptiles are represented by four orders of animals comprising approximately 5500 species. Species of reptiles belonging to the Chelonia (tortoises, terrapins, turtles) and Squamata, divided into the suborders Sauria (lizards), Serpentes (snakes), are increasingly kept and bred in captivity, both in zoological and private collections and kept as individual pets.

Reptiles in the wild are infected with a wide range of parasites, especially given the extremely varied range of prey animals, and their potential to act as intermediate hosts for many species of parasites. Generally though, if well fed and non-stressed, parasitised animals can remain comparatively healthy even when carrying burdens of several species of parasites. Parasites with heteroxenous life cycles, requiring two or more hosts, are only likely to be encountered in wild-caught animals.

Parasitic infections are frequently encountered in captive-bred reptiles and this section will concentrate only on these infections rather than wild-caught specimens. Given the range of reptile species kept in captivity, it is beyond the scope of this book to provide detailed descriptions of all the species of parasites that may be encountered. As such, only a general overview is provided with more detailed descriptions of those parasite species considered to be of importance.

It is not uncommon to encounter 'pseudoparasites', which may either be parasites of the prey host (e.g. the oxyurid parasite, *Syphacia* of rodents, seen in snake faeces) or normal commensals of the gut flora in herbivorous animals (e.g. the ciliate *Nyctotherus* in iguanas and tortoises). For this reason it is important to know both the taxonomic identification and the diet of captive reptiles prior to attempted parasite identification and instigation of potentially unnecessary treatment.

PARASITES OF THE DIGESTIVE SYSTEM

HELMINTHS

Whilst cestode, trematode and acanthocephalan parasites are commonly found in wild-caught reptiles, their complicated life cycles, which may involve one or more intermediate hosts, mean that they are rarely found in captive reptiles and as a consequence these parasite classes will not be discussed further.

Nematodes

Reptile digestive tracts can be infected with a wide range of trichostrongylid, strongylid, ascarid and other nematode superfamilies. Both strongyles and trichostrongyles can be found in the alimentary tracts of reptiles, especially snakes.

Kalicephalus spp

Predilection site: Small intestine

Parasite class: Nematoda

Superfamily: Strongyloidea

Description: Adult worms are 1–5 cm in length.

Hosts: Snakes

Life cycle: The life cycle is direct with a prepatent period of 2–4 months.

Pathogenesis and clinical signs: *Kalicephalus* causes a wide range of signs, including lethargy, regurgitation, diarrhoea, anorexia and debility. The larvae may undergo a visceral larva migrans and can cause respiratory problems.

Diagnosis: The embryonated eggs or larvae may be found in faecal smears or on microscopy of oral and oesophageal mucus, or tracheal washings.

Pathology: Adult worms embedded in the oesophageal, gastric and intestinal mucosa cause ulceration, usually with a secondary bacterial infection. Build-up of necrotic debris may cause occlusion of the oesophagus.

Epidemiology: Infection is by ingestion of contaminated food or water or percutaneously. There is a low host specificity and many species of snake can be infected, which is important where several species are kept together.

Treatment and control: Treatment is often unsuccessful, although fenbendazole (50–100 mg/kg) or oxfendazole (60 mg/kg) may be tried. Ivermectin at 200 μg/kg by subcutaneous injection has also been reported to be effective but should be used with caution in some species of reptiles. Recovery can be very protracted. Good husbandry is very important in controlling and preventing infection.

Within the Ascaridoidea, certain genera and species of these worms parasitise particular host groups. *Ophidascaris* and *Polydelphus* are found only in snakes; *Angusticaecum* and *Sulcascaris* are found in chelonia. The pathogenic effects of ascarid nematodes depend on parasite numbers, food availability and an infected animal's overall condition. Clinical signs, such as regurgitation and obstipation, may be seen. The presence of the worms in the gastrointestinal tract may cause gastritis, ulceration and perforation of the stomach wall; and in the intestines, intestinal obstruction, intussusception, necrotic enteritis leading to coelomitis and death. Such sequelae may be seen following treatment with anthelminitics in reptiles with heavy worm burdens.

Diagnosis of these infections is based on microscopic examination of eggs found in the faeces. Ascarid eggs are round with thick, heavily pitted walls. Control of ascarid nematodes depends on routine parasitological screening of all new arrivals and treatment of all infected animals with anthelmintics. Fenbendazole given at 50–100 mg/kg by mouth or stomach tube is generally reported to be effective.

Oxyurid parasites belonging to the superfamily Oxyuridoidea are commonly found in reptiles and at least 12 different genera have been described in snakes, lizards and chelonia. These small nematodes ('pinworms') may be present in large numbers in the large intestine, colon and rectum, causing discomfort. Some species are viviparous, but the majority are oviparous or ovovivaporous and a common feature of their eggs is an asymmetrical flattening on one side. Diagnosis of oxyurid infections is based on the identification of the characteristic eggs in faeces, or the adults from faeces or postmortem specimens. Treatment is as for ascarid infections.

Strongyloides and *Rhabdias* spp, belonging to the superfamily Rhabditoidea, are slender, hair-like worms. Only females are parasitic and these produce larvated, oval, thin-shelled eggs. After hatching, larvae may develop through four larval stages into free-living adult male and female worms and this can be followed by a succession of free-living generations. In *Strongyloides* infection, there is anorexia, weight loss, diarrhoea, dehydration and death. *Rhabdias* are primarily respiratory parasites but can be associated with enteritis. Treatment with fenbendazole, as for other worm species, is usually effective.

Several species of *Capillaria* (Trichuroidea) have been reported in reptiles. These are very fine filamentous worms found mainly in the gastrointestinal tract but may also infest other organs such as the liver and reproductive organs. Transmission is direct from one infected reptile to another via the larvated egg, which is barrel-shaped with bipolar plugs.

PROTOZOA

Flagellate protozoa (Zoomastigophorasida, Diplomonadidae) are commonly seen in the faeces of reptiles. *Spironucleus* (*Hexamita*) has been reported to cause fatal renal disease in aquatic chelonia (terrapins). A number of other flagellates have been reported in reptiles. These include *Chilmastix*, *Enteromonas*, *Eutrichomonas*, *Herpatamonas*, *Leptomonas*, *Trichomonas*, *Pentatrichomonas* and *Proteromonas*. *Monocercomonas* has been recorded in both Old and New World lizards and snakes of several different genera and species. Definitive diagnosis is made by identifying the organisms by their characteristic flagella, nuclear complement and other morphological characteristics. Most of these organisms are sensitive to oral metronidazole (dose rate 100–275 mg/kg).

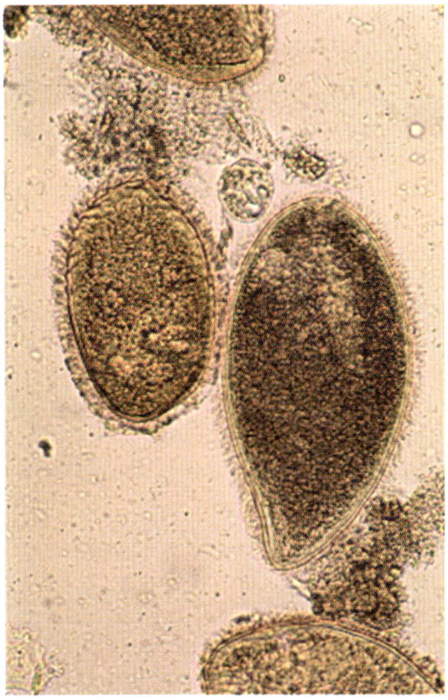

Fig. 10.4 *Nyctotherus* from an iguana.

Several protozoan species may often be present in clinically normal reptiles and may become pathogenic only if and when the host is stressed or becomes immunologically incompetent for one reason or another. *Nyctotherus* and other protozoa, such as *Balantidium* and *Paramecium*, are thought to serve as beneficial commencals required for the processing of dietary cellulose and complex carbohydrate constituents (Fig. 10.4). Correct identification is essential otherwise they become the objects of unnecessary (and possibly harmful) treatment. Neonatal common iguanas, for example, acquire their intestinal microflora by actively seeking out and ingesting the fresh stools of older lizards. When the normal microflora is substantially disturbed or destroyed, the gut must be re-inoculated with a culture or other source of bacterial and protozoan organisms from a healthy animal as close to the genus and species of the sick reptile as possible.

Entamoeba invadens

Predilection site: Large intestine

Parasite class: Sarcodina

Family: Endamoebidae

Description: Trophozoites are 11–20 μm and cysts approximately 16 μm.

Life cycle: Following ingestion of the infective cyst, it excysts and releases one quadrinucleate trophozoite which divides to produce eight uninucleate amoebae. These mature in the colon, eventually producing cysts which pass out in the faeces.

Pathogenesis: *E. invadens* usually lives as a commensal symbiont in turtles, some tortoises and crocodilians that serve as healthy reservoirs of the organism. Contamination of the water supply of snakes and lizards with *Entamoeba* can, on occasions, lead to enteritis, hepatitis and, occasionally, nephritis. It has been reported in cases of human and animal amoebic meningoencephalitis.

Clinical signs: There are few specific or pathognomonic signs attributable to amoebiosis in reptiles. The clinical signs of infection are usually related to regurgitation of undigested food, weight loss, dehydration, lethargy, severe diarrhoea, sometimes accompanied with blood or bile-tinged green mucus and/or tags of intestinal mucosa. Rupture of hollow viscus organs has been reported in some cases. Occasionally, rectal or cloacal prolapse occurs.

Diagnosis: Positive diagnosis of amoebiosis depends upon finding elongated uninucleate trophozoites and/or cysts containing four nuclei in the faeces. Cysts are more easily detected if stained with Lugol's iodine.

Pathology: Microscopically, the characteristic lesions produced by *E. invadens* are severe intestinal erosion, inflammation and, often, ulceration. The affected gut wall is thickened, ulcerated and focally necrotic, often a fibrinonecrotic pseudomembrane is found in the intestinal lumen overlying the foci of inflammation. Typically, the ileum and colon are the most severely affected intestinal segments. The liver shows focal areas of necrosis and evidence of fatty degeneration. Pulmonary abscessation has also been associated with more chronic infections.

Epidemiology: There does not appear to be any particular host susceptibility or resistance, although it is seen more commonly in captive boas and pythons. Cysts can survive for 7–14 days in the environment.

Treatment and control: Metronidazole at a single oral treatment of 275 mg/kg bodyweight has been reported to be effective. An alternative treatment is 160 mg/kg orally for 3 days. Supportive medical care, consisting of fluid and multivitamin complex therapy and increased ambient environmental temperature, should also be provided. Strict hygiene and quarantine are important in preventing the transmission of *E. invadens* cysts. All cages and water containers should be cleaned routinely with disinfectant.

Reptiles and amphibians may serve as natural hosts to other amoebae. *Acanthamoeba* have elongate filiform pseudopodia and a large nuclear karyosome. Some consider *Hartmannella* to be synonymous. Amoeboid forms of the genus *Naeglaria* have broad pseudopodia but may also exist as flagellate forms with two flagella and a large central nuclear karyosome. It is thought that the flagellate form is infective for both vertebrates and invertebrates.

Many of these organisms appear to share a commensal relationship with their hosts, but some infections have been associated with gastric, intestinal, hepatic, brain and renal lesions. Due to the potential for human infection, care must be taken when working with reptiles harbouring these organisms.

Several genera of coccidia (Eimeriidae) have been reported from reptiles. These include *Eimeria*, *Isospora*, *Caryosporai*, *Cyclospora*, *Hoarella*, *Octosporella*, *Pythonella*, *Weyonella*, *Dorisiella* and *Tyzzeria*. *Eimeria*, *Isospora* and *Caryospora* are the most frequently observed genera in reptiles, particularly in lizards and snakes. *Isospora* has also been reported in crocodilians. Only *Eimeria* have been found in chelonians. *Weyonella* has only been reported in snakes. Determining the number of sporocysts and sporozoites present within the sporulated oocysts is used for differentiating the genera (see Table 1.3).

It is important, however, to be aware that in some species of carnivorous snakes and lizards, some of the *Isospora* recorded may be *Toxoplasma* and *Sarcocystis*. *Eimeria* species recorded in snakes may similarly be parasites of the prey host.

Parasites of the genus *Cryptosporidium* are of increasing importance in reptiles. Two species have been reported: *C. serpentis* in snakes and lizards and *C. saurophilum* in lizards.

Cryptosporidium serpentis

Predilection site: Stomach

Parasite class: Sporozoasida

Family: Cryptosporidiidae

Description: Oocysts, passed fully sporulated, are ovoid, 5.9×5.1 μm, with a length:width ratio of 1.17.

Hosts: Snakes, lizards

Life cycle: The life cycle is unknown but is likely due to the ingestion of sporulated oocysts, each with four sporozoites. Following ingestion, the sporozoites appear to invade the microvillous brush border of the gastric glands to form meronts followed by gametogony and oocyst production. The prepatent period is unknown.

Geographical distribution: Presumed worldwide

Pathogenesis: Infection has been reported in snakes belonging to a number of species and genera with infected animals showing a severe chronic hypertrophic gastritis. Signs include postprandial regurgitation and firm midbody swelling. Infection usually occurs in mature snakes, the clinical course is usually protracted, and once infected most snakes remain infected. *C. serpentis* apparently also infects lizards and has been found in savannah monitors.

Clinical signs: Postprandial regurgitation, midbody swelling and chronic weight loss.

Diagnosis: Oocysts may be demonstrated using Ziehl–Nielsen-stained faecal smears in which the sporozoites appear as bright red granules. Speciation of *Cryptosporidium* is difficult, if not impossible, using conventional techniques. A range of molecular and immunological techniques has been developed, that includes the use of immunofluorescence (IF) or enzyme-linked immunosorbent assays (ELISA). More recently, DNA-based techniques have been used for the molecular characterisations of *Cryptosporidium* species.

Pathology: Oedema and thickening of gastric mucosa with exaggeration of normal longitudinal rugae with copious mucus adhesion. Histologically there is mucosal petechiation, ecchymotic haemorrhages and focal necrosis. There is hypertrophy of mucous neck cells with excess mucus in the gastric pits and adherent to the surface epithelium. The lamina propria is oedematous with lymphocyte and scattered heterophil infiltration. Trophozoites can be seen on the brush border of surface and glandular epithelial cells. In some animals there may be replacement of glandular cells by cuboidal or columnar epithelial cells, epithelial hyperplasia and mucosal necrosis with abscess formation and oedema.

Epidemiology: Transmission appears to be mainly by the faecal–oral route.

Treatment and control: There is no effective treatment. Strict hygiene and quarantine on imported or captive reptiles is required. Chronically infected animals showing weight loss, emaciation and gastric enlargement should be culled.

Cryptosporidium saurophilum

Predilection site: Intestine, cloaca

Parasite class: Sporozoasida

Family: Cryptosporidiidae

Description: Oocysts, passed fully sporulated, are ovoid, 4.4–5.6 × 4.2–5.2 μm (mean 5.0 × 4.7 μm), with a length:width ratio of 1.09.

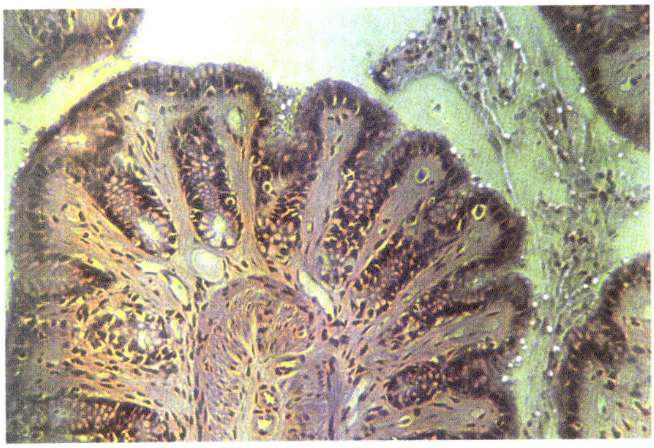

Fig. 10.5 *Cryptosporidium saurophilum* – lizard intestine.

Hosts: Lizards, snakes

Life cycle: The life cycle is unknown but is presumed similar to other species of *Cryptosporidium*.

Geographical distribution: Presumed worldwide

Pathogenesis: No pathological changes have been found in the intestine and cloaca of infected adult lizards, but weight loss, abdominal swelling and mortality have occurred in some colonies of juvenile geckos (*Eublepharis macularius*).

Clinical signs: Weight loss, abdominal swelling has been reported

Diagnosis: As for *C. serpentis*

Pathology: Cryptosporidia are found on the mucosal surfaces of the lower intestine and cloaca of lizards and are associated with mucosal thickening and hyperplastic and hypertrophic epithelia (Figs 10.5, 10.6).

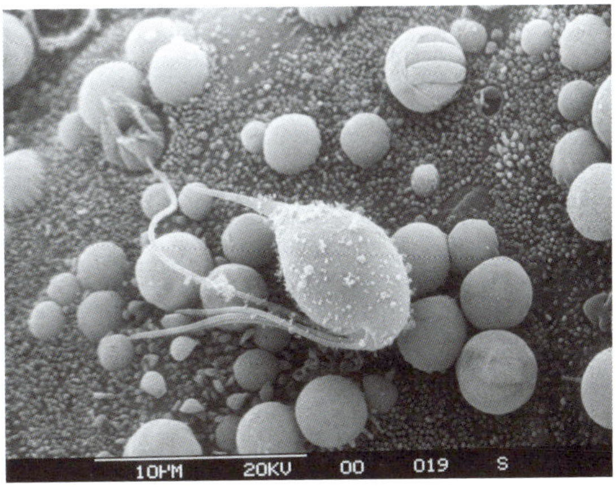

Fig. 10.6 Scanning electron micrograph of lizard intestine showing several stages of *Cryptosporidium saurophilum* and flagellated trichomonad (foreground).

C. saurophilum infection in snakes is not totally restricted to the intestine and may also infect the stomach.

Epidemiology: As for *C. serpentis*

Treatment and control: As for *C. serpentis*

PARASITES OF THE RESPIRATORY SYSTEM

Rhabdias spp

Predilection site: Lungs

Parasite class: Nematoda

Superfamily: Rhabditoidea

Hosts: Snakes

Life cycle: Only females are parasitic and these produce larvated, oval, thin-shelled eggs. After hatching, larvae may develop through four larval stages into free-living adult male and female worms and this can be followed by a succession of free-living generations. Infection is via the oral route, but percutaneous infection is also possible.

Pathogenesis and clinical signs: Infection causes minimal damage, but may result in inflammation and secondary bacterial infection of the oral mucosa with production of mucous exudate. Percutaneous infections may cause skin lesions.

Diagnosis: The larvae may be found in faecal smears or on microscopy of tracheal washings.

Treatment and control: Levamisole given at 10 mg/kg into the coelomic cavity and repeated after 2 weeks is effective. Ivermectin at 200 μg/kg by subcutaneous injection has also been reported to be effective.

PARASITES OF THE REPRODUCTIVE/UROGENITAL SYSTEM

Klossiella boiae

Predilection site: Kidney

Parasite class: Sporozoasida

Family: Klossiellidae

Description: Sporocysts contain about 30 sporozoites.

Hosts: Boa constrictor

Life cycle: The life cycle is not fully known. Development takes place within epithelial cells of kidney tubules. Mature sporocysts are surrounded by a thick wall and pass from the body in the urine. When ingested by another host, the sporozoites are released from the sporocyst, move to the kidney, where they enter epithelial cells and initiate the cycle.

Geographical distribution: Unknown

Pathogenesis and clinical signs: Not reported.

Diagnosis: Sporocysts may be detected in urine sediments or trophozoite stages may be found on postmortem in the kidney. The site and location are pathognomonic.

Pathology: Vegetative forms develop in renal tubular epithelial cells.

Epidemiology: Sporocysts are passed in the urine and infection takes place by the ingestion of the sporulated sporocysts.

Treatment and control: Not required, although some of the sulphonamide antibiotics, such as sulphaquinoxaline or sulphamethoxazole–trimethoprim, should be effective.

Sarcocystis, *Besnoitia* and *Toxoplasma* are occasionally found in reptiles in histological sections of postmortem material. Occasionally, oocysts of *Sarcocystis* are seen in the faeces of a predator reptile. The intermediate host is often a higher vertebrate such as a rodent, but can include other reptile species.

PARASITES OF THE CIRCULATORY SYSTEM

A wide range of haemoprotozoan parasites can be found in the blood of reptiles. The major genera found include *Haemoproteus*, *Leukocytozoon*, *Plasmodium*, *Schellakia*, *Trypanosoma*, *Hepatozoon* and *Haemogregarina*. As these parasites are transmitted by arthropod vectors they are unlikely to be found in captive reptiles unless recently caught from the wild.

ECTOPARASITES

A wide range of arthropods can affect reptiles in the wild. Both ticks and mites are frequently encountered in wild caught specimens but are generally less of a problem in captive-bred reptiles with a few exceptions.

MITES

Mesostigmata

One of the most commonly encountered mites is the snake mite, *Ophionyssus natricis*, which is described in detail below. Other species of mesostigmatid mites found on snakes and occasionally lizards include

Ophionyssus lacertinus, *O. mabuya* and *Neoliponyssus saurarum*.

Entonyssus, *Entophionyssus* and *Mabuyonyssus* mites belonging to the family Entonyssidae, are parasites of the trachea and lungs of snakes.

Ophionyssus natricis

Synonym: *Ophionyssus serpentium*, *Serpenticola serpentium*

Common name: Snake mite

Predilection site: Skin, scales

Parasite class: Arachnida

Sub-class: Acari

Order: Parasitiformes

Sub-order: Mesostigmata

Family: Macronyssidae

Description, gross: Adults are 0.6–1.3 mm long. Unfed females are yellow-brown; engorged females are dark red, brown or black (Fig. 10.7).

Description, microscopic: The cuticle bears only a few short bristle-like hairs.

Hosts: Snakes, lizards

Life cycle: The engorged female leaves the host and deposits eggs in cracks and crevices. The eggs hatch in 1–4 days, developing through larva, protonymph and deutonymph stages to the adult. Larvae do not feed but nymphs must feed before moulting to the next stage. The life cycle takes 13–19 days.

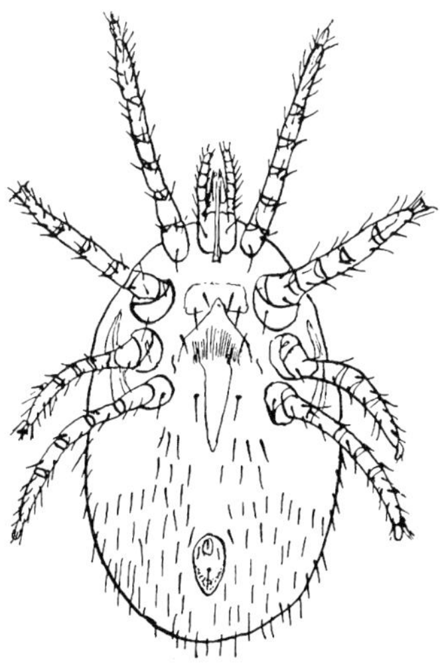

Fig. 10.7 *Ophionyssus natricis* (redrawn from Reichenbach-Klinke and Elkan, 1965).

Geographical distribution: Presumed worldwide

Pathogenesis and clinical signs: The number of mites on captive snakes is frequently large. The mites feed on blood and are found at several locations usually on the rim of the eye or beneath scales anterior to the neck. Heavy infestations are characterised by irritation, listlessness, debilitation, anaemia and death.

Diagnosis: Mite infestations are often diagnosed by direct visualisation of the mites or mite faeces on the snake.

Epidemiology: This mite is the most serious ectoparasite of captive snakes and lizards. The source of infection is other snakes or contaminated equipment or cages.

Treatment and control: Newly acquired snakes should be quarantined, inspected and placed in clean sterilised cages. If cages or cage contents become infested, thorough cleaning and treatment with acaricides or steam sterilisation are necessary. Infected animals may be treated with insecticides applied sparingly to skin by wiping with a cloth sprayed with an insecticidal flea spray preparation used on small animals, e.g. containing permetrin. Injectable ivermectin at 200 μg/kg has also been reported to be effective.

PROSTIGMATA

Trombiculid mites (family Trombiculidae) during their larval stages only, feed on reptiles for 2–10 days before dropping off, moulting to protonymphs and then deutonymphs, which feed on insects and spiders. The adult mites feed on detritus in the environment.

The family Pterygosamatidae are specialised parasitic mites of lizards, parasitising only certain species of lizards that include the agamids (Agamidae), geckoes (Gekonidae), iguanas (Iguanidae) and zonures (Zonuridae). *Geckobiella* and *Pimeliaphilus* infest primarily geckoes; *Hirstiella* infests iguanas and geckoes; *Ixodiderma* infests zonures; *Scapothrix* and *Zonurobia* infest zonures, with some infections causing severe dermatitis.

TICKS

At least seven genera of ticks have been found on reptiles and include *Amblyomma*, *Aponomma*, *Hyalomma*, *Haemaphysalis*, *Ixodes*, *Argas* and *Ornithodoros*. These tick genera are covered in more detail in Chapter 11.

Hyalomma aegyptium was seen frequently in northern Europe on tortoises imported from southern Europe for the pet trade. This practice has now ceased and there is no evidence of establishment outside its natural range.

The relapsing fever tick, *Ornithodoros turicata*, native to the USA and Mexico, has been reported on box turtles (*Terrepene* spp).

More detailed descriptions of these ticks are given in Chapter 11 (Facultative ectoparasites and arthropod vectors).

INSECTS

Several fly species are known to attack reptilian hosts and may be responsible for transmission of diseases in the wild. Phlebotomine sandflies are known to transmit *Leishmania* to reptiles, and mosquitoes transmit a range of haemoparasites, filarial worms and arboviruses to reptiles.

Myiasis has been reported in tortoises with blowfly larvae causing lesions especially around the cloaca, following diarrhoea or trauma to the cloaca. Treatment is by cleaning and debriding the lesion, followed by disinfection and application of a topical insecticide.

In the following checklists, the codes listed below apply:

Helminth classes:
N = Nematoda; T = Trematoda; C = Cestoda.

Arthropod classes:
I = Insecta; A = Arachnida.

Protozoal classes:
M = Mastigophora; S = Sarcodina; A = Apicomplexa; R = Rickettsia.

Pigeon parasite checklist.

Section/host system	Helminths		Arthropods		Protozoa	
	Parasite	(Super)family	Parasite	Family	Parasite	Family
Digestive						
Pharynx					*Trichomonas gallinae*	Trichomonadidae (M)
Oesophagus	*Dispharynx nasuta*	Spiruroidea (N)			*Trichomonas gallinae*	Trichomonadidae (M)
Crop	*Ornithostrongylus quadriradiatus*	Trichostrongyloidea (N)			*Trichomonas gallinae*	Trichomonadidae (M)
	Capillaria contorta	Trichuroidea (N)				
Proventriculus	*Ornithostrongylus quadriradiatus*	Trichostrongyloidea (N)			*Trichomonas gallinae*	Trichomonadidae (M)
	Tetrameres americana	Spiruroidea (N)				
	Tetrameres fissispina	Spiruroidea (N)				
	Dispharynx nasuta	Spiruroidea (N)				
Gizzard						
Small intestine	*Ornithostrongylus quadriradiatus*	Trichostrongyloidea (N)			*Eimeria labbeana*	Eimeriidae (A)
					Eimeria columbarum	Eimeriidae (A)
	Ascaridia columbae	Ascaridoidea (N)			*Wenyonella columbae*	Eimeriidae (A)
	Capillaria caudinflata	Trichuroidea (N)				
	Capillaria obsignata	Trichuroidea (N)			*Spironucleus columbae*	Diplomonadidae (M)
	Davainea proglottina	Davaineidae (C)				
	Raillietina tetragona	Davaineidae (C)				
	Echinoparyphium recurvatum	Echinostomatidae (T)				
	Hypoderaeum conoideum	Echinostomatidae (T)				
Large intestine	*Heterakis gallinarum*	Ascaridoidea (N)				
Caeca	*Capillaria anatis*	Trichuroidea (N)				
	Echinostoma revolutum	Echinostomatidae (T)				
	Brachylaemus commutatus	Brachylaemidae (T)				

(*continued*)

Pigeon parasite checklist (*continued*).

Section/host system	Helminths		Arthropods		Protozoa	
	Parasite	(Super)family	Parasite	Family	Parasite	Family
Respiratory						
Nares						
Trachea Bronchi	*Syngamus trachea*	Strongyloidea (N)				
Lung			*Laminosioptes cysticola*	Laminosioptidae (A)		
Air sacs			*Cytodites nudus*	Cytoditidae (A)		
Liver						
Pancreas						
Circulatory						
Blood					*Leucocytozoon marchouxi*	Plasmodiidae (A)
					Haemoproteus columbae	Plasmodiidae (A)
					Haemoproteus sacharovi	Plasmodiidae (A)
Blood vessels						
Nervous						
CNS						
Eye						

Reproductive/urogenital						
Oviduct						
Kidneys						
Locomotory						
Muscle						
Connective tissue					*Toxoplasma gondii*	Sarcocystiidae (A)
Integument						
Skin			*Dermanyssus gallinae*	Dermanyssidae (A)		
			Ornithonyssus sylvarium	Macronyssidae (A)		
			Ornithonyssus bursa	Macronyssidae (A)		
			Pseudolynchia canariensis	Hippoboscidae (I)		
			Colombicola columbae	Philopteridae (I)		
			Ceratophyllus columbae	Ceratophyllidae (I)		
Subcutaneous	*Pelecitus clavus*	Filarioidea (N)	*Laminosioptes cysticola*	Laminosioptidae (A)		
			Hypodectes propus	Hypoderatidae (A)		

Tick species found on pigeons.

Genus	Species	Common name	Family
Argas	*persicus*	Fowl tick	Argasidae
Argas	*reflexus*	Pigeon tick	Argasidae

Ratite parasite checklist – Ostrich (O), emu (E) and rhea (R).

Section/host system	Helminths		Arthropods		Protozoa	
	Parasite	(Super)family	Parasite	Family	Parasite	Family
Digestive						
Pharynx					*Trichomonas gallinae*	Trichomonadidae (M)
Oesophagus						
Crop						
Proventriculus	*Libyostrongylus douglassi* (O)	Trichostrongyloidea (N)				
	Libyostrongylus dentatus (O)	Trichostrongyloidea (N)				
	Spiruria uncinipenis (R)	Spiruroidea (N)				
	Spiruria zschokkei (R)	Spiruroidea (N)				
	Odontospiruria cetiopenis (R)	Spiruroidea (N)				
Gizzard	*Odontospiruria cetiopenis* (R)	Spiruroidea (N)				
	Libyostrongylus douglassi (O)	Trichostrongyloidea (N)				
	Libyostrongylus dentatus (O)	Trichostrongyloidea (N)				
Small intestine	*Hottuynia struthionis* (O), (R)	Davaineidae (C)			*Eimeria* sp (O), (R)	Eimeriidae (A)
	Deletrocephalus dimidiatus (R)	Strongyloidea (N)			*Isospora struthionis* (O)	Eimeriidae (A)
					Spironucleus meleagridis	Diplomonadidae (M)
	Paradeletrocephalus minor (R)	Strongyloidea (N)			*Cryptosporidium baileyi* (O)	Cryptosporidiidae (A)
	Ascaridia orthocerca (R)	Ascaridoidea (N)			*Retortamonas* spp	Retortamonadoridae (M)
	Trichostrongylus tenuis (E)	Trichostrongyloidea (N)				
Caeca	*Trichostrongylus tenuis* (E)	Trichostrongyloidea (N)			*Blastocystis galli* (O)	Blastocystidae (B)
Large intestine	*Codiostomum struthionis* (O)	Strongyloidea (N)			*Histomonas meleagridis* (O), (R)	Monocercomonadidae (M)
Cloacal bursa					*Trichomonas* spp	Trichomonadidae (M)
Rectum					*Balantidium coli* (O)	Balantiidae (C)
					Blastocystis galli (O)	Blastocystidae (B)
Respiratory						
Nares						
Trachea	*Syngamus trachea* (O, R, E)	Strongyloidea (N)				
Bronchi	*Cyathostoma variegatum* (E)	Strongyloidea (N)				
Lung						
Air sacs	*Paronchocerca struthionis* (O)	Filarioidea (N)				
	Dicheilonema spicularia (O)	Filarioidea (N)				
Liver						
Pancreas						

Circulatory						
Blood					*Plasmodium struthionis* (O)	Plasmodiidae (A)
					Plasmodium spp (O), (R)	Plasmodiidae (A)
					Leucocytozoon struthionis	Plasmodiidae (A)
Blood vessels					*Aegyptianella pullorum*	Anaplasmataceae (R)
Nervous						
CNS	*Baylisascaris procyonis* (O, E)	Ascaridoidea (N)				
	Chandlerella quiscali (E)	Filarioidea (N)				
Eye	*Philophthalmus gralli* (O)	Philophthalmidae (T)				
Reproductive/ urogenital						
Oviduct						
Kidneys						
Locomotory						
Muscle						
Connective tissue	*Dicheilonema spicularia* (O)	Filarioidea (N)				
	Dicheilonema rhea (R)	Filarioidea (N)				
Integument						
Skin			*Gabucinia sculpturata*	Pterolichidae (A)		
			Pterolichus bicaudatus	Pterolichidae (A)		
			Struthiolipeurus struthionis	Philopteridae (I)		
			Struthiolipeurus nandu	Philopteridae (I)		
			Struthiolipeurus stresemanni	Philopteridae (I)		
			Struthiolipeurus rheae	Philopteridae (I)		
			Meinertzhageniella lata	Philopteridae (I)		
			Meinertzhageniella schubarti	Philopteridae (I)		
			Dahlemhornia asymmetrica	Philopteridae (I)		
Subcutaneous						

B = Blastocystea.

Tick species found on ostrich.

Genus	Species	Common name	Family
Argas	*persicus* *walkerae*	Fowl tick Chicken tick	Argasidae (A)
Otobius	*megnini*	Spinose ear tick	
Amblyomma	*hebraeum* *gemma* *lepidum* *variegatum*	South African bont tick	Ixodidae (A)
Haemaphysalis	*punctata*		
Hyalomma	*dromedarii* *impeltatum* *marinatum* *rufipes* *truncatum*	Camel tick	Ixodidae (A)
Rhipicephalus	*sanguineus* *turanicus*	Brown dog or kennel tick	Ixodidae (A)

11
Facultative ectoparasites and arthropod vectors

TICKS

SOFT TICKS (ARGASIDAE)

In the soft ticks (Argasidae), the body is leathery and unsclerotised, with a textured surface. The cuticle in unfed ticks may be characteristically marked with grooves or folds. Argasids typically have a multi-host developmental cycle. The single larval instar feeds once, before moulting to become a first-stage nymph. There are between two and seven nymphal stages, each of which feed and then leave the host, before moulting to the next stage. Adults mate away from the host and feed several times. The adult female lays batches of 400–500 eggs after each feed. In contrast to the slow-feeding ixodids, argasid ticks feed for only a few minutes. Argasid, soft ticks are more common in deserts or dry conditions. In contrast to the hard ticks, argasid soft ticks tend to live in close proximity to their hosts: in chicken coops, pigsties, pigeon lofts, bird's nests, animal burrows or dens. In these restricted and sheltered habitats the hazards associated with host finding are reduced and more frequent feeding becomes possible.

Clinical signs: The adult ticks, particularly the engorged females, are easily seen on the skin, commonly beneath the wings. Egg laying decreases and may stop altogether as a result of the infestation. However, the ticks only feed for a limited period. Inflammation and raised areas will be present from tick bites.

Diagnosis: The parasites may be found on the host or found in cracks of the woodwork and walls around the animal housing. Microscopic examination may then be used to identify individual species.

Pathology: Small granulomatous reactions may form at the site of tick bites, consisting of a mixed inflammatory cell response with fibrosis.

Treatment: Argasid ticks, which exist in and around animal housing, poultry houses and enclosures, can be controlled by application of an acaricide to their environment coupled with treatment of the population on the host. Environmental treatment of roosts and poultry houses may be effected using acaricidal sprays or emulsions containing organophosphates and pyrethroids. All niches and crevices in affected buildings should be sprayed, and nesting boxes and perches in poultry houses should also be painted with acaricides. At the same time as premises are treated, birds should be dusted with a suitable acaricide or, in the case of larger animals, sprayed or dipped. Treatment should be repeated at monthly intervals.

Control: In poultry houses, all new birds should be treated prior to introduction into an existing flock. Control of argasid ticks can be assisted by elimination of cracks in walls and perches, which provide shelter to the free-living stages.

ARGAS

Species of the genus *Argas* are usually dorsoventrally flattened, with definite margins, which can be seen even when the tick is engorged. The cuticle is wrinkled and leathery. Most species are nocturnal and are parasites of birds, bats, reptiles or, occasionally, small insectivorous mammals. Most species seldom attack humans. Species of this genus are usually found in dry, arid habitats. Detailed description of only the major species of veterinary importance will be presented here.

Argas persicus

Common name: Fowl tick, chicken tick, adobe tick, blue bug

Predilection site: Skin

Parasite class: Arachnida

Sub-class: Acari

Order: Parasitiformes

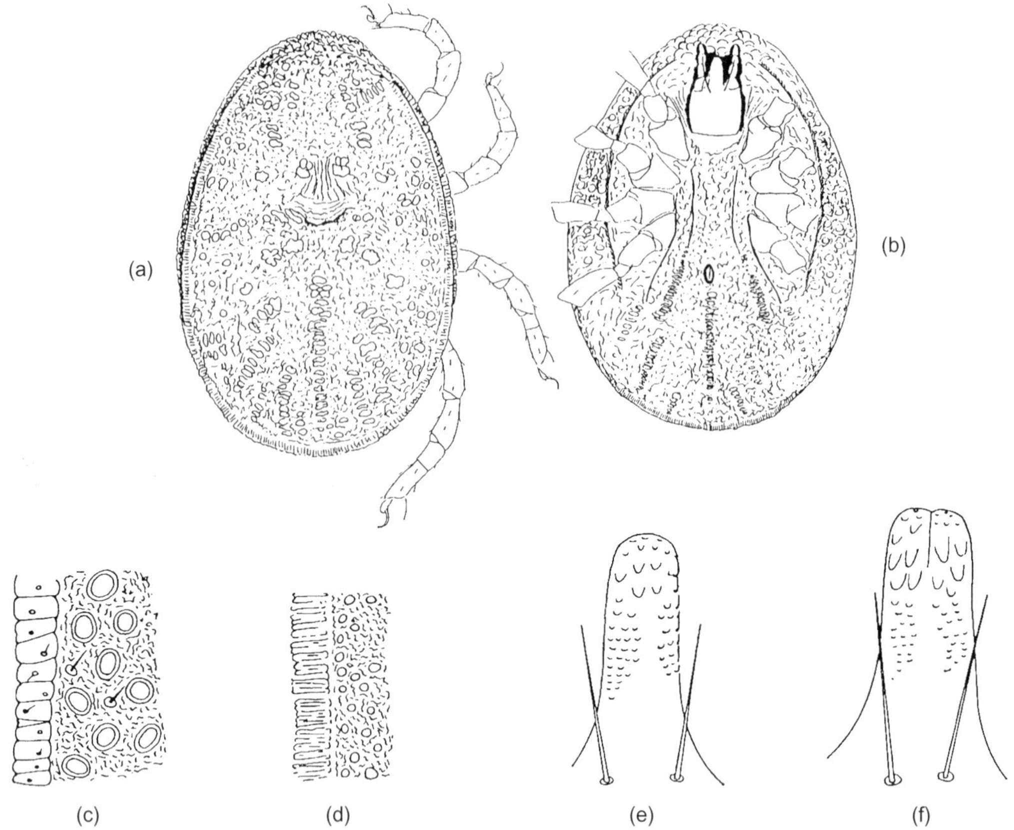

Fig. 11.1 Female *Argas reflexus* (a) dorsal and (b) ventral view (reproduced from Arthur, 1962). Margin of (c) *Argas reflexus* and (d) *Argas perscius*. Hypostome of female (e) *Argas reflexus* and (f) *Argas perscius* (reproduced from Arthur, 1962).

Sub-order: Ixodida (Metastigmata)

Family: Argasidae

Description: The unfed adult is reddish brown turning slate blue when fed. The female is about 8 mm in length and the male about 5 mm (Fig. 11.1). The margin of the body appears to be composed of irregular quadrangular plates or cells, and no scutum is present. Unlike hard ticks, the four segments of the pedipalps are equal in length. The stigmata are situated on the sides of the body above the third and fourth pairs of legs. The integument is granulated, leathery and wrinkled. The hypostome is notched at the tip, and the mouthparts are not visible when the tick is viewed from above.

Hosts: Chicken, turkey and wild birds

Life cycle: *Argas persicus* is nocturnal and breeds and shelters in cracks and crevices in the structure of poultry houses. Females deposit batches of 25–100 eggs in these cracks and crevices. Up to 700 eggs may be produced by a single female at intervals, each oviposition preceded by a blood-meal. After hatching, larvae locate a host and remain attached and feed for several days. After feeding they detach, leave the host and shelter in the poultry house structure. Several days later they moult to become first-stage nymphs. They then proceed through two or three nymphal stages, interspersed with frequent nightly feeds, before moulting to the adult stage. Adult males and females feed about once a month, but can survive for long periods without a blood-meal. Females can become completely engorged within 30–45 minutes. Under favourable conditions the life cycle can be completed in about 30 days. All stages of these ticks remain around the roosting area of poultry, quiescent in the day and actively feeding at night. *Argas persicus* can survive in empty poultry housing for years, and may travel long distances to find their hosts. This tick can undergo rapid increases in abundance, passing through one to ten generations per year, particularly in areas where birds are present all year round.

Geographical distribution: Worldwide, especially in the tropics

Pathogenesis: Though common pests of chickens and turkeys, they are not usually a significant veterinary problem, except in small, housed flocks. It will bite humans, particularly if living in proximity to an infested flock. Infestation may cause irritation, sleeplessness, loss of egg productivity and anaemia, which can prove fatal. Each tick requires a considerable quantity of blood for engorgement, and therefore heavy infestations can take enough blood to bring about the death of their host. Most species are nocturnal and are parasites of birds, bats, reptiles or, occasionally, small insectivorous mammals and seldom attack humans.

These ticks may transmit *Borrelia anserina*, the cause of fowl spirochaetosis, and *Aegyptianella pullorum*, a rickettsial infection. It is a vector of *Borrelia anserina* and *Aegyptianella pullorum* among poultry, as well as avian spirochaetosis. The spirochaetes may be passed from one generation of ticks to the next through the egg, and transmitted to the host by biting or by faecal contamination.

Argas reflexus

Common name: Pigeon tick

Predilection site: Skin

Parasite class: Arachnida

Sub-class: Acari

Order: Parasitiformes

Sub-order: Ixodida (Metastigmata)

Family: Argasidae

Description: The adult *Argas reflexus* is between 6 and 11 mm in length and may be distinguished from the fowl tick, *Argas persicus*, by its body margin, which is composed of irregular grooves, and the hypostome, which is not notched apically (Fig. 11.1). It is reddish brown in colour with paler legs.

Distribution: It is abundant in the Middle and Near East, from where it has spread into Europe and most of Asia.

Hosts: Pigeon

Life cycle: The life cycle is similar to that of *A. persicus.* The number of nymphal stadia ranges from two to four, with the fewest occuring in cooler temperatures. The egg to adult life cycle can take up to 11 years to complete. It is nocturnal and during the day lives in crevices in the pigeon house or nest material. It can withstand prolonged periods of starvation. Engorged females diapause during the summer months. If oviposition has already commenced, egg-laying stops and resumes the following year without the need for another blood meal.

Pathogenesis: Heavy infestations may cause death from anaemia. It may also transmit fowl spirochaetosis. This tick occasionally bites humans, causing allergy. Its northern distribution through Europe is limited by the temperature requirement of its eggs and oviposition in summer months, since *A. reflexus* eggs show low levels of cold tolerance. Typical winter temperatures of 3°C cause approximately 50% mortality in *A. reflexus* eggs.

Epidemiology: This species lives in close association with its host, *Columba livia.*

Argas walkerae

Common name: Chicken tick

Predilection site: Skin, commonly beneath the wings

Parasite class: Arachnida

Sub-class: Acari

Order: Parasitiformes

Sub-order: Ixodida (Metastigmata)

Family: Argasidae

Life cycle: Like most species of this genus: egg, larva, three nymphal stages and adult. It lives in crevices in the poultry house or nest material moving on to the host to feed.

Hosts: Chicken

Ditsribution: Southern Africa

Pathogenesis: It causes considerable economic losses, especially where it transmits *Aegyptianella pullorum* and *Borrelia anserina.* In addition, it may secrete a neurotoxin during feeding, frequently resulting in fatal paralysis.

Epidemiology: This species lives in close association with its poultry hosts and no wild hosts are known.

ORNITHODOROS

This genus includes about 90 species, almost all of which are found in tropical and subtropical habitats in both the Old and New World. Most *Ornithodoros* species are found in Africa, commonly in the burrows of warthogs and bush pigs, though other species may be found in Central and South America and the Rocky Mountain states of the USA. They are nocturnal and the mouthparts are well developed. The integument has a wrinkled pattern, which runs continuously over the dorsal and ventral surfaces (Fig. 11.2). There is no

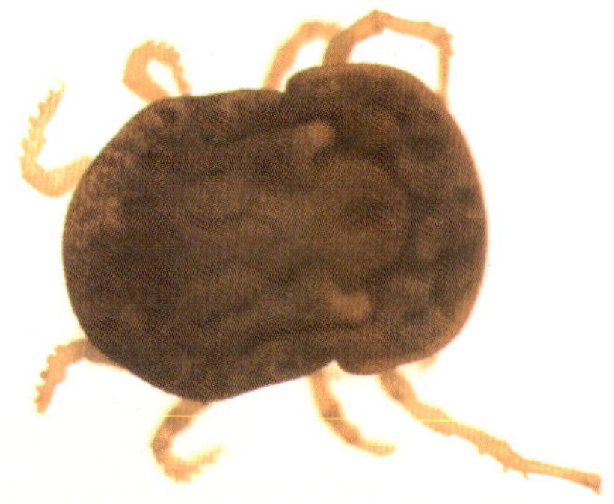

Fig. 11.2 *Ornithodoros* dorsal view.

distinct lateral margin to the body, which appears sac-like. Species of this genus are found largely in habitats such as dens, caves, nests and burrows, and so are not normally a problem for most domestic animals. Only the nymphs and adults are parasitic and may be responsible for considerable irritation; heavy infections can cause mortality of stock from blood loss.

Several species of *Ornithodoros* inflict painful bites and may be major vectors of relapsing fever. Detailed description of only the major species of veterinary importance will be presented here.

Ornithodoros erraticus

Synonym: *Ornothodoros marocanus*

Common name: Sand tampan

Predilection site: Skin

Parasite class: Arachnida

Sub-class: Acari

Order: Parasitiformes

Sub-order: Ixodida (Metastigmata)

Family: Argasidae

Hosts: Particularly small mammals, but also domestic livestock and humans

Life cycle: Females lay batches of approximately 100 eggs in the sand of the host den, cave, nest or burrow and remain with them until they hatch to produce larvae several days later. The larvae remain quiescent until they have moulted to the nymphal stage. There are several nymphal stadia. Both nymphs and adults only feed on their hosts for short periods of time.

Geographical distribution: Europe, Africa and the Middle East

Pathogenesis: *Ornithodoros erraticus* is a vector of the rickettsial parasite *Coxiella burnetii*, the causative agent of Q fever in cattle, sheep and goats. It also transmits *Borrelia hispanica* in the Spanish peninsula and adjacent North Africa, and *B. crocidurae* in Africa, the Near East and central Asia. These are both spirochaetes which cause tick-borne relapsing fever. This species also acts as a reservoir and vector for African swine fever and *Babesia*.

Ornithodoros hermsi

Common name: Sand tampan

Predilection site: Skin

Parasite class: Arachnida

Sub-class: Acari

Order: Parasitiformes

Sub-order: Ixodida (Metastigmata)

Family: Argasidae

Description: *Ornithodoros hermsi* is a pale, sandy coloured soft tick, which appears greyish blue when engorged. The adult female *O. hermsi* is typically 5–6 mm in length and 3–4 mm wide. The male is morphologically similar, though slightly smaller.

Hosts: Most mammals, particularly rodents

Life cycle: Females lay batches of approximately 100 eggs in the sand of the host den, cave, nest or burrow and remain with them until they hatch to produce larvae several days later. The larvae remain quiescent until they have moulted to the nymphal stage. There are several nymphal stadia. Both nymphs and adults only feed on their hosts for short periods of time, typically 15–30 minutes. This species is able to survive for long periods without feeding; juvenile stages may live as long as 95 days unfed, and the adults more than 7 months.

Geographical distribution: North America (Rocky Mountains and Pacific coast)

Pathogenesis: This species transmits *Borrelia hermsi*, the agent of tick-borne relapsing fever in America, and may also act as a vector for African swine fever. Rodents, including deer mice, squirrels and chipmunks, are the primary reservoir hosts for *B. hermsi.*

Epidemiology: *Ornithodoros hermsi* is found in rural areas that are usually mountainous and forested. They live in dark, cool places where rodents nest, such as woodpiles outside buildings, under houses, between walls or beneath floorboards inside cabins. They are most active during the summer months.

Ornithodoros moubata

Common name: Sand tampan

Predilection site: Skin

Parasite class: Arachnida

Sub-class: Acari

Order: Parasitiformes

Sub-order: Ixodida (Metastigmata)

Family: Argasidae

Hosts: Most mammals, birds and some reptiles

Geographical distribution: Africa and the Middle East

Pathogenesis: This species may be a reservoir host for the virus of African swine fever and for the spirochaete, *Borrelia duttoni*, which causes African relapsing fever in humans. *Ornithodoros moubata* is also a vector for viruses of Suidae (*Phacochoerus*, *Potamochoerus*, *Hylochoerus*) and for Q fever. It may transmit *Borrelia anserina* and *Aegyptianella pullorum* in fowl.

Ornithodoros porcinus porcinus

Synonym: *O. moubata porcinus*

Predilection site: Skin

Parasite class: Arachnida

Sub-class: Acari

Order: Parasitiformes

Sub-order: Ixodida (Metastigmata)

Family: Argasidae

Hosts: Warthogs, bushpigs, porcupines and domestic pigs

Geographical distribution: Africa, Madagascar, southern Europe

Pathogenesis: An important reservoir and vector of African swine fever

Epidemiology: This tick spends the day sheltered in the burrows of its natural hosts (warthogs), or the cracks and crevices of pig housing, emerging to feed at night.

Ornithodoros parkeri

Common name: Sand tampan

Predilection site: Skin

Parasite class: Arachnida

Sub-class: Acari

Order: Parasitiformes

Sub-order: Ixodida (Metastigmata)

Family: Argasidae

Hosts: Most mammals, particularly rodents

Geographical distribution: Western states and Pacific coast of North America.

Pathogenesis: The bite of this species can cause a severe toxic or allergic reaction in the host, which may involve skin rashes, fever, nausea, diarrhoea, shock and death. *Ornithodoros parkeri* transmits *Borrelia parkeri*, the agent of tick-borne relapsing fever in America, and may also act as a vector for African swine fever.

Ornithodoros savignyi

Common name: Sand tampan

Predilection site: Skin

Parasite class: Arachnida

Sub-class: Acari

Order: Parasitiformes

Sub-order: Ixodida (Metastigmata)

Family: Argasidae

Hosts: Most mammals, particularly camels, and poultry

Geographical distribution: Africa, India and the Middle East

Pathogenesis: Toxicosis may occur in response to the tick saliva, characterised by cutaneous oedema, haemorrhage, rapidly progressing weakness and prostration. Toxocosis can suppress the host's immune system, allowing the reactivation of chronic infections. Such toxicosis with *O. savignyi* occurs in young calves and lambs, especially when there are large tick populations and multiple bites.

Ornithodoros tholozani

Common name: Sand tampan

Predilection site: Skin

Parasite class: Arachnida

Sub-class: Acari

Order: Parasitiformes

Sub-order: Ixodida (Metastigmata)

Family: Argasidae

Hosts: Most mammals, birds and some reptiles

Geographical distribution: Africa and the Middle East

Pathogenesis: This species transmits *Borrelia persica*, the causative agent of Persian relapsing fever in northeast Africa and Asia.

Ornithodoros turicata

Common name: Sand tampan, relapsing fever tick

Predilection site: Skin

Parasite class: Arachnida

Sub-class: Acari

Order: Parasitiformes

Sub-order: Ixodida (Metastigmata)

Family: Argasidae

Hosts: Most mammals, particularly rodents

Geographical distribution: North America, particularly southern areas between Florida and California and northward to Colorado and Utah

Pathogenesis: The bite of this species can cause a severe toxic or allergic reaction in the host, which may involve skin rashes, fever, nausea, diarrhoea, shock and death. This species transmits *Coxiella burnetii*, the causative agent of Q fever in America, and *Borrelia turicatae*, the causative agent of tick-borne relapsing fever. It may also act as a vector for African swine fever.

Ornithodoros rudis

Predilection site: Skin

Parasite class: Arachnida

Sub-class: Acari

Order: Parasitiformes

Sub-order: Ixodida (Metastigmata)

Family: Argasidae

Hosts: Most mammals, particularly rodents and humans

Geographical distribution: Central and South America

Pathogenesis: A vector of *Borrelia* spp, pathogenic agents of relapsing fever.

Epidemiology: This tick spends its life in the burrows of its natural hosts, or cracks and crevices of human or animal housing in dry conditions. It emerges only to feed at night.

Ornithodoros lahorensis

Predilection site: Skin

Parasite class: Arachnida

Sub-class: Acari

Order: Parasitiformes

Sub-order: Ixodida (Metastigmata)

Family: Argasidae

Hosts: Wild sheep, domestic sheep and goats

Geographical distribution: Eastern Europe, northern India, southern former USSR, Middle East

Pathogenesis: An important vector of the agents of piroplasmosis, brucellosis, Q-fever, and tularaemia. Its feeding activity may also cause paralysis, anemia and toxicosis.

Epidemiology: This species is unusual because of its relatively prolonged contact with its host, to which it remains attached over winter. Large populations may build up on sheep and goats that are housed in infested stables and caves over winter.

OTOBIUS

This small genus contains only two species: *Otobius megnini* and *Otobius lagophilus*.

Otobius megnini

Common name: Spinose ear tick

Predilection site: Ears

Parasite class: Arachnida

Sub-class: Acari

Order: Parasitiformes

Sub-order: Ixodida (Metastigmata)

Family: Argasidae

Description: The adult body is rounded posteriorly and slightly attenuated anteriorly (Fig. 11.3). Adult females range in size from 5–8 mm in length; males are slightly smaller. They have no lateral sutural line, and no distinct margin to the body. Nymphs have spines. In adults the hypostome is much reduced and the integument is granular. The body has a blue–grey coloration with pale yellow legs and mouthparts. Larvae measure 2–3 mm in length and a fully-grown, engorged nymph measures 7–10 mm.

Hosts: Commonly infests wild and domestic animals, including sheep, cattle, dogs, horses and occasionally humans.

Life cycle: This species is a one-host tick. The larval and nymphal stages are parasites of a wide range of mammals, but the adults are not parasitic. Mating takes place off the host, and batches of eggs are laid

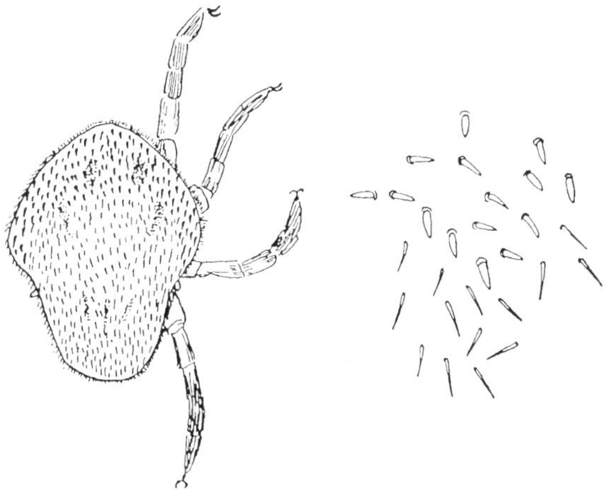

Fig. 11.3 Dorsal view of nymphal *Otobius megnini* and part of the integument showing hairs and spines (reproduced from Arthur, 1962).

in sheltered sites such as in cracks and crevices in the walls of animal shelters, under stones or the bark of trees. The larvae hatch within 3–8 weeks and attach to a host animal. They may survive without food for 2–4 months. The preferred predilection site for larvae is deep within the ear. The larvae moult in the ears and nymphs remain there for 1–7 months. When fully grown and engorged, the nymphs drop off the host and seek dry, sheltered sites, where they moult after a few days to become adults. The adults do not feed, and unmated females can survive in empty shelters and stables for over a year. Females lay 500–600 eggs; oviposition can last for up to 6 months.

Geographical distribution: North and South America, India and southern Africa

Pathogenesis: The larvae and nymphs feed in the external ear canal of the host, producing severe inflammation and a waxy exudate in the ear canals. Secondary bacterial infections can occur, which may extend up the ear canal. Infested hosts may scratch and shake their heads. Scratching can cause local skin trauma and occasionally perforate the eardrum. This can lead to infection, ulceration and in some cases meningitis. In horses, clinical signs may be mistaken for signs of colic.

Otobius lagophilus

Common name: Rabbit ear tick

Predilection site: Ears

Parasite class: Arachnida

Sub-class: Acari

Order: Parasitiformes

Sub-order: Ixodida (Metastigmata)

Family: Argasidae

Hosts: Rabbits

Life cycle: This species is a one-host tick. Only larvae and nymphs are parasitic.

Geographical distribution: North America, Canada

Pathogenesis: The larvae and nymphs feed in the external ear canal of the host, producing severe inflammation and a waxy exudate in the ear canals. Infested hosts may scratch and shake their heads. Scratching can cause local skin trauma.

HARD TICKS

Life cycle: The life cycles of ixodid ticks involve four instars: egg, six-legged larva, eight-legged nymph and eight-legged adult. During the passage through these stages ixodid ticks take a number of large blood meals, interspersed by lengthy free-living periods. They are relatively long-lived and each female may produce several thousand eggs.

Most hard ticks are relatively immobile and, rather than actively hunting for their hosts, the majority adopt a strategy known as questing, in which they wait at the tips of vegetation for an appropriate host to brush past. Once contact is made the ticks transfer to the host, and then move over the surface to find their preferred attachment sites, such as the ears. Preferred sites for attachment may be highly specific to the particular species of tick.

Ticks have developed a variety of complex life cycles and feeding strategies, which reflect the nature of the habitat, which the various species of tick inhabit, and the probability of contact with an appropriate host. For most a three-host life cycle has been adopted (Fig. 1.41). Larvae, nymphs and adults all feed on different hosts. Blood-feeding typically takes between 4 and 6 days after which they drop to the ground and either moult to the next life cycle stage or lay eggs. Ticks must then relocate a suitable host to feed and moult again or lay eggs. For a relatively small number of ixodid ticks, about 50 species, which inhabit areas where hosts are scarce and in which lengthy seasonal periods of unfavourable climate occur, two- and one-host feeding strategies have evolved.

In temperate habitats, feeding and generation cycles of hard ticks are closely synchronised with periods of suitable temperature and humidity conditions. Ticks, particularly in the immature stages, are very susceptible to desiccation, particularly when ticks are active. To minimise drying out they start questing when saturated with water and return to the humid ground level when dehydrated. Water may also be imbibed by drinking.

Clinical signs: There are no obvious signs of tick infestation other than the presence of the parasites and the local skin reactions to their bites.

Diagnosis: The adult ticks, particularly the engorged females, are easily seen on the skin, the predilection sites being the face, ears, axilla and inguinal region. Usually small, inflamed nodules are also seen in these areas. Ticks may be collected from the host or directly from the environment and microscopic examination used to identify individual species.

Pathology: The local reaction to tick bites varies considerably; commonly small granulomatous reactions may form at the site of tick bites consisting of a mixed inflammatory cell response with fibrosis.

Epidemiology: The distribution of ticks in a temperate climate with frequent and non-seasonal rainfall is closely linked with the availability of a microenvironment with a high relative humidity, such as occurs in the mat which forms under the surface of rough grazing. In contrast, in tropical grazing areas the grass cover on pastures is discontinuous and often interspersed with bare or eroded patches. Where suitable grass cover does exist it has been generally accepted, since temperatures are suitable for development throughout a large part of the year, that the distribution of ticks is mainly governed by rainfall, and with the exception of *Hyalomma* spp, a mean annual rainfall of more than 60 cm is required for survival.

However, recent studies have shown that the factors underlying the maintenance of the necessary microclimate with a high relative humidity are rather more complex, and depend on the transpiration of plant leaves. As long as this continues, adequate humidity is maintained in the microclimate despite the dryness of the general environment. However, when the rate of evaporation increases beyond a certain level, the stomata on the leaves close, transpiration ceases and the low humidity created in the microclimate rapidly becomes lethal to the ticks.

In the field, the stability of the microclimate is dependent on factors such as the quantity of herbage or plant debris and the grass species. The various genera of ticks have different thresholds of temperature and humidity within which they are active and feed, and these thresholds govern their distribution. Generally, ticks are most active during the warm season provided there is sufficient rainfall, but in some species the larval and nymphal stages are also active in milder weather. This affects the duration and timing of control programmes.

Treatment: The control of ixodid ticks is largely based on the use of chemical acaricides applied either by total immersion in a dipping bath or in the form of a spray, shower, spot-on or slow-release ear tags. A wide variety of formulations of organophosphate (e.g. malathion, chlorpyrifos, fenthion, dichlorvos, cythoate, diazinon, propetamphos, phosmet) and pyrethroid insecticides (e.g. permethrin, deltamethrin) are available for application as sprays, dips, spot-on or showers. Macrocyclic lactones or closantel given by the parenteral route have also been shown to be a useful aid in control of ticks. Where severely parasitised animals require individual treatment, special formulations of acaricides suspended in a greasy base may be applied to affected areas.

In companion animals, topical acaricidal compounds, such as fipronil (phenylpyrazole), imidacloprid (chloronicotinyl), selamectin (macrocyclic lactone), amitraz (formamidine) and the organophosphates (e.g. malathion, ronnel, chlorpyrifos, fenthion, dichlorvos, cythoate, diazinon, propetamphos, phosmet) and carbamates can be used to kill ticks on the host. Pyrethroids (e.g. permethrin, deltamethrin) should not be used in cats.

Control: The long-term control of three-host ticks is geared to the period required for the adult female stage to become fully engorged, which varies from 4–10 days according to the species. If an animal is treated with an acaricide which has a residual effect of, say, 3 days, it will be at least 7 days before any fully engorged female reappears following treatment (i.e. 3 days' residual effect plus a minimum of 4 days for engorgement). Weekly treatment during the tick season should therefore kill the adult female ticks before they are engorged, except in cases of very severe challenge when the treatment interval has to be reduced to 4 or 5 days.

Theoretically, weekly treatment should also control the larvae and nymphs, but in several areas the peak infestations of larvae and nymphs occur at different seasons to the adult females and the duration of the treatment season has to be extended.

Since many ticks occur on less accessible parts of the body, such as the anus, vulva, groin, scrotum, udder and ear, care must be exercised to ensure that the acaricide is properly applied.

Traditional control methods such as burning of cattle pastures are still used in some areas and are generally practised during a dry period before rains, when ticks are inactive. This technique is still a most useful one in extensive range conditions, and provided it is used after seeding of the grasses has taken place, regeneration of the pastures will rapidly occur following the onset of rains. Cultivation of land and, in some areas, improved drainage help to reduce the prevalence of tick populations and can be used where more intensive systems of agriculture prevail. Pasture 'spelling' in which domestic livestock are removed from pastures for a period of time has been used in

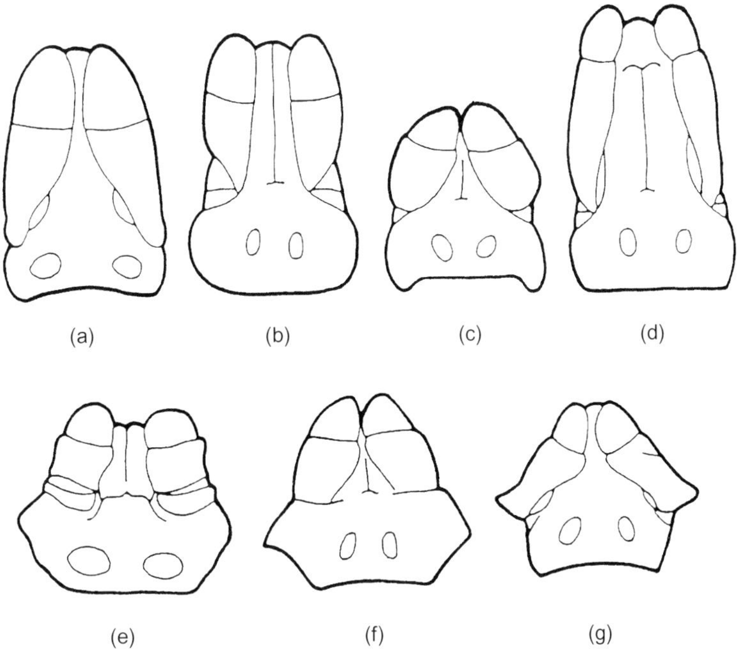

Fig. 11.4 Diagrammatic dorsal view of the gnathosoma of seven genera of ixodid ticks (from Smart, 1943). (a) *Ixodes*. (b) *Hyalomma*. (c) *Dermacentor*. (d) *Amblyomma*. (e) *Boophilus*. (f) *Rhipicephalus*. (g) *Haemaphysalis*.

semi-extensive or extensive areas, but often has the disadvantage that ticks can still obtain blood from a wide variety of other hosts.

IXODES

Ixodes is the largest genus in the family Ixodidae, with about 250 species. They are small, inornate ticks, which do not have eyes or festoons. The mouthparts are long and are longer in the female than male. The fourth segment of the palps is greatly reduced and bears chemoreceptor sensilla. The second segment of the palps may be restricted at the base, creating a gap between the palp and chelicerae (Fig. 11.4). Males have several ventral plates, which almost cover the ventral surface. *Ixodes* can be distinguished from other ixodid ticks by the anterior position of the anal groove. In other genera of the Ixodidae the anal groove is either absent or is posterior to the anus (see Fig. 11.8a).

Ixodes ricinus

Common name: Sheep tick; castor bean tick

Predilection site: Skin

Parasite class: Arachnida

Sub-class: Acari

Order: Parasitiformes

Sub-order: Ixodida (Metastigmata)

Family: Ixodidae

Description: The engorged adult female is light grey, up to 1.0 cm in length and bean shaped (Figs 11.5, 11.6). However, when engorged the legs are not visible when viewed from above. Adult male *Ixodes ricinus* are only 2.0–3.0 mm long, and because they take smaller blood meals than females, the four pairs of legs are readily visible from above. Nymphs resemble the adults but are less than 2.0 mm in length. The larvae, often described as 'seed ticks' or 'pepper ticks', are less than 1.0 mm in length and usually yellowish in colour.

In *I. ricinus*, as compared with *I. canisuga* and *I. hexagonus*, the tarsi are tapered (Fig. 11.7) and not humped and the posterior internal angle of the first coxa bears a spur, which overlaps the second coxa (Fig. 11.8).

Hosts: Sheep, cattle, goat, but can feed on all mammals and birds; juvenile stages may also feed on lizards.

Life cycle: *I. ricinus* is a three-host tick and the life cycle requires 3 years. The tick feeds for only a few days each year, as a larva in the first year, a nymph in the second and an adult in the third.

Mating takes place on the host. After attachment the female is inseminated once and subsequently

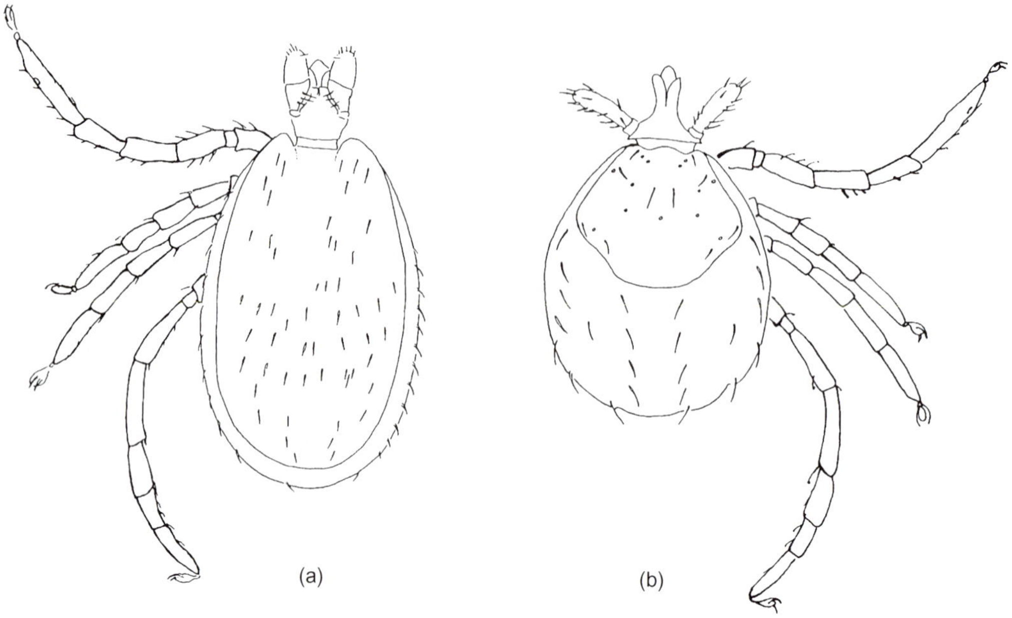

Fig. 11.5 Adult *Ixodes ricinus* in dorsal view. (a) Male. (b) Female (reproduced from Arthur, 1962).

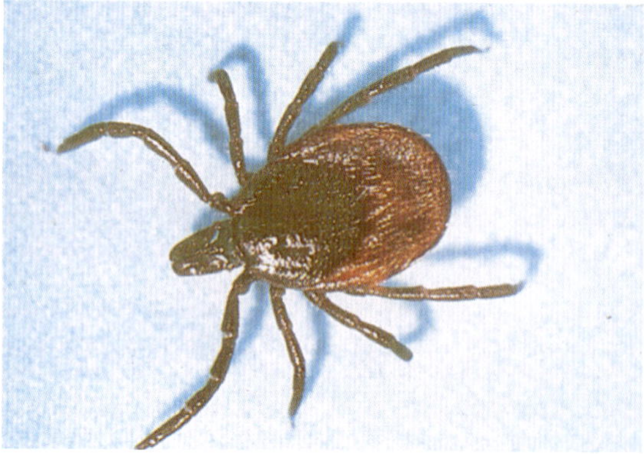

Fig. 11.6 Unfed female *Ixodes ricinus*. Note the relatively long mouthparts.

completes a single large blood meal; in contrast, the males feed intermittently and mate repeatedly. During mating, the male crawls under the female and, after manipulating the female genital opening with its mouthparts, transfers the spermatophore, a sac containing the spermatozoa, into the opening, with the aid of his front legs. Once fertilised, the female subsequently feeds for about 14 days and then drops to the ground to lay several thousand eggs in the soil in sheltered spots, over a period of about 30 days, after which it dies.

The eggs hatch to produce larvae. Larvae begin to quest several days to several weeks after hatching, the precise time depending on temperature and humidity. The larvae climb up the stems of vegetation ready to attach to a passing host. Once a host is located, larvae feed for 3–5 days, increasing their body weight by 10–20 times, then drop back on to the vegetation where they digest their blood meal and moult to become nymphs. The following year the nymphs begin to seek a new host, again feeding for 3–5 days, before dropping off the host and moulting into the adult stage.

The host on which nymphs feed is usually larger than that of the larvae, typically a bird, rabbit or squirrel. Twelve months later adults begin to quest for a host, on which they feed and mate. Adults feed on larger mammals, such as sheep, cattle or deer and achieve this selection by climbing to different levels in the vegetation while questing.

Although the life cycle takes 3 years to complete, the larvae, nymphs and adults feed for a total of only 26–28 days and *I. ricinus* is therefore a temporary parasite. Unfed larvae can survive for approximately 13–19 months, unfed nymphs for 24 months and unfed adults for 21–31 months, but the precise period over which they can survive depends on temperature and humidity.

Geographical distribution: Temperate areas of Europe, Australia, South Africa, Tunisia, Algeria and Asia. It

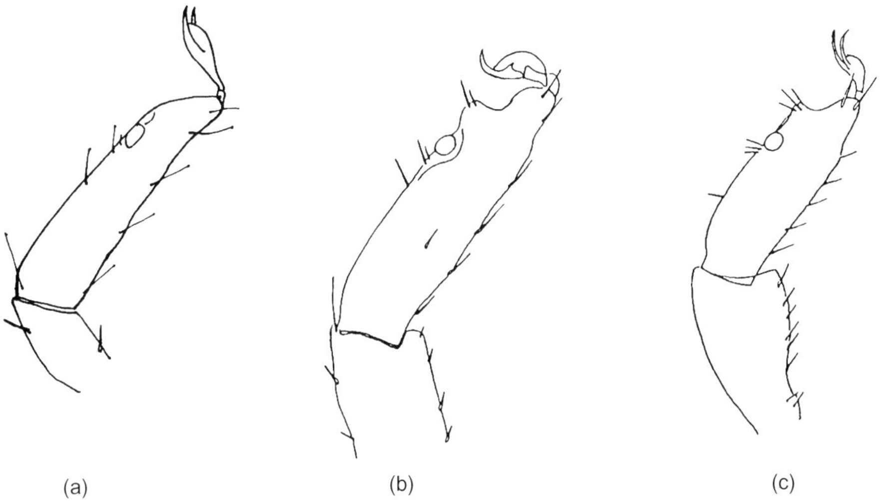

Fig. 11.7 The tarsi of adult male (a) *Ixodes ricinus*, (b) *Ixodes hexagonus* and (c) *Ixodes canisuga* (reproduced from Arthur, 1962).

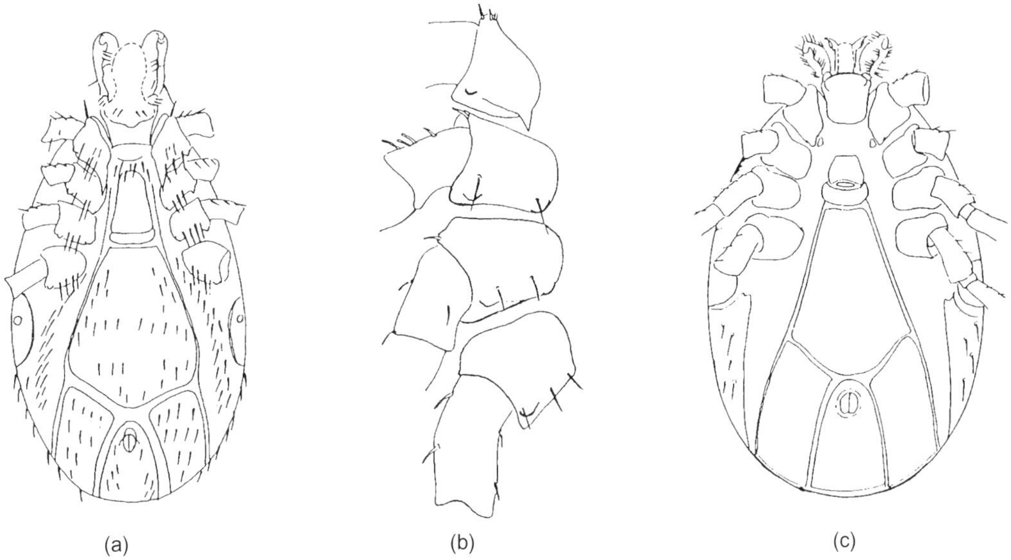

Fig. 11.8 Ventral view of the coxae of adult male (a) *Ixodes ricinus*, (b) *Ixodes hexagonus* and (c) *Ixodes canisuga* (reproduced from Arthur, 1962).

is more common in areas of rough grazing moorland and woodland.

Although recorded, this species has never become established in North America.

Pathogenesis: *Ixodes* ticks ingest blood and, occasionally, heavy infestations can cause anaemia. Tick bites may damage the host at the site of attachment causing local injury, which may predispose to secondary bacterial infection. The lesions caused during feeding may predispose to myiasis. Also at slaughter the value of the hide or fleece may be reduced.

Most significant of all, this tick transmits a range of pathogens. In western Europe, in cattle it transmits *Babesia divergens* and *B. bovis*, the causes of redwater fever and *Anaplasma marginale*, the cause of anaplasmosis in cattle. In sheep and cattle, it transmits the virus that causes louping-ill and the rickettsia responsible for tick-borne fever. It is also associated with tick pyaemia, caused by *Staphylococcus aureus*, in lambs in Britain and Norway.

Ixodid ticks also transmit *Borrelia burgdorferi*, the spirochaete responsible for Lyme disease in humans. *Ixodes ricinus* has been reported to cause tick paralysis and act as a vector for Czechoslovakian encephalitis, Russian spring–summer encephalitis and *Coxiella burnetii*. This tick may also transmit Bukhovinian haemorrhagic fever.

Ixodes canisuga

Common name: Dog tick

Predilection site: Skin

Parasite class: Arachnida

Sub-class: Acari

Order: Parasitiformes

Sub-order: Ixodida (Metastigmata)

Family: Ixodidae

Description: *Ixodes canisuga* is an inornate tick, without festoons or eyes. The palps are long and the ventral surface of the male is almost entirely covered with a series of plates. An anal groove is present anterior to the anus. The engorged female is light grey, up to 10 mm in length and bean-shaped, with four pairs of legs. The males are only 2.0–3.0 mm long, and the four pairs of legs are readily visible. *I. canisuga* can be differentiated from *I. ricinus* by the presence of humped tarsi (Fig. 11.7) and the absence of a spur on the posterior internal angle of the first coxa (Fig. 11.8). Nymphs resemble the adults and also have four pairs of legs, but are less than 2.0 mm in size. The larvae ('pepper ticks') are less than 1.0 mm, usually yellowish in colour and have only three pairs of legs.

Hosts: Mammals including dogs, foxes, sheep, horses and mules

Life cycle: *Ixodes canisuga* is a three-host tick and the life cycle requires approximately 3 years to complete. The tick feeds for only a few days each year; as a larva in the first year, a nymph in the second and an adult in the third. The life cycle is adapted to life in a lair or den. Mating takes place in the den and adult males are only rarely found on the host. Adult females lay relatively small numbers of eggs, probably about 400.

Geographical distribution: Throughout Europe, as far east as Russia

Pathogenesis: Infestation may cause dermatitis, pruritus, alopecia and anaemia, but it is not an important vector of disease. It may be a particular problem in packs of dogs in kennels.

Epidemiology: This species, sometimes called the British dog tick, has been found in a variety of hosts. It is particularly recognised as a problem in kennels, where the tick is capable of survival in crevices and cracks in the floors and walls.

Ixodes hexagonus

Common name: Hedgehog tick

Predilection site: Head, ears

Parasite class: Arachnida

Sub-class: Acari

Order: Parasitiformes

Sub-order: Ixodida (Metastigmata)

Family: Ixodidae

Description: Adults are red–brown, with legs that appear somewhat banded in colour. The scutum is broadly hexagonal (hence the name hexagonus) and, like *I. ricinus*, the coxae of the first pair of legs bear a spur. However, the spur is smaller than in *I. ricinus* and does not overlap the coxa of the second pair of legs (Fig. 11.8). When engorged the female may be up to 8 mm in length. Males are about 3.5–4 mm in length. The tarsi are long (0.8 mm in the female and 0.5 mm in the male) and sharply humped apically (Fig. 11.7).

Hosts: Hedgehog; other mammals, including dogs, cats, foxes, sheep, horse, moles

Life cycle: *Ixodes hexagonus* is a three-host tick adapted to live with hosts which use burrows or nests. It is primarily a parasite of hedgehogs but may also be found on dogs and other small mammals. The life cycle is similar to that of *I. ricinus*: egg, hexapod larva, octopod nymph and adult, occurring over 3 years. All life cycle stages feed on the same host for periods of about 8 days. After dropping to the ground adult females produce 1000–1500 eggs over a period of 19–25 days, before they die. The ticks may be active from early spring to late autumn, but are probably most active during April and May. This species inhabits sheltered habitats such as burrows and kennels and may infest pets in large numbers when they are exposed.

Geographical distribution: Europe and northwest Africa

Pathogenesis: On dogs and cats, adult females usually attach themselves behind the ears, on the jaws, neck and groin, causing localised dermatitis and the risk of wound infection. These ticks are often found to be responsible when dogs become repeatedly infested with ticks, particularly around the head area. It may also become a more significant pest in places where *I. ricinus* is absent. *Ixodes hexagonus* is a biological vector of *Borrelia* spp and tick-borne encephalitis.

Epidemiology: The main host is the European hedgehog, and the movement of this host to urbanised areas may increase the risk of both people and their animals being exposed to infectious diseases carried by *I. hexagonus*.

Ixodes holocyclus

Common name: Paralysis tick

Predilection site: Skin

Parasite class: Arachnida

Sub-class: Acari

Order: Parasitiformes

Sub-order: Ixodida (Metastigmata)

Family: Ixodidae

Description: The engorged adult female is light grey, up to 1.0 cm in length, bean shaped and has four pairs of legs. The males are only 2.0–3.0 mm long, and the four pairs of legs are readily visible. The palps are long and the ventral surface of the adult male is almost entirely covered with a series of plates. An anal groove is present anterior to the anus. Nymphs resemble the adults but are less than 2.0 mm in size while the larvae are less than 1.0 mm in length, and usually are yellowish in colour.

Hosts: Cattle, sheep, goat, dog, cat. All mammals and birds

Life cycle: This species is a three-host tick. The tick feeds for only a few days each year, as a larva in the first year, a nymph in the second and an adult in the third. Mating takes place on the host. After attachment the female is inseminated once and subsequently completes her single large blood meal; in contrast, the males feed intermittently and mate repeatedly. Once fertilised, the female subsequently feeds for about 14 days and then drops to the ground to lay several thousand eggs in sheltered spots, after which she dies. The larvae, which hatch from the eggs, will feed for about 6 days in the following year, then drop to the ground and moult to the nymphal stage. In the third year this stage feeds, drops off and becomes adult. Although the life cycle takes 3 years to complete, the larvae, nymphs and adults feed for a total of only 26–28 days.

Geographical distribution: Australia

Pathogenesis: *Ixodes holocyclus* is the main cause of tick paralysis in Australia. Its paralysing toxin has been reported to affect at least 20 000 domestic animals annually. Although infestations usually consist of relatively few individual ticks, *I. holocyclus* infestations can kill cattle, particularly calves, and small domestic animals. Fifty larvae or five nymphs will kill a 40 g rat, and larger numbers of either can cause paralysis in dogs and cats.

Generally only the adult stage infests cattle, with the worst outbreaks in late winter, spring and summer. *Ixodes holocyclus* is also a vector for *Coxiella burnetii* (Q fever) and *Rickettsia australis* (Queensland tick typhus).

Epidemiology: This species is most commonly found amongst low, leafy vegetation since this protects it against sun and wind exposure and maintains the high humidity required for development.

Ixodes persulcatus

Common name: Taiga tick

Predilection site: Skin

Parasite class: Arachnida

Sub-class: Acari

Order: Parasitiformes

Sub-order: Ixodida (Metastigmata)

Family: Ixodidae

Description: The taiga tick, *Ixodes persulcatus*, is morphologically very similar to *I. ricinus*; it is an inornate, red–brown coloured tick, without festoons or eyes. The palps are long and the ventral surface of the male is almost entirely covered with a series of plates. The engorged adult female is light grey and up to 10 mm in length. The major difference is that the female adult *I. persulcatus* has a straight or wavy genital opening rather than arched as in *I. ricinus*.

Hosts: Sheep, cattle, goat, horse, dog, other mammals, birds and man

Life cycle: The taiga tick has a similar life cycle to *Ixodes ricinus* although adults are rarely active during autumn.

Geographical distribution: It has a more easterly distribution than *Ixodes ricinus*, being widespread throughout eastern Europe, Russia and as far east as Japan.

Pathogenesis: *Ixodes persulcatus* is a major vector of the human diseases Russian spring–summer encephalitis virus and Lyme borreliosis.

Epidemiology: Taiga ticks may be dispersed by migrating birds.

Ixodes rubicundus

Common name: Karoo paralysis tick

Predilection site: Skin, neck, chest and belly

Parasite class: Arachnida

Sub-class: Acari

Order: Parasitiformes

Sub-order: Ixodida (Metastigmata)

Family: Ixodidae

Hosts: Domestic livestock and wild ungulates

Life cycle: This is a three-host tick species. The tick feeds for only a few days as a larva, a nymph and an adult. The life cycle of this species takes about 2 years. Mating takes place on the host. After attachment the female is inseminated once and subsequently completes her single large blood meal; in contrast, the males feed intermittently and mate repeatedly. Once fertilised, the female subsequently feeds for about 14 days and then drops to the ground to lay several thousand eggs in sheltered spots, after which she dies.

Geographical distribution: Southern Africa, particularly the Karrooveld

Pathogenesis: *Ixodes rubicundus*, the Karoo paralysis tick, parasitises domestic stock and wild ungulates in South Africa and may lead to serious losses. Ticks may cause damage at the site of attachment causing local injury, which may predispose to secondary bacterial infection. The adult tick produces a toxin that causes paralysis in sheep and goats. Affected animals become paralysed and some may show signs of incoordination and stumbling. Unless ticks are removed, the animal will remain paralysed and die within days. Most affected animals recover within 24 to 48 hours once the ticks have been removed or animals have been dipped.

Ixodes scapularis

Synonym: *Ixodes dammini*

Common name: Shoulder tick, black-legged tick

Predilection site: Skin

Parasite class: Arachnida

Sub-class: Acari

Order: Parasitiformes

Sub-order: Ixodida (Metastigmata)

Family: Ixodidae

Hosts: Deer. All mammals and birds

Life cycle: This is a three-host tick species. It feeds for only a few days each year, as a larva in the first year, a nymph in the second and an adult in the third. Mating usually takes place on the host. After attachment the female is inseminated and subsequently completes her single large blood meal. In contrast, the adult males feed intermittently and mate repeatedly. Once fertilised, the female subsequently feeds for about 14 days and then drops to the ground to lay several thousand eggs in sheltered spots, after which she dies. The following year, peak larval activity occurs in August, when larvae attach and feed on a wide variety of mammals and birds, particularly on white-footed mice (*Peromyscus leucopus*). After feeding for 3–5 days, engorged larvae drop from the host to the ground where they overwinter before moulting to become a nymph. In May of the following year, larvae moult to become nymphs, which feed on a variety of hosts for 3–4 days. Engorged nymphs then detach and drop to the forest floor where they moult into the adult stage, which becomes active in October. Adult ticks remain active through the winter on days when the ground and ambient temperatures are above freezing. The adult ticks feed on large mammals, primarily upon white-tailed deer, *Odocoileus virginianus*. Although the life cycle takes 3 years to complete, the larvae, nymphs and adults feed for a total of only 26–28 days.

Geographical distribution: North America, particularly in and around wooded areas

Pathogenesis: *Ixodes scapularis* inflicts a very painful bite. Nymphal and adult stages of this tick are the most common vector for Lyme disease in North America. They are also implicated in the transmission of *Francisella tularensis*. These ticks are major vectors for the transmission of human babesiosis and human granulocytic ehrlichiosis (HGE) and are responsible for the transmission of anaplasmosis and piroplasmosis.

Epidemiology: *Ixodes scapularis* requires a relative high humidity to survive, and its patterns of feeding activity reflect this requirement. With feeding restricted to times of year when conditions of temperature and humidity are appropriate, distinct restricted seasonal periods of activity result, usually in spring and autumn. As a result of its requirement for high humidity, in general, it is associated with areas of deciduous woodland containing small mammals and deer.

Ixodes pacificus

Common name: Western black-legged tick

Predilection site: Skin

Parasite class: Arachnida

Sub-class: Acari

Order: Parasitiformes

Sub-order: Ixodidia (Metastigmata)

Family: Ixodidae

Description: A very similar species to *Ixodes scapularis*. Adult ticks are red–brown in colour and about 3 mm in size. Larvae and nymphs are smaller and paler in colour.

Hosts: Rodents, lizards and large mammals, such as horses, deer and dogs

Life cycle: This is a three-host tick species.

Geographical distribution: Commonly found in the Western USA and British Columbia

Pathogenesis: It is known to be a vector of Lyme disease and the rickettsia responsible for equine granulocytic ehrliciosis.

Epidemiology: It is found in habitats with forest, north coastal scrub, high brush and open grasslands

Ixodes pilosus

Common name: Russet tick, bush tick

Predilection site: Skin

Parasite class: Arachnida

Sub-class: Acari

Order: Parasitiformes

Sub-order: Ixodida (Metastigmata)

Family: Ixodidae

Hosts: Cattle, sheep, goats, horses, dogs, cats and wild ungulates

Life cycle: This is a three-host tick species.

Geographical distribution: Most areas of South Africa

Pathogenesis: The feeding activity of this will cause bood loss, local dermatitis and may result in tick paralysis.

Several other species of *Ixodes* have been reported in North America and have been found mainly on dogs.

Species	Distribution	Comments
Ixodes angustus	Northeast USA	
Ixodes cookei	USA, southeastern Canada	Found on cattle, dogs and cats
Ixodes kingi	Western USA	Rotund tick
Ixodes rugosus	Western USA	
Ixodes sculptus	Northeast USA	
Ixodes muris	USA	Mouse tick
Ixodes texanus	Northern USA, Canada	

AMBLYOMMA

Members of this genus are large, often highly ornate ticks with long, often banded, legs. Unfed females may be up to 8 mm in length and when engorged may reach 20 mm in length. Eyes and festoons are present. Males lack ventral plates. They have long mouthparts (Fig. 11.4) with which they can inflict a deep, painful bite which may become secondarily infected. There are about 100 species of *Amblyomma*, largely distributed in tropical and subtropical areas of Africa. However, one important species is found in temperate North America. The identification of more than the major species is beyond the scope of this book and interested readers will need to consult a relevant taxonomic specialist.

Amblyomma americanum

Common name: Lone star tick

Predilection site: Ears, flanks, head and belly

Parasite class: Arachnida

Sub-class: Acari

Order: Parasitiformes

Sub-order: Ixodida (Metastigmata)

Family: Ixodidae

Description, adults: The lone star tick, *Amblyomma americanum*, is so called because of a single white spot on the scutum of the female (Fig. 11.9). These are large, usually ornate, ticks whose legs have bands of colour. Eyes and festoons are present. The palps and hypostome are long, and ventral plates are absent in the males. The engorged female is up to 10 mm in length, bean-shaped, and has four pairs of legs. The female is reddish-brown in colour, becoming light grey when engorged. On the scutum are two deep parallel cervical grooves and a large, pale spot at its posterior margin. The male is small with two pale symmetrical spots near the hind margin of the body, a pale stripe at each side, and a short oblique pale stripe behind each eye. The males are only 2–3 mm in length, and because of the small idiosoma the four pairs of legs are readily visible. In both sexes, coxa I has a long external spur and a short internal spur, and the mouthparts are much longer than the basis capituli.

Nymphs and larvae: Nymphs resemble the adults and also have four pairs of legs but are less than 2 mm in size, while the larvae ('pepper ticks') are less than 1 mm in length, usually yellowish in colour and have only three pairs of legs.

Hosts: Wild and domestic animals, particularly cattle; birds; larvae are most frequently found on wild small mammals.

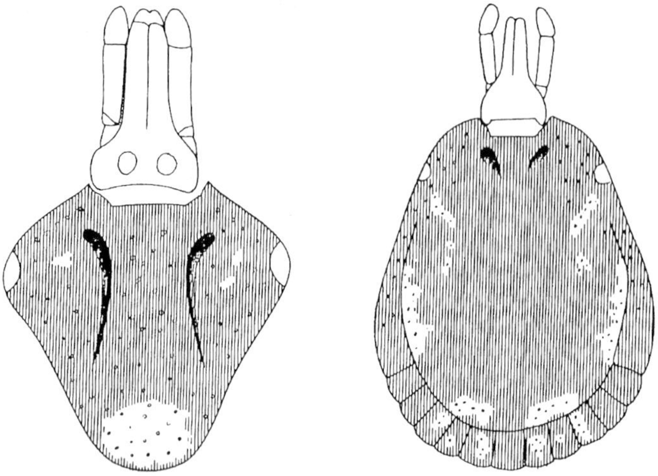

Fig. 11.9 Dorsal view of the gnathosoma and scutum of adult (a) female and (b) male *Amblyomma americanum* (from Arthur, 1963).

Life cycle: The life cycle is typical of a three-host tick. Adult females attach to a host and take a single large blood-meal over a period of 3–4 weeks, taking 0.5–2.0 ml of blood, during the course of which they mate once. In contrast, the males feed intermittently and mate repeatedly. Once fertilised, the female drops to the ground to lay several thousand eggs in sheltered spots, after which she dies. The larvae, which hatch from the eggs will feed for about 6 days in the following year, then drop to the ground and moult to the nymphal stage. In the third year this stage feeds, drops off and becomes adult. Although the life cycle takes 3 years to complete, the larvae, nymphs and adults feed for a total of only 26–28 days. Larvae and nymphs feed on rodents, rabbits and ground-inhabiting birds. Adults feed on larger mammals such as deer, cattle, horses and sheep.

Geographical distribution: Widely distributed throughout central and eastern USA

Pathogenesis: This tick is most commonly found on the ears, flanks, head and belly. Tick infestation is irritating and painful, and infestation has been shown to reduce weight gain in cattle. Each female ingests 0.5–2.0 ml of host blood, so large numbers can cause anaemia. Bites may cause tick paralysis. *Amblyomma americanum* is an important vector of *Rickettsia rickettsii* (Rocky Mountain spotted fever) and *Francisella tularensis* (tularaemia). It has also been implicated as a vector of *Borrelia burgdorferi* (Lyme disease), Q fever, canine ehrlichiosis and human monocytic ehrlichiosis.

Epidemiology: Feeding larvae, nymphs and adults are active between early spring and late summer in distinct periods corresponding with the feeding activity of each stage. There is usually a single generation per year. This species is particularly common in wooded areas, where hosts become infected as they brush against vegetation harbouring ticks.

Amblyomma variegatum

Common name: Bont ticks, variegated or tropical bont tick

Predilection site: Skin

Parasite class: Arachnida

Sub-class: Acari

Order: Parasitiformes

Sub-order: Ixodida (Metastigmata)

Family: Ixodidae

Description: Female *A. variegatum* are brown with a large pale patch on the posterior scutum while males are brightly ornamented with orange coloration and a dark brown border to the idiosoma (Fig. 11.10). Both sexes of *A. variegatum* have hemispherical eyes. *A. variegatum* and *A. hebraeum* can be distinguished from *A. americanum* and *A. cajennese* by the shorter external spur on coxa I, which is closely associated with the internal spur.

Hosts: Mammals, particularly cattle

Geographical distribution: Africa

Pathogenesis: *Amblyomma variegatum* transmit the important disease, heartwater, in cattle, caused by

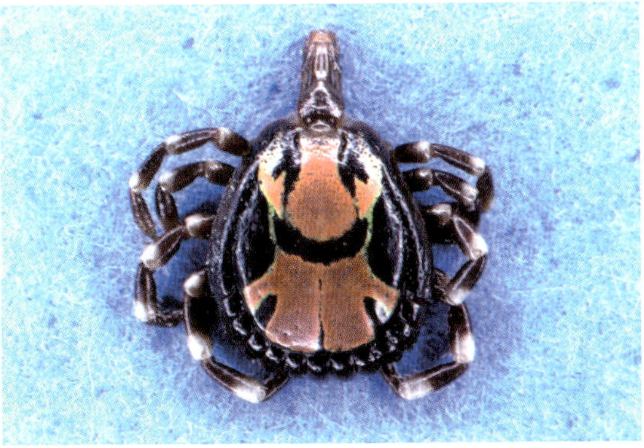

Fig. 11.10 Male *Amblyomma variagatum* (dorsal view).

the rickettsia, *Ehrlichia ruminantium*. It also transmits the viral Nairobi sheep disease and Q fever, caused by *Coxiella burnetii*.

Amblyomma cajennense

Common name: Cayenne tick

Predilection site: Skin, lower body surface, especially between the legs

Parasite class: Arachnida

Sub-class: Acari

Order: Parasitiformes

Sub-order: Ixodida (Metastigmata)

Family: Ixodidae

Description: In adults the scutum is usually very ornate, lattice patterned often with bright, multicoloured iridescent patterns. There may be pale central patches on the festoons.

Hosts: All mammals but most commonly equines

Geographical distribution: South and Central America, southern USA and the Caribbean

Pathogenesis: *Amblyomma cajennense* is an important tick in South America, the bites caused by this genus being particularly painful, probably due to the long mouthparts. In severe cases in South America this species has been reported to cause fever and weakness in cattle. The wounds created by this tick may create a suitable site for screwworm myiasis associated with *Cochliomyia* spp. This species transmits spotted fever in South America and *Leptospira pomona*.

Amblyomma hebraeum

Common name: Bont ticks

Predilection site: Skin

Parasite class: Arachnida

Sub-class: Acari

Order: Parasitiformes

Sub-order: Ixodida (Metastigmata)

Family: Ixodidae

Description: *A. variegatum* and *A. hebraeum* can be distinguished from *A. americanum* and *A. cajennese* by the shorter external spur on coxa I, which is closely associated with the internal spur.

Hosts: All mammals and birds

Geographical distribution: Mainly Africa

Pathogenesis: 'Bont ticks' transmit the important disease, heartwater, in cattle, sheep and goats; it is caused by the rickettsia, *Ehrlichia ruminantium*. This species also transmits *Rickettsia conorii*, the causative agent of Boutonneuse fever.

Amblyomma gemma

Predilection site: Skin

Parasite class: Arachnida

Sub-class: Acari

Order: Parasitiformes

Sub-order: Ixodida (Metastigmata)

Family: Ixodidae

Hosts: Mammals, particularly cattle, sheep and goats

Geographical distribution: Africa, particularly Kenya

Pathogenesis: *Amblyomma gemma* may be a vector for the transmission of heartwater in cattle, sheep and goats.

Amblyomma maculatum

Common name: Gulf coast tick

Predilection site: Skin, particularly the ears

Parasite class: Arachnida

Sub-class: Acari

Order: Parasitiformes

Sub-order: Ixodida (Metastigmata)

Family: Ixodidae

Table 11.1 Other *Amblyomma* tick species.

Species	Hosts	Geographical distribution	Pathogenesis
Amblyomma pomposum	Mammals, particularly cattle, sheep and goats	Africa, mainly western Zambia, southern DRC and Angola	All three species are involved in the transmission of heartwater (*Ehrlichia ruminantium*)
Amblyomma lepidum	Sheep, goats, cattle	Sudan	
Amblyomma astrion	Buffalo, cattle	West and central Africa	
Amblyomma sparsum	Reptiles, tortoise	Sub-Saharan Africa	These species are of particular importance because they are vectors of the rickettsia, *Ehrlichia ruminantium*, the causal agent of heartwater in cattle, sheep goats, deer and buffalo. Infected ticks may be present on imported reptiles, facilitating the transmission of disease into new areas such as the USA
Amblyomma marmorium	Tortoise tick	Sub-Saharan Africa	

Hosts: All mammals and birds

Geographical distribution: Southern USA, in regions of high temperature and humidity

Pathogenesis: The 'Gulf Coast tick', *A. maculatum*, is not known to transmit disease but does cause severe bites and painful swellings and has been associated with tick paralysis. The wounds created by this species may create a suitable site for screwworm myiasis associated with *Cochliomyia* spp.

BOOPHILUS

Ticks of the genus *Boophilus* are often known as 'blue ticks', and are important as vectors of *Babesia* spp and *Anaplasma marginale* in cattle in subtropical and tropical countries. The palps and hypostome are short. The males have adanal or accessory ventral shields. The basis capituli is hexagonal dorsally. The mouthparts are short and the compressed palps are ridged dorsally and laterally (Fig. 11.4). Unfed adults may be only 2 or 3 mm long, reaching lengths of up to 12 mm when engorged. The identification of more than the major species is beyond the scope of this text and interested readers will need to consult a relevant taxonomic specialist.

Control: The basis of successful control is to prevent the development of the engorged female ticks and so limit the deposition of large numbers of eggs. Since species of *Boophilus* have a parasitic life cycle, which requires 20 days before adult females become fully engorged, an animal dipped with an acaricide, which has a residual effect of 3–4 days should not harbour engorged females for at least 24 days (i.e. 20 + 4). In theory, therefore, treatment every 21 days during the tick season should give good control, but since the nymphal stages appear to be less susceptible to most acaricides, a 12-day interval is often necessary between treatments at the beginning of the tick season. The avermectins/milbemycins may play an increasing role in the control of one-host ticks. A single acaricide treatment can destroy all of the ticks on an animal, but will not prevent reinfestation. Hence, to effect long-term control, cattle that have had direct or presumed contact with *Boophilus* must be dipped at regular intervals for at least a year and the movement of animals into the affected farms or ranches strictly controlled.

Boophilus annulatus

Common name: Blue cattle tick, Texas cattle fever tick

Predilection site: Skin

Parasite class: Arachnida

Sub-class: Acari

Order: Parasitiformes

Sub-order: Ixodida (Metastigmata)

Family: Ixodidae

Hosts: Cattle, horse, goat, sheep, camel, dog. All mammals and birds

Life cycle: This is a one-host tick species. The larva, nymph and adult all attach to, and develop on, a single host. The engorged female drops off the host and lays between 2000 and 3000 eggs over a period of 14–59 days. The larvae hatch after 23–159 days depending on climatic conditions. The larvae then attach to the host, feed and moult to the nymph and then adult stage. Mating takes place on the host. The total period spent on the host is between 15 and 55 days, although unfed larvae can survive for up to 8 months before attachment to the host. Two to four generations may occur per year, depending on climatic conditions; the entire life cycle of this species can be completed in 6 weeks.

Geographical distribution: Central and South America, Africa, Mexico, Commonwealth of Independent States (former USSR), Africa, the Middle East, the Near East, the Mediterranean and Mexico. It has been largely eradicated from North America, but can be sometimes found in Texas or California, in a buffer quarantine zone along the Mexican border.

Pathogenesis: These ticks are most important vectors of *Babesia* spp and *Anaplasma marginale* in cattle in subtropical and tropical countries. *Boophilus annulatus* is an important vector of Texas cattle fever caused by *Babesia bigemina* and *B. bovis*. Skin irritation induces scratching and licking, sometimes leading to secondary infections. Severe infestations may cause anaemia.

Boophilus microplus

Common name: Tropical cattle tick, southern cattle tick

Predilection site: Skin

Parasite class: Arachnida

Sub-class: Acari

Order: Parasitiformes

Sub-order: Ixodida (Metastigmata)

Family: Ixodidae

Description: Adult *B. microplus* have a short, straight gnathosoma. The legs are pale cream. The body is oval to rectangular and the scutum is oval and wider at the front. The anal groove is obsolete in the female and is faint in the male and surrounds the anus posteriorly. Coxa I is bifid. The spiracles are circular or oval. The nymphs of this species have an orange–brown scutum. The body is oval and wider at the front. The body colour is brown to blue–grey, with white at the front and sides.

Hosts: Cattle, sheep, goat, wild ungulates

Life cycle: This species is a one-host tick. The larva, nymph and adult all attach to, and develop on, a single host. The engorged female drops off the host and lays between 2000 and 4500 eggs over a period of 4–44 days. The larvae hatch after 14–146 days depending on climatic conditions. The larvae then attach to the host, feed and moult to the nymph and then adult stages. From the attachment of larva to engorgement of the adult female requires 3 weeks. After engorging, females can weigh up to 250 times more than when unfed. Mating takes place on the host. The total period spent on the host is between 17 and 52 days, and the entire life cycle can be completed within 2 months, although unfed larvae can survive for up to 20 weeks before attachment to the host. Although present all year round, populations reach their peak in summer.

Geographical distribution: Asia, Australia, Mexico, Central and South America, West Indies, South Africa

Pathogenesis: *B. microplus* is widely distributed in the southern hemisphere and the southern states of the USA and is considered one of the most serious external parasites of Australian cattle. This tick species is an important vector for the transmission of *Babesia bigemina* and *Borrelia theileri* in South America, *Anaplasma marginale* in Australia and South America and *Coxiella burnetii* in Australia. Disease transmission can occur throughout all the parasite stages. Disease organisms may be passed transovarially to be transmitted by the next tick generation. Some disease organisms such as *Babesia* spp may remain in the body of the ticks for as many as five generations even when fed on non-infected, non-susceptible hosts.

Boophilus calcaratus

Common name: Blue tick

Predilection site: Skin

Parasite class: Acarhnida

Sub-class: Acari

Order: Parasitiformes

Sub-order: Ixodida (Metastigmata)

Family: Ixodidae

Hosts: Cattle, sheep, goat, wild ungulates

Life cycle: This is a one-host tick. The larva, nymph and adult all attach to, and develop on, a single host. Unfed larvae may survive 7 months. Development usually takes place in 1–2 months. Further details on the life cycle are lacking.

Geographical distribution: Asia, north Africa

Pathogenesis: *Boophilus calcaratus* transmits *B. bigemina* and *B. bovis* in North Africa and *Anaplasma marginale* in the northern Caucasus.

Boophilus decoloratus

Common name: Blue tick

Predilection site: Skin

Parasite class: Arachnida

Sub-class: Acari

Order: Parasitiformes

Sub-order: Ixodida (Metastigmata)

Family: Ixodidae

Description: The engorged females have 'slaty-blue' coloured bodies with pale yellow legs.

Hosts: Cattle, horse, donkey, sheep, goat, dog, wild ungulates

Life cycle: This is a one-host tick species. The larva, nymph and adult all attach to, and develop on, a single host. The engorged female drops off the host and lays and incubates approximately 2500 eggs over a period of 3–6 weeks. The larvae then attach to the host, feed and moult to the nymph and then adult stage. Mating takes place on the host. The total period spent on the host ranges between 21 and 25 days, although unfed larvae can survive for up to 7 months before attachment to the host.

Geographical distribution: Africa

Pathogenesis: *Boophilus decoloratus* is a vector *for Babesia bigemina*, *B. ovis* and *Anaplasma marginale* in cattle. It also transmits spirochaetosis, *Borrelia theileri*, in cattle, horses, goats and sheep and *Babesia trautmanni* in pigs in east Africa.

DERMACENTOR

Ticks of the genus *Dermacentor* are medium-sized to large ticks, usually with ornate patterning. The palps and mouthparts are short and the basis capituli is rectangular (Fig. 11.4). Festoons and eyes are present. The coxa of the first pair of legs is divided into two sections in both sexes. Coxae progressively increase in size from I to IV. The males lack ventral plates and, in the adult male, the coxa of the fourth pair of legs is greatly enlarged. The identification of more than the most important species is beyond the scope of this text and interested readers will need to consult a relevant taxonomic specialist.

Most species of *Dermacentor* are three-host ticks, but a few are one-host ticks. The genus is small with about 30 species, most of which are found in the New World. Several of the species are directly associated with Rocky Mountain spotted fever, Q fever, tularaemia and Colorado tick fever. The salivary secretions of some species may produce tick paralysis.

Dermacentor andersoni

Synonym: *Dermacentor venustus*

Common name: Rocky Mountain wood tick

Predilection site: All over the body but especially the axilla, inguinal region, face and ears

Parasite class: Arachnida

Sub-class: Acari

Order: Parasitiformes

Sub-order: Ixodida (Metastigmata)

Family: Ixodidae

Description, adults: *Dermacentor andersoni* is an ornate tick, with a base colour of brown and a grey pattern (Fig. 11.11). Males are about 2–6 mm in length and females about 3–5 mm in length when unfed and 10–11 mm in length when engorged. The mouthparts are short. The basis capituli is short and broad. The legs are patterned in the same manner as the body. The coxae of the first pair of legs have well developed external and internal spurs.

Hosts: Immature stages: small rodents; adults: wild and domestic herbivores

Life cycle: *Dermacentor andersoni* is a three-host tick. Immature stages primarily feed on small rodents, while adults feed largely on wild and domestic herbivores. Mating takes place on the host, following which females lay up to 6500 eggs over about 3 weeks. The eggs hatch in about 1 month, and the larvae begin to quest. Larvae feed for about 5 days, before dropping to the ground and moulting to the octopod nymphal stage. One- and 2-year population cycles may occur. Eggs hatch in early spring and individuals that are successful in finding hosts pass through their larval stages in spring, their nymphal stages in late summer and then overwinter as adults in a 1-year cycle. Nymphs that fail to feed have to overwinter, and form a spring-feeding generation of nymphs the following year. Unfed nymphs may survive for up to a year. *Dermacentor andersoni* is most common in areas of scrubby vegetation, since these attract both the small mammals required by the immature stages and the large herbivorous mammals required by the adults.

Geographical distribution: Widely distributed throughout the western and central parts of North America from Mexico as far north as British Columbia

Pathogenesis: High infestation levels may therefore cause anaemia. *Dermacentor andersoni* may cause tick paralysis, particularly in calves, and may be responsible for the transmission of bovine anaplasmosis, caused by *Anaplasma marginale*. It also transmits the Colorado tick fever virus, and the bacteria that cause tularaemia. *Dermacentor andersoni* is the chief vector of *Rickettsia rickettsii* (Rocky Mountain spotted fever) in western USA.

Epidemiology: Adult numbers peak in May, then decline by July. Larvae and nymphs appear later and

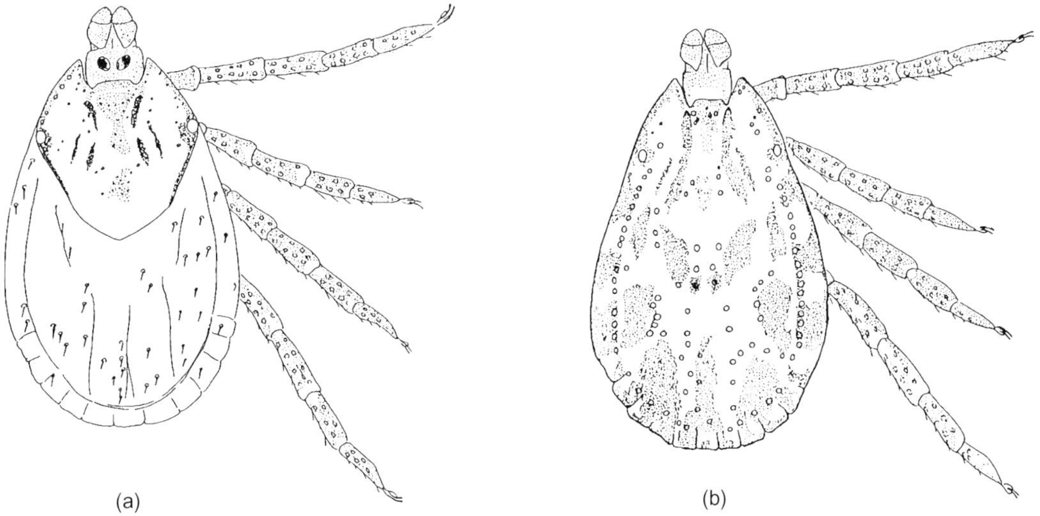

Fig. 11.11 Adult *Dermacentor andersoni*. (a) Dorsal view of male. (b) Dorsal view of female (reproduced from Arthur, 1962).

have usually disappeared by late summer. This species is particularly common amongst damp, grassy, brush-covered areas, since these attract both the small mammals required by the immature stages and the large herbivorous mammals required by the adults. Infection occurs when host animals brush against vegetation harbouring tick larvae.

Dermacentor variabilis

Common name: American dog tick, wood tick

Predilection site: Skin

Parasite class: Arachnida

Sub-class: Acari

Order: Parasitiformes

Sub-order: Ixodida (Metastigmata)

Family: Ixodidae

Description: These are ornate, pale brown and gray ticks with eyes and festoons present (Fig. 11.12). The basis capituli is rectangular and the palps short. The males lack ventral plates and the coxae of the fourth pair of legs are enlarged with external spurs. Adult males are about 3–4 mm in length and adult females about 4 mm in length when unfed and 15 mm in length when engorged.

Hosts: Dog, horse, cattle, man. This tick will feed on many species of domestic and wild mammals.

Life cycle: *Dermacentror variabilis* is a three-host tick, feeding once in each of the larval, nymphal and adult life cycle stages. After each feed it drops from the host. Mating takes place on the host. Once fertilised, the adult female feeds for 5–27 days before dropping to the ground to lay 4000–6000 eggs in sheltered spots, after which she dies. Oviposition may last 14–32 days, depending on temperature and humidity. The larvae hatch from the eggs after 20–57 days and feed for between 2 and 13 days on the host, then drop to the ground and moult to the nymphal stage. This stage feeds over a period of several days, drops off and moults to become an adult. Unfed larvae, nymphs and adults can survive for very long periods of time under appropriate environmental conditions. The larval and nymphal stages feed on wild rodents, particularly the short-tailed meadow mouse (*Microtus* spp), while the preferred hosts of adults are larger mammals, particularly wild and domestic carnivores.

Geographical distribution: North America

Pathogenesis: *Dermacentor variabilis* is an important parasite of wild and domestic carnivores. The feeding activity of *D. variabilis* may cause tick paralysis in dogs. In cattle it may transmit bovine anaplasmosis. It is also an important vector of *Rickettsia rickettsii* (Rocky Mountain spotted fever) in the USA and is able to transmit the bacteria which causes tularaemia (hunter's disease). It also transmits St Louis encephalitis virus and several studies have shown that it may carry the Lyme disease bacterium, *Borrelia burgdorferi*.

Dermacentor albipictus

Common name: Winter tick or moose tick

Predilection site: Skin

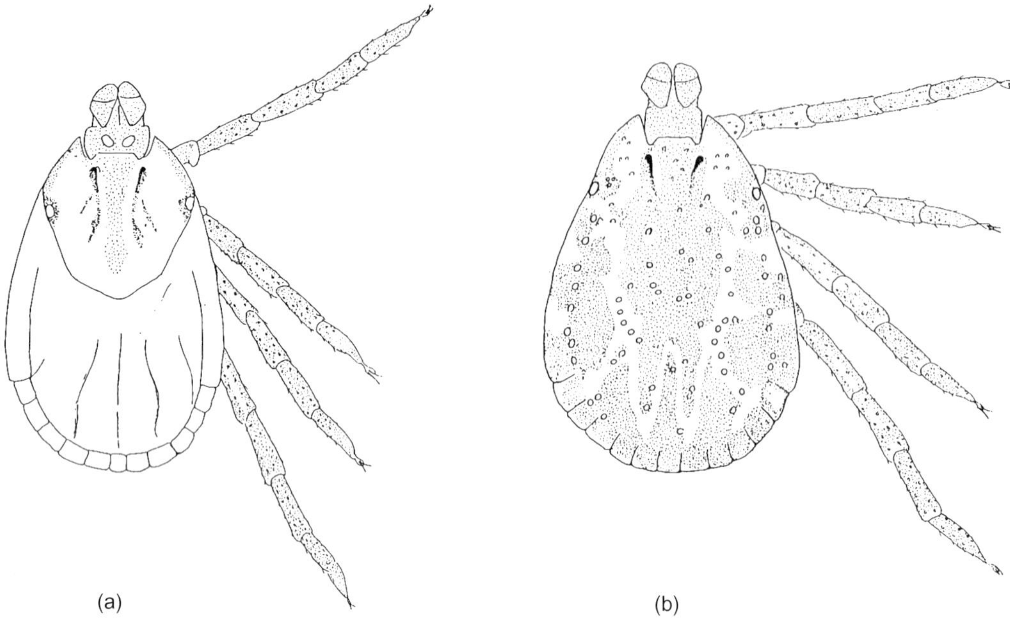

Fig. 11.12 Adult *Dermacentor variabilis*. (a) Dorsal view of male. (b) Dorsal view of female (reproduced from Arthur, 1962).

Parasite class: Arachnida

Sub-class: Acari

Order: Parasitoformes

Sub-order: Ixodida (Metastigmata)

Family: Ixodidae

Description: The adults are ornately patterened ticks with eyes and festoons present. The basis capituli is rectangular and the palps short. The males lack ventral plates and the coxae of the fourth pair of legs are enlarged. In the adults of both sexes the coxa of the first pair of legs has an enlarged spur (bidentate) and in the male, the coxae increase in size from I to IV.

Hosts: The preferred host is the moose but they will also feed on a wide variety of domestic and wild mammals, including horses, cattle and humans.

Life cycle: This is a one-host species of tick. The larva, nymph and adult all attach to, and develop on, a single host. This species feeds only in winter, usually between October and March/April, on horses, deer and related large mammals. The engorged female drops off the host in the spring and lays between 1500 and 4400 eggs over a period of 19–42 days. The eggs hatch within 33–71 days. The larvae remain inactive until autumn when they then attach to a host, feed and moult to the nymph stage in 10–76 days. The nymphs engorge and moult to the adult stage in 10–76 days. Mating takes place on the host. The total period spent on the host is between 28 and 60 days, although unfed larvae can survive for up to 12 months before attachment to the host. Under normal conditions this tick species produces one generation per year.

Geographical distribution: Northern USA and Canada, particularly upland and mountainous areas

Pathogenesis: *D. albipictus* may cause tick paralysis and is a vector of anaplasmosis, and possibly Rocky Mountain spotted fever. Heavy infestations with *D. albipictus* cause hair loss and a condition known as 'ghost moose' in northern parts of the USA. Heavy infection can occur in the long winter coats of mammals such as horses, deer, elk and moose, causing debilitation and anaemia, particularly when there are food shortages.

Dermacentor marginatus

Common name: Sheep tick

Predilection site: Skin

Parasite class: Arachnida

Sub-class: Acari

Order: Parasitiformes

Sub-order: Ixodida (Metastigmata)

Family: Ixodidae

Hosts: Adults feed largely on mammals: sheep, cattle, deer, dogs, humans, hares and hedgehogs. Nymphs and larva feed on small mammals, insectivores and birds.

Life cycle: This is a three-host tick.

Geographical distribution: Morocco, Spain, Italy, southern France, Switzerland, western Germany, Poland, eastwards to central Asia

Pathogenesis: This species is a vector for a wide range of diseases; in dogs, *Babesia canis*; in cattle, *Babesia divergens*; in sheep, *B. ovis*, *Theileria ovis* and *Anaplasma ovis*; in horses, *Babesia caballi*, *Theileria equi* and infectious encephalomyelitis. Also *Coxiella burnetii* (Q fever), *Francisella tularensis* (tularemia), *Brucella* spp and *Rickettsia conorii* (Boutonneuse fever)

Dermacentor nitens

Common name: Tropical horse tick

Predilection site: Skin. The preferred site of attachment is the ear; however, it may also infest nasal passages and the mane, ventral abdomen, and perianal area.

Parasite class: Arachnida

Sub-class: Acari

Order: Parasitiformes

Sub-order: Ixodida (Metastigmata)

Family: Ixodidae

Hosts: Horse, cattle, man, many domestic and wild mammals. Horses are the preferred host of this species.

Life cycle: This is a one-host tick species; the larva, nymph and adult all attach to, and develop on, a single host. The engorged female drops off the host, and lays up to 3500 eggs over a period of 15–37 days. The eggs hatch within 19–39 days. The larvae then attach to the host, feed and moult to the nymph stage in 8–16 days. The nymphs engorge and moult to the adult stage in 7–29 days. Mating takes place on the host. The total period spent on the host is between 26 and 41 days, although unfed larvae can survive for up to 117 days before attachment to the host. Under favourable tropical conditions this tick species can produce several generations per year.

Geographical distribution: Southern USA, Central and South America and the Caribbean

Pathogenesis: Heavy infections may lead to suppuration of the ears, and bite wounds may predispose the host to oviposition by screwworm flies. *Dermacentor nitens* is an important vector of *Babesia caballi*, resulting in equine babesiosis. It is able to transmit this pathogen transovarially to successive generations, and is important in the horse racing industry.

Dermacentor reticulatus

Synonym: *Dermacentor pictus*

Common name: Marsh tick, meadow tick or ornate cow tick

Predilection site: Skin

Parasite class: Arachnida

Sub-class: Acari

Order: Parasitiformes

Sub-order: Ixodida (Metastigmata)

Family: Ixodidae

Description: This species is an ornate tick with eyes and festoons present (Fig. 11.13). Both sexes are white with variegated brown splashes (Fig. 11.14). The basis capituli is rectangular and the palps short. The adult female is 3.8–4.2 mm when unfed and 10 mm in length when engorged. The adult male is approximately 4.2–4.8 mm in length. The males lack ventral plates, and the coxae of the fourth pair of legs are enlarged with a narrow, tapering external spur. In the adults of both sexes the coxa of the first pair of legs has an enlarged spur (bidentate). The other coxae have short internal spurs that become progressively smaller in legs II to IV. An unfed nymph is approximately 1.4–1.8 mm in length.

Hosts: Sheep, cattle, dog, horse, pig, human. Nymphs and larvae feed on smaller mammals, such as insectivores and occasionally birds.

Life cycle: *Dermacentor reticulatus* is a three-host tick, and the life cycle can be completed in only 1–2 years, depending on environmental conditions. The species feeds once in each of the larval, nymphal and adult life cycle stages, dropping from a host, moulting and then reacquiring a new host between feeds. Mating takes place on the host and once fertilised the adult female feeds for 9–15 days, before dropping to the ground to lay approximately 4000 eggs in sheltered spots, after which she dies. Oviposition may last for 6–40 days, depending on temperature and humidity, with oviposition rate peaking on about the 5th day. The larvae hatch from the eggs after 2–3 weeks and will feed for approximately 2 days on the host, then drop to the ground and moult to the nymphal stage. This stage feeds over a period of several days, drops off and moults to become an adult.

Geographical distribution: Europe (from the Atlantic coast to Kazakhstan) and central Africa

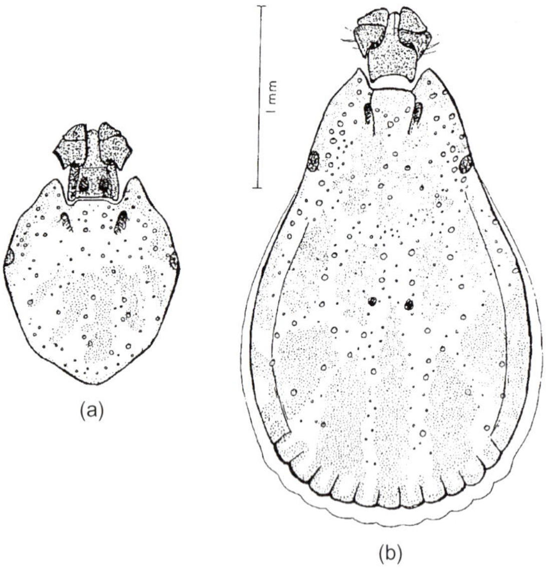

Fig. 11.13 Dorsal view of the gnathosoma and scutum of adult (a) male and (b) female *Dermacentor reticulatus* (reproduced from Arthur, 1962).

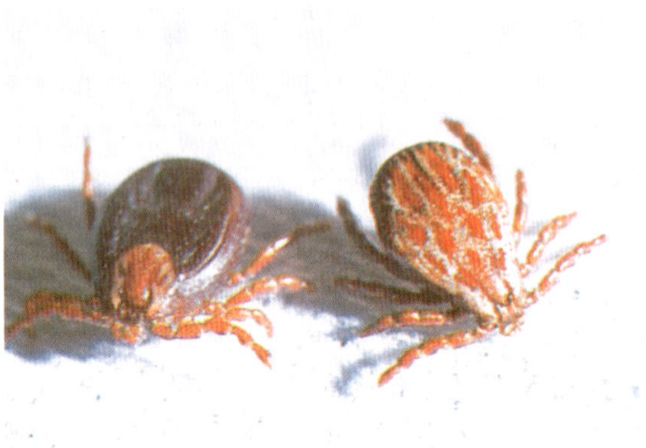

Fig. 11.14 Male and female *Dermacentor reticulatus*: ornate tick with festoons.

Pathogenesis: *D. reticulatus* is a vector for the transmission of a wide range of pathogens. It is particularly important as an ectoparasite of cattle and may be found along their backs in early spring. In cattle it is a vector for *Babesia divergens* (redwater), *B. ovis, Theileria ovis, Coxiella burnetii* (Q fever), *Francisella tularensis* (tularaemia), *Brucella, Rickettsia conorii* (Boutonneuse fever), *Anaplasma ovis.* In horses it is a vector of *Babesia caballi, Theileria equi* and infectious encephalomyelitis of horses. In dogs it is a vector for *Babesia canis.*

Dermacentor silvarum

Predilection site: Skin, all over the body but especially the axilla, inguinal region, face and ears

Parasite class: Arachnida

Sub-class: Acari

Order: Parasitiformes

Sub-order: Ixodida (Metastigmata)

Family: Ixodidae

Hosts: Cattle, sheep, horses, dogs, humans

Life cycle: This is a three-host species, feeding on a different host in each of its life cycle stages. Adult females and immature stages overwinter on the ground. However, some males may remain attached to the host during winter. Larvae and nymphs are active from spring to autumn, although there is a general peak in adult activity from early spring to summer with a second, lower peak in autumn. The development of *D. silvarum* from egg to adult may require as little as 45 days at 28°C and 50 days at 25°C. The threshold temperatures for larval and nymphal development are 8 and 10°C respectively. The life cycle may be completed in 1 year or, more usually in most parts of its range, it is extended by one or more summer or winter diapauses to 2–4 years.

Geographical distribution: Asia (central Siberia and northeastern China to Japan)

Pathogenesis: The salivary secretions of this species may also produce tick paralysis. *Dermacentor silvarum* is a vector for the transmission of Siberian tick typhus (*Rickettsia sibirica*) and also a vector of *Babesia bovis, B. caballi, Theileri equi, B. canis, Theileria ovis* and *Anaplasma ovis.*

Dermacentor nuttallii

Predilection site: Skin

Parasite class: Arachnida

Sub-class: Acari

Order: Parasitiformes

Sub-order: Ixodida (Metastigmata)

Family: Ixodidae

Geographical distribution: Siberia, northern Pakistan, China, Mongolia

Pathogenesis: *Dermacentor nuttallii* is a vector of *Rickettsia sibirica*

Dermacentor occidentalis

Common name: Pacific coast tick

Predilection site: Skin

Parasite class: Arachnida

Sub-class: Acari

Order: Parasitiformes

Sub-order: Ixodida (Metastigmata)

Family: Ixodidae

Hosts: Cattle, horse, other domestic animals and wild mammals

Life cycle: *Dermacentor occidentalis* is a three-host tick. The tick feeds for only a few days as a larva, a nymph and an adult, each on a different host. Mating takes place on the host. After attachment the female is inseminated once, subsequently completes her single large blood-meal, drops to the ground and lays her eggs.

Geographical distribution: Western USA (Sierra Nevada mountains and the Pacific coast from Oregon to southern California)

Pathogenesis: *Dermacentor occidentalis* is a vector of anaplasmosis, Colorado tick fever, Q fever and tularaemia and may cause tick paralysis.

HAEMAPHYSALIS

Ticks of the genus *Haemaphysalis* inhabit humid, well vegetated habitats in Eurasia and tropical Africa. They are three-host ticks, with the larvae and nymphs feeding on small mammals and birds and adults infesting larger mammals and, importantly, livestock. There are about 150 species, found largely in the Old World, with only two species found in the New World.

Most species of the genus are small, with short mouthparts and a rectangular basis capituli (Fig. 11.4). Ventral plates are not present in the male. Spiracular plates are rounded or oval in females and rounded or comma-shaped in males. Like *Ixodes* spp, these ticks lack eyes, but they differ in having festoons and a posterior anal groove. The identification of more than the major species is beyond the scope of this text and interested readers will need to consult a relevant taxonomic specialist.

Haemaphysalis punctata

Synonym: *Haemaphysalis cinnabarina punctata*

Predilection site: Skin

Parasite class: Arachnida

Sub-class: Acari

Order: Parasitiformes

Sub-order: Ixodida (Metastigmata)

Family: Ixodidae

Description: Small, inornate ticks with eyes and festoons absent (Figs 11.15, 11.16). The palps and hypostome are short. The adults of both sexes are about 3 mm in length, the female reaching about 12 mm in length when engorged. Sexual dimorphism is not pronounced, however. The basis capituli is rectangular, about twice as broad as long. The sensory palps are short and broad, with the second segment extending beyond the basis capituli. The anal groove is posterior to the anus. The coxae of the first pair of legs have a short, blunt internal spur, which is also present on the coxae of the second and third pair of legs and which is enlarged and tapering on the coxae of the fourth pair of legs. In the male the spur may be as long as the coxa.

Hosts: Cattle, sheep, goat, horse, deer, wolf, bear, bat, birds, rabbit. The larvae and nymphs may also be found on birds, hedgehogs, rodents and reptiles, such as lizards and snakes.

Life cycle: *Haemaphysalis punctata* is a three-host tick, feeding once in each of the larval, nymphal and adult life cycle stages. After each blood-meal it drops from the host. Engorgement on the host may take 6–30 days to complete. Once fed, each adult female lays 3000–5000 eggs on the ground, over a period of 10 days to 7 months. Unfed larvae can survive for up to 10 months, unfed nymphs and adults for 8.5 months.

Geographical distribution: Europe (including southern Scandinavia and Britain), central Asia and North Africa

Pathogenesis: *Haemaphysalis punctata* is responsible for the transmission of *Babesia major* and *Babesia bigemina*, *Theileria mutans* (*T. buffeli/orientalis*), *Anaplasma marginale* and *A. centrale* in cattle. In sheep, it transmits *Babesia motasi* and the benign *Theileria ovis*. It has also been reported to cause tick paralysis. In addition to transmitting *Anaplasma* and *Babesia* spp, different *H. punctata* populations are infected by tick-borne encephalitis virus, Tribec virus, Bhanja virus, and Crimean–Congo haemorrhagic fever virus.

Haemaphysalis leachi

Common name: Yellow dog tick

Predilection site: Head and body

Parasite class: Arachnida

Sub-class: Acari

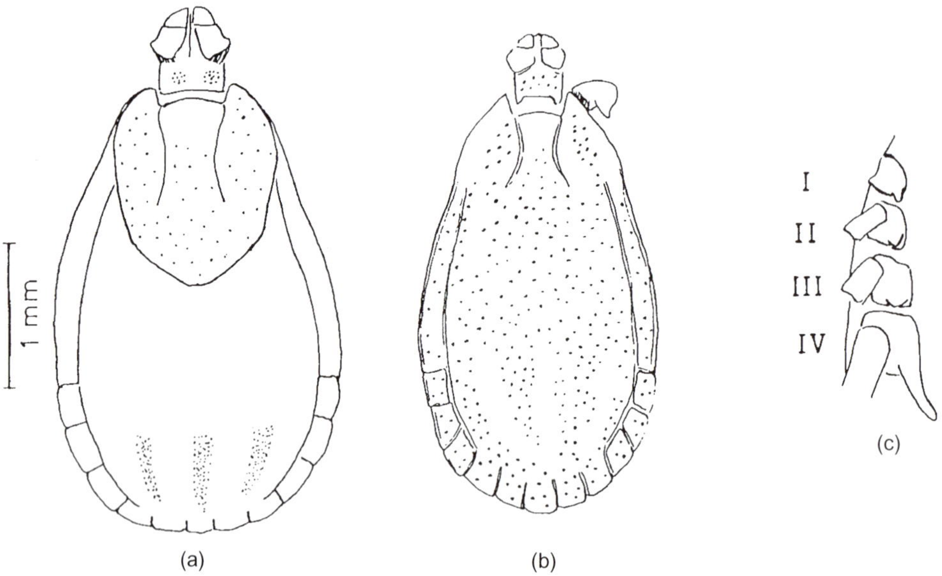

Fig. 11.15 Dorsal view of the gnathosoma and scutum of adult (a) male and (b) female *Haemaphysalis punctata*. (c) Ventral view of the coxae of an adult male (reproduced from Arthur, 1962).

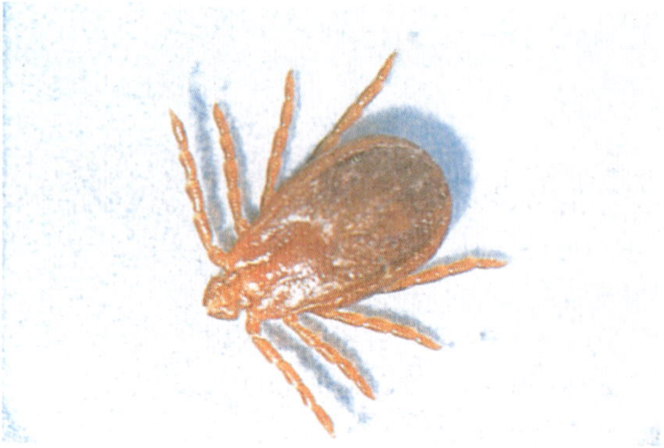

Fig. 11.16 Female *Haemaphysalis punctata*: note short mouthparts.

Order: Parasitiformes

Sub-order: Ixodida (Metastigmata)

Family: Ixodidae

Hosts: Dog, domestic and wild carnivores, small rodents and occasionally cattle

Life cycle: *Haemaphysalis leachi* is a three-host tick, feeding once in each of the larval, nymphal and adult life cycle stages. After each feed it drops from the host. Each female lays approximately 5000 eggs. The eggs hatch within 26–37 days, from where the emerging larvae attach to a host and engorge after 2–7 days. Unfed larvae can survive for over 6 months. The larvae drop off the host and moult to the nymphal stage after approximately 30 days. Nymphs attach to a host and become engorged after 2–7 days, after which they drop off and moult to become adult after 10–16 days. Unfed nymphs can survive for over 2 months. The adults attack a third host and engorge within 8–16 days, although they are able to survive unfed for over 7 months.

Geographical distribution: Africa, Australia and Asia

Pathogenesis: This species is responsible for the transmission of canine piroplasmosis (*B. canis*) in dogs, tick-bite fever (*Rickettsia conorii*) and *Coxiella burnetii*.

Haemaphysalis longicornis

Predilection site: Skin

Parasite class: Arachnida

Sub-class: Acari

Order: Parasitiformes

Sub-order: Ixodida (Metastigmata)

Family: Ixodidae

Hosts: Cattle. All mammals and birds

Life cycle: A three-host tick species. The larvae and nymphs primarily feed on small mammals and birds while adults infest larger mammals.

Geographical distribution: Widely distributed in the Far East and Australasia

Pathogenesis: The main result of infestation is tick worry. This lowers production in cattle and tick bites damage hides.

Haemaphysalis spinigera

Predilection site: Skin

Parasite class: Arachnida

Sub-class: Acari

Order: Parasitiformes

Sub-order: Ixodida (Metastigmata)

Family: Ixodidae

Hosts: Adults will feed on monkeys, birds and cattle; immatures feed on small mammals such as shrews and humans.

Life cycle: This species is a three-host tick feeding once in each of the larval, nymphal and adult life cycle stages. After each feed it drops from the host. The larvae and nymphs primarily feed on small mammals and birds while adults infest larger mammals.

Geographical distribution: Tropical evergreen/deciduous forests of southern and central India and Sri Lanka.

Pathogenesis: Kyasanur forest disease virus (KFD) which affects monkeys and humans. KFD virus has also been isolated from other species of *Haemaphysalis*, *Dermacentor* and *Ixodes* ticks.

Epidemiology: Cattle may be heavily parasitised by adults of *H. spinigera* and help to maintain the tick population, but neither cattle nor birds are thought to have any significant role in maintenance of the virus.

Haemaphysalis bispinosa

Common name: Bush tick

Predilection site: Skin

Parasite class: Arachnida

Sub-class: Acari

Order: Parasitiformes

Sub-order: Ixodida (Metastigmata)

Family: Ixodidae

Hosts: A variety of mammals; heavy infestations have been recorded on sheep and cattle.

Life cycle: A three-host tick species. Of interest is the suggestion that this tick may reproduce parthenogenetically.

Geographical distribution: Asia and Australasia, particularly problematic in coastal eastern Australia.

Pathogenesis: This species may act as a vector of *Babesia motasi* and *B. ovis* in sheep and goats, *Babesia equi* in horses and donkeys and *Babesia canis* and *Babesia gibsoni* in dogs.

Haemaphysalis concinna

Common name: Bush tick

Predilection site: Skin

Parasite class: Arachnida

Sub-class: Acari

Order: Parasitiformes

Sub-order: Ixodida (Metastigmata)

Family: Ixodidae

Hosts: A variety of mammals; particularly important as a parasite of sheep

Life cycle: A three-host tick species.

Geographical distribution: Eastern and central Europe, Russia east to China

Pathogenesis: This species may act as a vector of bunyavirus, the causative agent of Bunya fever.

Haemaphysalis cinnabarina

Synonym: *H. sanguinolenta*

Predilection site: Skin

Parasite class: Arachnida

Sub-class: Acari

Order: Parasitiformes

Sub-order: Ixodida (Metastigmata)

Family: Ixodidae

Hosts: A variety of ruminants

Life cycle: A three-host tick species.

Geographical distribution: Africa, southern Europe, Asia east to Japan

Pathogenesis: Anaplasmosis, Q-fever, babesiosis

Haemaphysalis leporispalustris

Common name: Rabbit tick

Predilection site: Skin

Parasite class: Arachnida

Sub-class: Acari

Order: Parasitiformes

Sub-order: Ixodida (Metastigmata)

Family: Ixodidae

Hosts: Rabbits, snowshoe hare, birds, rarely feeds on humans

Life cycle: A three-host tick species

Geographical distribution: North America, Canada

Pathogenesis: This species of of limited veterinary or public health concern, but may act as a vector of the Lyme disease spirochaete, *Borrelia burgdorferi.*

HYALOMMA

Species of this genus are medium-sized or large ticks, with eyes and long mouthparts. The males have ventral plates on each side of the anus. *Hyalomma* spp are usually two-host ticks, though some species may use three hosts. They are most commonly found on the legs, udder, tail or perianal region. There are about 20 species, found usually in semi-desert lowlands of central Asia, southern Europe and North Africa. They can survive exceptionally cold and dry conditions.

Species of *Hyalomma* are usually inornate, but with banded legs (the 'bont-legged tick'); eyes are present and festoons sometimes present. The palps and hypostome, as in *Amblyomma*, are long (Fig. 11.4). The males have adanal shields. The identification of more than the major species is beyond the scope of this text and interested readers will need to consult a relevant taxonomic specialist.

Hyalomma anatolicum

Sub-species: *anatolicum*

Common name: Bont-legged tick

Predilection site: All over the body but especially the axilla, inguinal region, face and ears

Parasite class: Arachnida

Sub-class: Acari

Order: Parasitiformes

Sub-order: Ixodida (Metastigmata)

Family: Ixodidae

Hosts: Cattle, horse; all mammals and birds

Life cycle: This species is a two- or three-host tick. Larvae acquire a host, feed and moult. Nymphs reattach to the same host soon after moulting. Following engorgement nymphs drop off the host, moult to the adult stage and then acquire a new second host where they feed. After attachment, mating occurs and the female completes her single large blood meal. Males feed intermittently and mate repeatedly. Once fertilised the female feeds for about 14 days and then drops to the ground to lay several thousand eggs in sheltered spots, after which she dies. The larvae and nymphs feed on birds and small mammals, and the adults on ruminants and equines. When larvae and nymphs infest smaller mammals, birds or reptiles, the life cycle may become a three-host model.

Geographical distribution: Steppe and semi-desert environments from central Asia to Bangladesh, the Middle and Near East, Arabia, southeastern Europe and Africa. *Hyalomma anatolicum* is believed to exist as two subspecies: *Hyalomma anatolicum excavatum* in the central European and Asiatic parts of its range and *Hyalomma anatolicum anatolicum* elsewhere. Some authors have suggested that these should be viewed as separate species.

Pathogenesis: This genus is mainly responsible for tick toxicosis, in parts of Africa and the Indian subcontinent. The 'toxin' produced by the adult tick causes a sweating sickness in ruminants and pigs characterised by a widespread hyperaemia of the mucous membranes and a profuse moist eczema. This is a highly damaging tick species. *Hyalomma anatolicum* transmits *Theileria annulata*, *T. equi*, *Babesia caballi*, *Anaplasma marginale*, *Trypanosoma theileri* and at least five arboviruses.

Notes: A closely related species, *H. lusitanicum*, replaces *H. anatolicum* from central Italy to Portugal, Morocco and the Canary Islands. It is believed to be a vector of equine and bovine babesiosis.

Hyalomma aegyptium

Common name: Tortoise tick

Predilection site: Skin

Parasite class: Arachnida

Sub-class: Acari

Order: Parasitiformes

Sub-order: Ixodida (Metastigmata)

Family: Ixodidae

Description: These are large brown ticks with eyes and long mouth parts. Females 5.5–20 mm; males 3–6 mm. Coxa I has a large divergent spur in females and a prominent, sharply-pointed spur in males.

Hosts: Tortoises (*Testudo* spp), lizards, dog, horse

Life cycle: This species is a two-host tick. The larval and nymphal stages engorge on the same host.

Geographical distribution: Southern Europe and southwest Asia

Epidemiology: *H. aegyptium* is found mainly in arid areas, sheltering in burrows of its tortoise host.

Treatment and control: Individual ticks can be removed carefully with forceps.

Hyalomma detritum

Subspecies: *scupense*

Subspecies: *mauretanicum*

Synonym: *Hyalomma volgense, Hyalomma uralense*

Common name: Bont-legged tick

Predilection site: Skin; all over the body but especially the axilla, inguinal region, face and ears

Parasite class: Arachnida

Sub-cass: Acari

Order: Parasitiformes

Sub-order: Ixodida (Metastigmata)

Family: Ixodidae

Hosts: Cattle, sheep, goat, horse. All mammals and birds

Life cycle: This species is a two-host tick. The larval and nymphal stages engorge on the same host. The female lays 5000 to 7000 eggs over a period of 37–59 days. These hatch in 34–66 days depending on the temperature and climatic conditions. Larvae and nymphs remain on the first host for between 13 and 45 days. Nymphs drop off the host and then moult to become adults. Subsequently the adult finds a second host where the adult female engorges in 5–6 days. Unfed larvae can survive for 12 months, unfed nymphs for 3 months and unfed adults for 14 months.

Geographical distribution: Africa

Pathogenesis: This genus is responsible for tick toxicosis in parts of southern Africa. The 'toxin' produced by the adult tick causes a sweating sickness in ruminants and pigs characterised by a widespread hyperaemia of the mucous membranes and a profuse moist eczema.

Hyalomma dromedarii

Common name: Camel tick

Predilection site: All over the body but especially the axilla, inguinal region, face and ears

Parasite class: Arachnida

Sub-class: Acari

Order: Parasitiformes

Sub-order: Ixodida (Metastigmata)

Family: Ixodidae

Description: *Hyalomma dromedarii* are usually inornate but with banded legs; eyes are present and festoons are sometimes present. The second segment of the palps is usually less than twice as long as the third segment, and the scutum has no pattern.

Host: Camels, but may also be of veterinary significance in ruminants and horses

Life cycle: This is predominantly a two-host species of tick. Larvae acquire a host, feed and moult. Nymphs reattach to the same host soon after moulting. Following engorgement nymphs drop off the host, moult to the adult stage and then acquire a new second host where they feed. After attachment, mating occurs and the female completes her single large blood-meal. Males feed intermittently and mate repeatedly. Once fertilised the female feeds for about 14 days and then drops to the ground to lay several thousand eggs in sheltered spots, after which she dies. In some circumstances, a variable life cycle has been reported for *H. dromedarii* with a three-host life cycle observed on sheep or cattle. It appears that the type of host, rearing conditions, density and age of the larvae may influence the life cycle adopted by this species.

Geographical distribution: India to Africa

Pathogenesis: Tick bites may cause damage at the site of attachment causing local injury, which may predispose to secondary bacterial infection. This genus is mainly responsible for tick toxicosis in parts of Africa and the Indian sub-continent. The 'toxin' produced by the adult tick causes a sweating sickness in ruminants and pigs characterised by a widespread hyperaemia of the mucous membranes and a profuse moist eczema.

Clinical signs: There are no obvious signs of tick infestation other than the presence of the parasites and the local skin reactions to their bites.

Diagnosis: The adult ticks, particularly the engorged females, are easily seen on the skin. The main predilection sites are the face, ears, axilla and inguinal region.

Pathology: Small granulomatous reactions may form at the site of tick bites consisting of a mixed inflammatory cell response with fibrosis.

Hyalomma excavatum

Synonym: *Hyalomma anatolicum excavatum*

Common name: Brown ear tick

Predilection site: Skin: all over the body but especially the axilla, inguinal region, face and ears

Parasite class: Arachnida

Sub-class: Acari

Order: Parasitiformes

Sub-order: Ixodida (Metastigmata)

Family: Ixodidae

Description: Usually with banded legs; eyes are present and festoons sometimes present. The palps and hypostome are long. The gnathosoma and coxae are dark, reddish or black–brown. The males have adanal shields. The second segment of the palps is less than twice as long as the third segment, and the scutum has no pattern.

Hosts: This species feeds primarily on burrowing rodents, particularly as larvae and nymphs. However, adults will also feed on ruminants and equines, where this species may be of veterinary significance.

Life cycle: Species of *Hyalomma* usually have a two-host life cycle, with larvae and nymphs remaining and feeding on the same host. The engorged nymphs drop to the ground and moult to become an adult. Subsequently the adult feeds and engorges on a second host. However, some populations may show a three-host feeding pattern.

Geographical distribution: Africa, Asia Minor and southern Europe

Pathogenesis: *Hyalomma excavatum* is a vector for the transmission of *Theileria annulata*, causing tropical theileriosis or Mediterranean coast fever in Bovidae species, and equine and bovine babesiosis.

Hyalomma marginatum

Subspecies: *marginatum*

Subspecies: *rufipes*

Subspecies: *turanicum*

Subspecies: *isaaci*

Common name: Bont-legged ticks

Predilection site: Skin, all over the body but especially the axilla, inguinal region, face and ears

Parasite class: Arachnida

Sub-class: Acari

Order: Parasitiformes

Sub-order: Ixodida (Metastigmata)

Family: Ixodidae

Description: Adult *Hyalomma marginatum* are usually inornate but with banded legs. Eyes are present and festoons sometimes present. The palps and hypostome are long. The males have adanal shields. The second segment of the palps is less than twice as long as the third segment, and the scutum has no pattern.

Hosts: Adults parasitise wild herbivores and livestock (particularly equines and ruminants). Immature stages primarily parasitise small wild mammals, lizards and birds.

Life cycle: The members of this species complex have a two-host life cycle, larvae and nymphs remaining and feeding on the same host. The engorged nymphs drop to the ground and moult to become an adult. Subsequently the adult feeds and engorges on a second host. The life cycle takes a minimum of 14 weeks from egg to adult.

Geographical distribution: Africa, Asia Minor and southern Europe:

- *H. marginatum marginatum* (Caspian area of Iran and CIS to Portugal and northwestern Africa)
- *H. marginatum rufipes* (south of the Sahara to South Africa, also Nile Valley and southern Arabia)
- *H. marginatum turanicum* (Pakistan, Iran, southern CIS, Arabia, parts of northeastern Africa)
- *H. marginatum isaaci* (Sri Lanka to southern Nepal, Pakistan, northern Afghanistan).

Pathogenesis: The salivary secretions of this species may also produce tick paralysis. *Hyalomma marginatum* subspecies are important vectors of disease: in dogs they transmit *Babesia canis*; in cattle *Babesia ovis*, *Rickettsia aeschlimanii* and Crimean–Congo haemorrhagic fever (CCHF); and in horses *Babesia caballi* and *Theileria equi*.

Hyalomma truncatum

Common name: Bont-legged ticks

Predilection site: Skin, all over the body but especially the axilla, inguinal region, face and ears

Parasite class: Arachnida

Sub-class: Acari

Order: Parasitiformes

Sub-order: Ixodida (Metastigmata)

Family: Ixodidae

Hosts: Cattle, sheep, goat, pig, horse. All mammals and birds

Life cycle: This species is a two-host tick.

Geographical distribution: Africa

Pathogenesis: This genus is responsible for tick toxicosis in parts of southern Africa. The 'toxin' produced by the adult tick causes a sweating sickness in ruminants and pigs characterised by a widespread hyperaemia of the mucous membranes and a profuse moist eczema. This species can act as a vector of *Babesia caballi*, *Theileria equi*, *Theileria parva*, *T. annulata*, *T. dispar*, *Coxiella burnetii*, *Rickettsia bovis* and *R. conorii*.

Hyalomma scupense

Common name: Bont-legged ticks

Predilection site: Skin, all over the body but especially the axilla, inguinal region, face and ears

Parasite class: Arachnida

Sub-class: Acari

Order: Parasitiformes

Sub-order: Ixodida (Metastigmata)

Family: Ixodidae

Hosts: Cattle, horses and antelope

Life cycle: This species is a one-host tick and is unusual in that it overwinters on the host.

Geographical distribution: Southwestern Russia and former USSR and southeastern Europe

Pathogenesis: It is a vector of *Theileria annulata* and *Babesia equi*.

Hyalomma impressum

Common name: Bont legged ticks

Predilection site: Skin, all over the body but especially the axilla, inguinal region, face and ears

Parasite class: Arachnida

Sub-class: Acari

Order: Parasitiformes

Sub-order: Ixodida (Metastigmata)

Family: Ixodidae

Hosts: Immature stages feed on small mammals and birds. Adults feed on large mammals, such as cattle and sheep

Geographical distribution: Central and west Africa

Pathogenesis: Of little known pathogenic significance, but may act as a vector of Crimean–Congo haemorrhagic fever virus.

RHIPICEPHALUS

The genus is composed of about 60 species, all of which were originally endemic to the Old World and, for the most part, distributed throughout sub-Saharan Africa. However, many species have now been introduced into a range of new habitats worldwide. They act as vectors of a number of disease pathogens. They infest a variety of mammals but seldom birds or reptiles. Most species are three-host ticks but some species of the genus are two-host ticks.

The basis capituli is hexagonal (Fig. 11.4) and, in the male, paired plates are found on each side of the anus. They are not ornate. Palps are short and eyes and festoons are usually present. Spiracular plates are comma-shaped. The identification of more than the major species is beyond the scope of this text and interested readers will need to consult a relevant taxonomic specialist.

Rhipicephalus appendiculatus

Common name: Brown ear tick

Predilection site: Skin; ears

Parasite class: Arachnida

Sub-class: Acari

Order: Parasitiformes

Sub-order: Ixodida (Metastigmata)

Family: Ixodidae

Description: Adult male *R. appendiculatus* are brownish, reddish brown, or very dark, with reddish brown legs. They vary from 1.8–4.4 mm in length. The scutal punctuations are scattered and of moderate size; they are evenly dispersed in the centre, but few or none may be found beyond the lateral grooves and in the lateral fields. The cervical grooves are moderately reticulate or non-reticulate. The postero-median and para-median grooves are narrow and distinct. The adanal shields are long and have slightly rounded angles, but can be somewhat variable.

Adult female *R. appendiculatus* are also brown, reddish brown, or very dark. The punctuations are small to moderate sized and are similar to those found in the male. The scutum is approximately equal in length and width; its posterior margin is slightly tapering or abruptly rounded. The lateral grooves are short, poorly defined or absent. The cervical grooves are long and shallow and almost reach the posterolateral margins.

Hosts: Cattle, horse, sheep, goat, deer, antelope, dog, rodents. This species of tick will feed on a wide variety of mammals and birds.

Life cycle: This species is a three-host tick and mating takes place on the host.

Geographical distribution: Africa, south of the Sahara. It occurs particularly in areas with substantial rainfall and shrub cover and it is absent in deserts.

Pathogenesis: This tick is considered a major pest in areas where it is endemic. Heavy infestations on cattle can result in severe damage to the ears and toxaemia. The excess blood excreted by the ticks may attract flies leading to secondary myiasis. Tick bites may become infected with bacteria. Tick salivary fluids and salivary toxins can produce host reactions such as toxicosis (sweating sickness and tick paralysis). Heavy infestations can result in fatal toxaemia and loss of resistance to other infections as well as severe damage to the host's ears, udder and tail. *R. appendiculatus* is a vector of east coast fever (*Theileria parva*), *T. lawrencei*, Nairobi sheep disease (NSD) virus, *Ehrlichia bovis*, *Hepatozoon canis*, *Rickettsia conorii* and Thogoto virus.

Epidemiology: Adults and immatures feed in the ears of cattle and other livestock and seasonal activity is closely associated with temperature and rain periods. *Rhipicephalus appendiculatus* is more abundant in cool, shaded shrubby or woody savannas with at least 60 cm of annual rainfall.

Control: Weekly dipping during the tick season should kill the adult female ticks before they are engorged, except in cases of very severe challenge when the dipping interval has to be reduced to 4 or 5 days. Dipping intervals of this latter frequency are also necessary for cattle infested with *R. appendiculatus* in areas where east coast fever is endemic so that the ticks are killed before the sporozoites of *T. parva* have time to develop to the infective stage in the salivary glands of the tick. Theoretically, weekly dipping should also control the larvae and nymphs, but in several areas the peak infestations of larvae and nymphs occur at different seasons to the adult females and the duration of the dipping season has to be extended.

Rhipicephalus bursa

Predilection site: Skin

Parasite class: Arachnida

Sub-class: Acari

Order: Parasitiformes

Sub-order: Ixodida (Metastigmata)

Family: Ixodidae

Hosts: Cattle, sheep, horse, dog. All mammals and birds

Life cycle: This is a three-host species of tick, feeding once in each of the larval, nymphal and adult life cycle stages. After engorging as a larva and nymph it drops from the host and then moults, before locating a further host. After engorging, adult females drop to the ground, lay their eggs and then die.

Geographical distribution: Africa (south of the Sahara), southern Europe

Pathogenesis: *Rhipicephalus bursa* is a major vector for the transmission of *Babesia bovis*, *Babesia ovis*, *Babesia motasi*, *Theileria equi*, *Babesia caballi*, *Theileria ovis*, *Anaplasma marginale*, *Anaplasma phagocytophilium*, *Coxiella burnetti*, Narobi sheep disease and Crimean–Congo haemorrhagic fever viruses.

Rhipicephalus capensis

Common name: Cape brown tick

Predilection site: Skin

Parasite class: Arachnida

Sub-class: Acari

Order: Parasitiformes

Sub-order: Ixodida (Metastigmata)

Family: Ixodidae

Hosts: Cattle, horse, sheep, goat, deer, antelope, dog. This species of tick will feed on a wide variety of mammals and birds.

Life cycle: This is a three-host species of tick. After locating a host, the adult female engorges in 4–21 days. It then drops to the ground where it lays 3000–7000 eggs before dying. The eggs hatch in 28 days to 3 months, depending on the temperature and climatic conditions. Subsequently the hexapod larvae locate a suitable host and engorge over a period of 3–6 days. They then drop to the ground before moulting 5–49 days later to become nymphs. The nymphs locate a further host where they engorge over a period of 3–9 days. Nymphs then drop to the ground and moult 10–61 days later to become adults.

Geographical distribution: Africa, south of the Sahara in afro-tropical, humid savannah or bush ecosystems, with temperatures under 30°C.

Pathogenesis: *R. capensis* is a major vector for the transmission of east coast fever (*Theileria parva*) and *Anaplasma marginale*.

Rhipicephalus evertsi

Common name: Red-legged tick

Predilection site: Skin

Parasite class: Arachnida

Sub-class: Acari

Order: Parasitiformes

Sub-order: Ixodida (Metastigmata)

Family: Ixodidae

Description: This species can be distinguished from other members of the genus by its red legs. It has a black scutum, which is densely pitted, and in the male leaves a red margin of the opisthosoma uncovered.

Hosts: Cattle, sheep, goat, horse, dog. All mammals and birds

Life cycle: This is a two-host species of tick. The larval and nymphal stages engorge on the same host. The female lays approximately 5000–7000 eggs over a period of 6–24 days. These hatch in 4–10 weeks depending on the temperature and climatic conditions. Larvae and nymphs remain on the host for between 10 and 15 days before dropping to the ground. Nymphs then moult after 42–56 days. Subsequently, adults locate a second host, when the adult female engorges in 6–10 days. The larvae and nymphs are commonly found in the ears or the inguinal region, while the adults are mainly found under the tail. Unfed larvae can survive for 7 months, while unfed adults can survive for 14 months.

Geographical distribution: Africa, south of the Sahara

Pathogenesis: *Rhipicephalus evertsi* is a major vector for the transmission of east coast fever, *Theileria parva*, redwater, *Babesia bigemina* and *T. mutans* of cattle. It also transmits *Borrelia* in various animals, and biliary fever, *Theileria equi*, in horses.

Rhipicephalus sanguineus

Common name: Brown dog tick, kennel tick

Predilection site: On dogs, *R. sanguineus* is often found in the ears and between the toes. Immature stages prefer the hair of the neck.

Parasite class: Arachnida

Sub-class: Acari

Order: Parasitiformes

Sub-order: Ixodida (Metastigmata)

Family: Ixodidae

Description: This species is yellow, reddish or blackish brown in colour and unfed adults may be 3–4.5 mm in length, although size is highly variable and engorged females may reach a length of 12 mm (Fig. 11.17). The palps and hypostome are short and the basis capituli hexagonal dorsally. The coxa of the first pair of legs has two spurs. The legs may become successively larger from the anterior to the posterior pair. The tarsi of the fourth pair of legs possess a marked ventral tarsal hook. The anal groove encircles only the posterior half of the anus and then extends into a median groove. The males have adanal plates and accessory shields. The six-legged larvae are small and light brown in colour, while the eight-legged nymphs are reddish brown in colour.

Hosts: Dog, other mammals and birds

Life cycle: This species has a three-host life cycle. Mating takes place on the host. Once fertilised, the female feeds for about 14 days and then drops to the ground to lay approximately 4000 eggs in sheltered spots, after which she dies. Egg masses are likely to be found in above-ground crack and crevices (for example, kennel roofs) due to the females' behavioural tendency to crawl upward. The eggs hatch after 17–30 days. The larvae, which hatch from the eggs, will feed for about 6 days the following year, then drop to the ground and moult to the nymphal stage over a period of 5–23 days. In the third year this stage feeds for 4–9 days, drops off the host and moults to the adult stage. Under favourable conditions the life cycle may require as little as 63 days, hence several generations may occur each year. However, under adverse conditions unfed larvae can survive for as long as 9 months, unfed nymphs for 6 months and unfed adults for 19 months.

Geographical distribution: Worldwide. This species is believed to have originated in Africa but is now considered to be the most widely distributed tick species in the world.

Pathogenesis: *Rhipicephalus sanguineus* is primarily parasitic on dogs and is responsible for the transmission of *Babesia canis* and *Ehrlichia canis* and can also cause tick paralysis in the dog. There seems little doubt that it can also transmit many protozoal, viral and rickettsial infections of animals and man. These include *Theileria equi* and *B. caballi* of equines, *Anaplasma marginale* in North America, *Hepatozoon canis* of dogs, *Coxiella burnetii*, *Rickettsia conorii*, *R. canis*, *R. rickettsii*, *Pasteurella tularensis*, *Borrelia hispanica* and the viruses that cause Nairobi sheep disease and other viral diseases of sheep in Africa. *Rhipicephalus sanguineus* is also a vector for east coast fever (*Theileria parva*) among cattle, *Babesia perroncitoi* and *Babesia trautmanni* among pigs, and transmits Rocky Mountain spotted fever in some areas of the USA and Mexico.

Rhipicephalus pulchellus

Common name: Ivory-ornamented tick

Predilection site: Ears and on the lower abdomen

Parasite class: Arachnida

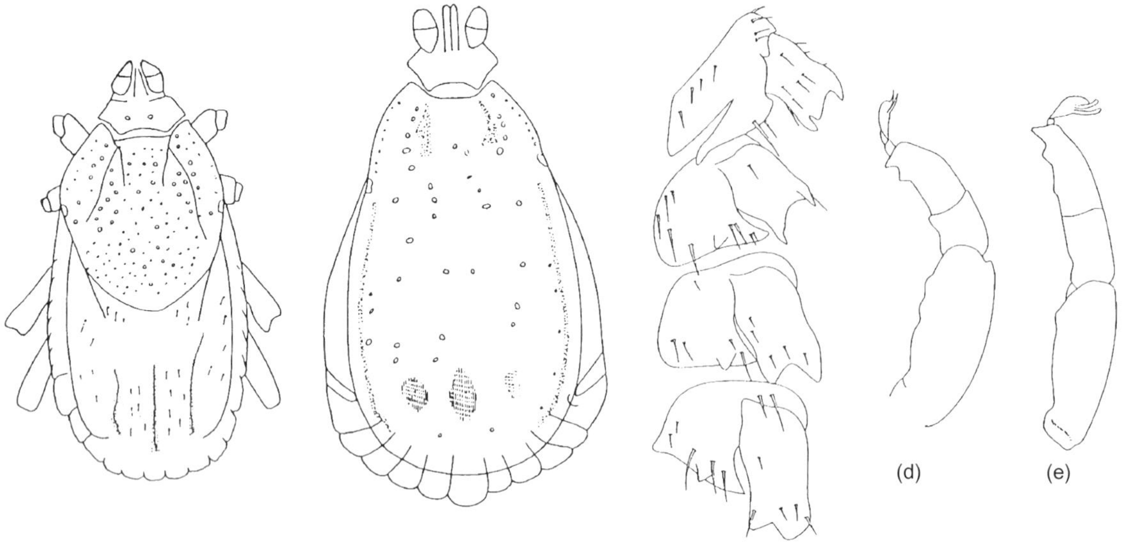

Fig. 11.17 Dorsal view of the gnathosoma and scutum of adult (a) female and (b) male *Rhipicephalus sanguineus*. (c) Ventral view of the coxae and trochanters of an adult male. Tarsi and metatarsi of the fourth pair of legs adult (d) male and (e) female (reproduced from Arthur, 1962).

Sub-class: Acari

Order: Parasitiformes

Sub-order: Ixodida (Metastigmata)

Family: Ixodidae

Hosts: Zebra, also infests livestock and game animals

Life cycle: Adults and immatures generally infest the same host; however, immatures also feed on small mammals

Geographical distribution: Africa: east of the Rift Valley from southern Ethiopia to Somalia and north-eastern Tanzania.

Pathogenesis: This tick is a vector of *Babesia equi*, *Theileria* spp, *Trypanosoma theileri*, *Rickettsia conorii*, several bunyaviridae (Crimean–Congo hemorrhagic fever virus, Nairobi sheep disease, kajiado, kismayo and dugbe viruses) and Barur virus.

Epidemiology: Found in savanna habitats with grass, bushes and scattered trees between 300 and 1300 m altitude where the annual rainfall is 250–600 mm. It feeds primarily during wet seasons.

Rhipicephalus simeus

Predilection site: Ears and on the lower abdomen

Parasite class: Arachnida

Sub-class: Acari

Order: Parasitiformes

Sub-order: Ixodida (Metastigmata)

Family: Ixodidae

Hosts: Dogs, wild carnivores, livestock, game animals and humans. Immature stages feed on the common burrowing savannah rodents.

Geographic distribution: Central and southern Africa

Pathogenesis: It is believed to act as a vector of *Anaplasma marginale*, *A. centrale*, *Rickettsia conorii* and *Coxiella burnetii*. It can also cause tick paralysis in humans.

Notes: In eastern and northern Africa *R. simeus* is replaced by *R. praetextatus*, which ranges from central Tanzania to Egypt and which is a vector of Thogoto virus. West of the Nile, these species are replaced by *R. senegalensis* and *R. muhsamae*.

MITES

Most mites are relatively host specific and are discussed in their relevant host chapter.

TROMBICULIDAE

Species of the family Trombiculidae are commonly known as chiggers, red bugs, harvest mites and scrub itch mites, and are unique, in that only the larval stage is ectoparasitic. In the adult and nymphal stages they are believed to be predators on the eggs and larvae of other arthropods. The principal species of veterinary interest are in the genus *Trombicula*.

They feed on blood, which they ingest by puncturing the skin.

Clinical signs: Infestation can result in pruritus, erythema, weals, papules and excoriation, leading to hair loss.

Diagnosis: Small clusters of orange larval mites may be seen on the skin surface. Microscopic examination may then be used to identify individual species.

Treatment: In most cases, the dermatitis should resolve a few days after the larvae have left the skin, however acarididal treatment may be necessary. Topical acaricides, such as organophosphates (e.g. phosmet, chlorpyriphos, malathion or diazinon), fipronil or lime–sulphur can be used, depending on the host infested.

Control: Environmental treatment with cyfluthrin, cyhalothrin, deltamethrin, carbaryl and deltamethrin may help to reduce mite abundance in areas such as back yards. However, area-wide control is usually impractical and unnecessary; problems should be managed by avoidance of sites of known mite prevalence.

Pathogenesis: Infestation causes pruritus, erythema and scratching, though there may be considerable individual variation in response. This variation may reflect the development of a hypersensitivity reaction to the mites, which may result in the development of weals, papules and excoriation leading to hair loss. In some cases, pruritus occasionally may continue long after the larvae have left, and heavy infestations may also induce systemic effects such as fever.

Neotrombicula autumnalis

Synonym: *Trombicula autumnalis*

Common name: Harvest mite

Predilection site: Harvest mites are commonly found in clusters on the foot and up the legs of dogs, on the genital area and eyelids of cats, on the face of cattle and horses and on the heads of birds, having been picked up from the grass.

Parasite class: Arachnida

Sub-class: Acari

Order: Acariformes

Sub-order: Trombidiformes (Prostigmata)

Family: Trombiculidae

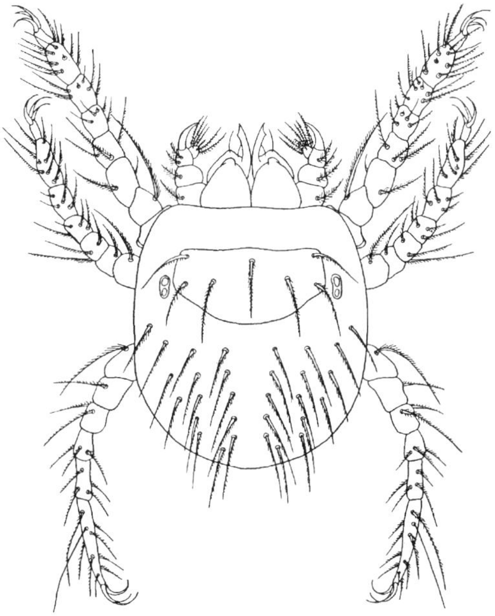

Fig. 11.18 Parasitic larval stage of the Harvest mite *Neotrombicula* (*Trombicula*) *autumnalis* (reproduced from Savory, 1935).

Description: The hexapod larvae are rounded, red to orange in colour and about 0.2 mm in length (Fig. 11.18). The scutum bears a pair of sensillae and five setae. In *N. autumnalis* the scutum is roughly pentangular and has numerous small punctuations. There are two simple eyes on each side of the scutum. The body is covered dorsally with 25–50 relatively long, ciliated, feather-like setae. The chelicerae are flanked by stout, five-segmented palps. The palpal femur and genu each bear a single seta. The palpal tibia has three setae and a thumb-like terminal claw, which opposes the palpal tarsus. The palpal claw is three-pronged (trifurcate). Adults and nymphs have a pronounced figure-of-eight shape. They have stigmata, which open at the base of the chelicerae and their bodies are covered with setae. Adults are about 1 mm in length.

Hosts: Dogs, cats, cattle, horses, rabbits and birds

Life cycle: They are parasitic only in the larval stage. Female adults lay their spherical eggs in damp but well drained soil. After about a week the hexapod larva hatches from the egg and begins to crawl about the soil, eventually climbing an object such as a grass stem. Here it awaits a passing host. Larvae of the species of veterinary interest are not highly host specific and may attach to a variety of domestic animals. The larva attaches itself by its blade-like chelicerae and feeds on the host's serous tissues for several days before falling from the host. After feeding, the larva enters a quiescent stage for a few days as a nymphochrysalis, before moulting to become the active octopod nymph. After a further inactive imagochrysalis nymphal stage, the adult emerges. The nymphal and adult stages are free-living, mobile and predatory. The life cycle typically requires 50–70 days. *Neotrombicula autumnalis* passes through only one generation per year and its abundance is usually strongly seasonal.

Geographical distribution: Europe

Epidemiology: In Europe the activity of *Neotrombicula autumnalis* is most pronounced in late summer and autumn, and larvae are most active on dry, sunny days. It will parasitise almost all domestic mammals, including humans and some ground-nesting birds. *N. autumnalis* may be particularly abundant in closely cropped chalk grassland, but it may also be found in wooded areas and scrub.

Eutrombicula alfreddugesi

Synonym: *Trombicula alfreddugesi*

Common name: Chigger mite

Predilection site: Commonly face, muzzle, thigh and belly

Parasite class: Arachnida

Sub-class: Acari

Order: Acariformes

Sub-crder: Trombidiformes (Prostigmata)

Family: Trombiculidae

Description: The larvae of *E. alfreddugesi*, known as chiggers, are similar in appearance to those of *N. autumnalis*. They are reddish orange and vary in length between 0.15 mm when not engorged to 0.6 mm when fully fed. However, for the larvae of *E. alfreddugesi* the palpal claws are two-pronged (bifurcate), the scutum is approximately rectangular and 22 dorsal setae are present.

Hosts: Dogs, cats, cattle, horses, rabbits, birds

Life cycle: The life cycle is similar to that described for *N. autumnalis*. Adult chiggers are free living while the immature stages are parasitic. Infestation is most common around the face, muzzle, thigh and belly. The resulting pruritus may persist for several days and is generally a hypersensitivity reaction to the mite saliva, occurring after the individual has detached.

Geographical distribution: *Eutrombicula alfreddugesi* is the most important and widespread of the trombiculid mites of veterinary interest in the New World. It is common from eastern Canada through to South America.

Epidemiology: *Eurombicula alfreddugesi* is particularly common at the margins of woodland, scrub and grassland, but is not highly habitat specific. In the northern parts of its range it may be most active between July and September, whereas in more southern habitats it may be active all year round. *E. alfreddugesi* parasitises a wide range of mammals and birds.

Eutrombicula splendens

Synonym: *Trombicula splendens*

Common name: Chigger mite

Predilection site: Commonly on the face, feet or legs

Parasite class: Arachnida

Sub-class: Acari

Order: Acariformes

Sub-order: Trombidiformes (Prostigmata)

Family: Trombiculidae

Description: *Eurombicula splendens* is morphologically similar and frequently sympatric with *E. alfreddugesi* in North America.

Geographical distribution: North America; generally confined to the east, from Ontario in Canada to the Gulf States, although it may also be abundant in Florida and parts of Georgia.

Epidemiology: This species generally occurs in moister habitats than *E. alfreddugesi*, such as swamps and bogs.

Eutrombicula sarcina

Synonym: *Trombicula sarcina*

Common name: Scrub itch mite, black soil itch mite

Predilection site: Commonly on the face, feet or legs

Parasite class: Arachnida

Sub-class: Acari

Order: Acariformes

Sub-order: Trombidiformes (Prostigmata)

Family: Trombiculidae

Description: The parasitic larvae are small (0.2 mm long), round mites with numerous setae.

Geographical distribution: Australasia

Epidemiology: The scrub itch mite *Eutrombicula sarcina* is an important parasite of sheep in Queensland and New South Wales of Australia. Its principal host, however, is the grey kangaroo. These mites prefer areas of savannah and grassland scrub.

They may be particularly abundant from November to February, after summer rain. The primary site of infestation is on the leg, resulting in intense irritation.

INSECTS

FLEAS: SIPHONAPTERA

The fleas are small, wingless, obligate, blood-feeding insects. Over 95% of flea species are ectoparasites of mammals, while the others are ectoparasites of birds. The order is relatively small with about 2500 described species, almost all of which are morphologically extremely similar.

Pathogenesis: The wounds created at the feeding site are usually seen as erythematous papules or wheals, surrounding the central puncture site. The wounds may develop a crust of dried exudate. The wheals may persist for several weeks. Pruritis may be intense, resulting in secondary traumatic lesions.

Clinical signs: Host animals scratch and bite at the affected area and the bite may produce a small, raised wheal on the skin.

Diagnosis: When the signs are indicative of flea infestation, but no parasites can be found, the host should be sprayed with an insecticide, placed on a large sheet of plastic or paper, and vigorously combed or groomed. The combings and debris should be examined for fleas or flea faeces, which show as dark brown–black crescentic particles. Consisting almost entirely of blood, these will produce a spreading reddish stain when placed on moist tissue.

Another technique is the use of a vacuum cleaner with fine gauze inserted behind the nozzle; the latter is applied to the host or its habitat and the fleas are retained on the gauze.

Treatment: In flea-bite allergy, where there is much distress, corticosteroids may be used topically or systemically as palliative treatment.

For specific treatment, insecticides are available, mainly in the form of powders, sprays, shampoos or spot-on preparations. These are generally organophosphorus compounds, pyrethrum and its derivatives, or carbamates. There are also oral and in-feed formulations of drugs for use against fleas in dogs and one of these is a benzoylurea derivative, lufenuron, which, when ingested by fleas during feeding, is transferred to the eggs and blocks the formation of chitin thereby inhibiting the development of flea larvae. Fipronil, one of a new generation of ectoparasiticides given by either spray or spot-on, has been licensed for use against fleas and ticks in dogs and cats and gives protection for 2–3 months. Imidacloprid is also a relatively new systemic neurotoxic insecticide, chemically related to the tobacco toxin, nicotine. It is highly effective at killing adult fleas for up to 1 month after application. Of importance is that fleas are not required to bite the animal to receive a lethal dose, which can be absorbed through the cuticle.

Since in-contact animals may also harbour fleas without developing allergy these should also be treated.

Control: For optimal control, the adults already infesting the host animal should be killed immediately and reinfestation from the environment prevented. A wide range of products is available. Many of the new chemicals with excellent long-acting flea adulticidal activity also have contact ovicidal and/or larvicidal activity. In addition, combination with insect growth regulators (chitin synthesis inhibitors, juvenile hormone analogues) applied directly to the animal, not only increases ovicidal and/or larvicidal activity but also delivers it effectively to the sleeping areas most likely to be infested without unnecessarily contaminating the environment. Insect growth regulators do not kill adult fleas and are not suitable by themselves for flea control, unless used in a completely closed environment. For flea infestations of domestic animals, frequent vacuuming can help to reduce environmental infestation and pet bedding should be washed at high temperatures.

Ctenocephalides felis

Subspecies: *felis*

Subspecies: *strongylus*

Subspecies: *damarensi*

Subspecies: *orientalis*

Common name: Cat flea

Predilection site: Skin

Parasite class: Insecta

Parasite order: Siphonaptera

Family: Pulicidae

Description: Cat fleas are dark brown–black, wingless insects, with laterally compressed bodies, which have a glossy surface. Females typically measure 2.5 mm in length; males are smaller, sometimes less than 1 mm in length. Eyes, are simply dark, photosensitive spots, and the antennae, which are short and club-like, are recessed into the head. In the female *C. f. felis* the head is twice as long as high and pointed anteriorly. In the male *C. f. felis* the head is as long as wide but is also slightly elongate anteriorly (Fig. 11.19). The third pair of legs is much longer than the others and, coupled to elaborate internal musculature, provide an adaptation for jumping to locate their host. The head bears at its posterior (pronotal) or ventral (genal)

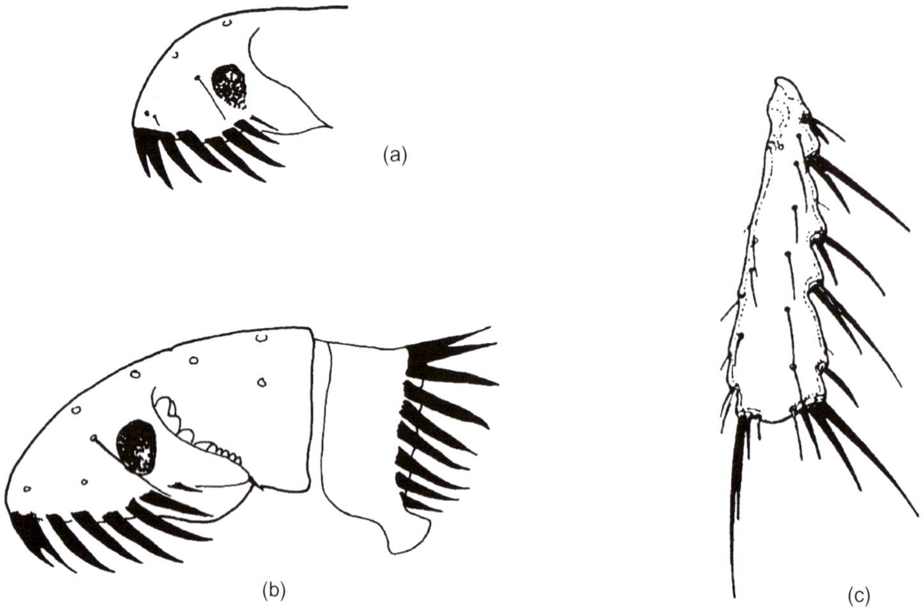

Fig. 11.19 The cat flea, *Ctenocephalides felis felis.* (a) Front of male head. (b) Female head and pronotum. (c) Hind tibia.

borders rows of dark spines called ctenidia or 'combs', and these are the most important features used in identification (Fig. 11.19). The genal ctenidium consists of 7–8 spines and the pronotal ctenidium about 16 spines. The teeth of the genal ctenidium are all about the same length. On the dorsal border of the hind (metathoracic) tibia in both sexes of *C. f. felis* there are only six notches bearing setae (Fig. 11.19). Between the postmedian and apical long setae there is a short, subapical spine.

Hosts: Cat, dog, human

Life cycle: Both sexes are blood feeders, and only the adults are parasitic. Once on its host *C. f. felis* tends to become a permanent resident. Within 24–48 hours of the first blood meal females begin to oviposit. The pearly white ovoid eggs (Fig. 11.20), which measure 0.5 mm in length, have smooth surfaces, and may be laid on the ground or on the host, from which they soon drop off. In the laboratory, an adult female *C. f. felis* can produce an average of about 30 eggs per day and a maximum of 50 eggs per day, over a life of about 50–100 days. However, on a cat, the average lifespan is probably substantially lower than this, possibly less than 1 week. The rate of oviposition is highest at times of day when cats normally rest, in the early morning and late afternoon. As a result, flea eggs are concentrated at host resting sites rather than over the large areas they roam. The eggs cannot withstand major climatic variations, particularly in temperature and humidity. Only those eggs that fall into an appropriate environment will ultimately develop into adults. At 70% relative humidity and 35°C, 50% of eggs hatch within 1.5 days. At 70% relative humidity and 15°C it takes 6 days for 50% of eggs to hatch. Eggs cannot survive below 50% relative humidity.

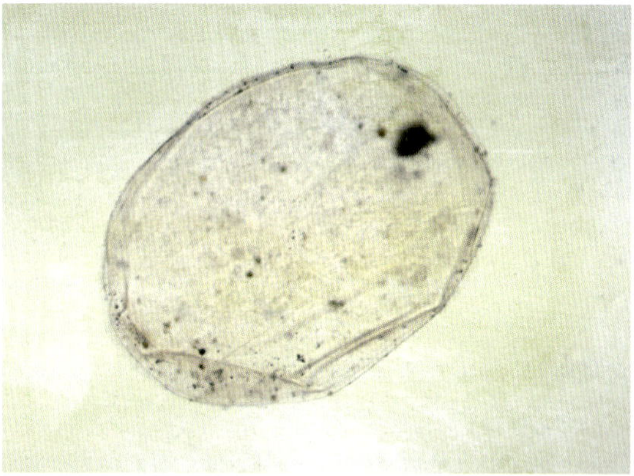

Fig. 11.20 Flea egg.

Hatching occurs in 2 days to 2 weeks, depending on the temperature of the surroundings. The creamy yellow larvae are elongate, slender and maggot-like (Fig. 11.21); each segment carries a ring of bristles. The last abominal segment bears two hooked processes

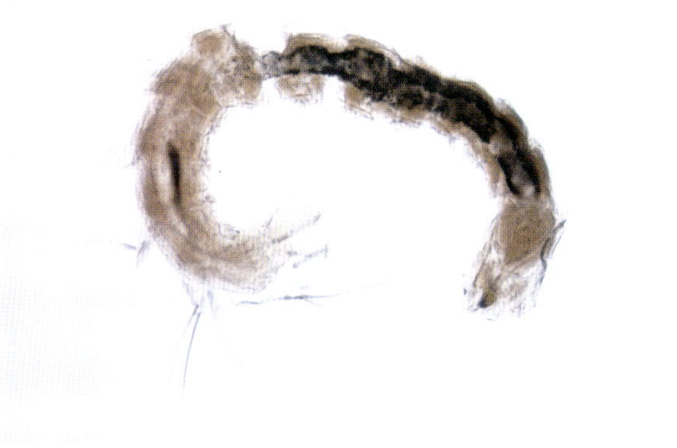

Fig. 11.21 Flea larva.

called anal struts, which are used for gripping in locomotion. They have chewing mouthparts and feed on debris and on the faeces of the adult fleas, which contain blood and give the larvae a reddish colour.

Within the host's bedding, den or lair the larvae of *C. f. felis* exist in a protected environment, with relatively high humidity, buffered from the extreme fluctuations of ambient temperatures and provided with detritus and a source of adult flea faecal blood. The larvae have limited powers of movement (probably less than 20 cm before pupation) and crawl about their environment largely at random, but they are negatively phototactic and positively geotactic. In the domestic environment this behaviour often takes them to the base of carpets where they can encounter food and are sheltered from light and mechanical damage. The larva moults twice, the final stage being about 5.0 mm long. At 24°C and 75% relative humidity, the duration of the three larval stages is about 1 week, but in unfavourable conditions, larvae may develop more slowly. At 13°C and 75% relative humidity larval development takes about 5 weeks, though the larval cycle can take up to 200 days. Larvae will only survive at temperatures between 13°C and 35°C. The larvae are extremely susceptible to desiccation and mortality is high below 50% relative humidity.

When fully developed, the mature third-stage larva empties its gut and spins a thin, silk cocoon. This process requires a vertical surface against which they can align themselves. Fragments of detritus adhere to the cocoon giving it some degree of camouflage. The larva pupates within the cocoon. At 24°C and 78% relative humidity the duration of the pupal stage is about 8–9 days. If the pupal stage is disturbed the larvae will either spin another cocoon or develop into naked pupae showing that the cocoon is not essential for development into an adult. When fully developed, adults emerge from the pupal cuticle but may remain within the cocoon. Adults may remain in this state for up to 140 days at 11°C and 75% relative humidity. At cooler temperatures, fully formed fleas may remain in their cocoons for up to 12 months.

The areas within a building with the necessary humidity for egg and larval development are limited. Sites outdoors are even less common and flea larvae cannot develop in arid areas exposed to the hot sun. If found outside they typically inhabit the top few millimetres of soil.

Emergence of the adult from the cocoon is triggered by stimuli such as mechanical pressure, vibrations or heat. Adult emergence may be extremely rapid, when provided with appropriate conditions. The ability to remain within the cocoon for extended periods is essential for a species such as *C. f. felis* since its mobile hosts may only return to the lair or bedding at infrequent intervals. The fully formed adults begin to feed almost as soon as they are on their host, though they can survive for several days without feeding, provided the relative humidity is above about 60%. Within 36 hours of adult emergence most females will have mated. Females will mate with several males and egg laying begins 24–48 hours after the first blood meal.

Within 10 minutes of feeding adults begin to produce faeces. Partially digested host blood forms a large component of the flea faeces. The faeces quickly dries into reddish black faecal pellets, known as 'flea dirt'.

It is important to recognise that most of the flea's life cycle is spent away from the host. This includes not only the eggs, larvae and cocoon, but also, if necessary, the adult flea.

Geographical distribution: Worldwide. However, there are four distinct subspecies of *C. felis*: *C. felis felis* is widespread, *C. f. strongylus* occurs in Africa, *C. f. damarensis* in southwestern Africa and *C. f. orientalis* in India, Sri Lanka and southeast Asia.

Pathogenesis: The response to a flea bite is a raised, slightly inflamed wheal on the skin, associated with mild pruritus, but though the animal will scratch intermittently there is little distress. However, after repeated flea bites over a period of several months a proportion of dogs and cats develop flea-bite allergy, which is often associated with profound clinical signs (Fig. 11.22).

Since each female *C. f. felis* can ingest as much as 13.6 μl of blood per day, severe infestations may lead to iron-deficiency anaemia. Anaemia caused by *C. f. felis* is particularly prevalent in young animals and has been reported in cats and dogs and, very rarely, goats, cattle and sheep.

Flea-bite allergy is a hypersensitive reaction to components of the flea saliva released into the skin during feeding. The allergy shows a seasonality in temperate areas, appearing in summer when flea activity is highest, though in centrally heated homes exposure may be continuous. In warmer regions, such as the western states of the USA, the problem occurs

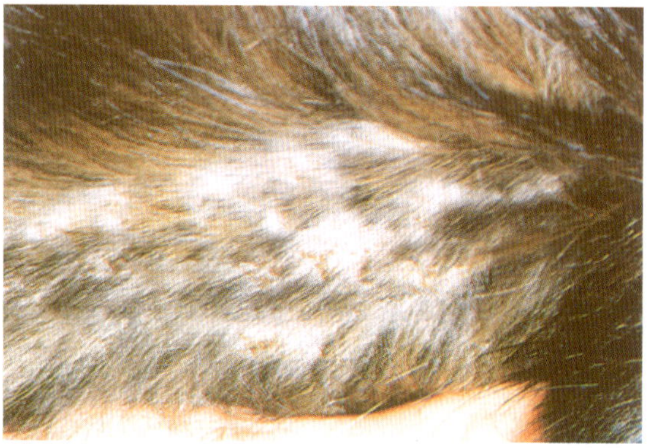

Fig. 11.22 The lesions of flea bite allergy in a cat.

throughout the year. As would be expected, the most commonly affected areas in both dogs and cats are the preferential biting sites of the fleas, which are the back, the ventral abdomen and the inner thighs. In the dog the primary lesions are discrete crusted papules which cause intense pruritus. The most important damage, however, is subsequently inflicted by the animals themselves, in scratching and biting the affected areas, to produce areas of alopecia or of moist dermatitis ('wet eczema'). In older dogs, which have been exposed for many years, the skin may become thickened, folded and hairless, and in these animals the pruritus is much less intense. In the cat, flea-bite allergy produces the condition commonly known as miliary dermatitis or eczema, readily detectable on palpation, in which the skin is covered with innumerable small, brown, crusty papules which cause marked pruritus. In cats, there are two distinct clinical manifestations associated with flea allergy: milary dermatitis and feline symmetrical alopecia.

Flea-allergy dermatitis is one of the most common causes of dermatological disease of dogs and cats. Dermatitis associated with allergy to flea bites is characterised by intense pruritus and reddening of the skin, with itching persisting up to 5 days after the bite. The resultant licking, chewing and scratching can lead to hair loss, self-induced trauma and secondary infection. Other symptoms include restlessness, irritability and weight loss, though the intensity of irritation varies greatly with the individual attacked.

All dogs can become allergic to fleas, though atopic dogs are predisposed to developing reactivity. One bite may be sufficient to cause an allergic reaction. Intermittent flea exposure encourages development of a flea allergy, while continual exposure appears to protect against it, as does contact with fleas at an early age. Though little is known about the allergens responsible for evoking the allergic response, recent findings suggest that multiple proteins are important in flea-bite hypersensitivity. In studies which have attempted to determine how flea antigens react with canine IgG or IgE, at least 15 different flea components have been found to bind IgE. No pattern of reactivity or differences in antibody structure have been observed which distinguish dogs with flea allergy from dogs without, suggesting that there is little association between particular antibody responses and allergic reactivity of dogs to fleas. Both immediate and delayed hypersensitivity can be observed, and individuals will vary in the strength and proportion of each type of sensitivity they express. Dogs chronically infested with *C. f. felis* rarely develop a state of natural tolerance resulting in loss of clinical signs.

Cats kept in a flea infested environment groom at twice the rate of cats in a flea-free environment. In normal grooming a cat may ingest almost 50% of its resident flea population within a few days and cats fitted with Elizabethan collars, which prevent grooming, harbour much greater populations of fleas than cats free to groom. The removal of fleas during grooming reduces the chance of finding them during a skin and coat examination. This is a particular diagnostic problem in cats with a low flea burden but marked flea-bite hypersensitivity. In such cases, since many of the groomed fleas are ingested, examination of the mouth may reveal fleas caught in the spines of the cat's tongue.

Fleas are vectors of a range of viruses and bacteria, and pathogen transmission is enhanced by their promiscuous feeding habits. Most species of flea are host-preferential rather than host-specific and will try to feed on any available animal. For example, *C. felis* has been found on over 50 different host species. Other factors which contribute to the potential of *C. felis* as a vector include transovarial transmission of some pathogens (*Rickettsia* species) and the transmission of pathogens such as *Bartonella henselae* through adult flea faeces.

Fleas act as intermediate hosts for the common tapeworm of dogs and cats, *Dipylidium caninum*. Though the adult flea can acquire the filarioid infection by intake of microfilariae in a blood meal, the specialised mouthparts do not allow the ingestion of the eggs of *Dipylidium*, and this infection can only be acquired by the flea larva. Tapeworm eggs, along with general organic debris, are ingested by flea larvae. The tapeworm eggs hatch in the midgut of the flea larva and the worm larvae penetrate the gut wall, passing into the haemocoel. The tapeworm larvae develop within the flea body cavity throughout larval, pupal and adult flea development, eventually encapsulating as an infective cysticercoid. After ingestion of the adult flea by the host, cysticercoids are

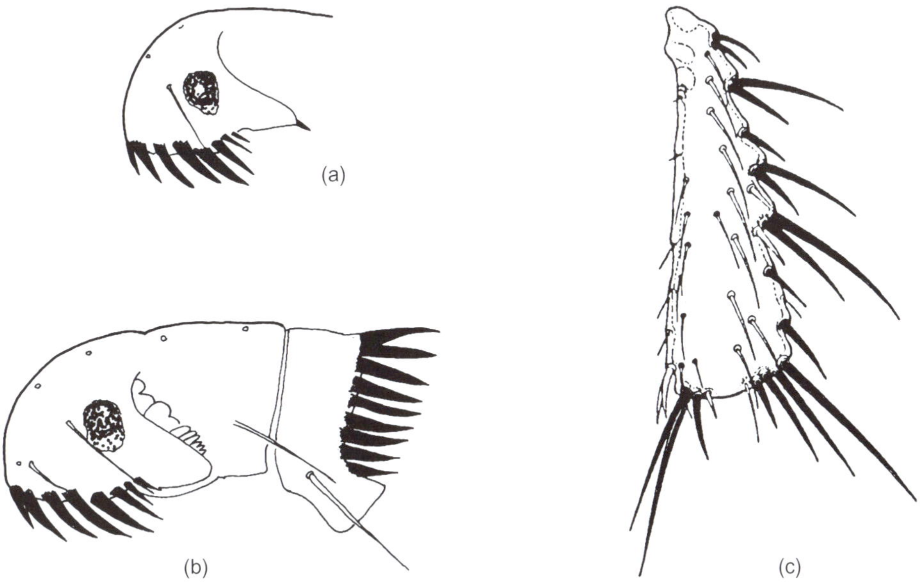

Fig. 11.23 The dog flea, *Ctenocephalides canis*. (a) Front of male head. (b) Female head and pronotum. (c) Hind tibia.

liberated and develop into tapeworms in the digestive tract.

Ctenocephalides felis felis also acts as an intermediate host of the non-pathogenic, subcutaneous filaroid nematode of dogs *Dipetalonema reconditum*, which adults may ingest during blood-feeding.

Epidemiology: The cat flea, *C. f. felis*, is the most common species of flea found on domestic cats and dogs throughout North America and northern Europe. Significantly more cats are infested with fleas than dogs, however, perhaps because of their tendency to roam, increasing their contact with other cats. Fleas may be found on pets throughout the year but, in the northern hemisphere, numbers tend to increase around late spring and early autumn when ambient conditions are favourable for larval development. Since *C. felis* are able to survive for long periods off the host they therefore do not require direct contact for transmission.

Ctenocephalides canis

Common name: Dog flea

Predilection site: Skin

Parasite class: Insecta

Parasite order: Siphonaptera

Family: Pulicidae

Description: The dog flea, *C. canis*, is closely related and is morphologically very similar to the cat flea, *C. f. felis*, although they cannot interbreed and, therefore, are truly distinct species. The head of the female dog flea is more rounded on its upper and anterior surface than that of the cat flea and less than twice as long as high (Fig. 11.23). Like *C. f. felis*, the dog flea has both genal and pronotal ctenidia (Fig. 11.24). The genal ctenidium consists of seven to eight spines and the pronotal ctenidium about 16 spines (Fig. 11.23). However, in both female and male *C. canis* the first spine of the genal ctenidium is shorter than the rest. On the dorsal border of the hind (metathoracic) tibia in both sexes of *C. canis* there are eight notches bearing stout setae (Fig. 11.23).

Hosts: Dogs, cats, rats, rabbits, foxes and humans have all been recorded as hosts of *C. canis*.

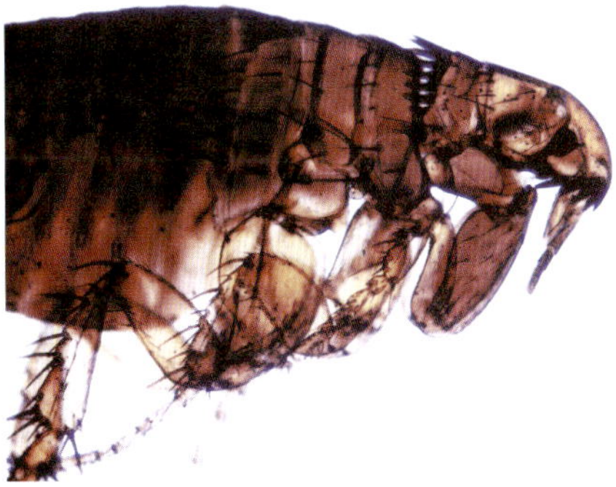

Fig. 11.24 Adult *Ctenocephalides canis*.

Life cycle: The life cycle of *C. canis* (egg, veriform larva, pupa and adult) is very similar to that of *C. f. felis*. Egg production commences 2 days after the male and female arrive on the dog. Eggs and larvae do not survive at temperatures of over 35°C, preferring a temperature range between 13 and 32°C and relative humidity between 50 and 90%. In these conditions even unfed adults can survive for many weeks. Pupae may remain dormant for a year or more, yet are able to hatch in 30 seconds when cues, such as vibration, indicate the presence of a suitable host. In an appropriate environment the total life cycle may take as little as 3 weeks.

Geographical distribution: Worldwide

Pathogenesis: Similar to that of *C. f. felis*.

Epidemiology: The behavioural differences between dog and cat fleas seem largely to involve the range of environmental conditions which their larvae are capable of tolerating. While household dogs in northern Europe and North America are more likely to be infested by the cat flea, working dogs in kennels and dogs in rural areas or at higher altitudes are more likely to be infested by *C. canis*.

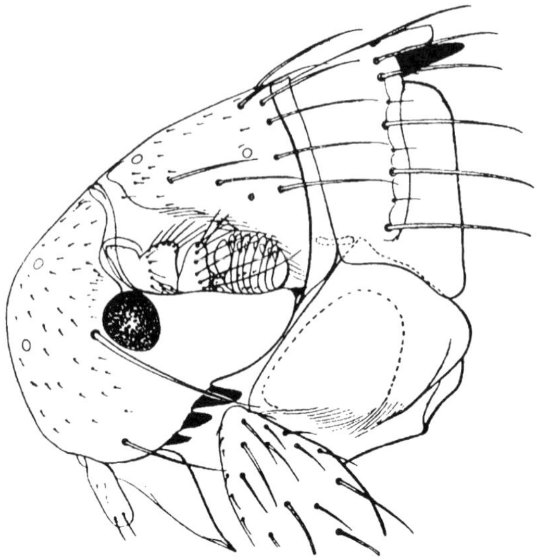

Fig. 11.25 The hedgehog flea, *Archaeopsylla erinacei*, female head (after Smart, 1943).

Archaeopsylla erinacei

Common name: Hedgehog flea

Predilection site: Skin

Parasite class: Insecta

Parasite order: Siphonaptera

Family: Pulicidae

Description: Adults are easily recognised, being 2–3.5 mm long with a genal comb of one to three short spines and a pronotal comb of one short spine (Fig. 11.25).

Hosts: Hedgehogs, dogs and cats

Life cycle: The life cycle is typical: egg, three larval stages, pupa and adult. Before the female can begin ovipositing she needs to feed on the host several times. Once on its host, *A. erinacei* tends to become a permanent resident.

Geographical distribution: Europe and North America

Epidemiology: *Archaeopsylla erinacei* occurs on hedgehogs and may be transferred to dogs and cats following contact.

Pulex irritans

Common name: Human flea

Predilection site: Skin

Parasite class: Insecta

Parasite order: Siphonaptera

Family: Pulicidae

Description: *Pulex irritans* has neither genal nor pronotal ctenidia (Fig. 11.26). The outer margin of the head is smoothly rounded and there is a pair of eyes. This species can be distinguished from *X. cheopis* by the presence of the single ocular bristle below the eye and the absence of a row of bristles along the rear margin of the head. The metacoxae have a patch of short spines on the inner side. The maxillary laciniae extend about halfway down the forecoxae, which distinguishes this species from the closely related *Pulex simulans* found in Hawaii (where the laciniae extend for at least three quarters the length of the forecoxae).

Hosts: Humans and pigs; may also occur on dogs, cats, rats and badgers

Life cycle: The life cycle is typical: egg, three larval stages, pupa and adult. It is thought that originally the principal hosts of this species were pigs. Each adult female *P. irritans* lays around 400 eggs.

Geographical distribution: Worldwide, but it is now uncommon in the USA and most of northern Europe.

Pathogenesis: The bites of *Pulex* can cause dermatitis and it may on occasion act as a vector of the plague pathogen of *Yersinia pestis*.

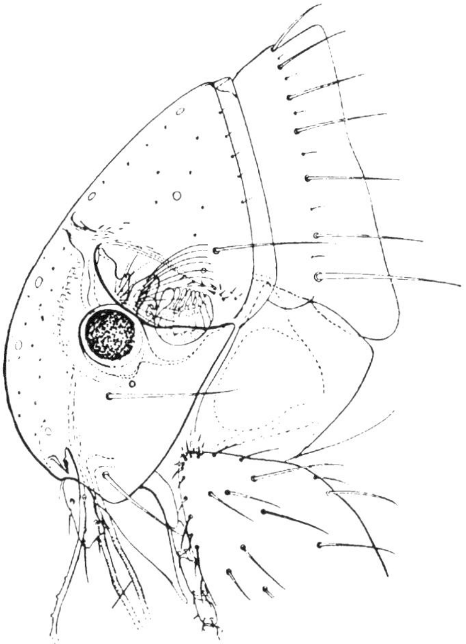

Fig. 11.26 The human flea, *Pulex irritans*, male head and pronotum (after Smart, 1943).

Epidemiology: Although described as the human flea, *P. irritans* can infest cats, dogs, and many other domestic animals, although it is probably most common on pigs. It breeds profusely in pigsties and is usually the most important species in farm areas. People working with infested pigs can also easily become infested and start infestations in their homes.

Spilopsyllus cuniculi

Common name: Rabbit flea, European rabbit flea

Predilection site: Ears

Parasite class: Insecta

Parasite order: Siphonaptera

Family: Pulicidae

Hosts: Rabbit, hare, dog, cat

Description: The rabbit flea, *S. cuniculi*, has both pronotal and genal ctenidia, the latter being composed of four to six oblique spines (Fig. 11.27). Adults are dark brown. Females are, on average, 1 mm in length; males are slightly smaller. Eyes are present and the frons at the front of the head is rounded with the frontal tubercle conspicuous. There are two stout spines beneath the eye.

Hosts: Rabbit, hare, dog, cat

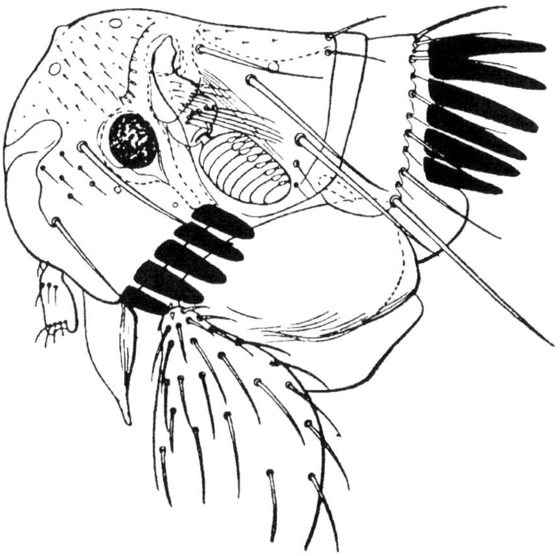

Fig. 11.27 Head and pronotum of the rabbit flea, *Spilopsyllus cuniculi*.

Life cycle: The rabbit flea, *S. cuniculi*, occurs largely on the ears. It is more sedentary than most other species of flea and remains for long periods with its mouthparts embedded in the host. These become increasingly active and mobile after feeding on a pregnant doe. Adults transfer to newborn young and lay eggs. The larvae feed on organic matter in the nest debris and mature 15–45 days later when they infest the host littermates before they disperse from the burrow. Populations of *S. cuniculi* may increase dramatically during the rabbit-breeding season.

Goegraphical distribution: Worldwide

Pathogenesis: When rabbits are not breeding, the distribution *of S. cuniculi* is related to skin temperature, with fleas usually congregating on the ears. Because they assemble here in large numbers, the intensity of bites may cause considerable irritation and tissue damage. Rabbit fleas may also be found on cats and dogs, which hunt or frequent rabbit habitats. On these hosts they are commonly found on the face and attached to the pinneal margin. *Spilopsyllus cuniculi* is the main vector of myxomatosis and it also transmits the non-pathogenic *Trypanosoma nabiasi*.

Echidnophaga gallinacea

Common name: Sticktight flea

Predilection site: Skin

Parasite class: Insecta

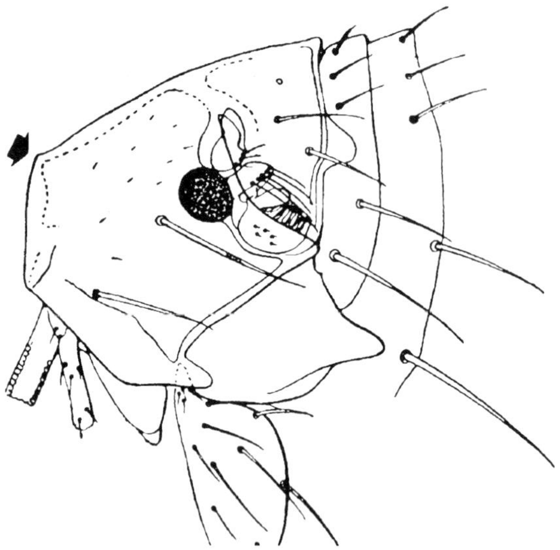

Fig. 11.28 The sticktight flea, *Echidnophaga gallinacea*, female head and thorax (arrow marking angulation of the frons) (after Smart, 1943).

Parasite order: Siphonaptera

Family: Pulicidae

Description: The sticktight flea, *E. gallinacea*, is a burrowing flea important mainly in domestic poultry. The adult sticktight flea is small: females are commonly about 2 mm in length and the males are less than 1 mm in length. The head is sharply angled at the front (frons). There are no genal or pronotal ctenidia (Fig. 11.28). On the head behind the antenna there are two setae and, in the female, usually a well developed occipital lobe. The thoracic segments are narrowed dorsally. Spiracles are present on the second and third abdominal segments. The mouthparts appear large, extending the length of the forecoxae, and project from the head conspicuously. The maxillary laciniae are broad and coarsely serrated. On the anteroventral surface of each hind coxa, there are three rows of minute spiniform bristles.

Hosts: Poultry, but may also attack cats, dogs, rabbits and humans

Life cycle: After host location, females aggregate on bare areas, often the head, comb or wattles. Newly emerged adults are active and move towards sunlight, which helps them accumulate on the wattles of cocks or hens. After feeding, females burrow into the skin where they attach firmly with their mouthparts. Each female may remain attached for between 2 and 6 weeks. Copulation then takes place. The skin around the point of attachment may become ulcerated. The female begins oviposition an average of 6–10 days after attachment, at a rate of about 1–4 eggs per day. Eggs are laid in the ulceration or dropped to the ground. If laid in the ulceration, larvae hatch, emerge from the skin and drop to the ground to complete their development. The incubation period may last from 4–14 days, though typically it takes 6–8 days. Eggs fail to survive temperatures of 43°C and above. The larvae feed on chicken manure and develop through three larval stages over a period of 14–31 days. The pupal period generally requires around 9–19 days and the entire life cycle may be completed in 30–60 days. Adults generally locate a new host and attach within about 5–8 days after emergence.

Geographical distribution: These fleas are most common in tropical areas throughout the world, but may also be found in many subtropical and temperate habitats.

Pathogenesis: The burrowing of adults and subsequent emergence of larvae through the skin tissue can result in areas of ulceration, leading to secondary bacterial infection. Sticktight fleas can occur at densities of over 100 individuals per bird, all concentrated on the head. As a result, infestation of poultry may reduce growth and egg production. Severe infestation can lead to anaemia. Ocular ulceration, caused by self-trauma, may result in blindness and starvation. The skin over the nodules often becomes ulcerated, and young birds may be killed by heavy infections.

Sticktight fleas may become abundant in poultry yards and adjacent buildings. They are potentially able to transmit the plague and murine typhus but, since the females spend most of their lives attached to a single host, they are not considered to be significant vectors of disease.

Clinical signs: Signs include restlessness and sratching of affected areas. The bites may be visible on the skin. Allergic dermatitis may be seen, but should be differentiated from other similar conditions such as sarcoptic mange.

Diagnosis: Diagnosis is not easy as adults may leave the host and eggs and larvae are difficult to find. Poultry sometimes have clusters of these fleas around the eyes, comb, wattles and other bare spots. These dark brown fleas have their heads embedded in the host's flesh and cannot be brushed off. Typically, on dogs and cats, the sticktight fleas will be found around the margin of the outer ear or occasionally between the toe pads.

Epidemiology: These fleas are not host specific and may attack any available mammal or bird for a blood meal. As they are able to survive off the host, transmission can occur from the bedding and housing. Primarily important as a parasite of birds, the adult sticktight flea is an especially serious pest of chickens.

However, it may also be found on humans, rats, cats, dogs, horses and larger insectivores. Infestations on dogs may be persistent if they are continually exposed to a source of infestation, and fleas are found on the poorly haired areas of the ventrum, scrotum, interdigital and periorbital skin and around the pinnae of the ears.

Treatment: Sticktight fleas can be removed with tweezers by grasping and pulling firmly. An antibiotic ointment should be applied to the area to prevent infection. If fleas are too numerous to remove individually, a flea product registered for on-animal use should be applied according to label instructions. Several organophosphorus, carbamate and pyrethrin-based insecticides are effective when applied as a solution.

Control: Should sticktight fleas become established in a poultry house, drastic measures may have to be adopted to get rid of them. All litter should be removed and burnt and the poultry house sprayed with an insecticide.

Ceratophyllus gallinae

Common name: European chicken flea

Predilection site: Skin

Parasite class: Insecta

Parasite order: Siphonaptera

Family: Ceratophyllidae

Description: Adults of *Ceratophyllus gallinae* are typically 2–2.5 mm long with no antennal fossae. Eyes are present. There is a pronotal comb, carrying more than 24 teeth, while the genal comb is absent (Fig. 11.29). There is a lateral row of four to six bristles on the inner surface of the hind femur and there are no spines on the basal section of the legs.

Hosts: Poultry, wild birds, dog, cat, humans

Life cycle: The life cycle is typical: egg, three larval stages, pupa and adult. Unlike most other fleas, which often remain on the host and feed for long periods, chicken fleas spend most of their time in the nest of the host, and only move on to the birds to feed for short periods.

The larvae feed on detritus amongst the nest material, chicken droppings and on undigested blood from the adult faeces. The larval stages are completed in a few weeks, before the pupal cocoon is spun. The flea overwinters in the cocoon and emerges in an old nest in spring as temperatures rise. Large numbers may occur in the nests of passerine birds and they may complete their life cycle during the period of nest occupation by these birds. Work has shown a negative correlation between flea abundance and mean body mass of the brood being parasitised.

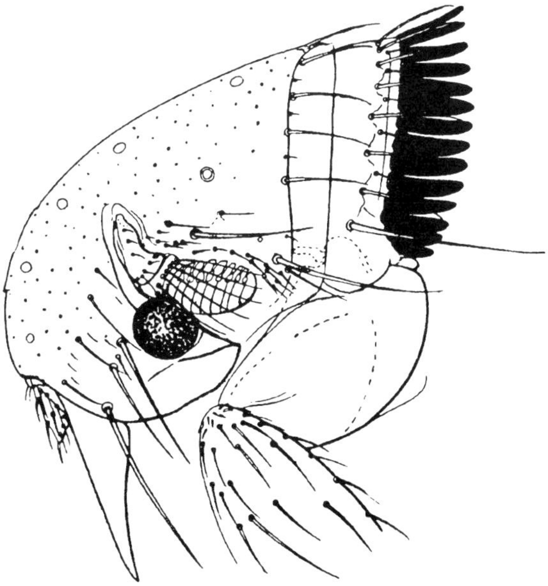

Fig. 11.29 Head and pronotum of a female chicken flea, *Ceratophyllus* (after Smart, 1943).

If the nest is reused by birds the following year, the newly emerged adults will attach to the new hosts and continue the cycle. If the nest is not reused, the newly emerged adults will make their way to the nest entrance, where they may be able attach to a bird that is examining the old nest as a potential nest site. Alternatively they may climb up trees and bushes; here they stop periodically and face the brightest source of light, jumping in response to a shadow passing in front of the light.

Geographical distribution: Found predominantly in the Old World but has been introduced into southeast Canada and northeast USA

Pathogenesis: *Ceratophyllus gallinae* is the commonest flea of domestic poultry. It is not however considered to be an important vector of disease. Feeding activity may cause irritation, restlessness and, with heavy infestations, anaemia.

Clinical signs: Symptoms include restlessness and scratching of affected areas. The bites may be visible on the skin. Allergic dermatitis may be seen, but should be differentiated from other similar conditions such as sarcoptic mange.

Diagnosis: Diagnosis is not easy as adults may leave the host and eggs and larvae are difficult to find.

Epidemiology: These fleas are not host specific and may attack any available mammal or bird for a blood meal. As they are able to survive off the host, transmission can occur from the bedding and housing. This flea is highly mobile on the host and can be especially common in host nesting material. It will feed readily on humans and domestic pets, and is often acquired in the handling of poultry and from injured wild birds brought into houses. It has also been known to migrate into rooms from nests under adjacent eaves. When such nests are removed they should be incinerated; otherwise the hungry fleas may parasitise domestic pets and humans. In wild birds, flea reproduction and feeding activity is synchronised with the breeding season of the birds; in domestic chickens, flea activity may continue all year round.

Notes: The European chicken flea, *Ceratophyllus gallinae*, is a very common flea of poultry and also infests more than 75 species of wild bird and some mammals. In Europe, the vast majority of its hosts are hole-nesting tits, particularly great tits and blue tits. This species originated in Europe and has spread with poultry operations round the world. It is difficult to eradicate, as it is able to feed on many different species and is highly adaptable.

Tunga penetrans

Common name: Chigger, jigger, chigoe, bicho do pé or sand flea

Predilection site: Skin

Parasite class: Insecta

Parasite order: Siphonaptera

Family: Pulicidae

Description: *Tunga penetrans* has no ctenidia and no spiniform bristles on the metathoracic coxae. The head is angular and has an acute frontal angle. The thorax is short and reddish brown. The female is about 1 mm long before a blood meal but may increase to a length of up to 7 mm when gravid. The male flea is smaller, about 0.5 mm long, and never embeds in the host.

Hosts: Humans and pigs. In addition, reservoir hosts include cattle, sheep, horses, mules, rats, mice, dogs, and other wild animals.

Life cycle: The fertilised female slashes the skin of the host with her mouthparts, then burrows into the wound, inserting her head and body until only the last two abdominal segments are exposed. Host skin proliferates and covers the flea, all bar the last abdominal segments. A free-living mobile adult male mates with the embedded female. The male possesses one of the longest intromittent organs relative to body size in the animal kingdom and mates from an inverted position. The female remains attached, feeding on host fluids and greatly expanding the size of the abdomen. The female often expands 80-fold to reach the size of a pea after 8–10 days. The embedded female produces a nodular swelling leaving only a small opening to the outside through which up to 200 eggs are passed and drop to the ground. The eggs hatch in 3 or 4 days, and the fleas moult through two larval stages. The entire life cycle requires about 17 days.

Geographical distribution: Parts of Africa, Asia and North and South America. The sand flea, jigger or chigoe, is an important parasite of humans in the Neotropical and Afrotropical regions.

Pathogenesis: Once *T. penetrans* becomes engorged with blood, its presence causes great pain, and may produce inflammation and localised ulcers. Tetanus and gangrene may result from secondary infections. Intense local irritation and pruritus are also symptomatic of more minor infestations.

Tunga penetrans may also pose significant problems in dogs, particularly in the interdigital spaces, under the pads and the scrotum, but infestation tends to be highly localised. The presence of a number of adult *T. penetrans* in the paws can be crippling.

The damage to the skin can facilitate the entry of other pathogens leading to secondary infection and ulceration.

Clinical signs: The presence of the female flea can cause extreme itching, pain, and inflammation, and secondary infections may occur. This flea occurs mainly on the feet of humans, causing severe irritation. In pigs the main sites of attachment are the feet and scrotum, but these animals tolerate the infection with no signs of distress.

Diagnosis: The swelling produced by the female is easily visible and often surrounded by eggs. The nodule (usually on the foot in humans) slowly enlarges over a few weeks in a patient who has recently been in an endemic area. The nodule can range from 4–10 mm in diameter. Sometimes, a serosanguinous exudate oozes from the central opening.

Epidemiology: The main habitat is warm, dry soil and sand of beaches, stables and stock farms. On contact, the fleas invade unprotected skin. The most common site of involvement is the feet (interdigital skin and subungual area). The flea has limited jumping ability.

Treatment: Reported topical treatments in humans include cryotherapy or electrodesiccation of the nodules. Application of formaldehyde, chloroform, or dichlorodiphenyltrichloroethane (DDT) to the infested skin has been used. Occlusive petrolatum suffocates the organism. These treatments do not remove the flea from the skin, and they do not result in quick relief from painful lesions. The flea may also be gently removed with a needle or a forceps. Surgical removal of the fleas is the recommended treatment. A number of surgical treatment methods are available. The flea can be removed from its cavity with sterile instruments, but this is more difficult when the flea is engorged. The orifice needs to be enlarged, and the entire nodule should be excised. An antibiotic ointment may be applied, along with systemic antibiotic therapy when indicated. Aggressive treatment of secondary infection, and tetanus prophylaxis are important. In dogs, foot-bathing with 0.2% trichlorphon or metriphonate has been shown to be effective, as has subcutaneous injection of ivermectin (0.2 mg/kg body weight).

Control: Tungiasis can be controlled by treating infested areas with pesticides (malathion and methoprene have been used sucesfully) and treating infected reservoir hosts.

BUGS: HEMIPTERA

Triatoma, Rhodnius

Common name: Assassin bugs, kissing bugs, conenoses

Predilection site: Skin

Parasite class: Insecta

Order: Hemiptera

Family: Reduviidae

Sub-family: Triatomatinae

Description, adult: The adults range in length from 10–40 mm; the majority of species are around 20–30 mm in length. They are usually dark brown to black in colour, with contrasting patterns of red, orange or yellow marks around the edge of the abdomen. The body is flattened and elongated. The forewings have a hardened basal section and a distal membranous section and overlie the entirely membranous hind wings. The antennae are elbowed with four segments. They also have a piercing proboscis that is three-segmented, tapered and slender and bent back under the body when not in use.

Description, nymphs: Nymphs are smaller than adults, lack mature genitalia or wings, but also blood-feed.

Hosts: Dog, cat, cattle, sheep, goat, man and wild mammals

Life cycle: All species are nocturnal, obligate blood-feeding bugs. Gravid females start to lay eggs about 2 weeks after mating. They then lay one or two eggs daily, each female producing about 200 eggs in total. Each egg is about 2 mm in length. Eggs hatch about 2 weeks after oviposition, although this is temperature dependent. There are five nymphal stages, all of which blood-feed. The entire egg to adult life cycle may take 2–3 months, but more usually 1–2 years.

Feeding is initiated by chemical and physical cues. Carbon dioxide causes increased activity and heat will stimulate probing. When probing is initiated, the rostrum is swung forward and the mandibular stylets are used to cut through the skin and then anchor the mouthparts. The maxillary stylets probe for a blood vessel and saliva, containing an anticoagulant, passes down the salivary canal while blood is pumped up the food canal. Feeding may take between 3 and 30 minutes. After engorging, the rostrum is removed from the host and the bug defecates after which it crawls away to find shelter.

Geographical distribution: Over 100 species are found in South and Central America, southern and the Midwest USA, predominantly in the tropical regions. However five species of *Linshcosteus* are found in India and seven species of *Triatoma* are found in southeast Asia and one in Africa.

Pathogenesis: Triatomines are important vectors of the protozoan *Trypanosoma cruzi*. This causes Chagas' disease in humans and a disease of similar pathology in dogs. Although cats are susceptible to infection there are no reports of clinical disease. As it feeds, the bug defecates and the parasite is transmitted in the faeces which is rubbed into the feeding-wound or into the eyes or the mouth. Infection may also be transmitted by the ingestion of infected bugs or infected prey.

Clinical signs: The bite causes irritation and swelling. Heavy infestations in poultry houses may result in chronic blood loss and mortality in young birds.

Diagnosis: Bugs may be found in cracks and crevices in the housing, or rarely may be seen on the host.

Pathology: The lesions produced at the feeding site may vary considerably between individual hosts. The wounds created are usually seen as erythematous papules or wheals, surrounding the central puncture site. The wheals may persist for several weeks. Pruritis may be intense, resulting in secondary traumatic lesions.

Epidemiology: Some species of tratomine bug, including *Triatoma infestans*, live in and near human dwellings and poultry houses where they hide in cracks and crevices in the structure. During the night, they emerge to search for warm-blooded hosts. The interval between feeding and defecation is critical in determining the effectiveness of disease transmission. Infected dogs provide a reservoir of infection for the vector and thus human infection.

Treatment: Dogs may be treated with pour-on formulations of pyrethroid insecticide to repel or kill host-seeking bugs.

Control: Long-term control of bugs in the domestic environment or animal house can be achieved by spraying dwellings with formulations of pyrethroid insecticide. This is often enough to eliminate existing populations of the bugs within a house, although reintroductions are possible.

Notes: Important species include *Triatoma infestans* and *Rhodnius prolixus*

DIPTERA

The Diptera is one of the largest orders in the class Insecta, with over 120 000 described species. All these species have a complex life cycle with complete metamorphosis. Hence, the larvae are completely different in structure and behaviour to the adults. As a result, dipterous flies can be ectoparasites as larvae or adults, but they are rarely parasites in both life cycle stages.

LARVAL PARASITES: MYIASIS

Myiasis is the infestation of the organs or tissues of host animals by the larval stages of dipterous flies, usually known as maggots or grubs. The fly larvae feed directly on the host's necrotic or living tissue. The hosts are usually mammals, occasionally birds and, less commonly, amphibians or reptiles. All the flies that act as economically important agents of veterinary myiasis are members of the superfamily Oestroidea. Within this superfamily there are three major families of myiasis-producing flies: Oestridae, Calliphoridae and Sarcophagidae. Oestridae are highly species specific and are dealt with in their respective host chapters. Calliphoridae and Sarcophagidae are generalists and so are dealt with here.

Description: The body of the larval myiasis species is usually clearly segmented, pointed anteriorly and truncated posteriorly (Fig. 1.29). However, this shape may be modified, with the larvae of some species being barrel-like or, occasionally, flattened. The cuticle is typically pale and soft but is often covered by spines or scales arranged in circular bands. Although legless, in some species, the body may have a number of fleshy protuberances, which aid in locomotion. The true head is completely invaginated into the thorax. The functional mouth is at the inner end of the pre-oral cavity, from which a pair of darkened mouth-hooks protrudes. The mouth-hooks are part of a complex structure, known as the cephalopharyngeal skeleton, to which muscles are attached. There is a pair of anterior spiracles on the prothoracic segment, immediately behind the head and a pair of posterior spiracles on the 12th segment. The structure of the posterior spiracles is of great taxonomic importance. They usually consist of a pair of sclerotised spiracular plates with slits or pores in the surface for gaseous exchange.

Life cycle: A small number of species are obligate agents of myiasis – that is, they require a living host for larval development. Adult females deposit approximately 200 eggs at a time on the host and the larvae hatch after 12–24 hours, moult once after 12–18 hours and a second time about 30 hours later. They feed for 3–4 days and then move to the soil to pupate for 7 days to several weeks depending on temperature. However, the vast majority of species are facultative agents of myiasis. In the latter case adult flies oviposit primarily in carrion, but also may act as secondary invaders of myiases on live mammals. The life cycle is identical to the obligate species, with three larval stages and the final larval stage migrating from the feeding site prior to pupation.

Clinical signs: Animals infested with fly larvae may appear dull and lethargic, and separate from the herd. They may cease feeding and show weight loss. Wounds with foul-smelling odour will be observed on inspection.

Diagnosis: Myiasis is diagnosed by the removal of the larvae and identification under a dissecting microscope. The larva possess a pair of oral hooks at the anterior extremity, spiracles on the anterior segment and, posteriorly, spiracular plates. The arrangement of the mouthparts and posterior spiracles serve to differentiate the species. However, identification of the larvae of most species is extremely difficult and, where possible, samples of live larvae should be retained until adult emergence to confirm the identification, which is more easily accomplished with the adult fly. The detailed description and identification of the larvae of most species is beyond the scope of this text and specimens should be referred to a relevant taxonomic specialist.

Pathology: The direct pathological effects of myiasis may vary considerably and depend on the species of ectoparasite, the number of larvae and the site of the infestation. In many cases infestation by small numbers of fly larvae may have little or no discernible clinical effect on the host. However, a heavier burden of parasites may produce effects including irritation, discomfort and pruritus, resulting in reduced feeding, weight loss, reduced fertility and loss of general condition. Ultimately, heavy infestation may lead rapidly to host death from direct tissue damage, haemorrhage, bacterial infection, dehydration, anaphylaxis and toxaemia. Myiasis from a range of species also has been shown to produce a marked immunological response in the host.

Treatment: For subdermal warble-forming larvae surgical removal of larvae may be required. Applying heavy oil or petrolatum jelly to the opening of the lesions will occlude the airway of the larvae and may cause them to exit the host. Applying a small amount of chloroform or ether to the opening may be helpful before removing the larva with forceps. Lidocaine hydrochloride can also be injected into the furuncular lesion to facilitate extraction of the larva. Antibiotics should be prescribed. Great care should be taken during the extraction process to avoid rupturing the larva in situ.

For cutaneous myiases, the larvae should also be removed and identified, and the wound should be thoroughly cleaned and disinfected. Topical organophosphate and pyrethroid insecticides are effective against newly hatched larvae, immature forms and adult flies. Larvae inside wounds must be treated with a suitable larvicide. Spraying or dipping animals with an approved insecticide and treating infested wounds can protect against new infestations for 7–10 days. Systemic insect growth regulators, cyromazine and dicyclanil, may give highly effective long-lasting prophylactic protection against cutaneous myiasis. The macrocyclic lacotones, ivermectin, eprinomectin, moxidectin and doramectin, may also be effective against cutaneous myiasis and are particularly effective against nasopharyngeal, subdermal and gastrointestinal myiases.

Control: Any wounds should be properly dressed to prevent infection. In areas where fly abundance is seasonal, operations such as branding, dehorning and ear marking should be avoided during the fly season. Given the high rates of reproduction, high rates of dispersal and multiple generations per year, area-wide control of most dipterous agents of myiasis is impractical. There are however, notable exceptions, which will be highlighted subsequently in this chapter.

Cochliomyia hominivorax

Synonym: *Callitroga hominivorax*

Common name: Screwworm

Predilection site: Skin

Parasite class: Insecta

Family: Calliphoridae

Description, adult: The adult fly has a deep greenish blue metallic colour with a yellow, orange or reddish face and three dark stripes on the dorsal surface of its thorax.

Description, larvae: Mature larvae measure 15 mm in length and have bands of spines around the body segments. The tracheal trunks leading from the posterior spiracles have a dark pigmentation extending forwards as far as the ninth or tenth segment (Fig. 11.30). This pigmentation is most conspicuous in fresh specimens.

Hosts: Commonly cattle, pigs and horses but may parasitise any mammals, including humans.

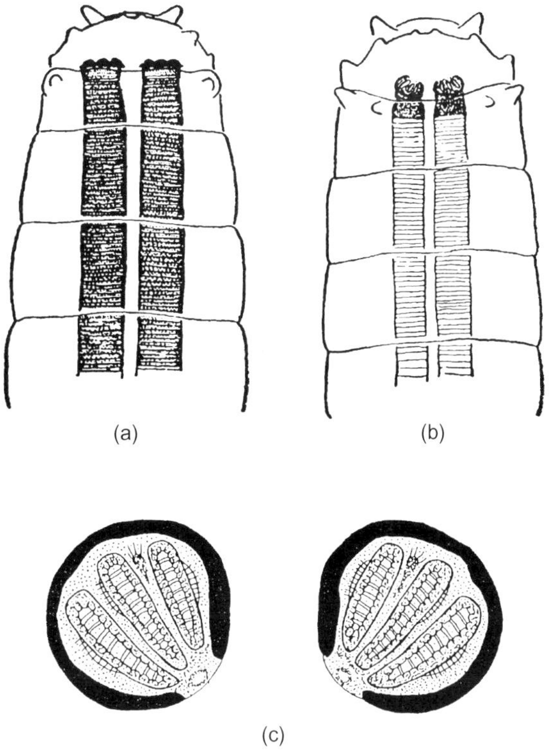

Fig. 11.30 (a) Pigmented dorsal tracheal trunks of *Cochliomyia hominivorax*. (b) Dorsal tracheal trunks. (c) Posterior spiracles of *Cochliomyia macellaria* (reproduced from Zumpt, 1965).

Life cycle: *Cochliomyia hominivorax* is an obligate parasite and cannot complete its life cycle on carrion. Female flies oviposit at the edge of wounds or in body orifices, in clusters of 150–300 eggs. Shearing, castration or dehorning wounds are common oviposition sites, as are the navels of newly born calves. Even wounds the size of a tick bite are reported to be sufficient to attract oviposition. The flies lay batches of this size every 2–3 days during adult life, which is on average 7–10 days in length. The larvae hatch in 10–12 hours and penetrate into the tissues, which they liquefy, and extend the lesion considerably. The wound may begin to emit a foul-smelling liquid attracting other female *C. hominivorax* and secondary agents of myiasis. The larvae become mature in 5–7 days, after which they leave the host to pupate in the ground. The pupal period lasts for between 3 days and several weeks, depending on temperature. There is no true diapause stage and *C. hominivorax* cannot survive over winter in cool temperate habitats. The entire life cycle may be completed in 24 days in optimum conditions.

Geographical distribution: *Cochliomyia hominivorax* occur primarily in tropical areas of southern and central America and the Caribbean islands. Its range formerly extended north into Mexico and the southern states of North America, from where it has now been eradicated.

Pathology and pathogenesis: In cattle, infestation initially causes intermittent irritation and pyrexia, followed by the production of a cavernous lesion. The tissue shows progressive liquefaction, necrosis and haemorrhage, before the larvae leave the wound. If untreated, repeated infestation by *C. hominivorax* and secondary fly species may quickly lead to the death of the host within 1–2 weeks.

Clinical signs: It may be difficult to see screwworm maggots at the wound surface because only the posterior spiracles are exposed. Larvae of other blowflies such as *Lucilia* do not feed in a vertical position or burrow deep into the wound, but instead feed more superficially.

Diagnosis: Screwworm larvae have distinct dorsal tracheal pigmentation that extends from the 12th somatic segment to the 10th or 9th segment.

Epidemiology: Adult females have been reported to fly up to 200 miles. The infestation can also be spread by the transport of animals and people from infested areas.

Control: As a result of the economic cost of this pest, large-scale screwworm fly control was initiated in the southeastern states of the USA in 1957–59. This was achieved by the release of large numbers of male *C. hominivorax*, which had been sterilised by radiation. Sterilised males mate with wild females, which are in turn rendered infertile. Subsequent control operations spread the area of sterile male release and by 1980 effective control of *C. hominivorax* in the USA was achieved. Despite a number of sporadic, but significant, outbreaks, effective control has been maintained. The eradication programme has subsequently been successfully directed against the fly in Mexico, Puerto Rico and as far as Panama.

Notes: In 1988, *C. hominivorax* were discovered in an area 10 km south of Tripoli in Libya. This was the first known established population of this species outside the Americas. The fly quickly spread to infest about 25 000 km^2. In 1989 there were about 150 cases of myiasis by *C. hominivorax* but by 1990, a total of 12 068 confirmed cases of screwworm fly myiasis were recorded and, at its peak, almost 3000 cases were seen in the single month of September 1990. It was estimated that if unchecked the infestation could cost the Libyan livestock industry about US$30 million per year and the north African region approximately US$280 million per year. This led to the implementation of a major international control programme, which successfully eradicated the fly from this area, again using the release of sterile males.

Cochliomyia macellaria

Synonym: *Callitroga macellaria*

Common name: Secondary screwworm

Predilection site: Skin

Parasite class: Insecta

Family: Calliphoridae

Description, adult: These blue–green flies have longitudinal stripes on the thorax and orange–brown eyes. Adults are extremely similar in appearance to *C. hominivorax*, but possess a number of white spots on the last segment of the abdomen.

Description, larvae: The larvae may be distinguished from those of *C. hominivorax* by the absence of pigmented tracheal trunks leading from small posterior spiracles (Fig. 11.30).

Hosts: Commonly cattle, pigs and horses but may parasitise a range of mammals including humans.

Life cycle: *Cochliomyia macellaria* is a ubiquitous carrion breeder. However, it can act as a secondary invader of myiasis, and is known as the secondary screwworm fly.

Geographical distribution: Neotropical and Nearctic, from Canada to Argentina, but it is more abundant in tropical parts of its range

Pathogenesis: Mechanical transmission of disease attributed to this species includes botulism in birds, 12 different Salmonella types including *Salmonella typhimurium*, poliomyelitis and swine influenza.

Epidemiology: *Cochliomyia macellaria* is often attracted to the wounds initiated by *C. hominivorax*. The two species are commonly found together.

Chrysomya bezziana

Common name: Old World screwworm

Predilection site: Skin wounds

Parasite class: Insecta

Family: Calliphoridae

Description, adult: These stout, blue–green flies have four longitudinal black stripes on the prescutum, orange–brown eyes and a pale coloured face. The flies have dark legs and white thoracic squamae. The anterior spiracle is dark orange or black–brown. The adult flies measure 8–10 mm in length.

Description, larvae: The first-stage larvae are creamy white and measure about 1.5 mm in length. The second- and third-stage larvae are 4–9 mm and 18 mm

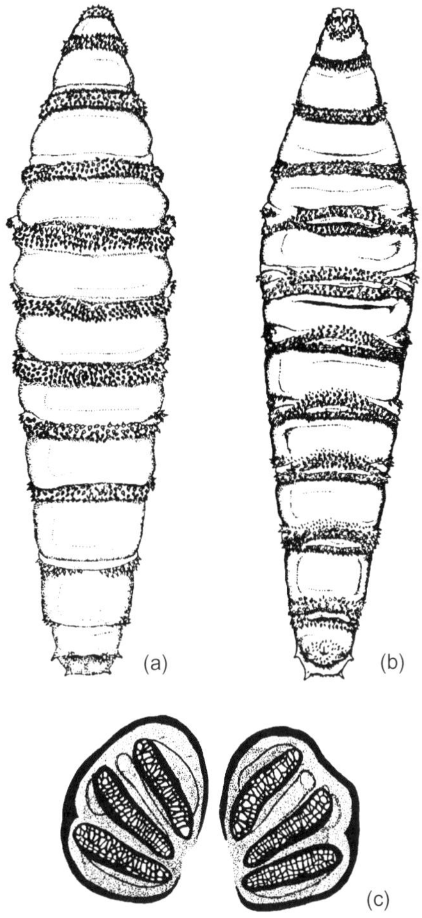

Fig. 11.31 Third stage larva of *Chrysomya bezziana*. (a) Dorsal, (b) ventral view, (c) posterior peritremes (reproduced from Zumpt, 1965).

in length respectively, and are similar in appearance; each segment carrying a broad, encircling belt of strongly developed spines (Fig. 11.31).

Hosts: Mammals including cattle, sheep, dogs and occasionally humans

Life cycle: *Chrysomya bezziana* is an obligate agent of myiasis. Gravid females are attracted to fresh open wounds and body orifices on any warm-blooded animal. Even small wounds resulting from thorn scratches and tick bites may be sufficient to attract oviposition. *C. bezziana* commonly infest the umbilicus of newborn calves. The female lays batches of 100–300 eggs on the dry perimeter around the wound. Each female produces several batches of eggs in her lifetime of about 9 days. The eggs hatch within 10–20 hours at 37°C and first-stage larvae begin to feed in the open wound or moist tissue, often penetrating deep into the host tissue.

Generally eggs are laid in the late afternoon, ensuring that their development is complete by the next morning, avoiding lethal exposure to direct sunlight and drying. The larvae mature in 4–12 days, after which they drop to the ground to pupate. Pupation lasts for approximately 7 days in optimum environmental conditions (28°C), but can take more than a month under cooler conditions. Adult *C. bezziana* may feed on honeydew, nectar and animal excrement in addition to decomposing corpses. The entire life cycle takes 2–3 weeks.

Geographical distribution: This species occurs primarily in tropical areas: Africa and southern Asia including India, the Arabian peninsula, southeast Asia, the Indonesian and Philippine islands and New Guinea.

Pathogenesis: Infestation by *Chrysomya bezziana* causes intermittent irritation and pyrexia, followed by the production of a cavernous lesion. Infested wounds often have a serosanguineous discharge and sometimes a distinctive foul-smelling odour. Sometimes, there may be large pockets of larvae with only small openings in the skin. The tissue shows progressive liquefaction, necrosis and haemorrhage, before the larvae leave the wound. Animals may die from secondary infection or toxicity in 1–2 weeks if the infestation is not treated.

Clinical signs: In the first day or two, screwworm infestations are difficult to detect. Often, all that can be seen is slight motion inside the wound. As the larvae feed, the wound gradually enlarges and deepens. Animals infested with screwworms may appear dull, lethargic and separate from the herd. They may cease feeding and show weight loss. Wounds with foul-smelling odour will be observed on inspection; however, it may be difficult to see the maggots at the wound surface because only the posterior spiracles are exposed. Larvae of other blowflies such as *Lucilia* do not feed in a vertical position or burrow deep into the wound, but instead feed more superficially. Screwworms may be particularly difficult to find inside the nasal, anal and vaginal openings.

Diagnosis: The larvae can be found packed deep inside the wound. Screwworms are diagnosed by the removal of the larvae and identification with a dissecting microscope.

Epidemiology: In temperate regions, screwworm attacks are restricted to the warm seasons, although may occur during mild winters. In the tropics they are continuous. Female screwworms are attracted to all warm-blooded animals. The distance a fly will travel can range from 10–20 km in tropical environments.

Notes: The precise status of *Chrysomya bezziana* as a clinical and economic pest is uncertain, particularly in sub-Saharan Africa, and few studies have been able to obtain quantitative estimates of myiasis incidence, its clinical or economic importance. The absence of livestock throughout much of its range in sub-Saharan Africa, due to the presence of trypanosomiasis and its vector the tsetse fly, may substantially limit its economic impact. However, *C. bezziana* has been inadvertently introduced into several countries in the Middle East, and such an introduction is believed to pose a major economic threat to the pastoral industry of Australia.

Chrysomya megacephala

Common name: Oriental latrine fly

Predilection site: Skin

Parasite class: Insecta

Family: Calliphoridae

Description, adults: Adults are medium-sized, stout, blue–green flies with longitudinal stripes on the thorax and orange–brown eyes (Fig. 11.32). *Chrysomya megacephala* can be distinguished from *Lucilia* by the broad bands on its rounder abdomen and by its black forelegs. The face is pale coloured. The anterior spiracle of the thorax of adults is dark coloured.

Description, larvae: The larvae are about 18 mm in length. They have hooked mouthparts and bands of small spines on each segment. There are four to six projections on the anterior spiracle with fleshy projections on the last segment only.

Hosts: A range of warm-blooded animals may be infested.

Life cycle: Flies oviposit primarily in carrion but also may act as secondary invaders of myiases on live mammals. Females lay batches of up to 250–300 eggs on carcases, faeces and other decomposing matter. The entire egg-to-adult life cycle takes about 8 days at 30°C. *Chrysomya megacephala* is commonly called the Oriental latrine fly because of its habit of breeding in faeces as well on carrion and other decomposing organic matter. It may occur in large numbers around latrines and may also become a nuisance in slaughterhouses, confined animal facilities and open-air meat and fish markets.

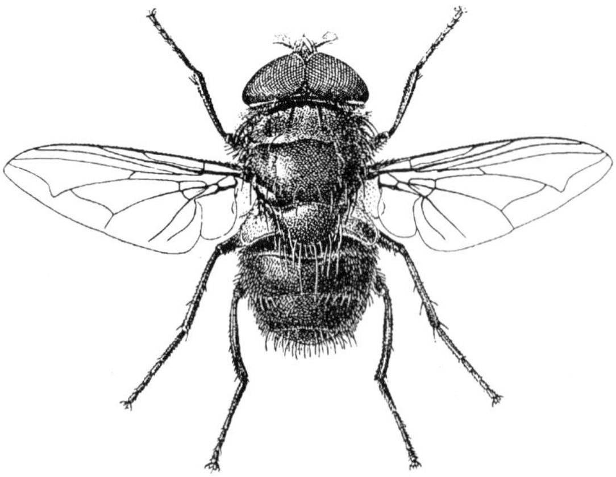

Fig. 11.32 Adult male of *Chrysomya megacephala* (reproduced from Shtakelbergh, 1956).

Geographical distribution: Worldwide. *Chrysomya megacephala* is a native of Australasian and Oriental regions. However this species has been introduced inadvertently into the New World and entered Brazil around 1975. Since then it has dispersed rapidly to reach Central and North America.

Chrysomya rufifacies

Common name: Hairy maggot blowfly

Predilection site: Skin wounds

Parasite class: Insecta

Family: Calliphoridae

Description, adult: These bluish green flies have longitudinal stripes on the thorax and orange–brown eyes. The hind margins of the abdominal segments have blackish bands and the anterior spiracle is white or pale yellow.

Description, larvae: The larvae bear a number of thorn-like, fleshy projections on most of the body segments, which give these species their common name of 'hairy maggot blowflies'. These projections become longer on the dorsal and lateral parts of the body. *C. rufifacies* larvae may be distinguished from *C. albiceps* by the presence of small spines on the stalks of the projections. Third-stage larvae are about 18 mm in length.

Hosts: A range of warm-blooded animals may be infested.

Life cycle: Flies oviposit primarily in carrion, but also may act as secondary invaders of myiases on live mammals. The larvae of this species will actively feed on other larvae in carcases.

Geographical distribution: *Chrysomya rufifacies* is an Australasian and Oriental species of tropical origin. This species and *C. albiceps* were inadvertently introduced in the Neotropical region in the 1970s and 1980s where, at a dispersal rate estimated at 1.8–3.2 km/day, they have quickly spread and become established throughout much of North and South America.

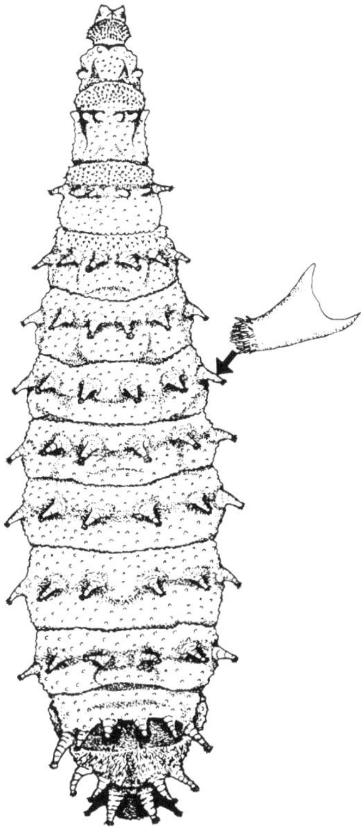

Fig. 11.33 Third-stage larva of *Chrysomya albiceps* (reproduced from Zumpt, 1965).

Chrysomya albiceps

Common name: Hairy maggot blowfly

Predilection site: Skin wounds

Parasite class: Insecta

Family: Calliphoridae

Description, adult: These bluish green flies have longitudinal stripes on the thorax and orange–brown eyes. The hind margins of the abdominal segments have blackish bands and the anterior spiracle is white or pale yellow.

Description, larvae: The larvae bear a number of thorn-like, fleshy projections on most of the body segments, which give these species their common name of 'hairy maggot blowflies' (Fig. 11.33). These projections become longer on the dorsal and lateral parts of the body. *C. albiceps* larvae may be distinguished from *C. rufifaces* by the absence of small spines on the stalks of the projections. Third-stage larvae are about 18 mm in length.

Hosts: A range of warm-blooded animals may be infested.

Life cycle: Flies oviposit primarily in carrion, but also may act as secondary invaders of myiases on live mammals. This species thrives in warm, humid conditions, at temperatures above 17°C but below 38°C.

Geographical distribution: *Chrysomya albiceps* is predominantly African and Mediterranean in its distribution. However, this species and *Chrysomya rufifaces* were inadvertently introduced in the Neotropical region in the 1970s and 1980s where, at a dispersal rate estimated at 1.8–3.2 km/day, they have quickly spread and become established throughout much of North and South America.

Calliphora vicina

Synonym: *Calliphora erythrocephala*

Common name: Bluebottle

Predilection site: Skin wounds

Parasite class: Insecta

Family: Calliphoridae

Description, adults: Bluebottles are stout and characterised by a metallic blue sheen on the body. The thoracic squamae have long dark hair on the upper surface. *Calliphora vicina* and *C. vomitoria* may be distinguished from each other by the presence of yellow–orange jowls with black hairs in the former and black jowls with predominantly reddish hairs in the latter.

Description, larvae: Smooth, segmented, and measure 10–14 mm in length. Posterior spiracles in a closed peritreme (Fig. 11.34).

Hosts: Predominantly colonisers of decaying carrion but may occasionally be found as a secondary invader of myiasis.

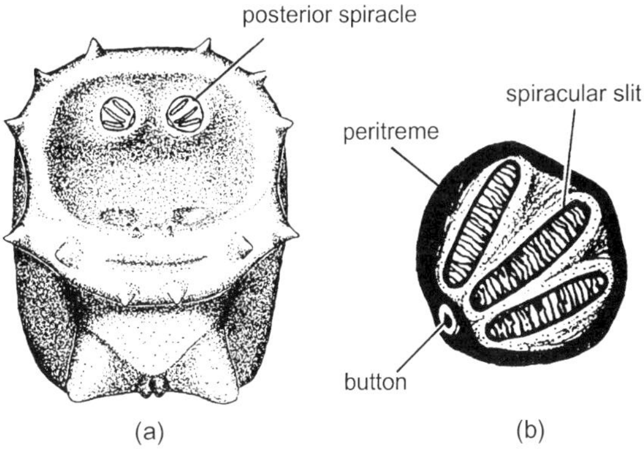

Fig. 11.34 (a) Posterior view of the last abdominal segment of *Calliphora vicina* and (b) detail of the posterior spiracles of a third-stage larva of *Calliphora vomitoria* (reproduced from Zumpt, 1965).

Life cycle: The gravid female blowfly is attracted by the odour of decomposing matter and lays clusters of yellow–cream eggs, usually on dead animals. Adults are commonly found around houses and livestock facilities, are attracted to faeces, and they will enter buildings.

Geographical distribution: Worldwide

Calliphora vomitoria

Common name: Bluebottle

Predilection site: Skin wounds

Parasite class: Insecta

Family: Calliphoridae

Description: See *Calliphora vicina*.

Hosts: Predominantly colonisers of decaying carrion but may occasionally be found as a secondary invader of myiasis.

Life cycle: The gravid female blowfly is attracted by the odour of decomposing matter and lays clusters of yellow–cream eggs, usually on dead animals. Adults are commonly found around houses and livestock facilities, are attracted to faeces, and they will enter buildings.

Geographical distribution: Worldwide

Calliphora augur

Common name: Lesser brown blowfly, blue-bodied blowfly

Predilection site: Skin wounds

Parasite class: Insecta

Family: Calliphoridae

Description, adults: The adult *Calliphora augur* is predominantly brown or brown–yellow in colour with a patch of metallic-coloured blue on the medial abdomen. The adult body is approximately 11 mm in length.

Description, larvae: The larvae are smooth, segmented and measure 10–14 mm in length.

Hosts: Mainly sheep, but any other animal may be affected.

Life cycle: Flies oviposit primarily in carrion, but also may act as secondary invaders of myiases on live mammals.

Geographical distribution: Australasia, mainly eastern Australia

Calliphora albifrontalis

Synonym: *Calliphora australis*

Common name: Western Australian brown blowfly

Predilection site: Skin wounds

Parasite class: Insecta

Family: Calliphoridae

Description, adult: In the adult *Calliphora albifrontalis* the thorax is non-metallic blue–black in colour but the abdomen is predominantly brown or brown–yellow.

Description, larvae: The larvae are smooth, segmented and measure 10–14 mm in length.

Hosts: Mainly sheep, but a range of other warm-blooded animals may also be infested.

Life cycle: Flies oviposit primarily in carrion but also may act as secondary invaders of myiases on live mammals.

Geographical distribution: Australasia

Calliphora nociva

Synonym: *Calliphora dubia*

Common name: Lesser brown blowfly

Predilection site: Skin wounds

Parasite class: Insecta

Family: Calliphoridae

Description, adults: The adult *Calliphora nociva* is predominantly brown or brown–yellow in colour and closely resembles *C. augur* except for the colour patch on the abdomen, which is a much brighter blue on *C. nociva* than on *C. augur*. *C. nociva* displaces *C. augur* in Western Australia.

Description, larvae: The larvae are smooth, segmented and measure 10–14 mm in length.

Hosts: Mainly sheep, but any other animal may be affected. It is important to note that only the larvae are responsible for myiasis.

Life cycle: Flies oviposit primarily in carrion, but also may act as secondary invaders of myiases on live mammals.

Geographical distribution: Australasia, mainly Western Australia

Calliphora stygia

Synonym: *Pollenia stygia*, *Calliphora laemica*

Common name: Eastern golden haired blowfly

Predilection site: Skin wounds

Parasite class: Insecta

Family: Calliphoridae

Description, adult: The adult *Calliphora stygia* is a large native Australasian blowfly with a grey thorax and yellow–brown mottled abdomen. It is one of the earliest flies to visit a corpse and will also feed on living sheep, causing fly strike.

Description, larvae: The larvae are smooth, segmented, and measure 10–14 mm in length.

Hosts: Mainly sheep, but any other animal may be affected. It is important to note that only the larvae are responsible for myiasis.

Life cycle: *Calliphora stygia* flies oviposit primarily in carrion, but also may act as secondary invaders of myiases on live mammals and may also sometimes be a primary initiator of myiasis.

Geographical distribution: Australasia

The appearance of adult flies of the genera *Calliphora*, *Lucilia*, *Phormia* and *Cochliomyia* is shown in Fig. 11.35.

Lucilia spp

Common name: Sheep blowflies

Synonym: *Phaenicia*

Predilection site: Skin

Parasite class: Insecta

Family: Calliphoridae

Geographical distribution: Worldwide

For detailed description see Chapter 3 (Sheep and goats).

Cordylobia anthropophaga

Common name: Tumbu fly

Predilection site: Skin

Parasite class: Insecta

Family: Calliphoridae

Description, adults: The adult is a stout, yellow–brown fly, 8–12 mm in length. It has a yellow face and legs and two black marks on the thorax. Adult flies feed on decaying fruits, carrion and faeces and have large, fully developed mouthparts. The arista of the antenna has setae on both sides. The thoracic squamae are without setae and the stem vein of the wing is without bristles.

Description, larvae: Third-stage larvae are 12–28 mm in length and are densely, but incompletely, covered with small, backwardly directed, single-toothed spines (Fig. 11.36). The posterior spiracles have three sinuous slits and a weakly sclerotised peritreme.

Hosts: Humans and other mammals. It is thought that the primary hosts of *C. anthropophaga* are rodents and that the flies have become secondarily adapted to parasitise many other animal species, including humans. The domestic dog is an important host.

Life cycle: The eggs are deposited singly in dry, sandy, shaded areas where animals lie, particularly areas contaminated with host urine or faeces. Females may also be attracted to dry, urine-soiled clothing. Eggs are laid in early morning or late evening. Up to 500 eggs are laid per female over their lifespan of 2–3 weeks. The eggs hatch after 2–4 days and the first-stage larvae wait in the dry substrate for a host. The larvae can remain alive, without feeding, for 9–15 days, hidden just beneath the soil surface. A sudden rise in temperature, vibration or carbon dioxide, which might signify the presence of a host, activates the larvae. They attach to the host and immediately burrow into the skin. Larvae develop beneath the skin and produce a swelling of approximately 10 mm in diameter at the point of entry. The swelling has a hole in the centre through which the larva breathes. The swellings may be found anywhere on the host animal's body but are most commonly found on ventral parts. The three larval stages are completed in the host and, when mature (7–15 days after infection), the larvae emerge out of this hole and pupate on the ground in surface debris. Adult flies emerge from the pupae after 3–4 weeks.

Geographical distribution: Sub-Saharan Africa

Pathogenesis: The larvae develop under the skin and produce a painful swelling, 10 mm in diameter, with a small central opening. The swelling is initially pruritic, becoming more painful as the larva grows. Serous fluid may exude from the lesion.

Cordylobia rodhaini

Common name: Tumbu fly, Lund's fly

Predilection site: Skin

Parasite class: Insecta

Family: Calliphoridae

Description, adult: This species closely resembles *C. anthropophaga* but is larger, measuring 12.5 mm in length. The adult is a stout, yellow–brown fly with a yellow face and legs and two black marks on the thorax. Adult flies feed on decaying fruits, carrion and

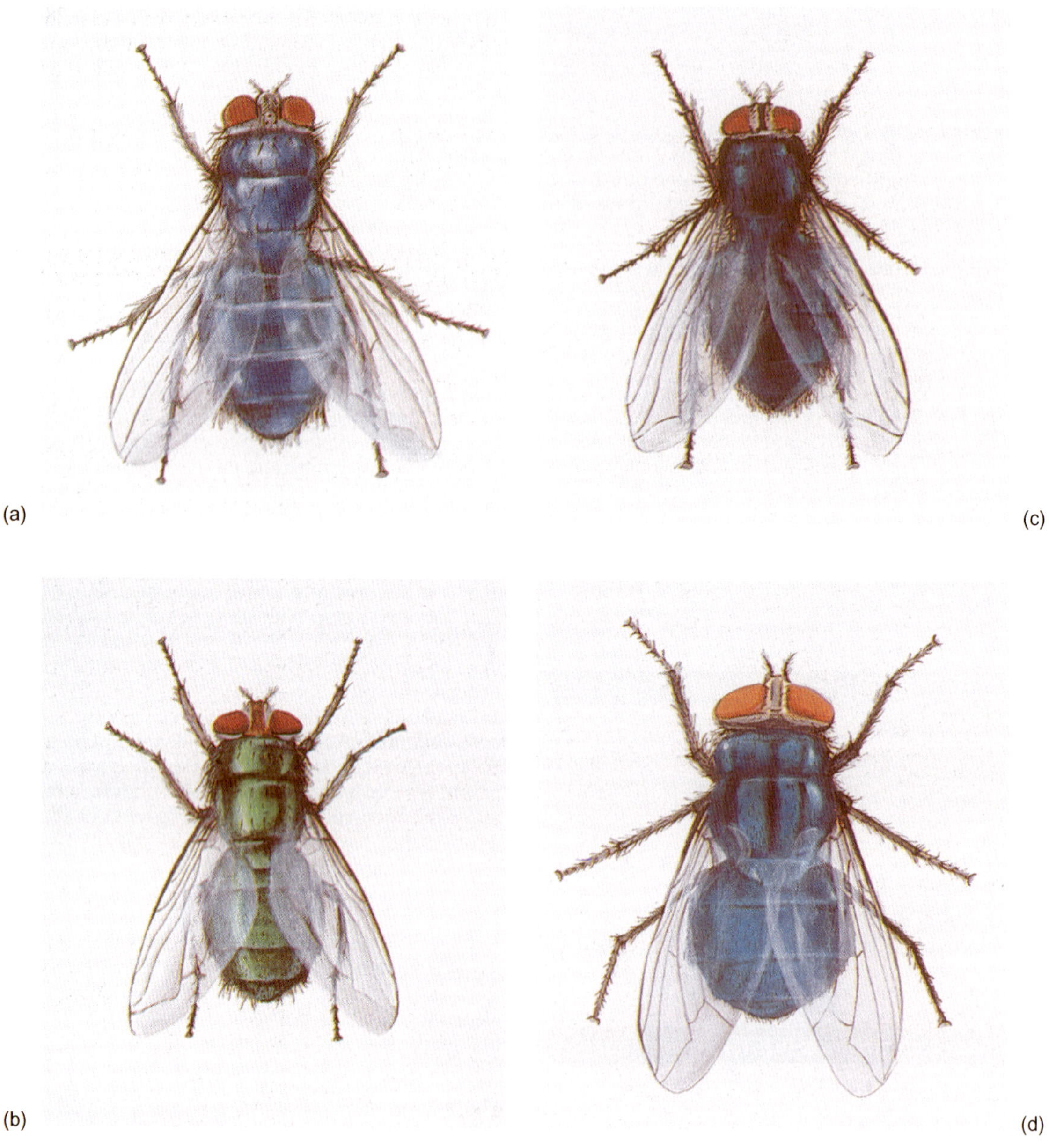

Fig. 11.35 Adult flies. (a) *Calliphora* spp. (b) *Lucilia* spp. (c) *Phormia* spp. (d) *Cochliomyia* spp.

faeces and have large, fully developed mouthparts. The arista of the antenna has setae on both sides. The thoracic squamae are without setae and the stem vein of the wing is without bristles.

Description, larvae: Third-stage larvae are 12–28 mm in length and are densely, but incompletely, covered with small, backwardly directed, single-toothed spines. On the posterior segment the larvae have a pair of spiracular plates and the arrangement of the posterior spiracles on these plates serves to differentiate the species. In *C. anthropophaga* the posterior spiracles have three sinuous slits and a weakly sclerotised peritreme.

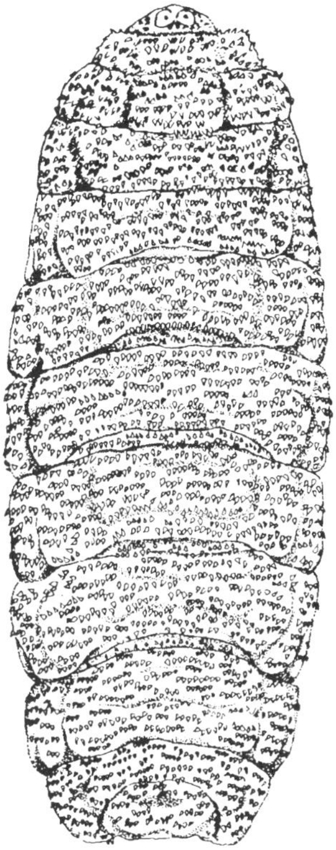

Fig. 11.36 Third-stage larva of *Cordylobia anthropophaga* (reproduced from Zumpt, 1965).

Hosts: Mainly antelope and rodents but may parasitise humans

Life cycle: The eggs are deposited singly in dry, sandy, shaded areas where animals lie, particularly areas contaminated with host urine or faeces. Females may also be attracted to dry, urine-soiled clothing. Eggs are laid in early morning or late evening. Up to 500 eggs are laid per female over their lifespan of 2–3 weeks. The eggs hatch after 2–4 days, and the first-stage larvae wait in the dry substrate for a host. The larvae can remain alive, without feeding, for 9–15 days hidden just beneath the soil surface. A sudden rise in temperature, vibration or carbon dioxide, which might signify the presence of a host, activates the larvae. They attach to the host and immediately burrow into the skin. Larvae develop beneath the skin and produce a swelling of approximately 10 mm in diameter at the point of entry. The swelling has a hole in the centre through which the larva breathes. The swellings may be found anywhere on the host animal's body, but are most commonly found on ventral parts. The three larval stages are completed in the host and, when mature (7–15 days after infection), the larvae emerge out of this hole and pupate on the ground in surface debris. Adult flies emerge from the pupae after 3–4 weeks.

Pathogenesis: See *Cordylobia anthropophaga*

Geographical distribution: Tropical Africa, particularly rainforest areas

Dermatobia hominis

Common name: Torsalo, berne, human bot fly, ura

Predilection site: Skin wounds

Parasite class: Insecta

Family: Oestridae

Description, adult: The adult *Dermatobia* fly resembles *Calliphora* in appearance, the short, broad abdomen having a bluish metallic sheen, but there are only vestigial mouthparts covered by a flap. The female measures approximately 12 mm in length. Adults have a yellow–orange head and legs, and the thorax possesses a sparse covering of short setae. The arista of the antennae has setae on the outer side only.

Description, larvae: Mature larvae measure up to 25 mm long and are somewhat oval. They have two to three rows of strong spines on most of the segments. Larvae are narrowed at the posterior end, particularly the second-stage larva. The third-stage larva is more oval in shape with prominent flower-like anterior spiracles (Fig. 11.37).

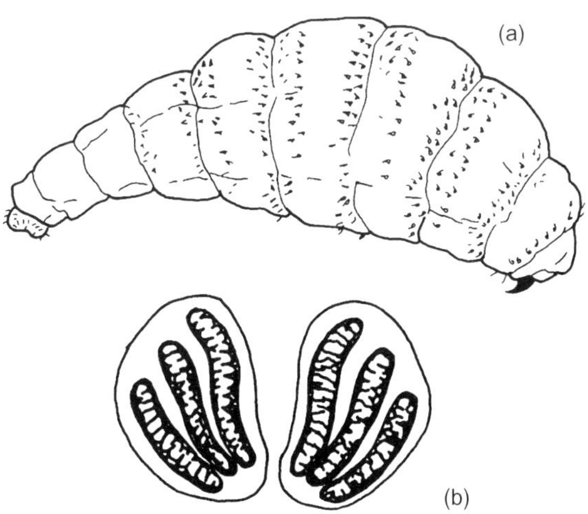

Fig. 11.37 *Dermatobia hominis*. (a) Third-stage larva. (b) Posterior spiracles.

Hosts: Humans, most domestic and wild mammals and many types of bird

Life cycle: *Dermatobia* is most common in forest and bush regions, the latter known in many parts of South America as the 'monte'. The adult flies do not feed; instead nourishment is derived from food stores accumulated during the larval stages. The female has a sedentary habit, resting on leaves until oviposition is imminent, when she catches an insect (usually a mosquito) and attaches a batch of up to 25 eggs to the underside of its abdomen or thorax. While attached to this transport host the L_1 develop within the eggs in about a week, but do not hatch until the carrier insect lands on a warm-blooded animal to feed. The first-stage larvae hatch in response to the sudden temperature rise near the host's body. The larvae then penetrate the skin (often through the opening made by the transport fly) and migrate to the subcutis, where they develop to the L_3 and breath through a skin perforation in the fashion of *Hypoderma*. The larvae do not wander. The mature larvae emerge after about 3 months and pupate on the ground for a further month before the adult flies emerge. There may be up to three generations each year.

Geographical distribution: Latin America from Mexico to northern Argentina and the island of Trinidad

Pathogenesis: The larvae occur in swellings in various parts of the body and these may suppurate and cause severe pain. In Latin America this condition is often known as 'ura'.

Dermatobia is a major problem in cattle in South America. Lesions are most numerous on the upper body, neck, back, flanks and tail, and are often grouped together to form large and often purulent swellings. As well as hide damage, the pain and distress of the lesions result in reduced time spent grazing, retarded growth and lowered meat and milk production. The exit holes made by the larvae may also attract myiasis-producing flies, including screwworms.

In humans the most common larval sites are the extremities of the limbs and the scalp. Fatal cerebral damage has occurred in children when larvae have migrated through the fontanelle into the cranial cavity.

Clinical signs: Symptoms include the swellings and lesions made by larvae. Infected animals show reduced weight gain and milk production.

Epidemiology: The most common vectors of *D. hominis* larvae are members of the genera *Psorophora*, *Culex* and *Stomoxys*. These flies breed in forest where both domestic and wild animals are commonly parasitised. Humans are usually infected through association with domestic animals; however, non-insect transmission may occur when *D. hominis* eggs are deposited on damp clothes or laundry.

Wohlfahrtia magnifica

Common name: Flesh fly, screwworm

Predilection site: Skin wounds

Parasite class: Insecta

Family: Sarcophagidae

Description, adult: The adult flies are large, measuring 8–14 mm in length, with elongated bodies. They are grey in colour and have three distinct, longitudinal, thoracic stripes. The abdomen is clearly marked with black spots (Fig. 11.38c). The flies have numerous bristles covering the body and long, black legs. The arista of the antennae does not possess setae.

Description, larvae: Larvae possess strongly developed oral hooks.

Hosts: Adult females will oviposit on any warm-blooded animal. This includes most livestock, particularly sheep and camels and also poultry, although cattle, horses, pigs, dogs and humans may also be infested.

Life cycle: *Wohlfahrtia magnifica* is an obligate agent of myiasis. Female flies deposit 120–170 first-stage larvae on the host, in wounds or next to body orifices. The larvae feed and mature in 5–7 days, moulting twice, before leaving the wound and dropping to the ground where they pupate.

Geographical distribution: Northern Africa, the Mediterranean, eastern Europe, Middle East and Russia

Pathogenesis: *Wohlfahrtia magnifica* can cause rapid and severe myiasis in most animals. Flies lay their larvae in sores (particularly around the eyes), body orifices, wounds or decomposing flesh. Infestation initially causes intermittent irritation and pyrexia, followed by the production of a cavernous lesion. The tissue shows progressive liquefaction, necrosis and haemorrhage, before the larvae leave the wound. If untreated, repeated infestation by *W. magnifica* and secondary fly species may quickly lead to the death of the host within 1–2 weeks.

Epidemiology: Levels of infestation appear to be high, particularly in sheep in eastern Europe. Faecal soiling in sheep has been recorded as an important predisposing factor for breech myiasis by *W. magnifica.* In a 4-year period, cases of myiasis by *W. magnifica* were recorded in 45 out of 195 sheep flocks in

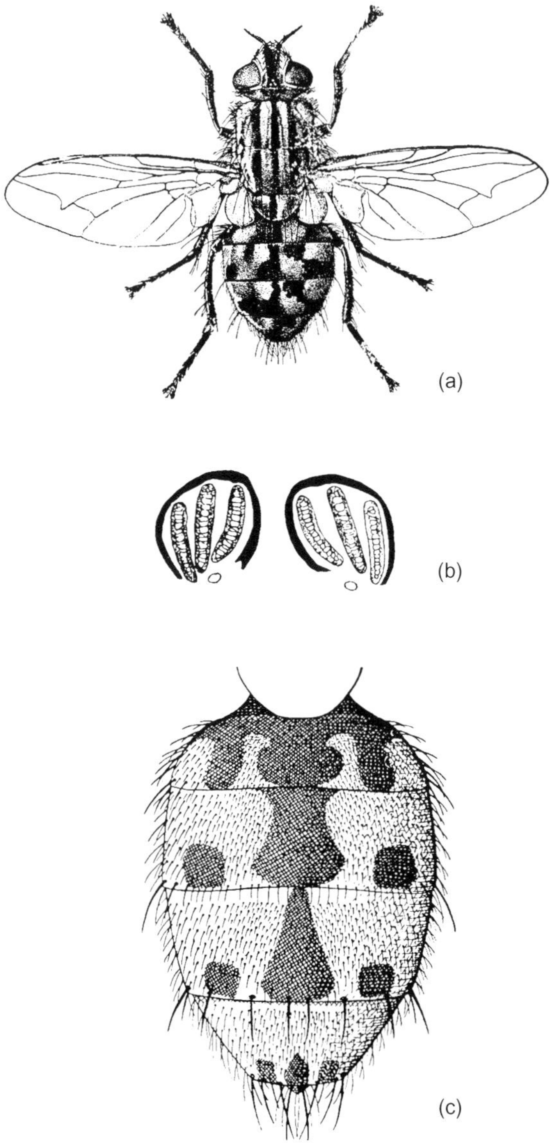

Fig. 11.38 (a) Adult of the flesh fly *Sarcophaga carnaria* (reproduced from Castellani and Chalmers, 1910). *Wohlfahrtia magnifica*, (b) posterior spiracles deeply sunk in a cavity and (c) abdomen of adult (reproduced from Smart, 1943).

Bulgaria, affecting between 23 and 41% of sheep each year. Only 0.5–1.0% of cows and goats were affected over the same period. In Romania, in one study 80–95% of sheep were infested, with 20% fatalities of newborn lambs.

Wohlfahrtia nuba

Common name: Flesh fly

Predilection site: Skin wounds

Parasite class: Insecta

Family: Sarcophagidae

Description: The adult flies are large, 8–14 mm in length, with elongated bodies, longitudinal black thoracic stripes and have a grey and black tessellated abdomen. Larvae possess strongly developed oral hooks.

Hosts: Camels

Life cycle: *Wohlfahrtia nuba* oviposit primarily in carrion, but they may also act as secondary invaders of myiases on live mammals in north Africa and the Near East. Females deposit live first-stage larvae rather than eggs. When fully mature, the third-stage larvae leave the feeding site to pupate in the ground.

Geographical distribution: Primarily north Africa and the Near East

Pathogenesis: When present in an infected wound or as a secondary invader at an existing myiasis, larvae extend and deepen the lesion. The irritation and distress caused by the lesion is extremely debilitating and the host animal can rapidly lose condition. If untreated, repeated infestation may quickly lead to the death of the host within 1–2 weeks.

Clinical signs: Animals infested by fly larvae may appear dull, lethargic, and separate from the herd or flock. They may cease feeding and show weight loss. Wounds with foul-smelling odour will be observed on inspection.

Diagnosis: Flesh fly larvae are diagnosed by the removal of the larvae and identification under a dissecting microscope.

Epidemiology: *Wohlfahrtia nuba* may be an occasional secondary facultative invader of wounds, particularly of camels, in north Africa and the Middle East.

Treatment and control: The larvae should be removed and identified and the wound thoroughly cleaned and disinfected. Organophosphate and pyrethroid insecticides are effective against newly hatched larvae, immature forms and adult flies. Larvae inside wounds must be treated with a suitable larvicide. Spraying or dipping animals with an approved insecticide and treating infested wounds can protect against new infestations for 7–10 days.

Wohlfahrtia vigil

Common name: Grey flesh fly

Predilection site: Skin wounds

Parasite class: Insecta

Family: Sarcophagidae

Description, adult: The adult flies are large, 8–14 mm in length, with elongated bodies, longitudinal black thoracic stripes and a grey and black tessellated abdomen.

Description, larvae: Larvae possess strongly developed oral hooks.

Hosts: Mink, fox, rabbit and other wild mammals. Dogs and cats may also occasionally be attacked.

Life cycle: The adult female of *Wohlfahrtia vigil* deposits active maggots on the host, often in wounds, body orifices or existing myiases. However, the larvae can penetrate intact skin if it is thin and tender; hence young animals tend to be most affected. Groups of larvae may be observed in boil-like swellings under the skin. The larvae feed and grow, moulting twice, before leaving the host and dropping to the ground where they pupate.

Geographical distribution: North, Central and South America

Pathogenesis: *Wohlfahrtia vigil* can cause rapid and severe myiasis in most animals. The myiasis caused is furuncular rather than cutaneous. Furuncles similar to those of *Dermatobia* are produced, although those of *W. vigil* can contain up to five larvae with a small pore opening to the outside.

Wohlfahrtia meigeni

Common name: Flesh fly

Predilection site: Skin wounds

Parasite class: Insecta

Family: Sarcophagidae

Description, adults: The adult flies are large, 8–14 mm in length, with elongated bodies, longitudinal black thoracic stripes and a grey and black tessellated abdomen.

Description, larvae: Larvae possess strongly developed oral hooks.

Hosts: Warm-blooded vertebrates, particularly mink and fox, may also infest rabbits and dogs

Life cycle: The adult female of *W. meigeni* deposits active maggots on the host, often in wounds, body orifices or existing myiases. However, the larvae can penetrate intact skin if it is thin and tender, hence young animals tend to be most affected. Groups of larvae may be observed in boil-like swellings under the skin. The larvae feed and grow, moulting twice, before leaving the host and dropping to the ground where they pupate.

Geographical distribution: Palearctic, primarily western USA

Pathogenesis: Flies lay their larvae in wounds, body orifices or existing myiases. The myiasis caused is furuncular rather than cutaneous. Furuncles similar to those of *Dermatobia* are produced, although those of *W. meigeni* can contain up to five larvae. This species may cause substantial mortality to young mink and foxes in fur farms.

Sarcophaga spp

Common name: Flesh flies

Predilection site: Skin wounds

Parasite class: Insecta

Family: Sarcophagidae

Description, adults: Adults are grey–black, non-metallic, medium to large flies with prominent stripes on the thorax and a checkered abdominal pattern (Fig. 11.38a).

Hosts: Cattle, sheep

Life cycle: All Sarcophagidae are larviporous; the ovulated eggs are retained within the oviduct of the adult female and batches of 30–200 larvae are deposited shortly after the eggs hatch. The larvae of *Sarcophaga* are normally associated with carrion but may occasionally infest wounds. They may extend the injury, increasing the severity of the infestation.

Geographical distribution: Worldwide

Notes: There are over 2000 species in the family, divided into 400 genera. Most species of the genus *Sarcophaga* are of no veterinary importance, breeding in excrement, carrion and other decomposing organic matter. One of the more widely distributed species is *Sarcophaga haemorrhoidalis*.

BITING AND NUISANCE FLIES

Adult flies may feed on blood, sweat, skin secretions, tears, saliva, urine or faeces of the domestic animals to which they are attracted. They may do this either by puncturing the skin directly, in which case they are known as biting flies, or by scavenging at the surface of the skin, wounds or body orifices, in which case they may be classified as non-biting or nuisance flies. These flies may act as biological and mechanical vectors for a range of pathogenic diseases. Mechanical transmission may be exacerbated by the fact that some fly species inflict extremely painful bites and, therefore, are frequently disturbed by the host while blood-feeding. As a result, the flies are forced to move from host to host over a short period, thereby increasing their potential for mechanical disease transmission.

Hosts: Flies may feed on almost all warm-blooded vertebrates, but are of particular veterinary importance in cattle and horses.

Pathogenesis: Very little is known about the pathology of the cutaneous lesions produced by most of these pests, which may vary considerably in character and severity. With biting flies, the wounds created are usually seen as erythematous papules or wheals, surrounding the central puncture site. The wounds may develop a crust of dried exudate. There may be epidermal necrosis or intraepithelial eosinophilic spongiform pustules. Pruritis may be intense, resulting in secondary traumatic lesions. The wheals may persist for several weeks.

Saliva injected during feeeding may be irritant and allogenic and hypersensitivity reactions may contribute to the severity of the local lesion.

Clinical signs: The activity of both biting and non-biting species of fly results in marked defensive behaviour, described as 'fly-worry' in livestock. This is the disturbance caused by the presence and attempted feeding behaviour of flies. Responses by the host may range from dramatic escape behaviour, in which self-injury can occur, to less or increased levels of tail twitching, licking, foot stamping and skin rippling; animals may bunch or seek the shelter of overhanging vegetation. All these changes in behaviour result in reduced time spent feeding and decreased performance. Flies may be observed, often in large numbers, feeding along the back, sides and ventral abdomen, particularly of cattle and horses. Irritation and blood loss can lead to a marked reduction in weight gain.

Diagnosis: Increased levels of disturbance in the host animals; observation of flies on the animals. Precise identification will require microscopic examination of specimens. Identification of the larvae of most species is extremely difficult and, where possible, adults should be collected or samples of live larvae should be retained until adult emergence to confirm the identification, which is more easily accomplished with the adult fly. The detailed description and identification of the larvae of most species is beyond the scope of this text and if identification to species level is required, specimens should be referred to a relevant taxonomic specialist.

Treatment: Insecticide-impregnated ear tags, tail bands and halters, mainly containing synthetic pyrethroids, together with pour-on, spot-on and spray preparations, are widely used to reduce fly annoyance in cattle and horses.

Control: Various types of screens and electrocution grids for buildings are available to reduce fly nuisance, but the best methods of control are those aimed at improving sanitation and reducing breeding places (source reduction). For example, in stables and farms manure should be removed, or stacked in large heaps where the heat of fermentation will kill the developing stages of flies, as well as eggs and larvae of helminths. In addition, insecticides applied to the surface of manure heaps may prove beneficial.

A range of insecticides and procedures is available for the control of adult flies. Aerosol space sprays, residual insecticides applied to walls and ceilings and insecticide-impregnated cards and strips may reduce fly numbers indoors. Insecticides may also be incorporated in solid or liquid fly baits, using attractants such as various sugary syrups or hydrolysed yeast and animal proteins.

Insecticide dust bags ('backrubbers') have been used to reduce the numbers of muscid flies associated with fly-worry. These consist of sacking impregnated with or containing insecticide, which is suspended between two posts at a height that allows cattle to rub and thus apply the insecticide to the skin.

However, given the high rates of reproduction, high rates of dispersal and multiple generations per year, area-wide control of most dipterous agents of myiasis is impractical.

The appearance of the adult flies *Musca domestica*, *Stomoxys calcitrans* and *Haematobia* (*Lyperosia*) spp is shown in Fig. 11.39.

Haematobia irritans

Subspecies: *irritans*

Synonym: *Lyperosia irritans*

Common name: Horn fly

Predilection site: Base of horns, back, shoulders and belly

Parasite class: Insecta

Family: Muscidae

Description: The adults are 3–4 mm in length and are the smallest of the blood-sucking muscids. They are usually grey, often with several dark stripes on the thorax. Unlike *Musca* the proboscis is held forwards

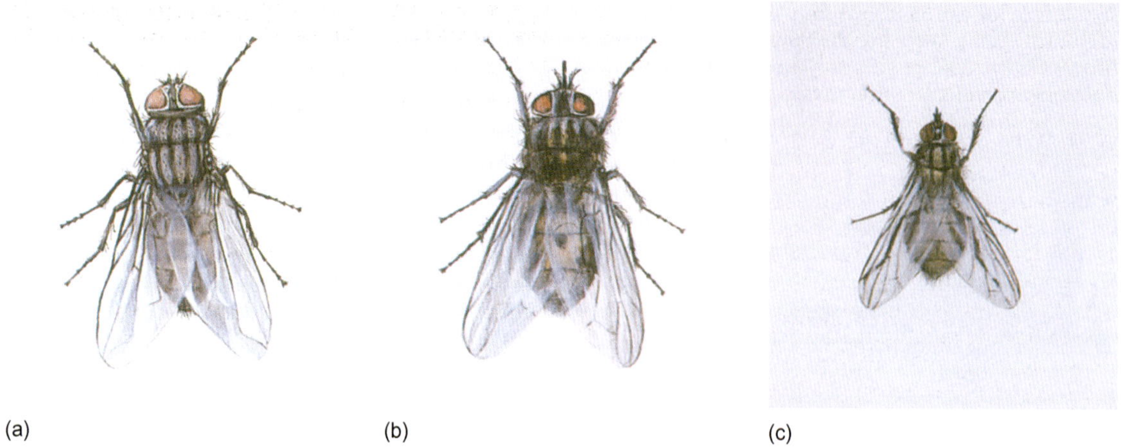

Fig. 11.39 Adult flies. (a) *Musca domestica.* (b) *Stomoxys calcitrans.* (c) *Haematobia* (*Lyperosia*) spp.

and unlike *Stomoxys* the palps are stout and as long as the proboscis (Fig. 11.40). In *H. irritans* the palps are dark greyish, whereas in *H. stimulans* they are yellowish in colour. Eggs are 1.0–1.5 mm long. The cylindrical larvae are yellow–white and generally about 7 mm long with two D-shaped posterior spiracles. Puparia are dull reddish brown and 3–4 mm long.

Hosts: Primarily cattle. They also occasionally attack horses, sheep and dogs.

Life cycle: In contrast to other muscids these flies generally remain on their hosts, leaving only to fly to another host or, in the case of females, to lay eggs in freshly passed faeces. Eggs are laid in groups of four to six, usually in the fresh faeces or in the soil immediately beneath it. These hatch quickly if the humidity is sufficiently high; larvae may be mature in as little as 4 days given adequate moisture and temperatures of around 27°C. Low temperatures and dry conditions delay larval development and kill the eggs. The pupal

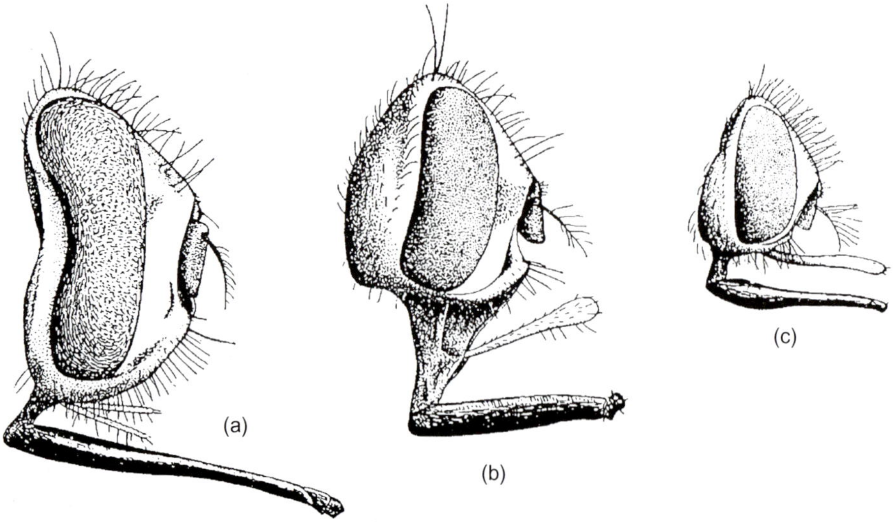

Fig. 11.40 Lateral views of the heads of blood-sucking Muscidae. (a) *Stomoxys calcitrans.* (b) *Haematobia stimulans.* (c) *Haematobia irritans* (reproduced from Edwards *et al.*, 1939).

period is around 6–8 days and on emergence the adult flies seek and remain on their cattle hosts. Horn flies overwinter as pupae in the soil below cowpats, emerging as adults the following spring.

Geographical distribution: Worldwide, particularly Europe, the USA and Australia

Pathogenesis: The adult flies feed on the host animal's blood, causing injury and irritation due to the constant piercing of the skin. Loss of blood due to horn flies can be considerable. In addition, during feeding the horn fly withdraws and reinserts its mouthparts many times, resulting in considerable irritation to the host. Although less important than many other muscid flies in disease transmission, *Haematobia* may transmit *Stephanofilaria*, the skin filarioid of cattle.

Epidemiology: Hot, humid weather, with a temperature of 23–27°C and a relative humidity of 65–90%, is ideal for horn fly activity. The flies may be more abundant on cattle with dark coats and dark-coloured areas of bicoloured cattle. When temperatures are above 29°C flies migrate to the shaded skin of the belly and udder.

Haematobia exigua

Synonym: *Haematobia irritans exigua*

Common name: Buffalo fly

Predilection site: Skin, withers, back and sides. Occasionally the belly in hot weather

Parasite class: Insecta

Family: Muscidae

Description: See *Haematobia irritans.*

Hosts: Buffalo and cattle

Life cycle: See *Haematobia irritans.*

Geographical distribution: Worldwide, particularly Asia and Australia

Pathogenesis: The buffalo fly has a pronounced effect on the health and productivity of buffalo and cattle. Significant blood loss can occur due to the high densities on the host (often several thousand) and the fact that both sexes feed several times per day. The bites are painful and irritating and may cause feeding lesions. Species of *Haematobia* may transmit *Stephanofilaria*, the skin filarioid of cattle.

Notes: The buffalo fly (*Haematobia irritans exigua*) and the horn fly (*H. irritans irritans*) were once recognised as two separate species. However, it has been concluded that they are probably best regarded as subspecies of *H. irritans.*

Haematobia minuta

Synonym: *Lyperosia minuta*

Predilection site: Skin, withers, back and sides. Occasionally the belly in hot weather

Parasite class: Insecta

Family: Muscidae

Description: The adults are up to 4 mm in length. They are usually grey, often with several dark stripes on the thorax. Unlike *Musca* the proboscis is held forwards, and unlike *Stomoxys* the palps are stout and as long as the proboscis.

Hosts: Cattle and buffalo

Life cycle: Eggs are 1.0–1.5 mm long and are laid in fresh faeces. These hatch quickly, and larvae may be mature in as little as 4 days given adequate moisture and temperatures. Low temperatures and dry conditions delay larval development and kill the eggs. After pupation in the ground, the newly emerged adult flies seek out and then remain on their cattle or buffalo hosts. Reproduction is continuous and populations are multivoltine.

Geographical distribution: Africa

Pathogenesis: Large numbers cause intense irritation, and the skin wounds made during feeding may attract other muscids and myiasis-producing flies. These flies may have a pronounced effect on the health and productivity of the cattle. Significant blood loss can occur due to the high densities on the host (often several thousand) and also the fact that both sexes feed several times per day. The bites are painful and irritating and may cause feeding lesions. It is difficult to assess the precise economic effect of these flies, but their effective control on grazing cattle can result in significant increases in production. Although less important than many other muscid flies in disease transmission, species of *Haematobia* transmit *Stephanofilaria*, the skin filarioid of cattle and, in some areas, camel trypanosomiasis.

Haematobia stimulans

Synonym: *Haematobosca stimulans*

Predilection site: Skin

Parasite class: Insecta

Family: Muscidae

Description, adult: *Haematobia stimulans* are slightly smaller than *Stomoxys calcitrans* at about 6 mm in length. They are usually grey, often with several dark stripes on the thorax. The proboscis is held forwards and, unlike *Stomoxys*, the palps are stout, as long as the proboscis and are club-shaped apically (Fig. 11.40b). In *H. stimulans* the palps are yellow in colour, whereas in *H. irritans* they are dark grey. The eggs are reddish brown and lack a terminal horn.

Description, larvae: The larvae are cylindrical and yellow–white in colour. They measure approximately 7 mm in length and have two D-shaped posterior spiracles. Puparia are dull reddish brown and 3–4 mm long.

Hosts: Cattle

Life cycle: *Haematobia stimulans* is less resident on its host than *H. irritans*, and more closely resembles *S. calcitrans* in its behaviour. The eggs are 1–1.5 mm in length and are laid in fresh faeces. Females require blood-meals for egg production and each female is capable of producing 300–400 eggs that are deposited in batches of 20–30. These hatch quickly and larvae may be mature in as little as 4 days given adequate moisture and temperatures. Pupation requires around 6–8 days. The egg-to-adult life cycle may be completed in as little as 10–14 days and three to four generations may occur in one summer.

Geographical distribution: Europe

Pathogenesis: The bites are painful and irritating and may cause feeding lesions. Although less important than many other muscid flies in disease transmission, species of *Haematobia* transmit *Stephanofilaria*, the skin filarioid of cattle.

Hydrotaea irritans

Common name: Sheep headfly

Predilection site: Skin wounds

Parasite class: Insecta

Family: Muscidae

Description: *Hydrotaea irritans* is generally similar in size and appearance to the various species of *Musca* and is characterised by an olive-green abdomen and an orange–yellow coloration at the base of the wings. The thorax is black with grey patches. Adults measure 4–7 mm in length. Specific identification of non-biting muscid flies requires specialist advice.

Hosts: Cattle, sheep and horses

Life cycle: Adult flies prefer still conditions and are found near woodlands and plantations, with peak numbers occurring in mid-summer. Eggs are laid in decaying vegetation or faeces; they hatch and develop into mature larvae by the autumn. Each female produces one or two batches of about 30 eggs in its lifetime. Third-stage larvae may be predatory on other larvae. These larvae then go into diapause (a temporary cessation of development) until the following spring when pupation and development is completed, with emergence of a new generation of adults in early summer. Thus there is only one generation of headfly each year with peak numbers occurring in mid-summer.

Geographical distribution: Widespread throughout northern Europe, but not believed to be present in North America.

Pathogenesis: Headflies are attracted to animals and feed on tears, saliva, sweat and wounds, such as those incurred by fighting rams. The mouthparts are adapted for feeding on liquids, but in addition they possess small teeth and the rasping effect of these during feeding leads to skin damage. They are facultative blood-feeders and will ingest blood at the edges of wounds if available. Horned breeds of sheep, such as the Swaledale and Scottish Blackface, are most susceptible to attack (Fig. 11.41). Swarms of these flies around the head lead to intense irritation and annoyance and result in self-inflicted wounds, which then attract more flies. Clusters of flies feeding at the base of the horns lead to extension of these wounds, and the condition may be confused with blowfly myiasis. Secondary bacterial infection of wounds is common, which may encourage blowfly strike. The economic losses due to headfly infection are difficult to assess, but are thought to be substantial.

In cattle, large numbers of *Hydrotaea irritans* have been found on the ventral abdomen and udder and, since the bacteria involved in 'summer mastitis' (*Corynebacterium pyogenes*, *Streptococcus dysgalactiae* and *Peptococcus indolicus*) have been isolated from these flies, there is strong presumptive evidence that they may transmit the disease. In addition, this species has been incriminated in the transmission of infectious bovine keratoconjunctivitis.

Epidemiology: Although commonly known as the sheep headfly, this species may be the most numer-

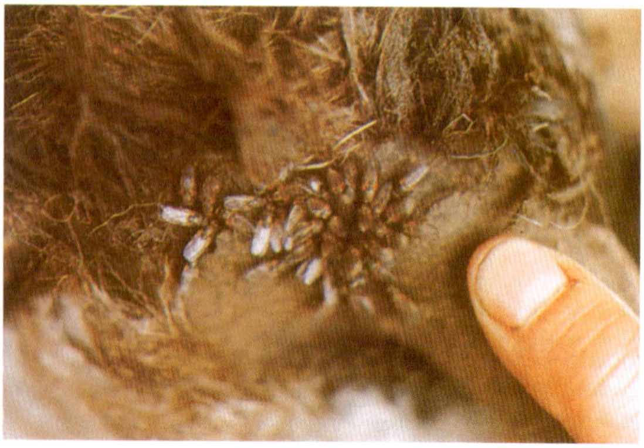

Fig. 11.41 *Hydrotaea irritans* clustered around the base of the horns in a sheep.

ous muscid species found on cattle and horses. The populations of *Hydrotaea irritans* peak during midsummer. Adult flies prefer still conditions and are associated with permanent, fairly sheltered pastures that border woodlands or plantations.

Musca autumnalis

Common name: Facefly

Predilection site: Skin, especially eyes, nose and mouth

Parasite class: Insecta

Family: Muscidae

Description: Female adults of *Musca autumnalis* are 6–8 mm in length, male adults 5–6 mm, and they vary in colour from light to dark grey. The thorax is usually grey with four dark longitudinal stripes, and there is a sharp upward bend in the fourth longitudinal wing vein. The abdomen is a yellowish brown background colour with a black median longitudinal stripe. The eyes are reddish and the space between them can be used to determine the sex of a specimen, since in females it is almost twice as broad as in males. The aristae are bilaterally plumose at the tip. The facefly, *M. autumnalis*, is very similar to *M. domestica* in size and appearance, although the abdomen of the female is darker, while in the male tergite two and three are typically yellowish orange along the sides. The detailed wing venation is of taxonomic importance in the differentiation of *Musca* from similar flies belonging to other genera such as *Fannia*, *Morellia* and *Muscina* and in the identification of different *Musca* species, but is beyond the scope of this text. The eggs of *M. autumnalis* bear a terminal respiratory horn.

Hosts: Cattle

Life cycle: The facefly, *Musca autumnalis*, congregates in large numbers around the faces of cattle. It feeds on secretions from the eyes, nose and mouth as well as from blood in wounds left by other flies, such as tabanids. It lays its eggs just beneath the surface of fresh cattle manure within about 15 minutes of the dung pats being deposited. The eggs of *M. autumnalis* are about 3 mm in length and possess a short respiratory stalk. They are arranged so that the respiratory stalk of each egg projects above the surface of the pat. Like *M. domestica*, the larvae pass throughout three stages within approximately 1 week, before entering the surrounding soil and pupariating to form a whitish coloured puparium. Summer generations require about 2 weeks to complete a life cycle. This allows several generations in any one season. Faceflies prefer bright sunshine and usually do not follow cattle into barns or heavy shade. Adults are strong fliers and can move between widely separated herds. Faceflies overwinter as adults, in response to short photoperiods, aggregating in overwintering sites such as farm buildings.

Geographical distribution: Worldwide. *Musca autumnalis* is widely distributed throughout Europe, central Asia and parts of Africa and, since its introduction in the 1950s, can now be found throughout North America.

Pathogenesis: The facefly feeds largely on secretions from the eyes, nose and mouth as well as on wounds left by biting flies. This is often the most numerous of the flies which worry cattle at pasture. These flies are considered to be important in the transmission of infectious bovine keratoconjunctivitis ('pink eye' or New Forest disease) due to *Moraxella bovis*, and they are also intermediate hosts of *Parafilaria bovicola*. Adults are developmental hosts for *Thelazia* (nematodes which live in the conjunctival sac of cattle and horses, causing conjunctivitis, keratitis, photophobia and epiphora).

Epidemiology: In northern Europe, *Musca autumnalis* may often be the most numerous fly worrying cattle in pasture. The eggs of *M. autumnalis* are usually laid in bovine faeces, and if conditions are suitable the resultant large fly populations can cause serious annoyance. This can lead to bunching and so interfere with grazing, contributing to reduced production rates.

Notes: *Musca autumnalis* is one of the most important livestock pests to invade North America. Its introduction from Europe was first detected in 1951 in Nova Scotia. From there it spread southward and, by 1959, many cases were being reported on cattle. It now occurs throughout cattle-rearing areas of the USA and Canada.

Musca domestica

Common name: Housefly

Predilection site: Skin

Parasite class: Insecta

Family: Muscidae

Distribution: Worldwide

Description: Female adults of *Musca domestica* are 6–8 mm in length, male adults 5–6 mm, and they vary in colour from light to dark grey. The thorax is usually grey with four dark longitudinal stripes, and there is a sharp upward bend in the fourth longitudinal wing vein (Fig. 11.42). The abdomen has a yellow–brown background colour with a black median longitudinal stripe. The eyes are reddish and the space between them can be used to determine the sex of a specimen, since in females it is almost twice as broad as in males. The aristae are bilaterally plumose at the tip. The

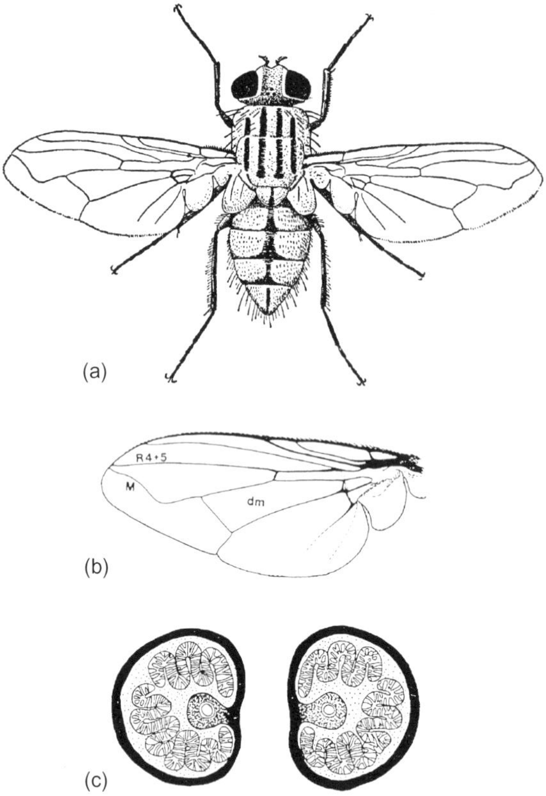

Fig. 11.42 (a) Female house fly, *Musca domestica*. (b) Wing venation typical of species of *Musca*, showing the strongly bent vein M ending close to R_{4+5}. (c) Posterior spiracles of a third-stage larva (after Smart, 1943).

detailed wing venation is of taxonomic importance in the differentiation of *Musca* from similar flies belonging to other genera such as *Fannia*, *Morellia* and *Muscina* and in the identification of different *Musca* species, but is beyond the scope of this text.

Hosts: Although *Musca domestica* is not itself a parasite of living animals, it is responsible for the transmission of a variety of important diseases and parasites, particularly to humans and a wide variety of domestic animals.

Life cycle: Female flies lay batches of up to 150 creamy white, 1.0 mm long, banana-shaped eggs in wet faeces or rotting organic material. The dorsal surface of the eggs has two curved, rib-like thickenings. Batches of eggs are laid at 3–4-day intervals throughout life. The eggs hatch (under optimal temperatures) in 12–24 hours to produce whitish coloured, segmented, cylindrical larvae with a pair of small anterior mouth hooks. High manure moisture favours their survival. At the posterior end of the larvae there are paired respiratory spiracles, the shape and structure of which allow generic and specific differentiation. The three larval stages feed on decomposing organic material and mature to 10–15 cm in length in 3–7 days under suitable conditions. Optimal temperatures for larval development are 30–37°C, although as the larvae mature their temperature tolerance increases. Mature larvae then move to drier areas around the larval habitat and pupate, forming a rigid and dark brown barrel-shaped puparium or 'pupal case'. The adult fly emerges after 3–26 days, depending on temperature. Mating and oviposition take place a few days after emergence. Total development time from egg to adult fly may be as little as 8 days at 35°C, but is extended at lower temperatures. In temperate areas, a small proportion of pupae or larvae may survive the winter, but more frequently the flies overwinter as hibernating adults.

Geographical distribution: Worldwide

Pathogenesis: Houseflies, as their name suggests, are closely associated with buildings inhabited by animals and humans. They are not only a source of annoyance, but may also mechanically transmit viruses, bacteria, helminths and protozoa due to their habit of visiting faecal and decaying organic material. Pathogens are either carried on the hairs of the feet and body or regurgitated as salivary vomit during subsequent feeding. A number of *Musca* spp. have been incriminated in the spread of diseases including mastitis, conjunctivitis and anthrax. In humans they are probably most important in the dissemination of *Shigella* and other enteric bacteria. Eggs of various helminths may be carried by the flies, and they also may act as intermediate hosts of a number of helminths such as *Habronema* spp and *Raillietina* spp. Deposition of *Habronema* larvae in wounds may give rise to skin lesions commonly termed 'summer sores' in horses. The housefly, *Musca domestica*, is closely associated with humans, livestock, their buildings and organic wastes. Although it may be of only minor direct annoyance to animals, its potential for transmission of viral and bacterial diseases and protozoan and metazoan parasites is of significance.

Musca sorbens

Common name: Bazaar fly

Predilection site: Skin

Parasite class: Insecta

Family: Muscidae

Distribution: In Africa, the Pacific islands and Oriental regions

Pathogenesis: *Musca sorbens* is a widespread species, largely replacing *M. domestica* where it occurs and is an important vector of disease in these regions (see *M. domestica*).

Musca vetustissima

Common name: Bush fly

Predilection site: Skin

Parasite class: Insecta

Family: Muscidae

Distribution: Australia

Pathogenesis: The bush fly, *Musca vetustissima*, which is very closely related to *M. sorbens*, is an important nuisance pest of humans and livestock. Bushflies have been known to transmit eye infections and other enteric diseases between other animals and humans.

Musca crassirostris

Predilection site: Skin

Parasite class: Insecta

Family: Muscidae

Description: *Musca crassirostris* are not obligatory parasites, but they can feed on a wide variety of animal secretions and are especially attracted to wounds. Adults are about 5.5–7.5 mm in length and vary in colour from light to dark grey. There are four distinct dark longitudinal stripes on the thorax and the greyish abdomen has various light and dark markings.

Life cycle: Female flies lay batches of up to 100 eggs in faeces or rotting organic material. Eggs hatch to produce whitish, segmented, cylindrical larvae (maggots). The three larval stages feed on decomposing organic material and mature within 3–7 days under suitable conditions. These then move to drier areas around the larval habitat and pupate. The adult fly emerges after 3–26 days, depending on temperature.

Geographical distribution: Mediterranean countries

Pathogenesis: *M. crassirostris* may use the prestomal teeth to rasp the skin and draw blood, which is then ingested. This species may act as a mechanical vector for a wide variety of viral and bacterial diseases and protozoan and metazoan parasites (see *M. domestica*).

Stomoxys calcitrans

Common name: Stable fly

Predilection site: Skin. Location depends on the host: on cattle the legs are preferred, on dogs the ears

Parasite class: Insecta

Family: Muscidae

Description, adults: Superficially, *Stomoxys calcitrans* resembles the housefly *M. domestica*, being similar in size (about 7–8 mm in length) and grey with four longitudinal dark stripes on the thorax. Its abdomen, however, is shorter and broader than *M. domestica* with three dark spots on the second and third abdominal segments. Probably the simplest method of distinguishing stable flies from *M. domestica* and other genera of non-biting muscid flies is by examination of the proboscis, which in *Stomoxys* is conspicuous and forward projecting (Fig. 11.40). When feeding, the proboscis swings downwards and skin penetration is achieved by the rasping action of fine teeth on the end of the labium. Stable flies can be distinguished from biting muscid flies of the genus *Haematobia* by the larger size and the much shorter palps of the former.

Description, larvae: Larvae of *Stomoxys* can be identified by examination of the posterior spiracles, which are relatively well separated and each has three S-shaped slits.

Life cycle: Both male and female flies feed on blood. The female lays batches of 25–50 eggs, resembling those of houseflies, in manure and moist, decaying vegetable matter, such as hay and straw contaminated with urine. The eggs are yellowish white with a longitudinal groove on one side, and measure approximately 1 mm in length. Eggs hatch in 1–4 days, or longer in cold weather, and the larvae develop in 6–30 days. Pupation occurs in the drier parts of the breeding material and takes 6–9 days or longer in cold weather. Optimal conditions for pupariation involve complete darkness and a temperature of about 27°C. The puparia are brown and about 6 mm in length. The complete life cycle from egg to adult fly may take 12–60 days depending mainly on temperature.

After emergence the adult females require several blood-meals before the ovaries mature and egg-laying can start (usually after about 9 days). If deprived of a blood-meal in the first few days after emergence, ovarian development is delayed and females produce fewer, smaller eggs. In temperate areas flies may overwinter as larvae or pupae, whereas in tropical climates breeding is continuous throughout the year.

Stable flies may double their body weight during feeding. After a blood-meal, flies move to a resting site on structures such as barn walls, fences or trees.

Geographical distribution: Worldwide

Pathogenesis: The salivary secretions of this species may cause toxic reactions with an immunosuppressive effect, rendering the host more susceptible to disease.

Stable flies may probe and attempt to feed on a number of hosts in rapid succession. They may therefore act as important mechanical vectors in the transmission of pathogens such as trypanosomes. *Trypanosoma evansi* (causing surra of equines and dogs), *T. equinum* (mal de caderas of equines, cattle, sheep and goats), *T. gambiense* and *T. rhodesiense* (human African trypanosomiasis) and *T. brucei* and *T. vivax* (nagana of equines, cattle, sheep and goats) are all mechanically transmitted by *S. calcitrans*. These flies also act as vectors for anthrax and *Dermatophilus congolensis*. *S. calcitrans* also serves as an intermediate host of the nematode *Habronema*.

Epidemiology: Approximately 3 minutes is required for a blood-meal during which time flies may almost double in weight. The bite of stable flies is painful and as such they are a serious pest of animals. In large numbers these flies are a great source of annoyance to grazing cattle and in some areas there are estimates of milk and meat production losses of up to 20%. Adult flies live for about 1 month and are abundant around farm buildings and stables in late summer and autumn in temperate areas. They largely remain in areas of strong sunlight and they bite mainly out of doors, although they will follow animals inside to feed. They will also enter buildings during rainy weather in the autumn. *S. calcitrans* are swift fliers but in general do not travel long distances.

Fannia canicularis

Common name: Lesser housefly

Predilection site: Skin, mouth, nose, eyes

Parasite class: Insecta

Family: Faniidae

Description, adult: Species of *Fannia* generally resemble houseflies in appearance but are more slender and smaller at about 4–6 mm in length. The fourth longitudinal vein is straight (not bent as in the house fly) (Fig. 11.43a). *Fannia canicularis* is greyish to almost black in colour, possessing three dark longitudinal stripes on the dorsal thorax. The palps are black. The aristae are bare.

Description, larvae: The larvae are easily recognised by the flattened shape and the branched, fleshy projections from the body (Fig. 11.43b). The brown-coloured puparium resembles the larva in shape.

Hosts: Cattle, poultry

Life cycle: *Fannia* breed in a wide range of decomposing organic material, particularly the excrement of chickens, humans, horses and cows. The life cycle is typical, with three larvae stages, followed by the pupa and adult. The complete life cycle requires from 15–30 days.

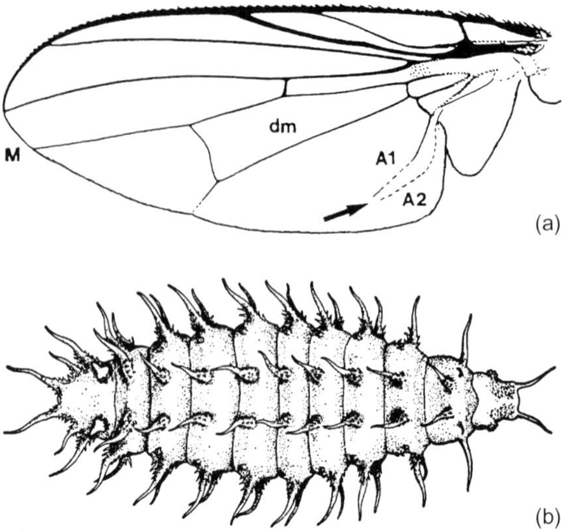

Fig. 11.43 (a) Wing venation typical of species of *Fannia*, showing the characteristic convergence of the anal veins. (b) Third-stage larva of the lesser house fly *Fannia canicularis* (from Zumpt, 1965).

Geographical distribution: Worldwide

Pathogenesis: Species of *Fannia* are of interest as nuisance pests of livestock and humans, especially in caged-layer poultry facilities, cattle-confinement areas and dairies. They rarely feed directly from animals; however, the few that do are attracted to smeared faeces, sweat, and mucus. Although it may be of only minor direct annoyance to animals, its potential for transmission of viral and bacterial diseases and protozoan and metazoan parasites is of significance, as for *Musca domestica*.

Epidemiology: Flies may be observed feeding on animal faeces, manure piles, garbage and other types of decomposing organic material, and seen attempting to land and feed on the liquid secretions of exudates of the eyes, nose and mouth. *Fannia canicularis* is the most cosmopolitan species and is commonly found breeding in animal manure and confined livestock facilities

In contrast to *Musca domestica*, the eggs and larvae of most species of *Fannia* are more susceptible to desiccation. Hence, they are more abundant in semi-liquid sites, especially pools of semi-liquid faeces. Adults are more abundant in the cooler months of spring and autumn, declining in midsummer. Adults of *Fannia* are readily attracted into buildings and adult males are familiar as the flies responsible for the regular triangular flight paths beneath light bulbs or shafts of sunlight from windows in buildings.

Fannia scalaris

Common name: Latrine fly

Predilection site: Mouth, nose, eyes

Parasite class: Insecta

Family: Faniidae

Description, adult: As for *F. canicularis* except the halteres are yellow.

Description, larvae: As for *F. canicularis*

Geographical distribution: Worldwide

Pathogenesis: This species may act as a mechanical vector for a wide variety of viral and bacterial diseases and protozoan and metazoan parasites (see *M. domestica*).

Fannia benjamini

Predilection site: Mouth, nose, eyes

Parasite class: Insecta

Family: Faniidae

Description, adult: As for *F. canicularis* except the palps are yellow.

Description, larvae: As for *F. canicularis*

Geographical distribution: North America

Pathogenesis: This species may act as a mechanical vector for a wide variety of viral and bacterial diseases and protozoan and metazoan parasites (see *M. domestica*).

Hippobosca equina

Common name: Forest fly, horse louse fly

Predilection site: Skin; perineum and between the hind legs

Parasite class: Insecta

Family: Hippoboscidae

Description: Adult flies are approximately 10 mm in length and are generally pale reddish brown with yellow spots on the indistinctly segmented abdomen. They have one pair of wings, the veins of which are crowded together towards the anterior margin (Fig. 11.44). The major part of the piercing proboscis is usually retracted under the head, except during feeding. Forest flies remain on their hosts for long periods and their preferred feeding sites are the perineum and between the hind legs. Both sexes of adult are blood feeders. The larvae are rarely seen and measure about 5 mm in length.

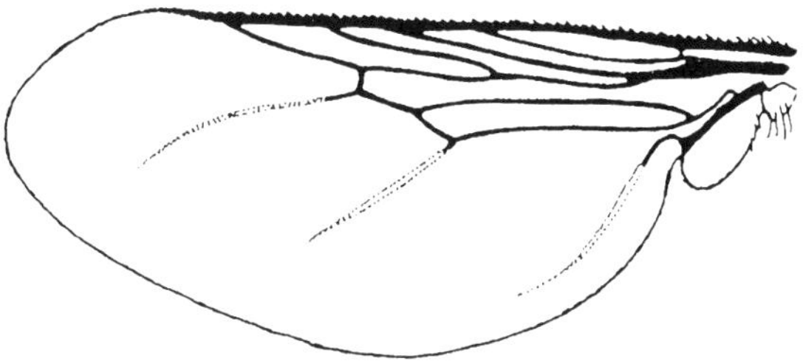

Fig. 11.44 Wing venation typical of species of *Hippobosca* showing the characteristic crowding of the veins into the leading half of the wings (reproduced from Smart, 1943).

Hosts: Mainly horses and cattle, but other domestic animals and birds may be attacked

Life cycle: Gravid female flies leave their hosts and deposit mature larvae singly in dry soil or humus. Each female can produce only five or six larvae in its lifetime. These larvae pupate almost immediately. When pupation is completed, the newly-emerged winged adults locate a suitable host animal on which they blood-feed, remaining on the host for long periods. In temperate areas, flies are most abundant in the summer months.

Geographical distribution: Worldwide

Pathogenesis: This species is primarily a nuisance and a cause of disturbance. Since they pierce the skin to suck blood they may be mechanical vectors of blood parasites such as the non-pathogenic *Trypanosoma theileri* in cattle, piroplasmosis of horses, Q fever and other types of rickettsioses. They may also transmit *Haemoproteus* species to birds.

Epidemiology: The adult flies are most abundant on the host during the summer months and attack more frequently in sunny weather.

Other common hippoboscids

These species are primarily a nuisance and a cause of disturbance; they may be mechanical vectors of pathogens such as *Trypanosoma*. The predilection site for these flies is the skin.

Hippobosca camelina

Common name: Camel fly

Parasite class: Insecta

Family: Hippoboscidae

Hosts: Camels

Geographical distribution: Worldwide in association with camels

Hippobosca maculata

Common name: Horse and cattle louse fly

Parasite class: Insecta

Family: Hippoboscidae

Hosts: Mainly horses and cattle, but other domestic animals and birds may be attacked.

Geographical distribution: Tropics and subtropics, particularly India and Africa

Hippobosca variegata

Common name: Horse louse fly

Parasite class: Insecta

Family: Hippoboscidae

Hosts: Mainly horses and cattle, but other domestic animals may be attacked.

Geographical distribution: Tropical Africa

Hippobosca rufipes

Common name: Cattle louse fly

Parasite class: Insecta

Family: Hippoboscidae

Hosts: cattle

Geographical distribution: Africa

Hippobosca longipennis

Common name: Dog fly

Parasite class: Insecta

Family: Hippoboscidae

Hosts: Dogs and wild carnivores

Geographical distribution: East and north Africa, but has been transported throughout the Mediterranean region.

Lipoptena spp

Common name: Deer keds

Parasite class: Insecta

Family: Hippoboscidae

Hosts: Deer, elk

Geographical distribution: Worldwide (*L. depressa* in North America, *L. cervi* in Europe and Asia, but has been introduced into North America)

Description: Wings are fully developed and function in newly emerged adults, but are shed once a suitable host has been located.

Life cycle: Like all Hippoboscids, adult females larviposit single, fully developed third-stage larvae while on the host. Pupae fall to the ground. Following pupation the newly emerged adult must find a suitable host, feed and mate. Both sexes are blood feeders.

Pathogenesis: These species are primarily a nuisance and a cause of disturbance.

TABANIDS: HORSEFLIES

Predilection site: Skin

Parasite class: Insecta

Family: Tabanidae

Hosts: Generally large domestic or wild animals and man, but small mammals and birds may also be attacked.

Description, adults: These are medium to large biting flies, up to 25 mm in length, with wingspans of up to 65 mm. The head is large and the proboscis prominent. They are generally dark coloured, but may have various stripes or patches of colour on the abdomen or thorax and even the large eyes, which are dichoptic in the female and holoptic in the male, may be coloured. The coloration of the wings and the short, stout, three-segmented antennae, which have no arista, are useful in differentiating the three major genera of Tabanidae (Fig. 11.45).

The mouthparts, which are adapted for slashing/sponging, are short and strong and always point downwards. Most prominent is the stout labium, which is grooved dorsally to take the other mouthparts, collectively termed the biting fascicle. The labium is also expanded terminally as paired large labella, which carry tubes called pseudotracheae, through which blood or fluid from wounds is aspirated. The biting fascicle, which creates the wound, consists of six elements, the upper sharp labrum, the hypopharynx with its salivary duct, paired rasp-like maxillae and paired broad pointed mandibles. Male flies have no mandibles and therefore cannot feed on blood. They instead feed on honeydew and the juice of flowers.

Description, larvae: These are spindle-shaped and off-white in colour and clearly segmented. The cuticle has distinct longitudinal striations. Mature larvae may be 15–30 mm in length. There is a distinct head capsule and strong biting mandibles. Abdominal segments have unsegmented leg-like structures (pseudopods)

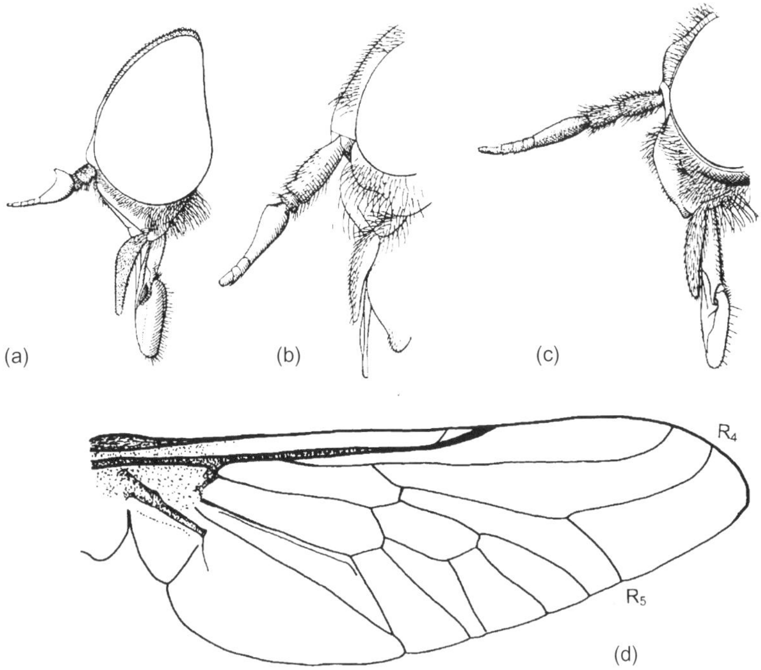

Fig. 11.45 Antennae of (a) *Chrysops*, (b) *Haematopota* and (c) *Tabanus*. (d) Wing venation of Tabanidae (reproduced from Smart, 1943).

for locomotion (four pairs in *Tabanus* and three pairs in *Chrysops*). A distinct posterior respiratory siphon is usually present, which may be greatly elongated.

Life cycle: After a blood meal the female lays batches of 100–1000 creamy white or greyish cigar-shaped eggs, 1.0–2.5 mm long, on the underside of vegetation or on stones, generally in muddy or marshy areas. The eggs hatch in 1–2 weeks, using a special spine to exit the egg case, and the cylindrical, poorly differentiated larvae drop into the mud or water. The larvae are 1.0–60 mm in length, and have 11 segments. They are recognised as tabanids by their small black retractable heads and the prominent raised rings around the segments, most of which bear pseudopods. They also have a structure in the last segment, unique to tabanid larvae, known as Graber's organ, the function of which may be sensory. They are sluggish and feed either by scavenging on decaying organic matter or by predation on small arthropods including other tabanid larvae. Optimally, larval development takes 3 months, but, if overwintering occurs, may extend for up to 3 years. The subcylindrical pupa is brown, the abdominal segments are movable and the anterior part of the appendages of the adult can be distinguished. Mature larvae pupate while partially buried in mud or soil and the adult fly emerges after 1–3 weeks. In most species, males complete their pupation before females. After emergence the male pursues the female and mating, initiated in the air, is completed on the ground. Adults are strong fliers and are usually diurnal. The whole life cycle takes a minimum of 4–5 months or longer if larval development is prolonged.

Populations of adult flies show seasonal fluctuations in both temperate and tropical areas. In temperate climates adults die in the autumn and are replaced by new populations the following spring and summer, whereas in tropical areas their numbers are merely reduced during the dry season with an increase at the start of the rainy season.

Although the female flies feed mostly on blood from their hosts, if a suitable host is unavailable they will consume honeydew and plant sap (the major food source of males who lack mandibles). They typically bite a number of times in different places before they are replete and the wounds created continue to bleed and may attract other flies. Adults feed approximately every 3 hours during the day and between feeding rest on the underside of leaves or on stones or trees.

Tabanus spp

Common name: Horseflies

Predilection site: Skin

Parasite class: Insecta

Family: Tabanidae

Description: Species of the genus *Tabanus* have transparent wings. Also useful in generic differentiation are the characteristics of short, stout, three-segmented antennae, which have no arista. In species of the genus *Tabanus* the first two antennal segments are small and the terminal segment has a tooth-like projection on its basal part and four annulations (Fig. 11.45).

Geographical distribution: Worldwide

Pathogenesis: The adult females locate their prey mainly by sight and their bites are deep and painful. They feed every 3–4 days causing a great deal of annoyance. The pain caused by their bites leads to interrupted feeding, and as a consequence flies may feed on a succession of hosts. They are therefore important in the mechanical transmission of a range of pathogens such as anthrax, pasteurellosis, trypanosomosis, anaplasmosis and the human filarial disease, loaosis.

Epidemiology: These powerful flies may disperse many kilometres from their breeding areas and are most active during hot, sunny days.

Notes: In North America in particular, several species of the genus *Tabanus* are particularly important pests. These are *Tabanus atratus* (the black horse fly), *Tabanus lineola* and *Tabanus similis* in the eastern states. In the western USA, *Tabanus punctifer* and *Tabanus sulcifrons* are of particular importance. Other common species are *Tabanus quinquevittatus* and *Tabanus nigrovittatus*, which are well known in North America as 'greenheads'.

Chrysops spp

Common name: Horseflies, deerflies

Predilection site: Preferred feeding sites are the underside of the abdomen, the legs, neck and withers.

Parasite class: Insecta

Family: Tabanidae

Description: *Chrysops* have dark banded wings, which are divergent when at rest. The wing venation is characteristic, especially the branching of the fourth-longitudinal vein (Fig. 11.45).

Geographical distribution: Worldwide, primarily in the Holarctic and Oriental regions

Pathogenesis: *Chrysops* species are responsible for the mechanical transmission of several diseases and pathogens. *Chrysops discalis* is a vector of *Pasteurella tularensis* in North America. *C. dimidiata*, the mango fly, and *C. siacea* are intermediate hosts of the filariid nematode, *Loa loa*. A number of *Chrysops* species also transmit *Trypanosoma evansi*, the causative agent of surra in equines and dogs; *T. equinum* the cause of mal de Caderas of equines; *T. simiae* of pigs; *T. vivax* and *T. brucei* which cause nagana of equines, cattle, sheep and other ungulates; and *T. gambiense* and *T. rhodesiense* which cause human African trypanosomiasis.

Haematopota spp

Common name: Horseflies, clegs

Predilection site: Skin

Parasite class: Insecta

Family: Tabanidae

Description: *Haematopota* have characteristically mottled wings that are held divergent when at rest. In *Haematopota* the first antennal segment is large and the second segment narrower, while the terminal segment has three annulations (Fig. 11.45).

Geographical distribution: Worldwide, although there are no *Haematopota* species in Australia. There are five species of *Haematopota* in the Nearctic region; *Haematopota americana* is of the greatest veterinary importance in America and *H. pluvialis* in Europe.

Pathogenesis: *Haematopota* species may feed on a number of hosts in rapid succession. They may therefore act as important mechanical vectors in the transmission of pathogens such as anthrax, pasteurellosis, trypanosomosis, anaplasmosis and the human filarial disease, loaosis.

Epidemiology: These powerful flies may disperse many kilometres from their breeding areas and are most active during hot, sunny days.

TSETSE FLIES

Glossina spp

Common name: Tsetse flies

Predilection site: Skin

Parasite class: Insecta

Family: Glossinidae

Description: In general, adult tsetse are narrow, yellow to dark brown flies, 6–15 mm in length, and have a long, rigid, forward-projecting proboscis (Fig. 11.46). There are 23 known species. When at rest, the wings are held over the abdomen like a closed pair of scissors. The thorax is a dull greenish brown colour and is marked with inconspicuous stripes and spots. The abdomen is brown, with six segments that are visible

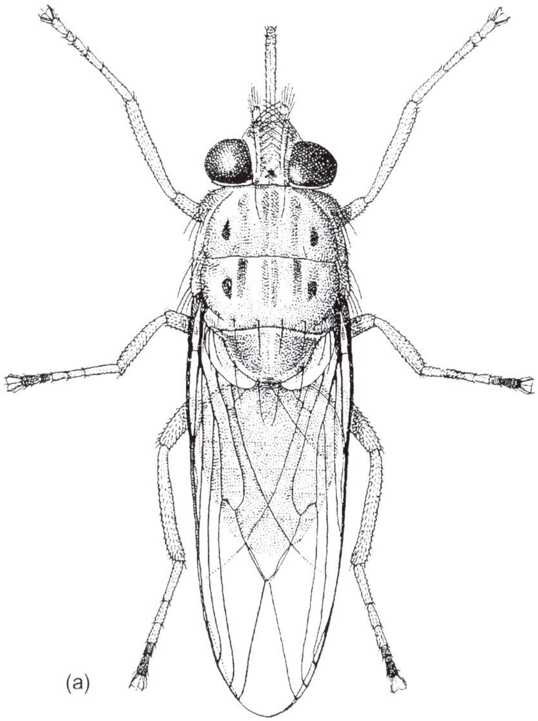

(a)

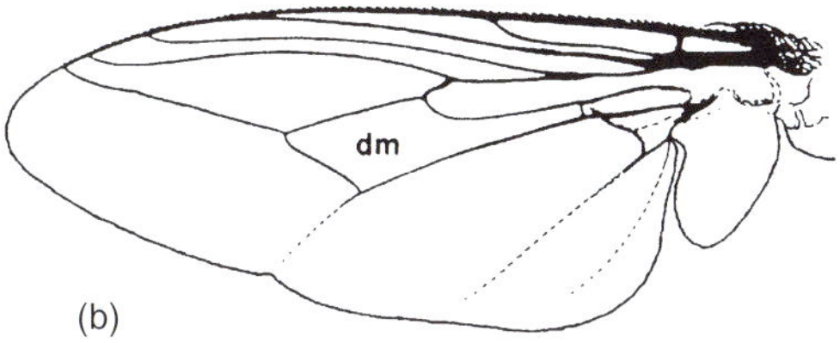

(b)

Fig. 11.46 (a) Male tsetse fly, *Glossina longipennis*. (b) Wing venation typical of species of *Glossina*, showing the characteristic hatchet shape of the cell dm (reproduced from Smart, 1943).

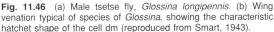

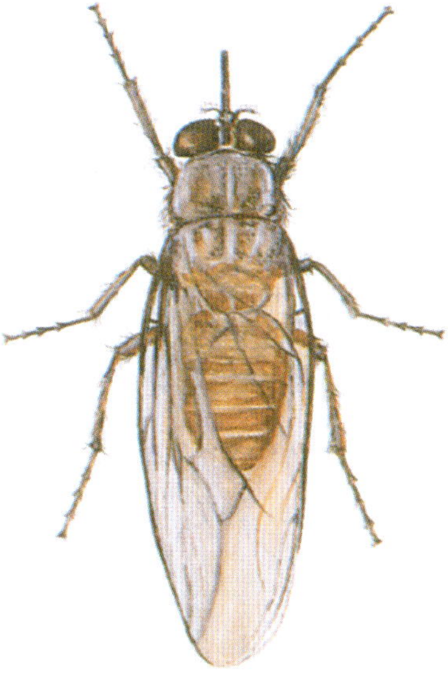

Fig. 11.47 *Glossina* spp.

form the dorsal aspect (Fig. 11.47). Tsetse flies are easily distinguished from all other flies by the characteristic hatchet-shaped medial cell in the wings. The antenna has a large third segment, with an arista that bears 17–29 dorsal branching hairs.

There are no maxillae or mandibles in the mouthparts of tsetse flies and the long proboscis is adapted for piercing and sucking. The proboscis is composed of a lower U-shaped labium with rasp-like labella terminally and an upper narrower labrum, which together create a food channel. Within this food channel sits the slender hypopharynx that carries saliva and anticoagulant down into the wound formed during feeding. The proboscis is held horizontally between long palps, which are of an even thickness throughout.

The 23 known species of tsetse flies can be divided into three groups, each with different habits and requirements. The *Glossina palpalis* group are riverine species, which feed primarily on reptiles and ungulates. Flies of the *G. morsitans* group are savannah and dry thorn-bush species, which feed mainly on large animals. Members of the *G. fusca* group occur in the rainforest, preferring dense shade and riverine thickets.

Hosts: Various mammals, reptiles and birds

Life cycle: Both male and female flies suck blood and although the various species of tsetse may have some host preferences, generally they will feed on a wide variety of animals.

The females, in contrast to other muscids, are viviparous. They ovulate a single egg at a time. The fertilised egg is retained in the oviduct, where it hatches after about 4 days at 25°C. The larva is retained in the common oviduct (uterus) where it is nourished with secretions from the highly specialised accessory glands. Maturation in the uterus from fertilised egg to the mobile, 8.0–10 mm long, third-stage larva takes approximately 10 days. At this stage the larva is creamy white, segmented and posteriorly has a pair of prominent dark ear-shaped protuberances known as polypneustic lobes. During the development of the third-stage larva these lobes protrude from the posterior abdomen of the adult female and have a respiratory function similar to the posterior spiracles of other muscid larvae.

When mature, the larva is deposited on to the ground by the adult female, usually into characteristic areas of bare, sandy soil under shade. After deposition the larva wriggles into loose soil to a depth of a few centimetres and forms a rigid dark brown, barrel-shaped puparium within 1–2 hours. The pupal period is relatively long, taking 4–5 weeks, or even more in cool weather. On emergence the adult is unable to fly until its wings have expanded. It takes at least a week for the complete endocuticle to be secreted and for the exocuticle to harden fully. The female fly may require several blood meals over a period of 16–20 days before producing her first larva. Once fully active the adult flies feed every 2–3 days and the first larviposition occurs 9–12 days after emergence.

Breeding generally continues throughout the year, with peak fly numbers occurring at the end of the rainy season. The longevity of adult flies in nature is variable, ranging from a few days to several months.

Geographical distribution: These flies are confined to a belt of tropical Africa extending from the southern Sahara (Lat. 5°N) in the north to Zimbabwe and Mozambique in the south (Lat. 20–30°S). The various species are restricted to different geographical areas according to habitat.

Pathogenesis: Although the bites of tsetse flies are very painful and cause marked irritation, their main significance is in the transmission of animal and human trypanosomiasis, described as nagana or sleeping sickness respectively. Flies become infected with protozoan trypanosome parasites during feeding and these then undergo multiplication and maturation within the fly. The fly is then infective to other hosts during subsequent feeding.

Clinical signs: Host animals may scratch and rub bite wound sites, which may result in significant skin trauma.

The symptoms of tsetse-transmitted trypanosomiasis include hyperthermia, anaemia, rapid emaciation, oedema of the lower parts of the abdomen and thorax, joints and genitalia, keratitis and nasal discharge. Paralysis may also occur.

Diagnosis: Observation and identification of the adult flies feeding on the host animal. The flies are most active at dawn and dusk.

Epidemiology: The normal hosts of tsetse flies are African wild, large mammals and reptiles, which experience few or no ill effects from the presence of the trypanosomes in their blood unless subject to stresses such as starvation. These wild animals act as reservoirs of the disease. When humans or domestic animals become infected, however, the pathogenic effects of the trypanosomes can be debilitating or fatal unless treated.

Treatment: Dipping cattle in pyrethroid insecticides such as deltamethrin can effectively protect against tsetse feeding. Trypanocidal drugs can be used to treat trypanosome infection.

Control: In the past, campaigns against tsetse flies to control trypanosomiasis both in humans and in animals depended mainly on large-scale killing of the game animals that act as reservoirs of trypanosome infection and as a source of blood for the flies. It was also common to clear large areas of bush in order to destroy the habitats of the adult flies. These methods were fairly successful, but are now largely unacceptable on ecological and economic grounds.

Currently, most anti-tsetse measures rely on the use of insecticides applied from the ground or by aircraft. When the objective is complete eradication of *Glossina*, residual formulations of insecticides are used. It is also essential that the area to be sprayed has economic potential and that agricultural development of the cleared area should proceed contemporaneously. Local eradication of tsetse populations is possible because of the relatively low rate of tsetse reproduction but, because of the inevitable reinvasion of tsetse from surrounding untreated areas, is uneconomic unless the selected area is on the edge of a tsetse belt where the fly population is already under stress because of relatively unfavourable climatic conditions. Advocates of insecticidal spraying argue that, since *Glossina* is highly susceptible to the insecticides used, the sophisticated and selective use of modern chemicals, usually on one occasion only, has no major and permanent effects on the environment. In fact they point out that the changes in land use which should ensue from successful control are much more significant in this respect.

Populations of tsetse flies have been reduced or eradicated in localised areas by the use of traps. These have the advantages of being cheap, can be used by local labour and are harmless to the environment. Essentially they depend on the presentation of a material, such as dark cloth, which attracts the flies and leads into a trap that often incorporates an insecticide. Volatile chemical odours, such as acetone octenol or cattle urine, placed in or near traps attract flies and increase the number caught. However, traps are relatively difficult to deploy and maintain in densely vegetated areas of bush.

Some breeds of domestic livestock such as N'dama cattle are relatively trypanotolerant.

Notes: Key species in the *fusca* and *palpalis* groups include *G. palpalis*, *G. austeni*, *G. fuscipes* and *G. tachinoides* while key species in the *morsitans* group include *G. morsitans and G. palidipes.*

CULICIDAE: MOSQUITOES

The mosquitoes, family Culicidae, are a diverse group of over 3000 species. They occur worldwide from the tropics to the arctic. There are three genera of medical and veterinary importance: these are *Anopheles*, *Aedes* and *Culex*. There are about 900 species in the genus *Aedes*.

Common name: Mosquito

Predilection site: Skin

Parasite class: Insecta

Family: Culicidae

Description: Mosquitoes vary from 2–10 mm in length and have slender bodies, prominent eyes and long legs (Fig. 11.48). The long, narrow wings are held crossed flat over the abdomen at rest and bear scales, which project as a fringe on the posterior margin. The mouthparts consist of a conspicuous, forward-projecting, elongated proboscis adapted for piercing and sucking. Individual elements comprise a long, U-shaped, fleshy labium containing paired maxillae, mandibles and a hypopharynx, which carries a salivary duct that delivers anticoagulant into the host's tissues (Fig. 1.25). The labrum forms the roof of the proboscis. All the elements, with the exception of the labium, enter the skin during feeding by the females, forming a tube through which blood is sucked. In the non-parasitic males the maxillae and mandibles are reduced or absent. The maxillary palps of different species are variable in length and morphology. Both sexes have long filamentous, segmented antennae, pilose in females and plumose in males.

Geographical distribution: Worldwide

Life cycle: The larvae of all species are aquatic and occur in a wide variety of habitats, ranging from extensive areas such as marshes to smaller areas; the edge of permanent pools, marshes, puddles, flooded treeholes and even, for some species, temporary water-filled containers (Fig. 11.49). However, they are usually absent from large tracts of uninterrupted water, such as lakes, and from fast-flowing streams or rivers. Mosquito larvae are known as wrigglers and require between 3 and 20 days to pass through four stadia. Hatching is temperature-dependent and occurs after several days or weeks, but in some temperate species eggs may overwinter. All four larval stages are aquatic. There is a distinct head with one pair of antennae, compound eyes and prominent mouth brushes, used in feeding on organic material (Fig. 11.48). Maturation of larvae can extend from 1 week to several months, and several species overwinter as larvae in temperate areas.

With the final larval moult, the pupal stage occurs. Mosquito pupae (known as tumblers) usually remain at the water surface, but when disturbed can be highly mobile. All mosquito pupae are aquatic, motile and

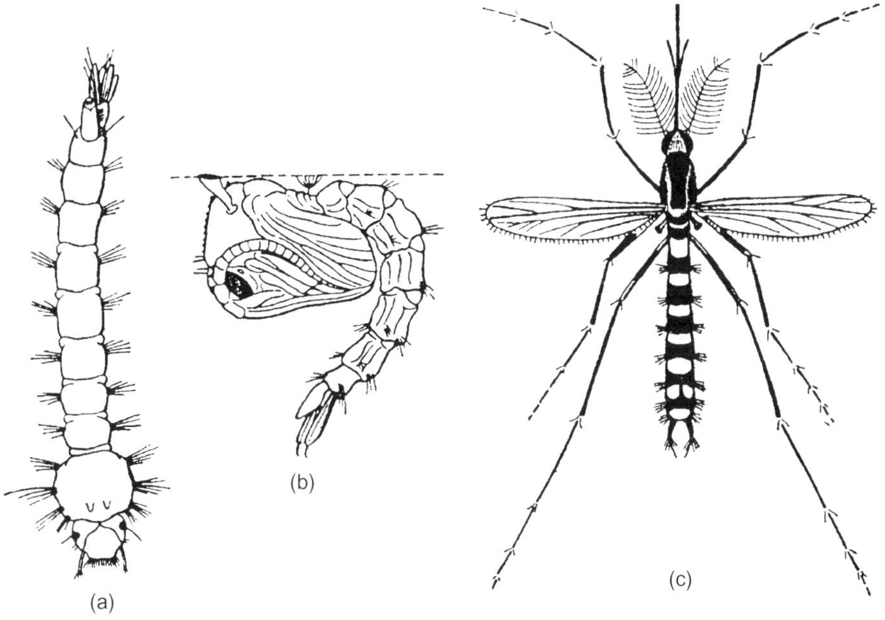

Fig. 11.48 *Aedes atropalpus*: (a) Larva. (b) Pupa. (c) Adult (reproduced from Eidmann and Kuhlhorn, 1970).

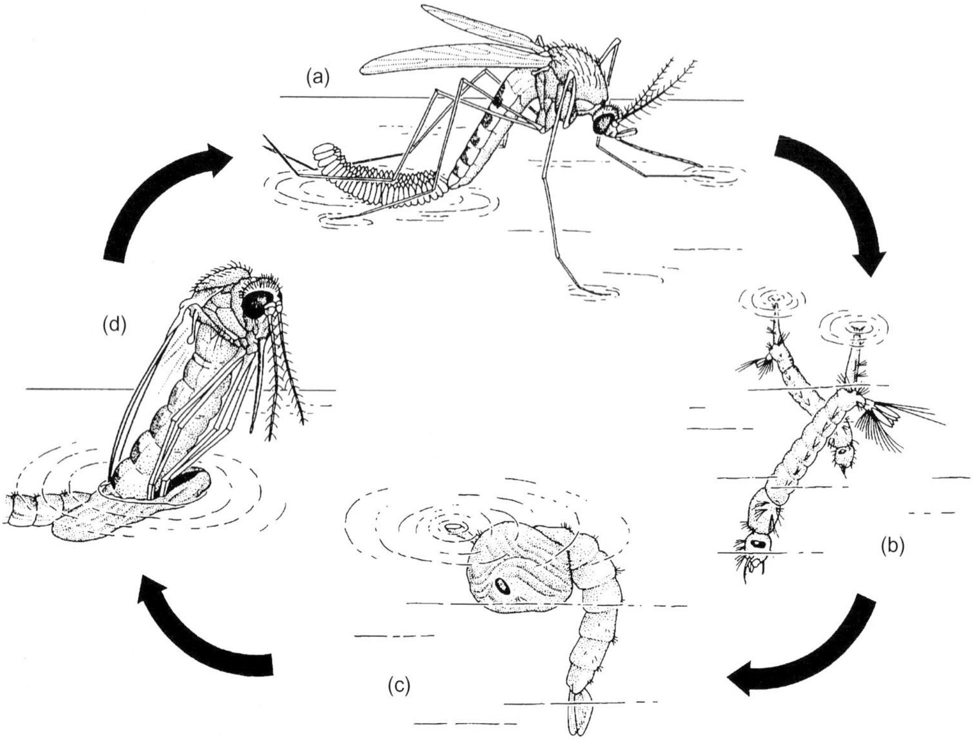

Fig. 11.49 Life cycle of the mosquito *Culex pipiens*. (a) Adult ovipositing. (b) Larvae at the water surface. (c) Pupa suspended from the water surface. (d) Adult emerging from its pupal case at the water surface (reproduced from Gullan and Cranston, 1994).

comma-shaped, with a distinct cephalothorax that bears a pair of respiratory trumpets (Fig. 11.48). The tegument of the cephalothorax is transparent and the eyes, legs and other structures of the developing adult are readily visible. The tapering abdominal segments have short hairs, and terminally there is a pair of oval, paddle-like extensions, which enable the pupa to move up and down in the water. Generally the pupal stage is short; only a few days in the tropics and several weeks or longer in temperate regions. The adult emerges through a dorsal split in the pupal tegument. Adults usually only fly up to a few hundred metres from their breeding sites, but may be dispersed long distances by winds. Although the lifespan of adult flies is generally short, some species can overwinter by hibernating.

When adult mosquitoes emerge from the pupal case they crawl to a nearby object, where they harden their cuticle and inflate their wings. Mating normally occurs within 24 hours of emergence and is completed in flight. One insemination is usually sufficient for the fertilisation of all eggs. For normal activity and flight, mosquitoes feed on nectar and plant juices, but females are anautogenous; they need an initial blood-meal to develop their ovaries and must feed again between each egg batch matured. A female mosquito will live for an average of 2–3 weeks, while the male's lifespan is shorter.

Mosquitoes are nocturnal or crepuscular feeders with a wide host range. Host selection is extremely opportunistic and is largely influenced by the relative abundance of hosts found in the habitat. Host location is achieved using a range of olfactory and visual cues, orientation to wind direction and body warmth. Oviposition begins as soon as a suitable site is located. Adult mosquitoes are strong fliers.

Pathogenesis: Mosquitoes may cause considerable annoyance by biting. Mosquito populations can reach large sizes, especially in parts of the southern USA, and the persistent feeding activity of adult females may cause considerable nuisance and reduce the productivity of livestock. Females preferentially feed on large mammals and are so persistent that livestock will be driven away from areas where they are numerous. Sensitivity to mosquito bites varies with individuals; most hosts will suffer only a minor reaction, showing local swelling, redness and irritation. Other hosts can exhibit severe hypersensitivity reactions to mosquito saliva and, if the bites are scratched, a secondary bacterial infection may ensue.

Epidemiology: In temperate climates the population size peaks during the summer, while in tropical countries large populations are usually present all year round.

Clinical signs: The bite of mosquitoes may cause a localised inflammatory reaction with intense itching. Sensitivity to mosquito bites varies with individuals; most hosts will suffer only a minor reaction, showing local swelling, redness and irritation. Other hosts can exhibit severe hypersensitivity reactions to mosquito saliva and, if the bites are scratched, a secondary bacterial infection may ensue.

Diagnosis: The bite appears as a reddened, raised area on the skin.

Treatment: Although synthetic pyrethroids have been available for some time as short-acting space sprays, some are now being developed as residual insecticides. Insecticides with a residual action are effective against the adult stages, particularly if applied indoors. Organophosphorous compounds and carbamates are recommended for this purpose.

Control: Measures, largely developed for the control of human malaria, are directed either against the developing larvae or adults, or against both simultaneously. The various measures used against larvae include the removal or reduction of available breeding sites by drainage or other means, which makes these sites unsuitable for larval development. This is not always practicable, economical or acceptable and the feasibility of these methods must always be assessed locally. Biological control has been attempted by, for example, introducing predatory fish into marshy areas and rice fields, but these methods are unsuitable for those mosquito species breeding in small temporary collections of water. The isolation and development of mosquito pathogens including microorganisms, protozoa and nematodes is mainly experimental at present, as are genetic methods of control.

Probably the most widely used measures against mosquito larvae are those which involve the repeated application of toxic chemicals, mineral oils or insecticides to breeding sites, but these have to be continuously applied. Since such measures may lead to environmental pollution and may also accelerate the development of insecticide resistance, the only permanent solution is the destruction of breeding sites. Essential water sources can be rendered unsuitable as breeding sites by spreading inert polystyrene beads to cover the surface of the water.

Fly-screens, nets and repellents are available for protection.

Aedes spp

Common name: Mosquito

Predilection site: Skin

Parasite class: Insecta

Family: Culicidae

Sub-family: Culicinae

Description: The genus *Aedes* belongs to the subfamily Culicinae. The culicine adult rests with its body angled and its abdomen directed towards the surface (Fig. 11.50). The palps of female culicine mosquitoes are usually only about one quarter of the length of the proboscis.

Hosts: A wide variety of mammals (including humans), reptiles and birds

Life cycle: After a blood meal the gravid female lays up to 300 eggs singly on the surface of water. The eggs are dark coloured, either elongate or ovoid, and cannot survive desiccation. Most species of *Aedes* lay their eggs on moist substrates rather than on the water itself, where they mature and await adequate water to stimulate hatching. In some cases the eggs may remain viable for up to 3 years. Despite some degree of temperature tolerance, freezing and temperatures in excess of 40°C will kill most eggs. In *Aedes* spp, larvae take in air through a pair of spiracles situated at the end of a small tube called the respiratory siphon.

Geographical distribution: Worldwide

Pathogenesis: More than 20 species of mosquito can be vectors of the dog heartworm, *Dirofilaria immitis*, although this occurs mainly in tropical and subtropical regions. Species of *Aedes* transmit avian malaria, caused by *Plasmodium*. Mosquitoes can act as vectors of various viral diseases, including arboviruses, such as equine encephalitis (a togavirus), rabbit myxomatosis and infectious equine anaemia (a retrovirus). *Aedes* spp transmit yellow fever and the human filarial nematodes, *Wuchereria* and *Brugia*.

Species of importance: *Aedes sierrensis* is one of the main carriers of *Dirofilaria immitis* and will attack mammals of all sizes. A particularly important aggressive biting species is *Aedes vigilex*. *Aedes taeniorhynchus*, *Ae. sollicitans*, *Ae. vexans* and *Ae. dorsalis* may be important vectors of the equine encephalitis virus.

Anopheles spp

Common name: Mosquito

Predilection site: Skin

Parasite class: Insecta

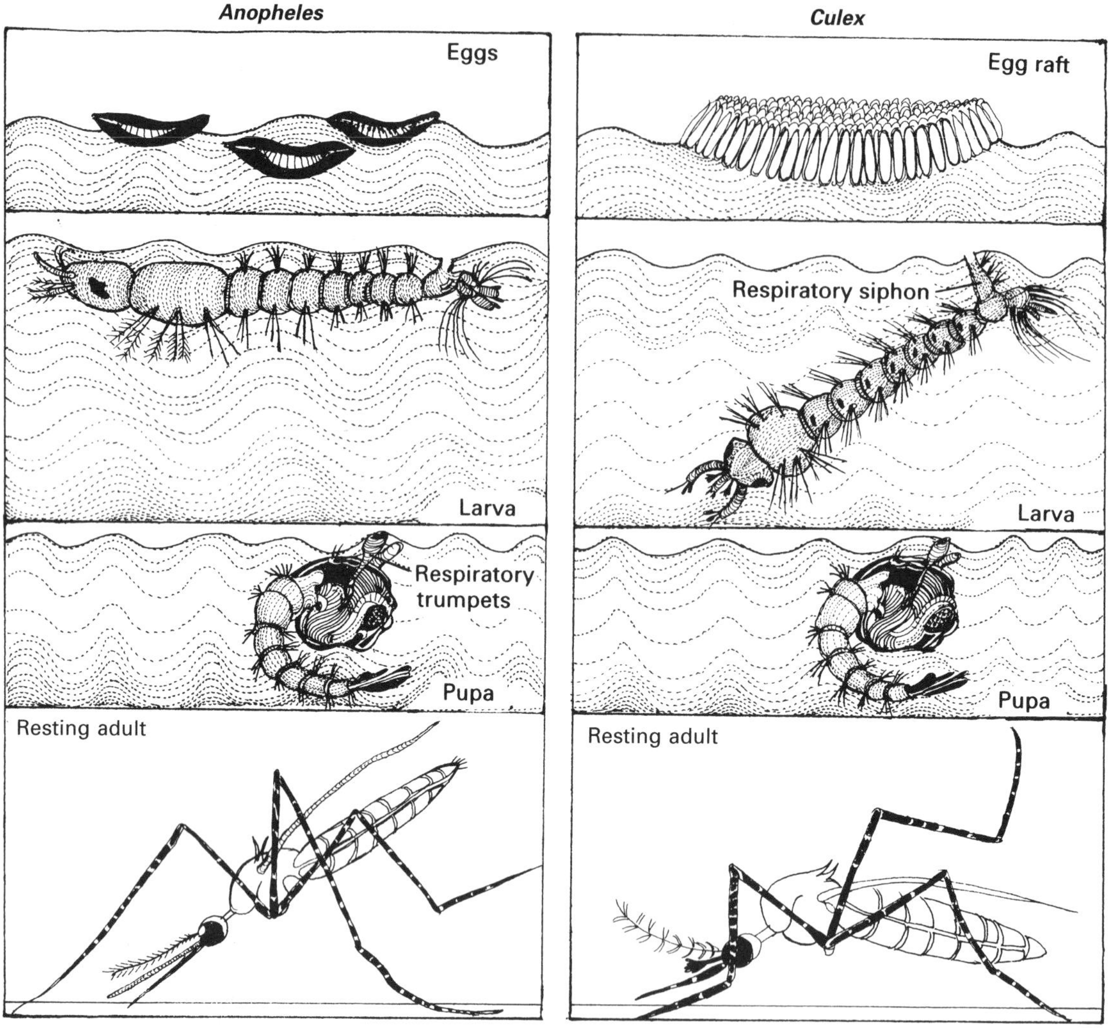

Fig. 11.50 The comparative life cycles of anopheline and culicine mosquitoes.

Family: Culicidae

Sub-family: Anophilinae

Description: Living anopheline adults can readily be distinguished from culicines, such as *Aedes* and *Culex*, when resting on a flat surface. On landing, anopheline mosquitoes rest with the proboscis, head, thorax and abdomen in one straight line at an angle to the surface (Fig. 11.50). The palps of female anopheline mosquitoes are as long and straight as the proboscis. The abdomen of *Anopheles* bears hairs but not scales.

Life cycle: The eggs are dark coloured, boat-shaped, and possess characteristic lateral floats that prevent them from sinking and maintain their orientation in the water. Such eggs usually hatch within 2 or 3 days and cannot survive desiccation. Most larvae of *Anopheles* lie parallel to the water surface and take in air through a pair of spiracles on the penultimate abdominal segment.

Pathogenesis: Species of *Anopheles* transmit the dog heartworm, *Dirofilaria immitis*. Mosquitoes are also important in the transmission of the arboviruses (arthropod-borne) causing eastern, western and Venezuelan encephalitis in horses and other arbovirus diseases of man and animals. The genus *Anopheles* contains the only known vectors of human malaria, and transmits the human filarial nematodes, *Wuchereria* and *Brugia*.

Culex spp

Common name: Mosquitoes

Predilection site: Skin

Parasite class: Insecta

Family: Culicidae

Sub-family: Culicinae

Description: The genus *Culex* belongs to the sub-family Culicinae. The culicine adult rests with its body angled and its abdomen directed towards the surface (Fig. 11.50). The palps of female culicine mosquitoes are usually only about one quarter of the length of the proboscis.

Life cycle: In species of the genus *Culex*, eggs are laid in groups forming 'egg-rafts'. A female *Culex* mosquito may lay a raft of eggs every third night during its lifetime, hence oviposition typically occurs around six or seven times. When the eggs mature they will hatch into larvae regardless of the availability of water. The eggs are dark coloured and either elongate or ovoid. Hatching is temperature-dependent and occurs after several days to weeks, but in some temperate species eggs may overwinter. All four larval stages are aquatic. In *Culex* spp larvae take in air through a pair of spiracles situated at the end of a small tube called the respiratory siphon.

Geographical distribution: Worldwide

Pathogenesis: Culicines are important vectors of a range of arboviruses. Species of *Culex* transmit both the dog heartworm, *Dirofilaria immitis* and avian malaria caused by *Plasmodium*. They also act as vectors for the filarid worm *Setaria labiatopapillosa*, cause of ovine abdominal filariosis, *Setaria equina*, the equine abdominal worm, and *Setaria congolensis* in pigs.

Species of importance: *Culex tarsalis* is the most important carrier of western equine and Saint Louis encephalitis in California and the western USA. It is frequently found living alongside wild birds, the natural reservoir of infection. *C. pipiens molustus* is a 'bridge vector' and can transmit west Nile virus (WNV) to mammals including humans.

CULICOIDES: MIDGES

Predilection site: Skin

Parasite class: Insecta

Family: Ceratopogonidae

Description: Insects within the large nematoceran family, the Ceratopogonidae, are known as the biting midges. The family contains one main genus of veterinary interest, *Culicoides*. *Culicoides* biting midges are among the most abundant of haematophagous insects, with over 1000 species that feed on birds or mammals, inflicting a painful bite. They transmit many disease pathogens and, most importantly, act as vectors of more than 50 arboviruses.

Culicoides midge adults are 1.5–5.0 mm in length with the thorax humped over a small head (Fig. 11.51). The wings are generally mottled in pattern, and at rest are held like a closed pair of scissors over the grey or brownish black abdomen. The legs are relatively short, particularly the forelegs, and the small mouthparts hang vertically. The short piercing proboscis consists of a sharp labrum, two maxillae, two mandibles, a hypopharynx and a fleshy labium, which does not enter the skin during feeding by the adult female. In the male, the long antennae are feathery or plumose, whereas those of the female possess only short hairs and are known as pilose antennae. Microscopic hairs cover the wings. Ceratopogonids have a forked medial vein (M_1, M_2) and species of the genus *Culicoides* usually have a distinct pattern of radial cells and an r-m cross-vein on their wings (Fig. 11.51).

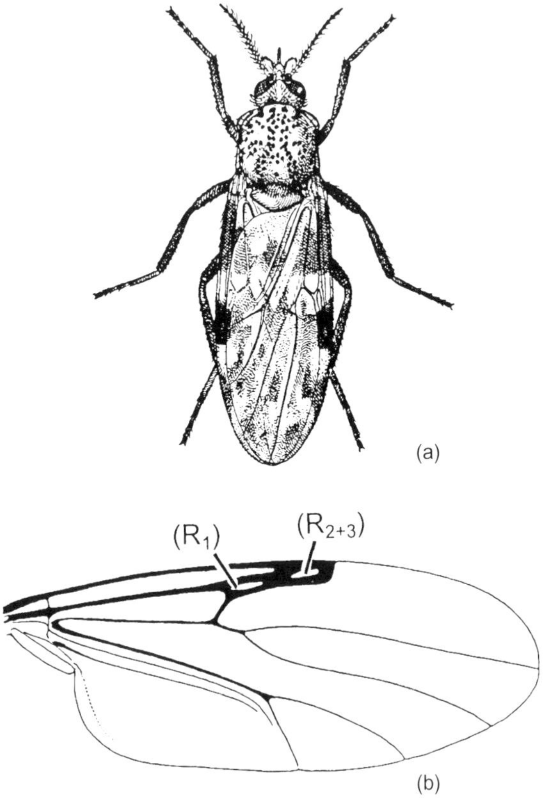

Fig. 11.51 (a) Adult female *Culicoides nebeculosus* at rest. (b) Wing venation typical of species of *Culicoides*, showing the two elongate radial cells (reproduced from Edwards *et al.*, 1939).

Hosts: All domestic animals and humans

Life cycle: The eggs, which are brown or black, are cylindrical or banana-shaped and 0.5 mm in length. Eggs are laid in damp marshy ground or in decaying vegetable matter near water. Hatching occurs in 2–9 days depending on the species and temperature, but temperate species may overwinter as eggs. There are four larval stages and these are characterised by having small dark heads, segmented bodies and terminal anal gills. They have a serpentine swimming action in water and feed on decaying vegetation. Larval development is complete in warm countries in 14–25 days, but in temperate areas this may be delayed for periods of up to 7 months. The less active brown pupae, 2.0–4.0 mm long, are found at the surface or edges of water and are characterised by a pair of respiratory trumpets on the cephalothorax and a pair of terminal horns that enable the pupa to move. Adult flies emerge from the pupae in 3–10 days.

Only females blood-feed and inflict a painful bite. Adult *Culicoides* are not strong fliers and they are usually found close to larval habitats in small and inconspicuous swarms. Adult *Culicoides* feed especially in dull, humid weather and tend to be crepuscular and nocturnal. Females are attracted to the smell and warmth of their hosts and different species may be host specific to varying degrees.

Geographical distribution: Worldwide

Pathogenesis: In large numbers, biting midges can be a serious source of irritation and annoyance to livestock. The main areas affected are usually the head and neck. The biting of midges has been linked to an immediate-type hypersensitivity reaction which causes an intensely pruritic skin disease of horses, described as seasonal equine pruritic dermatitis. Symptoms include pruritus, crusting and alopecia of the face, ears, withers, mane, rump and tail. The lesions are exacerbated by self-trauma and scratching, resulting in hyperpigmentation and skin thickening. This is one of the most common allergic skin diseases in horses worldwide; it is known as 'sweet itch' in the UK and 'Queensland itch' in Australia. In the UK, the disease is particularly a problem of native ponies and the tendency to develop a hypersensitivity reaction is likely to be inherited. Several species are involved in this condition, *C. pulicaris* in Europe, *C. robertsi* in Australia and *C. insignis*, *C. stelifer* and *C. venustus* in the USA.

Culicoides biting midges act as vectors of more than 50 arboviruses, which are transmitted across their broad host range, including those responsible for the important livestock diseases causing blue tongue in sheep, African horse sickness, bovine ephemeral fever and, in the USA, eastern equine encephalitis. Species of *Culicoides* may act as mechanical vectors for the filaroid nematodes *Onchocerca reticulata* and *Onchocerca gibsoni* to cattle, *Onchocerca cervicalis* to horses and several species of protozoa (*Haemoproteus*, *Leucocytozoon*) to poultry and other birds.

Clinical signs: The host animal's reaction to a bite of a *Culicoides* midge typically consists of a localised stinging or burning sensation and a well defined reddened area around the bite site. These may remain itchy from a few minutes to 2–3 days, and will cause the host animal to rub and scratch at the area.

Diagnosis: The bite of the adult flies leaves a characteristic reddened area and may remain itchy for several days. Flies may be seen on the host animal.

Epidemiology: *Culicoides* adults are crepuscular or nocturnal feeders, particularly prevalent in dull, humid weather. Flight activity can be influenced by temperature, light intensity, lunar cycles, relative humidity, wind velocity and other weather conditions. The mean distance travelled by *Culicoides* females is about 2 km, although males travel significantly shorter distances. Adult *Culicoides* are usually found close to larval habitats in small and inconspicuous swarms. Females are attracted to the smell and warmth of their hosts, and different species may be host specific to varying degrees, for example *C. brevitarsis* feeds mainly on cattle and *C. imicola* on horses.

There is a large number of species of *Culicoides* of varying importance as nuisance pests and vectors. Of particular note in Europe and Asia are *Culicoides pulicaris*, *Culicoides obsoletus* (a complex of four separate species), *Culicoides impunctatus* and *Culicoides sibirica*. *Culicoides imicola* is found throughout Africa and southern Europe and is the key vector of African horse sickness and blue tongue virus. In North America, *Culicoides furens* and *Culicoides denningi* inflict painful bites and *Culicoides variipennis* is the primary vector of blue tongue virus.

Treatment: Flies spend limited time on their hosts and are difficult to control using insecticides unless these have rapid killing or repellent ability. Applications of pyrethroid insecticides may give effective, though short-term, local control.

Control: This is difficult because of the usually extensive breeding habitat and depends on the destruction of breeding sites by drainage or spraying with insecticides. Repellents or screens may be used, but the latter have to be so fine that they may reduce air-flow, so screens impregnated with insecticides (originally designed to exclude larger flies) have been recommended instead. For 'sweet itch', antihistamine treatment may give immediate relief and the regular application of synthetic pyrethroid dressings may help prevent recurrence of the condition. It is also recommended that susceptible animals be housed when fly activity is maximal, usually in late afternoon and early morning.

Notes: Blue tongue virus (BTV) exists as a number of distinct serotypes, 24 of which have been recognised to date. These viruses can infect a wide range of ruminant species, but usually only cause severe disease in certain breeds of sheep, particularly the fine-fleeced species, such as Merino and Dorset Horn. In sheep it causes fever, enteritis, upper respiratory tract infection, ulceration of the tongue and lameness. BTV can cause very high mortality, in excess of 25%, and morbidity in excess of 75%. Blue tongue occurs generally in Africa, the Middle East, Asia, Australia and parts of North America, and serious outbreaks have occurred in the past 50 years in southern Europe. In one such outbreak, between 1956 and 1960, over 180 000 sheep died in Spain and Portugal. In the USA blue tongue is estimated to cost the livestock industry over US$100 million per year.

African horse sickness is caused by a retrovirus (AHSV) and is among the most lethal of equine diseases. It frequently causes mortality rates in excess of 90%. It is enzootic in Africa. A series of epizootics in Spain and Portugal from 1987 to the present have resulted in the deaths of over 3000 equines. *Culicoides imicola* is one of the members of the genus able to transmit the virus and occurs widely in Spain, Portugal and southern Greece.

Eastern equine encephalitis is a viral disease of horses and humans found only in the New World. It is caused by a species of the Alphavirus genus which is part of the Togaviridae. The disease is present throughout North and South America as far south as Argentina. The wild reservoir hosts are birds, and the primary midge vector is *Culicoides melanura*.

Bovine ephemeral fever, also known as 3-day sickness, is caused by an arbovirus. It is found throughout Africa, the Oriental region and occasionally causes epizootics in Australia. It affects cattle causing morbidity, but usually not mortality, resulting in reduced milk yields.

BLACKFLIES, BUFFALO GNATS

Simulium spp

Common name: Blackflies, buffalo gnats

Predilection site: Adult *Simulium* feed all over the body, but particularly the head, abdomen and legs.

Parasite class: Insecta

Family: Simuliidae

Description: More than 1700 species of blackflies have been described worldwide, although only 10–20% of these are regarded as pests of humans and their animals. As their common names indicate, these flies are usually black with a humped thorax. The adults are 1.5–5 mm in length, relatively stout-bodied, with broad, colourless wings that show indistinct venation and are held at rest like the closed blades of a pair of scissors. The wings are short, typically 1.5–6.5 mm long, broad with a large anal lobe and have veins, which are thickened at the anterior margin of the wing (Fig. 11.52). The first abdominal tergite is modified to form a prominent basal scale, fringed with fine hairs. Morphologically, adult male and female flies are similar, but can be differentiated by the fact that in the female the eyes are distinctly separated (dichoptic), whereas in males the eyes are very close together (holoptic) with characteristic enlarged ommatidia in

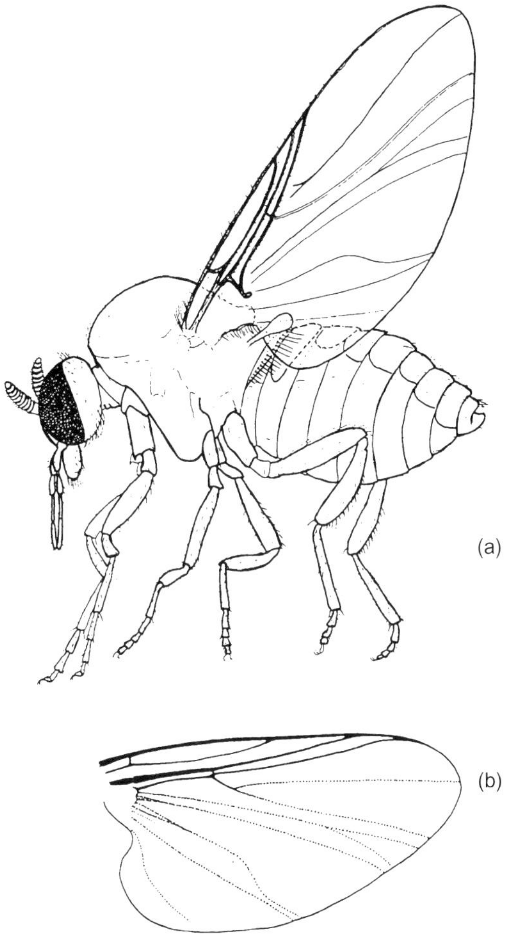

Fig. 11.52 (a) Adult female *Simulium*. (b) Wing venation typical of *Simulium*, showing the large anal lobe and crowding of the veins towards the leading edge (reproduced from Smart, 1943).

the upper part of the eye. This enables males to locate females against the blue backdrop of the sky. Compared with other closely related flies, the antennae, although 11-segmented, are relatively short, stout and devoid of bristles. The mouthparts resemble those of the biting midges except for the presence of conspicuous segmented maxillary palps. The body is covered with short golden or silvery hairs.

Hosts: Warm-blooded vertebrates

Life cycle: Eggs, 0.1–0.4 mm in length, are laid in sticky masses of 150–600 on partially submerged stones or vegetation in fast flowing water. Hatching takes only a few days in warm conditions, but may take weeks in temperate areas and in some species the eggs can overwinter. There may be up to eight larval stadia. The mature larvae are 5.0–13.0 mm long, light coloured and poorly segmented, and are distinguishable by a blackish head, which bears a prominent pair of feeding brushes (Fig. 11.53). The body is swollen posteriorly and just below the head is an appendage called the proleg, which bears hooks. Larvae normally remain attached to submerged vegetation or rocks by a circlet of posterior hooks, but may change their position in a looping manner by alternate use of the proleg and the posterior hooks. The larvae remain in areas of fast-flowing current, since they require highly oxygenated water to survive. They use the water current to passively filter feed on suspended debris and bacteria. In deoxygenated water, the larvae detach from their silken pads and drift downstream. Larval maturation takes from several weeks to several months, and in some species larvae can overwinter. Mature larvae pupate in a slipper-shaped brownish cocoon fixed to submerged objects. The pupa has prominent respiratory gills projecting from the cocoon. In the final stages of pupation, a film of air is secreted between the developing adult and the pupal cuticle. When the pupal case splits the emerging adult rises to the surface in a bubble of air and is able to fly away immediately. The pupal period is normally 2–6 days and a characteristic feature of many species is that there is simultaneous mass emergence of the adult flies, which gain the surface of the water and take flight. The duration of the life cycle, from egg to adult, is variable, depending on the species and water temperature. Typical longevity for adult blackflies ranges from 2–3 weeks to as long as 85 days. Adult flies feed on plant nectar, but in most species females require a blood-meal to obtain the protein necessary to mature their eggs.

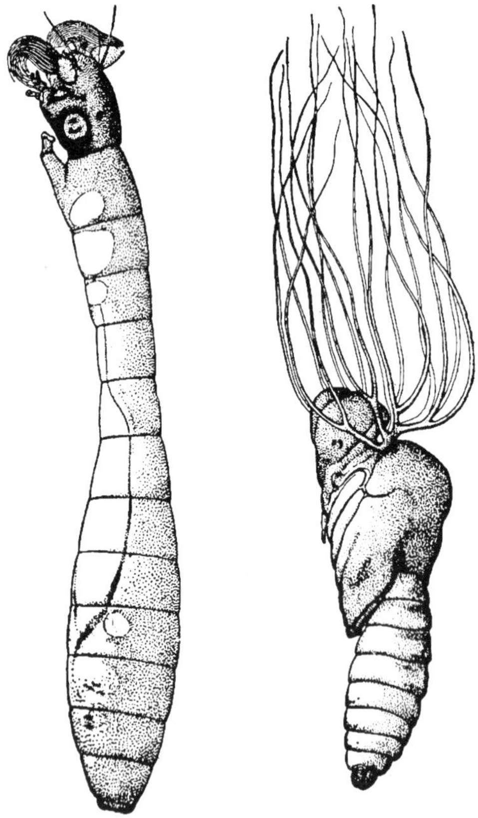
(a) (b)

Fig. 11.53 Immature stages of Simuliidae. (a) Larva. (b) Pupa. (Reproduced from Castellani and Chalmers, 1910.)

Geographical distribution: Worldwide except New Zealand, Hawaii and some minor island groups.

Pathogenesis and pathology: In domestic animals, especially cattle, mass attack by these flies may be associated with an acute syndrome characterised by generalised petechial haemorrhages, particularly in areas of fine skin, together with oedema of the larynx and abdominal wall. The painful bites of swarms of *Simulium* may interfere with grazing and cause production loss. In certain areas of central Europe it is often impossible to graze cattle during the spring due to the activity of these flies. Horses are often affected by the flies feeding inside the ears, and poultry may become anaemic from blood loss when attacked. Even at relatively low population densities the painful bites may cause considerable disturbance and reduced productivity. Some host animals may suffer from allergic reactions to saliva secreted by the flies as they feed. Certain areas of the tropics are rendered uninhabitable by *Simulium*.

Simulium spp may transmit the viruses causing eastern equine encephalitis and vesicular stomatitis and the avian protozoan *Leucocytozoon*. They also act as vectors for filarioid helminths, such as the nematodes *Onchocerca gutturosa* and *O. dukei* of cattle and *Onchocerca cervicalis* of horses. Bovine and equine onchocerciasis produce nodules containing adult worms in various regions of the skin, particularly the withers of cattle, resulting in hide damage. From a medical perspective Simuliidae are particularly important as vectors of the filaroid nematode *Onchocerca volvulus*, which causes river blindness in humans in Africa, Central and South America.

Clinical signs: Simulids cause severe irritation to livestock when they occur in large numbers and herds will often stampede. Bites are inflicted on all parts of the body and give rise to vesicles, which burst, exposing the underlying flesh. These skin wounds heal very slowly.

Diagnosis: The attacking swarms of adult flies are characteristic of most *Simulium* species. If the flies are seen on the host animal they may be collected and identified.

Epidemiology: Only the adult females blood-feed, and different species have different preferred feeding sites and times. Generally they feed on the legs, abdomen, head and ears, and most species are particularly active during the morning and evening in cloudy, warm weather. Although flies may be active throughout the year, there may be a large increase in their numbers in the tropics during the rainy season. In temperate and arctic regions the biting nuisance may be seasonal, since adults die in the autumn with new generations in spring and summer. The adult flies are found in swarms near free-running, well aerated streams, which are their breeding sites. Some rivers can produce nearly a billion flies per kilometre of riverbed per day. Adults are strong fliers and are highly responsive to carbon dioxide and other host-animal odours. They may fly as many as 4–8 miles in search of a host, before returning to the breeding site to commence oviposition.

Treatment: Flies spend limited time on their hosts and are difficult to control using insecticides unless these have rapid killing or repellent activity. Applications of pyrethroid insecticides may give effective, though short-term, local control.

Control: Blackfly control is extremely difficult since immature larval stages are found in running, well aerated water, often some distance from the farm or housing, and adult flies are capable of flying over 5 km. The most practical control method is the application of insecticides to breeding sites to kill larvae. This technique has been developed for the control of *Simulium* species, which are vectors of 'river blindness' in man in Africa, and entails the repeated application of insecticides to selected water-courses at intervals throughout the year. The insecticide is then carried downstream and kills larvae over long stretches of water.

Alternatively, bush clearing will remove adult resting sites and aerial application of insecticides may help in areas where breeding occurs in networks of small streams and watercourses. In horses, insecticides or repellents may be applied topically, and poultry can be provided with insecticidal dust baths.

Species of importance: Possibly the most damaging simuliid of temperate latitudes in the New World is *Simulium arcticum* which can be a major livestock pest in western Canada. Populations can reach densities which are high enough to kill cattle. In the USA, *Simulium venustum* and *Simulium vittatum* may be common and widespread pests of livestock, particularly common in June and July. *Simulium pecuarum*, the southern buffalo gnat, may cause losses in cattle in the Mississippi valley. The turkey gnat, *Simulium meridionale*, is common in southern USA and the Mississippi valley, where it may be a significant pest of poultry. *Simulium equinum*, *Simulium erythrocephalum* and *Simulium ornatum* may cause problems in western Europe and *Simulium kurenze* in Russia. Particularly damaging in central and southern Europe is *Simulium colombaschense*, which may cause heavy mortality of livestock.

SANDFLIES

Phlebotomus spp

Common name: Phlebotomine sandflies

Predilection site: Skin; sandflies primarily bite areas of exposed skin such as the ears, eyelids, nose, feet and tail

Parasite class: Insecta

Family: Psychodidae

Description, adults: These small flies, up to 5.0 mm long, are characterised by their hairy appearance, their large black eyes and long legs (Fig. 11.54). The wings, which, unlike those of other biting flies are lanceolate in outline, are also covered in hairs and are held erect over the body at rest. As in many other Nematoceran flies, the mouthparts are of short to medium length, hang downwards and are adapted for piercing and sucking. The maxillary palps are relatively conspicuous and consist of five segments. In both sexes the antennae are long, 16-segmented, filamentous and covered in fine setae.

Larvae: The mature larva is greyish white with a dark head. The head carries chewing mouthparts, which are used to feed on decaying organic matter. The antennae are small. The abdominal segments bear hairs and ventral, unsegmented leg-like structures (pseudopods) which are used in locomotion. A characteristic feature

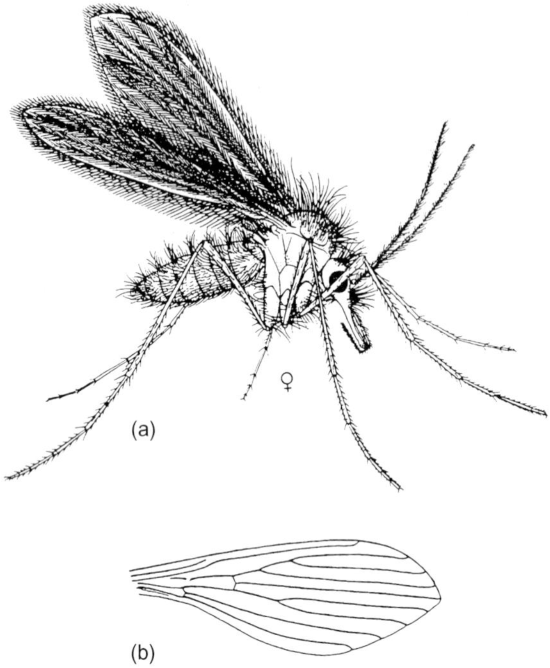

Fig. 11.54 (a) Adult female sandfly, *Phlebotomus papatasi*. (b) Wing venation typical of species of *Phlebotomus* (Psychodidae) (reproduced from Smart, 1943)

of phlebotomine larvae is the presence of long caudal setae; one pair in first-stage larvae and two pairs in second-, third- and fourth-stage larvae.

Hosts: Many mammals, reptiles, birds and humans

Life cycle: Up to 100 ovoid, 0.3–0.4 mm long, brown or black eggs may be laid at each oviposition in small cracks or holes in the ground, the floors of animal houses, or in leaf litter. Although not laid in water the eggs need moist conditions for survival, as do the larvae and pupae. A minimum temperature of 15°C is required for egg development. Under optimal conditions the eggs can hatch in 1–2 weeks, but this may be prolonged in cold weather. The larvae, which resemble small caterpillars, scavenge on organic matter and can survive flooding. There are four larval stages, maturation taking 3 weeks to several months, depending on species, temperature and food availability. In more temperate regions these flies overwinter as mature larvae. The mature larvae are 4–6 mm in length, have a well developed black head with eyespots, and a segmented greyish body, which is covered in bristles. The pupae attach themselves to the substrate in an erect position with the exuviae of the last larval instar attached at the caudal end. The adults emerge from pupation after 1–2 weeks. The whole life cycle takes 30–100 days, or even longer in cool weather.

Geographical distribution: Widely distributed in the tropics, subtropics and the Mediterranean area. Most species prefer semi-arid and savannah regions to forests.

Pathogenesis: These flies inflict a painful bite, causing irritation and blood loss, which may lead to a reduction in weight gain. Apart from their biting nuisance in localised areas, phlebotomine sandflies are important as known vectors of *Leishmania* spp which cause cutaneous and visceral leishmaniasis in humans. Dogs are important reservoir hosts in some regions.

Pathogenesis and pathology: Sandflies are important as vectors of various pathogens. Of particular importance is leishmaniasis in humans and dogs, caused by the protozoan *Leishmania* spp. The diseases caused in humans are commonly classified as either visceral (kala-azar) or cutaneous infections. Dogs, cats, rodents and other wild animals act as reservoirs of infection. Dogs affected with cutaneous leishmaniasis have a non-pruritic, exfoliative dermatitis with alopecia and peripheral lymphadenopathy. Systemic leishmaniasis leads to splenomegaly, hepatomegaly, generalised lymphadenopathy, lameness, anorexia, weight loss and death. The disease has also been reported in cats. In North America, sandflies may also act as vectors of vesicular stomatitis of cattle and horses, which is caused by a rhabdovirus.

Clinical signs: The bites of these flies are painful and irritating to the host, giving rise to weals in soft-skinned animals. Sandflies particularly bite areas of exposed skin such as the ears, eyelids, nose, feet and tail.

Diagnosis: Sandflies may be visible on the host during the night. During the day sandflies can most often be collected in the field and are not usually seen on animals.

Epidemiology: In common with many other small biting flies, only the females suck blood. They prefer to feed at night, resting in shaded areas during the day. Since they are capable of only limited flight, nuisance due to biting may be confined to certain areas near the breeding sites. There is some seasonality in activity, the numbers of flies increasing during the rainy season in the tropics, whereas they are only present during the summer months in temperate zones. Adults often accumulate in the burrows of rodents or in other shelters, such as caves, where the microclimate is suitable.

Treatment: The most effective method to prevent fly bites and transmission of infection is to ensure that animals avoid areas of high fly density and are kept indoors when fly activity is highest. Flies spend limited time on their hosts and are difficult to control using insecticides unless these have rapid killing or repellent activity. Permethrin and deltamethrin are the only insecticides with sufficient repellent activity and rapidity of action to make them suitable for the control of sandfly biting in dogs. Neither drug is suitable for cats.

Control: There have been few large-scale attempts to control phlebotomine sandflies, probably due to the fact that leishmaniasis has merited insufficient attention as a disease, and also because little is known in detail of the biology and ecology of the developing stages of these flies. The adults are, however, susceptible to most insecticides, and where there have been spraying campaigns to control the mosquito vectors of malaria these have effectively controlled *Phlebotomus*. Removal of dense vegetation may reduce the suitability of the environment for the breeding of these flies.

Notes: The large family Psychodidae, sub-family Phlebotominae, contains a single genus of veterinary importance in the Old World, *Phlebotomus*, and a single genus of veterinary importance in the New World, *Lutzomyia.* In some areas of the world, the term 'sandflies' includes some biting midges and blackflies, and should be distinguished by referring to them as 'phlebotomine sandflies'.

12
The epidemiology of parasitic diseases

Although the reasons for the occurrence of parasitic diseases are multiple and often interactive, the vast majority occur for one of four basic reasons. These are:

1. An increase in the numbers of infective stages.
2. An alteration in host susceptibility.
3. The introduction of susceptible stock.
4. The introduction of infection into a clean environment.

Each of these will be discussed in turn, giving examples.

AN INCREASE IN THE NUMBERS OF INFECTIVE STAGES

This category involves parasitic diseases which occur seasonally, and although more distinct in zones with a wide climatic variation, may also be observed in zones with minor variations in climate such as the humid tropics.

A multiplicity of causes is responsible for the seasonal fluctuations in the numbers, and availability of infective stages, and these may be conveniently grouped as factors affecting contamination of the environment, and those controlling the development and survival of the free-living stages of the parasites and, where applicable, their intermediate hosts.

CONTAMINATION OF THE ENVIRONMENT

The level of contamination is influenced by several factors.

BIOTIC POTENTIAL

This may be defined as the capacity of an organism for biological success as measured by its fecundity. Thus, some nematodes, such as *Haemonchus contortus* and *Ascaris suum*, produce many thousands of eggs daily, while others, like *Trichostrongylus*, produce only a few hundred. Egg production by some external parasites such as the blowfly, *Lucilia sericata*, or the tick, *Ixodes ricinus*, is also very high, whereas *Glossina* spp produce relatively few offspring.

The biotic potential of parasites which multiply either within an intermediate or final host is also considerable. For example, the infection of *Galba* (*Lymnaea*) with one miracidium of the trematode *Fasciola hepatica* can give rise to several hundred cercariae. Within the final host, protozoal parasites such as *Eimeria*, because of merogony and gametogony, also give rise to a rapid increase in the contamination of the environment.

STOCK MANAGEMENT

The density of stocking can influence the level of contamination and is particularly important in nematode and cestode infections in which no multiplication of the parasite takes place outside the final host. It has the greatest influence when climatic conditions are optimal for development of the contaminating eggs or larvae, such as in spring and summer in the northern hemisphere.

A high stocking density will also favour the spread of ectoparasitic conditions such as pediculosis and sarcoptic mange, where close contact between animals facilitates the spread of infection. This may occur under crowded conditions in cattle yards, or from mother to offspring where, for example, sows and their litters are in close contact.

In coccidiosis, where large numbers of oocysts are disseminated, management procedures which encourage the congregation of stock, such as the gathering of lambs around feeding troughs, may lead rapidly to heavy contamination.

In temperate countries, where livestock are stabled during the winter, the date of turning out to graze in spring will influence contamination of pasture with helminth eggs. Since many helminth infective stages, which have survived the winter, succumb during late spring, the withholding of stock until this time will minimise subsequent infection.

IMMUNE STATUS OF THE HOST

Clearly, the influence of stocking density will be greatest if all the stock are fully susceptible, or if the ratio of susceptible to immune stock is high, as in sheep flocks with a large percentage of twins or in multiple suckled beef herds.

However, even where the ratio of adults to juveniles is low it must be remembered that ewes, sows, female goats, and to a lesser extent cows, become more susceptible to many helminths during late pregnancy and early lactation due to the periparturient relaxation in immunity. In most areas of the world, parturition in grazing animals, synchronised to occur with the climate most favourable to pasture growth, is also the time most suitable for development of the free-living stages of most helminths. Thus, the epidemiological significance of the periparturient relaxation of immunity is that it ensures increased contamination of the environment when the number of susceptible animals is increasing.

There is some evidence that resistance to intestinal protozoal infections such as coccidiosis and toxoplasmosis is also lowered during pregnancy and lactation, and so enhances spread of these important infections.

On the credit side, host immunity will limit the level of contamination by modifying the development of new infections either by their destruction or arrest at the larval stages, while existing adult worm burdens are either expelled or their egg production severely curtailed.

Although immunity to ectoparasites is less well defined, in cattle it develops against most species of ticks, although in a herd this expression of resistance often inadvertently results in an overdispersed population of ticks with the susceptible young animals carrying most of the ticks.

In protozoal diseases, such as babesiosis or theileriosis, the presence of immune adults also limits the likelihood of ticks becoming infected; however, this effect is not absolute since such animals are often silent carriers of these protozoal infections.

HYPOBIOSIS/DIAPAUSE

These terms are used to describe an interruption in development of a parasite at a specific stage and for periods which may extend to several months.

Hypobiosis refers to the arrested development of nematode larvae within the host and occurs seasonally, usually at a time when conditions are adverse to the development and survival of the free-living stages. The epidemiological importance of hypobiosis is that the resumption of development of hypobiotic larvae usually occurs when conditions are optimal for free-living development and so results in an increased contamination of the environment. There are many examples of seasonal hypobiosis in nematodes including *Ostertagia*/*Teladorsagia* infections in ruminants, *Hyostrongylus rubidus* in pigs and *Trichonema* spp in horses.

Diapause in arthropods, like hypobiosis in nematodes, is also considered to be an adaptation phenomenon whereby ectoparasites survive adverse conditions by a cessation of growth and metabolism at a particular stage. It is most common in temporary arthropod parasites in temperate climates. In these, feeding activity is restricted to the warmer months of the year and winter survival is often accomplished by a period of diapause. Depending on the extremity of the northern or southern latitudes, this may occur after one or several generations. For example, the headfly, *Hydrotoea irritans*, in northern latititudes, has only one annual cycle and overwinters as a mature larva in diapause. Other insects, such as *Stomoxys calcitrans* or blowflies in these latitudes, have several generation cycles before entering diapause. Diapause occurs less in parasites which continuously infect the hosts, such as mange mites or lice.

To date, similar phenomena have not been ascribed to protozoa, although there is one report of latent coccidiosis occurring in cattle for which a similar hypothesis has been proposed.

DEVELOPMENT AND SURVIVAL OF INFECTIVE STAGES

The factors that affect development and survival are mainly environmental, especially seasonal climatic change and certain management practices. Current changes in the global climate are anticipated to influence the infective stages of many parasites and/or the prevalence of some intermediate hosts. For example, the trend towards warmer wetter seasons has been one factor attributed to the increase in prevalence of *Fasciola hepatica* infection in ruminants in some temperate regions.

THE MICROHABITAT

Several environmental factors which affect the microhabitats of free-living parasitic stages are vital for development and survival. Thus moderate temperatures and high humidity favour development of most parasites, while cool temperatures prolong survival. The microclimate humidity depends, of course, not only on rainfall and temperature, but on other elements such as soil structure, vegetation type and drainage. Soil type influences the growth and species composition of the herbage and this, in turn, determines the degree to which a layer of 'mat' is formed between the soil and the herbage. The mat is abundant in older pastures and holds a permanent store of moisture in which the relative humidity remains high even after weeks of drought. The presence of this moisture and pockets of air trapped in the mat limit the rate of temperature change and these factors favour the development and survival of helminth larvae, ticks, larval stages of insects and coccidial oocysts.

In contrast, the use of rotational cropping of pastures reduces the influence of 'mat' and therefore parasite survival. In the arid tropics pasture growth is usually negligible causing a similar effect.

In the same way, a high groundwater table is important for the development and survival of intermediate snail vectors of trematodes, such as liver and rumen flukes.

The development and survival of helminth eggs or larvae within faeces are also dependent on temperature and moisture. The host species may also influence this situation since normal cattle faeces remain in their original form for a longer time than, say, sheep pellets. Thus the moisture content at the centre of a bovine faecal pat remains high for several weeks or even months and so provides shelter for developing larvae until the outside environment is suitable.

Dictyocaulus larvae may also be distributed with the spores of the fungus *Pilobolus* which grow in bovine faeces, while several species of nematode larvae, including *Oesophagostomum* spp of pigs, are known to be spread mechanically by some dipteran flies.

SEASONAL DEVELOPMENT

In temperate countries with distinct seasons of summer and winter there is a limited number of generations and the same is true of countries with distinct dry and wet seasons. In Britain, for example, there has generally only been one, or at the most two, parasitic generations of the common trichostrongyle infections of ruminants, since larval development on the pasture occurs only from late spring through to early autumn, the peak levels of infective larvae being present from July until September. This pattern of events has changed in recent years with climate changes to milder and longer seasons. In tropical climates there may be numerous generations per year, but even in this case there are times when conditions for the development and survival of the free-living stages are optimal.

The development of large numbers of infective stages of parasites within distinct seasons is usually followed by a high mortality rate within a few weeks. However, considerable numbers survive for much longer than is commonly realised. For example, in the helminths, significant numbers of metacercariae of *Fasciola hepatica* and infective larvae of trichostrongyles are capable of survival for at least 9 months in Britain.

Dipteran fly populations also vary in the number of generations per year. Using the blowflies as an example, there are three or four generations, and therefore higher populations, in southern England, whereas in Scotland there are usually only two, temperature being the limiting factor. In the humid tropical or subtropical countries the development of trichostrongyle larvae or fly populations proceeds throughout most of the year and, although this may be slower at certain times, there will be numerous generations per annum.

Although the permanent ectoparasites, such as lice or mange mites, live on or in the skin of animals and, therefore, in an apparently stable environment, this is not really the case as the hair or wool alters in length due to seasonal factors or human intervention. In the northern hemisphere development of these parasites is optimal in the winter when the coat is long and the micro-environment humid and temperate.

Apart from the free-living stages of coccidian parasites, which have seasonal requirements similar to those of the trichostrongyles, the prevalence of other protozoan infections is related to the feeding activity of their arthropod vectors. For example, in Britain, babesiosis in cattle occurs at peak times of tick activity in the spring and autumn, although again in recent years climate changes have affected the seasons such that tick activity has become less confined to these times of the year.

STOCK MANAGEMENT

The availability of helminth infective stages is also affected by certain management practices. Thus, a high density of stocking increases the level of contamination, and, by lowering the sward height, enhances the availability of the larval stages largely concentrated in the lower part of the herbage. Also, the scarcity of grass may induce animals to graze closer to faeces than otherwise. However, against this, the microclimate in a short sward is more susceptible to changes in temperature and humidity and so the free-living stages may, on adverse occasions, be particularly vulnerable. This may explain why the helminth burdens of ruminants in close-cropped set-stocked pastures are often less than those in animals on rotated pastures.

Similarly, many pasture improvement schemes have direct or indirect effects on arthropod populations. Improved host nutrition results from pasture improvement and helps to maintain host resistance to parasitism. However, pasture improvement, particularly in the tropics, can increase the breeding success of ticks and of those dipteran flies which lay their eggs in faeces, by increasing the shelter available. Furthermore, the increased stocking rates on improved pastures may increase the chances of parasites finding a host.

The date of parturition in a flock or herd may also influence the likelihood of parasitic infection. Where livestock are born out of season the numbers of trichostrongyle infective stages are usually lower and the chance of infection is postponed until the young animals are older and stronger.

AN ALTERATION IN HOST SUSCEPTIBILITY

This may refer to existing infections or to the acquisition of new infections.

ALTERED EFFECTS OF AN EXISTING INFECTION

This is observed principally in adolescent or adult stock which are harbouring parasite populations below the threshold usually associated with disease and may be explained by various dietary and host factors.

DIET

It is well known that adequately fed animals are better able to tolerate parasitism than animals on a low plane of nutrition. Thus, ruminants affected with blood-sucking helminths, such as *Haemonchus contortus* or *Fasciola hepatica*, may be able to maintain their haemoglobin levels as long as their iron intake is adequate. However, if their iron reserves become low their haemopoeitic systems become exhausted and they may die. Similarly, cattle may grow at a reasonable rate with moderate trichostrongylid burdens even though some loss of protein is occurring through the alimentary mucosa. However, if there is a change in diet which reduces their protein intake, they are unable to compensate for the loss of protein and lose weight.

These deleterious effects of parasitism, without any change in the level of infection, are not uncommon in outwintered stock or, in the tropics, in animals during a period of drought.

Incidentally, the same effect is produced when food intake is not increased during pregnancy and lactation. Good examples of this are the accumulation of lice on poorly fed animals during the winter and the fact that the anaemia caused by ticks is greater in animals on poor nutrition.

Apart from protein and iron, dietary deficiencies in trace elements are also significant. Thus, trichostrongylosis in ruminants is known to impair the absorption of both calcium and phosphorus and, where the dietary intake of these is sub-optimal, osteoporosis can occur. Also, the deleterious effects of some abomasal parasites in sheep are greater where there is a cobalt deficiency and, in such animals, levels of parasitism generally considered to be non-pathogenic may be associated with severe diarrhoea and weight loss.

PREGNANCY AND LACTATION

In sheep, and to some extent in other livestock, there is a breakdown in immunity around the periparturient period and during early lactation. Recent studies support the hypothesis that there is competition between the immune system and the udder for nutrients, particularly metabolisable protein. This relaxation of immunity can be largely restored by supplementation with protein and is also influenced by the body protein status of the ewe.

The period of gestation in grazing livestock often coincides with that of inadequate nutrition and is geared to completion at a time when freshly growing pasture becomes available for their newborn progeny. In housed or outwintered livestock the cost of maintaining an adequate nutritional intake during pregnancy is often high and as a result the nutritional levels are often sub-optimal. If this occurs, quite low worm burdens can have a detrimental effect on the food conversion of the dam, which in turn influences fetal growth and subsequently that of the neonate through poor milk production by the dam. This has been clearly illustrated in sows infected with moderate burdens of *Oesophagostomum dentatum* and in ewes infected with helminths such as *Haemonchus* or *Fasciola*.

STEROID THERAPY

Steroids are widely used in therapy of both man and animals and it is known that they may alter the susceptibility to parasitism. A good example of this is in the cat infected with *Toxoplasma gondii*; excretion of oocysts usually occurs for only about 2 weeks, but may reappear and be prolonged following the administration of steroids. Egg production by nematodes is also known to increase following steroid treatment and so pasture contamination is increased.

ALTERED SUSCEPTIBILITY TO THE ACQUISITION OF NEW INFECTIONS

THE ROLE OF INTERCURRENT INFECTIONS

The interaction of various parasites, or a parasite with another pathogen, resulting in an exaggerated clinical disease, has been reported on several occasions. For example, in lambs, the nematode, *Nematodirus battus*, and the protozoan, *Eimeria*; in cattle, the trematode, *Fasciola hepatica*, and the bacterium, *Salmonella dublin*, and also *Fasciola hepatica* and the mange mite, *Sarcoptes*; in pigs, the nematode, *Trichuris suis*, and the spirochaete, *Serpula* (*Treponema*) *hyodysenteriae*.

THE EFFECT OF CHEMOTHERAPY

In certain instances, immunity to parasites appears to be dependent on the continuing presence of low threshold infections, commonly called premunity. If the balance between the host and the immunising infection is disturbed by therapy then reinfection of the host may occur, or in the case of helminths, an arrested larval population may develop to maturity from the reservoir of infection within the host. Thus, the use of anthelmintics, known to be effective against adult parasites, but not arrested nematode larvae, may precipitate development of the latter once the adults are removed; this is known to occur in infections with *Hyostrongylus rubidus* in the pig. Sometimes, also, the overzealous application of anthelmintics in grazing animals will result in the eventual establishment of higher numbers of trichostrongyles than were present prior to treatment. Excessive application of acaricides to control ticks may also lower herd immunity to babesial and theilerial infections, the so-called 'enzootic instability'.

HYPERSENSITIVITY

In many instances, at least part of the immune response to parasites is associated with a marked IgE response and a hypersensitivity reaction. Where this occurs in the gut, as in intestinal nematode infections, the reaction is associated with an increased permeability of the gut to macromolecules such as protein, and this may be a significant factor in immune animals under heavy larval challenge. In sheep, for example, relatively poor growth rates and poor wool production may result.

A stunting effect has also been observed in tick-resistant animals which are under constant challenge, while pet animals repeatedly exposed to mite infestations may have severely thickened, hyperaemic and sensitive skins, although only neglible numbers of mites are present.

THE INTRODUCTION OF SUSCEPTIBLE STOCK

Parasitism may result from the movement of susceptible stock into an infected environment due to the following factors.

ABSENCE OF ACQUIRED IMMUNITY

The common nematode diseases of ruminants provide the best examples of outbreaks of parasitic disease following the movement of calves into infected areas. For example, in western Europe the cattle lungworm, *Dictyocaulus viviparus*, is endemic; the most severe outbreaks are seen in calves born in early spring and turned out in late summer to graze alongside older batches of calves which have grazed from early spring. Overwintered larval populations have cycled in these older calves and when the fresh populations of infective larvae, which develop from these infections, accrue on pasture, the younger calves, with no previous experience of infection, are extremely susceptible.

The occurrence of 'cysticercosis storms' in adult cattle, grazed on fields contaminated with eggs of the human tapeworm, *Taenia saginata*, or handled by infected stockmen, are occasionally reported in Europe and the USA. This high degree of susceptibility is due to lack of previous exposure to infection. In contrast, in areas where cysticercosis is endemic, cattle are repeatedly infected and soon acquire a solid resistance to reinfection, only the cysts acquired in early life persisting in the muscles.

With protozoal diseases, such as babesiosis, theileriosis, coccidiosis and toxoplasmosis, caution has to be exercised in introducing naive animals into infected areas. In the case of toxoplasmosis, the introduction of female sheep into a flock in which the disease is endemic has to be carefully controlled and these should be non-pregnant when purchased and allowed to graze with the flock for some months prior to mating.

ABSENCE OF AGE IMMUNITY

A significant age immunity develops against relatively few parasites, and adult stock not previously exposed to many helminth and protozoal infections are at risk if moved into an endemic area.

LONGEVITY OF INFECTIVE STAGES

Especially in temperate zones and in parts of the subtropics, the free-living stages of most parasites will survive in the environment or in intermediate hosts for periods sufficiently long to reinfect successive batches of young animals and may cause disease in these animals within a few weeks of exposure.

THE INFLUENCE OF GENETIC FACTORS

BETWEEN HOST SPECIES

Most parasites are host specific and this specificity has been utilised in integrated control programmes, such as mixed grazing of sheep and cattle, to control gastrointestinal nematodes. However, some economically important parasites are capable of infecting a wide range of hosts which vary in their susceptibility to the effects of the parasite. For example, cattle seem able to cope with liver fluke infestations which would cause death in sheep, and goats appear to be very much more susceptible than cattle or sheep to their common gastrointestinal trichostrongyles.

BETWEEN BREEDS

Evidence is accumulating that the susceptibility of various breeds of animals to parasites varies and is genetically determined. For example, some breeds of sheep are more susceptible to the abomasal nematode, *Haemonchus contortus*, than others; *Bos indicus* breeds of cattle are more resistant to ticks and other haematophagous insects than *Bos taurus* breeds. In Denmark, the Black Pied cattle are genetically deficient in their cellular immune responses and have proved more susceptible to liver fluke, while the N'dama breed of cattle in west Africa is known to be tolerant to trypanosomosis.

Even within flocks or herds, individual responders and non-responders, in terms of their ability to develop resistance to internal and external parasites, are usually present and it is recommended by some experts that culling of the poorest responders should take place.

SEX

There is some evidence that entire male animals are more susceptible than females to some helminth infections. This could be of importance in countries where castration is not routinely practised, or where androgens are used to fatten castrates or cull cows.

STRAIN OF PARASITE

Although this aspect has received scant attention, except in protozoal infections, there is now evidence that strains of helminths occur which vary in infectivity and pathogenicity. The increasing prevalence of drug-resistant isolates of many parasites is another point which should be considered when disease outbreaks occur in herds, flocks or studs where control measures are routinely applied.

INTRODUCTION OF INFECTION INTO A CLEAN ENVIRONMENT

There are several ways in which a parasite may be introduced into an environment from which it has been eradicated or where it has never been found.

INTRODUCTION OF NEW STOCK

One of the current trends in the international livestock arena is the movement of breeding stock from country to country. Quarantine restrictions and vaccination requirements are stringent in relation to epidemic diseases, but limited or non-existent for parasitic diseases. When infected animals are moved into an area previously free from any given parasite the infection may cycle, provided suitable conditions exist, and the consequences for the indigenous stock can be extremely serious. Examples of this category include the introduction of *Toxocara vitulorum* into Britain and Ireland, the source of infection being Charolais heifers from mainland Europe and transmission occurring via the dam's milk. The spread of *Parafilaria bovicola* in Sweden, presumably introduced with cattle, or by the muscid intermediate hosts inadvertently transported from southern Europe, is another example. In the USA, Australia and Britain the increased movement of human populations and their pets has seen the spread of a number of diseases of dogs including heartworm, canine babeiosis and ehrlichiosis, infections previously limited to more tropical areas. In some of these situations, competent arthropod vectors suitable for transmission may have already been present in some areas. Psoroptic mange in cattle, originally confined to southern Europe, is now endemic in Belgium and Germany due to trade in breeds of cattle. Protozoal diseases, such as toxoplasmosis, have been introduced into sheep flocks in countries where it was previously absent, by the importation of infected sheep. Babesiosis has also spread where animals carrying infected ticks have moved into non-endemic areas where the ticks were able to become established.

THE ROLE OF EFFLUENT

The transfer of infection from one farm to another via manure has also been reported. Thus outbreaks of ostertagiosis have occurred in farms following the application of cattle slurry as a fertiliser, while cysticercosis 'storms' due to *Cysticercus bovis* have occurred in cattle following the application of human sewage to pastures. Finally, the application of pig slurry containing ascarid eggs to pastures subsequently grazed by sheep has resulted in pneumonia due to migrating ascarid larvae.

THE ROLE OF INFECTED VECTORS

Winged insects transmit a number of helminth and protozoal infections, and these can serve to introduce infection into areas previously free of infection. Migratory birds are known to carry larval or nymphal stages of potentially infected ticks. Occasionally also, birds may mechanically transport infective stages of parasites to a new environment. This has occurred in the Netherlands where the ditches and dykes surrounding reclaimed land have become colonised by *Lymnaea* (*Galba*) snails transported by wild birds. The introduction of livestock lightly infected with *Fasciola hepatica* resulted in the snails becoming infected and, subsequently, outbreaks of clinical fasciolosis.

13
Resistance to parasitic diseases

Broadly speaking, resistance to parasitic infections falls into two categories. The first of these, often termed innate resistance, includes species resistance, age resistance and in some cases breed resistance, which, by and large, are not immunological in origin. The second category, acquired immunity, is dependent on antigenic stimulation and subsequent humoral and cellular responses. Although, for reasons explained below, there are few vaccines available against parasitic diseases, natural expression of acquired immunity plays a highly significant role in protecting animals against infections and in modulating the epidemiology of many parasitic diseases.

SPECIES RESISTANCE

For a variety of parasitological, physiological and biochemical reasons, many parasites do not develop at all in other than their natural hosts; this is typified by, for example, the remarkable host specificity of the various species of *Eimeria*. In many instances however, a limited degree of development occurs, although this is not usually associated with clinical signs; for example, some larvae of the cattle parasite *Ostertagia ostertagi* undergo development in sheep, but very few reach the adult stage. However, in these unnatural or aberrant hosts, and especially with parasites which undergo tissue migration, there are occasionally serious consequences particularly if the migratory route becomes erratic. An example of this is visceral larva migrans in children due to *Toxocara canis*, which is associated with hepatomegaly and occasionally ocular and cerebral involvement.

Some parasites, of course, have a very wide host range, *Trichinella spiralis*, *Fasciola hepatica*, *Cryptosporidium parvum* and the asexual stages of *Toxoplasma* being four examples.

AGE RESISTANCE

Many animals become more resistant to primary infections with some parasites as they reach maturity. For example, ascarid infections of animals are most likely to develop to patency if the hosts are a few months old. If hosts are infected at an older age, the parasites either fail to develop, or are arrested as larval stages in the tissues; likewise, patent *Strongyloides* infections of ruminants and horses are most commonly seen in very young animals. Sheep of more than 3 months of age are relatively resistant to *Nematodirus battus*, and in a similar fashion dogs gradually develop resistance to infection with *Ancylostoma* over their first year of life.

The reasons underlying age resistance are unknown, although it has been suggested that the phenomenon is an indication that the host–parasite relationship has not yet fully evolved. Thus, while the parasite can develop in immature animals, it has not yet completely adapted to the adult.

On the other hand, where age resistance is encountered, most parasitic species seem to have developed an effective counter-mechanism. Thus, *Ancylostoma caninum*, *Toxocara canis*, *Toxocara mystax*, *Toxocara vitulorum* and *Strongyloides* spp all survive as larval stages in the tissues of the host, only becoming activated during late pregnancy to infect the young *in utero* or by the transmammary route. In the case of *Nematodirus battus*, the critical hatching requirements for the egg, i.e. prolonged chill followed by a temperature in excess of 10°C, ensure the parasites' survival as a lamb-to-lamb infection from one season to the next.

Oddly enough, with *Babesia* and *Anaplasma* infection of cattle, there is generally thought to be an inverse age resistance, in that young animals are more resistant than older naive animals.

BREED RESISTANCE

In recent years, there has been considerable practical interest in the fact that some breeds of domestic ruminants are more resistant to certain parasitic infections than others.

Probably the best example of this is the phenomenon of trypanotolerance displayed by west African humpless cattle, such as the N'dama, which survive in areas of heavy trypanosome challenge. The mechanism whereby these cattle control their parasitaemias is still not fully known, although it is thought that immunological responses may play a role.

In helminth infections, it has been shown that the Red Masai sheep, indigenous to east Africa, is more resistant to *Haemonchus contortus* infection than some imported breeds studied in that area, whilst in South Africa it has been reported that the Merino is less susceptible to trichostrongylosis than certain other breeds.

Within breeds, haemoglobin genotypes have been shown to reflect differences in susceptibility to *Haemonchus contortus* infection in that Merino, Scottish Blackface and Finn Dorset sheep which are homozygous for haemoglobin A, develop smaller worm burdens after infection than their haemoglobin B homozygous or heterozygous counterparts. Unfortunately, these genotypic differences in susceptibility often break down under heavy challenge.

Studies within a single breed have shown in Australia that individual Merino lambs may be divided into responders and non-responders on the basis of their immunological response to infection with *Trichostrongylus colubriformis* and that these differences are genetically transferred to the next generation.

The selection of resistant animals could be of great importance, especially in many developing areas of the world, but in practice would be most easily based on some easily recognisable feature such as 'coat colour' rather than be dependent on laboratory tests.

In Australia resistance to ticks, particularly *Boophilus*, has been shown to be influenced by genetics, being high in the humped, *Bos indicus*, Zebu breeds and low in the European, *Bos taurus*, breeds. However, where cattle are 50% Zebu, or greater, in genetic constitution, a high degree of resistance is still possible allowing a limited use of acaricides.

ACQUIRED IMMUNITY TO HELMINTH INFECTIONS

Immune responses to helminths are complex, possibly depending on antigenic stimulation by secretory or excretory products released during the development of the L_3 to the adult. For this reason it has only been possible to develop one or two practical methods of artificial immunisation of which the radiation-attenuated vaccine against *Dictyocaulus viviparus* is perhaps the best example.

Despite this, there is no doubt that the success of many systems of grazing management depend on the gradual development by cattle and sheep of a naturally acquired degree of immunity to gastrointestinal nematodes. For example, experimental observations have shown that an immune adult sheep may ingest around 50 000 *Teladorsagia* (*Ostertagia*) L_3 daily without showing any clinical signs of parasitic gastritis.

THE EFFECT OF THE IMMUNE RESPONSE

Dealing first with gastrointestinal and pulmonary nematodes, the effects of the immune response may be grouped under three headings, the sequence reflecting the usual progression of acquired immunity:

1. Initially, the host can attempt to limit reinfection by **preventing the migration and establishment of larvae** or, sometimes, **by arresting their development at a larval stage**. This type of inhibition of development should not be confused with the more common hypobiosis triggered by environmental effects on infective larvae on pasture or, in the present state of knowledge, with the arrested larval development associated with age resistance in, for example, the ascarids.
2. Adults that do develop may be **stunted in size or their fecundity may be reduced**. The important practical aspect of this mechanism is perhaps not so much the reduced pathogenicity of such worms as the great reduction in pasture contamination with eggs and larvae, which in turn reduces the chance of subsequent reinfection.
3. The development of immunity after a primary infection may be associated with an **ability to kill or expel the adult nematodes**.

Each of these mechanisms is exemplified in infections of the rat with the trichostrongyloid nematode *Nippostrongylus brasiliensis*, a much studied laboratory model, which has contributed greatly to our understanding of the mechanisms of host immunity in helminth infection. The infective stage of this parasite is normally a skin penetrator, but in the laboratory is usually injected subcutaneously for convenience. The larvae travel via the bloodstream to the lungs where, having moulted, they pass up the trachea and are swallowed. On reaching the small intestine they undergo a further moult and become adult, the time elapsing between infection and development to egg-laying adults being 5–6 days. The adult population remains static for about 5 more days. After this time the faecal worm egg output drops quickly, and the majority of the worms are rapidly expelled from the gut. This expulsion of adult worms, originally known as the 'self cure' phenomenon, has been shown to be due to an immune response.

If the rats are reinfected, a smaller proportion of the larval dose arrives in the intestine, i.e. their migration is stopped. The few adult worms which do develop in the gut remain stunted and are relatively infertile, and worm expulsion starts earlier and proceeds at a faster rate.

Under natural grazing conditions larval infections of cattle and sheep are acquired over a period, but an approximately similar series of events occurs. For example, calves exposed to *Dictyocaulus viviparus* quite rapidly acquire patent infections, readily recognisable by the clinical signs. After a period of a few weeks, immunity develops and the adult worm burdens are expelled. On subsequent exposure in succeeding years such animals are highly resistant to challenge, although if this is heavy, clinical signs associated with the reinfection syndrome, i.e. the immunological destruction of the invading larvae in the lungs, may be seen. With *Ostertagia* and *Trichostrongylus* infections, the pattern is the same with the build-up of an infestation of adult worms being followed by their expulsion and subsequent immunity; in later life only small, short-lived adult infections are established and eventually the infective larvae are expelled without any development at all. However, with gastrointestinal infections in ruminants, the ability to develop good immune responses is often delayed for some months because of immunological unresponsiveness.

The mechanism of immunity to luminal parasites is still not fully understood despite considerable research. However it is generally agreed that such infections produce a state of gut hypersensitivity associated with an increase of mucosal mast cells in the lamina propria and the production of worm-specific IgE, much of which becomes bound to the surface of the mast cells. The reaction of worm antigen, from an existing infection or from a subsequent challenge, with these sensitised mast cells releases vasoactive amines, which cause an increase in capillary and epithelial permeability and hyperproduction of mucus. Some workers have concluded that these physiological changes simply affect the well-being of the worms by, for example, lowering the oxygen tension of their environment, so that they become detached from the mucosa and subsequently expelled. Others have postulated that, in addition, the permeable mucosa allows the 'leakage' of IgG antiworm antibody from the plasma into the gut lumen, where it has access to the parasites.

Additional factors, such as the secretion of specific antiworm IgA on the mucosal surface and the significance of sensitised T cells, which are known to promote the differentiation of mast cells, eosinophils and mucus-secreting cells, are also currently under study.

With regard to tissue-invading helminths, the most closely studied have been the schistosomes. Schistosomulae of *Schistosoma mansoni* may be attacked by both eosinophils and macrophages, which attach to the antibody-coated parasite. Eosinophils, especially, attach closely to the parasites where their secretions damage the underlying parasite membrane. Attempts to find if a similar mechanism exists against *Fasciola hepatica* have indicated that although eosinophils do attach to parts of the tegument of the young fluke, the latter seems able to shed its surface layer to evade damage.

EVASION OF THE HOST'S IMMUNE RESPONSE

Despite the evidence that animals are able to develop vigorous immune responses to many helminth infections, it is now clear that parasites, in the course of evolution, have capitalised on certain defects in this armoury. This aspect of parasitology is still in its infancy, but three examples of immune evasion are described below.

NEONATAL IMMUNOLOGICAL UNRESPONSIVENESS

This is the inability of young animals to develop a proper immune response to some parasitic infections. For example, calves and lambs fail to develop any useful degree of immunity to reinfection with *Ostertagia* spp until they have been exposed to constant reinfection for an entire grazing season. Similarly, lambs remain susceptible to *Haemonchus contortus* infection until they are between 6 months and 1 year old. The cause of this unresponsiveness is unknown. However, while calves and lambs ultimately do develop a good immune response to *Ostertagia* or *Teladorsagia* infection, in the sheep/*Haemonchus contortus* system the neonatal unresponsiveness is apparently often succeeded by a long period of acquired immunological unresponsiveness, e.g. Merino sheep reared from birth in a *Haemonchus*-endemic environment remain susceptible to reinfection throughout their entire lives.

CONCOMITANT IMMUNITY

This term is used to describe an immunity which acts against invading larval stages, but not against an existing infection. Thus a host may be infected with adult parasites, but has a measure of immunity to further infection. Perhaps the best example is that found with schistosomes, which are covered by a cytoplasmic syncytium which, unlike the chitinous-like cuticle of nematodes, would at first seem to be vulnerable to the action of antibody or cells. However, it has been found that adult schistosomes have the property of being able to incorporate host antigens, such as blood group antigens or host immunoglobulin, on their surface membrane to mask their own foreign antigens.

Concomitant immunity does not appear to operate with *Fasciola hepatica* in sheep, in that they remain susceptible to reinfection. On the other hand, cattle not only expel their primary adult burden of *Fasciola hepatica*, but also develop a marked resistance to reinfection. Concomitant immunity also includes the situation where established larval cestodes may survive for years in the tissues of the host, although the latter is completely immune to reinfection. The mechanism is unknown, but it is thought that the established cyst may be 'masked' by host antigen or perhaps secrete an 'anti-complementary' substance which blocks the effect of an immune reaction.

POLYCLONAL STIMULATION OF IMMUNOGLOBULIN

As well as stimulating the production of specific IgE antibody, helminths 'turn on' the production of large amounts of non-specific IgE. This may help the parasite in two ways. First, if mast cells are coated by non-specific IgE they are less likely to attract parasite-specific IgE and so will not degranulate when exposed to parasite antigen. Secondly, the fact that the host is producing immunoglobulin in a non-specific fashion means that specific antibody to the helminth is less likely to be produced in adequate quantity.

THE DEBIT SIDE OF THE IMMUNE RESPONSE

Sometimes immune responses are associated with lesions that are damaging to the host. For example the pathogenic effects of oesophogostomosis are frequently attributable to the intestinal nodules of *Oesophagostomum columbianum*; similarly, the pathogenic effects of schistosomosis are due to the egg granulomata, the result of cell-mediated reactions, in the liver and bladder.

There is evidence from some studies for a negative genetic interaction between production traits and resistance to parasitism. Sheep which had been selected for their resistance to gastrointestinal nematode infection showed a higher incidence of scouring. This may be the result of an increased hypersensitivity to ingested larvae.

ACQUIRED IMMUNITY TO PROTOZOAL INFECTIONS

As might be anticipated from their microscopic size and unicellular state, immunological responses against protozoa are similar to those directed against bacteria. The subject is, however, exceedingly complex and the following account is essentially a digest of current information on some of the more important pathogens. As with bacterial infections, immune responses are typically humoral or cell-mediated in type and occasionally both are involved.

Trypanosomosis is a good example of a protozoal disease to which immunity is primarily humoral. Thus, *in vitro*, both IgG and IgM can be shown to lyse or agglutinate trypanosomes and *in vivo* even a small amount of immune serum will clear trypanosomes from the circulation, apparently by facilitating their uptake, through opsonisation, by phagocytic cells. Unfortunately, the phenomenon of antigenic variation, another method of immune evasion, prevents these infections being completely eliminated and typically allows the disease to run a characteristic course of continuous remissions and exacerbations of parasitaemia. It is likely, also, that the generalised immunosuppression induced by this disease, may, sooner or later, limit the responsiveness of the host.

It is also relevant to note that some of the important lesions of trypanosomosis, such as anaemia, myocarditis and lesions of skeletal muscle, are thought to be attributable to the deposition of trypanosome antigen or immune complexes on these cells leading to their subsequent destruction by macrophages or lymphocytes, a possible debit effect of the immune response.

Acquired immunity to babesiosis also appears to be mediated by antibody, perhaps acting as an opsonin, and facilitating the uptake of infected red cells by splenic macrophages. Antibody is also transferred in the colostrum of the mother to the new-born animal and confers a period of protection against infection.

Finally, in trichomonosis, antibody, presumably produced by plasma cells in the lamina propria of the uterus and vagina, is present in the mucus secreted by these organs and to a lesser extent in the plasma. This, *in vitro*, kills or agglutinates the trichomonads and is probably the major factor responsible for the self-limiting infections which typically occur in cows.

Of those protozoal infections against which immunity is primarily cell-mediated, leishmaniosis is of particular interest in that the amastigotes invade and proliferate in macrophages whose function, paradoxically, is the phagocytosis and destruction of foreign organisms. How they survive in macrophages is unknown, although it has been suggested that they may release substances which inhibit the enzyme activity of lysosomes or that the amastigote surface coat is refractory to lysosomal enzymes. The immunity that develops seems to be cell-mediated, perhaps by cytotoxic T cells destroying infected macrophages or by the soluble products of sensitised T cells 'activating' macrophages to a point where they are able to destroy their intracellular parasites. Unfortunately in many cases the efficacy of the immune response and the consequent recovery is delayed or prevented by a variable degree of immunosuppression of uncertain aetiology.

As noted above, sometimes both humoral and cell-mediated reactions are involved in immunity, and this seems to be the situation with coccidiosis, theileriosis and toxoplasmosis.

In coccidiosis, the protective antigens are associated with the developing asexual stages and the expression of immunity is dependent on T cell activity. It is thought that these function in two ways: first, as helper cells for the production of neutralising antibody against the extracellular sporozoites and merozoites and secondly, in a cell-mediated fashion, by releasing substances, such as lymphokines, which inhibit the multiplication of the intracellular stages. The net effect of these two immunological responses is manifested by a reduction in clinical signs, and a decrease in oocyst production.

As described earlier, the proliferative stages of theilerial infections are the merogonous stages, which develop in lymphoblasts and divide synchronously with these cells to produce two infected daughter cells. During the course of infection, and provided it is not rapidly fatal, cell-mediated responses are stimulated in the form of cytotoxic T cells which target on the infected lymphoblasts by recognising two antigens on the host surface. One of these is derived from the *Theileria* parasite and the other is a histocompatibility antigen of the host cell. The role of antibodies in protection is less clear, although it has been recently demonstrated, using an *in vitro* test, that an antibody against the sporozoites inoculated by the tick may be highly effective in protection.

In toxoplasmosis also, both humoral and cell-mediated components appear to be involved in the immune response. However, the relative importance of their roles remains to be ascertained, although it is generally believed that antibody formation by the host leads to a cessation in the production of tachyzoites and to the development of the latent bradyzoite cyst. It is also believed that recrudescence of tachyzoite activity may occur if the host becomes immunosuppressed as a consequence of therapy or some other disease.

ACQUIRED IMMUNITY TO ARTHROPOD INFECTIONS

It is known that animals exposed to repeated attacks by some insects gradually develop a degree of acquired immunity. For example, at least in man, over a period of time the skin reactions to the bites of *Culicoides* and mosquitoes usually decrease in severity. Likewise, after several attacks of calliphorine myiasis, sheep can develop a degree of resistance to further attack.

A similar sequence of events has been observed with many tick and mite infestations. The immune reaction to ticks, dependent on humoral and cell-mediated components to the oral secretions of the ticks, prevents proper engorgement of the parasites and has serious consequences on their subsequent fertility; dogs that have recovered from sarcoptic mange are usually immune to further infection. Sheep infected with sheep scab have developed a protective immunity to subsequent reinfections.

Although these immune responses must moderate considerably the significance of many ectoparasitic infections, their primary importance to date is largely concerned with their debit side, i.e. the unfortunate consequences which often occur when an animal becomes sensitised to arthropod antigens. Examples of this are flea dermatitis in dogs and cats, the pruritus and erythema associated with sarcoptic mange in the dog and pig and with psoroptic mange in sheep and cattle, and 'sweet itch' of horses due to skin hypersensitivity to *Culicoides* bites.

THE FUTURE OF PARASITE VACCINES

Early approaches investigating the use of live attenuated vaccines resulted in commercially available vaccines for the bovine lungworm, *Dictyocaulus viviparus*, and for *Eimeria* infections in poultry. Apart from *D. viviparus* there are no commercially produced vaccines for the control of helminth infections in ruminants. The increased prevalence of parasites which are resistant to drug therapy has led to further investment in vaccine development, particularly those based on recombinant parasite components, and considerable progress has been made in identifying candidate antigens for several important parasite species.

Vaccines have already been developed, for example, against *Taenia ovis* infection in sheep, for *Babesia canis* in dogs, and for *Babesia bovis* and *Boophilus microplus* in cattle. The commercial success of current experimental recombinant vaccines will depend not only on their efficacy in the protection against field challenge but also on factors such as effective, low-cost, delivery systems which will confer long-acting protection.

Two main approaches have been adopted for vaccine development: those based on 'natural antigens', which are recognised by the host during the course of infection, and those based on 'hidden' or 'covert' antigens. The latter strategy ignores the mechanisms of natural immunity and directs responses towards molecules located or secreted internally. There have been encouraging advances towards the aim of producing vaccines for the control of several parasitic diseases in the last decade. Recent research has identified and characterised protective antigens and the genes encoding several of these have been cloned.

NATURAL ANTIGENS

Protective effects have been reported against *Haemonchus contortus*, using adult worm excretory–secretory products comprising two proteins of 15 and 24 kd, and against *Fasciola hepatica* with excretory proteases; similarly, against the cestodes *Echinococcus granulosus*, *Taenia ovis* and *T. saginata* using molecules on the surface of the oncosphere stage. The recombinant *T. ovis* vaccine is not available commercially, mainly as it is not an ovine or human pathogen. The economic return for a recombinant cestode vaccine for developing countries needs to be further evaluated.

HIDDEN ANTIGENS

An important advantage of using 'covert' antigens in vaccine strategies is that they should be effective in those infections where natural immunity is poorly developed or is ineffective. A possible disadvantage is that immunity is not boosted by infection. However, it has been shown in *Haemonchus contortus* infection in lambs that vaccination with 'hidden' gut membrane antigens, which are predominantly proteases and which are not normally recognised by the host during infection, will provide protection and by the time this wanes sufficient natural immunity will have been acquired. The approach using 'hidden' gut antigens has been successful against some haematophagous nematodes but has been more limited against parasites which do not directly ingest blood. This gut membrane approach formed the basis of the recombinant vaccine against *Boophilus microplus*, the Australian cattle tick.

In conclusion, although considerable progress has been made towards the experimental production of some monovalent vaccines, it is likely to be several years before commercially produced recombinant vaccines are available.

14
Antiparasitics

INTRODUCTION

It is not practical to give full efficacy data and methods of application of the large number of drugs currently available against the vast range of parasites that parasitise domestic animals. As the number of compounds and their various formulations are continually changing it is perhaps more appropriate to discuss the use of antiparasitics in general terms, according to the groups of parasites they target. For the purposes of this chapter, antiparasitics are grouped as anthelmintics, ectoparasiticides or antiprotozoals. Details of their use against individual species or groups of parasites have been described under the appropriate sections of the main text.

ANTHELMINTICS

The control of parasitic helminths in domestic animals relies largely on the use of anthelmintic drugs. Although anthelmintics are used in all domestic species, the largest market is undoubtedly the ruminant market, especially cattle, where millions of pounds are spent annually in an effort to reduce the effects of parasitism.

ANTHELMINTICS AND THEIR MODE OF ACTION

The mode of action of many anthelmintics basically depends on interference with essential biochemical processes of the parasite, but not of the host.

The major groups of anthelmintics currently in use against nematodes, trematodes and cestodes are shown in Table 14.1.

BENZIMIDAZOLES/PRO-BENZIMIDAZOLES

The benzimidazoles include **thiabendazole**, **parbendazole**, **oxibendazole**, **fenbendazole**, **oxfendazole**, **albendazole**, **triclabendazole** and **ricobendazole** (albendazole oxide). Three other chemicals, **febantel**, **netobimin** and **thiophanate** (probenzimidazoles), are also included in this group because they are metabolised in the body to active benzimidazole metabolites. Modification of a particular benzimidazole can affect the pharmacokinetic behaviour of the drug through changes in relative insolubility, slowing the elimination of the parent drug and/or active metabolites. The greater efficacy, and wider spectrum of activity, of the

Table 14.1 Anthelmintic groups.

Chemical group	Nematodes	Trematodes	Cestodes	Ectoparasites
Broad spectrum				
Benzimidazoles and probenzimidazoles	+	±	±	–
Imidazothiazoles	+	–	–	–
Tetrahydropyrimidines	+	–	–	–
Avermectins/milbemycins	+	–	–	+
Narrow spectrum				
Salicylanilides and substituted phenols	±	+	±	±
Piperazines	±	–	–	–
Organophosphates	+	–	–	+
Arsenicals	+	–	–	–
Others	+	–	+	–

most recently introduced (second-generation) benzimidazoles appears to be due to the relative insolubility of these chemicals, which affects the absorption, transport and excretion of the anthelmintic compound from the host.

Benzimidazoles are poorly soluble and are generally given orally as a suspension. Netobimin can be solubilised and administered via drinking water. Benzimidazoles have also been incorporated into a range of controlled release devices for use in cattle. All are effective against nematodes affecting domestic animals and are ovicidal. Most are also effective against tapeworms and some have activity against adult liver fluke (*Fasciola*) in ruminants at increased dose rates.

All members of the benzimidazole class have a similar mode of action and act by disrupting energy metabolism in worms by binding to parasite tubulin, a constituent protein present in microtubules and in plasma and mitochondrial membranes. The formation of microtubules is a dynamic process involving the polymerisation of tubulin rings at one end and depolymerisation at the other end. Benzimidazole anthelmintics bind to ß-tubulin causing capping and inhibition of further microtubule formation. The resultant effect is starvation of the parasite due to inhibition of glucose uptake, protein secretion and microtubule production. There is also a reduction in enzyme activity such as acetylcholinesterase secretion, and carbohydrate catabolism by the fumarate reductase system. The mode of action of triclabendazole, on *Fasciola hepatica*, is at present unknown. It appears to have no tubulin-binding properties, unlike other members of this group, and it must therefore act along alternative pathways.

Benzimidazoles have a low toxicity, and in some cases can be used at over ten times the recommended dose rate. Parasite resistance to anthelmintics has most frequently been associated with repeated use of these drugs against nematodes of sheep, goats and horses and in many countries has limited both their effectiveness and use.

IMIDAZOTHIAZOLES/ TETRAHYDROPYRIMIDINES

The imidathiazole group contains two members, **tetramisole** and **levamisole**. Tetramisole is a racemic mixture of dextro and levo forms. Levamisole is the levo-isomer and it is with this form that anthelmintic potency resides. The dose rate of levamisole is therefore half that of tetramisole, and it has twice the safety index.

Levamisole is used mainly in cattle and sheep and has good activity against a range of gastrointestinal nematodes and is also highly effective against lungworms. Levamisole can be administered orally, by injection or pour-on, combined in a number of products with a specific flukicide (oxyclozanide or triclabendazole) to form a broad-spectrum drench for worms and fluke. Unlike the benzimidazoles it is not ovicidal. Levamisole is non-teratogenic and is therefore safe to use in pregnant animals. The therapeutic index in relation to other anthelmintics is, however, low. Animals given levamisole may be hyperactive for a few minutes after receiving the recommended therapeutic dose. Toxic signs, due to a stimulant effect on nerve ganglia, may manifest as salivation, bradycardia, muscular tremors and, in extreme cases, death from respiratory failure. Injectable levamisole may cause inflammation at the site of injection.

The drug is rapidly absorbed and excreted, most of the dose being lost from the system within 24 hours of administration. Because of the mode of action of these compounds nematode paralysis occurs quickly and removal of the worms is rapid. In addition to its anthelmintic properties, levamisole has been shown to stimulate the mammalian immune system by increasing cellular activity. The relationship between the immunostimulatory and nematocidal properties of levamisole is unknown.

Pyrantel and **morantel** are members of the tetrahydropyrimidine group. **Morantel** is used for the treatment of gastrointestinal worms of cattle and sheep but is not effective against mucosal or arrested stages or against established lungworm infections. Like levamisole, it has no activity against tapeworms and fluke. **Pyrantel** is used for the treatment and control of nematode and tapeworm infections in horses and nematodes in dogs. It is also active against nematodes in ruminants and pigs. Pyrantel salts (tartrate or pamoate) are active against adult and larval stages of large and small strongyles, ascarids, tapeworms (*Anoplocephala*) at double the regular dose, and benzimidazole-resistant strains of cyathostomes in the horse.

None of these drugs are particularly toxic and they can be used safely in pregnant and young animals.

The mode of action of these compounds appears to be as selective agonists, mimicking the action of acetylcholine (Ach), causing a rapid, reversible spastic paralysis. Paralysed worms are expelled by normal gut peristalsis.

AVERMECTINS/MILBEMYCINS

These are a series of macrocyclic lactone derivatives, which are fermentation products of the actinomycete *Streptomyces avermitilis* (avermectins) and *Streptomyces cyanogriseus* (milbemycins). Avermectins differ from each other chemically in side chain substitutions on the lactone ring, whilst milbemycins differ from the avermectins through the absence of a sugar moiety from the lactone skeleton. The avermectins include **abamectin**, **doramectin**, **eprinomectin** and **ivermectin**, and are active against a wide range of nematodes and arthropods. **Moxidectin** is a milbemycin and has a similar wide-ranging activity.

The macrocyclic lactones have been shown to have excellent activity, at very low dose rates, not only against a wide range of nematodes, but also against certain arthropod parasites and hence are sometimes referred to as endectocides. They are active against adult and larval gastrointestinal roundworms and lungworms of ruminants, horses and pigs, although none of these compounds have activity against tapeworms or liver fluke. Avermectins are also active against filarial worms (*Parafilaria*) in cattle, microfilariae of the canine heartworm (*Dirofilaria*) in dogs and spiruroid worms, including *Habronema* and *Draschsia*, in horses.

The ectoparasites these compounds have activity against include warbles (*Hypoderma* spp) in cattle, sucking lice (*Haematopinus*, *Linognathus*, *Solenopotes* spp) and mange mites (*Psoroptes*, *Sarcoptes*, *Chorioptes*) in cattle, sheep and pigs. More detailed information on the efficacy of the endectocides against ectoparasites is provided in the section on ectoparasiticides.

Selamectin is used as a preventative against heartworm disease in dogs and is effective against hookworms (*Ancylostoma*, *Uncinaria*) and ascarid roundworms (*Toxocara*, *Toxascaris*) in dogs and cats. Selamectin has been specifically developed for use in dogs and cats and is also active against fleas and mites in these hosts (see Ectoparasiticides).

Macrocyclic lactones are highly lipophilic and, following administration, are stored in fat tissue from where they are slowly released, metabolised and excreted. Ivermectin is absorbed systemically following oral, subcutaneous or dermal administration, but is absorbed to a greater degree, and has a longer half-life, when given subcutaneously or dermally. A temporary depot appears to occur in the fat and liver, from which there is a slow release. Excretion of the unaltered molecule is mainly via the faeces with less than 2% excreted in the urine. The reduced absorption and bioavailability of ivermectin when given orally in ruminants may be due to its metabolism in the rumen. The affinity of these compounds to fat explains their persistence in the body and the extended periods of protection afforded against lungworms and stomach worms in cattle and sheep. Individual variances in these periods of protection reflect differences in drug distribution, metabolism and excretion. In cattle, injectable and pour-on preparations provide protection for up to 42 days for lungworms and 35 days for stomach worms depending on the product and formulation. The prolonged half-life of these compounds also determines levels of residues in meat and milk, and subsequent compulsory withdrawal periods following treatment. With the exception of eprinomectin, which has a zero milk withdrawal period, treatment with this class of compounds cannot be given to lactating cattle, or during the last 2 months of pregnancy.

Their mode of action has been studied but has still not been completely elucidated. Ivermectin is known to act on γ-aminobutyric acid (GABA) neurotransmission at two or more sites in nematodes, blocking interneuronal stimulation of excitatory motor neurones and thus leading to a flaccid paralysis. It appears to achieve this by stimulating the release of GABA from nerve endings and enhancing the binding of GABA to its receptor on the post-synaptic membrane of an excitatory motor neurone. The enhanced GABA binding results in an increased flow of chloride ions (Cl^-) into the cell leading to hyperpolarisation. In mammals, GABA neurotransmission is confined to the central nervous system; the lack of effect of avermectin on the mammalian nervous system at therapeutic concentrations is probably because, being a large molecule, it does not readily cross the blood–brain barrier. More recent evidence suggests that ivermectin may exert its effect through action on glutamate-gated Cl^- conductance at the post-synaptic membrane or neuromuscular end-plate.

SALICYLANILIDES/SUBSTITUTED PHENOLS

The salicylanilides/substituted phenols can be regarded as close analogues and include the **bromsalans**, **clioxanide**, **oxyclozanide**, **brotianide**, **niclosamide**, **rafoxanide** and **closantel** (salicylanilides), **nitroxynil**, **disophenol**, **bithionol**, **hexachlorophene**, **niclofolan** (phenol derivatives). With the exception of niclosamide, the salicylanilides and substituted phenols are usually marketed as flukicides for cattle and sheep, being highly effective against adult, and to a lesser extent, immature flukes (*Fasciola*). Some also possess activity against blood-sucking nematodes such as *Haemonchus*. **Disophenol** has been used for treatment of dogs infected with hookworms, and is also effective against mature *H. contortus* and may be used in sheep for treatment of benzimidazole-resistant *H. contortus* infections. **Niclosamide** is highly effective against tapeworms in cattle, sheep, horses, poultry and possibly against immature paramphistomes in ruminants. In a number of countries, it is used mainly for the treatment of tapeworms in dogs and cats.

Salicylanilides and substituted phenols appear to be extensively bound to plasma proteins (>99%), which may explain their high efficacy against blood-feeding parasites. Fasciolicidal activity is dependent on the extent to which these drugs persist in the plasma. Rafoxanide and closantel have long plasma half-lives when compared with oxyclozanide. Evidence suggests that the apparent efficacy of these drugs, particularly against immature fluke (*Fasciola*), may be due more to their persistence in the plasma and the effect they have on maturing adult flukes when they reach the bile ducts, rather than the effect they have on the immature stages themselves. Young flukes probably ingest mainly liver cells, which contain little anthelmintic. As they grow and migrate through the liver they cause extensive haemorrhage and come into contact with anthelmintic. Finally, when the flukes reach the bile ducts they are in contact with even greater concentrations of anthelmintic as the bile ducts are important in the excretion of these compounds, as evidenced by the high proportion of these, and their metabolites, excreted in the faeces rather than the urine.

Salicylanilides and substituted phenols uncouple oxidative phosphorylation and therefore decrease the availability of high-energy phosphate compounds such as adenosine triphosphate (ATP) and reduced nicotinamide-adenine-dinucleotide ($NADH^-$) in the mitochondria. They have also been shown to inhibit succinate dehydrogenase activity and the fumarate reductase system, which is associated with oxidative phosphorylation. Because of the long half-life of the plasma protein-bound molecules, the parasites experience prolonged exposure to the drugs, which reduces the energy available to the parasites.

Plasma binding reduces incorporation of the drugs into host tissues and accounts for the selective parasite toxicity. Looseness of faeces and slight loss of appetite may be seen in some animals after treatment at recommended dose rates. High doses may cause blindness and signs of uncoupled oxidative phosphorylation, i.e. hyperventilation, hyperthermia, convulsions, tachycardia and ultimately death.

Dichlorophen is a chlorinated phenol and is active against tapeworms (*Dipylidium*, *Taenia*) in dogs and cats. Its mode of action is thought to be similar to that of the salicyclanides, interfering with oxidative phosphorylation.

PIPERAZINES

Piperazine salts are widely used against ascarids, particularly in dogs and cats, and act as GABA agonists, producing paralysis. Piperazine adipate has been widely used in horses and is effective against adult stages of small strongyles and *Parascaris*. In pigs, the drug is active against *Ascaris* and nodular worms *Oesophagostomum* spp after a single treatment.

Diethylcarbamazine is still marketed in certain parts of the world for the treatment of lungworm infections in cattle. It is primarily active against immature lungworms and because it has to be given over a period of 3 days to achieve its effect, it has been replaced by more modern anthelmintics. The action of diethylcarbamazine on immature lungworm larvae is thought to be a 'flaccid' paralysis due to hyperpolarisation of neuronal post-synaptic membranes resulting from an increased flow of Cl^- into the cell. It can be used as a preventive for heartworm disease when given to dogs in low daily doses throughout the mosquito season and for 2 months subsequently. The mode of action is incompletely understood, but it is thought to enhance phagocytosis of the microfilariae by the host immune system. It is, however, strictly contraindicated in microfilariae-positive dogs because of a possible but rare shock-type reaction that is sometimes fatal, produced by liberation of substances from dying or dead microfilariae following treatment. It has also been reported to be effective against the lungworm *Crenosoma vulpis* of dogs and farmed foxes.

ORGANOPHOSPHATES

Several organophosphorus compounds (see ectoparasiticides) are active against nematodes, but are becoming less widely available in many countries. Compounds used in the treatment of nematode infections include **coumaphos**, **trichlorophon**, **haloxon** and **dichlorvos**. They act by inhibiting cholinesterase resulting in a build-up of acetylcholine, which leads to neuromuscular paralysis of nematodes and their expulsion. This group of drugs is relatively toxic and has been used most frequently in horses, because of the additional insecticidal action against larvae of horse bots.

Coumaphos has been widely used as an ectoparasitic in livestock. It exhibits a cumulative effect on trichostrongyle nematodes if given in feed daily for 1 week; there is a good activity against *Haemonchus* spp and *Cooperia* spp in cattle and sheep, but it is less effective against *Trichostrongylus*, *Ostertagia* spp and *Oesophagostomum* spp. Anthelmintic activity can be enhanced if the drench passes via the closed oesophageal groove directly to the abomasum either with sodium bicarbonate in cattle, or copper sulphate in sheep. It is also effective against *Capillaria*, *Ascaridia* and *Heterakis* in chickens. The drug is toxic and may cause mortality in ruminants. Coloured breeds of egg-laying hens are more susceptible to the drug than white breeds and birds should not be treated while they are in lay.

Haloxon is still used in many countries for treatment of nematodes. In cattle, sheep and goats, there is good activity against adult *Haemonchus*; also *Cooperia* spp in sheep and *Neoascaris* in cattle. There is a moderate effect against *Ostertagia, Bunostomum*, *Trichostrongylus* and *Oesophagostomum* but little effect against *Nematodirus*, *Trichuris* and *Chabertia*. It is highly effective against adult stages of *Strongylus vulgaris*, most small strongyles (also benzimidazole-resistant strains), *Parascaris* and *Oxyuris* in the horse. Haloxon is also effective against *Capillaria* infections of birds (chicken, turkey, quail and pigeons) but is ineffective against *Heterakis*. In pigs, it is active against adult *Ascaris* and *Oesophagostomum* spp but there may be delayed neurotoxicity (posterior paralysis). It is used in some countries in chickens, turkeys, quail and pigeons against *Capillaria*. The recommended dose range for birds (50–100 mg/kg) is lethal for geese and possibly waterfowl.

Trichlorophon is effective against adult and immature *Parascaris*, adult pinworms (*Oxyuris*) and against bots (larvae of *Gasterophilus*) and, at higher doses, large strongyles (*S. vulgaris*) and small strongyles in horses. In some countries, trichlorphon is used in combination with various benzimidazoles, pyrantel pamoate or piperazine/phenothiazine for removal of ascarids, pinworms, small strongyles (cyathostomes) and all three species of large strongyles. It shows good efficacy against adults of *Ascaris*, *Trichuris* and *Hyostrongylus* in pigs. At therapeutic doses, there may be mild adverse effects such as transient softening of faeces and mild colic for several hours.

Dichlorvos has a similar spectrum of activity to trichlorophon in horses and pigs; formulation in a slow-release resin increases activity against large and small strongyles and safety in pigs. However, the resin pellets, which appear in the faeces, are toxic to other animals, especially chickens.

ARSENICALS

Thiocetarsamide is an arsenical compound that has been used for many years as an adulticidal drug for treatment of heartworm (*Dirofilaria*) in dogs. Its efficacy varies depending on the sex and age of worm, and there is a risk to treated animals of pulmonary embolism in the first month following treatment. The drug is highly irritant to subcutaneous tissues and is both hepatotoxic and nephrotoxic with mortality during or following therapy related to the degree of clinical manifestation of heartworm disease. It is now no longer available.

Melarsomine dihydrochloride is a new generation arsenical adulticide that can be used for treatment of canine heartworm disease. It is less nephrotoxic and hepatotoxic than thiocetarsamide and has a higher efficacy using a two-dose strategy. It is generally well tolerated causing only minor tissue reactions and is normally administered intramuscularly into the lumbar muscles.

OTHER DRUGS

Phenothiazine was the first broad-spectrum anthelmintic used for several years but it has now virtually disappeared. It is still available in some countries in combination with trichlorphon and piperazine and can be used for treating benzimidazole-resistant strains of small strongyles. The drug is active against adult stages of small strongyles but has little or no effect on large strongyles, immature stages of small strongyles and *Parascaris*. At therapeutic doses there may be side effects, such as anorexia, muscular weakness, icterus or anaemia, but seldom mortality.

Epsiprantel is a isoquinoline-pyrazine anthelmintic compound active against tapeworm infections in dogs and cats. It is generally formulated and administered with pyrantel pamoate to give a broader range of activity against both roundworms and tapeworms of dogs and cats.

Praziquantel is an aceylated quinoline-pyrazine and is active against a wide range of adult and larval tapeworms in dogs and cats and at higher dose rates against tapeworms of ruminants. It is the drug of choice against multilocular echinococcosis (*Echinococcus multilocularis*) and is also active against lung flukes (*Paragonimus*) and intestinal fluke (*Nanophyetus*) in dogs. Praziquantel modulates cell membrane permeability causing spastic paralysis of muscle cells in the parasite and, like a number of other cestodicidal drugs, causes damage to the parasite tegument.

Nitroscanate is marketed for treatment of common roundworm and tapeworm infections of dogs. Although active in cats its use in this species is contraindicated due to adverse side effects including posterior paralysis, inappetence and vomiting.

Emodepside is a semi-synthetic compound belonging to a new group of chemicals called the depsipeptides. The compound acts at the neuromuscular junction by stimulating secretin pre-synaptic receptors leading to paralysis and death of the parasites. Emodepside is active against roundworms of dogs and cats.

PROPERTIES OF ANTHELMINTIC COMPOUNDS

An ideal anthelmintic should possess the following properties:

1. **It should be efficient against all parasitic stages of a particular species**. It is also generally desirable that the spectrum of activity should include members of different genera, for example in dealing with the equine strongyles and *Parascaris equorum*. However in some circumstances, separate drugs have to be used at different times of year to control infections with unrelated helminths; the trichostrongyles responsible for ovine parasitic gastroenteritis and the liver fluke *Fasciola hepatica* are examples.
2. It is important that any anthelmintic **should be non-toxic to the host**, or at least have a wide safety margin. This is especially important in the treatment of groups of animals such as a flock of sheep, where individual body weights cannot easily be

obtained, rather than in the dosing of individual companion animals such as cats or dogs.

3. In general, an anthelmintic **should be rapidly cleared and excreted by the host**, otherwise long withdrawal periods would be necessary in meat- and milk-producing animals. However, in certain circumstances and in certain classes of animals, drug persistence is used to prophylactic advantage, for example the use of closantel to control *Haemonchus* in sheep.
4. Anthelmintics **should be easily administered**, otherwise they will not be readily accepted by owners; different formulations are available for different domestic animal species. Oral and injectable products are widely used in ruminants, and pour-on preparations are available for cattle. Anthelmintic boluses are also available for cattle and sheep. Palatable in-feed and paste formulations are convenient for use in horses, while anthelmintics are usually available as tablets for dogs and cats.
5. **The cost of an anthelmintic should be reasonable**. This is of special importance in pigs and poultry where profit margins may be narrow.

USE OF ANTHELMINTICS

Anthelmintics are generally used in two ways: therapeutically, to treat existing infections or clinical outbreaks, or prophylactically, in which the timing of treatment is based on knowledge of the epidemiology. Clearly prophylactic use is preferable where administration of a drug at selected intervals or continuously over a period can prevent the occurrence of disease.

THERAPEUTIC USAGE

When used therapeutically, the following factors should be considered:

- If the drug is not active against all stages it must be effective against the pathogenic stage of the parasite.
- Use of the anthelmintic should, by successfully removing parasites, result in cessation of clinical signs of infection, such as diarrhoea and respiratory distress; in other words, there should be a marked clinical improvement and rapid recovery after treatment.

PROPHYLACTIC USAGE

Several points should be considered where anthelmintics are used prophylactically:

- The cost of prophylactic treatment should be justifiable economically, by increased production in food animals, or by preventing the occurrence of clinical or subclinical disease in, for example, horses with strongylosis or dogs with heartworm disease.
- The cost–benefit of anthelmintic prophylaxis should stand comparison with the control, which can be achieved by other methods such as pasture management or, for example, in the case of dictyocaulosis, by vaccination.
- It is desirable that the use of anthelmintics should not interfere with the development of an acquired immunity, since there are reports of outbreaks of disease in older stock, which have been overprotected by control measures during their earlier years.
- Prolonged prophylactic use of one drug should be avoided as this may encourage the development of anthelmintic resistance.

METHODS OF ADMINISTRATION

Traditionally, anthelmintics have been administered orally or parenterally, usually by subcutaneous injection. Oral administration is common by drenching with liquids or suspensions, or by the incorporation of the drug in the feed or water for farm animals and by the administration of tablets to small animals. More recently, paste formulations have been introduced especially for horses and there are now several compounds which have systemic action when applied as pour-on or spot-on formulations to the skin. Methods for injecting compounds directly into the rumen of cattle have also been marketed. A number of rumen-dwelling boluses are available, mainly for cattle, and to a lesser extent for sheep. These are designed to deliver therapeutic doses of anthelmintic at intervals (pulse-release) or low doses over prolonged periods (sustained-release); both prevent the establishment of mature parasite populations and thus limit the contamination of pastures and the occurrence of disease. An apparatus for the delivery of anthelmintics into drinking water at daily or periodic intervals has also been developed.

Some products are marketed for cattle and sheep consisting of a mixture of a roundworm anthelmintic and a fluke drug, but the timing of treatments for roundworms or flukes, whether curative or prophylactic, is often different and the requirement for such combination compounds is therefore limited.

ECTOPARASITICIDES (INSECTICIDES/ACARICIDES)

The control of the ectoparasites found on animals, including fleas, lice, ticks, mange mites, warbles and nuisance flies, is largely based on the use of chemicals. There is a vast world market in these chemicals, with increasingly more spent on flea control products in companion animals.

ECTOPARASITICIDES AND THEIR MODE OF ACTION

Three main chemical groupings have been used as the basis for the common ectoparasiticides: the organochlorines, the organophosphates and the synthetic pyrethroids. Other groups that are also used include the carbamates (primarily in poultry), the formamidines, the triazines, benzyl benzoate and natural plant products such as pyrethrin. The avermectins and milbemycins have also been shown to have a high activity against a range of ectoparasites and these are increasingly used for ectoparasite control, for example mange in sheep, cattle and pigs. There are also compounds which affect the growth and development of insects. Based on their mode of action they can be divided into chitin inhibitors, chitin synthesis inhibitors and juvenile hormone analogues. Insect growth regulators (IGRs) are widely used for flea control in domestic pets and for blowfly control in sheep but have limited use in other host species. For example, lufenuron blocks the formation of larval chitin in fleas, and cyromazine disrupts growth regulation in blowfly larvae on sheep.

ORGANOCHLORINES (OCS)

Organochlorines are now banned in many countries on the grounds of both human and environmental safety. OCs fall into three main groups:

- *Chlorinated ethane derivatives.* Includes DDT (dichlorodiphenyltrichloroethane), DDE (dichlorodiphenyldichloroethane) and DDD (dicofol, methoxychlor). Chlorinated ethanes cause inhibition of sodium conductance along sensory and motor nerve fibres by holding sodium channels open, resulting in delayed repolarisation of the axonal membrane. This state renders the nerve vulnerable to repetitive discharge from small stimuli that would normally cause an action potential in a fully repolarised neurone.
- *Cyclodienes.* The cyclodienes include chlordane, aldrin, dieldrin, hepatochlor, endrin and tozaphene. They appear to have at least two component modes of action; inhibition of γ-amino butyric acid (GABA) stimulated Cl^- flux and interference with calcium ion (Ca^{2+}) flux. The resultant inhibitory post-synaptic potential leads to a state of partial depolarisation of the post-synaptic membrane and vulnerability to repeated discharge.
- *Hexachlorocyclohexanes (HCH).* Includes benzene hexachloride (BHC) and its γ-isomer, lindane. The mode of action is similar to the cyclodienes with the drug binding to the picrotoxin side of the GABA receptor resulting in an inhibition of GABA-dependent Cl^- flux into the neurone.

DDT and BHC were used extensively for flystrike control but were subsequently replaced in many countries by more effective cyclodiene compounds, dieldrin and aldrin. DDT and lindane (BHC) were widely used in dip formulations for the control of sheep scab but the organophosphates and synthetic pyrethroids have largely replaced them. They have the advantage that the effect of the drug persists for a longer time on the coat or fleece of the animal but the disadvantage, at least in food animals, is that they persist in animal tissues. If toxicity occurs the signs are those of central nervous system (CNS) stimulation with hypersensitivity, followed by increasing muscular spasm progressing to convulsions.

ORGANOPHOSPHATES (OPS)

These include a vast number of compounds of which **chlorfenvinphos**, **coumaphos**, **crotoxyphos**, **crufomate**, **cythioate**, **diazinon**, **dichlofenthion**, **dichlorvos**, **fenthion**, **iodofenphos**, **malathion**, **phosmet**, **propetamphos**, **ronnel**, **tetrachlorvinphos** and **trichlorphon** have been amongst the most commonly used. These can persist in the animals' coat or fleece for reasonable periods, but residues in animal tissues are short lived. Some have the ability to act systemically, given parenterally, orally or as a pour-on, but the effective blood levels of these are maintained for only 24 hours. The OPs are cholinesterase inhibitors; if acute toxicity occurs, the signs are salivation, dyspnoea, incoordination, muscle tremors and sometimes diarrhoea. There is also concern over chronic toxicity which may be associated with the use of these compounds and which is thought to be the result of inhibition of the enzyme neurotoxic esterase.

SYNTHETIC PYRETHROIDS (SPS)

The common SPs in use include **deltamethrin**, **permethrin**, **cypermethrin**, **flumethrin** and **fenvalerate**. The main value of these compounds lies in their repellent effect and since they persist well on the coat or skin, but not in tissue, they are of particular value against parasites which feed on the skin surface, such as lice, some mites and nuisance flies. Pyrethroids act as neurotoxins upon sensory and motor nerves of the neuroendocrine and CNS of insects. All the pyrethroids are lipophilic and this property helps them to act as contact insecticides. Some have the ability to repel and to 'knockdown', i.e. affect flight and balance without causing complete paralysis. Because the SPs have a strong affinity for sebum this property has been capitalised upon by incorporating the SPs into ear tags or tail bands. The SPs are fairly safe, but if toxicity does occur it is expressed in the peripheral nervous system as hypersensitivity and muscle tremors. SPs are also extremely toxic to fish and aquatic invertebrates and there are environmental concerns over their use.

CARBAMATES

Carbamate insecticides are closely related to the organophosphates (OPs) and are anticholinesterases, but unlike OP compounds they appear to cause a spontaneously reversible block on the enzyme acetylcholinesterase (AchE) without changing it. The two main carbamate compounds in use in veterinary medicine are **carbaryl** and **propoxur**, with **butocarb** and **carbanolate** also used in the control of poultry ectoparasites. Carbaryl has low mammalian toxicity but may be carcinogenic and is often combined with other active ingredients. **Fenoxycarb** is used for flea control and appears to have a mode of action closely related to the juvenile hormone analogues, preventing embryonic development in flea eggs, larval development and adult emergence (see Insect growth regulators). It has been formulated with permethrin or chlorpyrifos for use on animals or in liquid concentrate form for environmental flea control.

AVERMECTINS/MILBEMYCINS

These are effective at very low dose levels against certain ectoparasites when given parenterally and by pour-on preparations. They are particularly effective against ectoparasites with tissue stages, such as warbles, bots and mites, and have good activity against blood-sucking parasites such as lice and one-host ticks. As in nematodes, they are thought to affect cell function by direct action in Cl^- channels. They have a very wide safety margin. Some avermectins have a marked residual effect and a single treatment given parenterally is still effective against lice or mites hatching from eggs 3–4 weeks later.

Selamectin has high activity against fleas of cats and dogs (*Ctenocephalides*) and prevents flea infestations on dogs and cats for a period of 30 days. It is safe and effective in controlling mite (*Otodectes*, *Sarcoptes*) and tick (*Rhipicephalus*) infestations.

FORMAMIDINES

The main member of this group is **amitraz**, which acts at octopamine receptor sites in ectoparasites resulting in neuronal hyperexcitability and death. It is available as a spray or dip for use against mites, lice and ticks in domestic livestock. In cattle, for example, it has been widely used in dips, sprays or pour-on formulations for the control of single-host and multi-host tick species. In dipping baths, it can be stabilised by the addition of calcium hydroxide, and maintained by standard replenishment methods for routine tick control. An alternative method has been the use of total replenishment formulations whereby the dip bath is replenished with the full concentration of amitraz at weekly intervals prior to use. Amitraz has also been shown to have an expellent action against attached ticks. It has been shown to be effective on controlling lice and mange in pigs and psoroptic mange in sheep.

In small animals, amitraz is available for topical application for the treatment and control of ticks, and for canine demodicosis (*Demodex*) and sarcoptic mange (*Sarcoptes*). Amitraz is contraindicated in horses and in pregnant or nursing bitches and cats, although it has been used at a reduced concentration to treat feline demodicosis. Amitraz is also formulated in collars for tick control in dogs.

PHENYLPYRAZOLES

Fipronil is a phenylpyrazole compound which blocks transmission of signals by the inhibitory neurotransmitter, GABA, present in insects. The compound binds within the Cl^- channel and consequently inhibits the flux of Cl^- ions into the nerve cell resulting in hyperexcitation of the insect nervous system. Fipronil is used worldwide for the treatment and control of flea and tick infestations on dogs and cats and has reported activity against mange mites (*Sarcoptes*), ear mites (*Otodectes*), forage mites (*Trombicula*, *Cheyletiella*) and dog lice (*Trichodectes*). It is highly lipophilic and diffuses into the sebaceous glands of hair follicles that then act as a reservoir giving it a long residual activity. Sunlight, immersion in water and bathing do not significantly impact on the performance of products containing this compound. There is evidence that fipronil has an extremely rapid knock-down effect which occurs before the fleas have time to feed and hence it may be especially useful in cases of flea allergic dermatitis.

NITROGUANIDINES AND SPINOSYNS

Imidacloprid is a chloronicotinyl insecticide, a synthesised chlorinated derivative of nicotine. It specifically binds to nicotinic acetylcholine (Ach) receptors in the insect's CNS, leading to inhibition of cholinergic transmission resulting in paralysis and death. This mode of action is the same as nicotine, which has been used as a natural insecticide for centuries. The favourable selective toxicity of imidacloprid appears to be due to the fact that it only seems to bind to the Ach receptors of insects, having no effect on these receptors in mammals. Its activity appears to be mainly confined to insect parasites and it is available as a spot-on product in many countries for use in dogs and cats for the control of adult fleas providing protection against reinfestation for up to 4–5 weeks.

Spinosad is a fermentation product of the soil actinomycete, *Saccaropolyspora spinosa*, and has been developed in some countries for use on sheep in the control of blowfly strike and lice.

INSECT GROWTH REGULATORS

Several IGRs are used throughout the world, and represent a relatively new category of insect control agents. They constitute a group of chemical compounds that do not kill the target parasite directly, but interfere with growth and development. IGRs act mainly on immature stages of the parasite and as such are not usually suitable for the rapid control of established adult populations of parasites. Where parasites show a clear seasonal pattern, IGRs can be applied prior to any anticipated challenge as a preventative measure.

Based on their mode of action they can be divided into chitin synthesis inhibitors (benzoylphenyl ureas), chitin inhibitors (triazine/pyrimidine derivatives) and juvenile hormone analogues. IGRs are widely used for flea control in domestic pets and for blowfly control in sheep but have limited use in other host species.

Benzoylphenyl ureas

The benzoylphenyl ureas (**diflubenzuron**, **flufenoxuron**, **fluaxuron**, **lufenuron** and **triflumuron**) are chitin inhibitors, of which several have been introduced for the control of ectoparasites of veterinary importance. Chitin is a complex aminopolysaccharide and a major component of the insect's cuticle. During each moult it has to be newly formed by polymerisation of individual sugar molecules. Chitin molecules, together with proteins are assembled into chains, which in turn are assembled into microfibrils. The exact mode of action of the benzoylphenyl ureas is not fully understood. They inhibit chitin synthesis but have no effect on the enzyme chitin synthetase, and it has been suggested that they interfere with the assembly of the chitin chains into microfibrils. When immature insect stages are exposed to these compounds they are not able to complete ecdysis and as a consequence die during the moulting process. Benzyl phenylureas also appear to show a transovarial effect. Exposed adult female insects produce eggs in which the compound is incorporated into the egg nutrient. Egg development proceeds normally but the newly developed larvae are incapable of hatching. Benzoylphenyl ureas show a broad spectrum of activity against insects but have a relatively low efficacy against ticks and mites. The exception to this is fluazuron, which has greater activity against ticks and some mite species.

Benzoylphenyl ureas are highly lipophilic molecules and, when administered to the host, build up in the body fat from where they are slowly released into the bloodstream and excreted largely unchanged.

Diflubenzuron and **flufenoxuron** are used for the prevention of blowfly strike in sheep. Diflubenzuron is available in some countries as an emulsifiable concentrate for use as a dip or shower. It is more efficient against first-stage larvae than second and third instars and is therefore recommended as a preventative, providing 12–14 weeks' protection. It may also have potential for the control of a number of major insect pests such as tsetse flies. Fluazuron is available in some countries for use in cattle as a tick development inhibitor. When applied as a pour-on it provides long-term protection against the one-host tick, *Boophilus microplus*.

Lufenuron is administered orally and is used for the control of fleas of dogs and cats. The drug accumulates in fat tissue allowing subsequent slow release. Fleas take up the drug through the blood and transfer it to their eggs, which are non-viable within 24 hours of administration. The formation of larval chitin structures is blocked, thereby inhibiting the development of flea larvae and providing environmental control of the flea population. For oral administration, the drug must be administered in the food to allow sufficient time for absorption from the stomach. Injectable treatment is given at 6-monthly intervals whilst oral treatment is given once monthly during summer, commencing 2 months before fleas become active. As lufenuron has no activity against adult fleas, an insecticide treatment may be required if there is an initial heavy infestation or in cases of severe hypersensitivity.

Triflumuron is active against lice and fleas in dogs.

Triazine/pyrimidine derivatives

Triazine and pyrimidine derivatives are closely related compounds that are also chitin inhibitors. They differ from the benzylphenyl ureas both in chemical structure and in mode of action, in that they appear to alter the deposition of chitin into the cuticle rather than its synthesis.

Cyromazine, a triazine derivative, is effective against blowfly larvae on sheep and lambs and also against other Diptera, such as houseflies, mosquitoes, etc. At recommended dose rates, cyromazine shows only limited activity against established strikes and must therefore be used preventatively before anticipated challenge. Blowflies lay eggs usually on damp fleece of treated sheep. Although larvae are able to hatch out, the young larvae immediately come into contact with cyromazine, which prevents the moult to second instars. The use of a 'pour-on' preparation of cyromazine has the advantage that efficacy is not dependent upon factors such as weather, fleece length and whether the fleece is wet or dry. In addition, the persistence of the drug is such that control can be maintained for up to 13 weeks after a single pour-on application, or longer if applied by dip or shower.

Dicyclanil, a pyrimidine derivative, is highly active against dipteran larvae and is available as a pour-on formulation for blowfly control in sheep in some countries, providing up to 20 weeks protection.

Juvenile hormone analogues

The juvenile hormone analogues mimic the activity of naturally occurring juvenile hormones and prevent metamorphosis to the adult stage. Once the larva is fully developed, enzymes within the insect's circulatory system destroy endogenous juvenile hormones, and final development occurs to the adult stage. The juvenile hormone analogues bind to juvenile hormone receptor sites, but because they are structurally different are not destroyed by insect esterases. As a consequence, metamorphosis and further development to the adult stage does not proceed.

Methoprene is a terpenoid compound with very low mammalian toxicity that mimics a juvenile insect hormone and is regularly used for flea control. It is sensitive to light and will not persist outdoors. It has been used extensively and successfully in indoor environments and on pets in the form of collars, shampoos, sprays and dips and also as a feed through larvicide for hornfly (*Haematobia*) control on cattle. The other member of this group used for the control of fleas in dogs and cats is **pyriproxyfen**.

MISCELLANEOUS COMPOUNDS

Piperonyl butoxide (PBO) is a methylnedioxphenyl compound that has been widely used as a synergistic additive in the control of arthropod pests. It is commonly used as a synergist with natural pyrethrins, the combination having a much greater insecticidal activity than the natural product alone. The degree of potentiation of insecticidal activity is related to the ratio of components in the mixture, such that as the proportion of PBO increases, so the amount of natural pyrethrins required to evoke the same level of kill decreases. The insecticidal activity of other pyrethroids, particularly of knockdown agents, can also be enhanced by the addition of PBO. The enhancement of activity of synthetic pyrethroids is normally less dramatic but PBO may be included in several formulations. PBO inhibits the microsomal enzyme system of some arthropods and has been shown to be effective against some mites. In addition to having low mammalian toxicity and a long record of safety, PBO rapidly degrades in the environment.

Various products from natural sources, as well as synthetic compounds, have been used as insect repellents. Such compounds include cinerins, pyrethrins and jasmolins (see pyrethroids), citronella, indalone, garlic oil, MGK-264, butoxypolypropylene-glycol, **DEET** (N_1N-diethyl-M toluamide) and **DMP** (dimethylphthalate). The use of repellents is advantageous as legislative and regulatory authorities become more restrictive towards the use of conventional pesticides.

METHODS OF PESTICIDE APPLICATION AND USES

FARM ANIMALS

Traditionally, ectoparasiticides have been applied topically as dusts, sprays, foggers, washes, dips and occasionally used in baits to trap insects. However, with the advent of pour-on and spot-on formulations with a systemic effect, the parenteral administration of drugs such as the avermectins and closantel and the use of impregnated ear tags, collars and tail-tags, the methodology of control applications to animals has changed.

Traditional methods

To be successful, the use of insecticides in dusts, sprays or washes usually requires two or more treatments, since even the most diligent applicant is unlikely to be successful in applying these formulations at the right concentration to all parts of the animal's body. The interval between treatments should be linked to the persistence of the chemical in the skin, hair or wool and to the life cycle of the parasite, further treatment being given prior to completion of another cycle.

Dip baths or spray races containing the necessary concentration of insecticide are used to control mites, lice and ticks and certain dipterans such as blowflies on sheep on a worldwide basis and on cattle in tropical areas. This technique is more successful in sheep where the persistence of insecticide is greater in the wool fleece than in the hair coat found in cattle. It is important to remember that the concentration of insecticide in a dip bath is preferentially 'stripped' or removed as sheep or cattle are dipped, and so must be replenished at a higher than initial concentration, sufficient to maintain an adequate concentration of the active ingredient. Most dips are based on the organophosphate group and synthetic pyrethroids. Despite human and environmental safety concerns, some countries have reintroduced organochlorines because of developing resistance to organophosphates.

Insect control in dairies or stables may be aided by the use of various resins strips incorporating the insecticide; dichlorvos and trichlorfon are often used for this purpose. Sometimes baits containing synthetic pheromones, sugars or hydrolysed yeasts, plus insecticide are spread around animal premises to attract and kill dipterans.

Pour-on, spot-on or spray-on

Those available at present contain organophosphates with a systemic action such as fenthion or phosmet, the avermectins/milbemycins or the synthetic pyrethroids. They are recommended for the control of warbles and lice in cattle and lice and keds in sheep. A valuable development is that of pour-on phosmet for the control of sarcoptic mange in pigs and cattle. A single treatment in pigs gives very good results and, if used in sows prior to farrowing, prevents transmission to the litter; two treatments at an interval of 14 days are necessary in cattle. The synthetic pyrethroids are also available as sprays, pour-ons or spot-ons for the treatment of lice and the control of biting and nuisance flies in cattle, sheep and goats.

Ear tags, collars, leg and tail bands

These are based primarily on the synthetic pyrethroids and occasionally the organophosphates. They are recommended for the protection of cattle against nuisance flies. The tags are usually made of polyvinylchloride impregnated with the insecticide. When attached to an animal's ear the insecticide is released from the surface, dissolves in the sebum secreted by the skin and is then spread over the whole body by the normal grooming actions or ear flapping and tail swishing as well as by bodily contact between cattle. As the insecticide is rapidly bonded to the sebum on the animal's coat the treatment is rain-fast; also the tag or tail band continues to release a supply of chemical under all climatic conditions. Since the drugs are located in the sebum, they are not absorbed into the tissue so there is no need for a withdrawal period prior to slaughter, nor is it necessary to discard milk. The common SPs marketed for this purpose are cypermethrin and permethrin. Under conditions of heavy fly challenge a tag should be inserted in each ear, possibly augmented by a tail band.

Parenteral treatment

The avermectins/milbemycins and closantel may be given parenterally to control some ectoparasites. For example, the endectocides have good activity against warbles, lice, many mites and also the one-host tick *Boophilus*. Closantel is available in some tropical countries for use against one-host ticks and sucking lice.

COMPANION OR PET ANIMALS

Ectoparasiticides are mainly used as dusting powders, aerosols, washes/shampoos, spot-on preparations and impregnated collars, whilst some are available for oral use. They are mainly used for the control of fleas, lice and mange in dogs and cats and for lice, mange and nuisance flies in horses.

Dusting powders

The powders should be shaken well into the animal's fur or hair and, in the case of house pets, into the bedding. The powders commonly used contain pyrethroid-based insecticides with or without the synergist, piperonyl butoxide. These are particularly useful for fleas and lice and repeat treatments are generally recommended every 2–3 weeks.

Aerosols

Although easy to use, some of the noisier sprays can upset pets. Overzealous spraying in confined spaces, such as in a cat basket, may produce toxic effects. Sprays available are generally based on pyrethroids and carbamates or a mixture of organophosphates such as dichlorvos plus fenitrothion, or a mixture of the synergist piperonyl butoxide with OPs or pyrethroids. Depending on the spray, the aerosol container should be held at 15–30 cm from the animal and sprayed for up to 5 seconds for cats and a little longer for dogs. A repeat treatment is often recommended in 7–14 days; but only one spray application with fipronil can give up to 3 months' protection against reinfestation with fleas in dogs and cats. The aerosol sprays are very effective for fleas and lice, but several treatments may be necessary for mange mites. The synthetic pyrethroids are also available as a wash or spot-on for horses for the control of flies including midges, which are responsible for 'sweet-itch'.

Aerosols containing the insect growth regulator, methoprene, are available for the control of larval populations of fleas in the environment.

Baths

These are available as shampoos, emulsifiable concentrates, wettable agents or creams for the control of fleas, lice and mange mites. Most preparations are for dogs and care is needed if they are used for cats. Common ingredients are carbaryl, propoxur and the OP phosmet; amitraz is particularly useful for demodectic mange in dogs. The instructions for bathing should be carefully followed and, where necessary, care taken that the insecticide is properly rinsed from the coat. Organophosphate shampoos should not be used when dogs have insecticidal collars.

Insecticidal collars

These are used primarily for flea control and are based on the organophosphates, carbamates and synthetic pyrethroids. The period of protection is claimed to be 3–4 months, but the success of this method of application is variable. Occasional problems arise from contact dermatitis and care should be exercised that the animals do not receive other organophosphate treatments. Apart from collars, impregnated medallions are also available in some countries. Care should be taken with the use of collars in pedigree long-haired cats and greyhound dogs due to individual susceptibility to OP poisoning.

Collars have also been introduced containing deltamethrin for the control of biting flies, including sandflies, as a means of prevention of infection with transmissible diseases such as leishmaniosis.

Oral preparations

One organophosphate, cythioate, is marketed as an oral preparation. It is specifically for the treatment of demodectic mange and flea infestations in dogs and flea infestation in cats; the daily administration of tablets is recommended as a supplement to topical application.

Other preparations

Spot-on preparations containing fenthion, deltamethrin, fipronil, imidocloprid, emodepside and selamectin are now available for the control of fleas, and in some cases ticks, on dogs and cats. In horses, lice and areas of mange mite infestation can be treated topically, but the problem of nuisance or pasture flies remains. It has been suggested that ear tags impregnated with cypermethrin be attached to the saddle or mane as a possible means of incorporating the synthetic pyrethroid into the sebum.

POULTRY ECTOPARASITES

The carbamates and the organophosphate, malathion, are the most widely used. Individual birds are dusted and the insecticide applied in the poultry house, nesting boxes and litter. Cypermethrin is available for the environmental treatment of poultry red mites (*Dermanyssus*).

ANTIPROTOZOALS

Unlike other antiparasitic agents, for which a few chemical structural classes exhibit a wide spectrum of biological activity, antiprotozoal activity exists in a wide spectrum of chemical classes, each of which possess only a narrow spectrum of activity. The classification of antiprotozoal compounds is complex and for the purposes of this chapter they are divided into eight main groups, each of which may be further subdivided on the basis of structural similarities.

ANTIPROTOZOALS AND THEIR MODE OF ACTION

ANTIMONIALS AND ARSENICALS

Antimonials contain the group V metal, antimony, and have been used extensively for the treatment of leishmaniosis. The antimonials selectively inhibit enzymes that are required for glycolytic and fatty acid oxidation in tissue amastigotes found within macrophages.

Tartar emetic (**antimony potassium tartrate**) was the first antimonial used for this purpose in cases of human leishmaniosis. It was also used in the treatment of *Trypanosoma congolense congolense* and *T. v. vivax* infections in cattle and *T. b. evansi* infections in camels. Extravascular injection causes severe necrosis and the compound has a narrow chemotherapeutic index resulting in about 6% mortality during routine treatment.

Pentavalent antimony compounds **meglumine antimoniate** (**Glucantime** or N-methylglucamine antimoniate), **sodium antimony gluconate** and **sodium stibogluconate** (**Pentostam**) have been the first-line drugs for the treatment of leishmaniosis in humans and are the principal antimonials used for the treatment of canine leishmaniosis. The precise chemical structure of these drugs is difficult to identify. Drug tolerance to antimonials in human and canine leishmaniosis is known and there may be considerable rates of treatment failure and relapses. These drugs may show marked toxic effects such as arthralgia, nephrotoxicity and cardiotoxicity, leading rarely to sudden death. Antimonials are administered either by intralesional infiltration in simple single cutaneous lesions or by intramuscular injection in all cases with systemic involvement. Antimony is excreted quickly from the body so that daily treatment is necessary throughout each course of treatment. Meglumine antimoniate and allopurinol given simultaneously have been shown to maintain dogs in clinical remission.

Arsenicals are substituted benzene arsonic acid salts or esters and have been used in the treatment of trypanosomiosis (**tryparsamide**, **melarsamine**) and coccidiosis (**arsenilic acid, roxarsone**). **Melarsamine** is effective against trypanosomes of the *T. brucei* group (*T. b. evansi*). **Roxarsone** was used primarily as a growth promoter but had some activity against *Eimeria tenella* and *E. brunetti* in chickens when used alone or in combination with nitromide or dinitolmide. Arsenicals have a low safety index and have been superseded by comparatively less toxic compounds.

SUBSTITUTED AROMATICS

Amidines and diamidines

Pentamidine has the widest spectrum within the group with activity against *Leishmania*, *Trypanosoma*, *Babesia* and *Pneumocystis*, and is used mainly in human medicine. Stilbamidine has been used for the treatment of leishmaniosis. **Amicarbilide** is active against *Babesia* and **diminazene aceturate** is active against both *Babesia* and *Trypanosoma*. Very little is known about the mode of action of this class of compounds. Antiparasitic activity may be related to interference with aerobic glycolysis as well as interference with synthesis of parasite DNA.

Diminazene is highly active against babesiosis in cattle, sheep, pigs, horses and dogs although the small *Babesia* spp are generally more refractory to treatment than large ones. There appears to be a wide range of individual animal tolerance to the drug; it is well tolerated in horses at the recommended dose, although higher doses may cause severe side effects. Various treatment regimens are used for eliminating babesiosis in cattle, horses and dogs. In most cases the recommended dose is given in divided doses, e.g. 5 mg/kg, twice at 24-hour intervals, to eradicate *Babesia* spp infections in horses, or 1.75 mg/kg twice at 24-hour intervals to reduce or avoid neurotoxic side effects in horses (lethargy, incoordination and seizures) and dogs (ataxia, opisthotonus, nystagmus, extensor rigidity, coma and even death). Local reactions can occur in cattle and in horses there may be skin sloughing and abscessation following injection. In camels there may be mortality at the recommended dose rate.

Diminazine is also effective against *Trypanosoma congolense congolense* and *T. v. vivax*, but less active against *T. b. brucei* and *T. b. evansi* infections and shows no activity against *T. c. simiae*. Widespread use may lead to development of diminazene-resistant *T. v. vivax* and *T. c. congolense* strains. As a rule, diminazene-resistant strains are susceptible to isometamidium. Trypanosomes resistant to other drugs (except quinapyramine) are commonly susceptible to diminazene.

Phenamidine is used for treating canine and equine babesiosis and has also been used in *Babesia bigemina* infections in cattle. Frequent relapses may occur in *B. gibsoni* infections in dogs. The mechanism of drug action is uncertain but may be similar to that of pentamidine and diminazene.

Arylamides and urea derivatives

Nitolmide and **dinitolmide** are arylamides (nitrobenzamides) used as coccidiostats in poultry appearing to affect first-generation meronts; they are active against *Eimeria tenella* and *E. necatrix* infections but have limited activity against *E. acervulina*. Both drugs have been used in combination with roxarsone as in-feed coccidiostats for use in chickens.

Nicarbazin (phenyl urea) is also used as a coccidiostat in the control of coccidiosis in chickens and turkeys in shuttle programmes (starter feed only) usually in the winter and for that reason resistance of coccidia to nicarbazine is not yet widespread. It is also used in combination with narasin as it shows synergistic effect with the ionophores. It affects second-generation meronts, impairing oocyst formation and allowing treated birds to develop immunity against coccidia. There may be problems with side effects, as it can cause increased sensitivity to heat stress during summer, which results in growth depression and mortality in broilers. The drug should not be fed to laying hens because of toxic side effects (reduced hatchability, interruption of egg laying).

Imidocarb diproprionate is a phenyl urea and is the drug of choice for the treatment of babesiosis in cattle, horses and dogs. It appears to act directly on the parasite leading to an alteration in morphology, and is effective in both treatment and prevention without interfering with the development of immunity.

Ethopabate is an arylamide and has a similar mode of action to the sulphonamides acting as a para-aminobenzoic acid (PABA) agonist, blocking the utilisation of PABA into amino acids and DNA synthesis. It has been administered in combination with amprolium to achieve a broader spectrum of activity for the prophylaxis and treatment of coccidiosis in chickens and turkeys. With chicken coccidia, it has a good innate activity against *Eimeria acervulina*, is less active against *E. maxima* and *E. brunetti* and has no activity against *E. tenella*.

Quinuronium sulphate was for many years the drug of choice in treating bovine babesiosis (*B. bigemina*, *B. bovis*, *B. divergens*); and it is active against large *Babesia* spp of pigs, horses and dogs. The drug has a low therapeutic index and may stimulate the parasympathetic nervous system resulting in excessive salivation, frequent urination, or dyspnoea caused by anticholinesterase activity. The mode of action is unknown.

These compounds have similar modes of action and act by uncoupling oxidative phosphorylation through inhibition of glycerol phosphate oxidase and glycerol phosphate dehydrogenase, which prevents re-oxidation of NADH and decreased adenosine triphosphate (ATP) synthesis.

Sulphonic acids

Suramin and **trypan blue** were amongst the first antiprotozoals. **Suramin** was one of the first anti-trypanosomal drugs developed and shows high efficacy against trypanosomes of subgenus *Trypanozoon* (*T. b. brucei*, *T. b. evansi*, *T. equiperdum*) and is the drug of choice for *T. b. evansi* infections (surra) in camels and horses. The drug inhibits enzymes in the glucose metabolism pathway preventing re-oxidation of NADH and decreased ATP synthesis. It may be toxic in horses, causing oedema of sexual organs, lips and eyelids or painful hoofs. Intramuscular administration can cause severe necrosis at the injection site and sub-optimal dosing (less than 1 g/100 kg body weight) may lead to suramin-resistant strains.

Trypan blue is an azo-napthalene dye used for the treatment of babesiosis and was the first specific drug with activity against *B. bigemina* in cattle, but its use leads to blue staining of meat and milk, and it has been largely replaced by the diamidines.

Napthoquinones

Menoctone, **parvaquone** and **buparvaquone** are napthoquinones with marked anti-theilerial activity. They appear to block electron transport at the ubiquinone level. The mechanism of selective toxicity might be due to a difference between parasite and mammalian ubiquinone.

Menoctone was the first drug with high anti-theilerial activity, causing marked degeneration in appearance of macroschizonts and suppression of parasitaemia in established *Theileria parva parva* infections in cattle. Its use has now been discontinued.

Parvaquone is highly active against theileriosis (*Theileria p. parva* and *T. annulata*) infections in cattle when treatment is performed in the early stage of infection, allowing development of protective immunity without apparent clinical signs. **Buparvaquone** is an analogue of parvaquone with a substituted alkyl group, which slows down metabolic degradation of the parent compound, increasing efficacy against these species.

Miscellaneous diphenyls

Robenidine is a guanidine derivative and affects the late first-generation and second-stage meronts of *Eimeria*. It is both coccidiostatic and coccidiocidal and is used for the treatment of coccidiosis in chickens, turkeys and rabbits. It has a broad spectrum of activity but in rabbits it is active against intestinal *Eimeria* spp only. It is thought to interfere with energy metabolism by inhibition of respiratory chain phosphorylation and ATPase activity.

Dapsone and **acedapsone** are sulphones active against *Plasmodium* and are generally used in combination products only for treating human malaria. Their mode of action is similar to the sulphonamides, acting as antifolate drugs, blocking the incorporation of PABA to form dihydrofolic acid.

PYRIDINE DERIVATIVES

Decoquinate and **methylbenzoquate** are 4-hydroxyquinolones that act on the sporozoites and first-generation meronts of *Eimeria*, interfering with electron transport at the cytochrome B level and mitochondrial metabolism. Hydroxyquinolines are almost entirely coccidiostatic with activity against sporozoites and trophozoites of all *Eimeria* spp. As single compounds they have only limited success as a result of serious and immediate drug resistance in the field, such that methylbenzoquate-resistant *Eimeria* cannot be controlled by the drug at any level.

Decoquinate has been used for the control of coccidiosis in poultry and is used for the prevention and control of coccidiosis in cattle and sheep.

Methylbenzoquate is usually administered in combination with clopidol or meticlorpindol, mainly in shuttle or rotation programmes to achieve a broader spectrum of activity for the prophylaxis and treatment of coccidiosis in chickens and turkeys.

Iodoquinol is a 4-hydroxyquinolone that is active against Entamoeba.

Quinine, **chloroquine**, **droxycholoquine**, **primaquine** and **mefloquine** are quinolines used primarily as antimalarial treatments in human medicine, inhibiting electron transport processes by inhibiting pyrimidine synthesis.

Primaquine diphosphate is active against tissue stages of *Plasmodium*, but is much less active against erythrocytic stages. It has been shown to be active against *Babesia felis* in cats at 0.5 mg/kg by intramuscular injection, although doses above 1 mg/kg caused mortality. It has also been used in the treatment or prevention of avian malaria (100 mg/kg per os).

Clopidol and **meticlorpindol** are pyridinols and are active against first-generation meronts, arresting sporozoite and trophozoite development; they are effective against all *Eimeria* spp in chickens, although resistance problems limit their use to shuttle programmes. Both compounds need to be given before or shortly after exposure and are used as a coccidiostats. Clopidol is used in the prevention of coccidiosis in chickens, partridge, guinea fowl, pheasants and rabbits with a high safety index.

Emetine and **dehydroemetine** are isoquinolines with activity against *Entamoeba*. The acridine derivative, **quinacrine**, is active against *Plasmodium* and *Giardia*. **Acriflavine** hydrochloride is active against *Babesia bigemina* and other large *Babesia* spp.

PYRIMIDINE DERIVATIVES

Amprolium is structurally similar to thiamine (vitamin B1) and is a competitive thiamine antagonist. Because of the relatively high thiamine requirement of rapidly dividing coccidian cells compared with most host cells, the drug has a high safety margin. Amprolium acts on first-generation meronts, thereby preventing differentiation of merozoites, but has poor activity against some *Eimeria* spp. It is often used in combination with ethopabate but its use has declined in many countries for safety and tolerance reasons in food-producing animals. Amprolium, and amprolium + ethopabate, have been used as feed additives for use in chickens, guinea fowl and turkeys for the prevention of coccidiosis, showing activity against *Eimeria tenella* and *E. necatrix*, and to a lesser extent against *E. maxima* of chickens, and also the pathogenic *Eimeria* spp of turkeys.

Amprolium + ethopabate have been combined with sulphaquinoxaline and pyrimethamine to extend their activity spectrum and to improve efficacy against amprolium-resistant *Eimeria* spp, but such combinations have been discontinued in some countries because of residue problems.

Amprolium, and amprolium + ethopabate have also been used for the treatment and control of coccidiosis in pheasants (but are not active against all *Eimeria* spp); lambs and calves; sows to control disease in suckling pigs pre- and post-farrowing; and rabbits to control intestinal *Eimeria* spp, but they are ineffective against hepatic coccidiosis in rabbits.

Pyrimethamine and **trimethoprim** are both folate antagonists with activity against *Pneumocystis* and are useful for treating various types of coccidiosis (eimeriosis, toxoplasmosis, sarcocystosis, neosporosis), malaria and bacterial infections. These compounds target the enzyme dihydrofolate reductase, inhibit pyrimidine biosynthesis and DNA metabolism and are usually used in combination with long-acting sulphonamides. As antifolates they synergise the anticoccidial action of sulphonamides by blocking the same biosynthetic pathway.

Halofuginone is a quinazoline affecting first- and second-generation meronts of *Eimeria* and is used in the control of coccidiosis in chickens and turkeys. The drug has also been shown to possess marked antitheilerial activity in cattle, and is available in some countries for the prevention and treatment of cryptosporidiosis in calves. It has also been shown to be effective against acute sarcosporidiosis in goats and sheep (*Sarcocystis capracanis* and *S. ovicanis*, respectively at 0.67 mg/kg on two successive days). The therapeutic index of halofuginone is low and overdose may produce severe diarrhoea and cachexia.

Allopurinol is a pyrazolpyrimidine and is a xanthine oxidase inhibitor, used alone or in combination with meglumine antimonate for the treatment of leishmaniosis in dogs.

Aprinocid is no longer available due to the rapid emergence of resistant strains, but it was used a feed additive for the prevention of coccidiosis in broiler chickens with a broad spectrum of activity except against *Eimeria tenella*. The compound inhibits sporulation of oocysts and may be coccidiostatic after a short medication period or coccidiocidal after long periods of medication. Arprinocid acts against coccidia by inhibiting hypoxanthine transport.

PHENATHRIDIUMS

This group of compounds, which includes **isometamidium**, **homidium** and **quinapyrimine**, has been used exclusively in the treatment of trypanosomiosis. The mode of action appears to be interference with nucleic acid synthesis by intercalative DNA binding. Other drugs of this series, **pyrithridium**, **phenidium chloride** and **dimidium bromide**, were replaced because of a high incidence of delayed toxicity, including marked liver damage and severe local reaction at the injection site.

Isometamidium is a synthetic hybrid of the diazotised p-aminobenzamidine moiety of diminazene molecule linked with homidium chloride. The drug is highly active against *Trypanosoma vivax vivax* infections in ruminants and horses as well as against *T. c. congolense* infections in ruminants, horses and dogs. It is less active against *T. b. brucei* and *T. b. evansi* infections in horses, ruminants, camels and dogs. The recommended dose is usually well tolerated by cattle. However, intramuscular injection can cause severe local reactions at the injection site. Intravenous injection in horses and camels may avoid local reaction but may cause systemic toxicity (salivation, tachycardia, profuse diarrhoea, hindleg weakness and collapse due to histamine release).

Homidium salts (bromide or chloride) are effective against *T. v. vivax* infections in cattle but less so against *T. c. congolense* and *T. b. brucei*. Their limited protective activity in cattle depends on severity of challenge and may last 3–5 weeks. Homidium can also be used for treating *T. v. vivax* and *T. c. congolense* infections in horses and dogs. Widespread use in cattle resulted in appearance of resistant *T. c. congolense* strains in east and west Africa. Homidium-resistant trypanosomes can be controlled by diminazene or isometamidium at increased dose rates. The drug is generally well tolerated at the recommended dose and also at higher dose levels, but may be irritant at sites of injection. Deep intramuscular injection effectively reduces local irritations. Severe reactions may occur in horses after intramuscular injection, whereas intravenous injection seems to be well tolerated.

Quinapyrimine is highly active against *T. c. congolense*, *T. v. vivax*, *T. b. brucei* and *T. b. evansi* and reaches therapeutic levels quickly. The target of action of quinapyramine is protein synthesis, displacing magnesium (Mg^{2+}) ions and polyamines from cytoplasmic ribosomes, leading to an extensive loss of ribosomes and condensation of kinetoplast DNA. The drug can cause local and systemic reactions (salivation, shaking, trembling, diarrhoea, collapse) in cattle, horse, dogs and pigs within minutes of treatment. Unexpected acute toxicity and the rapid development of drug-resistant strains of *T. c. congolense* have limited its usefulness in treating trypanosomiosis in cattle. However, the drug seems to be safe and efficient for treating surra (*T. b. evansi*) in camels and horses as well as *T. b. evansi* infections in pigs. Quinapyramine-resistant strains are usually controlled by isometamidium. Quinapyramine is active against suramin-resistant strains of *T. b. evansi* and *T. b. brucei*.

TRIAZONES

Toltrazuril is a symmetrical triazone compound and is active against all intracellular stages of coccidia found in chicken, geese, ducks and cattle, sheep, goats and pigs. Toltrazuril is used therapeutically for the treatment of outbreaks of coccidiosis. It can be administered via drinking water and, because of its long residual activity, it can be used intermittently, allowing development of protective immunity.

Diclazuril and **clazuril** are asymmetrical triazones with a broad spectrum of activities against various coccidia in birds and animals at low concentrations (0.5–2 ppm in feed). **Diclazuril** has a strong anticoccidiocidal activity and has been developed as a feed additive for the prevention of coccidiosis in chickens and turkeys. It is active against developing first- and second-generation meronts and gamonts of *Eimeria tenella* and other pathogenic *Eimeria* spp of chickens; but developmental stages most affected by diclazuril varies with the *Eimeria* species. It is highly effective against all stages of *E. tenella* but only against gamont stages of *E. maxima*. Due to the development of resistance, it is used frequently in shuttle programmes. Diclazuril is also used for the treatment of rabbit coccidiosis, showing high activity against hepatic and intestinal coccidiosis, and in the treatment and prevention of coccidiosis in sheep.

Clazuril has only limited action against some chicken coccidia, but is highly active against coccidiosis in pigeons.

BENZIMIDAZOLES

The benzimidazoles have been described in more detail in the Anthelmintics section at the beginning of this chapter.

Benzimidazoles such as **mebendazole**, **fenbendazole** or **albendazole** are active against *Giardia* infections in man, farm animals and dogs; repeat treatments may be necessary, however, to eliminate parasites because of reinfection.

ANTIBACTERIALS

Sulphonamides

Sulphonamides, such as **sulphadimidine**, **sulphamethoxypyrizidine**, **sulphaguanidine**, **sulphaquinoxaline** and **sulphachloropyrazine**, are structural antagonists of para-aminobenzoic acid (PABA), which is incorporated into folic acid. They inhibit the conversion of dihydrofolic acid to tetrahydrofolic acid at the dihydropteroate synthase step. Tetrahydrofolate is an important cofactor in many active single carbon transfer reactions, required for the synthesis of certain amino acids, purines and especially the synthesis of de-oxythymidylate, required for DNA synthesis. Large doses used for therapeutic applications often cause toxicity (haemorrhagic syndrome, kidney damage and growth depression).

Sulphonamides were among the first anticoccidials and are active against first- and second-stage meronts, being coccidiostatic at low doses and coccidiocidal at higher doses. Many of the compounds used in chickens had a broad spectrum of activity against intestinal *Eimeria* spp but only a moderate effect on *E. tenella* in chickens, but their use has been stopped in many countries. Sulphonamides have also been used in the treatment of coccidiosis in cattle, sheep, pigs, dogs, cats and rabbits. When given in combination with pyrimethamine and other diaminopyrimidines, long-acting sulphonamides (e.g. sulphadoxine or sulphamethoxine) are highly active antibacterials, antimalarials and anticoccidials.

Nitroimidazoles

The nitroimidazoles include **dimetridazole**, **ornidazole**, **ronidazole**, **tinadazole**, **carnidazole** and **metronidazole**, which appear to interfere with RNA synthesis, and **nifursol**, which acts by causing damage to lipids and DNA within the cells.

These compounds exhibit potent activity against trichomonads, *Histomonas*, *Spironucleus* and *Giardia*, and were the drugs of choice for these infections in turkeys and gamebirds. Ronidazole, dimetridazole and nifursol were used in the treatment of *Histomonas* infections in turkeys and gamebirds (pheasants, partridge); however, because of concerns over mutagenicity their use has been suspended in many countries. Carnidazole is used for the treatment of trichomoniosis in pigeons. Metronidazole, ornidazole and tinazole are used in humans for the treatment of giardiosis and amoebiosis.

Nitrofurans

The nitrofurans, which include **furazolidone**, **nitrofurazone** and **nitrofurantoin**, are relatively broad-spectrum bactericidal drugs and have coccidiostatic activity; concerns over toxicity and carcinogenicity have restricted their widespread use and they are prohibited from use in many countries. **Furazolidone** has been used for the prevention and treatment of coccidiosis in chickens, turkeys and pigs and for the treatment of bacterial digestive tract infections and giardiosis. **Nitrofurazone** is active against second-generation meronts of *Eimeria tenella* and *E. necatrix* infections in poultry, and has been used for control of coccidiosis in lambs and goat kids.

Ionophores

The polyether ionophores are fermentation products of *Streptomyces* or *Actinomadura*. These are currently the most widely used anticoccidial compounds used mainly for the control of poultry coccidosis. **Monensin**, **narasin**, **salinomycin, maduramicin** and **semduramicin** are 'monovalent' ionophores preferentially binding to monovalent ions, sodium and potassium (Na^+, K^+), although divalent cations are also bound. **Lasalocid** has the ability to complex divalent cations (Ca^{2+}, Mg^{2+}) and is termed a 'divalent' ionophore. The effect is to destroy cross-membrane ion gradients. They may also block host carbohydrate transport and hence deprive carbohydrate supply from intracellular parasites.

Ionophores act upon the intestinal free forms of coccidian stages (sporozoites, merozoites and gametocytes) when the drug comes into contact with them in the intestinal lumen.

These compounds are extremely toxic to horses. Ionophores such as monensin, narasin and salinomycin may cause severe growth retardation when administered with tiamulin, and most of the ionophores may interact with sulphonamides, chloramphenicol and erythromycin.

Monensin has been used extensively in the broiler industry but drug tolerance, as with other ionophores, limits its use to shuttle programmes. It is effective against coccidia in cattle, sheep and rabbits when used prophylactically in feed.

Narasin is given in combination with nicarbazine to improve coccidiosis control, and the drug combination may be used in the starter phase of shuttle programmes followed by a different ionophore in the grower–finisher phase.

Salinomycin has broad-spectrum activity and better activity against *Eimeria tenella* and *E. acervulina* than other related ionophores, including drug-tolerant *Eimeria* spp in the field. In turkeys, it may cause severe toxicity with growth depression, excitement, paralysis of head and legs and death if feed containing recommended or lower doses is fed for long periods.

Lasalocid may alter water excretion in treated birds via dietary electrolytes to the extent that wet litter may be a problem at higher drug concentrations. At concentrations of 75 ppm activity against *E. tenella* is good but insufficient against *E. acervulina*. In the field, lasalocid may improve control of coccidiosis where *E. tenella* strains show tolerance to other ionophores.

Macrolide and lincosamide antibiotics

This group of compounds is better known and more widely applied for the treatment of bacterial and fungal infections. The mode of action appears to be an inhibition of protein synthesis. **Spiramycin** inhibits protein synthesis by inhibiting the translocation of peptidyl-t-RNA. It has been used for the treatment of *Toxoplasma* infections. **Clindamycin** is a lincosamide with a similar mode of action, and has been used to treat *Plasmodium*, *Babesia* and *Toxoplasma* infections.

Amphotericin B is a polyene macrolide antibiotic used mainly as an antifungal agent but is also used as a second-line drug for the treatment of *Leishmania*. The drug is extremely nephrotoxic but lipid and unilamellar liposome formulations of amphotericin B have been developed with lower toxicity.

Aminoglycoside antibiotics

Aminogycoside antibiotics are bactericidal agents and are widely applied for the treatment of Gram-negative bacterial infections. Aminoglycosides are not absorbed from the gastrointestinal tract and treatment via this route is reserved for the treatment of gastrointestinal infections. **Parmomycin** has activity against *Entamoeba*, *Giardia*, *Balantidium* and *Leishmania*.

Tetracycline antibiotics

The tetracyclines are broad-spectrum antibacterials active against a range of Gram-positive and Gram-negative bacteria, but also against the Rickettsiales (*Rickettsia*, *Ehrlichia*, *Anaplasma*), and *Mycoplasma* and *Chlamydia*. The mode of action is thought to be through inhibition of protein synthesis.

Oxytetracycline, **tetracycline** and **chlortetracycline** have similar properties and may be given orally or by intramuscular injection. **Doxycycline** is more lipophilic than the other tetracyclines and is better absorbed orally and penetrates better into the lung and cerebrospinal fluid. Members of this group exhibit the broadest antiprotozoal activity and have been used for the treatment of *Plasmodium*, *Balantidium*, *Theileria* and *Entamoeba*. Oxytetracycline has been shown to control active *Babesia divergens* infections in cattle by continuous administration of 20 mg/kg every 4 days.

USE OF ANTIPROTOZOALS

The use of antiprotozoals as therapeutic or prophylactic agents is similar to that described for anthelmintics.

METHODS OF ADMINISTRATION

Anticoccidials used for controlling enteric coccidia principally belonging to the genus, *Eimeria*, are administered in feed. In the poultry industry, it is usual to employ anticoccidials in broiler birds continuously in feed until just before slaughter. In layer replacement stock, pullets are medicated continuously until commencement of egg-laying. Continuous use of anticoccidials may lead to ineffective treatment due to drug resistance; as a consequence, various rotational programmes have been developed by the poultry industry to reduce or avoid this problem.

Antiprotozoals are generally used in two ways: therapeutically, to treat existing infections or clinical

Table 14.2 Trypanocidal drugs.

Generic name	Dosage rate (mg/kg)	Route	Remarks
Suramin	10	IV	Mainly used against *T. evansi* in camels. Some activity against *T. brucei* in camels and *T. equiperdum* in horses
Diminazene aceturate	3.5–7	IM	Mainly used in cattle and small ruminants against *T. vivax*, *T. congolense* and *T. brucei*
Homidium bromide	1	IM	Mainly used in cattle and small ruminants against *T. vivax*, *T. congolense* and *T. brucei*. Should be dissolved in hot water. Potentially carcinogenic
Homidium chloride	1	IM	Mainly used in cattle and small ruminants against *T. vivax*, *T. congolense* and *T. brucei*, but soluble in cold water
Quinapyramine methyl sulphate	5	SC	Active against *T. vivax*, *T. congolense* and *T. brucei* in cattle. Now mainly used against *T evansi*, *T brucei* in camels and horses; activity against *T. equiperdum* in horses
Isometamidium chloride	0.25–0.5	IM	Used mainly in cattle (*T. vivax*, *T. congolense*), as a curative at lower rates, as a prophylactic at higher rates. Also contains homidium, and is therefore to be considered as potentially carcinogenic

Not all trypanocides are available in every country and there is also no guarantee that production of all or any of them will economic reasons.

outbreaks, or prophylactically, in which the timing of treatment is based on knowledge of the epidemiology. Clearly prophylactic use is preferable where administration of a drug at selected intervals or continuously over a period can prevent the occurrence of disease.

Most other antiprotozoal agents, particularly those targeting haemoprotozoan infections, are given parenterally, either by subcutaneous or intramuscular injection.

RESISTANCE

ANTHELMINTIC RESISTANCE

Drug resistance is heritable and repeated dosing will therefore select for an increasing proportion of resistant individuals. The mechanisms involve either differences in drug metabolism within the parasite and/or mutations at the binding site of the drug. The prevalence and severity of anthelmintic resistance is increasing and leading to uncontrolled loss of production.

Helminth resistance to anthelmintics has been most frequently recorded in sheep and goats (mainly *Haemonchus* spp and *Trichostrongylus* spp in tropical and subtropical regions and *Teladorsagia* in temperate areas) and horses (mainly the small strongyles), and initially involved the benzimidazole group of compounds. Over the last decade resistance to all three chemical classes of broad-spectrum anthelmintics, 1-BZ (benzimidazoles and probenzimidazoles), 2-LM (levamisole/morantel) and 3-AV (avermectins/milbemycins), and in some cases to the narrow-spectrum anthelmintics, such as closantel, has become more widespread in nematode parasites of small ruminants. These multi-resistant isolates are particularly prevalent in countries in the southern hemisphere, such as Australia, New Zealand, South Africa and South American countries. The differences in the rate of emergence of anthelmintic resistance between these agroclimatic zones are considered to be due to the number of parasite generations and biotic potential of the parasite species involved and also to the proportion of the total population which is not exposed to the drug (i.e. left *in refugia*). Frequency of treatment and underdosing are considered to be the main cause of benzimidazole and levamisole resistance in *Haemonchus* and *Teladorsagia*. The timing of treatments and the presence of larvae *in refugia* may be particularly important in the development of macrocyclic lactone resistance. Trematode resistance to flukicides is currently at a considerably lower level.

Studies have shown minimal reversion to susceptibility in highly selected homozygous isolates following withdrawal of the selecting drug and, as a consequence, once resistant worms are present on a livestock enterprise they can be considered as permanent. Therefore, it is important to be able to detect the presence of emerging resistant isolates at an early stage. Unfortunately, the *in vivo* faecal egg count reduction test and the *in vitro* egg hatch assay, larval development assay and larval migration inhibition assay, used to detect the presence of resistant isolates, are insensitive and will only detect resistant parasites when resistant parasites comprise around 25% of the total population. The use of a discriminating dose of anthelmintic may increase the sensitivity. New molecular-based probes are more sensitive but to date are only available for the benzimidazoles and are mainly used as research tools.

Strategies to delay the development/transmission of anthelmintic resistance are discussed under Treatment, prevention and control of parasitic gastroenteritis in sheep (Chapter 3). No new anthelmintic families are expected to be licensed in the near future, partly due to cost, and partly as the sheep sector is a small global market. It is therefore essential that the sheep industry adopts control strategies that reduce the reliance on anthelmintics. Non-chemical approaches include:

1. The breeding of sheep that are able to resist or tolerate worm infections.
2. Feeding of nematophagous fungi which are able to trap larvae in the faeces and thus reduce pasture contamination.
3. Dietary supplementation with rumen bypass protein or forages rich in condensed tannins to increase the supply of protein to the small intestine and thus enhance the rate of acquisition of immunity.
4. Periodic grazing of pastures that contain forage species with anthelmintic properties.
5. The application of new molecular vaccines. These new approaches may initially need to be introduced in conjunction with limited chemotherapy to provide an integrated strategy for the control of PGE.

PESTICIDE RESISTANCE

At the recommended doses modern insecticides are highly effective at removing susceptible individuals, but they can impose strong selection pressure for the development of resistance. The development of resistance may reduce the effectiveness of the treatment applied and thereby increase the frequency of application and the dose required, in turn increasing the costs and adding to the environmental impact.

There are two major variables that determine the rate at which resistance is likely to spread throughout the population: its mechanism of inheritance and the severity of selective pressure (what percentage of susceptible individuals survive each generation). In general, resistance will spread through a population most rapidly when it is inherited as a single, dominant allele and selective pressure is high (meaning very few susceptible individuals escape and reproduce).

When an insect population develops resistance to one pesticide, it may also prove to be resistant to similar compounds that have the same mode of action. This phenomenon, known as class resistance, occurs frequently in pest populations that develop resistance to organophosphate, carbamate or pyrethroid insecticides. In some cases, a population may develop a form of resistance that protects it from compounds in more than one chemical class. This is known as cross-resistance, and may result in an ectoparasite population that can no longer be controlled with chemical insecticides.

Overall, resistance in the majority of ectoparasite species is not as severe or widespread a problem as that seen in endoparasites.

There are three general approaches that can be used to reduce the rate of resistance development:

1. **Management by saturation** involves heavy or frequent use of a pesticide that is designed to leave absolutely no survivors. It is most effective when the resistant gene is dominant and the target population is small, isolated or living in a limited habitat.
2. **Management by moderation** uses only the minimum control necessary to reduce a population below an acceptable level. This strategy tries to ensure that susceptible genes are never eliminated from the population. It works best when the susceptible trait is dominant over the resistant trait.
3. **Management by multiple attack** involves the use of several control tactics that work in different ways. By rotating insecticides with different modes of action or by alternating chemical with non-chemical control tactics, a pest population is exposed to selective pressures that change from generation to generation.

The approach adopted clearly also will depend on the parasite in question, the epidemiology of transmission and the farming environment. Permanent ectoparasites, or highly host-specific species which spend long periods on the host, and which have relatively low rates of transmission, such as bot and warble flies, can be susceptible to coordinated programmes of management by saturation because entire populations can be targeted and removed simultaneously. In general, however, for most ectoparasites, management by moderation and management by multiple attack are recommended. In addition, however, it is essential to ensure that manufacturer's recommendations are scrupulously followed and that all apparatus is calibrated correctly and working effectively.

For farmers wanting to reduce reliance on synthetic insecticides, a range of management practices and non-chemical methods may be utilised in an integrated manner to reduce ectoparasite prevalence. One or several techniques may be used, but importantly these should be integrated with each other to form components of a general livestock ectoparasite management programme. Such management is usually based on the use of control technologies which modify some aspect of the parasite's environment, on or off the host, either to increase pest mortality, to reduce fecundity or to reduce contact between the pest and host.

There can be little doubt that resistance to existing chemicals is unlikely to be reversed and indeed will become more widespread, and that new compounds developed in the future will also select for resistance. Probably the most optimistic prognosis is that appropriate management will allow the rate of development of resistance to be reduced.

ANTIPROTOZOAL RESISTANCE

Continuous use of antiprotozoals has also led to ineffective treatment due to drug resistance in the target parasite populations. This is perhaps best exemplified by the situation with anticoccidial compounds.

The control of avian coccidiosis (see Chapter 7: Poultry and gamebirds) relies almost entirely on chemotherapy, as is evident from the fact that most intensively reared chickens are fed an anticoccidial agent in the diet throughout their period of growth. Feed medication is a convenient and cost-effective method of enabling large numbers of chickens to be reared under intensive conditions. The practice of including drugs in the feed throughout the life of the bird has ensured that few parasites escape the effects of medication. In such an environment, parasites are exposed throughout their life cycle to agents designed for their removal and this has inevitably resulted in the development of resistance.

A succession of chemical compounds has been introduced and has been crucial in the successful control of coccidiosis in the rapidly expanding poultry industries throughout the world. However the emergence of resistance has been rapid and has limited the useful life of many chemical anticoccidials, although the speed at which resistance develops varies greatly between compounds. With the ionophorus antibiotics, which have dominated the scene for the last two decades, resistance has been considerably slower to develop. Nevertheless, resistance to this group has been reported in both Europe and the USA, with cross-resistance occurring notably among the monovalent cation group. Although ionophore-resistant strains may be present, it is possible that the numbers of oocysts are insufficient to cause clinical coccidiosis. Selection pressure is therefore probably lower than with many of the chemical anticoccidials. It has been suggested that this incomplete control of parasite development stimulates production of immunity in the host and this may be a major factor in the effectiveness of ionophores in the field.

Knowledge of the mode of action of anticoccidial compounds is necessary to understand the mechanisms of resistance. Although some information is available on the biochemical pathways inhibited by certain anticoccidial drugs, explanations for their selectivity are either circumstantial or unknown. As in other parasites, the most likely mechanism of resistance involves modification of the target receptor so that its sensitivity to inhibition is decreased. Compounds that share a similar mode of action may also share resistance (cross-resistance). This should be distinguished from multiple resistance in which resistance may be to several drugs with differing modes of action.

It has been shown that parasites resistant to the recommended levels of certain anticoccidial drugs may be suppressed if the concentration of drug is increased. Resistance to these higher concentrations, however, is likely to develop rapidly after further selection. Increasing the concentration of a drug may, therefore, only be of use in the short term and, in any case, would not be practical because most anticoccidial drugs are used at levels close to those that are toxic to the chicken.

Resistant strains may emerge if anticoccidial drugs have been employed at concentrations lower than those normally recommended for control. It would therefore appear to be important to maintain adequate drug levels in the field in order to reduce the possibility of selecting resistant strains. A reduction in the use of drugs is desirable since it is generally accepted that the selection of genes for resistance will occur more rapidly as the frequency of treatment is increased. Control of coccidiosis may be achieved by giving drugs intermittently; the objective being to prevent the build-up of infection in a poultry house. Such a policy would, however, be unacceptable to the poultry industry because of the impairment of food conversion etc. that would probably result.

The genetics of anticoccidial resistance in *Eimeria* are poorly understood. Most drugs inhibit the asexual stages of the life cycle. Many of the complexities involved in the selection of resistance in diploid organisms, such as the degree of dominance of resistance genes, are absent because these stages are haploid. Any resistant mutants will, therefore, be immediately selected at the expense of sensitive forms. Asexual division will ensure their rapid multiplication and resistance will rapidly become the dominant phenotype. It has been shown that resistance to certain drugs (e.g. decoquinate, methylbenzoquate) develops rapidly in a single step and may be due to a single mutation, whereas resistance to other drugs, such as amprolium and robenidine, develops more slowly, possibly as a result of a series of small discrete steps involving successive mutations. Information on the rate at which resistance develops may be helpful in selecting the most appropriate drugs for use in the field.

The control of coccidiosis is likely to continue to depend upon chemotherapy until alternatives, such as

Table 14.3 Insecticide resistance in the major ectoparasites of importance in cattle and sheep.

Family	Species	Primary host	Known resistance
Mites (Acari: Astigmata)	*Sarcoptes scabiei*	Pig	Ivermectin resistance in humans; not yet known in animal parasites
	Psoroptes ovis	Sheep (occasionally cattle)	Gamma-hexachlorohexane (OC), diazinon (OP), propetamphos (OP), flumethrin (SP), high-cis-cypermethrin (SP)
	Chorioptes bovis	Sheep	None recorded
Ticks (Acari: Ixodidae)	*Ixodes ricinus*	Sheep and cattle	None recorded
	Ixodes persulcatus	Sheep and cattle	None recorded
	Rhipicephalus sanguineus group, *R. bursa*, *R. turanicus*, *R. appendiculatus*	Sheep and cattle	Amitraz (Formamidine), dichlorfenvinphos (OP), cypermethrin (SP)
	Hyalomma marginatum	Sheep and cattle	None recorded
	Boophilus annulatus	Sheep and cattle	None recorded
	Dermacentor reticulatus, *D. marginatus*	Sheep and cattle	None recorded
	Haemaphysalis punctata	Sheep and cattle	None recorded
Sucking lice (Phthiraptera: Anoplura)	*Linognathus vituli*	Cattle	None recorded
	Linognathus pedalis, *L. ovillus*	Sheep	None recorded
	Haematopinus eurysternus	Cattle	None recorded
	Haematopinus quadripertusus	Cattle	None recorded
	Solenoptes capillatus	Cattle	None recorded
Chewing lice (Phthiraptera: Mallophaga)	*Bovicola bovis*, *B. ovis*	Cattle, sheep	Aldrin (OC), dieldrin (OC), gamma-hexachlorohexane (OC), diazinon (OP), deltamethrin (SP), high-cis-cypermethrin (SP)
Myiasis (Diptera: Calliphoridae)	*Lucilia* spp	Sheep	In Australia: dieldrin (OC), diazinon (OP), diflubenzuron (IGR)
Myiasis (Diptera: Sarcophagidae)	*Wohlfahrtia magnifica*	Sheep	None recorded
Myiasis (Diptera: Oestridae)	*Oestrus ovis*	Sheep	None recorded
	Hypoderma lineatum, *H. bovis*	Cattle	None recorded
Fleas: (Siphonaptera: Pulicidae)	*Ctenocephalides felis*	Sheep	Suspected but not yet confirmed

immunoprophylaxis, become a practical reality. Until now, as resistance has developed to the older compounds, new ones have been discovered to replace them. It is doubtful whether this situation will continue. It is important, therefore, that strategies be devised to obtain the best use of existing drugs.

Alternation of drugs (rotation) with different modes of action has been widely advocated in the poultry industry, but this has been based upon an empirical, rather than scientific, basis. It is not known for what duration (number of crops) a particular drug should be used before changing to another anticoccidial agent. Alternation of drugs within a single crop (shuttle programmes) has also been widely practised. It has been claimed that this may slow the development of resistance but no evidence to support this contention has been provided. The period of medication for the drugs in a shuttle may be too short to eliminate any resistant forms. Resistant parasites may survive in the litter for the life of the crop and the subsequent use of the same drugs would result in further selection pressure for resistance. A likely result of short periods of alternation between drugs is the development of strains resistant to several drugs (multiple resistance). Vaccines based upon live, attenuated parasites are a possible alternative to medication for the control of coccidiosis. Alternating cycles of planned immunisation and chemotherapy might result in the replacement of drug-resistant parasites by drug-sensitive strains with a reduced pathogenicity.

Reversion to sensitivity with older chemical compounds can eventually occur leading to their reintroduction in control programmes. The time interval, however, before a population recovers susceptibility to a drug is likely to be considerably longer than the time taken to acquire resistance. It is also probable that resistance will re-emerge more rapidly if older compounds are reintroduced. Various combinations of drugs have been employed to extend the spectrum of activity against different species of *Eimeria* rather than prevent the development of resistance (e.g. amprolium and ethopabate). Mixtures have also been used to reduce the risk of toxicity since, in some cases, adequate activity can be obtained with lower doses than if the drugs are used alone (e.g. naracin and nicarbazin). Even where these combination drug mixtures have been used, resistance has developed.

Another area in which resistance has become a problem is in the control of trypanosomiosis. Drug resistance was first noted in trypanosomes to the arsenicals and aromatic compounds. For example, diminazene-resistance in *Trypanosoma vivax vivax* and *T. c. congolense* strains is now widespread. As a rule, diminazene-resistant strains are susceptible to isometamidium. Widespread use of homidium and quinapyridine in cattle resulted in the appearance of resistant *T. c. congolense* strains in east and west Africa. Homidium-resistant trypanosomes can be controlled by diminazene or isometamidium at increased dose rates. Quinapyramine-resistant strains are usually controlled by isometamidium. Quinapyramine is also active against suramin-resistant strains of *T. b. evansi* and *T. b. brucei.*

15
The laboratory diagnosis of parasitism

HELMINTH INFECTIONS

Although there is much current interest in the use of serology and molecular methods as an aid to the diagnosis of helminthosis, particularly with the enzyme-linked immunosorbent assay (ELISA) test and the polymerase chain reaction (PCR), faecal examination for the presence of worm eggs or larvae is the most common routine aid to diagnosis employed.

COLLECTION OF FAECES

Faecal samples should preferably be collected from the rectum and examined fresh. If it is difficult to take rectal samples, then fresh faeces can be collected from the field or floor. A plastic glove is suitable for collection, the glove being turned inside out to act as the receptacle. For small pets a thermometer or glass rod may be used.

Ideally, about 5 g of faeces should be collected, since this amount is required for some of the concentration methods of examination.

Since eggs embryonate rapidly the faeces should be stored in the refrigerator unless examination is carried out within a day. For samples sent through the post, an anaerobic storage system in an air-tight container containing tap water will minimise development and hatching.

METHODS OF EXAMINATION OF FAECES

Several methods are available for preparing faeces for microscopic examination to detect the presence of eggs or larvae. However, whatever method of preparation is used, the slides should first be examined under low power since most eggs can be detected at this magnification. If necessary, higher magnification can then be employed for measurement of the eggs or more detailed morphological differentiation. An eyepiece micrometer is very useful for sizing populations of eggs or larvae.

DIRECT SMEAR METHOD

A few drops of water plus an equivalent amount of faeces are mixed on a microscope slide. Tilting the slide then allows the lighter eggs to flow away from the heavier debris, a cover slip is placed on the fluid and the preparation is then examined microscopically. It is possible to detect most eggs or larvae by this method, but due to the small amount of faeces used it may only detect relatively heavy infections.

FLOTATION METHODS

The basis of any flotation method is that when worm eggs are suspended in a liquid with a specific gravity higher than that of the eggs, the latter will float up to the surface. Nematode and cestode eggs float in a liquid with a specific gravity of between 1.10 and 1.20; trematode eggs, which are much heavier, require a specific gravity of 1.30–1.35.

The flotation solutions used for nematode and cestode ova are mainly based on sodium chloride or sometimes magnesium sulphate. A saturated solution of these is prepared and stored for a few days and the specific gravity checked prior to usage. In some laboratories a sugar solution of density 1.2 is preferred. For trematode eggs, saturated solutions of zinc chloride or zinc sulphate are widely used. Some laboratories use the more expensive and toxic potassium mercury iodine solution.

Whatever solutions are employed the specific gravity should be checked regularly and examination of the solution containing the eggs or larvae made rapidly, otherwise distortion may take place.

Direct flotation

A small amount of fresh faeces, say 2.0 g, is added to 10 ml of the flotation solution and, following thorough mixing, the suspension is poured into a test tube and more flotation solution added to fill the tube to the top. A coverslip is then placed on top of the surface of the liquid and the tube and coverslip are left standing for 10–15 minutes. The coverslip is then removed vertically and placed on a slide and examined under the microscope. If a centrifuge is available the flotation of the eggs in the flotation solution may be accelerated by centrifugation.

McMaster method

This quantitative technique is used where it is desirable to count the number of eggs or larvae per gram of faeces. The method is as follows:

1. Weigh 3.0 g of faeces or, if faeces are diarrhoeic, 3 teaspoonfuls.
2. Break up thoroughly in 42 ml of water in a plastic container. This can be done using a homogeniser if available or in a stoppered bottle containing glass beads.
3. Pour through a fine mesh sieve (aperture 205 μm, or 100 to 1 inch).
4. Collect filtrate, agitate and fill a 15 ml test tube.
5. Centrifuge at 2000 rpm for 2 minutes.
6. Pour off supernatant, agitate sediment and fill tube to previous level with flotation solution.
7. Invert tube six times and remove fluid with pipette to fill both chambers of McMaster slide (Fig. 15.1). Leave no fluid in the pipette or else pipette rapidly, since the eggs will rise quickly in the flotation fluid.
8. Examine one chamber and multiply number of eggs or larvae under one etched area by 100, or two chambers and multiply by 50, to arrive at the number of eggs per gram of faeces (epg):

If 3 g of faeces are dissolved in	42 ml
Total volume is	45 ml
Therefore 1 g	15 ml
The volume under etched area is	0.15 ml

Therefore, the number of eggs is multiplied by 100. If two chambers are examined, multiply by 50.

An abbreviated version of this technique is to homogenise the 3 g of faeces in 42 ml of salt solution, sieve and pipette the filtrate directly into the McMaster slide. Although a faster process, the slide contents are more difficult to 'read' because of their dark colour.

It is impossible to calculate from the epg the actual worm population of the host, since many factors influence egg production of worms and the number of eggs also varies with the species. Nevertheless, egg counts in excess of 1000 are generally considered indicative of heavy infections and those over 500 of moderate infection. However, a low epg is not necessarily indicative of very low infections, since patency may just be newly established; alternatively, the epg may be affected by developing immunity. The eggs of some species, such as certain ascarids, *Strongyloides*, *Oxyuris*, *Trichuris* and *Capillaria*, can be easily recognised morphologically. However, with the exception of *Nematodirus* spp, the common trichostrongyle eggs require measurement for differentiation.

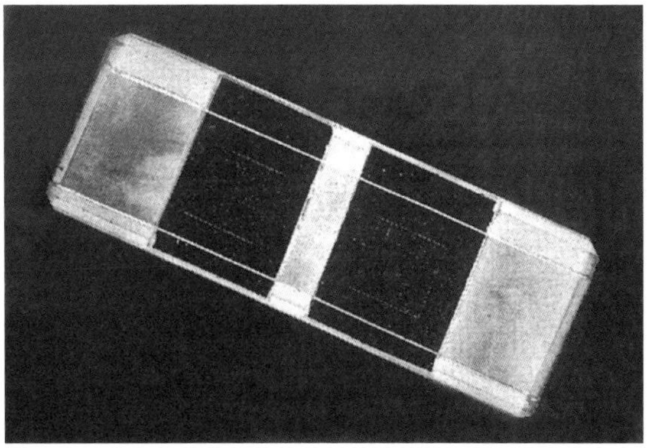

Fig. 15.1 McMaster slide for estimating numbers of nematode eggs in faeces.

While this technique will detect the eggs and larvae of most nematodes, cestodes and coccidia, it will not demonstrate trematode eggs, which have a higher specific density. For these, a flotation fluid of higher specific gravity such as a saturated solution of zinc sulphate has to be used or a sedimentation method employed as described below.

SEDIMENTATION METHODS

For trematode eggs:

1. Homogenise 3 g of faeces with water and pass the suspension through a coarse mesh sieve (250 μm). Thoroughly wash the material that is retained on this screen, using a fine water jet and discard the debris.
2. Transfer the filtrate to a conical flask and allow to stand for 2 minutes, remove the supernatant, and transfer the remainder (approximately 12–15 ml) to a flat-bottomed tube.
3. After sedimentation for a further 2 minutes the supernatant is again drawn off, a few drops of 5% methylene blue added and the sediment screened using a low power stereomicroscope. Any trematode eggs are readily visible against the pale blue background.

For lungworm larvae, the Baerman apparatus may be used. This consists of a glass funnel held in a retort stand. A rubber tube, attached to the bottom of the funnel, is constricted by a clip. A sieve (aperture 250 μm) is placed in the wide neck of the funnel, which has been partially filled with water, and a double layer of gauze is placed on top of the sieve.

Faeces are placed on the gauze and the funnel is slowly filled with water until the faeces are immersed. Alternatively, faeces are spread on a filter paper, which is then inverted and placed on the sieve. The apparatus is left overnight at room temperature during which the larvae migrate out of the faeces and through the sieve to sediment in the neck of the funnel. The clip on the rubber is then removed and the water in the neck of the funnel collected in a small beaker for microscopic examination in a petri dish.

A simple adaptation of the above method is to suspend the faeces enclosed in gauze in a wine glass filled with water and leave overnight. The larvae will leave the faeces, migrate through the gauze and settle at the bottom of the glass. After siphoning off the supernatant, the sediment is examined under the low power of the microscope as above.

CULTURE AND IDENTIFICATION OF LARVAE

Two techniques are widely used for the culture of infective larvae from nematode eggs.

In the first, faeces are placed in a jar with a lid and stored in the dark at a temperature of 21–24°C. The lid should be lined with moist filter paper and should not be tightly attached. After 7 days' incubation, the jar is filled with water and allowed to stand for 2–3 hours. The larvae will migrate into the water and the latter is poured into a cylinder for sedimentation. The larval suspension can be cleaned and concentrated by using the Baermann apparatus as described above and then killed by adding a few drops of Lugol's iodine and examined microscopically.

An alternative method is to spread faeces on the middle third of filter paper placed in a moistened petri dish. After storage at 21–24°C for 7–10 days, the dish is flooded with water and the larvae harvested as before.

The identification of infective larvae is a specialist technique and requires some experience. A key to the identification of infective larvae is provided in Table 15.4 and Figure 15.12.

RECOVERY OF ALIMENTARY NEMATODES

Details are given below of a technique for the collection, counting and identification of the alimentary nematodes of ruminants. The procedure is similar for other host species, information on identification being available in the text.

1. As soon as possible after removing the alimentary tract from the body cavity, the abomasal/duodenal junction should be ligatured to prevent transfer of parasites from one site to the other.
2. Separate the abomasum, small intestine and large intestine.
3. Open the abomasum along the side of the greater curvature, wash contents into a bucket under running water and make the total volume up to 2–4 litres.
4. After thorough mixing transfer duplicate 200 ml samples to suitably labelled containers and preserve in 10% formalin.
5. Scrape off the abomasal mucosa and digest in a pepsin/HCl mixture at 42°C for 6 hours; 200 g of mucosa will require 1 litre of mixture. Make digest up to a volume of 2 or 4 litres with cold water and again take duplicate 200 ml samples. Alternatively, the Williams technique may be used. In this, the washed abomasum is placed, mucosal surface down, in a bucket containing several litres of normal saline and maintained at 40°C for 4 hours. Subsequently, the abomasum is gently rubbed in a second bucket of warm saline. The saline from both buckets is poured through a sieve (aperture 38 μm, about 600 to 1 inch) and the residue examined.
6. Open the small intestine along its entire length and wash contents into a bucket. Treat as for the abomasal contents, but digestion of mucosal scrapings is unnecessary.
7. The contents of the large intestine are washed into a bucket, passed through a coarse mesh sieve (aperture 2–3 mm) and any parasites present collected and formalised.

WORM COUNTING PROCEDURE

1. Add 2–3 ml of iodine solution to one of the 200 ml samples.
2. After thorough mixing, transfer 4 ml of suspension to a petri dish, scored with lines to facilitate counting; add 2–3 ml sodium thiosulphate solution to decolourise debris. If necessary, worms may be preserved in an aqueous solution of 10% formalin or 70% alcohol. To clear large worms for microscopic examination, immerse in lactophenol for a suitable period prior to examination.
3. Examine for the presence of parasites using a stereoscopic microscope (×12 objective) and identify and count parasites as male, female and larval stages.

PREPARATION OF SOLUTIONS

- **Pepsin/hydrochloric acid** (HCl): dissolve 80 g of pepsin powder in 3 litres of cold water. Add 240 ml concentrated HCl slowly and stir well. Make final volume up to 8 litres. Store at 4°C.
- **Iodine solution**: dissolve 907 g of potassium iodide in 650 ml boiling water. Add 510 g iodine crystals and make up to 1 litre.
- **Sodium thiosulphate solution**: dissolve 100 g of sodium thiosulphate in 5 litres of water.

KEY TO THE IDENTIFICATION OF GASTROINTESTINAL NEMATODES OF RUMINANTS

Based on the characters described in Tables 15.1(a–c), the following key can be used to differentiate microscopically the genera of some common gastrointestinal nematodes of ruminants.

Body composed of a long filamentous anterior and a short broad posterior region .... ***Trichuris***

Body not so divided, oesophagus approximately one third of body length .... ***Strongyloides***

Short oesophagus and buccal capsule rudimentary .... **Trichostrongyloidea (A)**

Short oesophagus and buccal capsule well developed .... **Strongyloidea (B)**

(A) *TRICHOSTRONGYLOIDEA*

1. Distinct cephalic vesicle. Spicules very long uniting in a membrane at the tip........... ***Nematodirus***

   Cephalic vesicle small. Spicules relatively short and unjoined posteriorly .... ***Cooperia***

2. No cephalic vesicle. Excretory notch present in both sexes .... ***Trichostrongylus***

   Absence of excretory notch................................. **3**

3. Dorsal lobe of bursa asymmetrical, barbed spicules. Large prominent vulval flap in female .... ***Haemonchus***

   Dorsal lobe of bursa is symmetrical. Vulval flap small or absent...................................... ***Ostertagia***

(B) *STRONGYLOIDEA*

4. Buccal capsule cylindrical ..... ***Oesophagostomum***

   Buccal capsule well developed............................ **5**

5. Slight dorsal curvature of head and presence of cutting plates .... ***Bunostomum***

   Absence of teeth, rudimentary leaf crowns present .... ***Chabertia***

Table 15.1 Guide to adult alimentary nematodes of ruminants.

Table 15.1(a) Abomasal worms.

	Haemonchus contortus	*Ostertagia* spp	*Trichostrongylus axei*
Mature size	Large worms, reddish when fresh; easily seen, bursa visible with naked eye. Males 10–20 mm long Females 18–30 mm	Slender; reddish brown when fresh Males 7–8 mm long Females 9–12 mm long	Very small worms, less than 0.5 cm long, greyish when fresh, tapering to very fine anterior end Males 3–6 mm long Females 4–8 mm long
Head	Prominent large cervical papillae, distance from anterior end about 3 times diameter between papillae	Small cervical papillae set more posteriorly, distance from anterior end about 5 times diameter between papillae. Cuticle striations are longitudinal	No cervical papillae Excretory notch visible in oesophageal region Cuticle striations are annular
Female	In sheep, vulval flap, usually linguiform; gravid worm contains several hundred eggs; ovary coiled around intestine resembling 'Barber's pole' In cattle, vulval flap often bulb-shaped or vestigial	Small or no vulval flap. Under high magnification tip of tail shows annular rings. In cattle, female has vulval flap of variable size, but usually skirt-like	Simple genital opening with vulval flap absent; gravid worm contains four or five eggs, pole to pole
Male tail	Dorsal ray of bursa asymmetric. Spicules barbed near tips	Bursal lobes are symmetrical Spicules vary with species. In sheep species, spicules slender, rod-like (T. *circumcincta*) or stout with branch near middle (*O. trifurcata*) In cattle, male has stout, rod-like spicules with expanded tips (*O. ostertagi*) or very robust spicules, generally rectangular in outline (*O. lyrata*)	Bursal lobes are symmetrical Spicules unequal in length

Table 15.1(b) Small intestinal worms.

	Trichostrongylus	*Strongyloides*	*Cooperia*	*Nematodirus*	*Bunostomum*
Mature size	Very small worms, approx. 0.5 cm long, greyish when fresh, tapering to very fine anterior end. Males 4–5 mm long Females 5–7 mm long	Only females present Females 3–6 mm long	Approx. 0.5 cm long; slender; greyish; comma or watch-spring shape; coiled in 1 or 2 tight coils Males 4–6 mm long Females 5–7 mm long	Approx. 2 cm long; slender; much twisted, often tangled like cotton wool due to twisting of the 'thin neck' Males 10–15 mm long Females 15–25 mm long	Approx. 2 cm long; stout white worms; head bent slightly Male 12–17 mm long Female 19–26 mm long
Other features	Excretory notch present in oesophageal region. Vulval flap absent	Very long oesophagus, one third to half total length of worm	Small cephalic vesicle present, giving anterior end a cylindrical appearance; prominent cuticular striations in oesophageal region	Cephalic vesicle present	Large buccal cavity has prominent teeth. *B. trigonocephalum* of sheep and goats has one large and two small teeth *B. phlebotomum* of cattle has two pairs of subventral teeth
Female	Ovejectors present	Ovary and uterus show twisted thread appearance behind oesophagus; ovejectors absent. Eggs expressed from females have a fully developed larva in them	Body of female swollen at region of vulva	Female tail has prominent spine protruding from a blunt end Tip of tail is pointed (*N. battus*) or truncate with a small spine (other species) Large eggs present	
Male tail	Spicules leaf-shaped (*T. vitrinus*) or with 'step' near tip (*T. colubriformis*)		Male tail has short stout spicules; 'wing' at middle region, bearing striations (*C. curticei*) Spicules of *C. oncophora*, have a stout, bow-like, appearance, with small terminal 'feet'	Male tail has very long, slender spicules usually extended beyond the bursa Bursa shows two sets of parallel rays (*N. battus*) or four sets (other species). Spicules long, slender and fused, with expanded tip which is heart-shaped (*N. battus*); lanceloate (*N. filicollis*); bluntly rounded (*N. spathiger*) (sheep) In cattle, spicules of *N. helvetianus* have a spear-shaped expansion at the tips	*B. trigonocephalum* has short, twisted spicules *B. phlebotomum* has long, slender spicules

Table 15.1(c) Large intestinal worms.

	Trichuris	*Chabertia*	*Oesophagostomum*	*Skrjabinema*
Mature size	Up to 8 cm long; whip-like, with long filamentous anterior part twice as long as posterior part. Called the whipworm because of its shape Male 50–80 mm long Female 35–70 mm long	1.5–2 cm long; large buccal capsule Male 13–14 mm long Female 17–20 mm long	Up to 2 cm long approx. Male 11–16 mm long Female 13–24 mm long	Small spindle-shaped worm that is easily overlooked in contents Male 3 mm long. Female 6–7 mm long
Other features		*Chabertia* has a large bell-shaped buccal cavity that is visible to the naked eye in fresh specimens There are no teeth in the buccal cavity and rudimentary leaf crowns	Small buccal cavity surrounded by leaf crown. Cephalic vesicle with cervical groove behind it. Leaf crowns and cervical alae often present. Cervical papillae are situated posterior to the oesophagus	Prominent spherical bulb at posterior of oesophagus
Female	Female produces barrel-shaped eggs with a transparent plug at each end	Tail of female is bow-shaped		
Male tail	Male has single spicule in spine-covered protrusible sheath	Tail of male spirally coiled with one spicule		

IDENTIFICATION OF NEMATODE EGGS

The presence of nematode eggs in faeces is a useful aid to diagnosis of worm infections as they can be identified and counted in faecal samples (Figs 15.2–15.10). Strongyle eggs are approximately 60–80 μm long, oval, thin-shelled, contain 4–16 cells and are not easily differentiated; but eggs of *Trichuris*, *Nematodirus* spp and *Strongyloides* can be identified and may be counted and reported separately.

THIRD-STAGE LARVAL IDENTIFICATION

It is often useful to know whether faecal egg counts (FECs) are dominated by worms of one particular genus or not, particularly on farms where *Haemonchus* occurs. If so, larval culture and differentiation can be performed, usually using the faeces from the FEC. This technique takes a further 10–14 days, so results are not available for some time after the FEC is known.

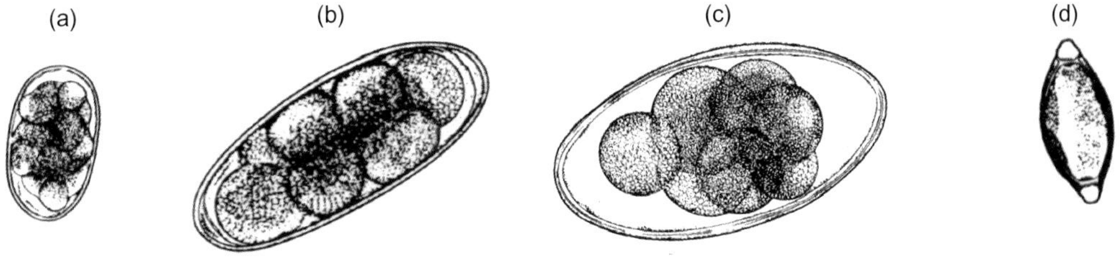

Fig. 15.2 Nematode eggs.

Table 15.2 Cattle worm egg counts – guide to interpretation.

Worm species	Degree of infestation		
	Light	Moderate	Heavy
Mixed infection	100	200–700	700+
Haemonchus	200	200–500	500+
Ostertagia ostertagi	150		500+
Trichostrongylus spp	50	50–300	500+
Bunostomum	20	20–100	100+
Cooperia	500	500–3000	3000
Fasciola hepatica	10	10–25	25–50

Larval differentiation (Table 15.4, Figs 15.11 and 15.12) requires the hatching of the eggs in the sample, culture in sterile faeces or peat, and the subsequent identification of the larvae. Usually, 50 or 100 larvae are counted, and the percentage of each genus reported. It should be noted that eggs of each genus do not always hatch at the same rate because of differences in temperature requirements for the different genera. Larval culture results should therefore be used as a general indication of the worm genera present, rather than a precise determination of the proportion of the FEC contributed by each genus.

Larvae can be identified in a similar manner for pasture samples (see later).

TECHNIQUE

A small drop of suspension of larvae is placed on a microscope and a drop of Gram's iodine added and a coverslip placed over the drops. The iodine kills the larvae and allows for easier identification of the salient features (Fig. 15.12).

RECOVERY OF LUNGWORMS

For *Dictyocaulus*, this is best done by opening the air passages starting from the trachea and cutting down to the small bronchi with fine, blunt-pointed scissors. Visible worms are then removed from the opened lungs and transferred to glass beakers containing saline. The worms are best counted immediately, failing which they should be left overnight at 4°C which will reduce clumping. Additional worms may be recovered if the opened lungs are soaked in warm saline overnight.

Another method is Inderbitzen's modification of the perfusion technique, described by Wolff *et al.* (1969), in which the lungs are perfused, is as follows. The pericardial sac is incised and reflected to expose the pulmonary artery in which a 2 cm incision is made. Rubber tubing is introduced into the artery and fixed *in situ* by double ligatures. The remaining large blood vessels are tied off and water from a mains supply allowed to enter the pulmonary artery. The water ruptures the alveolar and bronchiolar walls, flushes out the bronchial lumina, and is expelled from the trachea. The fluid is collected and its contents concentrated by passing through a fine sieve (aperture 38 μm). As before, this is best examined immediately for the presence of adult worms and larvae.

The smaller genera of lungworms of small ruminants are difficult to recover and enumerate, although the Inderbitzen technique may be of value.

Table 15.3 Sheep worm egg counts – guide to interpretation.

Worm species	Degree of infestation		
	Light	Moderate	Heavy
Mixed (*H. contortus* absent)	<150	500	1000
Haemonchus contortus	100–2500	2500–8000	8000+
Teladorsagia (*Ostertagia*) *circumcincta*	50–200	200–2000	2000+
Trichostrongylus spp	100–500	500–2000	2000+
Nematodirus spp	50–100	100–600	600+
Strongyloides			10 000
Fasciola hepatica	50–200	200–500	500+

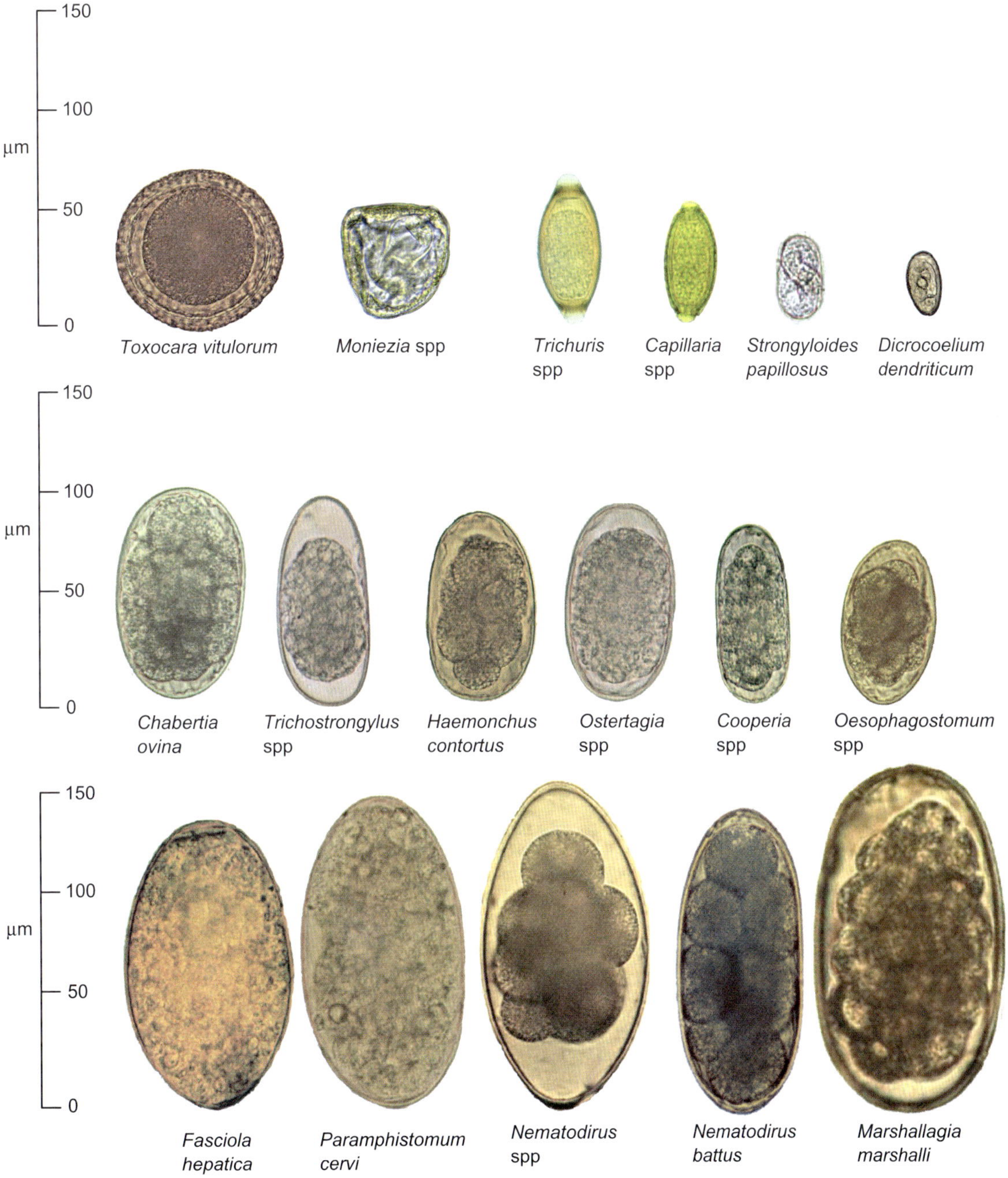

Fig. 15.3 Worm eggs from ruminants.

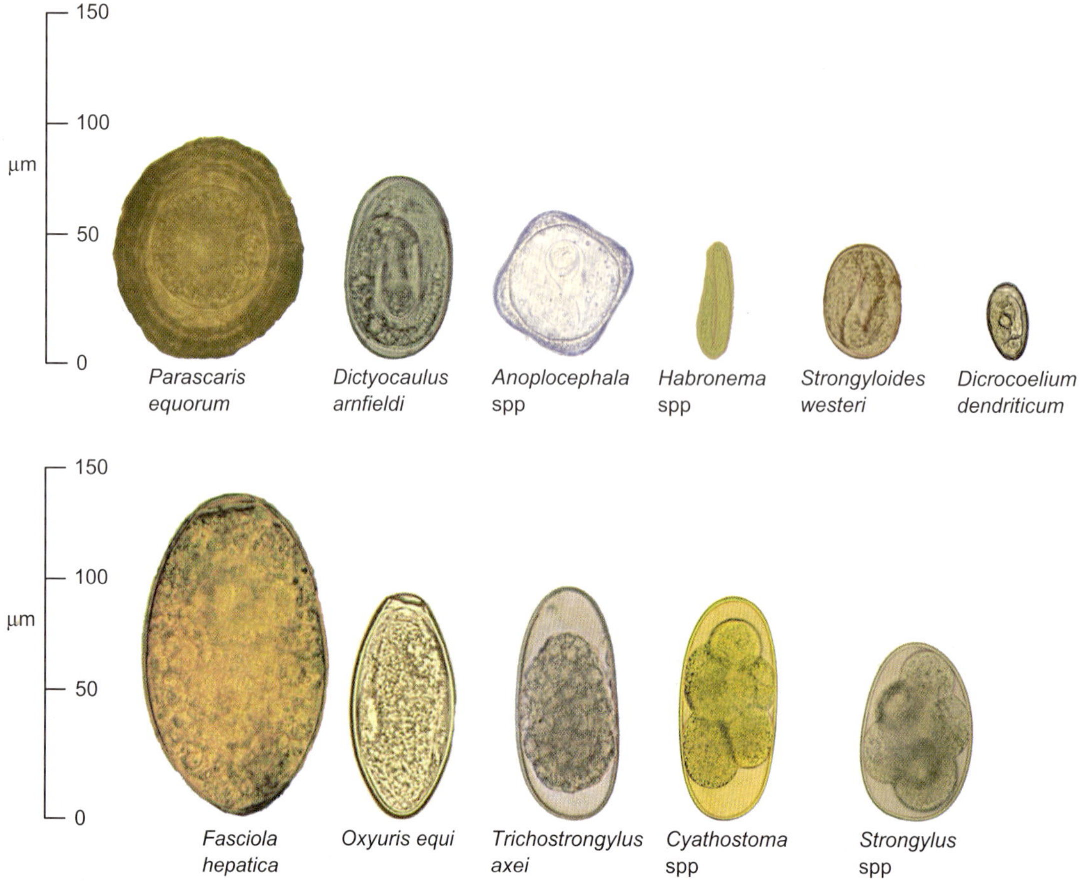

Fig. 15.4 Worm eggs from horses.

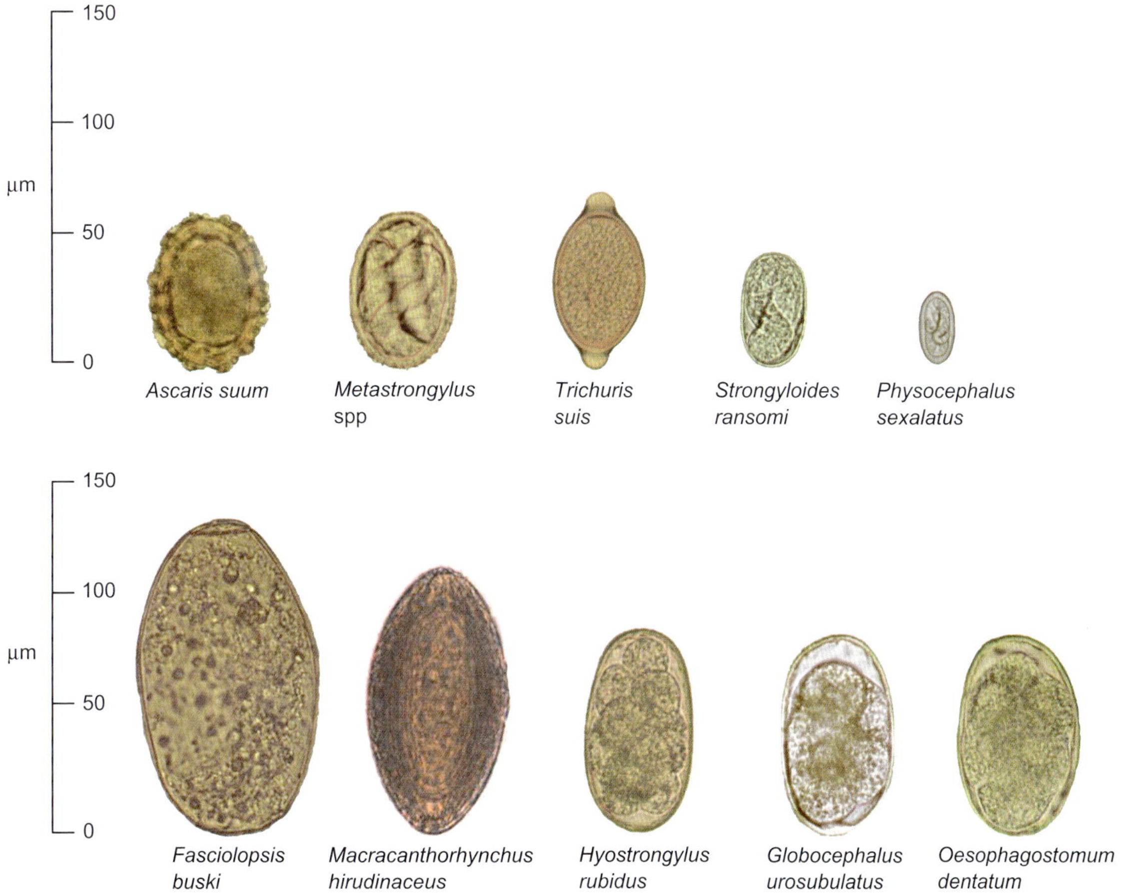

Fig. 15.5 Worm eggs from pigs.

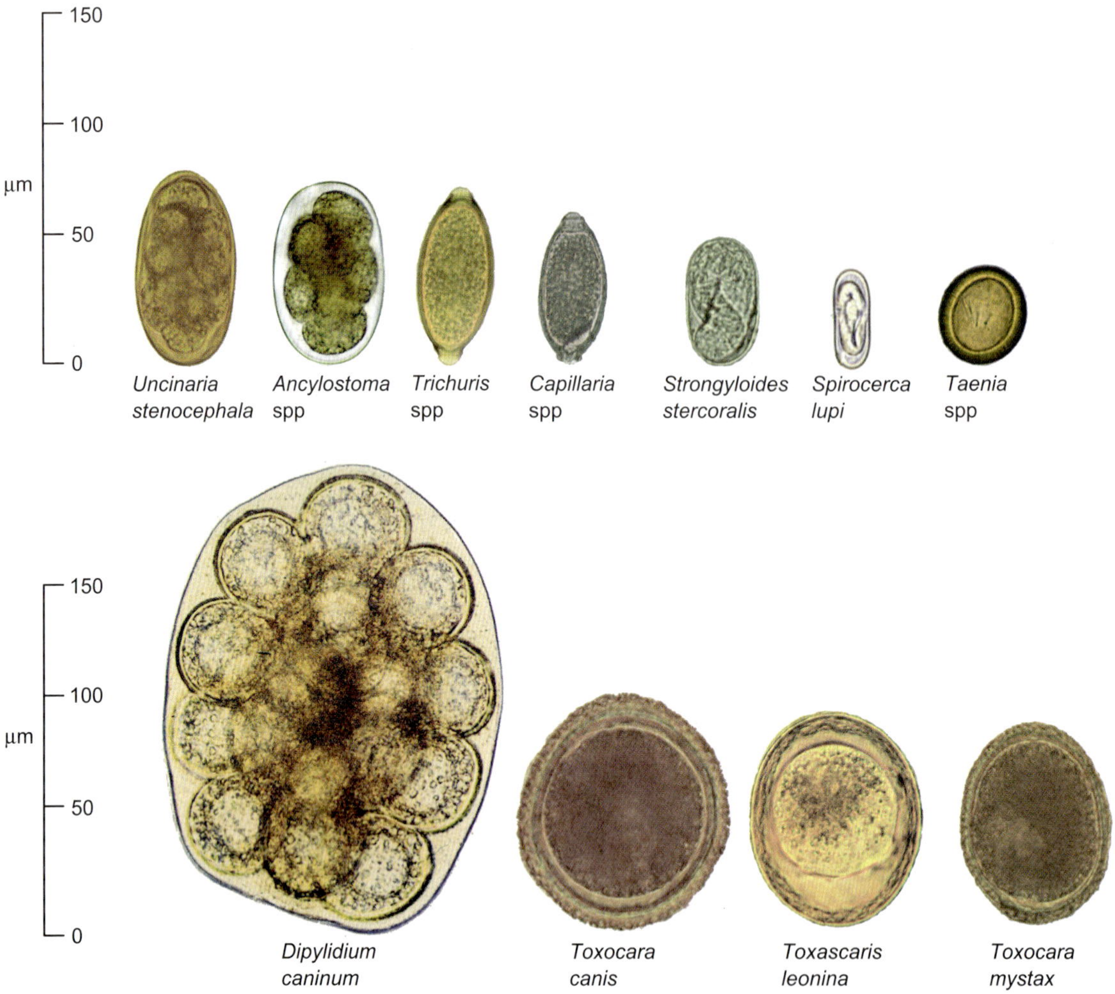

Fig. 15.6 Worm eggs from dogs and cats.

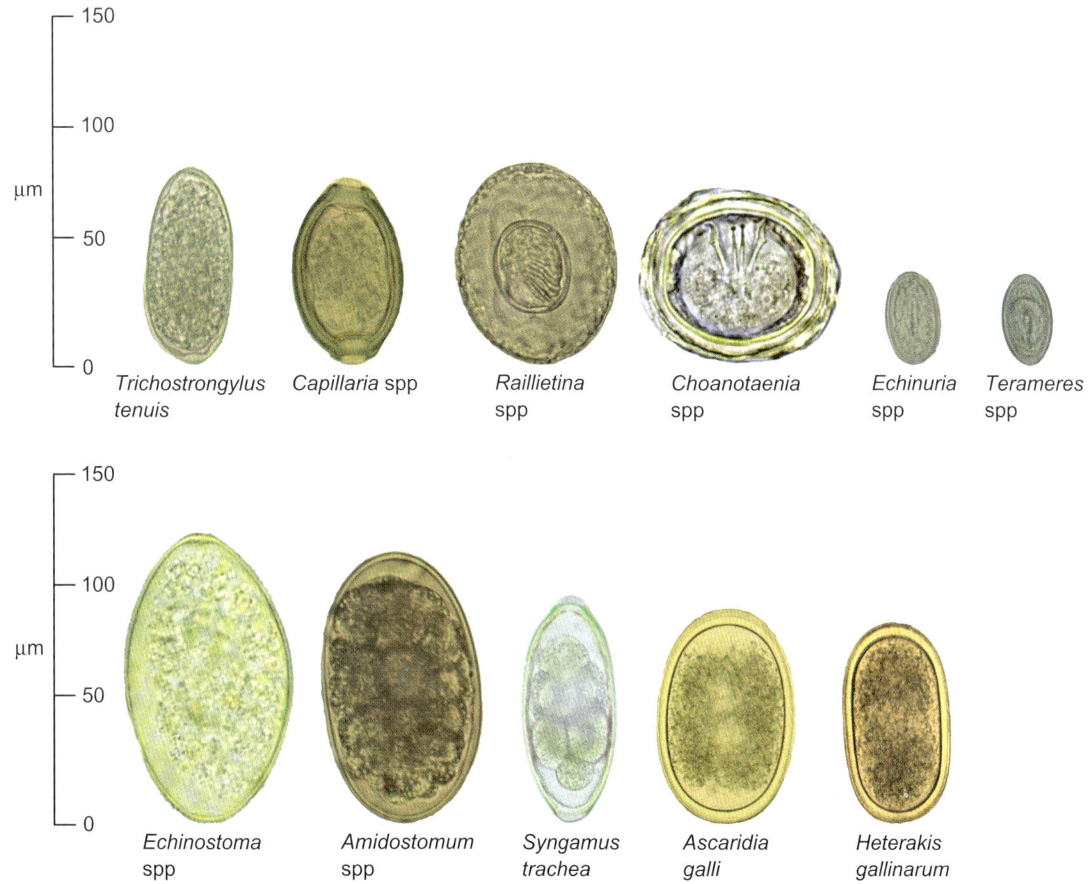

Fig. 15.7 Worm eggs from poultry.

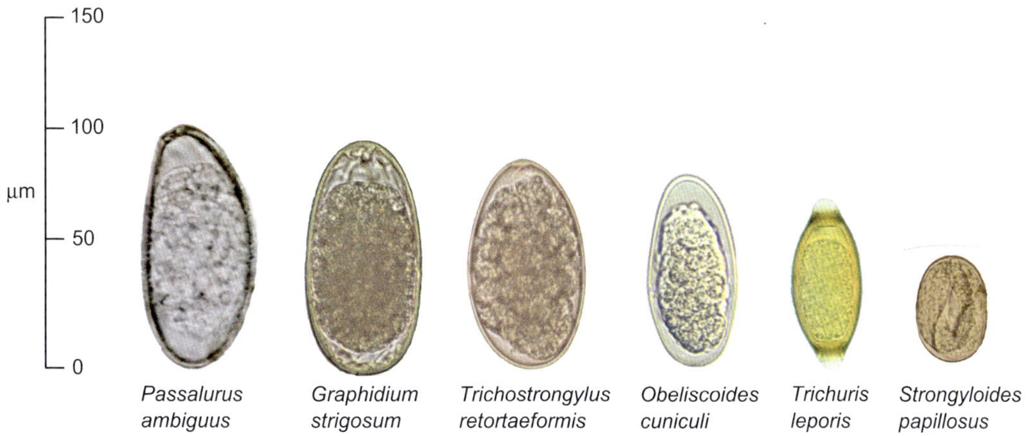

Fig. 15.8 Worm eggs from rabbits.

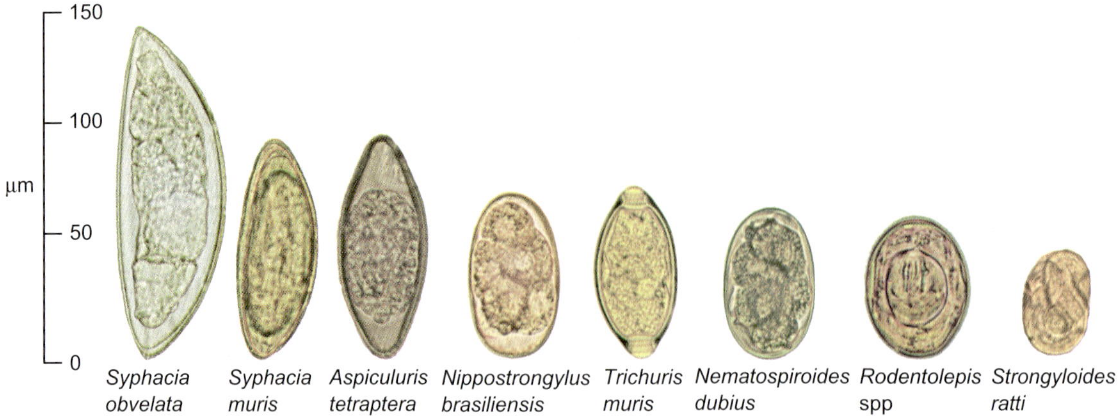

Fig. 15.9 Worm eggs from rodents.

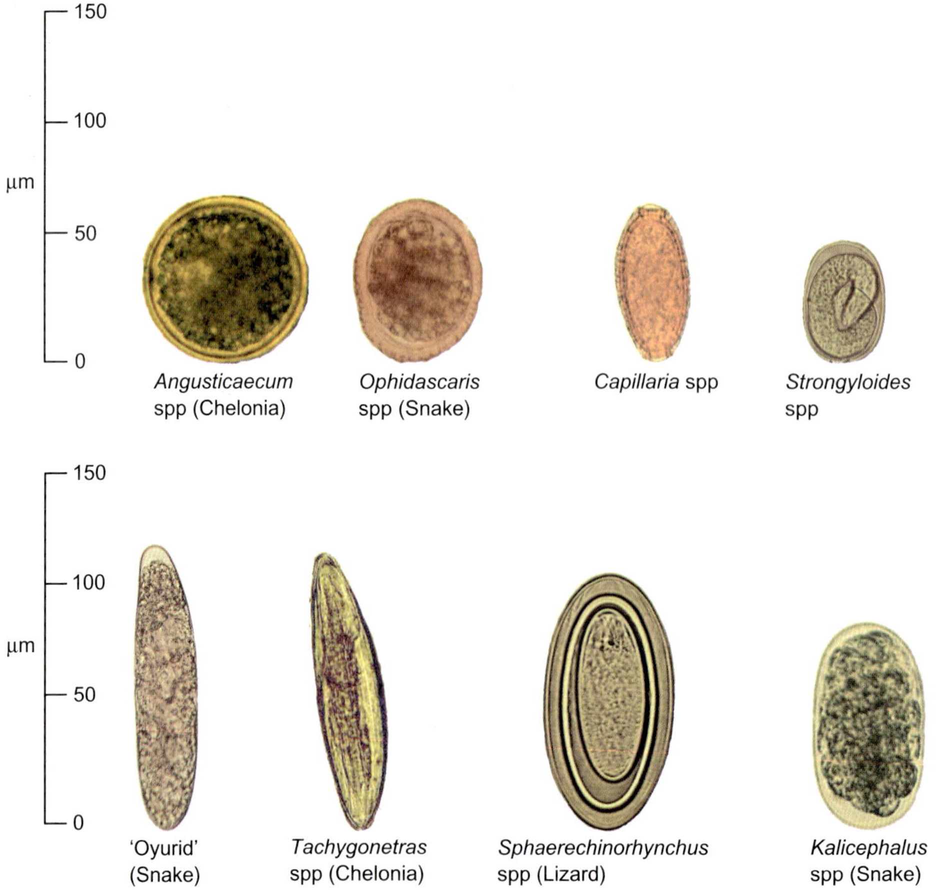

Fig. 15.10 Worm eggs from reptiles.

Table 15.4 Key characteristics used in the identification of third-stage larvae (see Figs 15.11 and 15.12).

Genus	Intestinal cell number	Head characteristics	Sheath tail characteristics
Nematodirus	8	Broad rounded	Filamentous sheath Speciated by shape of larval tail
Teladorsagia	16	Squared	Short sheath
Trichostrongylus	16	Tapered	Short sheath
Haemonchus	16	Narrow rounded	Medium offset sheath
Cooperia	16	Squared with refractile bodies	Medium tapering or finely pointed sheath
Bunostomum	16		Short filamentous
Oesophagostomum	32	Broad rounded	Filamentous sheath
Chabertia	32	Broad rounded	Filamentous sheath

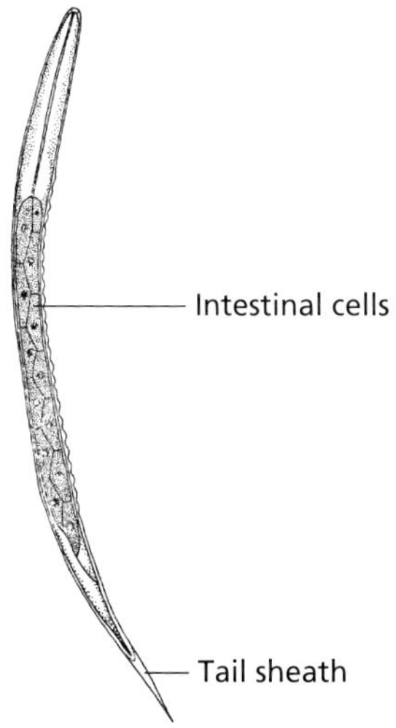

Fig. 15.11 Third-stage larva.

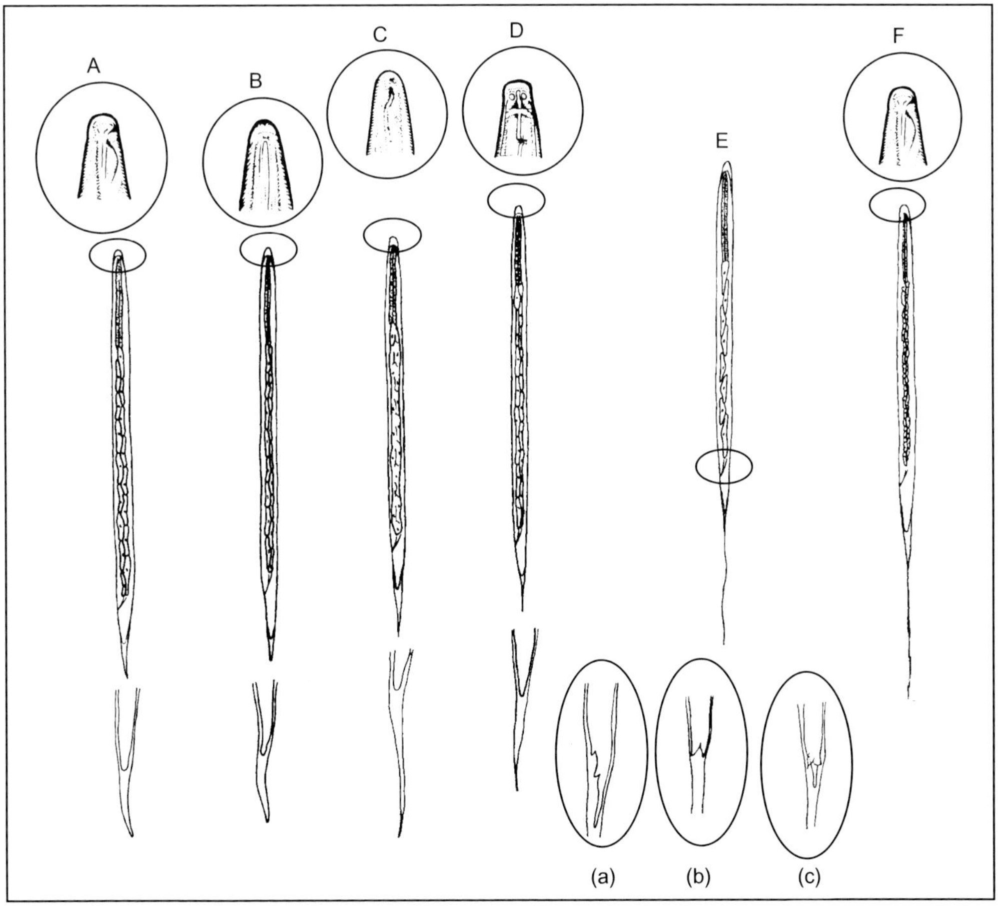

Fig. 15.12 Key to the identification of third-stage larvae of sheep gastrointestinal nematades. A, *Teladorsagia circumcincta*; B, *Trichostrongylus* spp; C, *Haemonchus contortus*; D, *Cooperia* spp; E, *Nematodirus*: (a) *battus*, (b) *filicollis*, (c) *spathiger*, F, *Oesophagostomum* spp.

RECOVERY OF TREMATODE AND CESTODE PARASITES

For both *Fasciola* and *Dicrocoelium* the livers are removed and cut into slices approximately 1 cm thick. On squeezing the liver slices, any flukes seen grossly are removed and formalised and the slices immersed in warm water overnight. The gallbladder should also be opened and washed, and any flukes removed.

After soaking, the liver slices are again squeezed, rinsed in clean water and discarded. Both washings are passed through a fine sieve (aperture 100 μm) and the material retained and formalised. In the case of intestinal paramphistomes, the first 4 m of duodenum should be tied off, opened, washed and examined for adherent trematodes.

Counts are carried out microscopically, entire flukes plus the numbers of heads and tails being recorded. The highest number of either of the latter is added to the number of entire flukes to give the total count.

Cestodes are usually readily visible in the intestine or liver, but whenever possible these should be removed intact so that, if necessary, the head and the mature and gravid segments are all available for specialist examination. In the case of *Echinococcus* in canids, however, the worms are so small that the more detailed examination described in the text should be undertaken.

OTHER AIDS TO DIAGNOSIS

There are two other techniques which are useful aids in the diagnosis of trichostrongyle infections in ruminants. The first is the plasma pepsinogen test and the second the estimation of infective larvae on herbage. Both of these techniques should be undertaken in a specialist parasitology laboratory, but a short account is given here of the material required for these tests, the basis of the techniques and how the results may be interpreted.

THE PLASMA PEPSINOGEN TEST

The estimation of circulating pepsinogen is of value in the diagnosis of abomasal damage, and is especially elevated in cases of ostertagiosis. Elevations also occur with other gastric parasites such as *Trichostrongylus axei*, *Haemonchus contortus* and, in the pig, *Hyostrongylus rubidus*.

The principle of the test, which is best carried out by a diagnostic laboratory, is that the sample of serum or plasma is acidified to pH 2.0, thus activating the inactive zymogen, pepsinogen, to the active proteolytic enzyme pepsin. This activated pepsin is then allowed to react with a protein substrate (usually bovine serum albumin) and the enzyme concentration calculated in international units (μmol tyrosine released per 100 ml serum per minute). The tyrosine liberated from the protein substrate by the pepsin is estimated by the blue colour, which is formed when phenolic compounds react with Folin–Ciocalteu's reagent. The minimum requirement for the test, as carried out in most laboratories, is 1.5 ml serum or plasma. The anticoagulant used for plasma samples is either EDTA or heparin.

In parasitic gastritis of ruminants due to *Ostertagia* spp and *T. axei* the levels of plasma pepsinogen become elevated. In parasite-free animals the level is less than 1.0 iu of tyrosine; in moderately infected animals, it is between 1.0 and 2.0 and in heavily infected animals it usually exceeds 3.0, reaching as high as 10.0 or more on occasion. Interpretation is simple in animals during their first 18 months, but thereafter becomes difficult as the level may become elevated when older and immune animals are under challenge. In such cases the absence of the classical clinical signs of diarrhoea and weight loss indicates that there are few adult parasites present.

PASTURE LARVAL COUNTS

For this technique, samples of grass are plucked from the pasture and placed in a polythene bag, which is then sealed and dispatched to a laboratory for processing. It is important to take a reasonable number of random samples, and one method is to traverse the pasture and remove four grass samples at intervals of about four paces until approximately 400 have been collected (Figure 15.13). Another, primarily for lungworm larvae, is to collect a similar number of samples from the close proximity of faecal pats. At the laboratory, the grass is thoroughly soaked, washed and dried and the washings containing the larvae passed

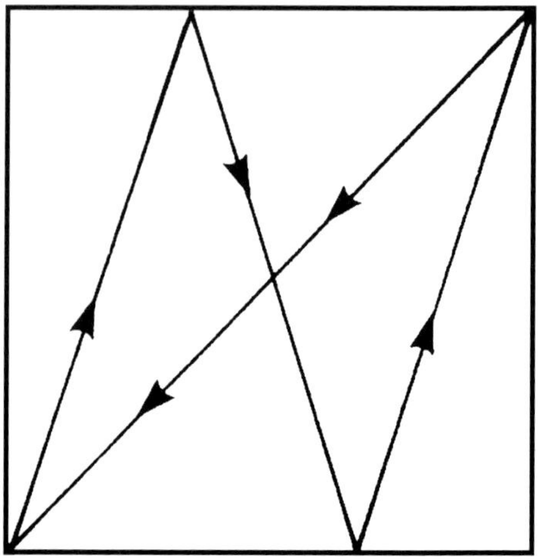

Fig. 15.13 Butterfly route.

through a sieve (aperture 38 μm; 600 to 1 inch) to remove fine debris. The material retained on the sieve is then Baermanised and the infective larvae are identified and counted microscopically under the high power. The numbers present are expressed as L_3 per kg of dried herbage.

Where counts in excess of 1000 L_3/kg of ruminant gastrointestinal trichostrongyles are recorded, the pasture can be regarded as moderately infective and values of over 5000 L_3/kg can be expected to produce clinical disease in young animals during their first season at grass.

Although this is a useful technique for detecting the level of gastrointestinal nematode L_3 on pastures, it is less valuable for detecting lungworm larvae because of the rapid fluctuations of these larvae on pastures.

A more sophisticated technique, the Jorgensen method, which depends on migration of larvae through an agar medium containing bile, is used in some laboratories for estimating *Dictyocaulus* larval populations on pasture; since most lungworm larvae are concentrated close to faeces, herbage samples should be collected from around faecal deposits. In the present state of knowledge, the detection of any lungworm larvae in herbage samples should be regarded with suspicion and even a negative finding does not necessarily imply that the pasture is free of infection.

ECTOPARASITES

Arthropods of veterinary interest are divided into two major groups, the Insecta and the Arachnida. Most are temporary or permanent ectoparasites, found either in or on the skin, with the exception of some flies whose larval stages may be found in the somatic tissues of the host. Parasitic insects include flies, lice and fleas, while the two groups of arachnids of veterinary importance are the ticks and mites. In all cases diagnosis of infection depends on the collection and identification of the parasite(s) concerned.

INSECTS

FLIES

Adult dipteran flies visiting animals are usually caught either by netting or after being killed by insecticides, while larvae may be collected in areas where animals are housed or directly from animals where the larval stages are parasitic. Identification of the common flies of veterinary interest, at least to generic level, is fairly simple, the key characters being described in the guide below. Identification of larvae to generic and species level is rather more specialised and depends on examination of certain features such as the structure of the posterior spiracles. Publications dealing with this may be found in References and further reading.

Guide to the families of adult Diptera of veterinary importance

1 Insects with one pair of wings on the mesothorax and a pair of club-like halteres on the metathorax **2**

Wingless insects; may be with or without halteres; body clearly divided into head, thorax and abdomen; three pairs of legs; dorsoventrally flattened; brown in colour; 5–8 mm in length; resident on sheep, horses, deer, goats or wild birds (Fig. 15.14) **5**

2 Antennae composed of three segments; third segment usually with an arista; foot with two pads (Fig. 15.15) .... **Cyclorrhapha 3**

Antennae composed of three sections; third antennal section enlarged and composed of four to eight segments; palps two-jointed with the second segment enlarged; foot with three pads; vein R_{4+5} forks to form a large 'Y' across the wing tip (Fig. 15.16); large, stout bodied flies with large eyes .... **Tabanidae 12**

Antennae long, slender and composed of many articulating segments; palps composed of four to five segments; small slender flies with long narrow wings .... **Nematocera 13**

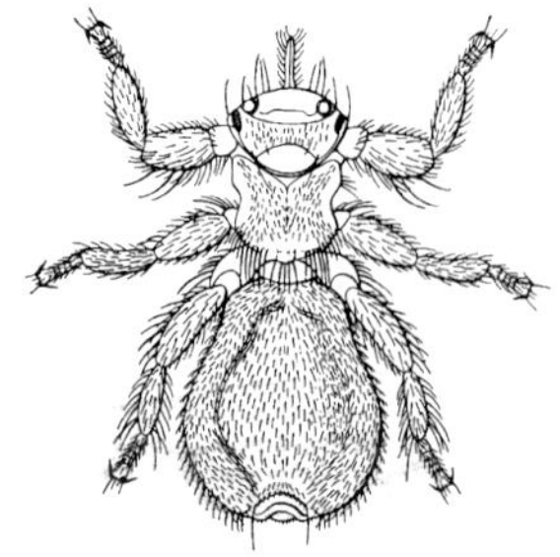

Fig. 15.14 Adult sheep ked, *Melophagus ovinus*.

3 Frons with ptilinal suture (Fig. 15.17) .... Series **Schizophora 4**

Frons without ptilinal suture .... Series **Aschiza**

4 Second antennal segment usually with a groove (Fig. 15.17); thoracic transverse suture strong (Fig. 15.19); thoracic squamae usually well developed (Fig. 15.20) .... **Calypterae 5**

Second antennal segment usually without a groove; thoracic transverse suture weak; thoracic squamae often vestigial .... **Acalypterae**

5 Thorax broad and dorsoventrally flattened; may appear spider or tick-like; often wingless (Fig. 15.14); wings when present with venation abnormal with veins crowded into leading half of wing .... **Hippoboscidae**

Wings with veins not crowded together towards the leading edge; thorax not dorsoventrally flattened **6**

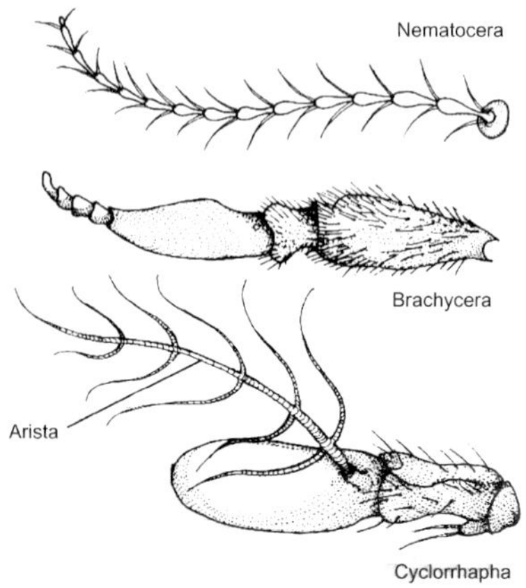

Fig. 15.15 Variations in the antennae found in the three suborders of Diptera.

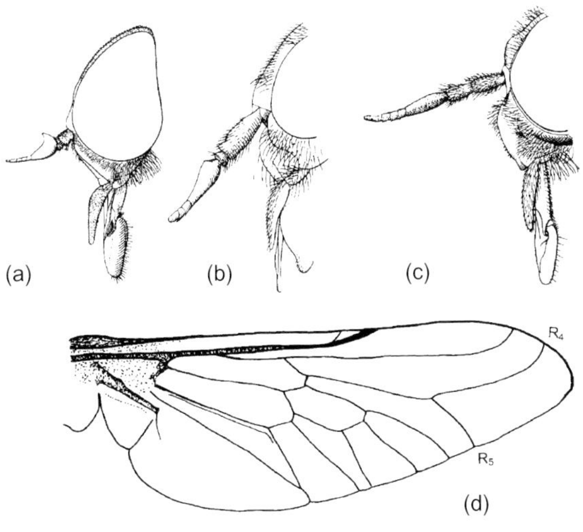

Fig. 15.16 Antennae of (a) *Chrysops*, (b) *Haematopota* and (c) *Tabanus*. (d) Wing venation of Tabanidae (reproduced from Smart, 1943).

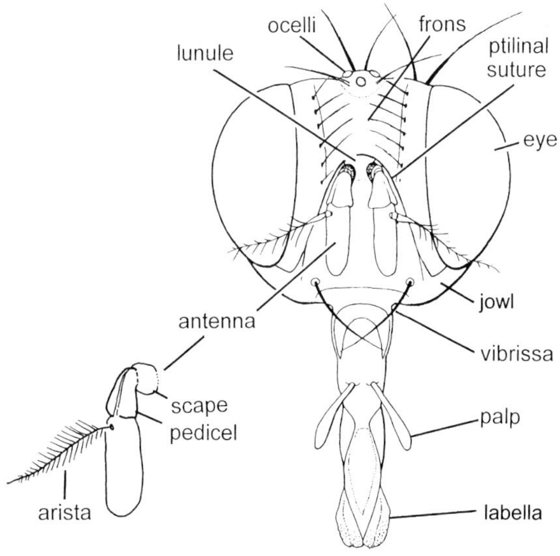

Fig. 15.17 The principal features of the dichoptic head of a typical adult Calypterate cyclorrhaphous dipteran (redrawn from Smart, 1943).

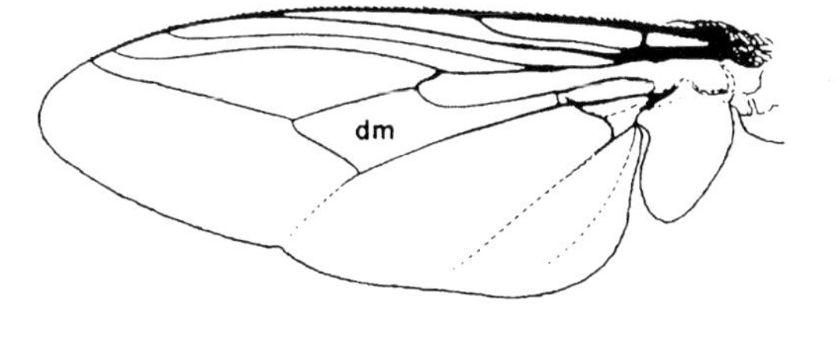

Fig. 15.18 Wing venation typical of species of *Glossina*, showing the characteristic hatchet shape of the cell dm.

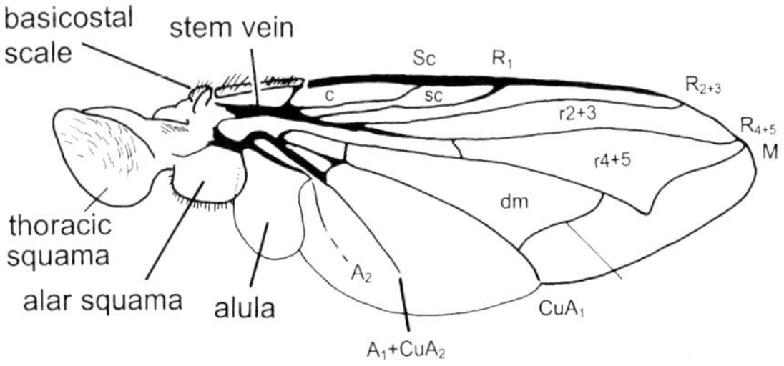

Fig. 15.20 The veins and cells of the wings of a typical calypterate dipteran, *Calliphora vicina*.

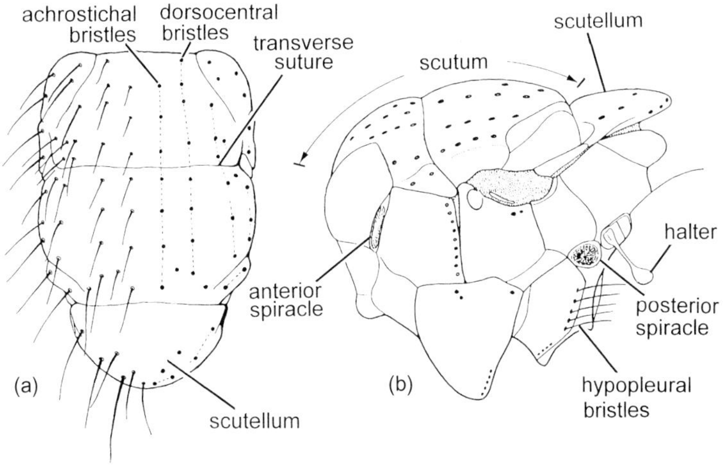

Fig. 15.19 The principal features of the generalised thorax of an adult Calypterate cyclorrhaphous dipteran. (a) Dorsal view. (b) Lateral view (redrawn from Smart, 1943).

6 Proboscis long, forwardly directed and embraced by long palps; arista with feathery short hairs present only on dorsal side; discal medial cell of wings characteristically 'hatchet' shaped (Fig. 15.18); found only in sub-Saharan Africa .... **Glossinidae**

Discal medial cell of wings widening gradually and more or less regularly from the base **7**

7 Mouthparts small, usually functionless; head bulbous; antennae small; flies more or less covered with soft hair; larval parasites of vertebrates....... .... **Oestridae**

Mouthparts usually well developed; antennae not small; flies with strong bristles **8**

8 Hypopleural bristles present (Fig. 15.19).......... **9**

Hypopleural bristles absent **11**

9 Post-scutellum strongly developed; larval parasitoids of insects .... **Tachinidae**

Post-scutellum weak or absent.......................... **10**

10 Dull grey appearance; three black stripes on the scutum; abdomen usually with chequered or spotted pattern (Fig. 15.21); larval parasites of vertebrates .... **Sarcophagidae**

Metallic, iridescent appearance (blue–black, violet–blue, green); larval parasites of vertebrates......... .... **Calliphoridae**

11 Wings with vein A_1 not reaching the wing edge; strong curved A_2 vein the tip of which approaches A_1 (Fig. 15.22); aristae bare.............. .... **Fanniidae**

Wings with vein A_1 not reaching the wing edge; A_2 vein not strongly curved (Fig. 15.23); aristae bilaterally plumose to the tip............... **Muscidae**

12 Antennal flagellum with four segments (Fig. 15.16); wings mottled; proboscis shorter than head........................... ***Haematopota* (Tabanidae)**

Antennal flagellum with five segments (Fig. 15.16); apical spurs on tibiae are small and may be hidden by hair; wings usually with costal region dark and a single dark broad transverse band; proboscis shorter than head........................ .... ***Chrysops* (Tabanidae)**

Antennal flagellum with five segments (Fig. 15.16); no apical spurs on hind tibiae; wings usually clear but may be dark or banded; proboscis shorter than head............. ***Tabanus* (Tabanidae)**

13 Small, hairy, moth-like flies; numerous parallel wing veins running to the margin; wings pointed at the tip...................................... **Psychodidae 14**

Not like this **15**

14 Palps five-segmented; biting mouthparts at least as long as head; antennal segments almost cylindrical; two longitudinal wing veins between radial and medial forks (Fig. 15.24)................................ .... **Phlebotominae**

15 Ten or more veins reaching the wing margin **16**

Not more than eight veins reaching the wing margin **17**

16 Wing veins and hind margins of wings covered by scales (Fig. 15.25); conspicuous forward-projecting proboscis.. **Culicidae**

17 Wings broad; wing veins thickened at the anterior margin; antennae not hairy; thorax humped; antennae usually with 11 rounded segments; palps long with five segments extending beyond the proboscis; first abdominal tergite with a prominent basal scale fringed with hairs (Fig. 15.26) .... **Simuliidae**

Wings not particularly broad, antennae hairy **18**

18 Front legs often longer than others; median vein not forked; (non-biting midges) .... **Chironomidae**

Front legs not longer than others; wings with median vein forked; antennae with 14–15 visible segments; palps with five segments; female mouthparts short; legs short and stout; two radial cells and cross vein r-m strongly angled in relation to media; at rest wings close flat over abdomen (Fig. 15.27) .... ***Culicoides* (Ceratopogonidae)**

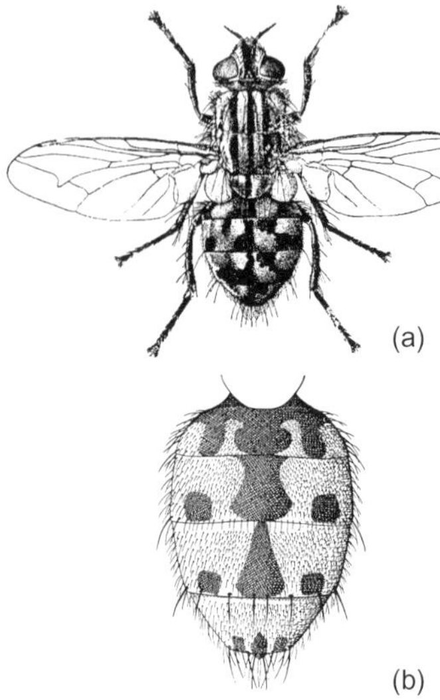

Fig. 15.21 (a) Adult of the flesh fly *Sarcophaga carnaria* (reproduced from Castellani and Chalmers, 1910). (b) *Wohlfahrtia magnifica*, abdomen of adult (reproduced from Smart, 1943).

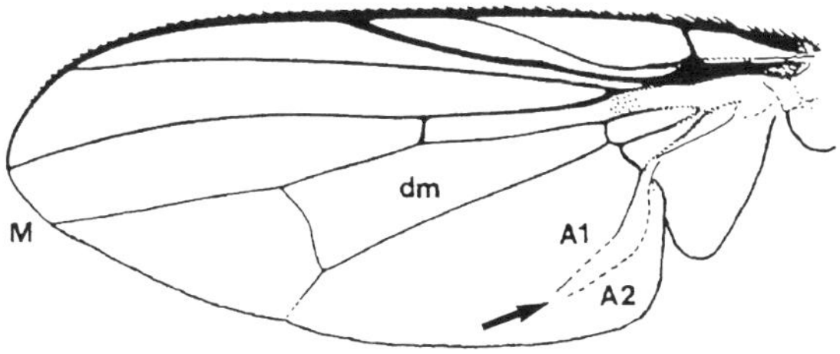

Fig. 15.22 Wing venation typical of species of *Fannia*, showing the characteristic convergence of the anal veins.

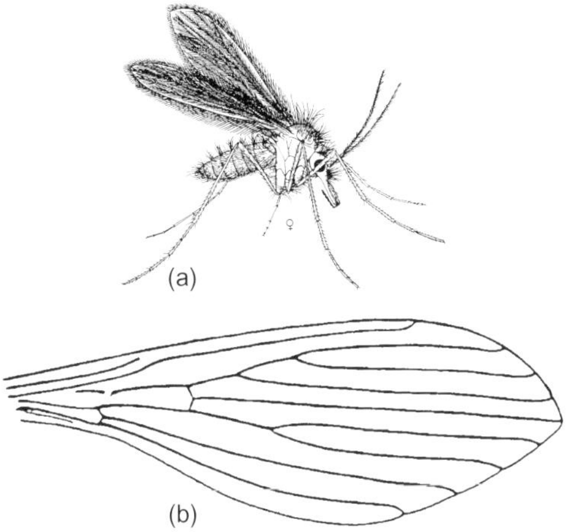

Fig. 15.24 (a) Adult female sandfly, *Phlebotomus papatasi*. (b) Wing venation typical of species of *Phlebotomus* (Psychodidae) (reproduced from Smart, 1943)

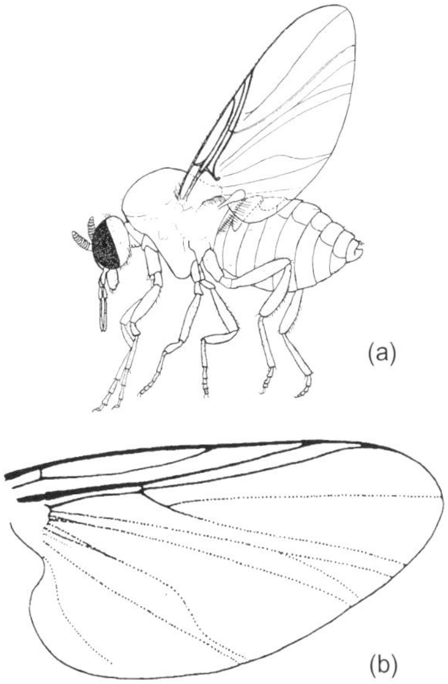

Fig. 15.26 (a) Adult female *Simulium*. (b) Wing venation typical of *Simulium*, showing the large anal lobe and crowding of the veins towards the leading edge (reproduced from Smart, 1943).

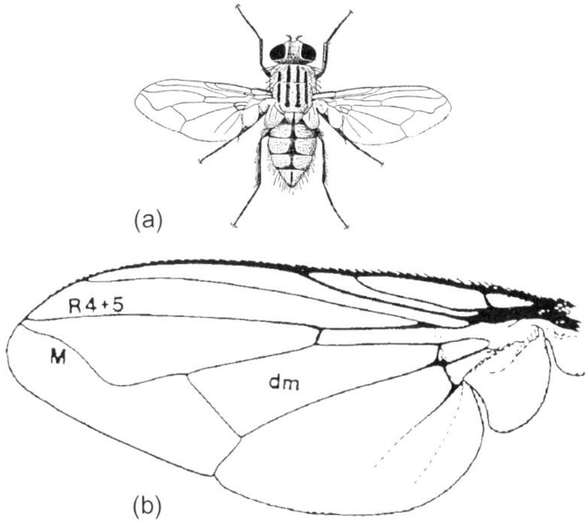

Fig. 15.23 (a) Female house fly, *Musca domestica*. (b) Wing venation typical of species of *Musca*, showing the strongly bent vein M ending close to R_{4+5} (after Smart, 1943).

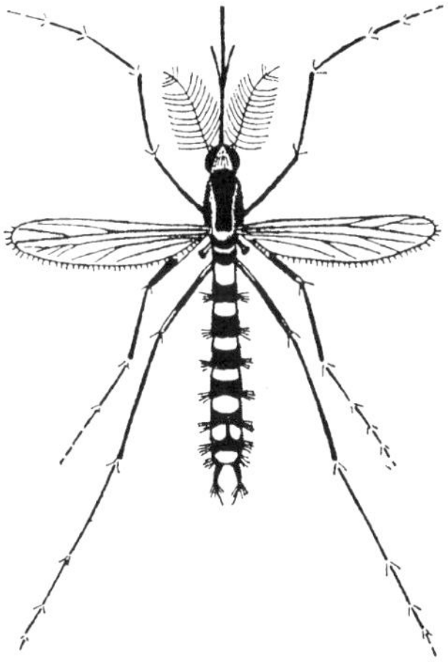

Fig. 15.25 *Aedes atropalpus*: adult (reproduced from Eidmann and Kuhlhorn, 1970).

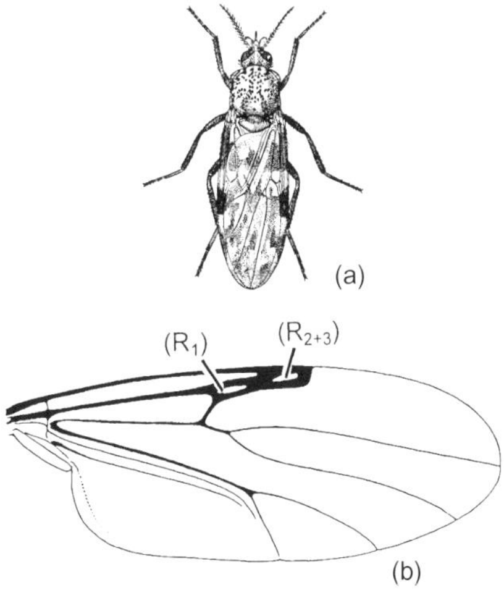

Fig. 15.27 (a) Adult female *Culicoides nebeculosus* at rest. (b) Wing venation typical of species of *Culicoides*, showing the two elongate radial cells (reproduced from Edwards *et al.*, 1939).

Guide to third-stage larvae causing myiasis in domestic animals

The guide to larvae presented below applies specifically to recognition of the third stage. This stage is usually of the longest duration and, since the larvae are approaching their maximum size or are beginning to wander, is usually the stage when they are most commonly observed. It should be noted, that because the external structure of larvae may change over the course of their growth and development, first- and second-stage larvae may not key out appropriately.

1 Body more or less cylindrical; no obvious head capsule **2**

Fly larvae with an obvious head capsule; rarely found associated with livestock myiasis ...... **Diptera, Nematocera or Brachycera**

2 Body with obvious fleshy processes **3**

Body without fleshy processes **4**

3 Third-stage larvae large, up to 18 mm long; large, pointed fleshy processes laterally and dorsally (Fig. 15.28); posterior spiracular plate without button (see Fig. 11.34); peritremes with a narrow opening; in carrion or secondarily in cutaneous myiasis of sheep; distribution, Afrotropical, Australasian and Oriental ...... ***Chrysomyia albiceps* and *C. rufifacies* (Calliphoridae)**

Third-stage larvae 7–8 mm in length; body flattened, with long processes (Fig. 15.29); posterior spiracles on short stalks on terminal segment; uncommon in livestock myiasis ...... **Fanniidae**

4 Posterior spiracles with a large number of small pores or many short intertwining slits arranged in three groups on each spiracular plate (e.g. Fig. 15.30) **5**

Posterior spiracles with up to three straight or curved slits (e.g. Fig. 15.31) **7**

5 Mouth-hooks well developed, strongly hooked **6**

Mouth-hooks poorly developed; third-stage larvae 20–30 mm in length (Fig. 15.32); in subcutaneous swellings or warbles (Fig. 15.33); on cattle or deer ...... ***Hypoderma* spp (Oestridae)**

6 Body with weak spines in distinct regions; posterior spiracles with many small pores (Fig. 15.30); in nasal myiasis of sheep; distribution, worldwide ...... ***Oestrus ovis* (Oestridae)**

Body spines stronger and more evenly distributed; posterior spiracles with many small slits; found in dermal myiases; in rodents and rabbits; distribution, New World ...... ***Cuterebra* spp (Oestridae)**

7 Posterior spiracles with straight or arced slits **8**

Posterior spiracles with serpentine slits; anterior spiracles in the form of membranous stalks bearing finger-like processes; body with obvious spines; furuncular myiases of dogs, rats and humans; distribution, sub-Saharan Africa ...... ***Cordylobia* spp (Calliphoridae)**

Posterior spiracles with serpentine slits (Fig. 15.34); anterior spiracles not as above; uncommon in livestock myiasis ...... **Muscidae**

8 Posterior spiracles sunk in a deep cavity which may conceal them (Fig. 15.35); slits more or less parallel **9**

Posterior spiracles visible, either exposed on surface or set in a ring of tubercles **11**

9 Body with strong spines **10**

Body with short spines; obligate agent of cutaneous myiasis; primarily in sheep and goats; distribution, worldwide ...... ***Wohlfahrtia* spp (Sarcophagidae)**

10 Posterior spiracles with slits bowed outwards at the middle; body oval; found in the pharynx or digestive tract of equids ...... ***Gasterophilus* spp (Oestridae)**

Posterior spiracles with slits relatively straight; body enlarged anteriorly and tapering posteriorly (Fig. 15.36); distribution, New World ...... ***Dermatobia hominis* (Oestridae)**

11 Posterior spiracles with straight slits (Fig. 11.30) **12**

Posterior spiracles with arced slits; uncommon in livestock myiasis ...... **Muscidae**

12 Posterior spiracles with a fully closed peritremal ring (Fig. 15.38) **13**

Posterior spiracles with an open peritremal ring (Fig. 15.37) **14**

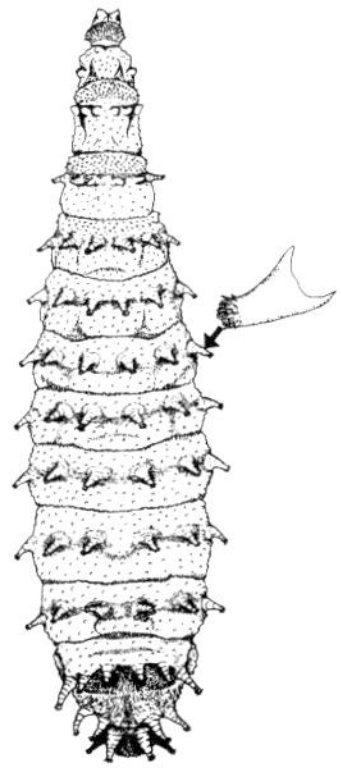

Fig. 15.28 Third-stage larva of *Chrysomya albiceps* (reproduced from Zumpt, 1965).

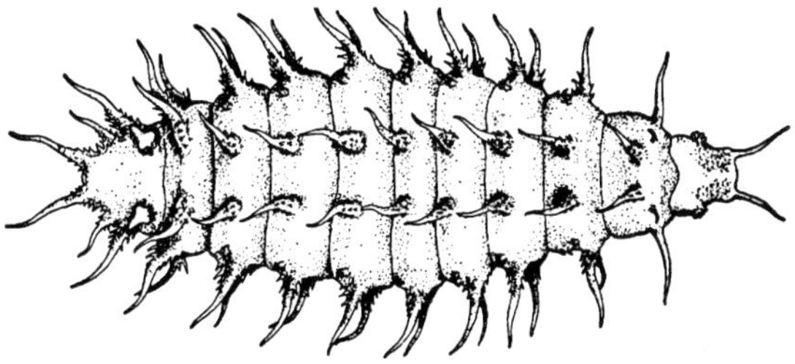

Fig. 15.29 Third-stage larva of the lesser house fly *Fannia canicularis* (from Zumpt, 1965).

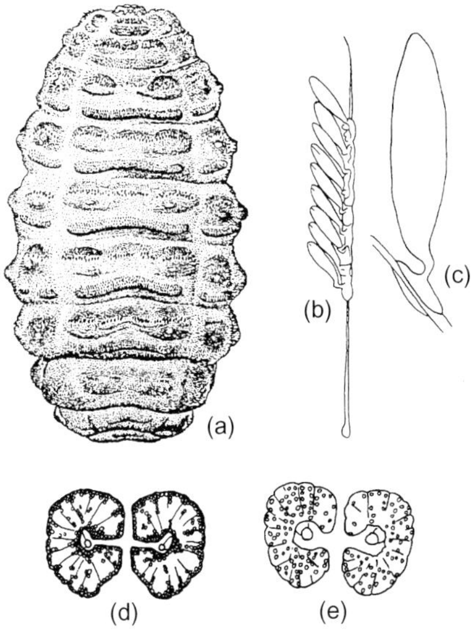

Fig. 15.32 (a) Third stage larva of *Hypoderma bovis*. Eggs of (b) *H. lineatum* and (c) *H. bovis*. Posterior spiracles of third stage larvae of (d) *H. bovis* and (e) *H. lineatum* (reproduced from Zumpt, 1965).

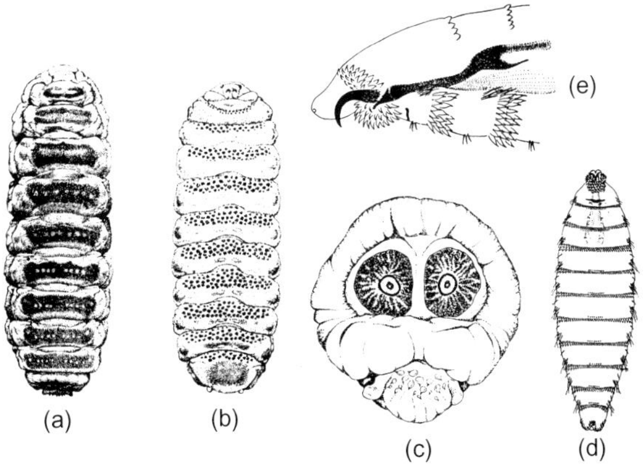

Fig. 15.30 *Oestris ovis*. (a) Ventral view and (b) dorsal view of third-stage larva. (c) Posterior-view of third-stage larva. (d) First-stage larva. (e) Mouthpart of first-stage larva in lateral view (reproduced from Zumpt, 1965).

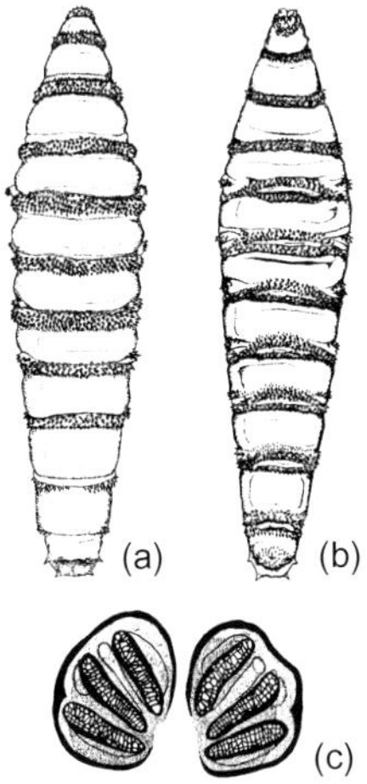

Fig. 15.31 Third-stage larvae of *Chrysomya bezziana*. (a) Dorsal, (b) ventral view and (c) posterior spiracles (reproduced from Zumpt, 1965).

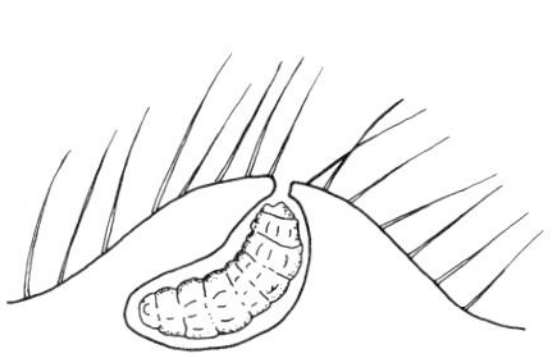

Fig. 15.33 Third stage *Hypoderma* larva in warble on the back of a cow.

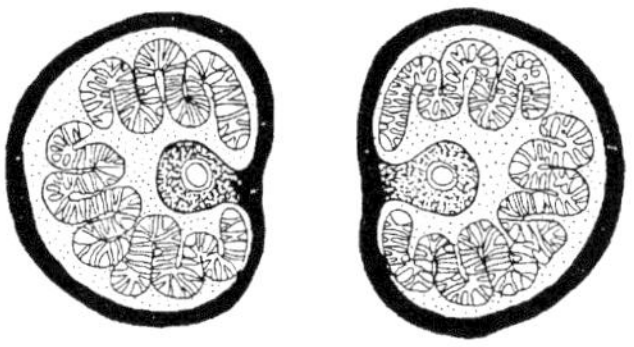

Fig. 15.34 Posterior spiracles of a third-stage larva of the house fly, *Musca domestica* (after Smart, 1943).

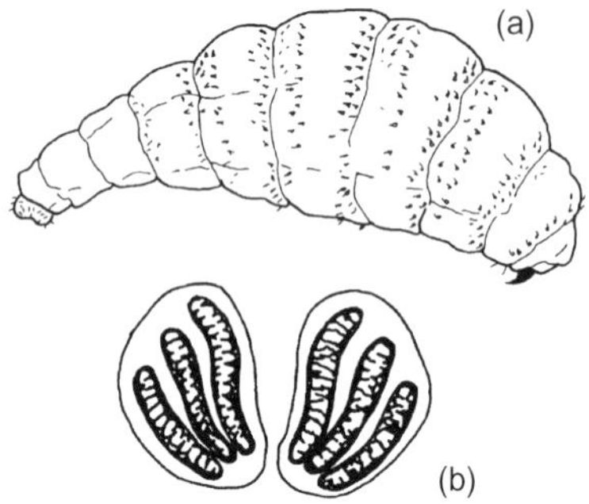

Fig. 15.36 *Dermatobia hominis*. (a) Third-stage larva. (b) Posterior spiracles.

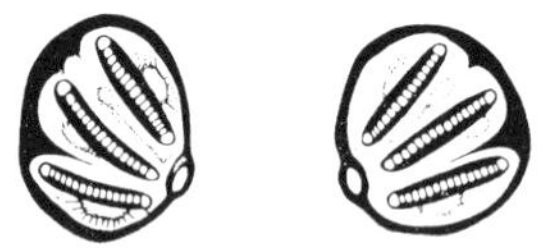

Fig. 15.38 *Lucilia sericata*. Posterior peritremes (reproduced from Zumpt, 1965).

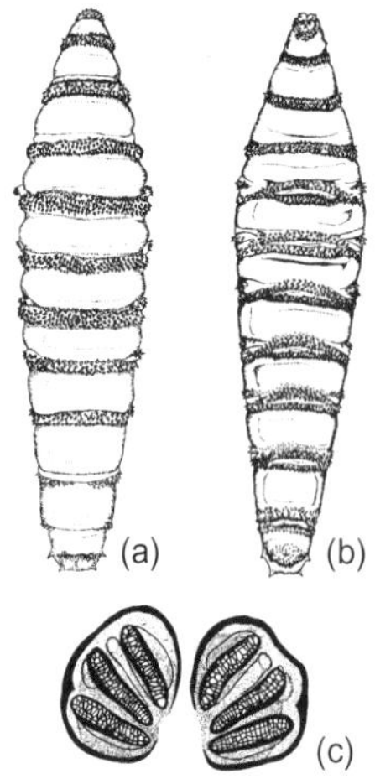

Fig. 15.40 (a) Posterior spiracles and (b) third-stage larvae of *Chrysomya bezziana* (reproduced from Zumpt, 1965).

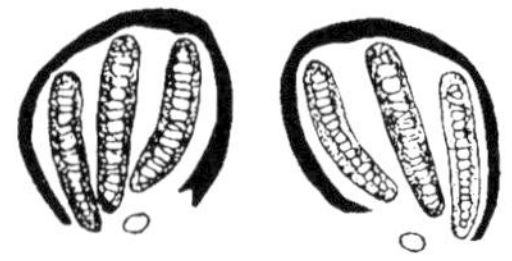

Fig. 15.35 *Wohlfahrtia magnifica*, posterior spiracles deeply sunk in a cavity.

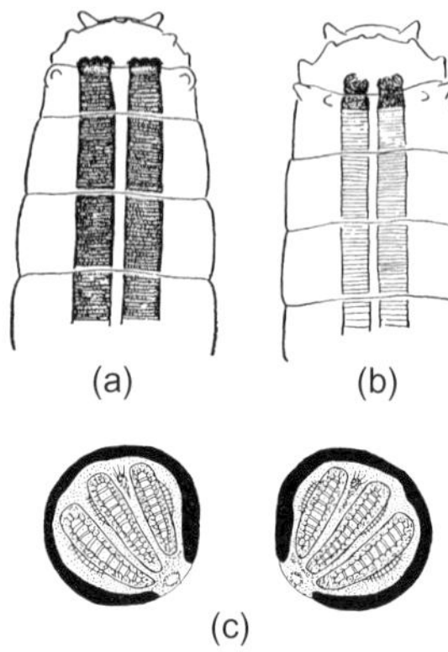

Fig. 15.37 (a) Pigmented dorsal tracheal trunks of *Cochliomyia hominivorax*. (b) Tracheal trunks and (c) posterior spiracles of *Cochliomyia macellaria* (reproduced from Zumpt, 1965).

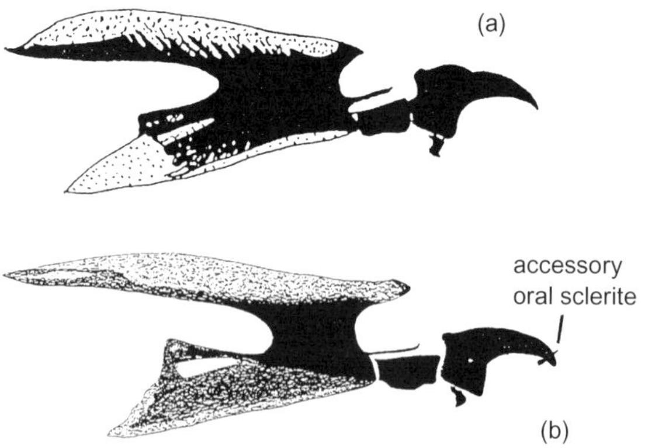

Fig. 15.39 Cephopharyngeal skeleton of (a) *Lucilia sericata* and (b) *Calliphora vicina*.

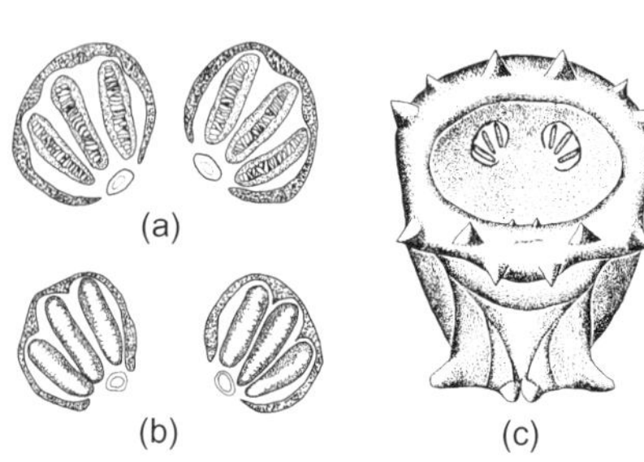

Fig. 15.41 Posterior spiracles of third-stage larvae of (a) *Protophormia terraenovae* and (b) *Phormia regina*. (c) Tubercles on the posterior face of the last segment of third-stage *Protophormia terraenovae* (reproduced from Zumpt, 1965).

13 Cephalopharyngeal skeleton with pigmented accessory oral sclerite (Fig. 15.39a); distribution, worldwide .... ***Calliphora* spp (Calliphoridae)**

Cephalopharyngeal skeleton without pigmented accessory oral sclerite (Fig. 15.39b); distribution, worldwide .... ***Lucilia* spp (Calliphoridae)**

14 Tracheal trunks leading from posterior spiracles without dark pigmentation **15**

Tracheal trunks leading from posterior spiracles with conspicuous dark pigmentation extending forwards as far as the 9th or 10th segment (Fig. 15.37); obligate, primary agent of traumatic livestock myiasis; distribution, Neotropical and Nearctic .... ***Cochliomyia hominivorax* (Calliphoridae)**

15 Posterior margin of segment 11 with dorsal spines **16**

Posterior margin of segment 11 without dorsal spines; a secondary facultative agent of cutaneous livestock myiasis; distribution, Neotropical and Nearctic .... ***Cochliomyia macellaria* (Calliphoridae)**

16 Posterior spiracles with distinct button **18**

Posterior spiracles without distinct button **17**

17 Body without fleshy processes; segments with belts of strongly developed spines (Fig. 15.40); anterior spiracle with four to six branches; an obligate, primary agent of cutaneous livestock myiasis; distribution, Afrotropical and Oriental .... ***Chrysomya bezziana* (Calliphoridae)**

Anterior spiracle with 11–13 branches; largely saprophagous; an occasional facultative ectoparasite causing cutaneous myiasis; distribution, Oriental and Australasian .... ***Chrysomya megacephala* (Calliphoridae)**

18 Posterior margins of segment 10 with dorsal spines; length of the larger tubercles on upper margin of posterior face of terminal segment greater than half the width of a posterior spiracle; causes facultative, cutaneous myiasis of cattle, sheep and reindeer (Fig. 15.41); distribution, northern Holarctic .... ***Protophormia terraenovae* (Calliphoridae)**

Posterior margins of segment 10 without dorsal spines; length of the larger tubercles on upper margin of posterior face of terminal segment less than half the width of a posterior spiracle (Fig. 15.41); distribution, Holarctic .... ***Phormia regina* (Calliphoridae)**

Guide to the adult Diptera causing myiasis in domestic animals

1 Insects with one pair of wings on the mesothorax and a pair of club-like halteres on the metathorax (Fig. 15.15); antennae composed of three segments, third segment usually with an arista (Fig. 15.17); foot with two pads; frons with ptilinal suture; second antennal segment usually with a groove; thoracic transverse suture strong; thoracic squamae usually well developed (Fig. 15.20) ....**Calypterate Diptera 2**

2 Mouthparts small, usually functionless; head bulbous; antennae small; flies more or less covered with soft hair **3**

Mouthparts usually well developed; antennae not small; flies with strong bristles; hypopleural bristles present (Fig. 15.19); post-scutellum weak or absent **7**

3 Vein M bent towards vein R_{4+5} **4**

Vein M not bent towards vein R_{4+5}; squamae small; cross-vein dm-cu absent; ovipositor strongly developed in female (Fig. 15.42) .... **Gasterophilinae spp (Oestridae)**

4 Sharp bend of vein M towards vein R_{4+5} but the two do not meet before the margin **5**

Vein M joins vein R_{4+5} before the margin; vein dm-cu in line with deflection of vein M; vein A_1+CuA_2 does not reach the margin (Fig. 3.20); frons enlarged; frons, scutellum and dorsal thorax bear small wart-like protuberances; eyes small (Fig. 15.43); abdomen brownish black .... **Oestrinae spp (Oestridae)**

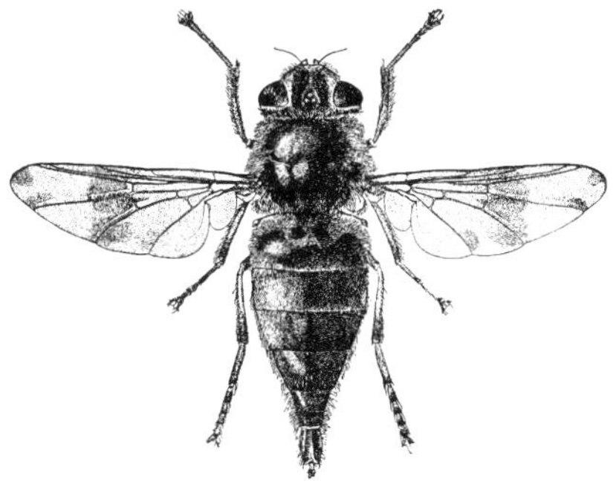

Fig. 15.42 Adult female *Gasterophilus intestinalis* (reproduced from Castellani and Chalmers, 1910).

5 Blue–black colour .... **Cuterebrinae spp**

Not blue–black **6**

6 Vein A_1+CuA_2 reaches the margin; vein dm-cu in line with deflection of vein M (Fig. 15.44); hairy bee-like flies with a light–dark colour pattern; fan of yellow hypopleural hairs; palps absent...... .... **Hypodermatinae spp (Oestridae)**

7 Metallic, iridescent appearance (blue–black, violet–blue, green) **8**

Dull grey appearance; three black stripes on the scutum; abdomen usually with chequered or spotted pattern.. **13**

Flies of predominantly reddish yellow or reddish brown colour, not metallic; distribution, tropical Africa .... ***Cordylobia* spp (Calliphoridae)**

8 Wing with stem vein (base of R) entirely bare **9**

Wing with stem vein with fine hairs along margin **10**

9 Flies with metallic green or coppery green thorax and abdomen; thoracic squamae bare; found in cutaneous myiasis, particularly of sheep; distribution, worldwide.. .... ***Lucilia* spp (Calliphoridae)**

Flies with black–blue thorax and blue or brown abdomen; thoracic squamae with long dark hair on upper surface; may be secondary invaders of cutaneous myiasis; distribution, worldwide .... ***Calliphora* spp (Calliphoridae)**

10 Head with almost entirely black ground colour and black hair; thoracic squamae bare; alar squamae hairy on outer half or dorsal surface.................**12**

Head with ground colour of at least lower half entirely or mainly orange or orange–red and with white, yellow or orange hair; thoracic squamae bare on dorsal surface **11**

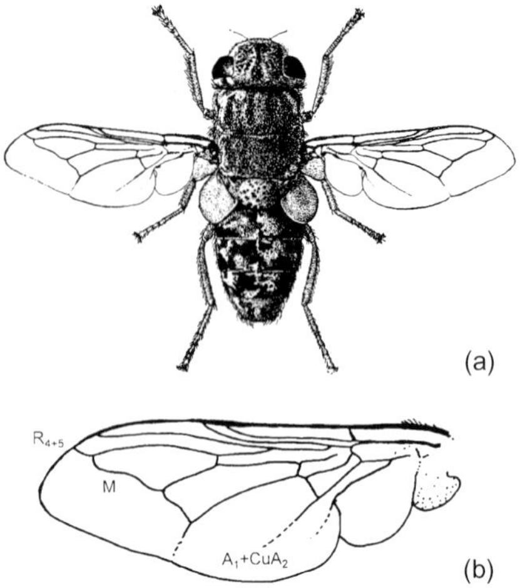

Fig. 15.43 (a) Adult female *Oestrus ovis* and (b) wing venation typical of *Oestrus*, showing the strongly bent vein M joining R_{4+5} before the wing margin (reproduced from Castellani and Chalmers, 1910).

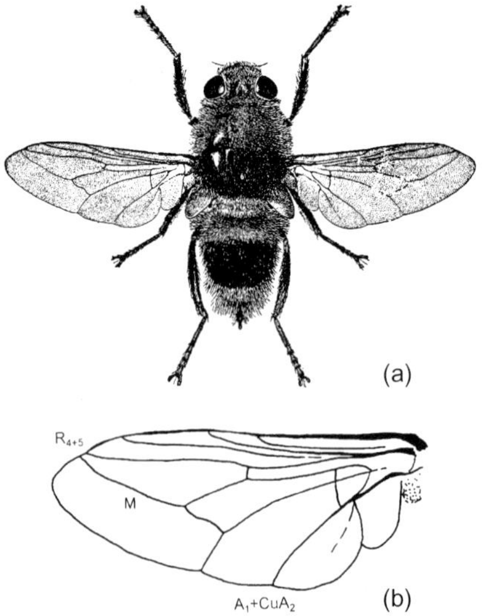

Fig. 15.44 (a) Adult female of *Hypoderma bovis* (reproduced from Castellani and Chalmers, 1910). (b) wing venation typical of *Hypoderma* showing the strongly bent vein M not joining R_{4+5} before the wing margin and vein A_1+CuA_2 reaching the wing margin.

11 Thoracic squamae hairy on whole dorsal surface; scutum of thorax without bold black stripes; distribution, Afrotropical, Oriental, Australasian, southern Palaearctic.. .... ***Chrysomya* spp (Calliphoridae)**

Thoracic squamae hairy only at the base, usually concealed by the alar squamae; scutum of thorax with three bold, black stripes; distribution: Nearctic and Neotropical .... ***Cochliomyia* spp (Calliphoridae)**

12 Thorax with anterior spiracle black or reddish brown; alar squamae with obvious dark hair dorsally; distribution, Palaearctic and Nearctic only .... ***Protophormia* spp (Calliphoridae)**

Thorax with anterior spiracle yellow or orange; thoracic squamae with white–yellow hair dorsally; distribution, Palaearctic and Nearctic only .... ***Phormia* spp (Calliphoridae)**

13 Arista almost bare; abdomen with pattern of black spots (Fig. 15.21) .... ***Wohlfahrtia* spp (Sarcophagidae)**

Arista with long and conspicuous hairs, at least on the basal half; abdomen with dark and light chequered pattern (Fig. 15.21) .... ***Sarcophaga* spp (Sarcophagidae)**

LICE AND FLEAS

The detection of small ectoparasites such as lice and fleas depends on close examination; in the case of lice, the eggs, commonly known as 'nits', may also be found attached to the hair or feathers. Fleas may be more difficult to detect, but the finding of flea faeces in the coat, which appear as small dark pieces of grit and which, on contact with moist cotton wool or tissue, produce a red coloration due to ingested blood, allow confirmation of infection. Collection may be straightforward as in the case of many lice, which may be brushed from the coat or removed by clipping hairs or feathers. Fleas may be removed by brushing or vacuum cleaning. Alternatively, in the case of small animals, the parasites may be readily recovered if the host is placed on a sheet of paper or plastic before being sprayed with an insecticide.The gross characteristics of biting and sucking lice, and a key to the fleas, which are commonly found on domestic animals are described below.

Guide to the recognition of common lice of veterinary importance

The identification of lice is complex and the features used to describe many genera are obscure. However, because lice in general are highly host specific, in many cases information relating to the species of host and the site of infestation will provide a reliable initial guide to identification. The various species of lice are usually found in all geographical regions of the world in which their host occurs.

1 Head broad, equal or almost equal in width to abdomen **2**

Head elongated, much narrower than abdomen **12**

2 Antennae hidden in antennal grooves; antennae four-segmented; maxillary palps present .... **Amblycera 3**

Antennae not hidden in grooves; antennae three- to five-segmented; maxillary palps absent .... **Ischnocera 6**

3 On birds **4**

On mammals **5**

4 Small lice, adults about 2 mm in length; abdomen with sparse covering of medium-length setae (Fig. 15.45); found on thigh or breast feathers; on birds, especially poultry .... ***Menopon* spp (Menoponidae)**

Large lice, adults about 3.5 mm in length; abdomen with dense covering of medium-length setae (Fig. 15.46); found on the breast, thighs and around vent; on birds, especially poultry............. .... ***Menacanthus* spp (Menoponidae)**

5 On guinea-pigs; oval abdomen, broad in middle; six pairs of abdominal spiracles are located ventrolaterally within poorly defined spiraclar plates (Fig. 15.47)................. ***Gyropus* spp (Gyropidae)**

On guinea pigs; slender body, with sides of the abdomen parallel; five pairs of abdominal spiracles located ventrally within distinct sclerotised spiraclar plates (Fig. 15.48) .... ***Gliricola* spp (Gyropidae)**

On dogs; relatively large, adults about 3 mm in length; abdomen with a dense covering of thick, medium and long setae (Fig. 15.49) .... ***Heterodoxus* spp (Boopidae)**

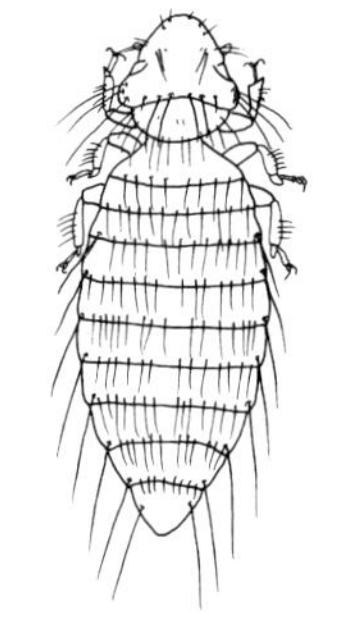

Fig. 15.45 Adult *Menopon gallinae* (dorsal view).

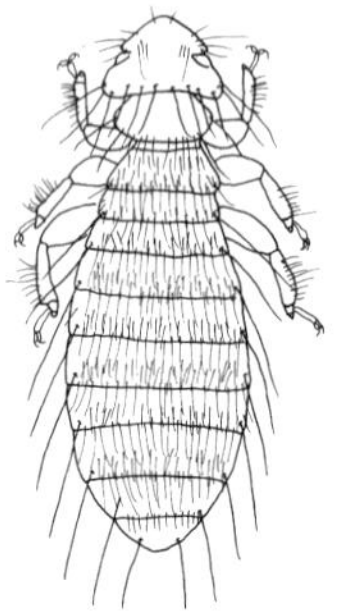

Fig. 15.46 Adult *Menacanthus stramineus* (dorsal view).

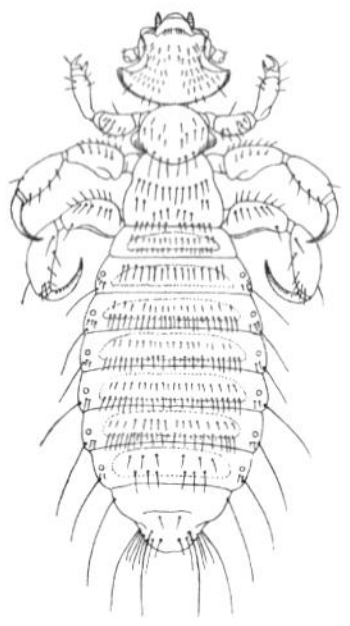

Fig. 15.47 Adult female *Gyropus ovalis* (from Séguy, 1944).

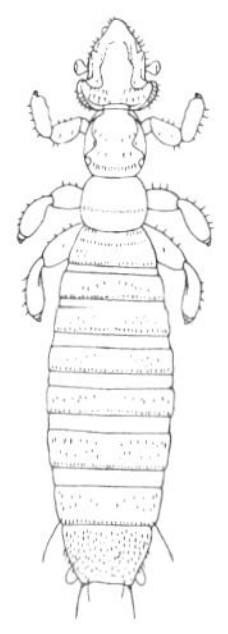

Fig. 15.48 Adult female *Gliricola porcelli* (from Séguy, 1944).

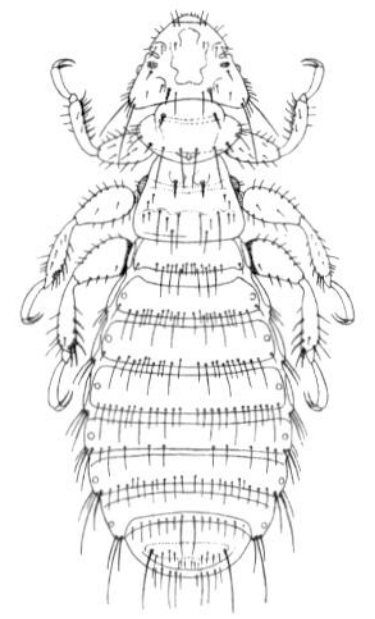

Fig. 15.49 Adult female *Heterodoxus* in ventral view (reproduced from Séguy, 1944).

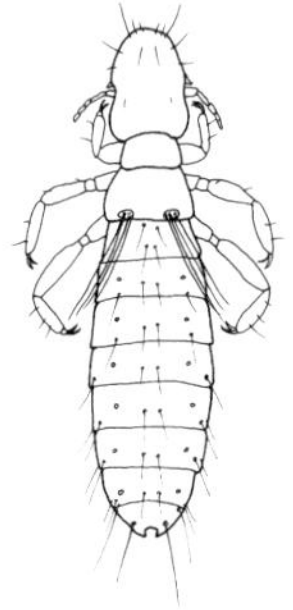

Fig. 15.50 Adult *Lipeurus caponis* (dorsal view).

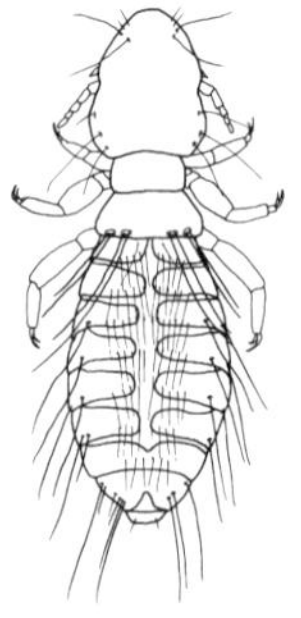

Fig. 15.51 Adult female *Cuclotogaster heterographus* (dorsal view).

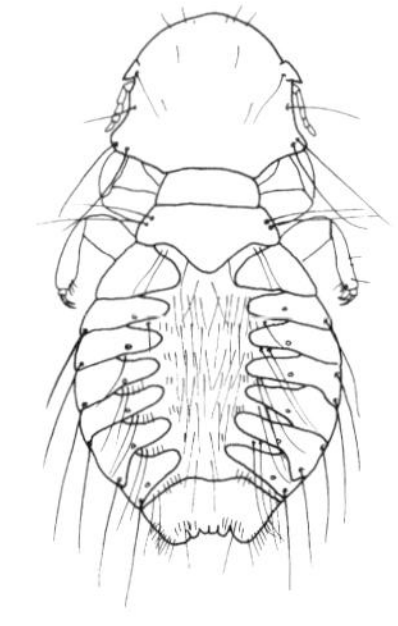

Fig. 15.52 Adult female *Goniodes disimilis* (dorsal view).

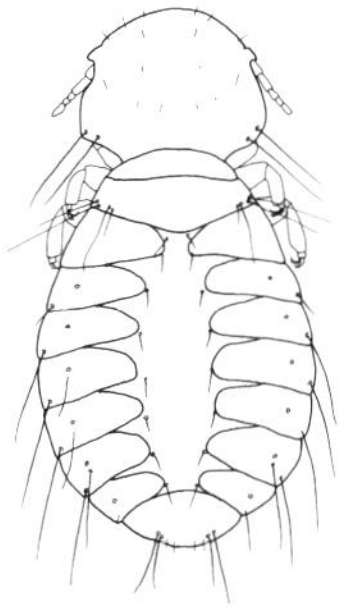

Fig. 15.53 Adult female *Goniocotes gallinae* (dorsal view).

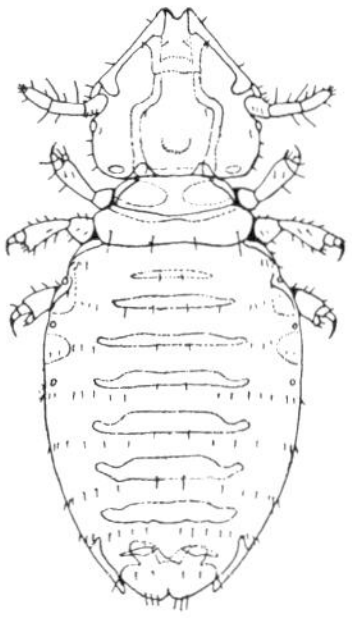

Fig. 15.54 Adult female *Felicola* in ventral view (reproduced from Séguy, 1944).

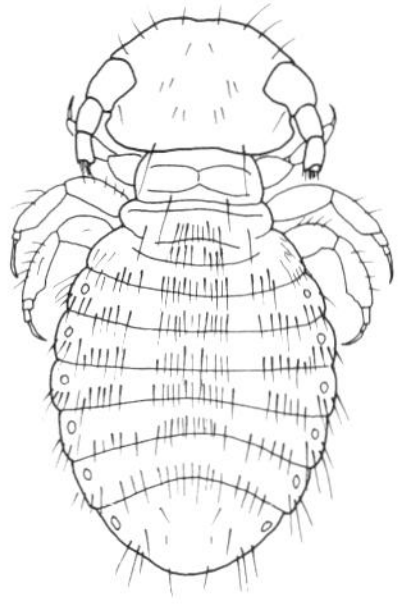

Fig. 15.55 Adult female *Trichodectes* in ventral view (from Séguy, 1944).

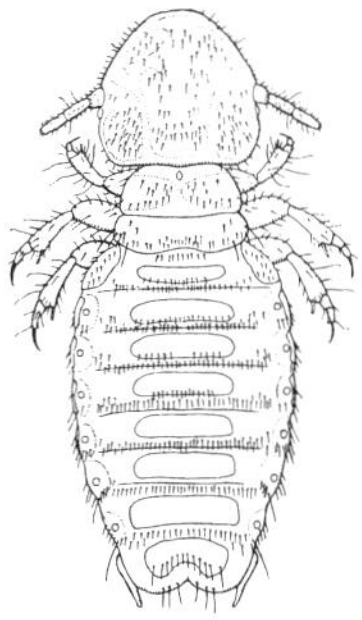

Fig. 15.56 Dorsal view of adult female *Bovicola* (reproduced from Séguy, 1944).

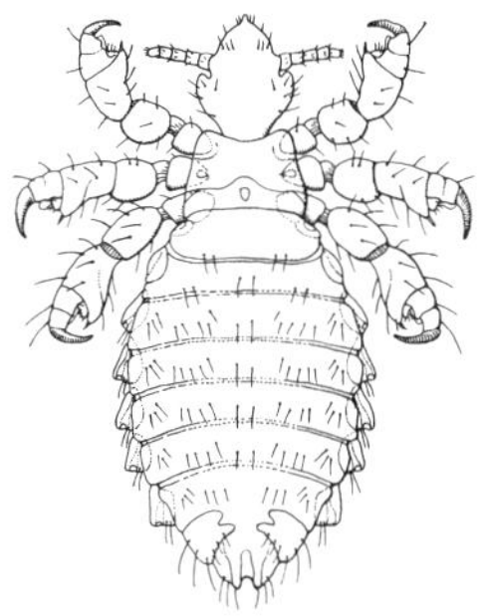

Fig. 15.57 Dorsal view of adult *Haematopinus* (reproduced from Séguy, 1944).

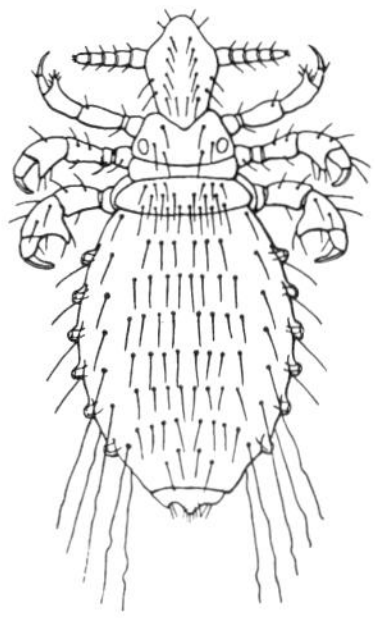

Fig. 15.58 Dorsal view of adult female *Solenopotes* (reproduced from Séguy, 1944).

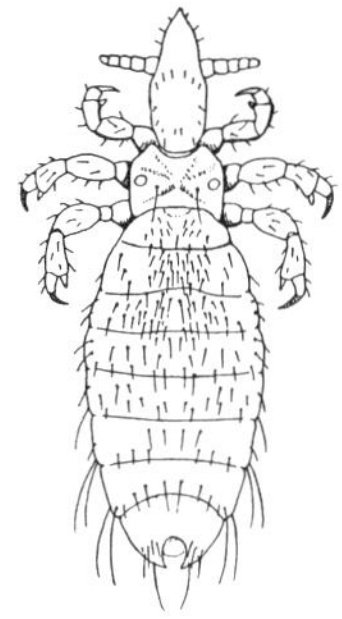

Fig. 15.59 Dorsal view of adult female *Linognathus* (reproduced from Séguy, 1944).

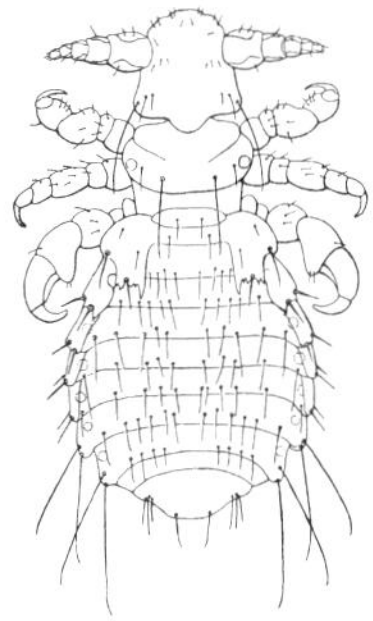

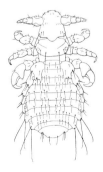

Fig. 15.60 Adult female *Polyplax* in dorsal view.

6 On birds; antennae five-segmented; tarsi with paired claws .... **Philopteridae 7**

On mammals; antennae three-segmented; tarsi with single claws .... **Trichodectidae 10**

7 Hind legs similar in length to first two pairs **8**

Hind legs at least twice as long as first two pairs; body long and narrow; head with small narrow projections in front of antennae; first segment of antennae considerably longer than following four segments (Fig. 15.50); on poultry; distribution, worldwide .... ***Lipeurus* (Philopteridae)**

8 Three long bristles projecting from each side of the dorsal surface of the head; rounded body; adult about 2 mm in length (Fig. 15.51); on poultry .... ***Cuclotogaster* (Philopteridae)**

Two long bristles projecting from each side of the dorsal surface of the head.................................. **9**

9 Head with prominent angles and a distinct hollow margin posterior to the antennae; adult about 5 mm in length (Fig. 15.52); on poultry .... ***Goniodes* spp (Philopteridae)**

Head lacking prominent angles; adult about 2 mm in length (Fig. 15.53); on poultry............... .... ***Goniocotes* (Philopteridae)**

10 Head rounded anteriorly **11**

Head sharply angled anteriorly; legs small; abdomen smooth, with only three pairs of spiracles (Fig. 15.54); on cats .... ***Felicola* spp (Trichodectidae)**

11 Setae of abdomen large and thick (Fig. 15.55); on dogs .... ***Trichodectes* spp (Trichodectidae)**

Setae of abdomen small or of medium length (Fig. 15.56); on mammals....................................... .... ***Bovicola* spp (Trichodectidae)**

12 Distinct ocular points present behind the antennae; all legs of similar size; adult up to 5 mm in length; distinct paratergal plates visible on abdominal segments; ventral surface of the thorax with a dark coloured plate (Fig. 15.57)................ .... ***Haematopinus* spp (Haematopinidae)**

No ocular points behind the antennae; forelegs small **13**

13 Two rows of ventral setae on each abdominal segment **14**

One row of ventral setae on each abdominal segment; paratergal plates absent; spiracles on tubercles which protrude from the abdomen; distinct five-sided sternal plate on the ventral surface of the thorax (Fig. 15.58); on cattle .... ***Solenopotes* spp (Linognathidae)**

14 Paratergal plates absent; ventral sternal plate of thorax is narrow or absent (Fig. 15.59); on cattle, sheep, goats and dogs .... ***Linognathus* spp (Linognathidae)**

Paratergal plates present; ovoid sternal plate on the ventral surface of the thorax (Fig. 15.60); on rodents .... ***Polyplax* spp (Polyplacidae)**

Guide to the flea species of veterinary importance

The physical differences between flea species and even between families tend to be small and there may be considerable variation between individuals within a species. Identification, therefore, is often difficult. The following is a general diagnostic guide to the adults of the most common species of veterinary importance found as parasites on domestic and companion animals.

1 Ctenidia absent... **2**

Ctenidium present, at least on the pronotum..... **4**

2 Pleural ridge absent **3**

Pleural ridge present...............***Xenopsylla cheopis***

3 Frons sharply angled (Fig. 15.61); head behind the antenna with two setae and, in the female, usually with a well developed occipital lobe; the maxillary laciniae are broad and coarsely serrated; adult females embedded in the skin in aggregations on bare areas; found on birds, especially poultry, also on cats, dogs, rabbits and humans.................. .... ***Echidnophaga gallinacea***

Frons smoothly rounded; head behind antennae with only one strong seta; conspicuous ocular seta below the eye; a single, much reduced spine on the genal margin (Fig. 15.62); on pigs, badgers, humans .... ***Pulex irritans***

4 Genal ctenidium present **5**

Genal ctenidium absent; pronotal ctenidium with 18–20 spines; head with a row of three strong setae below the eye (Fig. 15.63); frontal tubercle on head of both sexes conspicuous; 3–4 conspicuous bristles on the inner surface of the hind femur; on rodents .... ***Nosopsyllus fasciatus***

Genal ctenidium absent; pronotal ctenidium with more than 24 spines; head with a row of three strong setae below the eye (Fig. 15.64); on poultry .... ***Ceratophyllus* spp**

5 Genal ctenidium formed of eight or nine spines oriented vertically **6**

Genal ctenidium with four to six oblique spines; frontal tubercle conspicuous on head of both sexes (Fig. 15.65); on rabbits .... ***Spilopsyllus cuniculi***

Genal ctenidium with three very short oblique spines; single vestigial spine on the genal lobe; single short pronotal spine (Fig. 15.66); on hedgehogs, dogs and cats .... ***Archaeopsylla erinacei***

6 Head strongly convex anteriorly in both sexes and not noticeably elongate; hind tibia with eight seta-bearing notches along the dorsal margin (Fig. 15.67); on cats and dogs................ ***Ctenocephalides canis***

Head not strongly convex anteriorly and distinctly elongate, especially in the female; hind tibia with six seta-bearing notches along the dorsal margin (Fig. 15.68); on cats and dogs .... ***Ctenocephalides felis***

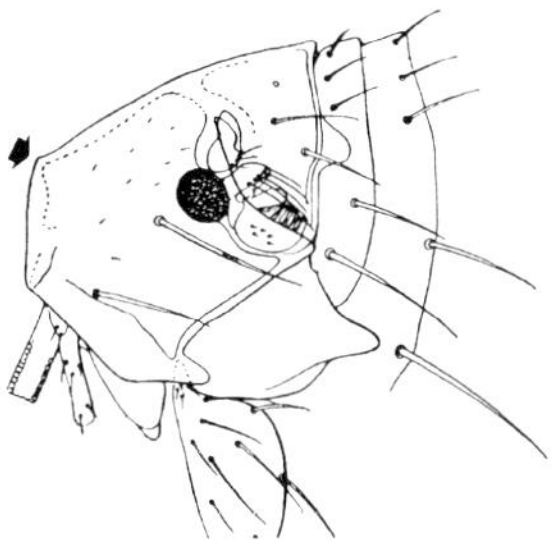

Fig. 15.61 The sticktight flea, *Echidnophaga gallinacea*, female head and thorax (arrow marking angulation of the frons) (after Smart, 1943).

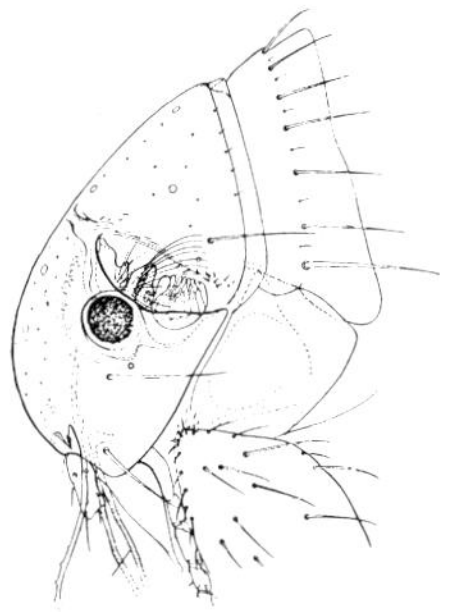

Fig. 15.62 The human flea, *Pulex irritans*, male head and pronotum (after Smart, 1943).

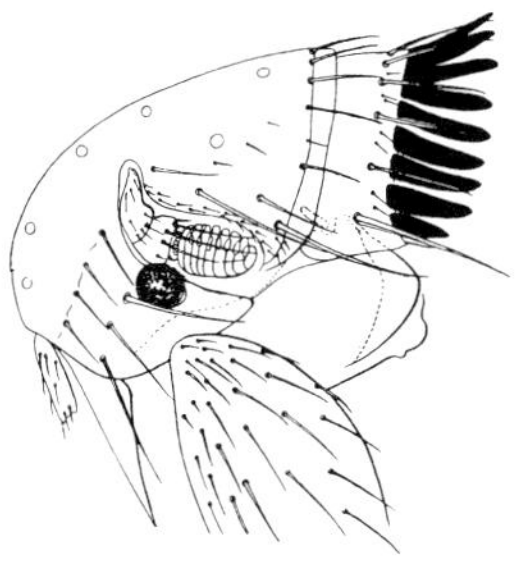

Fig. 15.63 The northern rat flea, *Nosopsyllus fasciatus*, male head (after Smart *et al.*, 1943).

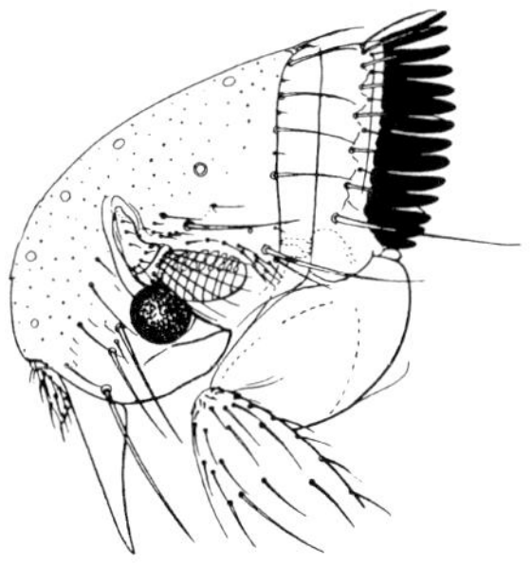

Fig. 15.64 Head and pronotum of a female chicken flea, *Ceratophyllus* (after Smart, 1943).

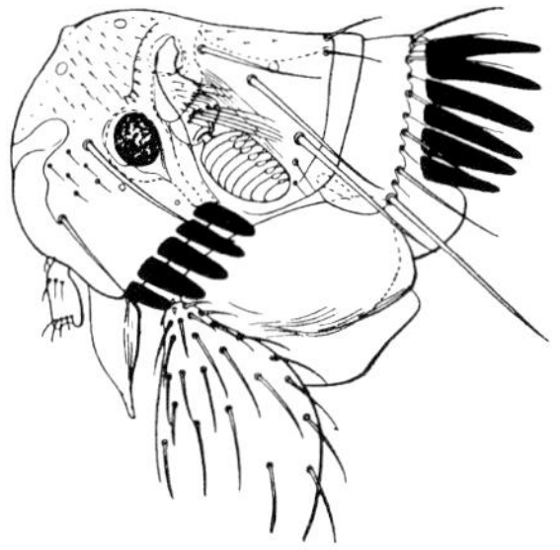

Fig. 15.65 Head and pronotum of the rabbit flea, *Spilopsyllus cuniculi*.

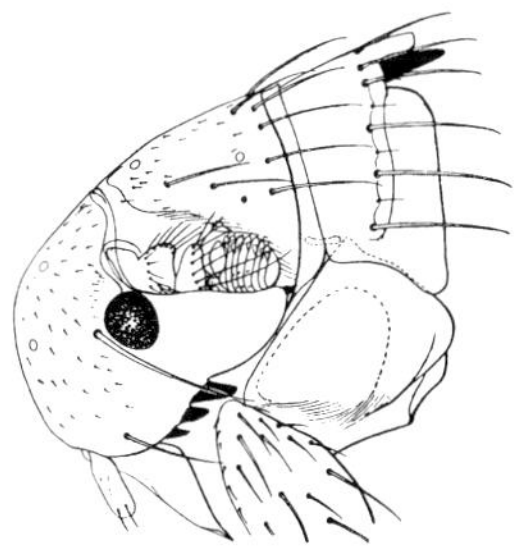

Fig. 15.66 The hedgehog flea, *Archaeopsylla erinacei*, female head (after Smart, 1943).

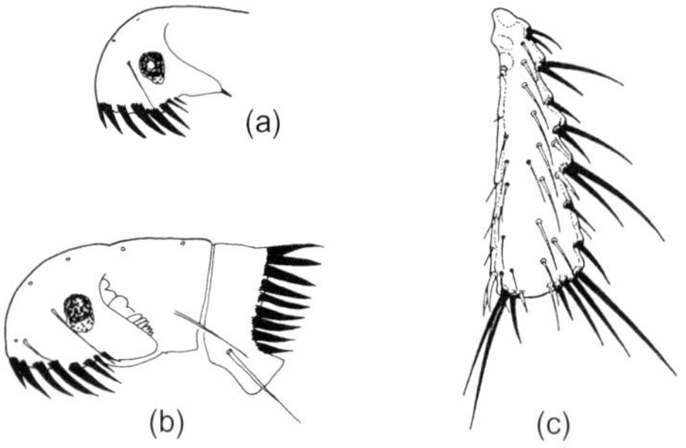

Fig. 15.67 The dog flea, *Ctenocephalides canis*. (a) Front of male head. (b) Female head and pronotum. (c) Hind tibia.

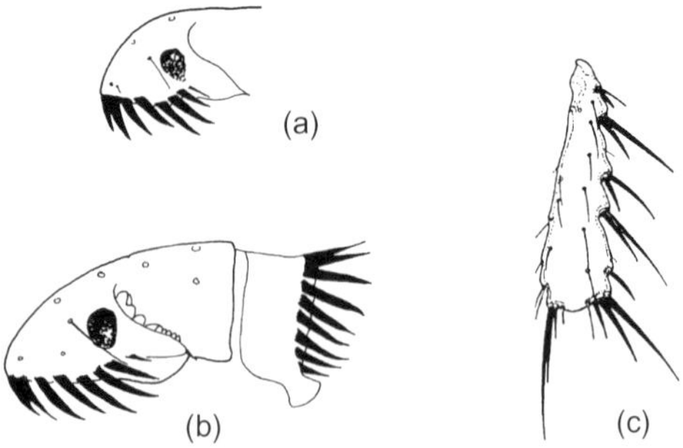

Fig. 15.68 The cat flea, *Ctenocephalides felis felis*. (a) Front of male head. (b) Female head and pronotum. (c) Hind tibia.

TICKS AND MITES

Ticks and mites belong to the Class Arachnida; subclass **Acari** (sometimes also called Acarina).

GUIDE TO THE SUB-ORDERS OF ACARI

1 Hypostome of the gnathosoma without backwardly directed barbs. Stigmata present or absent, when present not opening on stigmatal plates; if stigmata lateral to coxae 2 and 3 then with peritremes. Tarsi of first pair of legs without sensory pit **2**

Hypostome of the gnathosoma with backwardly directed barbs. Stigmatal shields present behind coxae of the fourth pair of legs or laterally above the coxae of legs 2 or 3: stigmata without peritremes. Tarsi of the first pair of legs with a sensory pit .... **Ixodida (Metastigmata)**

2 Idiosoma without conspicuous shields. Legs with coxae fused to body wall. Palps without an apotele **3**

Idiosoma with sclerotised areas forming distinct shields (darkened brown colour). Legs with free coxae articulated to the idiosoma. Palps with an apotele .... **Gamesid mites (Mesostigmata)**

3 Stigmata absent. Palps small, inconspicuous and pressed against the sides of the hypostome. Legs usually with three claws and with a complex pulvillus (varying from pad-like to trumpet like). Body never worm-like .... **Sarcoptiformes (Astigmata)**

Palps usually well developed. Chelicerae usually adapted for piercing, sometimes pincer-like. Legs with one or two claws, without a complex pulvillus. Body sometimes worm-like. Stigmata present or absent; when present positioned between the bases of the chelicerae or on the upper surface of the propodosoma .... **Trombidiformes (Prostigmata)**

TICKS

Ticks are easily recognised, on their hosts, especially when they are engorged, but care should be taken in their removal since their mouthparts are usually firmly embedded in the skin. The tick may be persuaded to withdraw its mouthparts if a piece of cotton wool, soaked in anaesthetic, is placed around it or, alternatively, if something hot is held near its body.

One of the simplest methods used to recover ticks from pasture is to drag a blanket over the ground to which the unfed ticks become attached as they would to a host. Specific identification of the large variety of ticks which parasitise domestic animals is a specialised task.

Guide to the ticks of veterinary importance

The guide presented below and the species descriptions given in the following pages are intended as a general guide to the ticks of veterinary interest only. Specialist texts are required for more detailed descriptions of species and their immature stages.

1 Hypostome with backwardly directed barbs; stigmatal shields present behind coxae of the fourth pair of legs or laterally above the coxae of legs 2 or 3; stigmata without peritremes; tarsi of the first pair of legs with a sensory pit.. **Metastigmata (Ixodida)**

Gnathosoma projecting anteriorly and visible when specimen seen from above; scutum present, covering the dorsal surface completely (male) or the anterior portion only (female); stigmatal plates large, situated posteriorly to the coxae of the fourth pair of legs (Figs 15.69, 15.70)..**Ixodidae 2**

Gnathosoma ventral and not visible when adult is viewed from above; scutum absent; dorsal integument leathery; stigmatal plates small, situated anteriorly to the coxae of the fourth pair of legs; eyes, if present, in lateral folds .... **Argasidae 11**

2 Anal groove surrounding the anus distinct, both anteriorly and posteriorly (Figs. 15.69, 15.70) .... ***Ixodes***

Anal groove entirely posterior to the anus....... **3**

3 Eyes absent **4**

Eyes present.. **5**

4 Palps short and broad, about twice as wide as segment 2 with obvious outer angulation at the base (Figs. 15.71, 15.72) .... ***Haemaphysalis***

5 Palps wider than long or, at most, only slightly longer than their width **6**

Palps much longer than wide **10**

6 Basis capituli usually hexagonal dorsally (Fig. 15.71); medium-sized or small ticks, usually without colour patterns... **7**

Basis capituli rectangular dorsally (Fig. 15.71); large ticks with definite colour patterns (Fig. 15.73) .... ***Dermacentor***

7 Festoons absent; stigmatal plates round or oval; anal groove faint or obsolete **8**

Festoons present; stigmatal plate with a tail-like protrusion; anal groove distinct **9**

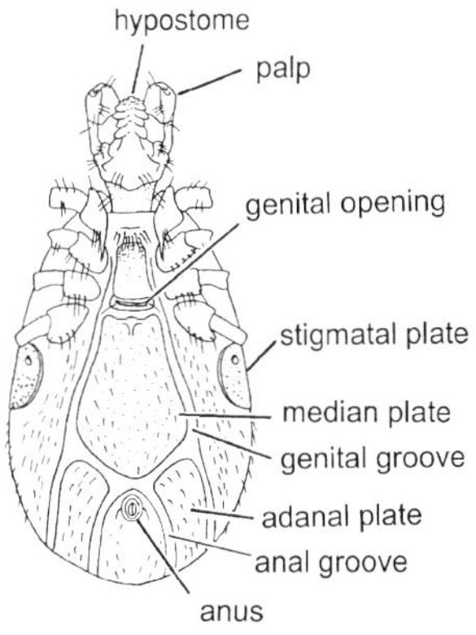

Fig. 15.69 Ventral view of a generalised male, ixodid tick.

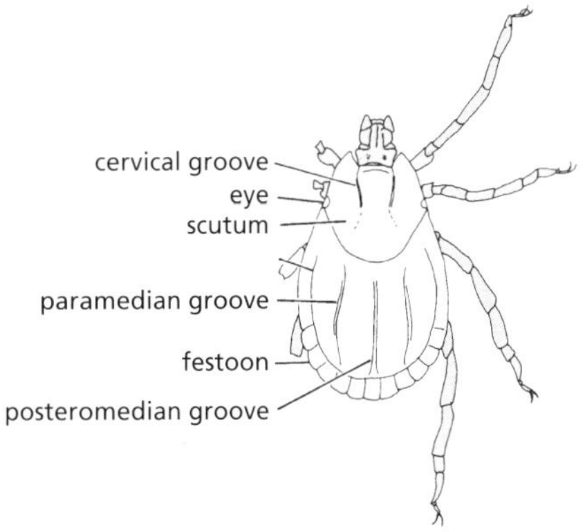

Fig. 15.70 Dorsal view of a generalised female, ixodid tick.

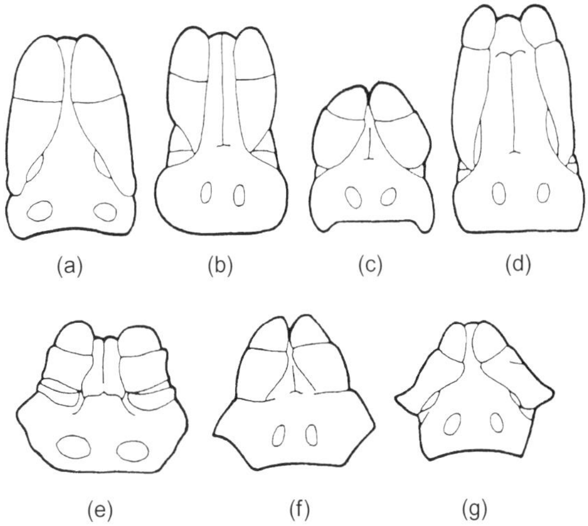

Fig. 15.71 Diagrammatic dorsal view of the gnathosoma of seven genera of ixodid ticks (from Smart, 1943). (a) *Ixodes*. (b) *Hyalomma*. (c) *Dermacentor*. (d) *Ambylomma*. (e) *Boophilus*. (f) *Rhiphicephalus*. (g) *Haemaphysalis*.

8 Palps with dorsal and lateral ridges; male with normal legs .... ***Boophilus***

9 Basis capituli without pronounced lateral angles (Fig. 11.4); males with ventral plates; males with coxae of fourth pair of legs normal (Fig. 15.71) .... ***Rhipicephalus***

10 Palps with second segment less than twice as long as third segment (Fig. 15.71); scutum without pattern... ***Hyalomma***

Palps with second segment more than twice as long as third segment (Fig. 15.71); scutum with pattern; male without ventral plates... ***Amblyomma***

11 Body periphery undifferentiated, without a definite suture distinguishing the dorsal from ventral surface.. **12**

Body surface flattened and usually structurally different from the dorsal surface, with a definite suture distinguishing dorsal and ventral surface (Fig. 15.74)... ***Argas***

12 Adult integument is granular; hypostome vestigial; nymphal integument spiny; hypostome well developed .... ***Otobius***

Adult and nymph integument leathery (Fig. 15.75); hypostome well developed............ ***Ornithodoros***

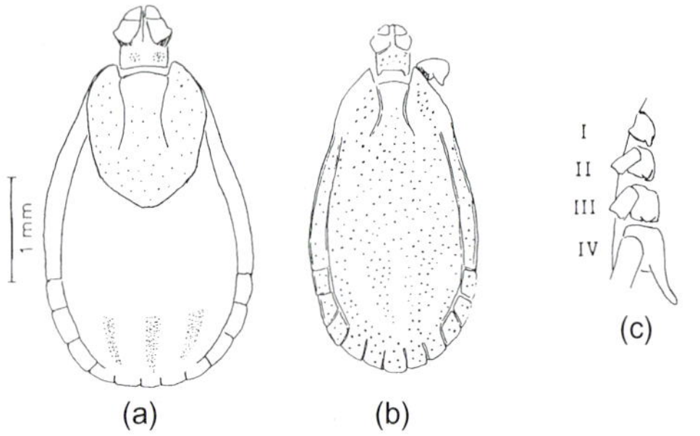

Fig. 15.72 Dorsal view of the gnathosoma and scutum of adult (a) female and (b) male *Haemaphysalis punctata*. (c) Ventral view of the coxae of an adult male (reproduced from Arthur, 1962).

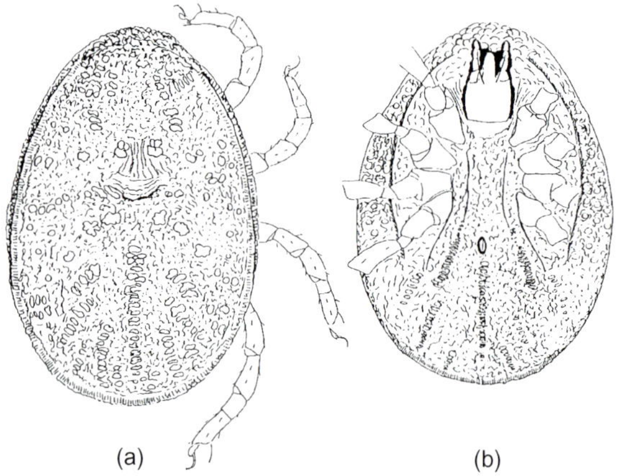

Fig. 15.74 Female *Argas reflexus* (a) dorsal and (b) ventral view (reproduced from Arthur, 1962).

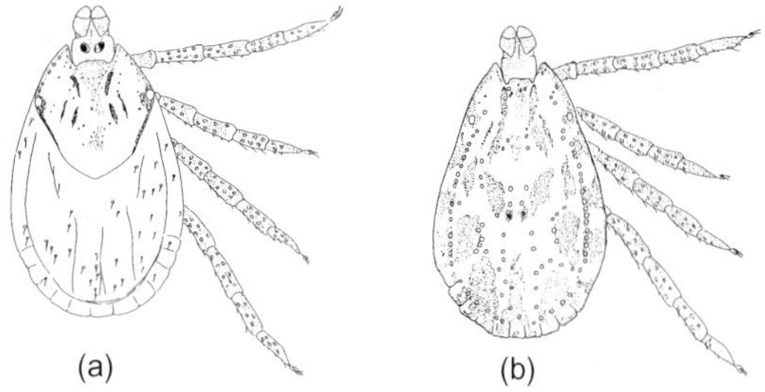

Fig. 15.73 Adult *Dermacentor andersoni*. (a) Dorsal view of female. (b) Dorsal view of male (reproduced from Arthur, 1962).

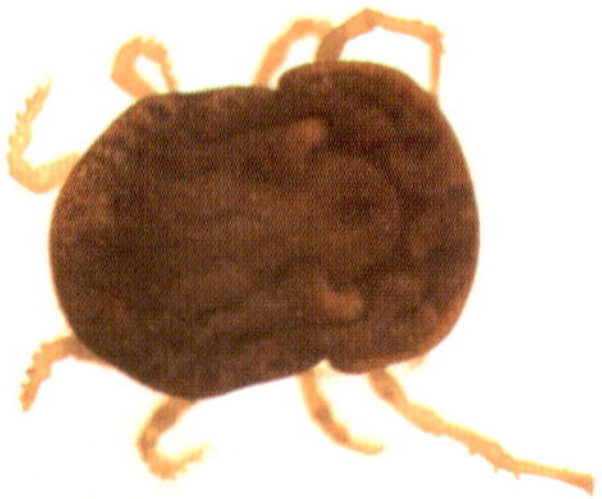

Fig. 15.75 *Ornithodoros* dorsal view.

MITES

Some non-burrowing mites such as *Otodectes* and *Cheyletiella* can be found by close examination. For example, *Otodectes* may be seen either on examination of the external auditory canal using an auroscope or on microscopic examination of ear wax removed by means of a swab; likewise, rigorous brushing of the coat and subsequent microscopic examination of this material will usually confirm infection with *Cheyletiella*. For the demonstration of some non-burrowing and burrowing mites it is often necessary to obtain a skin scraping which is subsequently examined microscopically. The area selected for scraping should be at the edge of a visible lesion and the hair over this area should be clipped away. A drop of lubricating oil such as liquid paraffin is placed on a microscope slide and a clean scalpel blade dipped in the oil before using it to scrape the surface of a fold of affected skin. Scraping should be continued until a slight amount of blood oozes from the skin surface and the material obtained then transferred to the oil on the slide. A coverslip should then be applied and the sample examined under low magnification (×100). If during this initial examination no mites are detected a further sample may be heated on a slide with a drop of 10% caustic potash. After allowing this preparation to clear for 5–10 minutes it should be re-examined.

Guide to the mite species and families of veterinary importance

The identification of mites can be difficult. However, since mites in general tend to be relatively host specific, a good first practical indication of the likely identity of any species in question can be the species of host and the location of the mite on that host. The following is a general guide to the adults of the most common species and genera of ectoparasitic mites likely to be encountered. It is important to note that this guide is not comprehensive and if in doubt more specialist keys should be used.

1 Stigmata absent posterior to the second pair of legs **2**

Stigmata present as one lateral pair between the bases of legs II and IV **3**

2 Legs without claws; palps with two segments; stigmata absent **14**

Some or all legs with claws; palps with more than two segments; stigmata present or absent, when present they open on the gnathosoma or the anterior part of the idiosoma (Fig. 15.76) **20**

3 Genital plate rudimentary or absent **4**

Genital plate well defined **5**

4 Genital plate present although rudimentary; in lungs of canary .... ***Sternostoma tracheacolum* (Rhinonyssidae)**

Genital plate absent; palps elongated with five segments; in nasal passage of dogs .... ***Pneumonyssus caninum* (Halarachnidae)**

5 Chelicerae long and whip-like; chelae at tips absent or very small **6**

Chelicerae not long and whip-like, shorter and stronger; chelae blade-like at tips **7**

6 Dorsal surface of body with one shield; anal shield not egg shaped and with anal opening at posterior end (Fig. 15.77); parasite of birds .... ***Dermanyssus gallinae* (Dermanyssidae)**

7 Dorsal shield not nearly covering dorsal body surface; genitoventral shield narrowed posteriorly; chelicerae with toothless chelae **8**

Dorsal shield virtually covering dorsal body surface; genitoventral shield not narrowed posteriorly; chelicerae usually with toothed chelae **10**

8 Dorsal shield broad, its setae short **9**

Dorsal shield narrow and tapering posteriorly, its setae long; parasite of rats, mice, hamsters ....***Ornithonyssus bacoti* (Macronyssidae)**

9 Sternal shield with two pairs of setae (Fig. 15.78); parasite of birds .... ***Ornithonyssus sylviarum* (Macronyssidae)**

Sternal shield with three pairs of setae; parasite of birds........ ***Ornithonyssus bursa* (Macronyssidae)**

10 Genitoventral shield widened posteriorly, with more than one pair of setae **11**

Genitoventral shield not widened posteriorly, one pair of setae; on small rodents, weasels and moles............ .... ***Hirstionyssus isabellinus* (Laelapidae)**

11 Body densely covered in setae **12**

Body with few setae (these arranged in transverse rows) **13**

12 Genitoventral shield with pear-shaped outline; on rodents .... *Haemogamasus pontiger* **(Laelapidae)**

Genitoventral shield with large subcircular outline; on rodents .... *Eulaelaps stabularis* **(Laelapidae)**

13 Genitoventral shield with concave posterior margin, surrounding anterior part of anal shield; on rodents .... *Laelaps echidninus* **(Laelapidae)**

14 Legs short and stubby; genital opening of female a transverse slit paralleling body striations; dorsal striations broken by strong pointed scales; dorsal setae strong and spine-like; anus terminal (Fig. 15.79); on mammals .... *Sarcoptes scabiei* **(Sarcoptidae)**

Dorsal setae not spine-like **15**

Legs not short and stubby **17**

15 Anus terminal; tarsi claw-like, with terminal setae **16**

Anus dorsal; dorsal striations broken by many pointed scales; dorsal setae simple, not spine-like (Fig. 15.80); on rats and guinea pigs .... *Trixicarus caviae* **(Sarcoptidae)**

Anus dorsal; dorsal striations not broken by pointed scales; dorsal setae simple, not spine-like; tarsi with long pretarsi on legs I and II (Fig. 15.81); on cats .... *Notoedres cati* **(Sarcoptidae)**

16 Dorsal striations simple, unbroken (Fig. 15.82); on poultry .... *Knemidokoptes gallinae* **(Knemidokoptidae)**

Dorsal striations broken, forming scale-like pattern; on poultry .... *Knemidokoptes mutans* **(Knemidokoptidae)**

Dorsal striations broken, forming scale-like pattern; on caged birds .... *Knemidokoptes pilae* **(Knemidokoptidae)**

17 Pretarsi with short stalks **18**

In the adult female, pretarsi of I, II and IV with three-jointed long stalks; tarsi III with two long terminal whip-like setae; legs of equal sizes; genital opening an inverted U. In the adult male, pretarsi on legs I, II and III with three-jointed long stalks; long setae on legs IV which are smaller than others (Fig. 15.83); on domestic mammals .... *Psoroptes* **spp (Psoroptidae)**

18 In the adult female, tarsi I, II and IV with short-stalked pretarsi; tarsi III with a pair of long terminal whip-like setae; legs I and II stronger than the others; legs III shortest; legs IV with long slender tarsi; genital opening almost a transverse slit. In the adult male all legs with short-stalked pretarsi; fourth pair of legs short (Fig. 15.84); on domestic animals .... *Chorioptes bovis* **(Psoroptidae)**

Legs I and II with short-stalked pretarsi; legs III and IV with a pair of terminal whip-like setae; legs IV much reduced; genital opening transverse (Fig. 15.85); found in the ears of cats and dogs .... *Otodectes cynotis* **(Psoroptidae)**

19 Mouthparts not well developed, reduced; small oval, nude mites; all tarsi with pretarsi (Fig. 15.86); in the tissues of birds .... *Cytodites nudus* **(Cytoditidae)**

Mouthparts well developed; elongated mites; body setae long; tarsi I and II claw-like distally; tarsi III and IV with long, spatulate pretarsi (Fig. 15.87); in the tissues of birds .... *Laminosioptes cysticola* **(Laminosioptidae)**

20 Body not unusually elongated, with setae **21**

Body unusually elongated and crocodile-like with annulations, without setae (Fig. 15.88); in skin pores of mammals .... *Demodex* **spp (Demodicidae)**

21 Gnathosoma and palps conspicuous; body with feathery setae; three pairs of legs when attached to host (larval forms) (Fig. 15.89) .... species of **Trombiculidae**

Gnathosoma and palps conspicuous; body not with feathery setae; stigma opening at base of chelicerae **22**

Gnathsoma and palps inconspicuous; body with simple non-feathery setae; not ectoparasitic .... *Pyemotes tritici* **(Pyemotidae)**

22 Palps with thumb–claw complex **23**

Palps without thumb–claw complex **24**

23 Chelicerae fused with rostrum to form cone; palps opposable, with large distal claws; peritreme obvious, M-shaped on gnathosoma (Fig. 15.90)

On rabbits .... *Cheyletiella parasitivorax* **(Cheyletiellidae)**

On cats .... *Cheyletiella blakei* **(Cheyletiellidae)**

On dogs .... *Cheyletiella yasguri* **(Cheyletiellidae)**

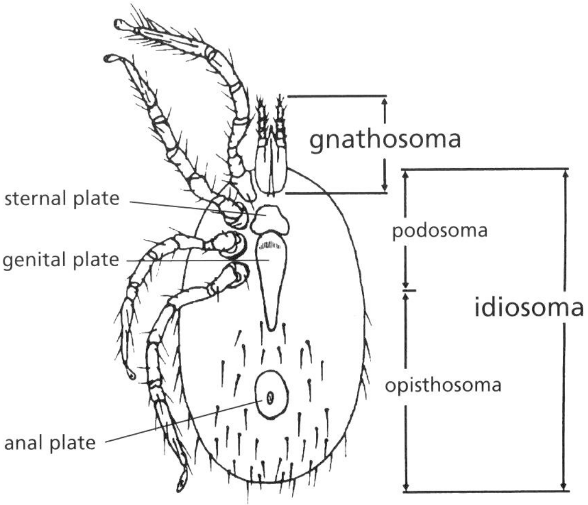

Fig. 15.76 The body of a generalised mite, ventral view.

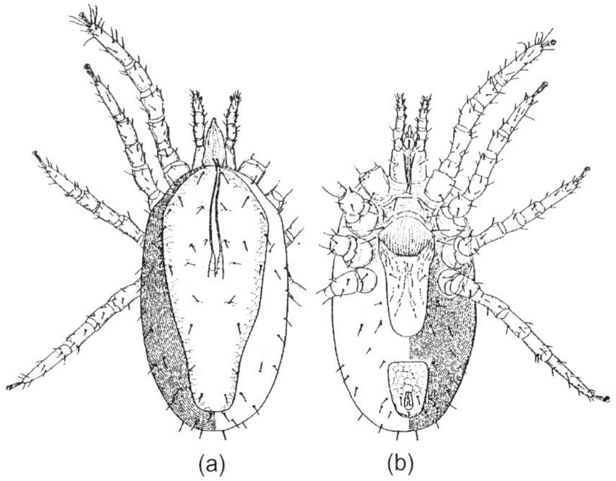

Fig. 15.77 Adult female of the red mite, *Dermanyssus gallinae*. (a) Dorsal view. (b) Ventral view (reproduced from Baker *et al*., 1956).

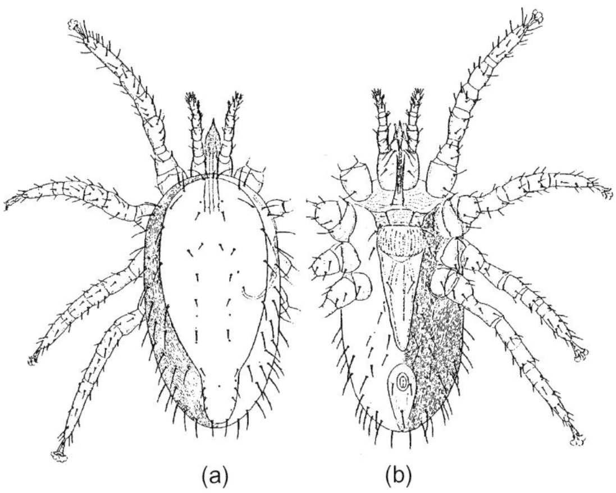

Fig. 15.78 Adult females *Ornithonyssus sylviarum* (northern fowl mite). (a) Dorsal view. (b) Ventral view (reproduced from Baker *et al*., 1956).

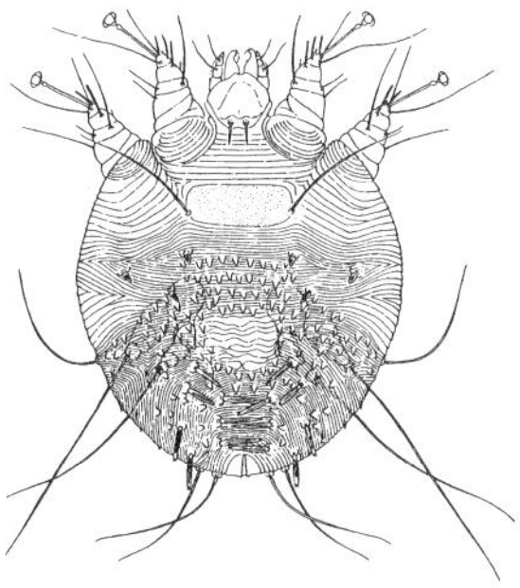

Fig. 15.79 Adult female of *Sarcoptes scabiei*, dorsal view (reproduced from Baker *et al*., 1956).

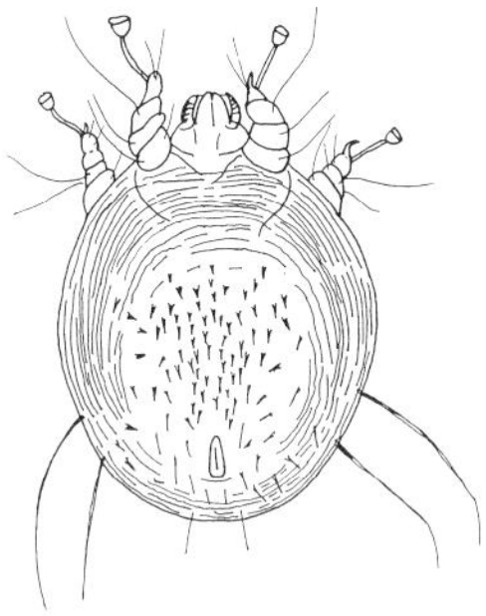

Fig. 15.80 Adult female of *Trixicarus caviae* (dorsal view).

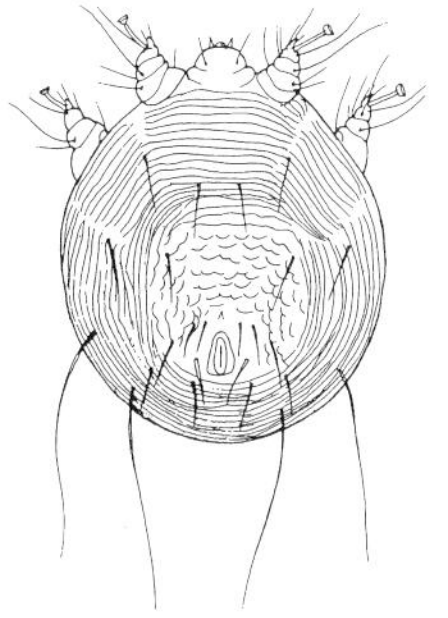

Fig. 15.81 Adult female *Notoedres cati* in dorsal view.

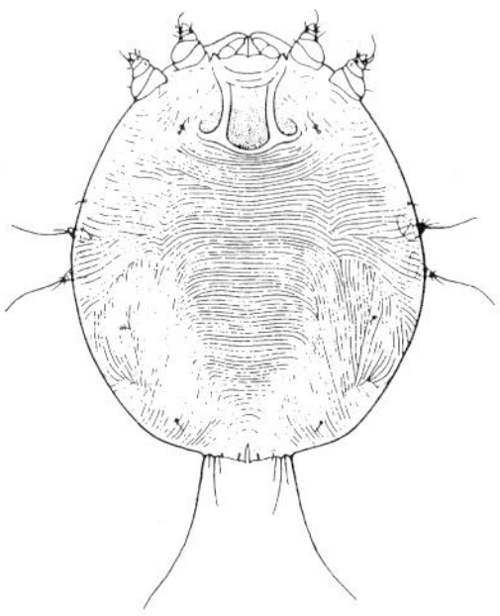

Fig. 15.82 Adult female of *Knemidokoptes gallinae*, dorsal view (reproduced from Hirst, 1922).

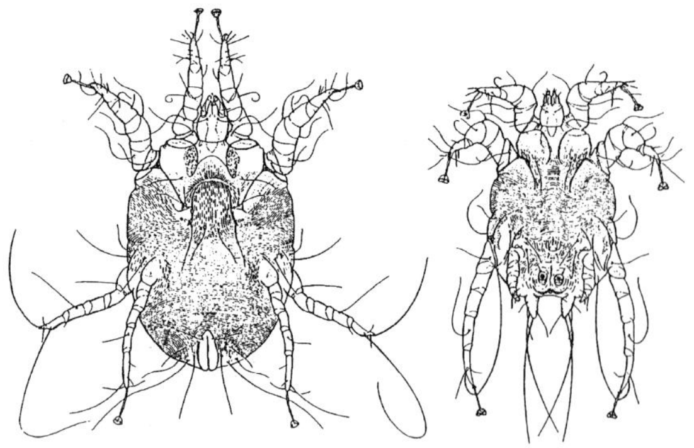

(a) (b)

Fig. 15.83 Adult *Psoroptes ovis*, ventral views. (a) Female. (b) Male (reproduced from Baker *et al.*, 1956).

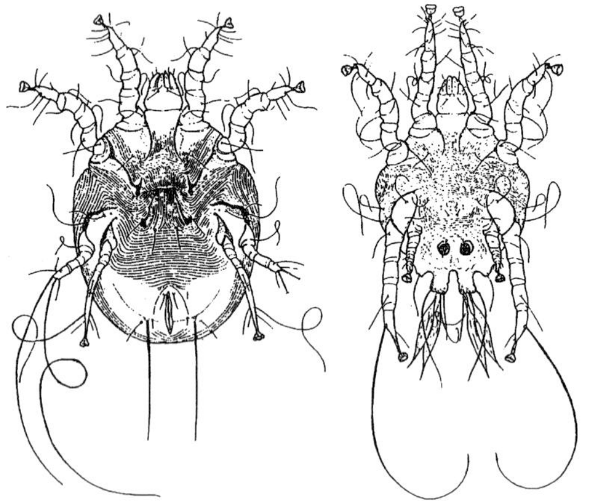

(a) (b)

Fig. 15.84 Adult *Chorioptes bovis*, ventral views. (a) Female. (b) Male (reproduced from Baker *et al.*, 1956).

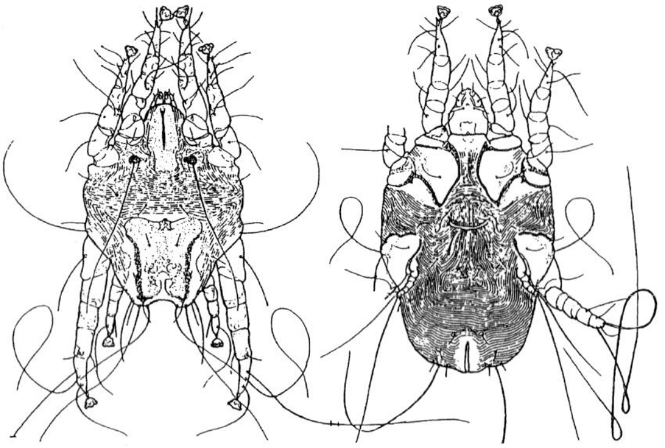

(a) (b)

Fig. 15.85 Adult *Otodectes cynotis*. (a) Male, dorsal view. (b) Female ventral view (reproduced from Baker *et al.*, 1956).

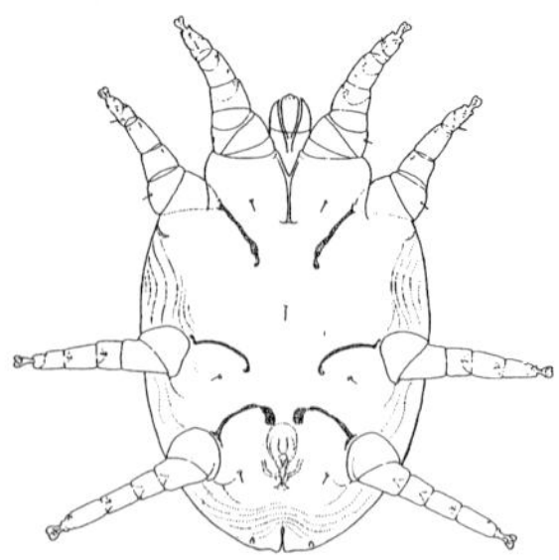

Fig. 15.86 Adult *Cytodites nudus*, ventral view (reproduced from Baker *et al.*, 1956).

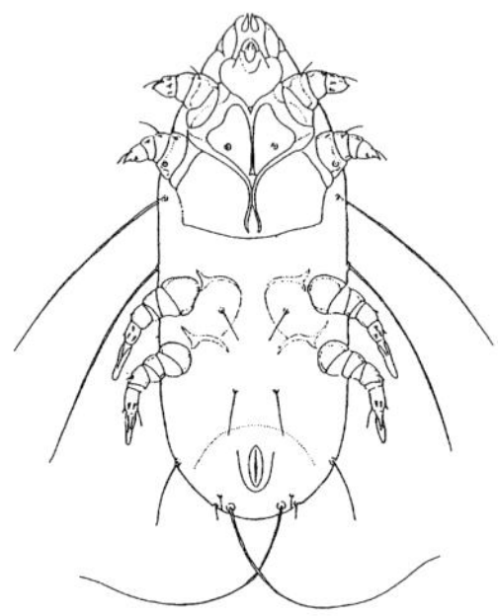

Fig. 15.87 Adult female *Laminosioptes cysticola*, ventral view (reproduced from Baker *et al.*, 1956).

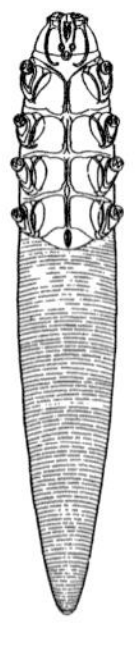

Fig. 15.88 Adult *Demodex* spp ventral view (reproduced from Baker *et al.*, 1956).

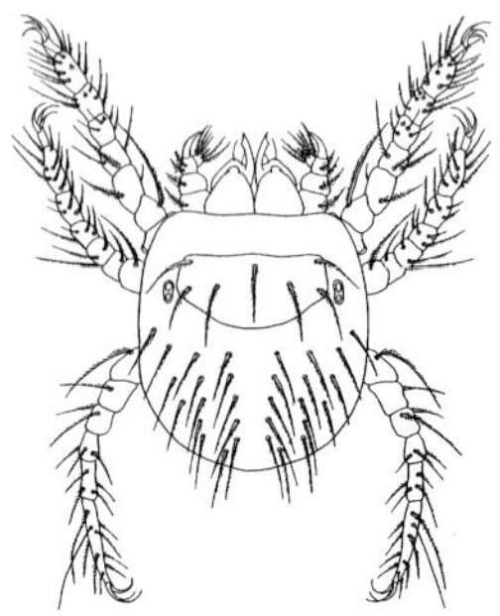

Fig. 15.89 Parasitic larval stage of the Harvest mite *Neotrombicula* (*Trombicula*) *autumnalis* (reproduced from Savory, 1935).

24 Legs normal, for walking **25**

First pair of legs highly modified for clasping hairs of host; body elongate, with transverse striations; on mice and rats .... **Myobidae**

Legs I and II and tarsi IV adapted for clasping hairs (Fig. 15.91); on guinea pigs .... ***Chirodiscoides caviae* (Listrophoridae)**

Legs III and IV of female modified for clasping hairs (Fig. 15.92); on mice .... ***Myocoptes musculinus* (Listrophoridae)**

25 Small, round mites with short stubby, radiating legs, each with a strong hook; female with two pairs of posterior setae, male with a single pair of posterior setae (Fig. 15.93)

On sheep .... ***Psorergates ovis* (Psorergatidae)**

On mice .... ***Psorergates simplex* (Psorergatidae)**

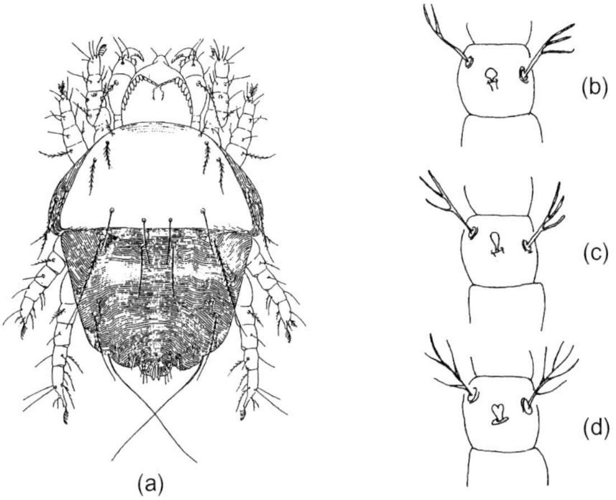

Fig. 15.90 (a) Adult female *Cheyletiella parasitovorax*, dorsal view (reproduced from Baker *et al.*, 1956). Genu of the first pair of legs of adult females of (b) *Cheyletiella parasitovorax*, (c) *Cheyletiella blakei* and (d) *Cheyletiella yasguri*.

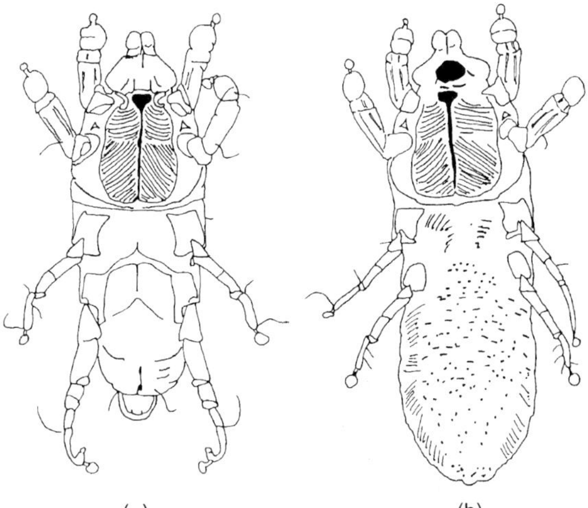

Fig. 15.91 Adults of *Chirodiscoides caviae*. (a) Male ventral view. (b) Female ventral view.

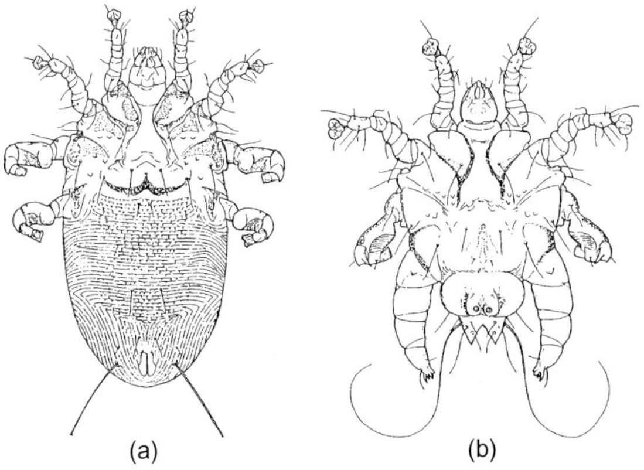

Fig. 15.92 Adults of *Mycoptes musculinus*. (a) Female ventral view. (b) Male ventral view (from Baker *et al.*, 1956).

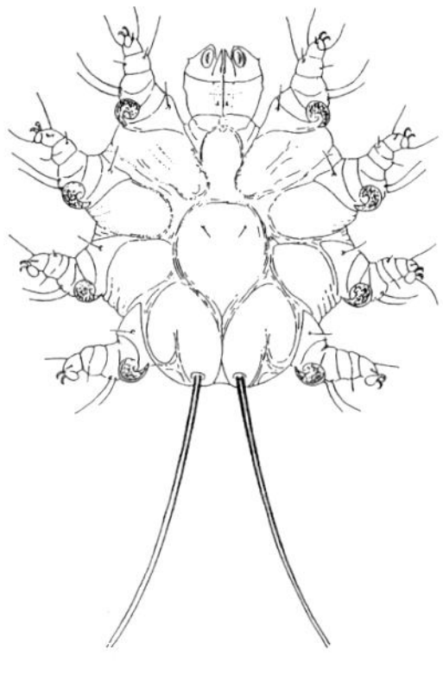

Fig. 15.93 Adult female *Psorergates* (reproduced from Baker *et al.*, 1956).

PRESERVATION

Most adult arthropods and their developing stages may be preserved satisfactorily in 70% alcohol in small glass or plastic tubes. A plug of cotton wool should be pushed down the tube to limit damage during transit and the tube firmly corked and labelled. Otherwise, the specimen may be pinned through the thorax on to the cork stopper of a specimen tube, but this is best left to the specialist for all but the largest flies.

PROTOZOAL INFECTIONS

The laboratory diagnosis of protozoal diseases is often relatively straightforward and well within the scope of the general practitioner, athough on other occasions it may require specialised techniques and long experience. This section is concerned primarily with the former and supplements the information already given in the general text.

EXAMINATION OF FAECAL SAMPLES

The McMaster flotation method is the simplest technique for detecting the presence and estimating the number of coccidial oocysts in faeces. The technique is exactly the same as that described for helminthological diagnosis although the small size of the oocysts makes the microscopic examination more prolonged. If the animal has acute clinical signs of coccidiosis, such as blood-stained faeces, and many thousands of oocysts are present, one may reasonably consider that the diagnosis is confirmed. Unfortunately, with the more pathogenic species of coccidia, clinical signs may appear during the meroogonous phase or when oocyst production has just started, so that a negative or low oocyst count does not necessarily indicate that the clinical diagnosis was wrong. The oocyst count is also of little value in the less acute coccidial infections associated with production losses. In general, because of the limitations of the oocyst count, a postmortem examination, at least on poultry, is always advisable.

For the detection of intestinal protozoa such as *Entamoeba*, *Giardia* or *Balantidium*, a small amount of fresh faeces may be mixed with warm saline and examined under a warm-stage microscope for the presence of trophozoites or cysts. However, their identification requires considerable experience and faecal samples preserved in formalin or polyvinyl alcohol may be sent to a specialist laboratory for confirmation.

The diagnosis of suspected *Cryptosporidium* infection depends on the examination of faecal smears stained by the Ziehl–Nielsen technique, the small thin-shelled oocysts appearing bright red.

EXAMINATION OF BLOOD AND LYMPH

Thin blood smears stained with Romanowsky dyes, such as Giemsa or Leishmann, and examined under an oil immersion lens are commonly used for the detection of trypanosomes, babesial and theilerial piroplasms and rickettsial infections such as anaplasmosis, ehrlichiosis and eperythrozoonosis. On other occasions, needle biopsies of enlarged lymph nodes may be similarly stained for the detection of trypanosomes (especially *Trypanosoma brucei* or *T. vivax*) or theilerial schizonts.

In trypanosomosis, the parasitaemia may be light and the chance of a positive diagnosis is increased if a thick blood film, dehaemoglobinised by immersing the slide in water before eosin staining, is used. For this a drop of fresh blood, with no added anticoagulant, is gently stirred on a slide to cover an area of about 10 mm diameter and allowed to dry. Subsequently it may be stained by Field's technique as follows.

Preparation of solutions:

Solution A	Methylene blue	0.4 g
	Azure I	0.25 g
	Solution B	250 ml
Solution B	$Na_2HPO_412H_2O$	25.2 g
	KH_2PO_4	12.5 g
	Distilled water	1000 ml
Solution C	Eosin	0.5 g
	Solution B	250 ml

These solutions do not keep and should be freshly prepared each day.

(1)	Dip slide in solution A	1–3 seconds
(2)	Rinse in solution B	2–3 seconds
(3)	Dip slide in C	1–3 seconds
(4)	Rinse in tap water	2–3 seconds
(5)	Stand upright to drain and dry.	

This technique is commonly used in large-scale survey work in the field.

A particularly efficient diagnostic technique for trypanosomosis, described earlier in the text, is the examination, under darkground illumination, of the expressed buffy coat of a microhaematocrit tube for the detection of motile trypanosomes.

The inoculation of mice with fresh blood from suspected cases of *Trypanosoma congolense* or *T. brucei* infection is another common technique practised in the field. Three days later the tail blood of such mice should be examined and subsequently daily thereafter for about 3–4 weeks to establish if trypanosomes are present.

The detection of specific antibody in a specialist laboratory may also be useful in the diagnosis of several protozoal diseases such as theileriosis, trypanosomosis, including *T. cruzi* infection, babesiosis, cryptosporidiosis and rickettsial infections such as anaplasmosis and ehrlichiosis. However a positive result does not necessarily imply the presence of a still active infection, but simply that the animal has at some time been exposed to the pathogen. An exception to this interpretation is the diagnosis of suspected toxoplasmosis in sheep, where rising antibody levels over a period of several weeks are reasonable evidence of recent and active infection.

EXAMINATION OF SKIN

Histological examination of skin biopsies or scrapings from the edges of skin ulcers, suspected to be due to leishmaniosis, may be used to demonstrate the amastigote parasites in the macrophages.

In dourine, caused by *Trypanosoma equiperdum*, fluid extracted from the cutaneous plaques usually offers a better chance of detecting trypanosomes than blood smears.

Finally, although not within the province of the general practitioner, the use of **xenodiagnosis** as a diagnostic technique should be noted. This is used to detect protozoal infections such as babesiosis, theileriosis or *Trypanosoma cruzi* infection where the parasite cannot be found easily. It consists of allowing the correct intermediate host, such as a tick or a haematophagous bug, to feed on the animal. These arthropod vectors have, of course, to be reared in the laboratory so that they are free from infection. After feeding, the arthropod host is maintained for several weeks to allow any ingested organisms to multiply, after which it is killed and examined for evidence of infection. Although a valuable technique, especially for the detection of carrier states, the method has the disadvantage that the diagnosis may take several weeks.

Table 15.5 Identification key for sporulated oocysts of *Eimeria* from cattle (see Fig. 15.94).

Species	Oocyst	Mean size (μm)	Sporulation time (days)
Pathogenic species			
Eimeria bovis	Ovoid or subspherical, colourless, and have a smooth wall with inconspicuous micropyle, no polar granule or oocyst residuum	27.7 × 20.3	2–3
E. zuernii	Subspherical, colourless, with no micropyle or oocyst residuum	17.8 × 15.6	2–3
E. alabamensis	Usually ovoid with a smooth, colourless wall with no micropyle, polar body or residuum	18.9 × 13.4	5–8
Non-pathogenic species			
E. auburnensis	Elongated, ovoid, yellowish brown, with smooth or heavily granulated wall with a micropyle and polar granule, but no oocyst residuum	38.4 × 23.1	2–3
E. brasiliensis	Ellipsoidal, yellowish brown, with a micropyle covered by a distinct polar cap. Polar granules may also be present, but there is no oocyst residuum	37 × 27	12–14
E. bukidnonensis	Pear-shaped or oval, tapering at one pole, yellowish brown, with a thick, radially striated wall and micropyle. A polar granule may be present but there is no oocyst residuum	48.6 × 35.4	4–7
E. canadensis	Ovoid or ellipsoidal, colourless, or pale yellow, with an inconspicuous micropyle, one or more polar granules and an oocyst residuum	32.5 × 23.4	3–4
E. cylindrica	Elongated, cylindrical with a colourless, smooth wall, no micropyle, and no oocyst residuum	23.3 × 12.3	2–3
E. ellipsoidalis	Ellipsoidal to slightly ovoid, colourless, with no discernible micropyle, polar granule or oocyst residuum	23.4 × 15.9	2–3
E. pellita	Egg-shaped, very thick, brown wall with evenly distributed protruberences, with a micropyle and polar granule consisting of several rodlike bodies but no oocyst residuum	40 × 28	10–12
E. subspherica	Round or subspherical, colourless, with no micropyle, polar granule or oocyst residuum	11 × 10.4	4–5
E. wyomingensis	Ovoid, yellowish brown, with a thick wall, a wide micropyle but no polar granule or oocyst residuum	40.3 × 28.1	5–7

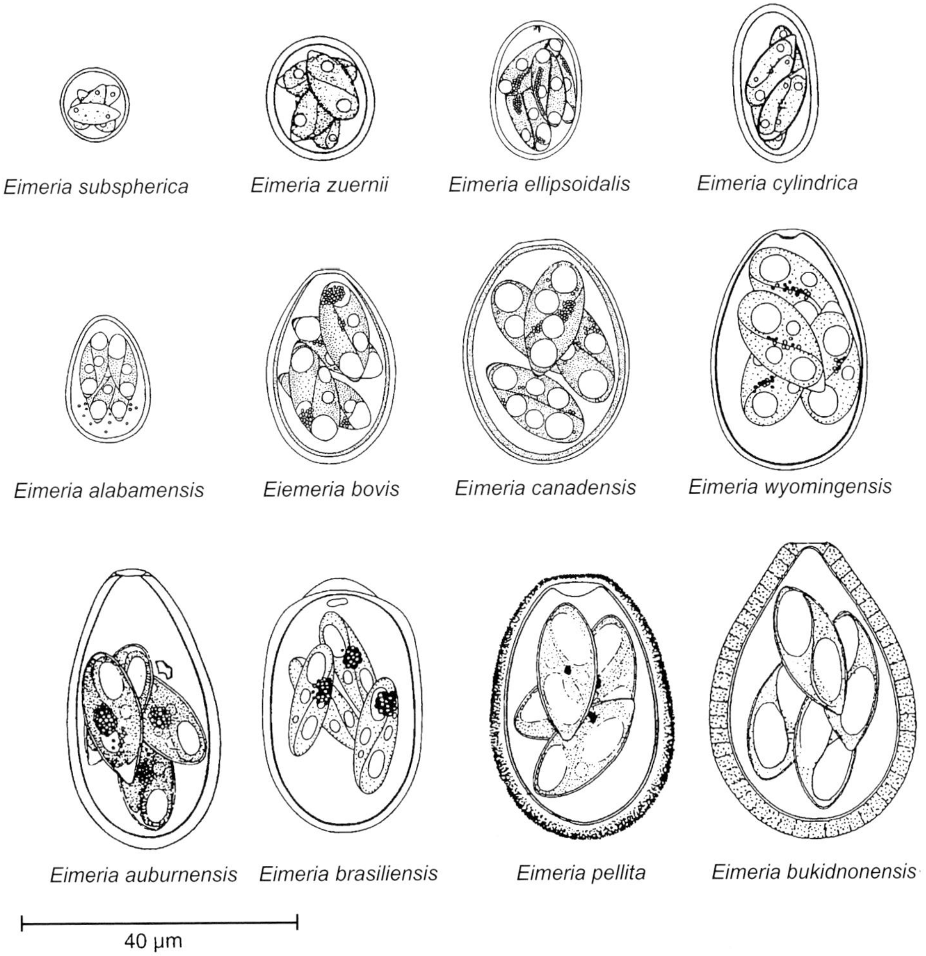

Fig. 15.94 Sporulated oocysts from cattle.

Table 15.6 Identification key for sporulated oocysts of *Eimeria* from sheep (see Fig. 15.95).

Species	Oocyst	Mean size (μm)	Sporulation time (days)
Pathogenic species			
E. crandallis	Broadly ellipsoidal or subspherical, with or without polar cap, without oocyst residuum, sporocysts very broad, with sporocyst residuum	21.9 × 19.4	1–3
E. ovinoidalis	Ellipsoidal, indistinct micropyle, colourless or pale yellow, without oocyst residuum, with sporocyst residuum	23 × 18	1–3
Non-pathogenic species			
E. ahsata	Ovoid with distinct polar cap, yellowish brown, no oocyst residuum	33.4 × 22.6	2–3
E. bakuensis	Ellipsoidal, with polar cap, pale yellowish brown, without oocyst residuum, with sporocyst residuum	31 × 20	2–4
E. faurei	Ovoid, pale yellowish brown, without oocyst residuum or sporocyst residuum	32 × 23	1–3
E. granulosa	Urn-shaped with large micropolar cap at broad end, yellowish brown, without oocyst residuum	29.4 × 20.9	3–4
E. intricata	Ellipsoidal, thick and striated wall, brown no oocyst residuum	48 × 34	3–7
E. marsica	Ellipsoidal, with inconspicuous micropyle, colourless or pale yellow, without oocyst or sporocyst residuum	19 × 13	3
E. pallida	Ellipsoidal, thin-walled, colourless to pale yellow, without oocyst residuum, but with sporocyst residuum	14 × 10	1–3
E. parva	Spherical to subspherical, colourless, no oocyst residuum, sporocyst residuum composed of few granules	16.5 × 14.0	3–5
E. weybridgensis	Broadly ellipsoidal or subspherical, micropyle with or without polar cap, without oocyst or sporocyst residuum	24 × 17	1–3

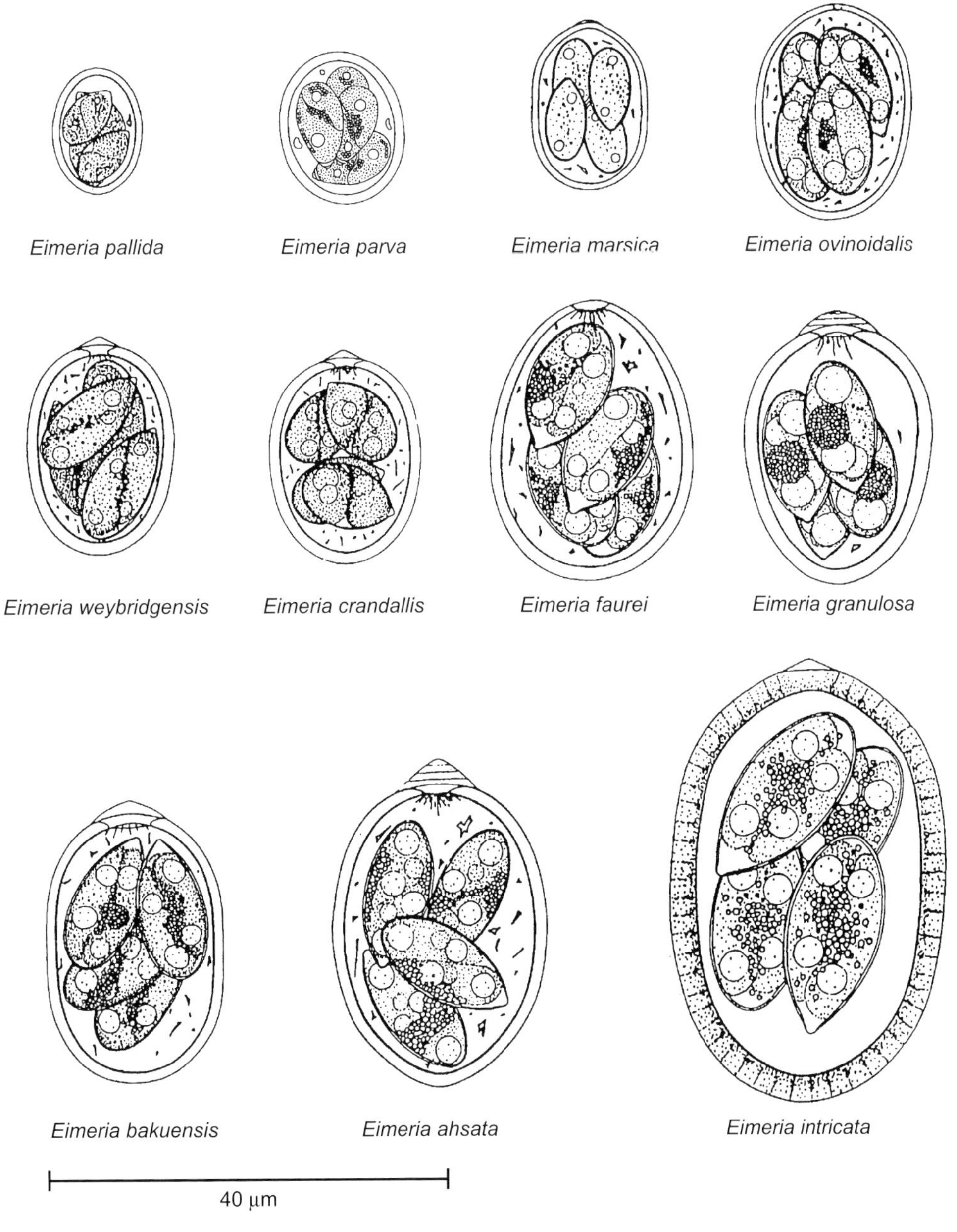

Fig. 15.95 Sporulated oocysts from sheep.

Table 15.7 Identification key for sporulated oocysts of *Eimeria* of goats (see Fig. 15.96).

Species	Oocyst	Mean size (μm)	Sporulation time (days)
Pathogenic species			
E. caprina	Ellipsoidal, dark brown to brownish yellow, with micropyle, without oocyst residuum but with sporocyst residuum	32 × 23	2–3
E. ninakohlyakimovae	Ellipsoidal, thin walled, colourless, micropyle absent or indistinct, without oocyst residuum but with sporocyst residuum	20.7 × 14.8	1–4
E. christenseni	Ovoid, thick wall, colourless to pale yellow, with micropyle and polar cap, without oocyst residuum but with sporocyst residuum	38 × 25	6
E. hirci	Roundish oval, light yellow, with micropyle and polar cap, no oocyst residuum, sporocysts broadly oval with small residuum	20.7 × 16.2	2–3
Non-pathogenic species			
E. alijevi	Ovoid or ellipsoidal, with inconspicuous micropyle, colourless or pale yellow, without oocyst residuum but with sporocyst residuum	17 × 15	1–5
E. arloingi	Ellipsoidal, thick wall with micropyle and polar cap, without oocyst residuum but with sporocyst residuum	27 × 18	1–2
E. aspheronica	Ovoid, greenish to yellow–brown, with micropyle, without oocyst residuum but with sporocyst residuum	31 × 32	1–2
E. caprovina	Ellipsoidal to subspherical, colourless, with micropyle, without oocyst residuum but with sporocyst residuum	30 × 24	2–3
E. jolchijevi	Ellipsoidal or oval, pale yellow, with micropyle and polar cap, without oocyst residuum but with sporocyst residuum	31 × 22	2–4

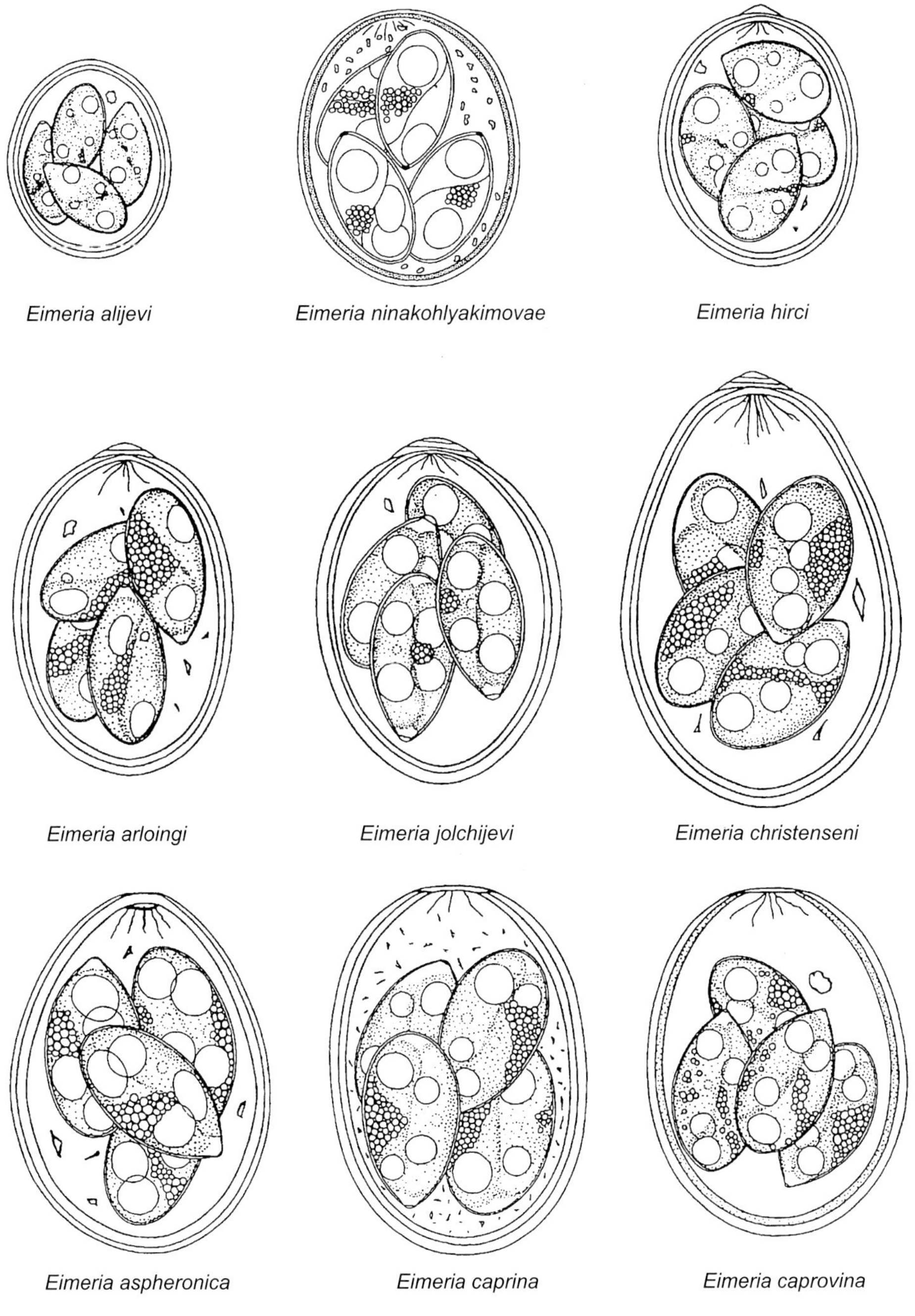

Fig. 15.96 Sporulated oocysts from goats.

Table 15.8 Identification key for sporulated oocysts of pigs (see Fig. 15.97).

Species	Oocyst	Mean size (μm)	Sporulation time (days)
Oocysts without micropyle			
Isospora suis	Spherical to subspherical, wall colourless and thin without a micropyle or residuum and when sporulated contains two sporocysts each with four sporozoites	20.6 × 18.1	1–2
Eimeria perminuta	Ovoid to subspherical, yellow in colour, and wall with a rough surface. A polar granule is present but no micropyle or oocyst residuum	13.3 × 11.7	10–12
E. suis	Ellipsoidal, wall smooth and colourless with a polar granule but no micropyle or oocyst residuum	18.2 × 14.0	5–6
E. spinosa	Ovoid with a thick, rough, brown wall with long spines. There is a polar granule but no micropyle or oocyst residuum	20.6 × 16.2	9–10
E. neodebliecki	Ellipsoid; wall smooth and colourless with no micropyle or oocyst residuum but there is a polar granule	21.2 × 15.8	13
E. debliecki	Ellipsoid or ovoid; wall smooth and colourless with no micropyle or oocyst residuum but with a polar granule	18.8 × 14.3	5–7
E. polita	Ellipsoidal or broad ovoid with a slightly rough yellowish brown wall with no micropyle, oocyst residuum, although a polar granule may be present	25.9 × 18.1	8–9
Oocysts with micropyle			
E. porci	Ovoid, colourless to yellowish brown, with an indistinct micropyle, a polar granule but no oocyst residuum	21.6 × 15.5	9
E. scabra	Ovoid or ellipsoidal, with a thick rough, striated wall, yellow brown in colour with a micropyle and polar granule, but no oocyst residuum	31.9 × 22.5	9–12

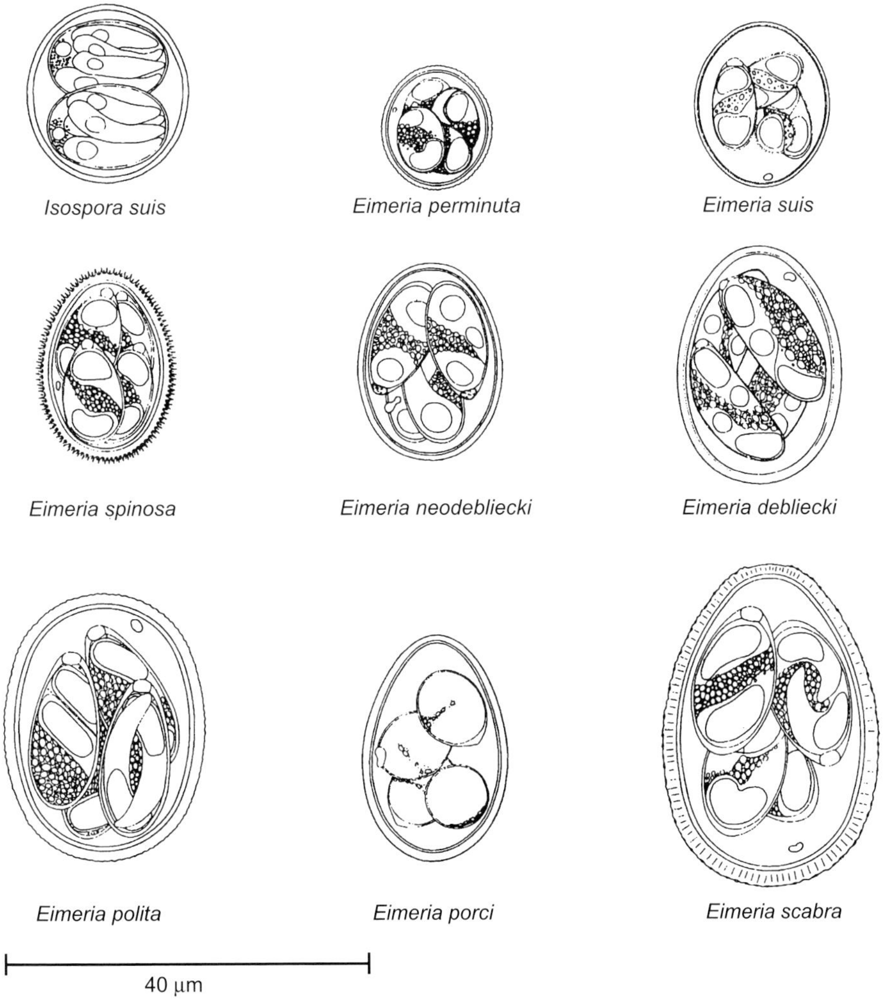

Fig. 15.97 Sporulated oocysts from pigs.

Table 15.9 Identification key for sporulated oocysts of *Eimeria* of rabbits.

Species	Oocyst	Mean size (μm)	Sporulation time (days)
Oocysts without micropyle			
E. exigua	Spherical or subspherical, colourless, with no micropyle, polar granule or oocyst residuum	15.1 × 14.0	1
E. perforans	Ellipsoidal to sub-rectangular, smooth, colourless with a uniformly thin wall. There is an inconspicuous micropyle and an oocyst residuum but no polar granule	22.2 × 13.9	1.5–2
Oocysts with micropyle			
E. piriformis	Piriform, often asymmetrical, yellowish brown, with a prominent micropyle but no polar granule or oocyst residuum	29.5 × 18.1	4
E. flavescens	Ovoid, yellowish, with a prominent micropyle at the broad end. There is no polar granule or oocyst residuum	30 × 21	4
E. irresidua	Ovoid, barrel-shaped, smooth, yellowish, with a wide micropyle. A residuum may be present but there are no polar granules	39.2 × 23.1	4
E. stiedai	Slightly ellipsoidal, colourless or pinkish orange, with an inapparent micropyle and no oocyst residuum	36.9 × 19.9	2–3
E. intestinalis	Pyriform, yellowish brown, with a micropyle at the narrow end, a large oocyst residuum but no polar granule	26.7 × 18.9	3
E. media	Ovoid or ellipsoidal, smooth, light pink with a micropyle with a pyramidal-shaped protuberance, a medium to large oocyst residuum and no polar granule	31.1 × 17.0	2
E. vejdovsyi	Elongate or ovoid, micropyle present without collar-like protrusion, and with medium size oocyst residuum	31.5 × 19.1	2
E. coecicola	Ellipsoidal, light yellow to light brown in colour, with a smooth wall, a distinct micropyle with a slight collar-like protrusion, an oocyst residuum but no polar granule	34.5 × 19.7	4
E. magna	Ovoid, dark yellow, truncated at micropylar end with marked collar-like thickening around micropyle, with very large oocyst residuum but no polar granules	36.3 × 24.1	2–3

Table 15.10 Identification key for sporulated oocysts of *Eimeria* of chickens.

Species	Oocyst	Mean size (µm)	Sporulation time (hours)
Oocysts without micropyle			
E. acervulina	Ovoid, smooth without a micropyle or residuum but with a polar granule	18 × 14	24
E. brunetti	Ovoid, smooth without a micropyle or residuum but with a polar granule	26 × 22	24–48
E. maxima	Ovoid, yellowish and smooth without a micropyle or residuum but with a polar granule	30 × 20	30–48
E. mitis	Subspherical, smooth without a micropyle or residuum but with a polar granule	16 × 15	18–24
E. necatrix	Ovoid, smooth, colourless without a micropyle or residuum but with a polar granule	20 × 17	18–24
E. praecox	Ovoid, smooth, colourless without a micropyle or residuum but with a polar granule	21 × 17	48
E. tenella	Ovoid, smooth, colourless without a micropyle or residuum but with a polar granule	25 × 19	18–48

Table 15.11 Identification key for sporulated oocysts of *Eimeria* of turkeys.

Species	Oocyst	Mean size (µm)	Sporulation time (hours)
E. adenoides	Ellipsoidal or ovoid, smooth, colourless with a micropyle, one to three polar granules but with no oocyst residuum	26 × 17	24
E. dispersa	Ovoid, smooth with no micropyle, polar granule or oocyst residuum	26 × 21	48
E. meleagridis	Ellipsoidal, smooth with no micropyle and no oocyst residuum but with one to two polar granules	23 × 16	15–72
E. meleagrimitis	Subspherical, smooth, colourless with no micropyle or oocyst residuum, but with one to three polar granules	19 × 16	24–72
E. gallapovonis	Ellipsoidal, smooth, colourless without a micropyle or oocyst residuum, but with one polar granule	27 × 17	24
E. innocua	Subspherical, smooth, without a micropyle or polar granules	22 × 21	48
E. subrotunda	Subspherical, smooth, without a micropyle or polar granules	22 × 21	48

References and further reading

Anderson, R.C. (1992) *Nematode Parasites of Vertebrates. Their Development and Transmission.* CAB International, Wallingford.

Arthur, D.R. (1962) *Ticks and Disease.* International Series of Monographs on Pure and Applied Biology, Pergamon Press, London, Vol. 9.

Arthur, D.R. (1963) *British Ticks.* Butterworths, London.

Aubertin, D. (1933) Revision of the genus *Lucilia* R.-D. (Diptera, Calliphoridae). *Journal of the Linnean Society*, **33**, 389–436.

Axtell, R.C. and Arends, J.J. (1990) Ecology and management of arthropod pests of poultry. *Annual Review of Entomology*, **35**, 101–126.

Baker, A.S. (1999) *Mites and Ticks of Domestic Animals. An Identification Guide and Information Source.* The Natural History Museum, London.

Baker, E.W., Camin, J.H., Cunliffe, F. *et al.* (1958) *Guide to the Families of Mites*, Contribution No. 3. Institute of Acarology, University of Maryland.

Baker, E.W., Evans, T.M., Gould, D.J. *et al.* (1956) *A Manual of Parasitic Mites of Medical or Economic Importance.* National Pest Control Association, New York.

Burgess, I. (1994) *Sarcoptes scabiei* and scabies. *Advances in Parasitology*, **33**, 235–293.

Campbell, W.C. and Rew, R.S. (1986) *Chemotherapy of Parasitic Diseases.* Plenum Press, Iowa.

Castellani, A. and Chalmers, A.J. (1910) *Manual of Tropical Medicine.* Bailliere, Tindall & Cox, London.

Chapman, R.F. (1971) *The Insects: Structure and Function.* English Universities Press, London.

Clutton-Brock, J. (1987) *A Natural History of Domesticated Mammals.* Cambridge University Press, Cambridge.

Colebrook, E. & Wall, R. (2004) Ectoparasites of livestock in Europe and the Mediterranean region. *Veterinary Parasitology*, **120**, 251–274.

Cox, F.E.G. (1993) *Modern Parasitology.* Blackwell Scientific Publications, Oxford.

Diseases of camels. Scientific and Technical Review (1987) Vol. 6, No. 2, Office International des Epizooties, Paris.

Dryden, M.W. and Rust, M.K. (1994) The cat flea: biology, ecology and control. *Veterinary Parasitology*, **52**, 1–19.

Dunn, A.M. (1980) *Veterinary Helminthology.* Second edition. Heinemann Medical Books, London.

Edwards, F.W., Oldroyd, H. and Smart, J. (1939) *British Blood-Sucking Flies.* British Museum, London.

Edwards, K., Jepson, R.P. & Wood, K.F. (1960) Value of plasma pepsinogen estimation. *British Medical Journal*, **1**, 30.

Ewald, P.W. (1993) The evolution of virulence. *Scientific American*, **268**, 56–62.

Fain, A. (1994) Adaptation, specificity and host–parasite coevolution in mites (Acari). *International Journal for Parasitology*, **24**, 1273–1283.

Georgi, J.R. and Georgi, M.E. (1990) *Parasitology for Veterinarians.* W.B. Saunders Company, Philadelphia, Pennsylvania.

Gullan, P.J. and Cranston, P.S. (1994) *The Insects. An Outline of Entomology.* Chapman & Hall, London.

Hall, M.J.R. and Wall, R. (1994) Myiasis of humans and domestic animals. *Advances in Parasitology*, **35**, 258–334.

Harwood, R.F. and James, M.T. (1979) *Entomology in Human and Animal Health.* Macmillan, New York.

Hirst, S. (1922) *Mites Injurious to Domestic Animals.* Economic Series No. 13, British Museum, Natural History, London.

Jacobs, D.E. (1986) *A Colour Atlas of Equine Parasites.* Bailliere Tindall, London.

Jorgensen, R. (1975) Isolation of infective *Dictyocaulus* larvae from herbage. *Veterinary Parasitology*, **1**, 61.

Kassai, T. (1999) *Veterinary Helminthology.* Butterworth-Heinemann, Oxford.

Kaufmann, J. (1996) *Parasitic Infections of Domestic Animals: A Diagnostic Manual.* Birkhausse Verlag, Basel.

Kettle, D.S. (1984) *Medical and Veterinary Entomology*. Croom Helm, London.
Lane, R.P. and Croskey, R.W. (eds) *Medical Insects and Arachnids*. Chapman & Hall, London.
Levine, N.D. (1985) *Veterinary Protozoology*. Iowa State University Press, Ames.
Long, P.L. (ed.) (1990) *Coccidiosis of Man and Domestic Animals*. CRC Press, Inc., Boca Raton, Boston.
Manual of Veterinary Parasitological Laboratory Techniques (1986) Reference Book 418. Ministry of Agriculture, Fisheries and Food, Her Majesty's Stationery Office, London.
Mullen, G. and Durden, L. (2002) *Medical and Veterinary Entomology*. Academic Press, Amsterdam.
Newstead, R., Evans, A.M. and Potts, W.H. (1924) Guide to the study of tsetse flies. In: *Liverpool School of Tropical Medicine Memoirs*. University of Liverpool Press, Liverpool, and Hodder and Stoughton, London.
Palmer, S.R., Soulsby, E.J.L. and Simpson, D.I.H. (1998) *Zoonoses: Biology, Clinical Practice and Public Health Control*. Oxford Medical Publications, Oxford.
Reichenbach-Klinke, H. and Elkan, E. (1965) *The Principal Diseases of Lower Vertebrates. Book III. Diseases of Reptiles*. T.F.H. Publishing Inc., Hong Kong.
Reinecke, R.K. (1983) *Veterinary Helminthology*. Butterworths, Durban, Pretoria.
Rothschild, M. (1965) Fleas. *Scientific American*, **213**, (6), 44–53.
Savory, T.H. (1935) *The Arachnida*. Edward Arnold & Co., London.
Séguy, E. (1944) *Insectes Ectoparasites: Mallophages Anopioures, Siphonapteres*. Lechevalier, Paris.
Shtakelbergh, A.A. (1956) *Diptera Associated with Man from the Russian Fauna*. Moscow.
Smart, J.A. (1943) *Handbook for the Identification of Insects of Medical Importance*. British Museum (Natural History), London.
Smith, K.G.V. (1989) An introduction to the immature stages of British flies: Diptera larvae, with notes on eggs, puparia and pupae. *Handbooks for the Identification of British Insects*, **10**, (14), 1–280.
Smyth, J.D. (1994) *Introduction to Animal Parasitology*. Third edition. Cambridge University Press, Cambridge.
Snodgrass, R.E. (1935) *Principles of Insect Morphology*. McGraw-Hill, New York.
Sonenshine, D.E. (1986) Tick pheromones. *Current Topics in Vector Research*, **2**, 225–263.
Soulsby, E.J.L. (1982) *Helminths, Arthropods and Protozoa of Domesticated Animals*. Baillière Tindall, London.
Vercruysse, J. and Rew, R.S. (2002) *Macrocyclic Lactones in Antiparasitic Therapy*. CABI Publishing, Wallingford.
Wakelin, D. (1996) *Immunity to parasites: how parasitic infections are controlled*. Second edition. Cambridge University Press, Cambridge.
Walker, A. (1994) *Arthropods of Humans and Domestic Animals*. Chapman & Hall, London.
Wigglesworth, V.B. (1972) *The Principles of Insect Physiology*. Chapman & Hall, London.
Williams, J.C., Knox, J.W., Sheehan, D. & Fuselier, R.H. (1977) Efficacy of albendazole against inhibited early 4th stage larvae of *Ostertagia ostertagi*. *Veterinary Record*, **101**, 484.
Woldehiwet, Z. and Ristic, M. (1993) *Rickettsial and Chlamydial Diseases of Domestic Animals*. Pergamon Press, Oxford.
Wolff, K., Ruosch, W. & Eckert, J. (1969) Perfusionstechnik zur Gewinnung von *Dicrocoelium dendriticum* aus Schaf- und Rinderlebern. *Zeitschrift für Parasitenkunde*, **33**, 85.
Zinser, H. (1934) *Rats, Lice and History*. Little, Brown, Boston.
Zumpt, F. (1965) *Myiasis in Man and Animals in the Old World*. Butterworths, London.

Index

Note: page numbers in *italics* refer to figures and those in **bold** to tables, but note that figures and tables are only indicated when they are separated from their text references.